Instruments for Clinical Health-Care Research

Jones and Bartlett Series in Oncology

2004 Oncology Nursing Drug Handbook, Wilkes/Barton-Burke

American Cancer Society Patient Education Guide to Oncology Drugs, Second Edition, Wilkes/Ades/Krakoff

American Cancer Society Consumer's Guide to Cancer Drugs, Second Edition, Wilkes/Ades/Krakoff

A Step-by-Step Guide to Clinical Trials, Mulay

Biotherapy: A Comprehensive Overview, Second Edition, Rieger

Blood and Marrow Stem Cell Transplantation, Second Edition, Whedon

Cancer and HIV Clinical Nutrition Pocket Guide, Second Edition, Wilkes

Cancer Chemotherapy: A Nursing Process Approach, Third Edition, Barton-Burke/Wilkes/Ingwerson

Cancer Nursing: Principles and Practice, Fifth Edition, Yarbro/Frogge/Goodman/Groenwald

Cancer Symptom Management, Third Edition, Yarbro/Frogge/Goodman

Chemotherapy Care Plans Handbook, Third Edition, Barton-Burke/Wilkes/Ingwersen

Clinical Guide to Cancer Nursing, Fifth Edition, Yarbro/Frogge/Goodman

Clinical Handbook for Biotherapy, Rieger

Contemporary Issues in Breast Cancer: A Nursing Perspective, Second Edition, Hassey Dow

Contemporary Issues in Colorectal Cancer: A Nursing Perspective, Berg

Contemporary Issues in Lung Cancer: A Nursing Perspective, Haas

Contemporary Issues in Prostate Cancer: A Nursing Perspective, Held-Warmkessel

Fatigue in Cancer: A Multidimensional Approach, Winningham/Barton-Burke

Handbook of Oncology Nursing, Third Edition, Johnson/Gross

Homecare Management of the Bone Marrow Transplant Patient, Third Edition, Kelley/McBride/Randolph/Leum/Lonergan

Making the Decision: A Cancer Patient's Guide to Clinical Trials, Mulay

Oncology Nursing Review, Second Edition, Yarbro/Frogge/Goodman

Outcomes in Radiation Therapy: Multidisciplinary Management, Bruner/Moore-Higgs/Haas

Physicians' Cancer Chemotherapy Drug Manual 2004, Chu

Pocket Guide to Colorectal Cancer, Berg

Pocket Guide to Colorectal Cancer Drugs and Treatment, Wilkes

Pocket Guide to Breast Cancer, Second Edition, Hassey Dow

Pocket Guide to Lung Cancer, Haas

Pocket Guide to Prostate Cancer, Held-Warmkessel

Pocket Guide for Women and Cancer, Moore-Higgs/Almadrones/Colvin-Huff/Gossfield/Eriksson

Progress in Oncology 2003, Devita/Hellman/Rosenberg

Quality of Life: From Nursing and Patient Perspectives, Second Edition, King/Hinds

Women and Cancer: A Gynecologic Oncology Nursing Perspective, Second Edition, Moore-Higgs/Almadrones/Colvin Huff/Gossfield/Eriksson

Instruments for Clinical Health-Care Research

Third Edition

Editors

Marilyn Frank-Stromborg, EdD, RN, JD, FAAN
Chair and Presidential Research Professor
School of Nursing
Northern Illinois University
DeKalb, Illinois

Sharon J. Olsen, MS, RN, AOCN
Assistant Professor
School of Nursing
The Johns Hopkins University
Baltimore, Maryland

JONES AND BARTLETT PUBLISHERS
Sudbury, Massachusetts
BOSTON   TORONTO   LONDON   SINGAPORE

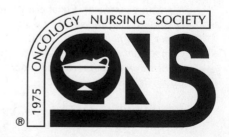

World Headquarters
Jones and Bartlett Publishers
40 Tall Pine Drive
Sudbury, MA 01776
978-443-5000
info@jbpub.com
www.jbpub.com

Jones and Bartlett Publishers Canada
2406 Nikanna Road
Mississauga, ON L5C 2W6
CANADA

Jones and Bartlett Publishers International
Barb House, Barb Mews
London W6 7PA
UK

Library of Congress Cataloging-in-Publication Data

Instruments for clinical health-care research / [edited by] Marilyn Frank-Stromborg and
    Sharon J. Olsen.—3rd ed.
        p. ; cm.
    Includes bibliographical references and index.
    ISBN 0-7637-2252-9 (pbk.)
        1. Nursing—Research. I. Frank-Stromborg, Marilyn. II. Olsen, Sharon J.
    [DNLM: 1. Nursing Research—methods. WY 20.5 I59 2004]
    RT81.5.I57 2004
    610.73'072—dc22

                                                                    2003015429

Acquisitions Editor: Penny M. Glynn
Production Manager: Amy Rose
Associate Production Editor: Jenny L. McIsaac
Editorial Assistant: Amy Sibley
Associate Marketing Manager: Joy Stark-Vancs
Marketing Associate: Elizabeth Waterfall
Manufacturing Buyer: Amy Bacus
Cover Design: Kristin E. Ohlin
Composition: Publishers' Design and Production Services, Inc.
Printing and Binding: Malloy Inc.
Cover Printing: Malloy Inc.

Printed in the United States of America
07 06 05 04 03   10 9 8 7 6 5 4 3 2 1

This book is dedicated to our fathers . . .

The words that a father speaks to his children in the privacy of home are not heard by the world, but, as in whispering galleries, they are clearly heard at the end, and by posterity.

—Ricther

Irving Frank, MD, EdD

My father was a Family Practitioner for over 60 years. His love of medicine was legendary and he considered his life blessed being a doctor and living in a small rural town. Every young person he encountered was encouraged to further their education and consider medicine as a career. He transmitted to his children a deep love and respect for learning and the belief that there wasn't anything that his two daughters couldn't accomplish. One of the best experiences of my father's life was teaching nursing students "Growth and Development" at the Northern Illinois University School of Nursing. He is truly missed.

Marilyn Frank-Stromborg

Eugene J. Meyer

My father was an engineer and computer programmer at Sandia National Laboratories. It seemed a lot of what he did was classified. He was a quiet, steadfast man who taught me to fish and to read the stars. He taught me perseverance by example and to appreciate the quiet internal reward that comes from personal achievement. To this day I remember spending hours on my math homework—if he couldn't get it across one way he'd try another. These were the seeds of today's personal love for teaching and the sense of accomplishment I get from doggedly doing it my way. I thank him and I miss him.

Sharon J. Olsen

Contents

Preface

With health care expenditures rising once again and evidence-based decision-making guiding care management, it is incumbent upon healthcare professionals to act collectively to ensure the provision of high quality, cost effective, sociologically and politically conscientious care. Well designed clinical research using culturally sensitive instruments with valid and reliable psychometric properties can contribute in significant ways to collect the data with which clinical outcomes studies are conducted and evidence-based recommendations are designed.

Throughout the 15 years of this book's existence, it has been the editors' experience that healthcare professionals continue to show significant interest in and need for information on clinical research tools. Therefore, the goals of this third edition remain the same as the first and second editions: review key critical issues that influence the design, development and utilization of clinical research instruments, review available instruments that measure select clinical phenomena, describe available psychometric properties for each tool, review selected studies employing the tool, identify instrument strengths and weaknesses, and discuss the relevance of each instrument for health–care research.

The first edition selectively addressed concepts that measured holistic dimensions of human functioning and client status associated with common clinical problems. The second edition was expanded to include fourteen new chapters. In that publication, the title was changed to *Instruments for Clinical Health-Care Research* to reflect the national emphasis on the new U.S. health-care agenda for the 1990s for a "team" approach to health care. In this, the third edition, one new chapter has been added, and all, but Chapter 32, have been significantly updated. Where appropriate, references to relevant internet sites have been added.

The *intended audience* for this book includes healthcare professionals in educational, clinical, and research settings who are interested in conducting clinical research. Those with at least one beginning-level research course should have no difficulty understanding and utilizing the material in this book.

Organization of the Text

Section I provides an overview of generic issues related to clinical research. Seven chapters address many of the unique measurement issues associated with research with diverse populations and varying age groups. The first chapter is devoted to the rigorous evaluation of research instruments. The sixth chapter addresses the unique problems associated with physiologic measurement. Attention to the growing diversity in the U.S. population is acknowledged by chapters that address the adaptation of instruments for socioeconomically disadvantaged populations and guidelines for translating instruments. Chapter 7, Cultural Considerations in Research Instrumentation Development, is new and provides a step-by-step framework for developing instruments for cross-cultural research. Its co-author, Dr. Miyong Kim, came highly recommended having recently completed post doctoral study in cross-cultural instrumentation at the National Institutes of Health.

The unique issues of doing research with children and the elderly are addressed in two additional chapters in this section.

Chapters in Sections II, III and IV selectively address clinical outcomes commonly related to health and function, health promotion activities, and clinical problems, respectively. In general, the format for each chapter is standardized. The target concept is defined and a brief history of its evolution is reviewed. This is followed by an overview of existing research using instruments that measure the concept; a discussion of related psychometric properties (e.g., reliability and validity measures) and strengths and weaknesses are included. At the end of each chapter the reader will find a published exemplar, a brief summary of a study that thoughtfully and rigorously examines the concept of interest. Finally, an appendix presents critical information about each available instrument. Research in seventeen conceptual areas is addressed in Section II: function, cognitive status, quality of life, social support, stress, coping, hope, spirituality, body image, sexuality, diet, sleep, attitudes toward chronic illness, cancer attitudes, family outcomes, anxiety, and depression. The national movement from acute care management to greater chronic care management necessitates a stronger personal commitment to health maintenance. As such, Section III provides an overview of research concepts important in health promotion: healthy lifestyle, self-care activities, breast and colorectal cancer screening beliefs and practices, information seeking and decision making preferences. Finally, a body of research continues to expand around a number of select clinical problems. These are reviewed in Section IV: alterations in taste and smell, bowel elimination, cardiac parameters, physiologic parameters in obstetric nursing, dyspnea, fatigue, mobility and falls, nausea, vomiting and retching, problems of the oral cavity, pain, skin integrity, and vaginitis.

A consequence of the clinical outcomes movement of the past few years has been the development as well as expanded use of research tools in a number of clinical areas. Past users of this book will find that authors may have deleted a number of older, less used instruments in favor of adding more recent resources and/or updated reliability and validity measures.

The reader will also notice that many chapters are authored by prominent researchers. Clearly, their chapters reflect both their scholarship and clinical research expertise. As these individuals have contributed to this body of research, so too have they mentored new investigators. Readers will commonly find the contributions of new co-authors who are continuing to move a particular area of research forward.

How to Use the Book

This book may be used in two different ways. The first is to select a concept and read the related chapter. The second way is to peruse the index for a specific instrument or a group of instruments that measure a concept or topic of interest or identify one tool that measures multiple concepts. Readers will find some instruments (e.g., Sickness Impact Profile-SIP) are explored in several chapters because they measure more than one concept. Historical experience has taught us that most readers select a specific chapter that describes the concept they are interested in studying.

This book will be useful to both the novice and the experienced researcher, though each may use the information somewhat differently. For the novice, concepts are defined and historically situated. Many instruments are critiqued and sample populations are suggested. For the expert, this book offers a ready reference to the ever-expanding database of clinical instruments and their available psychometric testing qualities.

Clinical researchers increasingly must balance clinical responsibilities, teaching, and research activities. We hope that *Instruments for Clinical Health-Care Research* will ease the burden of researching clinical concepts and variables of interest and enhance focus on linking clinical variable assessment with routine measurement of everyday clinical interventions.

Marilyn Frank-Stromborg, EdD, RN, JD, FAAN
Sharon J. Olsen, MS, RN, AOCN

About the Authors

Marilyn Frank-Stromborg, EdD, RN, JD, FAAN

Professor Frank-Stromborg is Chair and Distinguished Research Professor in the School of Nursing at Northern Illinois University (NIU), DeKalb, Illinois. She completed a doctoral degree in Educational Psychology from NIU, a Masters of Science degree in nursing from the New York Medical College, New York City, and undergraduate studies in Biology/Chemistry at NIU. In 1991, she returned to school to obtain her juris doctorate. Dr. Frank-Stromborg is also a licensed advanced practice nurse having obtained her Adult Nurse Practitioner certificate from Rush College of Nursing, Chicago. Her clinical background includes 17 years in a part-time nurse practitioner role in rural northern Illinois.

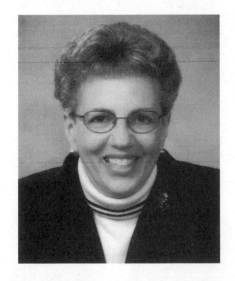

Dr. Frank-Stromborg has published extensively and has 7 books, 79 articles and 34 book chapters to her credit. She is the recipient of many national honors and awards including: the Oncology Nursing Society/Chiron Excellence of Scholarship and Consistency of Contribution to the Oncology Nursing Literature Award, NIU Award for Outstanding Grant Acquisitions, and Outstanding Nurse Researcher for Alumni from Pace University. She has received over 3 million dollars of funding from local, state, and federal sources including NINR, NCI, Illinois Department of Nuclear Safety, Helene Fuld Health Trust, and the Department of Defense.

Dr. Frank-Stromborg has been appointed to serve on multiple state and national committees. She was appointed a permanent member of the NCI Scientific Review Group-Subcommittee H, state of Illinois Board of Nursing, Chair of the Research Committee of the American Board of Nursing Specialties, and the National Advisory Council for Nursing Research.

Sharon J. Olsen, MS, RN, AOCN

Sharon Olsen is an assistant professor in the graduate nursing program in the School of Nursing at The Johns Hopkins University, Baltimore, Maryland. She has a joint appointment with The Sidney Kimmel Comprehensive Cancer Center, School of Medicine, The Johns Hopkins University.

Her academic and research interests in genetics were augmented by the completion of a two month summer fellowship in genetics sponsored by the National Institute for

Nursing Research, NIH and a two month summer short course at The Jackson Laboratory in Bar Harbor, Maine. Ms Olsen is continuing this area of research as a doctoral student at The Catholic University of America, Washington DC. She completed a Masters of Science degree in nursing from the University of Wisconsin-Madison and undergraduate nursing studies at Texas Woman's University, Denton Texas.

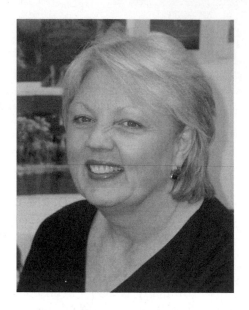

Her current sponsored research, through the National Cancer Institute and the National Human Genome Research Institute, addresses public and professional education in cancer genetics and minority recruitment to a national cancer genetics registry. She has published over 30 manuscripts, book chapters and books in the areas of ethnic diversity and cancer prevention, screening, and genetics.

Ms Olsen is a member of numerous nursing organizations including the American Nurses Association, the International Society of Nurses in Genetics, the Oncology Nursing Society and Sigma Theta Tau International.

Contributors

Ann Malone. Berger, PhD, RN, AOCN
Associate Professor and Advanced Practice Nurse, College of Nursing, University of Nebraska, Omaha, Nebraska

Nancy Bergstrom, PhD, RN, FAAN
Theodore J. and Mary E. Trumble Professorship in Aging Research and Associate Director of Aging Research, The University of Texas Health Science Center at Houston, Houston, Texas

Angela D. Berry, BSN
Staff Nurse, Wake Forest Baptist Hospital, Winston-Salem, North Carolina

Marlyn D. Boyd, PhD, RN, CHES
Adjunct Associate Professor, Department of Health Promotion and Education, College of Nursing, University of South Carolina, Columbia, South Carolina

Barbara Braden, PhD, RN, FAAN
Dean, Graduate School and University College, Creighton University, Omaha, Nebraska

Caroline Bagley Burnett, ScD, RN
Visiting Professor, Department of Psychiatry, Institute for Ethics, University of New Mexico, Albuquerque, New Mexico

Nancy Burns, PhD, RN, FAAN
Jenkins Garrett Professor, Evaluation Coordinator, School of Nursing, The University of Texas at Arlington, Arlington, Texas

Kathryn K. Chambers, MS, ARNP, OCN
Education Specialist, St. Joseph's Baptist Health Care, Tampa, Florida

Victoria L. Champion, DNS, RN
Associate Dean for Research, Mary Margaret Walther Distinguished Professor of Nursing, Department of Environments for Health, School of Nursing, Director of Cancer Control, Indiana University. Affiliated Scientist, Indiana University Center for Aging Research, Indianapolis, Indiana

Rebecca F. Cohen, EdD, RN, MPA, CPHQ
Co-Project Director, Adult Nurse Practitioner Grant, School of Nursing, Northern Illinois University, DeKalb, Illinois

Sue B. Davidson, PhD, RN, CNS
Nursing Practice Director, Oregon Nurses Association, Tualatin, Oregon

Hannah Dean, PhD, RN, CPHQ
Providence St. Joseph Medical Center, Quality Improvement/Outcomes Research, Burbank, California

Marylin J. Dodd, PhD, RN, FAAN
Professor and Associate Dean of Academic Personnel, Director for the Center for Symptom Management, School of Nursing, University of California in San Francisco, San Francisco, California

Jan M. Ellerhorst-Ryan, MSN, RN, CS
Vitas Hospice Group, Norwood office, Cincinnati, Ohio

Jacqueline Fawcett, PhD, RN, FAAN
Professor, College of Nursing and Health Sciences, University of Massachusetts, Boston, Massachusetts

Betty R. Ferrell, PhD, RN, FAAN
Research Scientist, Department of Nursing Research and Education, City of Hope Medical Center, Duarte, California

Marquis D. Foreman, PhD, RN, FAAN
Associate Professor, Department of Biobehavioral Nursing Science, College of Nursing, University of Illinois at Chicago, Chicago, Illinois

Marilyn Frank-Stromborg, EdD, RN, JD, FAAN
Chair and Distinguished Research Professor, School of Nursing, Northern Illinois University, DeKalb, Illinois

Rita A. Frantz, PhD, RN, FAAN
Professor and Area Chair of Biobehavioral Nursing, College of Nursing, University of Iowa, Iowa City, Iowa

Freda DeKeyser Ganz, PhD, RN
Hadassah-Hebrew University School of Nursing, Jerusalem, Israel

Marcia Grant, DNSc, RN, FAAN
Research Scientist, Director of Nursing Research and Education, City of Hope Medical Center, Duarte, California

Patricia M. Grimm, PhD, RN, APRN, BC
Formerly, Associate Professor, School of Nursing, The Johns Hopkins University, Baltimore, Maryland

Hae-Ra Han, PhD, RN
Assistant Professor, School of Nursing, The Johns Hopkins University, Baltimore, Maryland

JoAnne Herman, PhD, RN
Associate Professor, College of Nursing, University of South Carolina, Columbia, South Carolina

Sharon Ann Hyland, MS, RN, ANP
James P. Wilmot Cancer Center, University of Rochester, Rochester, New York, Roswell Park Cancer Institute

Debra P. Hymovich, PhD, RN
Consultant and Professor Emeritus, College of Nursing and Health Professions, University of North Carolina, Charlotte, North Carolina

Sharol F. Jacobson, PhD, RN, FAAN
Professor and Associate Dean for Research and Practice, Capstone College of Nursing, University of Alabama, Tuscaloosa, Alabama

Gloria Juarez, PhD, RN
Assistant Research Scientist, Nursing Research and Education, City of Hope Medical Center, Duarte, California

Hee-Ju Kim, MSN, RN
Doctoral Student, School of Nursing, University of Pennsylvania, Philadelphia, Pennsylvania

Miyong T. Kim, PhD, RN
Associate Professor, School of Nursing, The Johns Hopkins University, Baltimore, Maryland

Setsuko Koresawa, MSN, RN
Doctoral Student, School of Nursing, University of California in San Francisco, San Francisco, California

Xiaotao Lang, MSN, RN
Doctoral Student, School of Nursing, University of Pennsylvania, Philadelphia, Pennsylvania

Felissa R. Lashley, PhD, RN, ACRN, FAAN
Dean and Professor, College of Nursing, Rutgers, The State University of New Jersey, Newark, New Jersey

Jana Lauderdale, PhD, RN
School of Nursing, Vanderbuilt University, Nashville, Tennessee

Ada M. Lindsey, PhD, RN
Dean, College of Nursing, University of Nebraska Medical Center, Omaha, Nebraska

Ruth McCorkle, PhD, RN, FAAN
The Florence S. Wald Professor of Nursing, Director, Center for Excellence in Chronic Illness Care, Chair, Doctoral Program, School of Nursing, Yale University, New Haven, Connecticut

Roxanne W. McDaniel, PhD, RN
Associate Professor and Associate Dean of Undergraduate and Master's Programs, School of Nursing, University of Missouri-Columbia, Columbia, Missouri

Deborah B. McGuire, PhD, RN, FAAN
Associate Professor, Director, Adult Oncology Nursing Program, University of Pennsylvania, School of Nursing, Philadelphia, Pennsylvania

Kimberly McClaine, PhD, RN
Lecturer, Division of Nursing, California State University, Carson, California

Susan C. McMillan, PhD, RN, FAAN
Professor of Oncology Nursing, American Cancer Society, College of Nursing, University of South Florida, Tampa, Florida

Sharon Fish Mooney, PhD, RN, MSN
Adjunct Faculty for Parish Nursing, McMaster Divinity College, Ontario, Canada

Sharon J. Olsen, MS, RN, AOCN
Assistant Professor, School of Nursing, The Johns Hopkins University, Baltimore, Maryland

Anna K. Omery, DNSc, RN
Nurse Scientist, Kaiser Permanente, California Division, Pasadena, California

Geraldine V. Padilla, PhD
Associate Dean for Research, School of Nursing, University of California in San Francisco, San Francisco, California

Jeannie V. Pasacreta, PhD, RN, CS
Associate Professor, School of Nursing, Yale University, New Haven, Connecticut

Barbara F. Piper, DNSc, RN, AOCN, FAAN
Associate Professor, College of Nursing, University of Nebraska Medical Center, Omaha, Nebraska

Linda C. Pugh, PhD, RNC
Associate Professor and Director of the Baccalaureate Program, School of Nursing, The Johns Hopkins University, Baltimore, Maryland

Susan J. Quaal, PhD, APRN
Salt Lake VA Healthcare System, Salt Lake City, Utah

Joyce H. Rasin, PhD, RN
Associate Professor, The University of North Carolina at Chapel Hill, Chapel Hill,
North Carolina

Susan M. Rawl, PhD, RN
Assistant Professor, School of Nursing, Indiana University, Indianapolis, Indiana

Michelle Rhiner, MS, RN, NP, CHPN
Patient Coordinator/Manager, Supportive Care, Pain and Palliative Medicine, City
of Hope Medical Center, Duarte, California

Verna A. Rhodes, EdD, RN, FAAN
Associate Professor Emeritus, School of Nursing, University of Missouri, Columbia,
Missouri

Therese Richmond, PhD, CRNP, FAAN
Associate Professor, School of Nursing, University of Pennsylvania, Philadelphia,
Pennsylvania

Julie F. Robertson, EdD, RN
Associate Professor, School of Nursing, Northern Illinois University, DeKalb, Illinois

Judith W. Ryan, PhD, RN, CRNP
President, Nurse Practitioners & Consultants, P.C., Owings Mills, Maryland

Mary L. Scott, MS, RN, OCN
Director, Oncology Nursing, Huntsman Cancer Research Hospital, Salt Lake City,
Utah

Margaret S. Soderstrom, PhD, RN, CS-P, ARNP, PHM
Assistant Professor, School of Nursing, The Johns Hopkins University, Baltimore,
Maryland

Ann Marie Spellbring, PhD, RN
Nursing Coordinator, Gerontology, University of Maryland at Baltimore, Baltimore,
Maryland

Martha H. Stoner, PhD, RN
Associate Professor Emeritus, School of Nursing, University of Colorado Health
Sciences, Denver, Colorado

Nancy A. Stotts, EdD, RN
Professor, Department of Physiological Nursing, School of Nursing, University of
California in San Francisco, San Francisco, California

Roberta Anne Strohl, MN, RN, AOCN
Patient Care Consultant, Schering Plough, Baltimore, Maryland

Siew Tzah Tang, DNSc, RN
Assistant Professor, National Ying-Ming University, Taiwan

Lorraine Tulman, DNSc, RN, FAAN
Associate Professor, School of Nursing, University of Pennsylvania, Philadelphia,
Pennsylvania

Claudette Varricchio, DSN, RN, FAAN
Chief, Office of Extramural Programs, National Institute of Nursing Research,
National Institutes of Health, Bethesda, Maryland

Patricia E. H. Vermeersch, PhD, RN
Wright State University- Miami Valley, College of Nursing and Health, Dayton, Ohio

Susan Noble Walker, PhD, RN, FAAN
Professor, College of Nursing, University of Nebraska Medical Center, Omaha, Nebraska

Jo Ann Wegmann, PhD, RN
Professor, Division of Nursing, School of Nursing, California State University-Dominguez Hills, Carson, California

Sally P. Weinrich, PhD, RN
Professor, School of Nursing, University of Louisville, Louisville, Kentucky

Margaret Chamberlain Wilmoth (formerly Metcalfe), PhD, RN, MSS
Associate Professor, Department of Adult Health Nursing, College of Nursing and Health Professions, University of North Carolina at Charlotte, Charlotte, North Carolina

Bernice C. Yates, PhD, RN
Associate Professor and Associate Dean for Research, College of Nursing, University of Nebraska Medical Center, Omaha, Nebraska

I

Overview

1

Evaluating Instruments for Use in Clinical Nursing Research

Sharol F. Jacobson

This chapter provides a brief review of key concepts in measurement and a summary of current recommendations for the selection, use, and continued development of existing instruments in clinical nursing research. The emphasis is on practical information for decision making. The chapter is aimed at health-care professionals who have had at least one course in research methods and statistics but whose background in measurement and research may be neither extensive nor recent. It is not the purpose of the chapter to serve as a comprehensive research or measurement text. This chapter uses the terms *measure, test*, and *instrument* interchangeably to refer to the measuring device; the terms *concept, construct*, and *attribute* refer to what is being measured.

The State of the Art of Measurement in Nursing Research

The state of measurement in nursing research has improved considerably since Waltz and Strickland's critical appraisal in the 1980s.[1,2] At that time they found that the conceptual basis of tools was identified only 20% of the time, that no reliability data were reported for 38% of the measures, and no validity data were reported for 58% of the measures. Only about 2% of reports provided reliability and validity data from both the current and previous studies.

Norbeck's proposed standards for what constitutes a publishable report of instrument development[3] were another important influence on measurement reports. She identified the essential descriptive information about an instrument as its conceptual basis, the methods of item generation and refinement, characteristics for the intended respondents, details of administration, method of scoring, type of data obtained, and any other instrument-specific information. Means, standard deviations, and ranges of scores should be provided so that users may compare their study samples with others. Initial reports also should provide examples of the tool format and sample items or a complete copy of the instrument in an appendix. The minimal standard for publishing psycho-metric testing should include test-retest reliability, internal consistency reliability, and at least one type each of content- and construct- or criterion-related validity, each of which should meet the minimal acceptable levels specified by current measurement theory. Use of these standards reduces premature and fragmented publication and aids evaluation of the adequacy of an instrument's development.

Despite improvements in instrument development and reporting, the prospective instrument user (*user/s* hereafter) still needs to read widely and think critically. A common error in selecting an instrument is to assume that it is sound if it has been published or widely used. This is not necessarily true, as standards for measurement adequacy change over time,[4] and journals vary in the rigor demanded to publish instrument development reports. Users should be aware that there is a relationship between the amount of relevant psychometric information provided by the developer or publisher of an instrument and its quality. Missing data should be assumed to be negative. Users also should continue to review the literature *after* reading a report of a promising instrument. Instruments can fall from favor rapidly if their psychometric properties are not supported by other users or if superior instruments are developed.

Users should be wary of tools developed on small samples. Small samples are, by nature, less representative of the population and more prone to sampling error (the tendency for statistics to fluctuate from one sample to another) than large samples are.[5] Therefore, one cannot be as confident that an instrument developed on a small sample will perform the same way again.

Assessing the Conceptual Basis of Instruments

Increasingly, instruments are being based on conceptual or theoretical models from nursing or related disciplines, such as psychology. When considering instruments based on models from other disciplines or older instruments from any discipline, users should ascertain through reflection, concept analysis, or extensive literature review that the instrument's conceptual basis is at least compatible with, if not identical to, their individual and professional perspectives on the problem and that the instrument is current.[6] The authors of a recent evaluation of the 20-year-old Organizational Job Satisfaction Scale noted that its items did not reflect the contemporary issues of shared governance, institutional respect for nursing, or interdisciplinary interaction.[7] If those issues are part of users' conceptualization of job satisfaction, researchers should select another instrument or locate supplementary items.

Failure to assess the adequacy or currency of the conceptual framework and the fit of framework and items is more than a personal matter: It creates a validity problem in that the findings obtained with a particular instrument cannot be interpreted adequately.[6]

Measurement Frameworks

Two major frameworks guide the design and interpretation of measurement.[8] The *norm-referenced framework* discriminates among individuals and spreads people across a range of scores, ideally, normally distributed. The majority of personality, affective, attitudinal, and cognitive constructs used in nursing employ this framework.

The *criterion-referenced framework* determines what a person knows or can do in relation to a specified domain or fixed performance standard. How one person compares with others is irrelevant in this framework. Criterion-referenced measures (CRMs) produce classifications or judgments, such as satisfactory/unsatisfactory or met/not met. Scores from a CRM have a narrower range than those from a norm-referenced measure and are skewed (clustered) toward one end of the scale. Criterion-referenced measures often are useful in clinical research that requires measuring a process or attaining outcome variables. For example, the Denver Developmental Screening Test and the National Cancer Institute's criteria for the proper performance of breast self-examination are useful CRMs. Space limitations do not permit further discussion of this measurement framework, but a comprehensive description can be found in Waltz et al.[8]

Choosing a Data-Collection Method

Every instrument uses one or more methods of data collection to operationalize the variables of interest. Each method has its own advantages and disadvantages for certain purposes and populations and its special reliability and validity problems. For example, because semantic differentials are rapid to complete, many items can be used.[9] Q sorts are time-consuming and are best suited to intensive analysis of individuals or small samples.[9] Instruments whose items use identical response formats, such as Likert or numerical rating scales, are prone to response sets, in which subjects respond to items in characteristic ways regardless of the item content; such tendencies are threats to validity.[5] Useful information about the features of methods of data collection can be found in basic research texts.[5,9] Research articles also increasingly comment on the practical, as well as the theoretical, aspects of different data collection methods.

Item Generation and Analysis

Reports of instrument development should contain some description of how items were developed and refined. Items can be generated by reviews of the literature, clinical observations and interviews, qualitative methodologies such as grounded theory, selection from existing instruments, or by combinations of these strategies. Some form of item analysis, which is an examination of the pattern of responses to each item to assess its effectiveness and provide guidelines for its revision, also should be described. The results of item analysis affect both reliability and validity by manipulating the variability of scores, eliminating the extraneous effects of very easy or very difficult items, and strengthening the relationship between items and an external criterion.[8]

Several statistical procedures are widely used in item development and analysis. Item intercorrelations (the correlation of each item with every other item) and item-total correlations (the correlation of each item with the total score for the entire instrument) are often used to decide which items to retain, revise, or delete. A common rule of thumb for such correlations is that they should be between 0.30 and 0.70. Those below 0.30 are not contributing much to measurement of the concept, and those above 0.70 are probably redundant.[10]

Item difficulty and discrimination are also relevant to instrument development and refinement in both norm- and criterion-referenced measurement. Item difficulty (ID), also called *item p level*, is the percentage of correct responses to the item. Item difficulty can range from 0 to 100. The closer it is to zero, the more difficult the item is. Average item difficulties, around 50 or with a range of 30 to 70, are generally sought to promote variability of scores and, hence, reliability.[8]

The discrimination power or index (D) represents the degree to which an item distinguishes high and low achievers on the test or to which performance on any one item predicts performance on the entire test. D scores can range from −1.00 to +1.00. Positive D scores are desirable and indicate that the item is discriminating in the desired direction.

Those who answer the item correctly tend to do well on the test or to have a large amount of the measured attribute. D scores near zero mean that the item is not discriminating and serves no useful purpose in the test. Negative D scores mean that respondents who answer the item correctly tend to do poorly on the total test. Such items need major revision. D scores of +0.30 are generally accepted as adequate.[8]

Item response charts display the response patterns to items and allow the inspection, comparison, and chi-square testing of differences between high- and lower-scoring groups. An explanation of how to perform the various item analysis calculations can be found in Waltz et al.[8]

Psychometric Characteristics of Instruments

In classic measurement theory, an observed score on any measure is seen as a combination of a true score (what the subject would get if the instrument were perfect) and random and systematic error. Random error results from chance variations in the instrument (the directions may not be clear), the subject (he or she may have a headache today), or the conditions of the test administration (the room may be very hot, or all administrators may not use the same instructions). By sometimes raising and sometimes lowering the observed score, random error reduces the consistency of measurements and, indirectly, makes it difficult to know what exactly is being measured. Systematic error results from the presence of some extraneous factor that affects all measurements made with the tool in the same way. For example, a scale that reads 3 pounds high is systematically upwardly biased. Systematic bias compromises *validity*, or the extent to which an instrument measures what it is intended to measure. The aim of all reliability and validity measures is to minimize the portion of the observed score that is due to error and to maximize the portion that is true. The larger the portion of random error in a score, the lower the reliability coefficient of the instrument. The lower the reliability coefficient, the lower the confidence that can be placed in any subsequent judgments or relationships using that instrument.[5,8]

Reliability

Concerns about reliability involve the consistency or repeatability of measurements made with the instrument. Reliability can be conceptualized in terms of stability, equivalence, or internal consistency. It often is possible and desirable to use more than one approach.[5] The most common estimate of reliability is a correlation coefficient. Theoretically, correlation coefficients may range between −1.00 and +1.00, but in reliability assessment, they usually fall between 0.0 and 1.0. The closer the correlation coefficient is to 1.00, the more reliable the tool.[5]

Reliability as Stability

Reliability as stability takes two forms. Test-retest reliability is the correlation between scores from the same subjects tested at two different times. The interval between testings should not be so short that subject's recall of items can spuriously inflate the reliability coefficient or so long that one is studying the stability of the characteristic over time rather than the performance of the instrument.[11] Two to four weeks is a suitable interval for most uses of stability estimates. Test-retest reliability is more useful for measures of enduring attributes than for changeable states and for affective rather than cognitive measures.[8] For example, a test-retest correlation is better suited to a measure of introversion/extroversion (an enduring affective attribute) than to a measure of knowledge of the warning signals of cancer (a changeable cognitive state).

The second form of reliability as stability is *intrarater reliability*, or the consistency with which one rater assigns scores to a single event on two different occasions. The correlation is calculated from the scores of the same observer at time 1 and time 2.[8]

Reliability as Equivalence

Reliability as equivalence has two forms. Parallel (or alternate) forms reliability requires the development of two different tests that measure the same trait in the same way. The correlation coefficient is based on the scores of the same individuals taking test A and test B sequentially. This procedure overcomes the problem of specific recall associated with the administration of a single test twice. Thus, parallel forms are useful for studies using repeated measures. The disadvantage is that parallel tests are very difficult to construct.[5] The chief application of parallel forms reliability has been with standardized tests in education.

The second form of reliability as equivalence, much more common in nursing research than parallel forms, is interrater (or interobserver) reliability. Here, two or more trained observers watch an event simultaneously and score it independently, using established scoring criteria.[8] Training raters to achieve adequate interrater reliability is considerably more complex than it may first appear. Washington and Moss[12] identified six essential aspects: (1) understanding the theoretical perspective, (2) familiarization of raters with the instrument, (3) selection of an adequate number of subjects (a minimum of 10 is recommended), (4) use of a set time frame for observance, (5) concern for interfering variables, and (6) completing scoring and discussion soon after the observation session. An excellent description of training raters to use an instrument for assessment of patient intensity can be found in Castorr et al.[13]

Various procedures besides the Pearson r (for interval data) are available for assessing intrarater and interrater reliability. For nominal dichotomous data, the percentage of agreement is easy to compute and provides useful information (e.g., two raters agreed 90% of the time), but it is easily inflated by agreements as a result of chance.[5] Cohen's kappa controls for the amount of agreement that may have occurred by chance and can be extended to cases with more than two raters;[14] weighted kappa also allows assessment of the relative seriousness of disagreement among raters.[15] Because kappa controls for chance agreement, kappa reliabilities are likely to be lower than the reliability based on other estimates. Topf[16] provides an example showing a kappa of 0.59 and total percentage agreement of 80% for the same data.

Reliability as Internal Consistency

The third approach to reliability, internal consistency, is perhaps the most widely used today. Internal consistency is concerned with the degree to which a set of items designed to measure the same concept are intercorrelated. An instrument is said to be internally consistent (or homogeneous) to the extent that all items demonstrate desirable intercorrelations, thus appearing to measure the concept of interest and nothing else.[8]

Historically, the oldest method of assessing internal consistency is the split-half technique. The items of a single test are divided into halves—usually odd- and even-numbered items—and scored separately. The correlation coefficient is calculated from the scores on each half of the test. Although splitting the test avoids the need to create two tests, it creates another problem. Because reliability is related to test length, a correlation coefficient based on split-halves systematically underestimates the reliability of the entire scale. A statistical correction known as the Spearman-Brown prophecy formula is used to adjust (prophesy) the split-half correlation coefficient for the full-length test. The chief disadvantage of the split-half technique is that different splits (e.g., odd-even, first half–second half) yield different reliability estimates.[9] Because of this problem, psychometricians have developed reliability coefficients that do not require item repetition or splitting.

The most widely used measure of internal consistency is the Cronbach coefficient alpha, called alpha hereafter. Alpha—not to be confused with alpha meaning the level of significance—measures the extent to which performance on any one item in an instrument indicates performance on any other item in that instrument.[8] Alpha can range from 0.00 to 1.00, indicating very low to very high internal consistency.[9] Alpha has many strengths as an indicator of internal consistency. It addresses the sampling of content, which is the major source of measurement error, as well as the sampling of the situational factors that accompany individual items. Because it is equal to the average of all possible split-halves, it subsumes the Spearman-Brown prophecy formula.[17]

Unfortunately the Cronbach alpha is misused. It is not appropriate for instruments like life events scales or risk factor scales, in which items are a collection of discrete events rather than representatives of a single domain and are unlikely to occur together consistently or at all.[18] The Cronbach alpha is also unsuited for scales of fewer than five items.[19]

The Kuder-Richardson formulas (KR 20 and KR 21) are two other measures of internal consistency. They are special cases of alpha developed for dichotomous responses.[8]

Interpretation of Reliability Coefficients

Reliability is a matter of degree rather than an all-or-nothing affair, and it is not a self-contained property of an instrument but of an instrument when administered to certain people under certain conditions. For all types of reliability, users must ascertain the characteristics of the group on or for whom the instrument was developed. The more similar the original group to the user's group, the more likely that the instrument will perform reliably for the new study. Reliability is increased by longer test length (up to a point), by speeded conditions in which all subjects do not finish, by heterogeneous samples, and by variability of the scores on the total test.[19]

Other things being equal, the instrument with the highest reliability is best,[5] subject to the caution that very high reliabilities may indicate redundant items. Because reliability coefficients are not automatically generalizable, they should be recalculated each time an instrument is used, particularly if used on a different population. This increases the research community's knowledge of instrument quality and aids appropriate interpretation of the data.[4]

"How high is high?" is a common question about reliability coefficients. There is no simple answer. The judgment depends on what is being measured, the stage of development of the instrument, and the procedure used to estimate reliability. The reliability of physiologic measures often is generally higher than that of attitudinal measures. Acceptable standards for interrater reliability using percentage agreement range from 70% to 90%.[20] Standards for kappa reliabilities are virtually none, 0.00–0.10; slight, 0.11–0.40; fair, 0.41–0.60; moderate, 0.61–0.80; and substantial, 0.81–1.00.[21] Nunnally and Bernstein's guidelines,[22] propose that an alpha coefficient of 0.70 is acceptable but modest for an instrument in the early stages of development but that 0.80 is desirable for a more developed instrument and when the purpose is to compare groups. If the research purpose is to make important decisions about individuals, a reliability of 0.90 is minimal and a reliability of 0.95 is desirable. It is noteworthy that the standards given here for kappa[21] and alpha coefficients[22] represent increases over earlier guidelines—it is important for tool users to realize that psychometric standards change (rise) over time as measurement sophistication increases.[4]

If an instrument contains subscales that are analyzed, the reliability of each subscale must be assessed as well as that of the total instrument. Because they are shorter, the reliability of subscales is often lower than that of the total instrument.

Generalizability Theory

Generalizability theory (G theory) is an extension and liberalization of classic measurement theory. Although classic theory recognizes that there are multiple sources of measurement error, it deals with them collectively. Generalizability theory identifies and disentangles them. A generalizability (G) study estimates sources of error; uses analysis of variance procedures to provide separate, simultaneous estimates of the effects of different sources of error; and, in the process, provides a summary coefficient reflecting the level of dependability of the instrument. Decision (D) studies use information from G studies to design highly reliable instruments for certain purposes.[23,24] Although not yet common in the nursing measurement literature, use of this approach to assess measurement error is likely to increase.

Validity

The second characteristic of a measuring instrument is validity, commonly and briefly defined as whether a tool measures what it claims to measure. The most recent (1999) *Standards for Educational and Psychological Testing*[25] present a major reconceptualization of validity that has yet to be reflected in most nursing measurement literature. Instead of the former three types or aspects of validity (content, criterion-related, and construct), which tended to compartmentalize validity and focus on the test rather than on the uses of test scores, the new definition is "the degree to which evidence and theory support the interpretations of test scores entailed by proposed uses of tests."[25] Within this definition all validity is construct validity, for which five categories of validity evidence exist. These categories will be discussed briefly, inserting the familiar terminology and procedures of validity "types" into the new "categories of evidence."

Evidence based on test content corresponds to the former *content validity*. Content validity is concerned with whether or not instrument items adequately measure the content area: Are they representative and comprehensive? Evidence about test content may come from the literature, representatives of the target population, and consensual judgments by experts in the theory.[9] Once reported with a simple statement that a panel of judges agreed that the items possessed content validity, content validity is now seen as a two-stage process of development and judgment quantification by carefully selected experts.[26–28] In the developmental stage the characteristics of the content domain are identified and items are generated, sampled, and assembled into a useable form. In the judgment-quantification stage, five to ten experts who meet detailed criteria for expertise respond to specific questions about the content relevance of each item and the total scale, suggest revisions, and identify omissions. An index of content validity (the CVI) showing the proportion of agreement among judges can be calculated for each item and the full instrument.[26–28]

Content validity is essential for all instruments and should not be seen as less important than other forms of validity evidence.[29] However, because it is by definition focused on the test content rather than the meaning and use of test scores, it should be obvious that content judgments alone are insufficient for assuming that scores on instruments are valid for a certain use. Unfortunately some published tool descriptions continue to report content validity as the only category of validity evidence.

Evidence based on response processes deals with the fit between the measured construct and participants' responses. Activities that provide this kind of evidence include interviewing test takers about their performance strategies and the effects of extraneous factors like social desirability on their responses and observations or interviewing judges to determine if and how they applied the appropriate criteria. Such analyses were one part of the former "type" of construct validity.[25]

Evidence based on internal structure encompasses various factor analysis and item analysis procedures formerly called statistical or correlational construct validity.[25] Conceptually, the many varieties of factor analysis all aim to reduce a set of variables (the instrument items) to smaller clusters of correlated items called factors. The content of the items within a factor and the mathematical weights of the factors are then used to define the concept or to support prior theorizing about its nature. By identifying items that do not fall into a cluster (do not *load*, in factor analysis jargon), factor analysis is useful in refining an instrument. It also sheds light on whether a construct is unidimensional or multidimensional, that is, whether a construct has subparts and whether subscale scores should be calculated. To be credible, factor analysis requires a minimum of five subjects per variable (test item) for shorter tests; Froman cites recommendations for samples ranging from 100 to "several hundred" for longer tests in her lucid, nonstatistical introduction to factor analysis.[30] This guideline is frequently violated in published reports, especially older ones. *Confirmatory factor analysis* is a newer, more powerful procedure that requires researchers to specify in advance and test hypotheses about relationships between factors, and which items will load on which factors, while (very importantly) taking measurement error into consideration.[22] An example of its use can be found in Wineman, Durand, and McCulloch.[31]

Evidence based on relations to other variables addresses the relationships of test scores to scores on other tests, the ability of the test to predict external criteria, and the evaluation of group differences logical in light of the proposed test interpretation.[25] This evidence is usually obtained through correlational and group comparison studies.[32]

The relationship of test scores to scores on other tests can be assessed by convergent and discriminant or divergent validity. Scores from two anxiety scales should converge and be positively and at least moderately correlated. Scores from a depression measure and a happiness measure should diverge and have a low or negative correlation. A more elaborate technique is the multitrait-multimethod (MTMM) approach of Campbell and Fisk.[33] Scores from at least two constructs, each measured in at least two different ways, are entered into a correlation matrix. By reading different diagonals of the matrix, one can obtain separate correlations for reliability and for convergent, discriminant, and construct validity. The technique is informative but is often difficult to carry out. A clear example of the procedure is found in Burns and Grove.[9]

Two designs have historically been used to assess test-criterion relationships (previously called criterion validity). They differ on when the criterion data are collected. In concurrent validity, data from the test and the criterion measure are collected at the same time and indicate the person's present standing on the criterion. For example, a measure of patients' perceived readiness for discharge could be correlated with caregivers' perceptions of their readiness. A high correlation between the scores of the two samples would support concurrent test-criterion relationships. For predictive validity, data on the criterion are collected from the same subjects at a future date.[25] The predictive validity of the Graduate Record Examination for success in graduate study could be evaluated by correlating entering students' scores on the test with their final grade point averages.

In principle, test-criterion relationships are a strong form of validity. In practice, there are some important problems.[8] Often, identification of an adequate criterion is not possible, or if a criterion can be identified, reliable measures for it may not be available. Validity coefficients based on a criterion measure with low reliability will underestimate the true strength of the predictor-criterion relationship. Underestimates of validity also will occur if the sample is not random or representative.[8] The validity coefficient may be falsely high if criterion contamination occurs, that is, if raters or judges know how members of the sample performed on the predictor.[8] Consumers of measurement literature should look for wording that the judges or collectors of criterion data were blind to (unaware of) participants' group assignments to rule out this possibility. In addition, a coefficient from a single criterion-related study will tend to inflate the predictor-criterion relationship. Ideally, cross-validation should occur, a procedure in which the predictor-criterion relationship is developed on one sample and tested on a second independent sample from the same population. The cross-validation correlation usually is a lower, more accurate estimate of the true predictor-criterion relationship.[8]

Evidence about group differences that support relations between the test scores and other variables is collected in two ways. First, the instrument can be administered to two groups known to be high and low on the measured concept (the former *known groups* approach to construct validity). If the groups' scores differ significantly in the expected direction, construct validity is supported. Second, one can conduct experimental studies to test hypotheses about the effects of specific interventions on test scores (the former *experimental* or *hypothesis-testing* approach to construct validity).[32] For example, an intervention to teach stress management strategies to patients might logically be expected to reduce scores on perceived stress. If that hypothesis is borne out, construct validity is supported.

Evidence based on the consequences of testing provides information about the anticipated and unanticipated benefits and harm resulting from testing and whether test use results in differential consequences for different identifiable groups.[25] This newest addition to the *Standards for Educational and Psychological Testing*[25] is controversial. To many it crosses the line between science and sociopolitical concerns;[34] to others, the task is overwhelmingly large or too lacking in strategies for accomplishment.[32] No other reference to this standard was found in the nursing measurement literature.

Item Response Theory: A Nonclassic Approach to Test Construction and Construct Validation

In classic measurement theory, respondent characteristics and test characteristics cannot be separated from each other. Test scores depend on the specific items administered and there is no way to predict how likely an individual test taker is to answer a certain item in a certain way. Item response theory (IRT)[35] was developed to address these limitations.

On the assumption that a test taker's response to an item reflects her standing on the concept of interest (called a latent trait), IRT models let one measure the difficulty of each item and each item's relationship to the trait and arrange large numbers of items from least to most difficult. One can then focus on the contributions of individual items as they are added to or removed from a test and conduct rigorous tests of measurement equivalence across groups.[36] By providing data on predicted and unpredicted responses and on expected performance of both high- and low-scoring test takers, IRT improves the users' understanding of the meaning of scores,[37] thus advancing construct validity.

IRT also has greatly facilitated computer adaptive testing, in which test takers' answers to preceding items determine which items they will see next and how many in order to determine their status on the underlying latent trait.[38] The NCLEX (National Council Licensure Examination) examination uses the form of IRT known as Rasch measurement to assess the latent trait of entry-level nursing competency and does so with high validity.[39]

Although it was developed more than 25 years ago, IRT is still rare in the nursing literature. Its prominence may increase as more nurse researchers learn of its value for developing affective instruments and about the availability of computer programs for data analysis.[37]

Interpretation of Validity Evidence

Establishing validity is more difficult than establishing reliability for at least three reasons. First, whereas reliability involves some form of correlation of the test with itself, many validity assessments are based on measures or outcomes *external* to the test and require evaluating the meaning of logical, but indirect, relationships. Second, because many logical relationships may need to be examined to support validity, validation often requires the completion of several distinct studies, which can use any research design.[25] Third, validation often involves the use of more and more complex statistical procedures than does estimation of reliability.

Validity coefficients are usually lower than those for reliability. In contrast to reliability coefficients of 0.70 to 0.90, validity coefficients of 0.30 to 0.60 may be entirely satisfactory.[22] Unlike reliability coefficients, some validity coefficients will be negative. Tool users should ask: What is being correlated (statistically or logically) with what? How strong can the relationship reasonably be expected to be? Is use of the tool an improvement over use of previous tools or of no measurement at all? How similar is the proposed use to conditions under which the available validity evidence was obtained? What use will be made of the scores?

Evidence for the validity of a test should be viewed as a cumulative pattern. Each positive study results in greater confidence that the test scores are useful for a given purpose. On the other hand, despite many previous successes, one strong negative finding can destroy confidence in the test. Because validity evidence is specific to a use of the test scores for a certain group and purpose rather than to the instrument itself, users should plan to provide additional evidence of validity from their studies.[8]

Other Desirable Tool Characteristics

Sensitivity is the ability of an instrument to make discriminations of the needed fineness. Often, instruments with yes/no categories will not allow many subjects to respond accurately. Expanding the response options to five categories ranging from "strongly approve" to "strongly disapprove" will increase its sensitivity. Sensitivity is especially important when physiologic measurements are being monitored, when measurements will be used to make decisions about an individual rather than a group, and when the experimental and control conditions are not drastically different.[8,9] These are all common conditions in clinical research. Unnecessary sensitivity may be expensive to achieve and burdensome for either the respondent or the investigator.

Comprehensibility is the extent to which subjects can meet the requirements of the instrument. Comprehensibility often involves the reading level of an instrument and its fit to the demographic and cultural backgrounds of the intended subjects.[5] An incomprehensible tool will produce invalid responses or refusals to complete it.

Objectivity is the extent to which the data obtained reflect what is being measured rather than some outside influence. Common threats to objectivity are the influence of the race or sex of an interviewer on the subject, instructions that suggest what the answers should be, and observation guides that require the researcher to judge behavior.

The *feasibility* of an instrument is assessed in terms of the time, cost, and skill needed for the study and in terms of the instrument's acceptability to potential subjects. Cost factors include the time and expense of obtaining subjects, and the purchase price of the instrument, printing, photocopying, postage, clerical help, computer time, and consultation. Other things being equal, a short, machine-scorable instrument would be more feasible than a longer one that must be hand-scored or interpreted by a specialist.

Choosing Instruments for Intervention Studies

Most descriptions of psychometric properties of instruments deal with the ability of instruments to assess individual differences reliably and validly. Much less attention has been given to evaluating instruments for use in intervention studies, now a rapidly growing focus of nursing research.[40]

For intervention studies the most important characteristic of the instruments used to measure the dependent variables is sensitivity: the instrument must be able to detect changes that result from the intervention. An instrument that is not adequately sensitive may lead to the false conclusion that the intervention was ineffective.[40,41]

Although a full description of this issue is beyond the scope of this chapter, there are several strategies for promoting sensitive measurement in intervention research. Examining the conceptual fit between the intervention and candidate measures is essential. This means asking oneself whether the proposed outcome variable is indeed changeable and how much, whether the outcome variable is influenced by many factors other than the intervention, and whether the content of the instrument items is closely related to the content of the intervention.[40,41] In an intervention to lower dietary cholesterol, life satisfaction would be a poor choice for a dependent variable. It is not closely related to the intervention, the intervention is not likely to change it, and it is affected by many factors outside of the study.

Users seeking instruments for intervention research should search for literature dealing with measurement of change. Reports that an instrument has successfully detected change and change of a certain magnitude in other interventions, reports that compare the ability of several measures to detect change, and reports that compare groups known to be very different on the clinical outcome measure are powerful evidence of construct validity for dealing with change.[40,42]

More strategies for sensitive measurement include the use of disease- or condition-specific measures rather than or in addition to generic measures (such as a scale measuring diabetes-related quality of life rather than a general measure of quality of life),[43] use of measures based on the criterion-referenced measurement framework,[41] and the use of procedures designed to establish individual norms for research participants, such as magnitude estimation and goal attainment scaling. Magnitude estimation[44] obtains participants' quantitative estimates of the intensity of a stimulus, such as breathlessness, fatigue, or pain in a proportional manner, yielding ratio-level data. In a study of breathlessness and various airway resistances, participants assign numbers above or below a personally set average value to different levels of airway resistance ("This is a 4.0, twice as hard as the 2.0."). Magnitude estimation requires extensive preparation of the investigator and careful training of participants to be able to make proportional judgments. Goal attainment scaling (GAS)[45] is a means of comparing individuals' relative success in achieving personal goals for an intervention. Advantages of GAS include sensitivity, overcoming floor and ceiling effects that set limits on change in some other measurement strategies,[40] and suitability for assessing changes in lifestyles and behavioral skills.[45]

The interpretation of reliability as stability over time for instruments in intervention research has no simple answer. High test-retest reliability ($r = 0.90$) over a short period of time does not necessarily mean that the instrument would not detect change, but high stability correlations over longer periods of time may. Lower correlations (r = 0.30–0.60) over short intervals may not be a problem for intervention studies if between-subject variability on the instrument is also low.[42]

Psychometric Properties of Biophysiologic Measures

Although data obtained from bioinstrumentation and laboratory procedures are generally accurate, sensitive, and objective, several threats to their reliability and validity (more often referred to as precision and accuracy in physiologic measurement) do exist.[9] Most involve human error (e.g., improper use or calibration of equipment, failure to follow established procedures, or clerical errors in reporting results) or equipment failure. Users of biophysiologic measures often must employ quality-control strategies, such as regular calibrations of equipment and random checks of adherence to procedures. Although biophysical measures are relatively immune to subjects' distortions of readings, the measurement process itself can alter the variable of interest. For example, the presence of a transducer in the bloodstream can reduce the blood flow in the vessel.[8] Other considerations with biophysiologic instruments include direct versus indirect measurement, invasive versus noninvasive measurement, single versus multiple measures, and sensitivity.[5]

Some biophysiologic phenomena (pain, nausea, fatigue) are more subjective than objective and can be assessed by paper-and-pencil instruments. The chief consideration in choosing the data collection method is the conceptualization of the phenomenon being studied. If a visual analog scale or short questionnaire captures the variable of interest and adequate psychometric data are available, there is no point in using an expensive, invasive physiologic procedure.[5,9]

Other Helpful Procedures in Instrument Evaluation

Pretesting and Piloting an Instrument

Pretesting (trying out an instrument with a few volunteers) and piloting (trying out the research procedure as a small-scale trial run) can be useful in choosing and using an instrument. The following instrumentation issues can be addressed in a pretest or pilot study.[46]

- Perform reliability and validity checks.
- Reduce random error by assessing subjects' response to the instrument. Are the instructions clear? Do subjects understand the questions and answer them correctly? Do some questions cause embarrassment or resistance? Is cheating or unwanted collaboration among subjects a problem?
- Obtain accurate estimates of the time required to complete the instrument and of the cost of data collection.
- Determine that the tool will indeed yield the needed data and eliminate the collection of unnecessary data.
- Gain staff experience and confidence in working with the subjects and the tool.
- Standardize rater, interview, and other measurement techniques.
- Compare two or more instruments to aid one's final choice.

Subjects for a pilot study should be as similar as possible to those in the eventual study group. Some researchers are content to obtain only the views of fellow nurses or graduate students or faculty; although their evaluations may be helpful, they are no substitute for representatives of the study populations. For most trial runs, a sample size of 10 to 20 should suffice. More may be needed if the measurement procedure is complex or if the sample is heterogeneous.

For maximum benefit from a pilot study, the investigator should observe subjects as they complete the instrument and then interview them about their reactions. The meaning of subjects' nonverbal responses should be explored. Do frowns, fidgets, and many erasures indicate item ambiguity, resistance to the content or circumstances of administration, or genuine involvement? Because of the small sample size and the relative artificiality of the situation, a pilot study cannot anticipate or solve all the problems.[46] Nevertheless, few research procedures are as useful.

Putting It All Together

These are important questions to consider when evaluating existing instruments:

- *Purpose.* Is the purpose of the instrument clearly defined? Is the purpose of the study to identify differences between persons or to evaluate an intervention? Is the purpose similar to that of my study?
- *Measurement framework.* Is the measurement framework specified? Is it appropriate for my study?
- *Conceptual base.* Is the conceptual base stated? Implied? If not a match, is it at least compatible with my orientation to the problem?
- *Subjects.* Are the intended subjects clearly described? How similar or different are they to those in my study? How many subjects have contributed to the development of this tool?
- *Data-gathering method.* What method is used? Is the method properly used? What are the advantages and disadvantages of this method?
- *Content.* Is the content dated or current? Is a rationale apparent for each item?
- *Administration and scoring.* Are these clearly described? Will the conditions of administration be similar in my study? Will I need help in scoring or interpreting the results?
- *Reliability and validity.* Are multiple and appropriate forms of reliability and validity reported? Are reliability and validity methods and coefficients appropriate for the concept being measured and the study purpose? Can responses be faked or distorted easily (a threat to validity)?
- *Sensitivity.* Will this instrument make discriminations of the necessary fineness? If selecting instruments for an intervention, is there evidence that this instrument detected change in other studies?
- *Comprehensibility.* Is the reading level suited to the intended subjects? Do assumptions made about things like standard of living or cultural background fit the intended subjects?
- *Feasibility.* How much time will subjects need to complete this tool? Will subjects be able to do this task under the conditions for my study? Can I afford to use this tool? Does this tool need to be modified before I can use it? Do I have the expertise to make these modifications? If not, can I find help to do this?

Because few instruments have model histories, the evaluation of instruments always is a judgment call. If you answered most questions positively and you generally believe that the instrument meets your needs, use it. If there are major doubts, look for another instrument or conduct a pilot study. A helpful hint: Saving the written assessment of instruments will result in a useful instrument file. Instruments not used for one study may suit another.

Ethical and Legal Aspects of Instrument Use

The ethical and legal use of instruments places obligations on the investigator to the subjects, the developer or publisher, and the professional and scientific communities. Because obligations to subjects are described in most research texts or can be clarified by research review boards, this discussion will focus on the obligations to the developer and the larger community.

Ethical considerations are inherent in the measurement considerations just discussed. The thoughtful selection of an appropriate instrument and its proper use are themselves ethical acts. Failure to perform them is at best a waste of time and at worst a hindrance to the advancement of nursing knowledge.

Obligations to the Instrument Developer

The user's first obligation to the developer is to obtain his or her written permission to use the tool. Doing so may or may not be simple. Because research literature gives very little guidance about this, the following experiential suggestions are offered.

Ideally, the developer will be at the institution named in the source of instrument information. If not, an address may sometimes be obtained from a later publication by the developer, from another user of the instrument, or from a test publisher. Membership directories of professional organizations, conference brochures, lists of conference participants, and one's own network may also be helpful.

The letter to the instrument developer should be short and simple. The user should state that he or she wishes to use Instrument X described in Journal Y for Purpose Z. (The name and the source are important because authors may have published more than one instrument in more than one source.) A short abstract or a three- or four-sentence description of the project should be provided. It is permissible to ask authors whether they have more recent information about the instrument to share, but they should not be expected to supply a review of literature. The letter should close with an offer to share the findings, an indication of when they may be available, and a statement that full credit will be given to the developer. If 6 weeks pass without a reply, a courteous second letter may be sent, inquiring whether the previous one was received and requesting a prompt reply.

Although most authors are delighted when people wish to use their instruments, the replies are not always favorable. Some authors do not release their tools until they are highly developed or until they have written a certain article or grant proposal. Others grant permission for use but attach a list of conditions. For example, they may charge for the instrument's use, limit the number of copies allowed, stipulate that the instrument may not be altered, request a report of the results, or ask that the responses be shared for the ongoing development of the instrument. Users are obligated to fulfill those conditions unless they can negotiate otherwise.

The user's second obligation to the instrument developer is to report the results of the instrument's use to the developer, whether or not such feedback was requested. Information about difficulties encountered, additional determinations of reliability and validity, and suggestions for modification or future use help the developer to improve the instrument and aid the accumulation of knowledge about it.[8]

Obligations to a Test Publisher

Some instruments are available from commercial test publishers. The publisher can be identified in the publication describing the instrument, by the author, or by the publisher's catalog. In this case, users purchase the manual and copies. Some publishers request documentation of users' qualifications for using the instrument properly. Acceptable documentation may consist of a graduate degree in a field that emphasizes measurement, the titles and credit hours of measurement courses, membership in a professional organization concerned with measurement, a brief list of one's research activities, or supervision from a qualified individual who consents to oversee the use of the instrument.

Obligations to the Scientific and Professional Communities

Knowledge about instruments and their applications cannot accumulate if the research is never published. The most available and enduring form of publication is a journal article.

The goal of a report on instrument use is to provide enough information so that readers can determine that sound measurement principles were observed and reach justified conclusions about the findings. In these reports, full credit must be given to the original developer. Any modifications in tool content, administration, scoring, or interpretation must be clearly described, along with psychometric data about the changes. Information about extraneous or confounding variables that might have influenced subjects' scores and reliability and validity assessments within the study should be provided. Reports of problems with an instrument are as useful to other investigators as reports of success.[3,4]

Copyright Considerations

Because of widespread Internet access and the surge of various electronic technologies with which existing copyright laws were never designed to deal,[47] it is difficult to provide comprehensive guidance about copyright concerns. The safest advice to users is never to use an instrument if permission cannot be obtained from the original author or a legal designee, such as the publisher. According to the Copyright Clearance Center,[48] the old doctrine of *fair use*, in which one may use portions of copyrighted materials in research, is increasingly unclear and is being tested in the courts. The absence of a copyright notice or symbol on a tool does not mean that it may be freely used, because copyright notices have not been mandatory since 1989. Moreover, the most recent U.S. copyright laws have automatically renewed copyright protection for many works for which it had lapsed and extended its duration to either life-plus-70 years or to 95 or 120 years after the author's death, depending on the date of creation.[49] Giving credit to the author or publisher or the fact that the user makes no money from using another's material does not free one of possible charges of copyright infringement. Last, to be safe in using tools believed to be in the public domain, researchers should use only those for which a notice to that effect appears in the article or on the instrument or for which the author or the sponsoring governmental unit confirms that it is indeed in the public domain. This will avoid problems with distinguishing between works *by* the federal government that are in the public domain and works prepared *for* the government, which may or may not be in the public domain.[48] Reference librarians or the legal counsel of a clinical agency or school of nursing also may give advice on these matters.

Useful Websites for Measurement

A very large compilation of full-text instruments (80 sources containing 8,089 measures) compiled and updated by Helen Hough, a health sciences reference librarian, can be found at libraries.uta.edu/helen/Test&meas/testframed.htm.[50]

The U.S. Copyright Office is also helpful for detailed copyright information. A particularly comprehensive circular, *How to Investigate the Copyright Status of a Work*, can be found at www.copyright.gov/circs/circ22.html.[49]

References

1. Waltz, C.F., & Strickland, O.L. Measurement of nursing outcomes: State of the art as we enter the eighties. In W.E. Field (Ed.), *Measuring outcomes of nursing practice, education, and administration: Proceedings of the First Annual Southern Council on Collegiate Education for Nursing Research Conference.* Atlanta: Southern Regional Education Board, 1982, p. 47.

2. Strickland, O.L., & Waltz, C.F. Measurement of research variables in nursing. In P.L. Chinn (Ed.), *Nursing research methodology: Issues and implementation.* Rockville, MD: Aspen, 1986, p. 79.

3. Norbeck, J.S. What constitutes a publishable report of instrument development? *Nurs Res,* 1986, 34(6):380-382.

4. Froman, R.D. Measuring our words on measurement. *Res Nurs Health,* 2000, 23(6):421-422.

5. Polit, D., & Hungler, B. *Nursing research: Principles and methods* (6th ed.). Philadelphia: Lippincott, 1999.

6. Strickland, O.L. An instrument's conceptual base: Its link to theory. *J Nurs Measurement,* 2001, 9(1):3-4.

7. Sauter, M.A., Boyle, D., Andrews, J.L., et al. Psychometric valuation of the Organizational Job Satisfaction Scale. *J Nurs Measurement,* 1997, 5(1):53-69.

8. Waltz, C.F., Strickland, O.L., & Lenz, E.R. *Measurement in nursing research* (2nd ed.). Philadelphia: Davis, 1991.

9. Burns, N., & Grove, S.K. *The practice of nursing research: Conduct, critique, and utilization* (4th ed.). Philadelphia: Saunders, 2001.

10. Ferketich, S. Aspects of item analysis. *Res Nurs Health,* 1991, 14(2):165-168.

11. Knapp, T.R. Validity, reliability, and neither. *Nurs Res,* 1985, 34(3):189-192.

12. Washington, C.C., & Moss, M. Pragmatic aspects of establishing interrater reliability in research. *Nurs Res,* 1988, 37(3):190-191.

13. Castorr, A.H., Thompson, K.O., Ryan, J.W., et al. The process of rater training for observational instruments: Implications for interrater reliability. *Res Nurs Health,* 1990, 13(5):311-318.

14. Cohen, J.A. A coefficient of agreement for nominal scales. *Educ Psychol Measurement,* 1960, 20(1):37-46.

15. Cohen, J. Weighted kappa: Nominal scale agreement with provision for scaled disagreement or partial credit. *Psychological Bulletin,* 1968, 70(4):213-220.

16. Topf, M. Three estimates of interrater reliability for nominal data. *Nurs Res,* 1986, 36(4):253-255.

17. Ferketich, S. Internal consistency estimates of reliability. *Res Nurs Health,* 1990, 13(6):437-440.

18. Strickland, O.L. When is internal consistency reliability assessment inappropriate? *J Nurs Measurement,* 1999, 7(1):3-4.

19. Zeller, R.P., & Carmines, E.G. *Measurement in the social sciences.* Cambridge, England: Cambridge University Press, 1980.

20. Hartmann, D. Considerations in the choice of interobserver reliability estimates. *J Appl Behav Anal,* 1977, 10(1):103-116.

21. Shrout, P.E. Measurement reliability and agreement in psychiatry. *Stat Meth Med Res,* 1998, 7:301-317.

22. Nunnally, J.C., & Bernstein, R.L. *Psychometric theory* (3rd ed.). New York: McGraw-Hill, 1994.

23. Shavelson, R.J., & Webb, N. *Generalizabilty theory: A primer.* Newbury Park, CA: Sage, 1991.

24. Burns, K.J. Beyond classical reliability: Using generalizability theory to assess dependability. *Res Nurs Health,* 1998, 21(1):83-90.

25. American Psychological Association, American Educational Research Association, & National Council on Measurement in Education. *Standards for educational and psychological testing.* Washington, D.C.: American Psychological Association, 1999.

26. Lynn, M.R. Determination and quantification of content validity. *Nurs Res,* 1986, 35(6):382-385.

27. Gable, R.K., & Wolf, J.W. *Instrument development in the affective domain: Measuring attitudes and values in corporate and school settings.* Boston: Kluwer Academic, 1993.

28. Grant, J.S., & Davis, L.L. Selection and use of content experts for instrument development. *Res Nurs Health,* 1997, 20(3):269-274.

29. Berk, R.A. Importance of expert judgment in content-related validity evidence. *West J Nurs Res,* 1990, 12(5):659-671.

30. Froman, R.D. Elements to consider in planning the use of factor analysis. *South Online J Nurs Res,* 2001, 2(5). Access date 3 March 2003. www.snrs/org/members/journal.html.

31. Wineman, N.M., Durand, E.J., & McCulloch, B.J. Examination of the factor structure of the ways of coping questionnaire with clinical populations. *Nurs Res,* 1994, 43(5):268-273.

32. Goodwin, L.D. Changing conceptions of measurement validity: An update on the new *Standards. J Nurs Ed,* 2002, 41(3):100-106.

33. Campbell, D.T., & Fiske, D.W. Convergent and discriminant validity in the multitrait-multimethod matrix. *Psychol Bull,* 1959, 56(2):81-105.

34. Crocker, L. Editorial: The great validity debate. *Edu Measurement: Issues and Practice,* 1997, 16(2):4.

35. Hambleton, R., Swaminathan, H., & Rogers, H.J. *Fundamentals of item response theory.* Newbury Park, CA: Sage, 1991.

36. Uebersax, J.S. *Latent trait analysis and item response theory (IRT) models.* Updated 30 June 2003. Access date 3 March 2003. www.ourworld.compuserve.com/homepages/jsuebersax/etc.htm.

37. Beck, C.T., & Gable, R.K. Item response theory in affective instrument development: An illustration. *J Nurs Measurement,* 2001, 9(1):5-22.

38. University of Illinois at Urbana-Champaign. Item Response Theory Laboratory, 2001. Access date 3 March 2003. www.work.psych.uiuc.edu/irt/intro_main.asp.

39. National Council of State Boards of Nursing. Testing services, NCLEX Psychometrics, 1996-2001. Access date 3 March 2003. www.nscbn.org/public/testing/info_dvlpmnt.htm. Click on "NCLEX Reliability and Validity."

40. Lipsey, M.W. *Design sensitivity: Statistical power for experimental research.* Newbury Park, CA: Sage, 1990.

41. Stewart, B.J., & Archbold, P.G. Nursing intervention studies require outcome measures that are sensitive to change: Part One. *Res Nurs Health,* 1992, 15(6):477-481.

42. Stewart, B.J., & Archbold, P.G. Nursing intervention studies require outcome measures that are sensitive to change: Part Two. *Res Nurs Health,* 1993, 16(1):77-81.

43. Kane, R.L. *Understanding health care outcomes research.* Gaithersburg, MD: Aspen, 1997.

44. Meek, P.M., Sennott-Miller, L., & Ferketich, S.L. Scaling stimuli with magnitude estimation. *Res Nurs Health,* 1992, 15(1):77-81.

45. Becker, H., Stuifbergen, A., Rogers, S., & Timmerman, G. Goal attainment scaling to measure individual

change in intervention studies. *Nurs Res*, 2000, 20(3):176-180.

46. Fox, R.N., & Ventura, M. Small scale administration of instruments and procedures. *Nurs Res*, 1983, 32(2):122-125

47. Goudreau, K.A. The copyright quagmire on the Internet. *Comput Nurs*, 1999, 17(2):82-85.

48. Copyright Clearance Center, Inc. *Copyright law: Who needs it?*, 1995-2002. Access date 7 February 2003. www.copyright.com/Copyright_Resources/default.asp.

49. United States Copyright Office. *How to investigate the copyright status of a work*, June 2002. Access date 3 March 2003. www.copyright.gov/circs/circ22.html.

50. University of Texas at Arlington. An index to assessment instruments as found fulltext in printed texts and journals. Updated December 2002 by Helen Hough. Access date 7 February 2003. www.libraries.uta.edu/helen/Test&meas/testframed.htm.

2

Tool Adaptation to Reduce Health Disparities

Sally P. Weinrich, Marlyn D. Boyd, and JoAnne Herman

Health Disparities

Ethnic minorities and medically underserved populations, who have disproportional rates of disease, have been underrepresented in research.[1] Today, increased emphasis on reducing health disparities is mandating that research instruments be developed and adapted for these populations. *Medically underserved* refers to populations that have inadequate access to or reduced utilization of cancer prevention, screening, early detection, treatment, or rehabilitation services.[2] The term includes people underinsured or uninsured, those with little formal education, rural and inner-city populations, the unemployed, and those with low socioeconomic status (SES).[1] Each tool should operationally define the specific medically underserved population because there is no consistent definition.

There has been a significant increase in the number and type of instruments useful for nursing research, but few instruments have been designed specifically for or adapted for medically underserved populations.[2] This chapter provides guidelines for the evaluation and adaptation of instruments for use with medically underserved populations.

More than 11% of the population lived at the poverty level in 2000.[3] The highest poverty levels are in African Americans (22.1%) and Hispanics (21.2%).[3] Many researchers have made the mistake of attributing the health disparities between groups to race or ethnicity without paying close attention to income or socioeconomic variability. Socioeconomic variability is often more relevant than race or ethnicity in assessing health.[4] In 2002, 12% of the population was covered by Medicaid.[5] More than 30% of the poor had no health insurance of any kind during 2001.[3]

Between 21% and 24% of United States adults have low literacy skills (reading below the eighth-grade level).[6] A high school diploma does not mean that a person is literate.[7] Although grade completed of formal schooling and reading ability are not synonymous, there is some correlation. Most studies have found that people tend to read three to five grade levels below the last grade completed.[9,10] If reading is not used in work or leisure activities, reading skills deteriorate over time.[9,11,12] It is important for the researcher to remember that impaired literacy does *not* mean *below-normal intelligence*. Instead, a study participant with low literacy abilities has a deficit in the use of written and oral language in a literate society. These limitations can greatly affect test outcomes. High literacy level of patient education materials, including instruments, has been documented in several studies.[11–16]

The medically underserved participant may have difficulty in a number of areas that can affect the validity and reliability of instruments. Impaired language skills, including a limited vocabulary, can mean that the study participant's viewpoint is limited to his or her own personal experience.[8] Extrapolating to an unknown may be an impossible task for the medically underserved participant. For example, if a medically underserved participant is asked, "What would you do if you started having bad headaches?" he or she might answer, "No, I don't never get bad headaches." The person may not be able to think abstractly outside of his or her present state.

Another limitation may be that the medically underserved participant may not comprehend the rationale for questions. When asked, "Tell me how you fix your meals," the medically underserved participant may say, "Well you know, just like I always done." The rationale for attitude or opinion questions can be especially confusing. For example, in response to questions about fear of cancer, respondents have responded to the authors with "Are you trying to trick me?" Similarly, the rationale for mental status questions can be confusing to older medically underserved people. The 10 mental status questions include questions such as "Who is the current president, and who was the past president?" Noninstitutionalized, well, elderly participants asked these questions responded with "I'm not crazy," "Don't you think I know what I'm doing?" and even "I'm not going to answer anymore." The authors have reduced the 10 mental status questions to two questions dealing with date and location. Experience has shown that these two questions are reliable indicators of mental status in older, *noninstitutionalized* medically underserved populations.

Similarly, a medically underserved study participant may have difficulty categorizing data. Asking participants to choose foods low in fat or to list several aerobic exercises may result in no response or a jumbled list of several foods and activity items. Literacy-impaired individuals may also have difficulty with abstract concepts, synthesizing data, and problem solving. Asking a cardiac rehabilitation patient to describe how the heart works may net the interviewer a prolonged silence from someone who cannot conceptualize the heart's physiology.

The literacy-impaired study participant usually has a very limited vocabulary and is not capable of distinguishing between nuances of terms or distinguishing between spectrums of options. For example, asking a medically underserved individual to describe pain in terms such as burning, stabbing, or radiating may only confuse the respondent. Similarly, a Likert-type scale may be too confusing for the literacy-impaired adult to respond to with accuracy or reliability. Because reading and listening can be difficult for medically underserved study participants, they may be easily distracted, have short attention spans, and refuse to complete a tool, or they can become irritable or angry.

Tools Designed to Reduce Health Disparities

The majority of published literature on research that has used tools for medically underserved populations concerns women[17–25] or children.[26–32] Less research on low-income men has been published.[33-38] African Americans are underrepresented in research instrument studies.

Three tools that have been developed for medically underserved populations are the Dartmouth Primary Care Cooperative Information scales (COOP),[39-42] the John Henryism Scale for Active Coping,[43,38] and the Knowledge of Colorectal Cancer Questionnaire.[36]

Adaptation of Existing Tools

Existing instruments can and should be pilot tested and adapted when used with a medically underserved population that is different from the population on which the instrument was developed.[44] For example, an instrument first used with low-income urban residents can be used for low-income migratory farm workers. Potential changes in the instrument include reducing the literacy level, changing individual words, changing response options, and shortening the instrument. A comprehensive assessment of the medically underserved population is the initial step. Focus groups that are similar in demographic characteristics to the population who will be surveyed are also excellent sources for evaluating and modifying questionnaires.[45]

Several studies have adapted instruments for medically underserved populations.[40,42,46-52] Adaptations have included adjustments for literacy level and cultural level and pilot testing of the instrument. The studies of Bill-Harvey et al.[50] with arthritic patients are examples of studies that have adapted a tool for a medically underserved population.

Assessment of the Medically Underserved

Assessment of the specific population and pilot studies are crucial first steps in the development of a valid and reliable instrument.[53] Data on the population to be studied can be obtained from a variety of sources such as patient records, databases, and individuals. Data such as age, gender, educational attainment, ethnicity, and work history can be obtained from records or databases. A small sample of the study population should be interviewed to assess factors such as readability (if tool is to be self-administered), oral comprehension (if interview format is to be used), and slang or regional terms used for concepts that are being measured.

Reducing Literacy Level

The subjects' reading abilities, as well as the literacy level of the instrument, should be assessed.[8,13,54] Every subject's reading level does need to be tested, but rather, a random sample of the typical client population should be tested to establish a baseline or profile for the study population. One quick, easy, and accurate method of testing a subject's reading ability is to use the reading subtest of the Wide Range Achievement Test (WRAT). This brief test (5 minutes or less) is normed on age versus grade levels and is a good clinical tool for assessing reading ability.[55] It is noteworthy that the authors of this chapter have found major inconsistencies with medically underserved populations in self-reported educational level and actual reading level when using the WRAT.

An assessment of the medical reading level is critical. The Test of Functional Health Literacy in Adults (TOFHLA) is an instrument designed to assess the ability of individuals to understand and act on common instructions given to patients.[56] The instrument has two parts: Comprehension and Numeracy. Both parts contain passages from common instructions. After the participant reads the passage, the researcher asks questions about actions that are required. For example, the Comprehension TOFHLA contains x-ray preparation instructions, Medicaid rights and responsibilities, and informed consent. The Numeracy TOFHLA is similarly designed but the content includes numbers, such as instructions on how to take medications. Participant scores are calculated by adding up the correct responses to the questions. The scores are combined to determine the total health literacy score. Norms have been developed to use in interpretation of scores. A score of 0–59 indicates inadequate functional health literacy. A score of 60–74 indicates marginal health literacy and a score of 75–100 indicates adequate functional health literacy. The TOFHLA is available in both English and Spanish.

Measurement of a subject's reading level is only one step in the process of developing valid and reliable instruments. Measurement of the literacy level of the instrument with a readability formula is also important. Readability formulas are mathematical equations that predict the level of reading ability needed to understand a printed piece. Readability formulas measure various grammatical components such as sentence length, the number of syllables, and word familiarity. The SMOG, Fry Formula, FOG Index, and the Flesch-Kincaid are common readability formulas.[12,57–60] They are accurate to within 1.5 to 2 grade levels.[58] Appendix 2A and Appendix 2B provides guidelines for using the SMOG formula. Today, many computer word processing programs have readability assessment programs that are easily used. However, they often yield significantly different reading grade level scores.[61]

Reducing the literacy level of an instrument includes using short words and avoiding the use of words with three or more syllables; using short sentences; using active rather than passive voice; using boldface, serif type, italics, or underline for emphasis; using pictures to illustrate concepts; using analogies or examples for abstract terms; and giving simple directions (Exhibit 2.1).[62] Consider the differences in wording in the following:

- *College Reading Level.* With the onset of nausea, diarrhea, or other gastrointestinal disturbances consult your physician immediately.
- *Twelfth Grade Reading Level.* If you experience nausea, diarrhea, or other stomach or bowel problems, call your physician immediately.
- *Eighth Grade Reading Level.* If you start having nausea, loose bowel movements, or other stomach or bowel problems, call your doctor immediately.
- *Fourth Grade Reading Level.* If you start having an upset stomach, loose bowel movements, or other problems, call your doctor right away.[9]

The effectiveness and reliability of pictures to measure functional status has been documented. In a study by Larson et al.[63] no response differences occurred between patients who received functional questions that were depicted with pictures and those who received written text and no pictures.

Wording Changes

Individual words may have different meanings for various populations. Some participants in the authors' study of colorectal cancer[64] thought *stool* meant bar stool and were quite puzzled when asked if they had ever had their stool tested for hidden blood. There are no set guidelines for what medically underserved persons will and will not understand. The instrument must be pilot tested and changes made based on the feedback from the target population. Medically underserved persons often hide the fact that they do not understand. They have had a lifetime of reading incomprehensible material and are not used to an environment in which they can feel safe in admitting their confusion or lack of understanding. The misinterpretation of *stool* in the above example was identified by another medically underserved person who was hired as a research assistant in the Colorectal Cancer Project.[65] Of special significance was the fact that the researcher failed to detect this misunderstanding in the pilot studies, even though a special effort was made to check for literacy levels and understanding.

Exhibit 2.1   Reduction of Literacy Level[62]

- Avoid words with three syllables or more. For example, use *doctor* rather than *physician*, and use *cut* instead of *laceration*.
- Use shorter words for longer ones. For example, *give* versus *administer* or *wipe clean* versus *thoroughly cleanse*.[44]
- Use short sentences of about 10 words or less.
- Avoid complex sentence structures.
- Use the active rather than the passive voice.
- Make directions simple.
- Assess your population and use words that have meaning to your population.
- Use concrete examples rather than abstract whenever possible.
- Use boldface type, italics, or underlining for emphasis.
- Use pictures to illustrate concepts whenever possible.
- Use analogies or examples for abstract terms.
- Avoid medical abbreviations such as MI, SCAN, or TRP.
- Pilot test the instrument with a representative sample of the population.
- Use white space to rest the eyes (double spacing and margins).
- Use upper and lower case letters. ALL CAPS MAKES TEXT HARDER TO READ.
- Use type appropriate for age and vision (8- to 10-point type for patients with normal vision, 12- to 14-point type or larger for children or those with failing vision).

  This is 8 point type

  This is 10 point type

  This is 12 point type

  This is 14 point type

Serif type (letters with horizontal strokes at the bottoms and tops of letters) should typically be used; it is easier to read than sans serif. However, sans serif type is easier to read for those with poor vision, blurring, or distortion because it is a clearer, cleaner type.

Medical jargon is usually not understood by the general population, including medically underserved populations. For example, diabetes is often referred to as "sugar," hypertension as "high blood pressure," and anemia as "low blood." Commonly used examples heard by these authors are listed in Table 2.1. Again, the *specific* medically underserved population must be interviewed and words that they use identified for each questionnaire.

Medically underserved people think primarily in concrete terms and may have difficulty understanding abstract concepts. For example, a medically underserved participant may have great difficulty understanding the heart's need for oxygen (air), until it is compared to a car engine's need for gas. Testing the meaning of abstract terms usually takes more time; however, without this step of the process, the instrument may not be valid.

Identifying confusing and misunderstood words in a group setting is usually ineffective because people do not like to admit in public what they do not understand. Pilot testing should include individual questioning of study participants in a nonthreatening and private setting. An example of a method to encourage pilot study participants to help identify confusing words, concepts, or sentences is, "We will be asking many people like you these questions. Will you help me find questions that are not clear?" Or "Will you tell me what this means to you?" If the answer is yes, the questions should be read one at a time and the goal (identification of confusing words and concepts) repeated often. Asking about a specific word is also effective. For example, "Many people do not know what *bran* means. What does it mean to you?"

TABLE 2.1 Lay Terms for Common Medical Conditions

Medical Condition	Lay Terms
Anemia	Low blood, poor blood, tired blood
Arthritis	Stiffness, old joint disease, bursitis, gout, joint misery, old stiffness, rheumatism, Arthur
Cardiovascular disease	Heart trouble, bad heart
Constipation	Stopped up, bowels locked, bowel misery
Diabetes	Sugar, rot, high sugar
Diarrhea	Runs, outhouse trot, runny bowels
Hypertension	High blood pressure, high blood
Migraine headache	Sick headache, period headache
Sickle cell anemia	Blood disease, black curse
Syphilis	Bad blood
Pulmonary disease	The wheeze, breathing disease, bad lungs
Urinary retention	Kidneys won't act, water backed up, can't make water
Impotence	Trouble with my nature
Urinate	Pee, make water, make kidneys act, locked kidneys, piss

Changes in Response Options

Many instruments use Likert-type responses that have four to five options for answering. Some medically underserved persons think in terms of yes or no rather than variations of yes and no. The researcher should try to encourage an answer first by asking such things as "Is that a strong yes or a weak yes?" because Likert-type responses are more desirable. Results need to be analyzed. If all the responses fall into two categories rather than four, the instrument may need to be changed to yes/no responses. For example, in development of the Knowledge of Colorectal Cancer Questionnaire,[37] five response items were originally used: strongly agree, agree, disagree, strongly disagree, and don't know. In the pilot studies, respondents would answer yes or no. Trying to force a response by asking, "Is that a strong yes or just a yes?" resulted in confusion and misunderstanding among the participants. From their concrete perspective, they had already answered yes or no, and did not understand why they were being asked the same question again. Repeating and trying to force an answer to cover all the questions was a deterrent to the interview process, not an enhancing factor. When the response options were changed to yes or true and no or false, the interviewing process ran much more smoothly. The yes or no responses were used by most of the respondents. However, a small minority of about 15% would answer true or false. So both options were retained on the questionnaire, with the true/false option being placed in parentheses under the yes/no option.[37]

    Bowel cancer is always a deadly disease.
    Yes   No   Don't Know
    (True)   (False)

The key point here is to measure what works in *each* individually selected medically underserved population. Research studies are needed to document the effect of changes in response options on the sensitivity and reliability of instruments.

Awareness of Socially Desirable Answers

Medically underserved people may have a greater tendency to answer in terms of socially desirable answers. For example, questions that measure instrumental activities of daily living (dressing, cooking, shopping, cleaning house, and phone use)[66] were used in a research project involving older medically underserved people.[62] Most of the older people wanted to be independent in their activities of daily living, and data analyses revealed that the majority of the participants had answered that they were independent in their activities of daily living. Experience had taught these authors that the participants were more dependent than the data revealed. Changing the stem from "Can you fix your meals?" to "Tell me what problems you have with fixing your meals" resulted in answers that reflected greater levels of dependence. Also, the researcher should not assume anything. For example, regarding activities of daily living, the researcher should make sure to assess the study participants and determine whether they shower or bathe or use a broom or a vacuum cleaner. When one participant was asked how often he took a shower, he looked puzzled and replied, "Never." When the interviewer looked surprised, the study participant said, "I take a bath every day. The last time I took a shower was when I visited my sister."

Shortening the Instrument

Many medically underserved people have not had previous or recent experience with questionnaires. It is important to measure the time needed to administer the instrument with *your* medically underserved population. Fatigue and disinterest can be a factor with lengthy tools. This information is best gathered through a pilot test and observation. The researcher should look for changes in behavior from the beginning to the end of the tool administration. Examples of fatigue and disinterest can include looking up frequently, squirming, gazing out a window, and failure to complete the questionnaire. In addition, test-retest procedures can be used to check for the effect of test fatigue. For this assessment, the position of items are switched to determine if items answered at the end of the instrument are answered in a significantly different manner from items answered at the beginning of the instrument. If items are eliminated from an instrument, reliability and validity analyses[67] are critical.

Pilot Studies and Reliability and Validity of Instrument

Reliability and validity analyses are mandatory in using instruments with medically underserved populations, even at the pilot study phase (see Chapter 1, "Evaluating Instruments for Use in Clinical Nursing Research"). Reliability is affected by the number of items: The shorter the instrument, the lower the reliability. Frequently, short instruments are needed for medically underserved populations. Principal component analyses[68] or Spearman-Brown prophecy formula[69] can be used to obtain improved scores with shorter instruments. Time must be allocated to revise the instrument and make changes *before* beginning the main research.[44]

Few research studies contrast reliability analyses of medically underserved populations and non–medically underserved populations. It has been the experience of these authors that medically underserved populations tend to have lower reliabilities than non–medically underserved populations. Additional research is needed in this area.

Administration of Instruments to Medically Underserved Populations

Questionnaires must be given differently to a medically underserved population. These differences include interviewing, considering environmental conditions, collecting sensitive data, and wording of informed consent. Medically underserved persons may not be able to read, in which case the instrument must be read to the subject and responses scored by an interviewer. Uniform procedures are needed for administration of the instrument and training of the interviewers. Individual variations in interviewing can have significant effects on responses. Data analyses should include analyses by the interviewer to detect if trends or consistent differences in responses are occurring. Environmental conditions that reduce noise and provide privacy are important.

Certain data, such as income, is sensitive regardless of the socioeconomic background of the population. If this information must be collected in a group setting, identify ways to maintain the respondents' privacy. For example, in the Colorectal Cancer Project, which included reading and scoring of the instrument by an interviewer, the income options were typed in large print on a separate piece of paper. The respondent was asked to point to the monthly income that was most similar to his or her income. The respondent's privacy was maintained, and the income answer was never said out loud by the interviewer.

Informed consent usually accompanies instrument administration. Unfortunately, most informed consent statements have a reading level of 12th grade or college level.[70-72] The preceding discussion about assessing and reducing the literacy level of an instrument to match each medically underserved population applies equally to informed consent.

Using the Internet/Computer for Data Collection with Low Literacy Individuals

Although those with low incomes, minorities, and those in rural areas are less likely to have easy access to a computer and the Internet, these tools hold promise for research with the medically underserved. The Internet is in its infancy, yet it is clear that the telecommunication revolution is transforming health care. As Internet interventions increase, data collection via the Internet will increase. The Internet holds great promise as a method of obtaining participant information, directly downloading scores into a database, and entering into a statistical program seamlessly. This process eliminates many sources of error. In addition, collecting data on the Internet will save precious research dollars because no data collectors are used.

Some realities of the Internet must be taken into consideration before designing Internet instruments. First, reading from a computer screen is 25% slower than reading a paper document. Second, reading comprehension is 20% less on a computer screen. Third, users do not read Web pages the same way they usually read. Instead, they scan, look for titles or headings, skip sections that do not grab their attention, and selectively search for needed information.[73,74] For low-literacy persons, these characteristics have the potential to accentuate their reading and comprehension deficits. In contrast, Lewis[75], who conducted a review of the literature on Internet interventions, concluded that these interventions worked especially well for low-literacy individuals because of the individualized pace and nonthreatening environment.

The basic principles for designing instruments for low-literacy individuals apply to Internet data collection. The reading level, font size, word selection, level of abstraction, and response options must be appropriate for the literacy level of research participants. However, even more scrupulous attention must be given to writing in the simplest, most direct way to compensate for the increased reading time and decreased comprehension. Advantages of the Internet for low-literacy individuals include color, white space, graphic layout, and voice-over.

To use colors as an organizing framework for the data collection instrument, construct a complete layout of the instrument, including background, font, instructions, question format, and response options. Next, select specific colors for each of these items and use these colors consistently throughout the instrument. Remember, users search for headings when reading on a computer screen, so use colored headings to draw attention to the task at hand. The use of color, however, is not helpful for those with color blindness.

Web sites are usually designed to have a lot of pizzazz, with movement, clutter, pop-up boxes, overlays, and fancy fonts. When designing for low-literacy participants, you must resist the urge to make the screen very busy. Rather, the focus should be on presenting the instrument items in a simple, clear format. This means using white space generously.

A long list of questions will not work for low-literacy participants. They need a layout that will help them understand where to focus their attention. One scheme is to have questions appear on the screen individually. The questions may even be boxed to provide further focus. Pictures or graphics that match the text are very helpful. For example, a graphic of a ethnically or gender appropriate person scratching his or her head might be used with each question. Another option is to use a graphic that matches the content of each question.

Sound is a great asset for assisting low-literacy participants to understand the written text. You can use voice-over to give basic instructions, introduce a new item, draw attention to a specific area of the instrument, or lead the participant through the steps of an instrument. Sound is especially useful to alert participants to a problem with an answer that requires attention. For example, if a participant answered a question that was not one of the expected answers, a voice could suggest that the person check the answer. All voice-over text must conform to the principles of plain language used in written material.

Adaptations in literacy and content are essential with medically underserved populations.

References

1. Haynes, A.M. *The unequal burden of cancer.* Washington, D.C.: National Academy Press, 1999. Committee on Cancer Research Among Minorities and Medically Underserved: *The unequal burden of cancer.* Washington D.C.: National Academy Press, 1999.
2. Weinrich, S. The high risk of low literacy. *Reflections,* (Sigma Theta Tau, nursing's honor society magazine), 1999, Fourth Quarter, 22-24.
3. U.S. Census Bureau. *Current population survey 2001 annual demographic supplement, 1990 based controls* [On-line]. www.census.gov/prod/2002pubs, 2001. Accessed December 2002.
4. Lillie-Blanton, M., & Laveist, T. Race/ethnicity, the social environment, and health. *Soc Sci Med,* 1996, 43(1):83-91.
5. Medicaid. Medicaid Information [On-line]. www.cms.hhs.gov/medicaid/, 2002. Accessed November 2002.
6. National Institute for Literacy, www.nifl/gov. Accessed October 2002.
7. National Center for Education. *Adult literacy in Americans.* Washington D.C.: Educational Testing Service, Department of Education, 1993.
8. Doak, C.C., Doak, L.G., & Root, J.H. *Teaching patients with low literacy skills.* Philadelphia: Lippincott, 1985.
9. Boyd, M.D., & Feldman, H.L. Information seeking and reading and comprehension abilities of cardiac rehab patients. *J Cardiac Rehab,* 1984, 4:343-347.
10. Boyd, M.D. Patient education literature: A comparison of reading levels and the reading ability of patients. In J.H. Humphrey (Ed.), *Advances in health education: Current research.* New York: AMS Press, 1988, pp. 101-110.
11. Whitman, N.I., Graham, B.A., Gelit, C.J., & Boyd, M.D. *Teaching in nursing practice: A professional model.* Norwalk, CT: Appleton & Lange, 1992.
12. Doak, C.C., Doak, L.G., Friedell, G.H., & Meade, C.D. Improving comprehension for cancer patients with low literacy skills: Strategies for clinicians. *CA Cancer J Clin,* 1998, 48(3):151-162.
13. Meade, C., Diekman, J., & Thornhill, D. Readability of American Cancer Society patient education literature. *Oncol Nurs Forum,* 1992, 19(1):51-55.
14. Stephens, S. Patient education materials: Are they readable? *Oncol Nurs Forum,* 1992, 19(1):83-85.
15. Michielutte, R., Bahnson, J., & Beal, P. Readability of the public education literature on cancer prevention and detection. *J Cancer Educ* 1990, 5(1):55-61.
16. Kahn, R.L., Goldfarb, A.I., Pollack, M., & Peck, A. Brief objective measure for the determination of mental status in the aged. *Am J Psychiatry,* 1960, 117:326.
17. Curry, M.A., Burton, D., & Fields, J. The Prenatal Psychological Profile: A research and clinical tool. *Res Nur Health,* 1998, 21(3):211-219.
18. Flaskerud, J.H., Nyamathi, A.M., & Uman, G.C. Longitudinal effects of an HIV testing and counseling programme for low-income Latina women. *Ethn Health,* 1997, 2(1-2):89-103.
19. Harper, C., Balistreri, E., Boggess, J., et al. Provision of hormonal contraceptives without a mandatory

pelvic examination: The first stop demonstration project. *Fam Planning Perspect*, 2001, *33*(1):13-18.

20. Lindenberg, C.S., Solorzano, R., Kelley, M., et al. Competence and drug use: Theoretical frameworks, empirical evidence, and measurement. *J Drug Edu*, 1998, *28*(2):117-134.

21. Logsdon, M.C., & Usui, W. Psychosocial predictors of postpartum depression in diverse groups of women. *West J Nurs Res*, 2001, *23*(6):563-574.

22. Lutenbacher, M. Psychometric assessment of the Adult-Adolescent Parenting Inventory in a sample of low-income single mothers. *J Nurs Measurement*, 2001, *9*(3):291-308.

23. Midanik, L.T., Zahnd, E.G., & Klein, D. Alcohol and drug CAGE screeners for pregnant, low-income women: The California Perinatal Needs Assessment. *Alcoholism: Clin Exp Res*, 1998, *22*(1):121-125.

24. Weinreb, L., Goldberg, R., Lessard, D., et al. HIV-risk practices among homeless and low-income medically under-served mothers. *J Fam Pract*, 1999, *48*(11):859-867.

25. Williams, R.D., Lethbridge, D.J., & Chambers, W.V. Development of a health promotion inventory for poor rural women. *Fam Community Health*, 1997, *20*(2):13-23.

26. Asmussen, L., Olson, L.M., Grant, E.N., et al. Use of the child health questionnaire in a sample of moderate and low-income inner-city children with asthma. *Am J Respiratory Crit Care Med*, 2000, *162*(4 Pt 1):1215-1221.

27. Bassuk, E.L., Weinreb, L.F., Dawson, R., et al. Determinants of behavior in homeless and low-income medically underserved preschool children. *Pediatrics*, 1997, *100*(1):92-100.

28. Knitzer, J. Federal and state efforts to improve care for infants and toddlers. *Future Choices*, 2001, *11*(1):78-97.

29. Li, X., Feigleman, S., & Stanton, B. Perceived parenting monitoring and health risk behaviors among urban low-income African-American children and adolescents. *J Adolesc Health*, 2000, *27*(1):43-48.

30. Robinson, J., Herot, C., Haynes, P., & Mantz-Simmons, L. Children's story stem responses: A measure of program impact in developmental risks associated with dysfunctional parenting. *Child Abuse Negl*, 2000, *24*(1):99-110.

31. Tymchuk, A.J., Lang, C.M., Dolyniuk, C.A., et al. The home inventory of dangers and safety precautions—2: Addressing critical needs for prescriptive assessment devices in child maltreatment and in healthcare. *Child Abuse Negl*, 1999, *23*(1):1-14.

32. Weinreb, L., Goldberg, R., Bassuk, E., & Perloff, J. Determinants of health and service use patterns in homeless and low-income medically under-served children. *Pediatrics*, 1998, *102*(3 Pt 1):554-562.

33. Caron, J., Tempier, R., Mercier, C., & Leouffre, P. Components of social support and quality of life in severely mentally ill, low-income individuals and a general population group. *Community Ment Health J*, 1998, *34*(5):459-475

34. Gray-Donald, K., O'Loughlin, J., Richard, L., & Paradis, G. Validation of a short telephone administered questionnaire to evaluate dietary interventions in low income communities in Montreal, Canada. *J Epidemiol Community Health*, 1997, *51*(3):326-331.

35. Sharp, L.K., Knight, S.J., Nadler, R., et al. Quality of life in low-income patients with metastatic prostate cancer: Divergent and convergent validity of three instruments. *Qual Life Res*, 1999, *8*(5):461-470.

36. Weinrich, S., Weinrich, M., Boyd, M., & Atkinson. C. The impact of prostate cancer knowledge on cancer screening. *Oncol Nurs Forum*, 1998, *25*(3):527-534.

37. Weinrich, S.P., Weinrich, M.C., Boyd, M.D., et al. Knowledge of colorectal cancer among older persons. *Cancer Nurs*, 1992, *15*(5):322-330.

38. Weinrich, S.P., Keil, J.E., Gazes, P.C., et al. The John Henryism and Framingham Type A Scales: Measurement properties in elderly blacks and whites. *Am J Epidemiol*, 1988, *128*(1):165-178.

39. Nelson, E., Wasson, J., Kirk, J., et al. Assessment of function in routine clinical practice: Description of the COOP chart method and preliminary findings. *J Chron Dis*, 1987, *40*:55S-63S.

40. Nelson, E.C., Landgraf, R.D., Hays, J.W., et al. The COOP function charts: A system to measure patient function in physicians' offices. In WONCA Classification Committee (Eds.) *Functional status measurement in primary care*. New York: Springer-Verlag, 1990, pp. 97-131.

41. WONCA Classification Committee. *Functional status measurement in primary care*. New York: Springer-Verlag, 1990.

42. Nelson, E.C., Landgraf, J.M., Hays, R.D., et al. The functional status of patients: How can it be measured in physicians' offices? *Med Care*, 1990, *28*(12):1111-1126.

43. James, S.A., Hartnett, S.A., & Kalsbeek, W.D. John Henryism and blood pressure differences among black men. *J Behav Med*, 1983, *6*:259-278.

44. U.S. Department of Health and Human Services. *Pretesting in health communications: Methods, examples, and resources for improving health messages and materials* (NIH Publication No. 83-1493). Bethesda, MD: National Cancer Institute, 1982.

45. Ford M.E., Hill D.D., Blount A., et al. Modifying a breast cancer risk factor survey for African American women. *Oncol Nurs Forum*, 2002, *29*(5):827-834.

46. Ammerman, A.S., DeVellis, B.M., Haines, P.S., et al. Nutrition education for cardiovascular disease prevention among low income populations—Description and pilot evaluation of a physician-medically under-served model. *Patient Educ Couns*, 1992, *19*:5-18.

47. Reis, J. Medicaid maternal and child health care: Prepaid plans vs. private fee-for-service. *Res Nurs Health*, 1990, *13*:163-171.

48. Flaskerud, J.H., & Nyamathi, A.M. Black and Latina women's AIDS-related knowledge, attitudes, and practices. *Res Nurs Health*, 1989, *12*:339-346.

49. Reis, J., Sherman, S., & Macon, J. Teaching inner-city mothers about family planning and prenatal and pediatric services. *J Pediatric Health Care*, 1989, *3*(5):251-256.

50. Bill-Harvey, D., Rippey, R., Abeles, M., et al. Outcome of an osteoarthritis education program for low-literacy patients taught by indigenous instructors. *Patient Educ Couns*, 1989, *13*:133-142.

51. Brannan, J.E. Accidental poisoning of children: Barriers to resource use in a black, low-income community. *Public Health Nurs*, 1992, *9*(2):81-86.

52. Meyboom-de-Jong, B., Smith, R.J. Studies with the Dartmouth COOP Charts in General Practice: Comparison with the Nottingham Health Profile and the General Health Questionnaire. In WONCA Classification Committee (Eds.). *Functional status measurement in primary care.* New York: Springer-Verlag, 1990, pp. 132-149.

53. Weinrich, S.P., Weinrich, M.C., Boyd, M.D., *Effective approaches for increasing compliance with ACS's screening recommendations in socioeconomically disadvantaged populations.* Atlanta: American Cancer Society, 1992, pp. 1-8.

54. Davis, T. C., Williams, M. V., Marin, E., et al. Health literacy and cancer communication. *CA Cancer J Clin,* 2002, *52*(3):134-149.

55. Wide Range Achievement Test. Wilmington, DE: Jastak Associates Inc., 1978.

56. Parker, R.M., Baker, D.W., Williams, M.V., Nurss, J.R. Test of Functional Health Literacy in Adults (TOFHLA): A new instrument for measuring patient's literacy skills. *J General Intern Med,* 1995, *10*(10):537-541.

57. McGraw, H.C. SMOG testing. In C. Doak, L.G. Doak, & J.H. Root (Eds.), *Teaching patients with low literacy skills.* Philadelphia: Lippincott, 1985, pp. 36-37.

58. McLaughlin, G.H. SMOG grading—a new readability formula. *J Reading,* 1969, *12*:639-646.

59. Fry, E. A readability formula that saves time. In *Classroom strategies for secondary reading.* Newark, DE: International Reading Association, 1977, pp. 29-35.

60. Fry, E. Fry's Readability Graph: Clarifications, validity, and extension to level 17. *J Reading,* 1977, December:242-252.

61. Mailloux, S.L., Johnson, M.E., Fisher, D.G., & Pettibone, T.J. How reliable is computerized assessment of readability? *Comput Nurs,* 1995, *13*(5):221-225.

62. Weinrich, S.P., & Boyd, M. Education in the elderly: Adapting and evaluating teaching tools. *J Gerontol Nurs,* 1992, *18*(1):15-20.

63. Larson, C.O., Hays, R.D., & Nelson, E.C. Do the pictures influence scores on the Dartmouth COOP charts? *Qual Life Res,* 1992, *1*:247-249.

64. Weinrich, S.W., Weinrich, M.C., Stromborg, M., et al. The elderly educator method. *Gerontologist,* 1993, *33*(4):401-406.

65. Garrison, C.Z., Schoenbach, V.J., Schluchter, M.D., & Kaplan, B.H. Life events in early adolescence. *J Am Acad Child Adol Psychiatry,* 1987, *26*:865-872.

66. Duke University Center for the Study of Aging and Human Development. *Multidimensional functional assessment: The OARS methodology.* Durham, NC: Duke University Medical Center, 1978.

67. Jacobson, S.F. Evaluating instruments for use in clinical nursing research. In M. Frank-Stromborg (Ed.), *Instruments for clinical nursing research* (2nd ed.). Norwalk, CT: Appleton & Lange, 1988, pp. 3-20.

68. Carmines, E.G., & Zeller, R.A. *Reliability and validity assessment.* Newbury Park, CA: Sage, 1979.

69. Sax, G. *Principles of educational and psychological measurement and evaluation.* Belmont, CA: Wadsworth, 1980.

70. Berg, A., & Hammilt, K.B. Assessing the psychiatric patient's ability to meet the literacy demands of hospitalization. *Hosp Community Psychiatry,* 1980, *31*:266-268.

71. Bergler, J.H., Pennington, C., Metcalf, M., & Freis, E.D. Informed consent: How much does the patient understand? *Clin Pharmacol Ther,* 1980, *27*:435-439.

72. O'Connor, R.G. Informed consent: Legal, behavioral, and educational issues. *Patient Couns Health Educ,* 1991, *3*:49-55.

73. Howles, L., & Howles, D. Writing for the Web. Proceedings of the 17th Annual Conference on Distance Teaching and Learning, Madison, WI, August 8-10, 2001.

74. Moore, M.G. Surviving as a distance teacher. *Am J Distance Ed,* 2001, *15*(2):1-6.

75. Lewis, D. Computer based approaches to patient education. *J Am Med Inform Assoc,* 1999, *6*(4):272-282.

Appendix 2A SMOG Readability Formula: Samples with at Least 30 Sentences

1. Select a total of 30 sentences: 10 consecutive sentences from the beginning, 10 from the middle, and 10 from the end of the written piece. A sentence is any string of words punctuated by a period, an exclamation point, or a question mark.
2. Count the words containing *three or more syllables*, including repetitions in the 30 sentences.
   * Hyphenated words are one word.
   * For numerals, pronounce them aloud and count the syllables pronounced for each numeral (e.g., for the number 573, five = 1, hundred = 2, seventy = 3, and three = 1, or 7 syllables).
   * Proper nouns should be counted.
   * If a long sentence has a colon, consider each part of it as a separate sentence. However, if possible, avoid selecting that segment of the passage.
   * The words for which the abbreviations stand should be read aloud to determine their syllable count (e.g., Oct. = October = 3 syllables).
3. Obtain the nearest perfect square root of the total number of words of three or more syllables and then add a constant of 3 to the square root to obtain the grade level. Or you can use the convenient conversion method in the SMOG conversion table, which ends this appendix.

Example:	First 10 sentences	= 23 polysyllabic words
	Second 10 sentences	= 22 polysyllabic words
	Third 10 sentences	= 22 polysyllabic words
	Total	67 polysyllabic words

Square root of 67 = 8.
Add the constant of 3.
8 + 3 = 11th grade.

You can also use the conversion method shown in the following table.

SMOG Conversion Table[58]

Word Count	Grade Level	Word Count	Grade Level
0–2	4	73–90	12
3–6	5	91–110	13
7–12	6	111–132	14
13–20	7	133–156	15
21–30	8	157–182	16
31–42	9	183–210	17
43–56	10	211–240	18
57–72	11		

Developed by Harold C. McGraw, Office of Educational Research, Baltimore County Public Schools, Towson, Maryland. There is not a copyright on the SMOG Conversion Table. You are welcome to use the table.

Appendix 2B Sample with Fewer Than 30 Sentences

Number of Sentences	Word Count A (Example = 6)	Conversion Number B	Reading Level = A × B*
29	6	1.03	7
28	6	1.07	6
27	6	1.1	7
26	6	1.15	6
25	6	1.2	7
24	6	1.25	8
23	6	1.3	8
22	6	1.36	9
21	6	1.43	9
20	6	1.5	9
19	6	1.58	10
18	6	1.67	10
17	6	1.76	11
16	6	1.87	11
15	6	2.0	12
14	6	2.14	12
13	6	2.3	14
12	6	2.5	15
11	6	2.7	16
10	6	3.0	18

*Reading levels rounded to nearest grade level.
Directions: Use this table for instruments with less than 30 sentences.

3

Measurement Issues with Children and Adolescents

Debra P. Hymovich

This chapter provides an overview of issues involving research and measurement, selection of appropriate instruments, and ethical and legal aspects of research with children and adolescents. Most studies related to children and adolescents involve direct observation, interview, completion of questionnaires or other instruments, or indirect observation through data collected by significant others, such as the child's parents, teachers, or peers. In this chapter, measurement issues are limited to children from birth through 18 years of age who are studied directly. The terms *measure*, *tool*, and *instrument* are used interchangeably.

Considerations in selecting research instruments are (1) the conceptual or theoretical base and its consistency with the proposed study; (2) appropriateness for the child's age, including available norms for children of the same age and sex in the proposed study; (3) length of time needed to complete the instrument; (4) whether the instrument is norm-referenced or criterion-referenced; and (5) the validity and reliability of the instrument.

Ethical Issues

Obtaining informed consent and assent for research involving children in numerous research studies and weighing the physical and psychosocial risks and benefits of conducting studies with children are ethical considerations for researchers.[1,2]

Informed Consent
Parent Consent

Voluntary and informed consent is one of the most difficult aspects of child research. Parental or guardian consent is required to safeguard the rights of children and adolescents.[3] Traditionally, researchers relied on proxy consent from parents as a substitute for obtaining informed consent from children. However, proxy consent does not fully meet the requirements for informed consent.[4]

Because parents are legally responsible for all matters pertaining to their children, parental consent to permit children to participate in a study is mandatory in research ethics codes. In studies of minimal risk, permission from one or both parents is usually sufficient, but both parents must give their permission if the study involves greater risk and there is no prospect of benefit to the child. Exceptions to this requirement would be if one parent is deceased, incompetent, the parent's whereabouts are unknown, or when only one parent has legal responsibility for the child.[5] Parents may refuse to permit their children to participate in even the most innocent study for a variety of reasons. Parents may distrust scientists in general or a particular researcher; they may not want strangers to talk to their children; or they may be unwilling to endure any inconvenience to themselves.[6] Liaschenko and Underwood[7] found that a "fatal diagnosis and the sense of urgency obliterated any meaningful sense of choice for parents."

Child Assent

Although parents have the legal consenting responsibility regarding their children's participation in research, the child who has reached the "age of understanding" has the right to assent.[8] Assent has been referred to as knowledgeable agreement. Children 7 years of age and older with normal cognitive development are capable of giving a degree of informed consent, subject to developmental constraints. It is the researcher's responsibility to ensure that the child's rights are respected. The child must be given complete information about the study, including the purpose, methods to be used (e.g., demonstrations, peer discussion, videotapes), risks, and benefits. The child should be given an assent form to sign. Throughout the study, the child must be given opportunities to ask questions and to withdraw at any time.[8] Equally important is the child's right to dissent without coercion. The parent's permission may override the child's dissent only if participation may provide direct therapeutic benefit to the child that would not otherwise be available.[9]

There are limited data regarding children's ability to consent to research. Abramowitz and colleagues[10] describe four studies, using a total of 148 subjects ranging in age from 7 to 12 years, to obtain data on children's ability to consent to psychologic research. Subjects were from suburban, relatively affluent families whose parents were willing to have them participate in the research. Most subjects understood all or most of what they were asked to do in a psychology study, but few younger than 12 years understood or believed that their performance would be confidential. Study results imply that 7- to 12-year-old children have the capacity to assent meaningfully to participation in research, but problems exist in guaranteeing that they make this decision freely. Frame and Strauss[11] investigated the possibility of sample bias resulting from parental consent in 308 grade-school children for whom sociometric and teacher ratings were available prior to requesting parental consent for a research project. Parental consent was lower for socially rejected and neglected students and those who had significantly lower academic performance. Social withdrawal and poor academic performance were the best independent predictors of nonconsent, accounting for 10% of the variance. Teacher ratings of various psychological characteristics failed to differentiate children who gave consent from those who did not. Sussman et al.[12] compared the views of children and physicians related to the consent process. They found that the majority of children understood the benefits to themselves, the limitations of the research, and the freedom to ask questions. However, less than half understood they were free to withdraw, that alternative treatments existed, or that others might benefit from the study.

Recommendations and procedures for obtaining informed consent or assent from children to participate in research generally vary somewhat among institutions. Federal guidelines for research with minors[13] allows institutional review boards (IRBs) to determine the conditions under which parental consent is required. Currently, there is discussion regarding adolescents' rights to consent to participate in research without parental consent or knowledge. All states allow adolescents to be treated for venereal disease without guardian consent, and some states allow independent decision making about other treatments as well. As Fisher pointed out, "Decisions regarding whether adolescents should participate in research without parental consent should be based on the potential benefits to the participant rather than the utility needs of the researcher."[3]

It often is a challenge for the researcher to explain the study at the child's level of understanding. Obtaining a child's assent requires time, effort, and respect for the youngster's autonomy. Strategies for obtaining consent are provided by Lindeke, Hauck, and Tanner[14] and Hughes and Helling,[15] who highlight the following ethical issues:

- Being sensitive and responsible
- Considering the child's intellectual maturity and comprehension level
- Avoiding taking advantage of subjects' immaturity
- Being sure that children understand that they can refuse or quit at any time (repeat this more than once)
- Realizing that, although the children may enjoy the increased attention, most do not see their role in contributing to a knowledge base
- Determining whether some features of the research can be rewarding to the child
- Giving certificate of acknowledgment to the child for participating
- Offering tangible gifts (pens/pencils, stickers, tape recording) as a surprise after the study so that they are not construed as bribes
- Weighing the risks and benefits carefully (physical and psychologic harm, social injury against scientific validity of study)
- Ensuring that child is not involved in numerous research studies

Theoretical Model

Investigators need a clear theoretical foundation to conceptualize a study.[16] The majority of nursing studies with children and adolescents have been guided by theories of development. These theories, emerging from the mechanistic and organismic world views, include Piaget's cognitive development and Erikson's psychologic development. However, these traditional theories are limited in their ability to inform about the influences of history, culture, and environment on behavioral change.[17] Weekes[17] recommends using the lifespan developmental framework perspective rather than traditional approaches for research with chronically ill adolescents. She believes this permits an understanding of events preceding adolescence. For example, Weekes's study of adolescents with cancer did not support the hypotheses based on Piagetian theory. Similarly, a cross-sequential study of adolescents by Nesselroade and Baltes[18] did not support the age-related developmental changes suggested by Erikson's and Piaget's theories.

The lifespan developmental framework emerges from the dialectic world view. "The basic aims of the life span perspective are to describe, explain, and modify developmental change across the lifespan."[17] This theoretical approach may be useful in studying younger children, as well as adolescents. With this approach, the researcher would not only consider children at different stages in their development but also how the developmental, cognitive, and social or emotional changes that occur before and after the study period influence their responses. An array of theoretical models and outcome measures are available for situations in which the contextual nature of child health is considered as part of the study.[19] Newer models based on neuropsychology, such as Als' synactive model for premature infant development, may become increasingly useful for child and adolescent testing.[20]

Design

The research designs used most often for developmental research have been the traditional longitudinal and descriptive designs. Issues in designing a study include the following:

- The need to be efficient and economical without giving a static picture
- Cost (time, money, effort, subject attrition)
- Difficulty in recruiting an adequate number of subjects
- Nonrandom loss of subjects through experimental mortality (refusal, death)
- The need for comparison groups
- Flaws in cross-sectional and longitudinal designs, so that uncontrolled influences (i.e., maturation, new technology, contextual factors) cannot be attributed to random occurrences; viable alternative explanations exist for differences between measurement groups other than age[21]
- The lifespan developmental model, which can be helpful in addressing developmental change in responses to health, illness, and influence of age, time, and cohort on this change[21–23]
- Shaie's redefinition of cohort, time of measurement, and age:[23] *Cohort:* all persons experiencing a particular event at some point in time (age-graded, history-graded, nonnormative); *Time of measurement:* time an event has had the opportunity to have an impact on individuals or group (nature of an event rather than time); *Age:* not a threat to validity because maturational effects are considered age effects

Longitudinal data usually are essential for direct investigation of issues of lifespan development. According to Wohlwill,[24] longitudinal data are necessary (1) to preserve information related to the shape of the function of the developmental response, (2) to provide information on change and the patterning of change, (3) to relate earlier behavior to later behavior, and (4) to relate earlier conditions of life to subsequent behavior.

Weekes[17] suggests that there are sound shortcuts to longitudinal research. Weekes identifies retrospective data collection, despite its problems, as a useful method with adolescents over about 13 years of age. Problems associated with retrospective data collection include inaccurate recall, selective remembering, distortion, projection of the present into the past, and age of child. Another strategy, sequential data collection, involves combining cross-sectional and longitudinal data-collection methods to expedite the collection of developmental data.[25,26] Sequential design strategies can be used to answer questions related to influences of age, cohort, and time of measurement on intraindividual change in behavior. These strategies may be especially useful to researchers who are interested in age and time, or time and cohort influences on developmental change in response to numerous health and illness situations. Problems associated with using sequential designs include the potential for lack of availability of large sample sizes and inability to control for age and time of induction to the study. Certain adjustments may have to be made, such as oversampling certain age groups.

Outcome studies with children are problematic because of the many developmental and contextual issues involved.[27] The priorities given to various health outcomes will differ depending on the child's age, developmental stage, and the expectations of family and community. Interpreting outcome data for children is especially difficult because of the influence of developmental change, as well as the effects of current health care on health outcomes for later years, including adulthood.

Sampling

Sample size and rigor of sampling methodology are important. Equally important are the developmental level and ethnicity of subjects in considering generalizability. Small, single-hospital samples are likely to provide limited data because protocols differ among institutions.[27]

Beal and Betz[28] evaluated the sample size, study setting, age, and cultural background of subjects of research published in parent-child health nursing journals from 1980 to 1989. In their analysis of 322 articles from 7 journals, 25% had sample sizes of fewer than 30 subjects, and 66% had sample sizes under 100 subjects. In 5 studies, it was not clear how many subjects were sampled. Nonprobability sampling was the principal technique, with 91% using samples of convenience and only 3% using random sampling. Forty-seven percent of the studies were conducted in the hospital, 12% in the home, and 37% in outpatient clinics and physicians' offices. The remaining studies were conducted in schools ($n = 36$), camps ($n = 3$), and a homeless shelter ($n = 1$). In 3 studies it was unclear where data were collected. In many cases it was difficult to differentiate the age groups of the samples. The majority of studies ($n = 116, 37\%$) used parents as samples. Neonates were sampled in 33 studies, and 21 studies sampled toddlers. Overall, Beal and Betz found small sample sizes accessed through nonprobability sampling techniques, which render generalizability difficult. Generalizability is further limited when examining ethnicity data. Nonwhite samples were studied in 35% of the 322 studies. In 32 studies, no reference was made to ethnicity. The major focus of the studies was on individual parental response to child behavior, but only 12 studies had a family focus and few studies targeted young children. Beal and Betz[28] suggest that nursing research move into the community to study health promotion issues in high-risk groups. Increasing the sample size and ethnic heterogeneity will further enhance the generalizability and relevance of findings to pediatric practice.

Methodologic Issues

Methodologic issues specifically related to research with children include smaller and more heterogeneous populations compared to the adult population, as well as the difficulty in identifying objective and clinically relevant outcome measures related to this diversity.[29] In addition, consideration must be given to the confounding issues of the child's current age, age of onset of the condition, and disease duration.[30] Children may be assessed directly through observation or by having them complete questionnaires or answer questions. They can be measured indirectly by asking parents, teachers, or other significant individuals to complete measures about the children. Several studies indicate that parents' perceptions and children's perceptions differ. For example, studies suggest that children and adults (e.g., parents, caretakers, teachers) frequently disagree about children's health and quality of life.[20] Research involving children requires an exploration of the child's beliefs, thoughts, feelings, and knowledge rather than just those of the adults. Existing measures of concepts often are completed by parents or other adult observers. Although these instruments may be valid and reliable, they provide information only from the adult's perspective, thus missing the child's perception. Data obtained directly from children and data obtained indirectly from parents are each types of data that might shed light on the issue under study. Whenever possible, researchers should consider collecting data from the perspective of both the children and significant adults.

Instrument Reliability and Validity

Psychometrically sound methods are needed for measuring variables. Because of the wide developmental differences that must be addressed in conducting studies with children and adolescents, the issue of measurement and assessment is complex. Although some measures have been developed for this population, it is still necessary to develop others. Carpenter[31] noted that the use of different measuring techniques with younger and older children creates serious problems for interpreting study results. He recommends that instruments be developed that can be applied across the child and adolescent developmental spectrum.

Because reliability estimates vary from sample to sample, instrument reliability should be reestimated for each study. Validity usually is sample invariant; it should be a relatively stable property as long as the technique is used appropriately to derive the type of data for which it was developed. Commonly used measures for assessing validity are correlations with other measures, cluster analyses, and factor analyses. In addition, developmental differences are used as evidence of construct validity, especially to assess instruments devised to evaluate the performance of children.[32]

Developmental Considerations

Although instruments designed for use with adult populations can be used with adolescents, there are very few for use with young children. Tools used with children may have been developed for populations that have little in common with those being studied (sensitivity). Because the items are not sufficiently sensitive, researchers who try to use these instruments may be unable to discriminate important differences between groups or detect changes over time. For example, standardized tests of children's intelligence and academic performance are available and appropriate to study the long-term effects of neurotoxic therapy for childhood leukemia.[33] However, available instruments are not sufficiently sensitive to measure other aspects of cognition, such as information processing speed, concentration, and attention. In some cases all that is needed may be simply to adapt an existing tool and validate it by obtaining appropriate normative data.

The age and developmental level of the child or adolescent are important considerations in developing or selecting data-collection instruments. The younger the child, the more complex measurement issues become. Cognitive capabilities, psychomotor abilities, and attention span must be considered when selecting and developing instruments for children and adolescents. Appendix 3A highlights developmentally specific measures.[34-45]

Adapting Standardized Instruments

Brown and Haylor identified four areas of development as "most important" when considering how to use standardized tests with young children: (1) psychosocial and emotional development, (2) perceptual-motor development, (3) cognitive development, and (4) linguistic development.[39] Appendix 3B illustrates the steps recommended to adapt standardized tests for preoperational children.

Issues with Special Children

Special children are those who have conditions, impairments, or disabilities that significantly interfere with normal development and psychologic adaptation. These impairments may be cognitive, sensory, motor, developmental, or related to chronic illnesses or learning disabilities. These impairments can interfere with a child's ability to complete many instruments standardized with nonhandicapped children. Several issues require consideration when using psychometric measures with special children.[46] The first issue of a conceptual nature has to do with age equivalence. Although the use of age equivalents makes it easy to summarize and communicate test performance, a direct correspondence of test ages to chronological ages should not be assumed. Two other issues are methodologic in nature. The first concerns the comparability of instruments with similar labels. Identical test ages derived from different tests should not be assumed to be identical conceptually because they may not necessarily measure the same characteristics and may differ in content and comprehensiveness. Another methodologic issue relates to the concept of standardization and its implications for assessing and interpreting psychometric test results. Most of the tests used with special children have not been standardized with this population.

Measurement Limitations

Characteristics that limit the utility of instruments with special children often are those of reliability and validity. The technical adequacy of instruments is important. Salvia and Ysseldyke[47] presented various tables for instruments they judge to be inadequate on the basis of reliability and validity as well as those judged inadequate in terms of descriptions or construction of norms.

The psychometric base for psychological testing of many special children is inadequate.[34] Many tests present stimuli of a visual or auditory nature that cannot be perceived by a child with sensory impairment. Responses requiring speech or manipulation may not be possible for children with hearing or motor impairments. A measurement limitation of a psychomotor nature is the failure to include special children in standardization samples, thus placing restrictions on inferences and generalizations. The lack of comparability of scores for tests with similar content, purpose, and truncated normative tables are other limiting factors. Ramsey and Fitzhardenge[48] have shown that Bayley Scales of Infant Development and the Griffiths Developmental Scales[49] yielded substantially different scores for 50 high-risk infants. In another study of infants with Down syndrome,[50] the Bayley Scales and Gessell Developmental Schedules did not yield similar results.

Instrument labels are not always descriptive of the domain they represent. Instruments labeled as intelligence tests, for example, may vary widely in content. Tests with similar labels also may differ dramatically in the nature and comprehensiveness with which a particular domain is assessed.

A final limitation of measurement involves the methodology employed. Diebold, Curtis, and DuBose[51] compared performance of handicapped youngsters using data derived from observation and from testing. In spite of the similarity of the domains being assessed, marked differences were found as a function of methodologies. Performance based on testing was lower than by observation.

Reducing the limitations associated with inappropriate materials can take many forms. The major strategies are to modify, expand, or vary the instruments (such as test stimuli and format) or to modify the testing procedures.[46] Simeonsson et al.[46] advocate using a multivariate approach and recognizing that there are problems in assessing special children that require flexible, rather than rigid, standards of reliability and validity.

Minority Children

Another group of special children are those from minority ethnic, racial, or cultural groups. When planning studies with minority subjects, the researcher needs to consider the client, the instruments, and the evaluator. Few instruments available for children have been normed on these minority groups.[52] Children who differ culturally from the predominant society do not necessarily have a deficit.[53] Most minority parents and children have experienced prejudice, and they bring these previous experiences to the testing situation.

The problem of instrument bias is multifaceted. Instrument bias can exist at the content level, as decisions are made about what items to include in a test, and at the level of standardization, where decisions are made about the population for whom the test is appropriate[54] Most standardized tests reflect largely white, middle-class values and attitudes. They are biased and unfair to people from cultural and socioeconomic minorities because they do not reflect the experience and linguistic, cognitive, and other cultural styles and values of minority group persons. The Denver Developmental Screening Test (DDST)[55,56] is an example of an instrument that has been criticized for its cultural bias. The recent revision, DDST II, was standardized on sample subgroups divided by age, gender, and ethnicity (Anglo, African-American, Hispanic), and age-adjusted norms were determined for items in which significant differences exist.[56] In addition, to improve the preparation of screeners, a two-day training course was developed for master trainers. Further documentation is needed to resolve the issue of cultural bias with the revised instrument.

Bias can occur when instruments are administered by researchers who are unfamiliar with the patterns of language, behavior, and customs of the person being examined.[54] When data are collected by those who do not understand the culture and language of minority group children, they are unable to elicit a level of performance that accurately reflects the child's underlying competence.[54]

Projective techniques frequently used in research with children are detailed in Appendix 3C.[57–60] The most common tests are presented in Appendix 3D.[61–74]

Summary

Much of the research involving child and adolescent subjects is still plagued by sampling bias and design flaws. Most of the nursing research with children and adolescents involves small, nonrepresentative samples; a lack of comparison groups; and the absence of a conceptual framework. Researchers need more valid and reliable instruments; improved designs (qualitative, experimental, multivariate) guided by conceptual or theoretical models; and more representative and larger samples that include minorities, males, and lower-class youth.[75] The content validity, construct validity, and stability of instruments need to be extended and improved for descriptive studies.

References

1. Assent of children 21 CFR 50.25 Elements of informed consent. Food and Drug Administration. Information Sheets: Guidance for Institutional Review Boards and Clinical Investigators, September 1998. Access date 20 February 2003. www.fda.gov/oc/ohrt/irbs/informedconsent.html#children.

2. Sales, B.D., & Folkman, S. (Eds.). *Ethics in research with human participants.* Washington, D.C.: American Psychological Association, 2000, Appendixes B & C.

3. Fisher, C.B. Integrating science and ethics in research with high-risk children and youth. *Soc Pol Rep: Soc Res Child Devel*, 1993, 7(4):1-26.

4. Committee on Bioethics. Informed consent, parental permission, and assent in pediatric practice. *Pediatrics*, 1995, 95(2):314-317.

5. National Institutes. of Health. *OHSR*, 1991, 45CFR, Section 46.408b.

6. Keith-Spiegel, P. Children's rights as participants in research. In G.P. Koocher (Ed.), *Children's rights and the mental health professions.* New York: Wiley, 1976, pp. 53–81.

7. Liaschenko, J., & Underwood, S.M. Children in research: Fathers in cancer research—meanings and reasons for participation. *J Fam Nurs*, 2000, 7:71-91.

8. Broome, M.E. Consent (assent) for research with pediatric patients. *Sem Pediatr Nurs*, 1999, 15(2):96-103.

9. Weithorn, L.A., & Scherer, D. Children's involvement in research participation decisions: Psychological considerations. In M. Grodin & L. Glantz (Eds.), *Children as research subjects: Science, ethics, and law*. New York: Oxford University Press, 1994, pp. 133-179.

10. Abramowitz, R., Freedman, J.L., Thoden, K., & Nikolich, C. Children's capacity to consent to participate in psychological research: Empirical findings. *Child Dev*, 1991, 62(5):1100-1109.

11. Frame, C.L., & Strauss, C.C. Parental informed consent and sample bias in grade-school children. *J Soc Clin Psychol*, 1987, 5(2):227-236.

12. Sussman, E.J., Dorn, D.L., Fletcher, J.C. Participation in biomedical research: The consent process as viewed by children, adolescents, young adults, and physicians. *J Pediatr*, 1992, 124:547-552.

13. U.S. Department of Health and Human Services. Additional protection for children involved as subjects of research. *Federal Register*, 1983, 48(46):9814-9820.

14. Lindeke, L.L., Hauck, M.R., & Tanner, M. Practical issues in obtaining child assent for research. *J Pediatr Nurs*, 2000, 15(2):99-104.

15. Hughes, T., & Helling, M.K. A case for obtaining informed consent from young children. *Early Childhood Res Q*, 1991, 6(2):225-232.

16. Ramsay, M.C., & Reynolds, C.R. Development of a scientific test: A practical guide. In G. Goldstein & M. Hersen (Eds.), *Handbook of psychological assessment* (3rd ed.). Oxford, UK: Elsevier Science, 2000, pp. 21-42.

17. Weekes, D.P. Application of the life-span developmental perspective to nursing research with adolescents. *J Pediatr Nurs*, 1991, 6(1):38-48.

18. Nesselroade, J.R., & Baltes, P.B. Adolescent personality development and historical change: 1970-1972. *Monographs of the Society for Research in Child Development*, 1974, 39:1-80.

19. Christakis, D.A., Johnston, B.D., & Connell, F.A. Methodological issues in pediatric outcomes research. *Ambulatory Pediatrics*, 2001, 1(1):59-62.

20. Bernstein, J.H., & Wieder, M.D. "Pediatric neurological assessment" examined. In G. Goldstein & M. Hersen (Eds.), *Handbook of psychological assessment* (3rd ed.). Oxford, UK: Elsevier Science, 2000, pp. 263-300.

21. Kosloski, K. Isolating age, period, and cohort effects in development research. *Res Aging*, 1987, 8(4):461-479.

22. Weekes, D.P., & Rankin, S.H. Life-span developmental methods: Application to nursing research. *Nurs Res*, 1988, 37(6):380-383.

23. Schaie, K.W. Beyond calendar definition of age, time, and cohort: The general developmental model revisited. *Dev Rev*, 1986, 6(3):252-277.

24. Wohlwill, J.F. *The study of behavioral development*. San Diego, CA: Academic Press, 1973.

25. Schaie, K.W. A general model for the study of developmental problems. *Psychol Bull*, 1965, 64(2):92-107.

26. Schaie, K.W., & Baltes, P.B. On sequential strategies in developmental research. *Hum Dev*, 1975, 18(5):384-390.

27. Aylward, G.P. Methodological issues in outcome studies with at-risk infants. *Pediatr Psychol*, 2002, 27(1):37-45.

28. Beal, J.A., & Betz, C.L. Sampling issues in parent-child nursing research: Implications for nursing practice. *J Pediatric Nurs*, 1993, 8(4):261-262.

29. Smyth, R.I., & Weindling, A.M. Research in children: Ethical and scientific aspects. *Lancet*, 1999, 354 (Suppl II):21-24.

30. Johnson, S.B., & Meltzer, L.J. Methodological issues involve the confounding of current age, onset age, and disease duration. *J Pediatr Psychol*, 2002, 27(1):77-86.

31. Carpenter, P.J. Scientific inquiry in childhood cancer psychosocial research. *Cancer*, 1991, 67:833-838.

32. Goldman, J., Stein, C.L., & Guerry, S. *Psychological methods of child assessment*. New York: Brunner/Routledge, 1984.

33. Challinor, J., Miaskowski, C., Moore, I., et al. Review of research studies that evaluated the impact of treatment for childhood cancers on neurocognition and behavioral and social competence: Nursing implications. *J Soc Pediatr Nurs*, 2000, 5(2):57-74.

34. Moore, I.M., & Ruccione, K. Challenges to conducting research with children with cancer. *Oncol Nurs Forum*, 1989, 16(4):587-589.

35. Keefe, M., Kotzer, A.M., Reuss, J.L., & Sander, L.W. The development of a system of monitoring infant state behavior. *Nurs Res*, 1989, 38(6):344-347.

36. Achenbach, T.M. *Manual for the Youth Self-Report and 1991 Profile*. Burlington, VT: University of Vermont Department of Psychiatry, 1991.

37. Bordens, K.S., & Abbott, B.B. *Research designs and methods: A process approach* (5th ed.). Mountain View, CA: Mayfield, 2001.

38. Hester, N.K. The preoperational child's reaction to immunization. *Nurs Res*, 1979, 28(4):250-254.

39. Brown, M.S., & Haylor, M. Nursing research with preoperational age children: The use of standardized tests. *J Pediatr Nurs*, 1989, 4(1):19-25.

40. Hetherington, E.M., & Parke, R.D. *Child psychology: A contemporary viewpoint* (2nd ed.). San Francisco: McGraw-Hill, 1993.

41. Kotzer, A.M. Cognitive strategies for pediatric nursing research: Data collection. *J Pediatr Nurs*, 1990, 5(1):50-53.

42. Romero, I. Individual assessment procedures with preschool children. In E.V. Nuttall, I. Romero, & J. Kalesnik (Eds.), *Assessing and screening preschoolers: Psychological and educational dimensions* (2nd ed.). Boston: Allyn and Bacon, 1999, pp. 59-71.

43. Henker, B., Whalen, C.K., Jamner, L.D., & Delfino, R.J. Anxiety, affect, and activity in teenagers: Monitoring daily life with electronic diaries. *J Am Acad Child Adolesc Psychiatry*, 2002, 41(6):660-670.

44. Savedra, M., & Highly, B. Photography: Is it useful in learning how adolescents cope with hospitalization? *J Adolesc Health Care*, 1988, 9(3):219-224.

45. Hinds, P.S., Weekes, D.P., & Zeltzer, L.K. Identifying threats to data integrity in studies of adolescents with cancer. *Oncology Nursing Forum*, 1988, 15(6):821-824.

46. Simeonsson, R.J., Cook, C., & Hill, S. Quantitative assessment. In R.J. Simeonsson & S.L. Rosenthal (Eds.), *Psychological and developmental assessment:*

Children with disabilities and chronic conditions. New York: Guilford Press, 2001, pp. 53-82.

47. Salvia, J., & Ysseldyke, J.E. Assessment (8th ed.). Boston: Houghton Mifflin, 2001.

48. Ramsey, M., & Fitzhardenge, P.M. Comparative study of two developmental scales: The Bayley and the Griffiths. *Early Hum Dev*, 1977, *1*:151-157.

49. Griffiths, R. *The abilities of young children.* Chard, England: Young & Son, 1970.

50. Eippert, D.S., & Azen, S.P. A comparison of two developmental instruments in evaluating children with Down's syndrome. *Physical Ther*, 1978, *58*:1066-1069.

51. Diebold, M.H., Curtis, W.S., & DuBose, R.F. Relationships between psychometric and observational measures of performance in low-functioning children. *American Association for the Education of the Severely/Profoundly Handicapped Review*, 1978, *3*:123-128.

52. Suzuki, L.A., Ponterotto, J.G., & Meller, P.J. (Eds.), *Handbook of multicultural assessment: Clinical, psychological, and educational applications* (2nd ed.). San Francisco: Jossey-Bass, 2001.

53. Li, C., Walton, J.R., & Nuttal, E.V. Preschool evaluation of culturally different children. In E.V. Nuttall, I. Romero, & J. Kalesnik (Eds.), *Assessing and screening preschoolers: Psychological and educational dimensions* (2nd ed.). Boston: Allyn and Bacon, 1999, pp. 296-317.

54. Jones, R.L. Psychoeducational assessment of minority group children: Issues and perspectives. In R.L. Jones (Ed.), *Psychoeducational assessment of minority group children: A casebook* (2nd. ed.). Berkeley, CA: Cobb & Henry, 1998, pp. 13-35.

55. Brachlow, A., Jordan, A.E., & Tervo, R. Developmental screenings in rural settings: A comparison of the child development review and the Denver II Developmental Screening Test. *J Rural Health*, 2001, *17*(3):156-159.

56. Wade, G.H. Update on the Denver II. *J Pediatr Nurs*, 1992, *18*(2):140-141.

57. Krahn, G.L. The use of projective assessment techniques in pediatric settings. *J Pediatr Psychol*, 1985, *10*(2):179-193.

58. Lynn, M.R. Projective technique: A way of getting "hidden" information: Part I. *J Pediatric Nurs*, 1986, *1*(6):407-408.

59. Johnson, B.H. Children's drawings as a projective technique. *J Pediatric Nurs*, 1990, *16*(1):11-17.

60. Poster, E.C. The use of projective assessment techniques in pediatric research. *J Pediatric Nurs*, 1989, *4*(1):26-35.

61. Peterson, C., & Schilling, K. Card pull and projective testing. *J Pers Assess*, 1983, *47*:265-275.

62. Waechter, E.H. Children's awareness of fatal illness. *Am J Nurs*, 1971, *71*(6):1168-1172.

63. Bellak, L., & Abrams, D.M. *The thematic apperception test, the children's apperception test, and the senior apperception technique in clinical use* (6th ed.). Boston: Allyn & Bacon, 1997.

64. Poster, E., Betz, C.L., McKenna, A., & Mossar, M. Children's attitudes toward the mentally ill as reflected in their human figure drawings and stories. *J Am Acad Child Psychiatry*, 1986, *25*(5):680-686.

65. Scavnicky-Mylant, M. The use of drawings in the assessment and treatment of children of alcoholics. *J Pediatr Nurs*, 1986, *1*(3):178-184.

66. Burgess, A.W. Sexually abused children and their drawings. *Arch Psychiatr Nurs*, 1988, *2*(2):65-73.

67. Engle, P.L., & Suppes, J.S. The relation between human drawing and test anxiety in children. *J Projective Tech*, 1970, *34*:223-231.

68. Rubin, J.A., Schacter, J., & Ragins, N. Intra-individual variability in human figure drawings: A developmental study. *Am J Orthopsychiatry*, 1983, *53*(4):654-657.

69. Blau, T.H. *The psychological examination of the child.* New York: Wiley, 1991.

70. Farel, A.M., Freeman, V.A., Keenan, N.L., & Huber, C.J. Interaction between high-risk infants and their mothers: The NCAST as an assessment tool. *Res Nurs Health*, 1991, *14*:109-118.

71. Coppens, N.M., & Gentry, L.K. Video analysis of playground injury-risk situations. *Res Nurs Health*, 1991, *14*:129-136.

72. Medinnus, G.R. *Child study and observation guide.* New York: Wiley, 1976.

73. Lobo, M.L. Observation: A valuable data collection strategy for research with children. *J Pediatr Nurs*, 1992, *7*(5):320-328.

74. Pellegrini, A.D. *Applied child study: A developmental approach* (2nd ed.). Hillsdale, NJ: Lawrence Erlbaum, 1991.

75. Opie, N.D. Childhood and adolescent bereavement. In J.J. Fitzpatrick, R.L. Taunton, & A.K. Jacox (Eds.), *Annual review of nursing research* (Vol. 10). New York: Springer, 1992, pp. 127-141.

Appendix 3A Strategies for Measurement across Childhood

Infant (Preverbal)

The following strategies can be used with preverbal children.[34]

Habituation technique. This technique tests discrimination as the infant becomes bored with the repeated presentation of the same stimulus; once the infant no longer looks at it, a different stimulus is presented. If the infant looks at the second stimulus, it is inferred that the infant can discriminate.

Preference. The infant is presented with two objects simultaneously, and the length of time the infant looks at each is measured. The infant looks at the preferred object longer.

Discriminant learning. This strategy attempts to have the infant respond differently to different stimuli.

Other measures. Other interventions that can be carried out include assessment of heart rate, cry, sleep–wake patterns before and after an intervention; videotaping or tape recording of behavior or vocalization; non-invasive computerized monitoring.[35]

Preschool-Age Children

Challenge. The lack of adequate instruments and cognitive and social immaturity limit recall and ability to report feelings and behavior,[36] and so does the inability to respond to measures designed for older individuals.

Children egocentric. Those aged 4 to 7 years are able to quantify, classify, and relate objects but are unaware of underlying principles.

Strategies.
- Establish and maintain rapport (developmentally appropriate).
- Be sensitive to nonverbal communication.
- Adapt perceptual-motor aspects to developmental level.
- Be flexible and creative (give child maximum opportunity to respond—children will differ in their fatigue and anxiety levels, as well as length of testing time they can tolerate).
- Make measures concrete.[37,38]
- Videotape the child's interaction with the environment, recording behavioral and verbal communication.
- Maximum testing time with best time 9:00 A.M. to 11:00 A.M. Worst times are nap time and before and after meals.[39]

School-Age Children

Capacities. School-age children can use instruments requiring concrete or abstract Likert-type responses (e.g., rank-ordering objects),[40] self-administered questionnaires, and qualitative interviews.

Other techniques. A child's drawings of human figures, storytelling, using dolls and puppets to elicit information,[41] autobiographical scrapbook,[42] diary or semistructured journal[43] can all be used.

Pilot testing. It is important to pilot test questions to ensure understanding and to assure the child that there are no right or wrong answers and that it is okay to say no.

Adolescence

Capacities. Adolescents can describe feelings and behaviors across situations (self-reports).

Other perspectives. Reports of others who see the adolescent in a different context should be considered.

Other techniques. Journals, self-recorded interviews, and photography[44] can be used.

Reliability and validity. The reliability and validity of adolescent-reported data can be threatened by the researcher, the adolescent, and the nature of the research question. For instance, how valid are data gathered when the parent is present?[45]

Appendix 3B Adapting Standardized Tests for Preoperational Children

The following adaptations with preoperational children can be considered:[39]

1. Identify and adapt the perceptual-motor appropriateness of the test.
   Use heavy black or colored lines separating every five questions.
   Use cartoons (preferably animals) to illustrate questions.
   Develop alternate forms for Asian and African-American children.
2. Identify and adapt cognitive appropriateness of the test.
   Phrase questions in concrete language.
   Deal with only one variable at a time.
   Avoid words involving time and sequence.
   Use words appropriate for various age groups.
3. Identify and adapt linguistic appropriateness of the test.
   Use simple sentence structure and a sentence length no longer than 12 to 14 words.
   Avoid double negatives and prepositional and adverbial phrases with more than 5 words, including exceptions (e.g., "All of the following EXCEPT").
   Use pictures to replace words when needed.
4. Restandardize the measure.
   Assess child's ability to comply.
   Individualize the research approach (this may threaten the internal validity of the study, but the responses may be a more accurate reflection of the child's feelings, attitudes, or beliefs and thus may enhance the external validity of the findings).

Appendix 3C Projective Testing with Children

Projective Techniques

Projective techniques include the presentation of ambiguous (nonspecific) material or stimuli to enable the child to disclose verbally or nonverbally images or ideas previously undisclosed;[57,58] based on psychoanalytic view of an individual. Useful with child who cannot verbalize.[59]

Categories

A number of categories can be distinguished.[60]

Associative. The child is expected to respond quickly to stimuli word or image (i.e., Rorschach ink-blot technique).

Construction. The child is asked to make up or to create response to stimulus (i.e., Child Apperception Test [CAT]).

Completion. The child completes a partially developed sentence or story.

Expressive. The child uses drawings or play.

Tests

- The most commonly used tests are Thematic Apperception Test (TAT), CAT, Rorschach, and human figure drawings (HFDs).
- Tests require specially trained individuals to administer and score.
- Overall, there is a lack of reliability and validity data. Many tests are developed to diagnose emotionally disturbed individuals; additional study with comparable "normal" children must be done.
- Results are interpreted based on psychoanalytic theory, so accuracy, quality, and utility of data must be considered.

Techniques for Personality Appraisal

- Structured or unstructured: investigator interprets response in broad psychological terms and behavior dynamics.
- Verbal: word association tests, sentence completion tests, or child asked to tell a story about a picture.
- Nonverbal: expressive or productive, involving children's drawings (i.e., human figures).

Appendix 3D Projective Tests Used in Research with Children

Thematic Apperception Test (TAT)

Administration. The child is given ambiguous pictures and asked to make up a story or fantasy, including what is happening, what led up to it, and what will happen in the future.[61]

Results. It is assumed that the child will project motives, emotions, and attitudes about self, significant adults, the world, and expectations.

Comments. Requires skillful and sensitive researcher. The TAT was adapted by Waechter[62] to study death anxiety in children.

Child's Apperception Test (CAT)

Administration. Children aged 3 to 10 years old are given cards with pictures of animals that illustrate themes of sibling rivalry, nighttime loneliness, attitudes toward parents, toileting behavior, aggression, and oral problems.[63]

Results. It is assumed that the child will project feelings and attitudes onto animals;[64] various scoring methods can be used (few validity or reliability studies).

Human Figure Drawing (HFD) Tests

Administration. Draw-a-Person (DAP), Kinetic Family Drawing (KFD), and House-Tree-Person (HTP) tests have been used to measure children's perception of mental illness,[64] as well as measuring children of alcoholics[65] and sexually abused youngsters.[64,66]

Results. Scoring is subjective, depending on the skills, knowledge of child development, and experience of the researcher. Many scoring systems exist[67] that provide evidence of interrater reliability. Test–retest reliability and validity are questionable.[67] It is difficult to compare study findings because of the differences in subjects, scoring systems, and test environments.[60]

Comments. Complex, so caution should be used with neurologically impaired or developmentally disabled children. Increase reliability and validity by controlled administration; standardize instructions; use together with other measures; obtain at least three drawings from each child; and use concurrent comparison groups.[60] Limit interpretation only to aspects selected for evaluation. Scoring should be done by raters blind to study details and data collection.

Sentence Completion

Administration. Children are asked to complete incomplete sentences, drawing from their own experiences (e.g., "My mother . . .").[69]

Results. These tests have considerable face validity, but other psychometric properties are questionable.

Comments. There are many differences in stimulus sentences presented to children and adolescents.

Children's Drawings

Administration. Based on psychoanalytic theory, these demonstrate a child's usual presentation of self to the world and the nature of his or her inner personality.[62]

Results. Interpretation is most valid when based on a *series* of drawings. It should be used in conjunction with other available information about the child. Free drawings are more physically meaningful than assigned drawings. When drawing, the sex of the figure the child draws first is related to his or her concept of sex role. The child adapts his or her own drawing style (psychologically significant). The manner that elements are portrayed may be a useful indicator of psychological state. Drawings may be interpreted as a whole rather than segmentally or analytically.

Comments. Drawings constitute a valuable tool in the hands of an expert; ideally, the child should validate the researcher's interpretation.[65]

Observation

Administration. Observation is used for a child's interaction with animate or inanimate environment.[70,71] A child's behavior is recorded without the use of predetermined categories or arbitrary time intervals (*naturalistic*). It is important not to modify the behavior of the observed child. *Time sampling* can be used to determine the frequency of certain behaviors; the reliability of behaviors is established by observation over time. There is some difficulty in identifying interrelationships among a number of behaviors because the researcher is studying only one behavior.[72] *Event sampling* describes a behavior sequence.

Results. Many rating scales and checklists exist to quantify observations, but these do not provide data about causes or management of the behavior.

Comments. Major concerns[73] include definition, reliability, validity of coding categories, identification of unit of measurement (molar or molecular), method of recording the observation, sampling strategies, observer training, interrater reliability, taxonomy of behaviors (motor or vocal), and instrument and observer reliability. Children's play can be observed in controlled situations where specific materials are provided to elicit specific responses.[74]

Questionnaires and Inventories

Administration. These tools measure personality and intellectual ability: A child's behavior and responses when presented with various materials and tasks are observed and recorded.

Results. Tests of ability are more precise, highly developed, and accurate in predicting behaviors (e.g., school achievement) than personality measures. *Psychometric tests of intelligence* are highly reliable and valid (scores agree with other estimates of intellectual ability and predict school achievement), but they are affected more by the child's motivation, rapport with examiner, physical health, mood, attention, and familiarity with the testing situation.

4

Measurement Issues with the Elderly

Joyce H. Rasin

The number of older adults is increasing in this country. In 2000, there were 35 million persons 65 years or older, representing 12.4% of the population.[1] By 2030, it is projected that there will be approximately 70 million older adults, comprising almost 20% of the population. The fastest-growing group of elders are those 85 years and older. Their numbers by the year 2030 will be double that of 2000. With more persons in the old-old group, there will also be more persons with disabilities. Seventy-four percent of people aged 80+ have at least one disability versus 45% of those aged 65–69.

Elders are overrepresented in the health care system and, unless specifically excluded, will be selected as subjects in any study that focuses on adults, given that everyone older than 18 or 21 years of age is grouped into the category of adult. There are, however, biopsychosocial factors that make elders different from their younger counterparts. Some of these factors can influence the measurement of study variables in a research project. And, because elders are heterogeneous, the influence of these factors cannot be automatically generalized to all elders. Most elders are healthy and are primarily adapting to changes associated with aging. Some elders are frail because of the interplay of pathologic and age-related changes.

In this chapter, factors that should be considered when developing a measurement plan for elders are discussed. Specifically, concerns about the purpose, conceptualization, and threats to the psychometric properties of instruments are explored. Except for illustrative purposes, instruments to measure specific concepts are not reviewed because they will be discussed in the chapters that follow.

Purpose

Congruence between the purpose for which the researcher will use an instrument and the purpose for which the instrument was originally developed is crucial. An instrument is created for a particular population and a particular setting. Many researchers do not consider the heterogeneity within the population of elders because of the general propensity to group all adults together. If an instrument is not carefully matched to the population, a ceiling or floor effect may result. It will not be sensitive to changes in the variable of interest. With a ceiling effect the scores will cluster in the high range because the questions are too easy. The opposite occurs with a floor effect: The questions are too difficult for the sample and the scores are low. The Mini-Mental State Examination (MMSE), a test for cognitive impairment, has floor effects for people with severe impairment. Other instruments, such as the Test for the Severely Impaired, have been developed to evaluate the cognitive abilities of those with low scores on the MMSE.[2] Another example of not matching the instrument to the sample would be to assess the functional status of a nursing home resident with an instrumental activities of living (IADL) scale developed for individuals living in their own homes. The nursing home residents will be unable to do the same tasks as elders living independently and will have low scores. For example, ability to do shopping is not relevant to a nursing home resident. Overall, if the setting and the sample of the investigation do not match those for which the instrument was developed, the reliability and validity of the data collected will be compromised.

Conceptualization

The conceptualization of research variables guides the selection of the appropriate measures for operationalization. The complexity of elder-related concepts is continuously being discovered, and operationalization must reflect this complexity. For example, measures of cognition have been used as indicators of severity of dementia and subsequent ADL and IADL functioning. Reed et al.[3] demonstrated that dementia severity is a complex concept and that the relationship between cognition and ADL function varies by level of cognition. In their study, they found that for subjects with MMSE scores less than 14.5, there was a significant relationship between MMSE scores and both instrumental and physical ADLs. In the group with greater cognitive functioning (MMSE scores > 14.5), MMSE and ADL scores were independent.

For research that has a direct impact on gerontologic clinical practice, recognizing the complexity of conceptualization is necessary but not sufficient; clinical relevance must also be reflected in the conceptualization. This is a particularly salient issue for researchers interested in measuring elder outcomes. For example, when the improvement of cognitive functioning is the focus, effectiveness should not be limited to the cognitive dimensions of attention and memory because they can be very sensitively measured. Drug (trials) research tells us that additional criteria for success that are related to the impact on everyday life must be added.[3] This focus is particularly relevant to health care providers whose interest is to assist older people to function at their highest level. A significant change in a memory test is not very important if there is no other change in the level of functioning that can be recognized by the patient, family, or caregiver.

Psychometric Properties

Reliability and validity are fundamental characteristics of an instrument's measurement qualities.[4] *Reliability* is the consistency or stability of measurement. *Validity* refers to the degree to which the instrument actually reflects the concept of interest. There are two different perspectives regarding the definition of validity. According to the revised Standards for Educational and Psychological Testing, validity is a unitary concept, and content, criterion, and construct validity are types of evidence rather than types of validity.[5] Alternatively, Messick, a measurement theorist, argues for the integration of the validity concept and considers content- and criterion-related validity as *evidence* of construct *validity*.[6]

Validity varies from situation to situation and sample to sample. Validity testing validates an instrument with a specific group, not the instrument itself, so any instrument used with elders must be validated with this group. Psychometrically sound measurement instruments are essential for any type of research. Outcomes from a relevant question and a perfectly designed study are useless if the data collected are not accurate and meaningful.

To enhance both reliability and validity, researchers need to minimize both random and systematic measurement error. Random error threatens measurement reliability.[5] Systematic error threatens validity. The following section discusses the potential sources of random and systematic error (1) within the elder respondent, (2) within the measuring device, and (3) related to the instrument administration.

Characteristics of Respondent

Anxiety and primary or secondary physiologic age changes may be sources of error in the measurement process. Primary age changes are those that result from the aging process that all individuals will experience if they live long enough. Secondary age changes are those ensuing from disease processes. Not all older adults experience secondary age changes.

Anxiety

Testing situations can be stressful to elders. Their perception and appraisal of stress depends on personality, health, education, and previous experiences.[7] Many elders were educated in a system that did not use Likert scales, semantic differentials, or multiple-choice questions; they may feel more anxious when confronted with these formats. High anxiety has been associated with decreased memory function for elders without diagnosable psychopathology. Eisdorfer et al. demonstrated that deficits in verbal learning were associated with heightened autonomic nervous system receptor activity.[8] An experimental group of elders was given an intravenous solution of propranolol, to dampen their autonomic response, while learning a verbal task. The experimental group had significantly higher learning scores than the placebo group, demonstrating that high anxiety impedes the performance of older adults on memory tasks.

Conversely, to determine whether a reduction in anxiety would improve performance, Yesavage taught relaxation techniques to elders before memory training began.[9] Both the experimental and the control groups showed improvements in memory, but improvement was significantly greater in the experimental group receiving relaxation training. Lower anxiety scores at final testing were significantly correlated with recall. These studies indicate the potential effect of anxiety on responses. To obtain reliable data, researchers must create a calm, relaxing atmosphere for test taking.

Primary Age Changes

Primary age changes (also known as age-related changes) in vision and hearing can significantly affect the measurement process. Research has demonstrated that visual and hearing quality may decrease in old age even when pathology is not found.[10] However, one cannot generalize about the specific changes that might occur because of the intraindividual differences in patterns of change and variations in the time of sensory decline. For every physiologic function, some elders consistently score within the normal range of young adults, whereas others show severe deficits.

Vision. Kosnik et al.[11] conducted a survey of adults 18–100 years of age to determine the impact of age-related changes on everyday visual performance. They found that five visual dimensions declined with age: visual processing speed, light sensitivity, near vision, dynamic vision, and visual search. The older adults took longer to carry out visual tasks and had more trouble with glare, dim illumination, and near-visual tasks. They also had more difficulty locating a target in a cluttered visual scene. These changes in visual performance are caused by (1) the cornea becoming slightly thicker and more likely to scatter light; (2) the lens becoming denser, more yellow, and less elastic; (3) the pupil becoming smaller, admitting less light; (4) the vitreous gel condensing and collapsing with bits of dense gel appearing as floaters; and (5) a gradual decrease in the number of nerve cells in the retina.[10] Older individuals also have increased difficulty differentiating between blue and green, the short light wavelengths, as opposed to red and yellow, which have longer wavelengths.

These age-related visual changes must be considered in instrument development and administration. To enhance near-visual tasks the type size is important. Printed materials should be in large type, at least 14 or 16 point.[12] Because low contrast negatively affects acuity, the color of both the paper and the type is important.[13] Black lettering on white paper provides a very high degree of contrast, whereas the contrast of yellow letters on green paper is much lower. Visual acuity is diminished in conditions of low illumination, so the testing environment must be well lit. The type of lighting also may be significant. According to Marmor, "warm" incandescent lighting is often more comfortable than "cold" fluorescent lighting.[14] Although lighting is important, glare also needs to be prevented. Close lighting should be directed onto the reading material, and the elder should not face a window with unfiltered sunlight. Nongloss paper should be used for the self-report instrument. Vision can be quite good when lighting is optimal and the words are sharply defined.[14] To compensate for decreased visual processing speed, the research protocol must provide enough time for elders to read self-report instruments.

Hearing. Hearing impairment is more likely to go undetected than visual problems and has been associated with decreased performance on certain cognitive tests.[15,16] In a nationally representative sample of community-dwelling people aged 70 years and older, 25% rated their hearing as fair or poor.[17] Age-related changes in the anatomy and physiology of the ear result in a change in the quality of hearing—the older person can usually hear but not understand what is being said. Elders have decreasing (1) sensitivity to high-frequency tones (presbycusis), (2) ability to hear rapid speech, and (3) ability to discriminate sounds in the presence of background noise. The researcher should make sure that the subject's attention is obtained before starting to talk. To improve the understanding of speech, stand facing the elder as he or she might be lip-reading. The researcher should not stand so that a bright light is behind him or her as the elder's vision may be diminished. Researchers must also eliminate or minimize background noise and avoid rapid, loud speech as volume and speed can distort sounds.

Secondary Age Changes

Chronic illnesses increase with age. The effects of primary aging are complicated by these pathologic processes or secondary aging. The interaction of pathology with age-related changes enhances heterogeneity among elders. The specificity of the health problem will determine the nature of any impairment that may affect the measurement process. For example, a person with arthritis may have difficulty writing or may be uncomfortable sitting for a long time. The elder with a genitourinary problem or who is taking diuretics may need frequent bathroom breaks. Individual physical and mental limitations must be assessed. However, two factors that should be considered with all frail elders are fatigue and the need for proxy respondents.

Fatigue should be considered when working with the frail elderly because it has implications for the item format of a written instrument and/or its administration. Depending on the extent of the fatigue, closed-ended questions that require short answers or just checking off items may be preferable to open-ended questions.[18] If an interview is used, it should be no longer than one to 1–1.5 hours.

Proxy respondents may need to be used when frail elders, particularly the cognitively impaired, are involved. In a study of Medicare beneficiaries, 75% of those with cognitive impairment had a proxy respond for them.[19] In order to have reliable and valid data, the validity of proxy responses needs to be considered. A review of 24 clinical studies listed in Medline from 1900 to 1999 that used proxy respondents for elders revealed that the validity of the proxy response varied by the area assessed.[20] There was generally good agreement in describing overall health, physical symptoms, chronic physical conditions, and settings of care, but proxies tended to identify more functional impairment among persons with dementia. The proxy's responses were influenced by their relationship to the subject, co-residence, and their level of burden.

Characteristics of a Measuring Device

When developing a measuring device, two questions must be answered: (1) What is the domain to be measured? and (2) How will the domain be measured? Embedded in the answers to these questions are potential sources of systematic error that can threaten validity.

What Is to Be Measured?

What an instrument measures depends on the definition of the concept. The definition delineates the scope of the content domain. Evidence for content validity is demonstrated when the test items are representative of the content domain.[4] Problems can occur when an instrument created for one age group is used for another. Age-related differences in what comprises the content domain of interest can threaten content validity.[20] One example is in the measurement of depression.[21,22] Although somatic symptoms are common among the young, they are not sensitive indicators of early depression in elders as many elders without depression have the same somatic complaints. One reason the Geriatric Depression Scale was created was to eliminate the somatic items included in earlier depression scales.[23] Resnick also found that many items on an instrument used to measure self-motivation in the young-old were not indicators of motivation for the old-old. [24]

Threats to validity are not limited to content domain differences between elders and younger people. Threats to content validity can also occur because of gender differences. Males and females may differ on IADLs.[25] A scale that includes items about cooking, cleaning, and shopping may not be appropriate for the present cohort of married elderly men because they do not usually perform these tasks. In addition, with couples, there may be dependence not because of inability to function but because the couple voluntarily shares household functions.[26]

How Is the Domain Measured?

Once the appropriate content domain has been delimited, the specific questions to evaluate that domain have to be developed. Item content, word clarity, readability, and item format can all be potential sources of error that can threaten reliability and validity.

The instrument developer and content experts determine if item content adequately reflects the domain. However, the viewpoint of the elder test taker also is important. Items that are not relevant and that appear childish will not encourage elder participation even if they accurately measure the domain. Elders will not perform tasks that seem trivial or ridiculous.[27] Tasks that are realistic and that seem to be related to real-life activities in daily functioning have face validity.[28] Face validity also has been called ecologic validity by some psychologists and psychiatrists.[29] An ecologically valid memory task should appear to relate to the memory tasks faced by elders in their daily lives.[28] Activities such as repeating progressively longer strings of numbers or learning nonsense syllables are frequently taken from neuropsychological test batteries. For example, a method frequently used to assess secondary memory is to ask the person to repeat three words and then later in the interview to ask the person to recall the same three words. If this task seems unimportant, the elderly may not even try to remember the words. Alternatively, the elder may become antagonistic, anxious, and unmotivated. If cooperation diminishes, performance also decreases.

Crook and colleagues[30,31] have developed a number of ecologically valid memory tests. To measure primary memory, instead of being asked to repeat a series of digits, the elder is asked to remember a telephone number or a telephone number with an area code. An ecologically valid test to measure secondary memory is called the misplaced object test.[30] The subject is presented a board showing various rooms of a house. He is given 10 objects and asked to place them in various rooms. After 30 minutes, he is asked to indicate where the objects were placed. These types of ecologically valid tasks should produce less anxiety and higher motivation, resulting in more reliable data.[32]

Lack of *clarity in wording* will threaten validity. Words have different meanings to different groups of people, and the researcher should confirm that there is congruence in meaning between the subject and the researcher and within the subject population itself. In a project to identify cognitive problems with survey questions, using questions from the National Health Interview Survey,[33] it was determined that elders interpreted some words differently. For example, in the question "Do you have any difficulty sitting for two hours?" some elders interpreted sitting as including standing for short periods whereas others did not include standing in their definition. Another important feature of this special project was that it identified a method to judge the understandability of questions. Usually an indicator of a problematic survey item is a large number of "I don't know" or "no response" answers. In this project unclear items would not have been detected during a routine instrument administration because elders answered promptly and the responses sounded plausible. Problems were recognized only when probe questions were used to ascertain how questions were answered. Jobe and Mingay[33] recommended that pretesting of new questions be augmented with cognitive interviews.

Low readability of items will influence validity. Although the number of years of formal education of older adults is increasing, there still are a large number of elders of low literacy. Between 1970 and 2000, the percentage who had completed high school rose from 28% to 70%.[1] Among ethnic and racial elderly groups, there are broad differences. In 2000, 74% of whites, 63% of Asians and Pacific Islanders, 46% of African Americans, and 37% of Hispanics had a high school education. Because education levels are still quite variable, it is difficult to develop or select one set of measurement procedures that all elders can use. The researcher cannot automatically assume that if the sample respondents are old and African American or Hispanic that they will not be able to read. It is possible to have a group of high school and college graduates or a group containing individuals who have only an elementary school education. The researcher must estimate the mean educational level of the elderly population of interest so that measurement procedures are neither too difficult nor too basic. For example, an interview rather than a written format will be needed if the elder has minimal to no literacy skills. When many of the elders have low education levels, evaluating the readability of written material will provide a more objective assessment of difficulty. Several readability formulas are available, but one that has been recommended for patient education materials is the SMOG formula that assesses reading grade level for written text.[34] Many word processing software programs, such as Microsoft Word and Wordperfect, can calculate readability levels.

An instrument developer has to make many decisions about *item format*: open-ended versus closed-ended questions and if closed, the specific type. Closed-ended questions with their preset response options may be problematic for some elders because of difficulty categorizing their responses. This was illustrated in Jobe and Mingay's project[33] to evaluate survey questions. When elders were asked how frequently they had attended the senior center during the previous 12 months, many would provide a narrative answer that included frequency information instead of selecting a category (frequently, sometimes, never) as requested. The authors noted that younger respondents did not usually have difficulty selecting categories and attributed this difference to the younger respondents' testing experiences in school. Actually, the older respondent is providing a more accurate response as the categories could be defined differently by each respondent. Because the operationalization of the categories is really the researcher's decision, this type of question could be open-ended rather than fixed choice. Categorization of the response would then be a coding task of the research staff.

Visual Analog Scales (VASs) can threaten validity, as many elders have trouble using them. A VAS is used to measure subjective experiences such as dyspnea, mood, anxiety, and pain.[35] Elders have some difficulty with use of the VAS. Herr and Mobily compared a horizontal verbal descriptor scale and a horizontal VAS with a sample of 49 elderly patients.[36] The rate of failure for correct completion was 7.1% for the VAS and 2% for the verbal descriptor scale. With 53 geriatric patients (mean = 82 years) Bergh et al. compared four rating scales with a verbal report of the effectiveness of analgesics.[37] One of the scales was a VAS. The ability to complete any of the scales diminished with age, and the verbal reports were often directly opposite the rated pain.

Administration

When it is anticipated that the subjects are not highly educated, the quality of the data may be improved by administering the instruments one to one or in a small group. Giving subjects the option to either complete the instruments independently or have the investigator read the instruments to them while they follow along allows those with no or low literacy skills to "save face."[38] It also is less anxiety provoking and allows for immediate detection of misinterpretations by the data gatherer.[39] The disadvantage to this approach is the increased cost in time and money for trained data gatherers. However, the success of a scientific investigation depends on the quality of the data, so these costs should be considered in the planning stages.

The time allowed to complete instruments is very important. More time is needed for one-on-one than for group administration. Elders should also be allowed to work at their own pace. Kim[40] found that when testing knowledge, self-paced elders performed better than those in the experiment-paced response conditions. The time for administration also must take into account the subject's priorities, which may be different from that of the data collector.[41]

Any interaction with the data collector could be viewed as a time for socializing. When asked a question, the elder may provide much more information than is required or may initiate another topic. Data collectors must be skilled interviewers experienced in working with elders. Data collection is more than just filling out forms. Data collectors must know how to maintain flexibility while completing the session in a timely fashion. If the data collectors are not familiar with the instruments, a training session should be conducted. Role-playing possible subject reactions and potential responses will help make the actual testing process pleasant for both the data collector and the subject.[42] Response burden also is a concern. Several long instruments can create excessive subject burden. Although longer instruments increase internal consistency,[4] they may not be the best choice for elders who are physically or mentally frail. A person with dementia may become unmotivated, uncooperative, or fatigued if the testing sessions are too long. Data-collection sessions should be between 1[32] and 2 hours long.[43] To further ease the burden, either rest periods or two very short data-gathering sessions could be offered to the elders.

Summary

Because of the interplay of normal age-related changes and pathology for older adults, particular attention must be paid to instrument selection and administration. The conceptualization of the study variables, the purpose of the instruments, and any threats to reliability and validity must be considered. Instruments are being developed specifically for elders that consider age-related changes and deal with age-related measurement problems. The Delayed Word Recall Test and the Geriatric Depression Scale[44] are two examples of these instruments. The Delayed Word Recall Test, which measures secondary memory, integrates the concept that healthy elders benefit from encoding enhancement. The subject creates sentences for each of 10 words supposed to improve the encoding of these words. After a short time, the subject is asked to recall the words freely. A normal older person is supposed to do very well on this task, whereas one with dementia would not. The Geriatric Depression Scale[44] was developed to deal with domain, item format, and item acceptability issues of preexisting self-report depression scales.

Several collections of instruments are available for use with older adults. Examples include *Assessing the Health Status of Older Adults*,[45] *Practical Geriatric Assessment*,[46] *Comprehensive Geriatric Assessment*,[47] *Handbook of Geriatric Assessment*,[48] and *Assessing Older Persons: Measures, Meaning, and Practical Applications*.[49] Much research is still needed regarding the health needs of elders. Being cognizant of and attending to the potential measurement issues associated with this population will help to ensure the acquisition of high-quality data.

References

1. Administration on Aging. A Profile of Older Americans: 2002. Access date 28 January 2003. www.aoa.gov/aoa/stats/profile/2002/.
2. Albert, M., & Cohen, C. The test for severe impairment: An instrument for the assessment of patients with severe cognitive dysfunction. *J Am Geriatr Soc*, 1992, 40:449-453.
3. Reed, B.R., Jagust, W.J., & Seab, J.P. Mental status as a predictor of daily function in progressive dementia. *Gerontology*, 1989, 29:804-807.
4. Waltz, C.F., Strickland, O.L., & Lenz, E.R. *Measurement in nursing research* (2nd ed.). Philadelphia: Davis, 1991.
5. American Educational Research Association, American Psychological Association & National Council on Measurement in Education. *Standards for educa-

tional and psychological testing*. Washington, D.C.: American Educational Research Association, 1999.
6. Messick, S. Validity. In R.L. Linn (Ed.), *Educational measurement* (3rd ed.). New York: Macmillan, 1989, pp. 13-104.
7. Eisdorfer, C. Stress, disease and cognitive change in the aged. In C. Eisdorfer & R. Friedel (Eds.), *Cognitive and emotional disturbance in the elderly*. Chicago: Year Book Medical, 1977.
8. Eisdorfer, C., Nowlin, J., & Wilkie, F. Improvement of learning in the aged by modification of autonomic nervous system activity. *Science*, 1970, 170:1327-1329.
9. Yesavage, J.A. Relaxation and memory training in 39 elderly patients. *Am J Psychiatry*, 1984, 141:778-781.

10. Kalina, R.E. Aging and visual function. In W.R. Hazard, J.P. Blass, W.H. Ettinger, et al. (Eds.), *Principles of geriatric medicine and gerontology*. New York: McGraw-Hill, 1999, pp. 603-604.

11. Kosnik, W., Winslow, L., Kline, D., et al. Visual changes in daily life throughout adulthood. *J Gerontol*, 1988, 43:63-70.

12. Weinrich, S.P., Boyd, M., & Nussbaum, J. Continuing education: Adapting strategies to teach the elderly. *J Gerontol Nurs*, 1989, 15:17-21.

13. Arditi, A. *Making text legible: Designing for people with partial sight*. New York: Lighthouse International, 1999.

14. Marmor, M.F. Age-related eye diseases and their effects on visual function. In E.E. Faye & C.S. Stuen (Eds.), *The aging eye and low vision*. New York: The Lighthouse, 1992, pp. 11-21.

15. Pearman, A., Friedman, L., Brooks, J.O. Hearing impairment and serial word recall in older adults. *Exp Aging Res*, 2000, 26:383-391.

16. van Boxtel, M.P., vanBeijsterveldt, C.E., Hous, P.J., et al. Mild hearing impairment can reduce verbal memory performance in a healthy adult population. *J Clin Exp Neuropsychol*, 2000, 22:147-154.

17. Lee P., Smith, J.P., & Kington, R. The relationship of self-rated vision and hearing to functional status and well-being among seniors 70 years and older. *Am J Ophthalmol*, 1999, 127:447-452.

18. Sexton, D.L. Some methodological issues in chronic illness research. *Nurs Res*, 1983, 32:378–380.

19. Corder, L.S., Woodbury, M.A., & Manton, K.G. Proxy response patterns among the aged: Effects on estimates of health status and medical care utilization from the 1982-84 Long-term Care Surveys. *J Clin Epidemiol*, 1996, 49:173-182.

20. Neumann, P.J., Araki, S.S., & Gutterman, E.M. The use of proxy respondents in studies of older adults: Lessons, challenges, and opportunities. *J Am Geriatr Soc*, 2000, 48:1646-1654.

21. Kasniak, A.W. Psychological assessment of the aging individual. In J.E. Birren & K.E. Schaie (Eds.), *Handbook of psychology of aging* (3rd ed.). Boston: Academic Press, 1990, p. 432.

22. Phillips, L.R. Challenges of nursing research with the frail elderly. *West J Nurs Res*, 1992, 14:721-730.

23. Bolla-Wilson, K., & Bleecker, M.L. Absence of depression in elderly adults. *J Gerontol*, 1989, 2:53-55.

24. Resnick, B. Measurement tools: Do they apply equally to older adults? *J Gerontol Nurs*, 1995, 21(7):18-22.

25. Pearson, V.I. Assessment of function in older adults. In R.L. Kane & R.A. Kane (Eds.), *Assessing older persons*. New York: Oxford University Press, 2000, pp. 17-48.

26. Fillenbaum, G.C. Screening the elderly: A brief instrumental activities of daily living measure. *J Am Geriatr Soc*, 1985, 33:698-706.

27. Cunningham, W.R. Psychometric perspectives: Validity and reliability. In L.W. Poon (Ed.), *Clinical memory assessment of older adults*. Washington, D.C.: American Psychological Association, 1986, pp. 27-31.

28. Ferris, S.H., Reisberg, B., deLeon, M., & Crook, T. Recent developments in the assessment of senile dementia. In J.P. Abrahams & V. Crooks (Eds.), *Geriatric mental health*. New York: Grune & Stratton, 1984.

29. Woods, R.T., & Britton, R.G. *Clinical psychology with the elderly*. Rockville, MD: Aspen, 1985.

30. Crook, T., Ferris, S.H., & McCarthy, M. The misplaced objects test: A brief test for memory dysfunction in the aged. *J Am Geriatr Soc*, 1979, 27:284-287.

31. Crook, T., Ferris, S.H., McCarthy, M., & Rae, D. The utility of digit recall tasks for assessing memory in the aging. *J Consult Clin Psychol*, 1980, 48(2):228-233.

32. Ferris, S.H., Crook, T., Flicker, C., et al. Assessing cognitive impairment and evaluating treatment effects: Psychometric performance tests. In L.W. Poon. (Ed.), *Clinical memory assessment of older adults*. Washington, D.C.: American Psychological Association, 1986, pp. 139-148.

33. Jobe, J.B., & Mingay, D.J. Cognitive laboratory approach to designing questionnaires for surveys of the elderly. *Public Health Rep*, 1990, 105:518-524.

34. McLaughlin, G.H. SMOG grading: A new readability formula. *J Reading*, 1969, 12:639-646.

35. Wewers, M.E., & Lowe, N.K. A critical review of visual analogue scales in the measurement of clinical phenomena. *Res Nurs Health*, 1990, 13:227-236.

36. Herr, K.A., & Mobily, P.R. Comparison of selected pain assessment tools for use with the elderly. *Appl Nurs Res*, 1993, 6:39-46.

37. Bergh, I., Sjostrom, B., Oden, A., & Steen, B. Assessing pain and pain relief in geriatric patients with non-pathological fractures with different rating scales. *Aging*, 2001, Oct; 13(5):355-361.

38. Rasin, J.H. The relationship between confusion and blood pressure in black, community elders. *Dissertation Abstracts International*, 1989, 50:2663B.

39. Gueldner, S.H., & Hanner, M.B. Methodological issues related to gerontological nursing research. *Nurs Res*, 1989, 38:183-185.

40. Kim, K.K. Response time and health care learning of elderly patients. *Res Nurs Health*, 1986, 9:233-239.

41. Zimmer, A.W., Calkins, E., Hadley, E., et al. Conducting clinical research in geriatric populations. *Ann Intern Med*, 1985, 2:276-283.

42. Kane, R. Accomplishments, problems, trends and future challenges. In R.L. Kane & R.A. Kane (Eds.), *Assessing older persons*. New York: Oxford University Press, 2000, pp. 519-529.

43. Applegate, W.B., & Curb, J.D. Designing and executing randomized clinical trials involving elderly persons. *J Am Geriatr Soc*, 1990, 8:943-950.

44. Yesavage, J.A., & Brink, T.L. Development and validation of a geriatric depression screening scale: A preliminary report. *J Psychiatry Res*, 1983, 17:37-49.

45. Andresen, E., Rothenberg, B., & Zimmer, J. G. (Eds.) *Assessing the health status of older adults*. New York: Springer, 1997.

46. Fillit, H. *Practical geriatric assessment*. London: Greenwich Medical Media, 1998.

47. Osterweil, D., Brummel-Smith, K., & Beck, J.C. (Eds.). *Comprehensive geriatric assessment*. New York: McGraw-Hill, 2000.

48. Gallo, J.J., Fulmer, T., Paveza, G.J., & Reichel, W. *Handbook of geriatric assessment*. Gaithersburg, MD: Aspen, 2000.

49. Kane, R.L., & Kane, R.A. (Eds.). *Assessing older persons*. New York: Oxford University Press, 2000.

5

Measurement Issues Concerning Linguistic Translations

Claudette G. Varricchio

The current research climate emphasizes the inclusion in clinical research of representative samples of all ethnic and cultural groups, thereby reflecting the composition of the U.S. population. Many researchers are interested in the cross-cultural aspects of illness and wellness phenomena, symptoms, and other variables. For these reasons, it is important to consider linguistic translations and the cultural appropriateness of research tools. This chapter addresses the issues, controversies, and techniques used for translating and determining the cultural appropriateness of measurement instruments.

Many instruments that assess physical symptoms, functional status, psychologic state, and social interactions, as well as more global constructs, have been developed and validated. If these instruments are considered for cultural adaptation or linguistic translation, a researcher must have operationally defined the concepts. The researcher must then determine whether the concepts exist in the target culture and whether they can be operationalized in the same way. Few existing methods of assessment of health–illness concepts are appropriate for, or have been validated with, subjects from diverse cultural backgrounds. This problem is compounded by the practical difficulties of language barriers, cultural differences, and economic constraints in addition to the cultural and ethnic diversity of the subjects. Thought must be given to the validity of cultural equivalence of meaning when interpreting the scores. Decisions regarding treatment and supportive care or other interventions for persons from special populations often are based on clinical research that includes few participants from these groups.

Language is one of the most obvious barriers to assessment. Simple, direct translation of standardized or new instruments will not solve this problem.[1-5] Psychosocial and other concepts do not necessarily have a one-to-one correspondence between languages, or within a language from dialect to dialect.[6,7] Measures of health-related concepts must be sensitive to these subtle language differences, as well as to cultural differences that influence understanding of the constructs. The development or modification of instruments for people from non-English-derived cultures requires knowledge of the customs, beliefs, and traditions the target subjects practice related to health, illness, independence, and decision making. Methods and instruments must be validated in the target population to ensure that the concepts of interest have the same meaning as in the original language and culture. There is no reason to expect that a reliable and valid research instrument in one language will accurately measure the phenomenon as experienced by people from another culture.[1]

The underlying questions are whether the research stimuli are presented in equivalent ways to all the individuals included in a study, and whether conclusions from a study using a specific set of measures in a primarily white, middle-class U.S. sample can be generalized or compared to conclusions derived from, or applied to, subgroups of Americans or to subjects from other ethnic or cultural groups. The methods of approaching cross-cultural research and the translation, cultural appropriateness, and adaptation of existing instruments are the focus of this chapter.

Instrument Translation

The recommended procedure for translating research instruments is known as back-translation.[1,2] The goal is to ensure the equivalent meaning of items in both languages. This is accomplished by having questions in the source language translated by a bilingual person, preferably from the target culture, into the target language. Another bilingual individual then translates the items from the target language back to the source language. The two source-language versions are then compared for equivalence. This process can be repeated until satisfactory equivalence is obtained.

When the original English version is revised to ensure conceptually identical items in the target language and back-translated versions, the result is known as *decentering*. In this process, no one language is the center of attention. Both languages are equally important during the translation procedure. In decentering, both languages contribute to the final set of questions, and both are open to revisions.[8]

Researchers are cautioned not to become overly confident in the outcome of the initial efforts at back-translation. In some instances, seeming equivalence between versions may be the result of factors other than good translations. Brislin[8] suggests that the following factors must be considered when judging the adequacy of a translation: Translators may have a shared set of rules for translating certain nonequivalent words and phrases; some back-translators may be able to make sense out of a poorly written target-language version; and the bilingual translating from the source to the target may retain many of the grammatical forms of the source. In such situations, the translated document may be worthless for the purpose of asking questions of target-language monolinguals because it uses grammar common to the source, not the target group.

A second issue to consider in translation is that of etic versus emic concepts. *Etic* refers to phenomena that are universal or have a common meaning across the cultures of interest. If a concept survives repeated rounds of translation and back-translation, it can be considered etic. An etic concept can be expressed with readily available words and phrases in the languages of the two cultures. *Emic* concepts are group specific or are not readily expressed in the different cultures and do not survive back-translation in a consistent, common interpretation.[1,2] Emic concepts are not readily expressed in one of the languages or do not have a word form with equivalent meaning in both languages.

An ideal translation contains etic concepts, with emic concepts added to ensure that the questionnaire is culturally relevant. This process works best when adjustments are made in the wording of the source-language items. Some suggestions for successful translation efforts follow:[1] pp. 144–149

- Use short, simple sentences of less than 16 words with one dominant idea per sentence.
- Use active rather than passive voice.
- Repeat nouns rather than using pronouns.
- Avoid metaphors and colloquialisms.
- Avoid the subjunctive (verb forms with *could*, *should*, or *would*).
- Add sentences to provide a context for key ideas.
- Avoid adverbs and prepositions telling where or when. There often are no direct equivalents for these words, and the meaning of the entire item may be changed.
- Avoid possessive forms whenever possible. The concept of ownership may differ in different cultures.
- Use specific rather than general terms.
- Avoid vague terms regarding some event or thing, such as *probably*, *maybe*, or *perhaps*.
- Use words that are familiar to the translator.
- Avoid sentences with two different verbs if the verbs suggest two different actions.

Often a discussion of etic versus emic leads to a philosophic discussion concerning the desired outcome: linguistic equivalence or conceptual equivalence. In a linguistically equivalent item, there is a word-for-word translation. If no equivalent word is available in the target language, the item may be dropped or a word is chosen that conveys, as closely as possible, the same idea even if this concept has no meaning to the target group. In a conceptually equivalent translation, an item may use different words, but the intent is to convey an equivalent idea that has meaning and relevance to the target population.

Concept equivalence as a goal may necessitate adaptation of source-language items and changes in an existing instrument. This works best when applied to the translation of new instruments or if the researcher is willing to make changes in the choice of words in an existing instrument and validate both versions of the instrument in the appropriate targeted populations. The intent of the item is maintained, not the exact content. In this situation, the final back-translated version may serve as the source-language version in the research setting because it is most likely to be equivalent to the target-language version. Some authors of established tools resist any changes in their instruments made by others working on translations or cultural adaptations. Some recommendations for the back-translation process can be followed:[8]

- If possible, the translators should be familiar with the content (disease vocabulary, psychosocial concepts, etc.) in the source language and in the target language.
- Use words in the source language that have similar frequency of use in the target language.
- Translators and back-translators should work independently of each other.
- Test the translation on bilinguals. The researcher could use a split-half arrangement, in which one group takes the first half of the test in the source language and the second half in the target language. The process is reversed for group two.
- Refine translations on items for which there is ambiguity or discrepancy in responses.
- Discard items in which agreement on the wording or meaning cannot be achieved. Modification of the wording of items in the source language may be necessary at this point.
- Test with focus groups or a small pilot group of the target population to ensure that people representative of the target group understand the items. Administer the items to bilingual subjects: Some see the source-language version, some see the target-language version, and some see both. Responses should be similar across groups.

Cultural Appropriateness

Accurate translations can result in linguistic equivalence, but they may not elicit accurate responses from subjects using the target-language version because appropriate attention was not given to culture-specific aspects in tool development. Cultural or linguistic subgroups may preferentially use different words for an object or an idea. If the word or phrase commonly used by the target population is not used, the translation may be stilted, foreign, or meaningless for those responding.[9] A detailed discussion of this topic can be found in Marin and Marin.[2] A given translation may meet one or many criteria for cross-cultural equivalence. One technique for judging the adequacy of the translation is presented here. The following five criteria are often used:[10]

1. *Content equivalence.* The content of each item of the instrument is relevant to the phenomena of each culture being studied.
2. *Semantic equivalence.* The meaning of each item is the same in each culture after translation into the language and idiom of each culture.
3. *Technical equivalence.* The method of assessing the concept is comparable in each culture with respect to the data that it yields.
4. *Criterion equivalence.* The interpretation of the findings remains the same when compared with the norm for each culture studied.
5. *Conceptual equivalence.* The instrument is measuring the same theoretical construct in each culture.

An instrument may be cross-culturally equivalent by one of the criteria and not by the others. The goal of true cultural and language equivalence is that an instrument be equivalent in all five criteria.[10] This approach to cross-cultural validity is similar in concept to the more familiar types of validity used in research (i.e., face validity, construct validity).

One way to evaluate cultural appropriateness or relevance is to convene a focus group representative of the target population and ask participants to review the proposed items and comment on their meaning, clarity, and currency. Another way is to ask selected individuals in an interview setting, "What does the item mean to you?" and "What ideas are conveyed by this item?" This process is particularly relevant when dealing with translations of standardized instruments that have been normed on English-speaking groups.

The psychometric characteristics of the target-language version also must be established. It has been reported that the internal structure of an instrument changes when it is adapted and translated.[2] Different factor structures in a factor analysis may mean that different constructs are being tapped in the two versions.[10] As with the adaptation of all research instruments, any changes in the wording or structure of an instrument requires that validity and reliability be established for the new version.

Acculturation

The culture learning that occurs when immigrants come into contact with a new group, nation, or culture has been labeled *acculturation*.[2,11,12] The degree to which people from one culture assume the thoughts, behaviors, beliefs, and values of the host culture is a measure of their acculturation. Berry[13] suggested that acculturation involves change in any or all of six areas of psychologic functioning: language use, cognitive style, personality, identity, attitudes, and stress.

Measures of acculturation should go beyond demographic information. Self-identity of the subjects, as an outsider or a member of the culture, is an important aspect of this construct. Diversity within cultural or ethnic communities must not be overlooked.

Assumptions of homogeneity cannot be made. Varying degrees of acculturation are likely in any given cohort of subjects and are based on the degree of exposure and interaction of the individual or group with the new culture. The researcher must decide to what extent the degree of acculturation is likely to affect the variables of interest in any research study. Excellent discussions of the assessment of acculturation and of existing acculturation scales are available in Marin and Marin.[2,11]

Is it necessary and cost-effective to measure acculturation in the planning phase of the research? Will acculturation be taken into consideration when choosing how to measure the research variables? These questions are increasingly relevant given the current requirement to include women, minorities, and subpopulations in clinical research. The costs of producing appropriate measurement tools must be included in calculating research budgets. The time required for translations and cultural adaptations must be planned into research, and pilot studies for validation of the adapted research tools will be necessary preliminary work until a critical mass of validated and reliable instruments is available.

Additional Resources

Researchers who are considering translating or adapting an existing instrument or creating a new one will find the Additional Readings section at the end of this chapter useful. Translation and cultural sensitivity in research are areas that are developing rapidly and where new information is constantly becoming available. Many of the currently available instruments have had limited validity testing in culturally diverse populations. The researcher is cautioned about the need to establish validity and other parameters in the target population before making assumptions or interpreting the data. The list of Internet sites provides sources of information about instruments that have been translated or culturally adapted. In some cases the validity of the translated version is still under investigation.

References

1. Brislin, R.W. The wording and translation of research instruments. In W.J. Lonner & J.W. Berry (Eds.), *Field methods in cross-cultural research*. Beverly Hills, CA: Sage, 1986, pp. 137-164.
2. Marin, G., & Marin B.V. *Research with Hispanic populations*. Newbury Park, CA: Sage, 1991.
3. Montero, D. Research among racial and cultural minorities: An overview. *J Soc Issues*, 1977, 33(4):1-10.
4. Hayes-Bautista, D.E., & Chapa, G. Latino terminology: Conceptual bases for standardized terminology. *Am J Pub Health*, 1987, 77(1):61-68.
5. Hendricson, W.D., Russel, L.J., Prihoda, T.J., et al. An approach to developing a valid Spanish language translation of a health status questionnaire. *Med Care*, 1989, 27(10):959-966.
6. Schur, C.L., Bernstein, A.B., & Berk, M.L. The importance of distinguishing Hispanic subpopulations in the use of medical care. *Med Care*, 1987, 25(7):627-641.
7. Trevino, F.M. Standardized terminology for Hispanic populations. *Am J Pub Health*, 1987, 77(1):69-72.
8. Brislin, R.W. Back-translation for cross-cultural research. *J Cross-Cultural Psychol*, 1970, 1(3):185-216.
9. Bravo, M., Canino, G.J., Rubio-Sitpec, M., & Woodburry-Farina, M. A cross-cultural adaptation of a psychiatric epidemiologic instrument: The diagnostic interview schedule's adaptation in Puerto Rico. *Culture, Med Psychiatry*, 1991, 15(1):1-18.
10. Flaherty, J.A., Gavira, M.F., Pathak, D., et al. Developing instruments for cross-cultural psychiatric research. *J Nerv Mental Dis*, 1988, 176(5):257-263.
11. Marin G., Sabogal, F., Marin, BY., et al. Development of a short acculturation scale for Hispanics. *Hispanic J Behav Sci*, 1987, 9(2):183-205.
12. Berry, J.W., Trimble, J.E., & Olmedo, E.L. Assessment of acculturation. In W.L. Lonner & J.W. Berry (Eds.), *Field methods in cross-cultural research*. Beverly Hills, CA: Sage, 1986, pp. 291-324.
13. Berry, J. Acculturation as varieties of adaptation. In A.M. Padilla (Ed.), *Acculturation: Theory, models and some new findings*. Boulder, CO: Westview, 1980, pp. 9-25.

Additional Readings

Information on Specific Measurement Tools That Have Been Translated

Bravo, M., Canino, G.J., Rubio-Stipec, M., & Woodbury-Farina, M. A cross-cultural adaptation of a psychiatric epidemiologic instrument: The diagnostic interview schedule's adaptation in Puerto Rico. *Culture Med Psychiatry*, 1991, 15:1-18.

Bundek, N.I., Marks, G., & Richardson, J.L. Role of health locus of control beliefs in cancer screening of elderly Hispanic women. *Health Psychol*, 1993, 12(3):193-199.

Canino, G.J., Bird, H.R., Shrout, P.E., et al. The Spanish diagnostic interview schedule. Reliability and concordance with clinical diagnoses in Puerto Rico. *Arch Gen Psychiatry*, 1987, 44:720-726.

Cervantes, R.C., Padilla, A.M., & Salgado de Snyder, N. Reliability and validity of the Hispanic stress inventory. *Hispanic J Behav Sci*, 1990, 12(1):76-82.

Deyo, R.A. Pitfalls in measuring the health status of Mexican Americans: Comparative validity of the English and Spanish Sickness Impact Profile. *Am J Pub Health*, 1984, 74(6):569-573.

De Benedittis, G., Massei, R., Nobili, R., & Pieri, A. The Italian pain questionnaire. *Pain*, 1988, 33:53-62.

DeVogler-Ebersole, K.L., & Ebersole, P. Meaning in life depth test "Spanish." In D. Jenerson-Madden, P. Ebersole, A.M. Romero (Eds.), Personal life meaning of Mexicans. *J Soc Behav Personality*, 1992, 7:151-161.

Erkel, E.A. Conceptions of community health nurses regarding low-income Black, Mexican American, and white families: Part I. *J Comm Health Nurs*, 1985, 2(2):99-107.

Evers, G.C.M., Isenberg, M.A., Philipsen, H., Senten, M., & Brouns, G. Validity testing of the Dutch translation of the appraisal of the self-care agency A.S.A.Scale. *Int J Nurs Stud*, 1993, 30(4):331-342.

Flaherty, J.A., Gaviria, F.M., Pathak, D., et al. Developing instruments for cross-cultural psychiatric research. *J Nerv Ment Dis*, 1988, 176(5):257-263.

Franks, F., & Faux, S.A. Depression, stress, mastery, and social resources in four ethnocultural women's groups. *Res Nurs Women's Health*, 1990, 13:283-292.

Garcia, H.B., & Lee, P.C.Y. Knowledge about cancer and use of health care services among Hispanic- and Asian-American older adults. *J Psychosoc Oncol*, 1988, 6(3/4):157-177.

Gaston-Johansson, F., Albert, M., Fagan, E., & Zimmerman, L. Similarities in pain descriptions of four different ethnic-culture groups. *J Pain Symptom Man*, 1990, 5:(2):94-100.

Gilson, B.S., Gilson, J.S., Bergner, M., et al. Sickness Impact Profile. In W.D. Hendricson, I.J. Russell, T.J. Prihoda, et al. (Eds.), An approach to developing a valid Spanish language translation of a health status questionnaire. *Med Care*, 1989, 27:959-966.

Gilson, B.S., Erickson, D., Chavez, C.T., et al. A Chicano version of the Sickness Impact Profile (SIP). *Culture Med Psychiatry*, 1980, 4:137-150.

Gonzales, J.T., & Gonzales, V.M. Initial validation of a scale measuring self-efficacy of breast self-examination among low-income Mexican American women. *Hispanic J Behav Sci*, 1990, 12(3):277-291.

Guarnaccia, P.J., Angel, R., & Worobey, J.L. The factor structure of the CES-D in the Hispanic health and nutrition examination survey: The influences of ethnicity, gender and language. *Soc Sci Med*, 1989, 29(1):85-94.

Guillemin, F., Bombardier, C., & Beaton, D. Cross-cultural adaptation of health-related quality of life measures: Literature review and proposed guidelines. *J Clin Epidemiol*, 1993, 46:1417-1432.

Hendricson, W.D., Russell, L.J., Prihonda, T.J., et al. Sickness Impact Profile—San Antonio format. In W.D. Hendricson, I.J. Russell, T.J. Prihoda, et al. (Eds.), An approach to developing a valid Spanish language translation of a health-status questionnaire. *Med Care*, 1989, 27(10):959-966.

Lobo, A., Perez-Echeverria, M.J., & Artal, J. Validity of the scaled version of the General Health Questionnaire (QHQ-28) in a Spanish population. *Psychol Med*, 1986, 16:135-140.

Lobo, A., Perez-Echeverria, M.J., Jimenez-Aznarez, A., & Sancho, M.A. Emotional disturbances in endocrine patients. Validity of the scaled version of the General Health Questionnaire (GHQ-28). *Br J Psychiatry*, 1988, 152:807-812.

Lopez-Aqueres, W., Kemp, B., Plopper, M., et al. Health needs of the Hispanic elderly. *J Am Geriatr Soc*, 1984, 32(3):191-198.

Lorensen, M., Holter, L.M., Evers, G.C.M., et al. Cross-cultural testing of the "appraisal of self-care agency: ASA scale" in Norway. *Int J Nurs Stud*, 1993, 30(1):15-23.

Madiros, M. A view toward hospitalization: The Mexican American experience. *J Adv Nurs*, 1984, 9:469-478.

Meenan, R.F., Gertman, P.M., & Mason, J.M. Arthritis Impact Measurement Scale. (AIMS). In W.D. Hendricson, I.J. Russell, T.J. Prihoda et al. (Eds.), An approach to developing a valid Spanish language translation of a health-status questionnaire. *Med Care*, 1989, 27:959-966.

Meister, J.S., Warrick, L.H., de Zapien, J.G., & Wood, A.H. Using lay health workers: Case study of a community-based prenatal intervention. *J Comm Health*, 1992, 17(1):37-51.

Moinpour, C.M. Quality of life assessment in Southwest Oncology Group Clinical Trials translating and validating a Spanish questionnaire. In Quality of Life Assessment: International Perspectives. Orley j, Kuyken W, (Eds.), 1994. Springer Verlag, Berlin, 83-97.

Naughton, M.J., & Wiklund, I. A critical review of dimension-specific measures of health-related quality of life in cross-cultural research. *Qual Life Res*, 1993, 2(6):397-432.

Nielsen, B.B., McMillan, S., & Diaz, E. Instruments that measure beliefs about cancer from a cultural perspective. *Cancer Nurs*, 1992, 15(2):109-115.

Park, K.B., Upshaw, H.S., & Koh, S.D. East Asians: Response to Western health items. *J Cross-Cultural Psychol*, 1988, 19(1):51-63.

Patrick, D.L., Sittamplam, Y., Somesville, S.M., et al. Cross-cultural comparison of health status values. *Am J Pub Health*, 1985, *75*(12):1402-1407.

Spinetta, J.J. Measurement of family function, communication, and cultural effects. *Cancer*, 1984, *53910* (suppl):2330-2337.

Salek, S. *The compendium of quality of life instruments.* (RA 407.C651, latest edition.) NY: Wiley. (Contains over 150 questionnaires and translations).

Vallerand, R.J., & Halliwell, W.R. Vers une methodologie de validation trans-culturelle de questionnaires psychologiques: Implications pour la psychologie du sport. *Can J Appl Sport Sci*, 1983, *8*(1):9-18.

Walker, S.N., Kerr, M.J., Pender, N.J., & Sechrist, K.R. A Spanish language version of the health-promoting lifestyle profile. *Nurs Res*, 1990, *39*(5):268-273.

Warrick, L.H., Wood, A.H., Meister, J.S., & de Zapien, J.G. Evaluation of a peer health worker prenatal outreach and education program for Hispanic farm worker families. *J Comm Health*, 1992, *17*(1):13-26.

World Health Organization Quality of Life Assessment (WHOQOL): Development and general psychometric properties. *Soc Sci Med*, 1998, *46*:1569-1585.

Zapka, J.G., Harris, D.R., Hosmer, D., et al. Effect of a community health intervention on breast cancer screening among Hispanic American women. *Health Serv Res*, 1993, *28*(2):223-235.

Cultural Issues

AAN Expert Panel on Culturally Competent Nursing Care. AAN expert panel report: Culturally competent health care. *Nurs Outlook*, 1992, *40*(6):277-283.

Eliason, M.J. Ethics and transcultural nursing care. *Nurs Outlook*, 1993, *41*(5):225-228.

Ell, K.O., Mantell, J.E., & Hamovitch, M.B. Socioculturally sensitive interventions for patients with cancer. *J Psychosocial Oncol*, 1989, *6*(3/4):141-155.

Fong, C.M. Ethnicity and nursing practice. *Topics Clin Nurs*, 1985, *7*(3):1-10.

Frank-Stromborg, M., and Olsen, S. (2001). Cancer prevention in diverse populations. Cultural implications for the multidisciplinary team. Pittsburgh, PA: Oncology Nursing Society.

Harwood, A. (Ed.) *Ethnicity and medical care*. Cambridge, MA: Harvard University Press, 1984.

Henderson, G., & Primeaux, M. (Eds.). *Transcultural health care*. Menlo Park, CA: Addison-Wesley, 1981.

Lipson, J.G., & Meleis, A.I. Culturally appropriate care: The case of immigrants. *Topics Clin Nurs*, 1985, *7*(3):48-56.

Porter, C.P., & Villarruel, A.M. Nursing research with African American and Hispanic people: Guidelines for action. *Nurs Outlook*, 1993, *41*(2):59-67.

Reinert, B.R. The health care beliefs and values of Mexican-Americans. *Home Healthcare Nurse*, 1986, *4*(5):23-31.

Rogler, L.H. The meaning of culturally sensitive research in mental health. *Am J Psychiatry*, 1989, *146*(3):296-303.

Seachrest, L., Fay, T.L., & Zaidi, S.F.H. Problems of translation in cross-cultural research. *J Cross-Cult Psychol*, 1972, *3*:41-56.

Sprangers, M., Cull, A., & Groenvold, M., on behalf of the EORTC. *EORTC quality of life study group guidelines for developing questionnaire modules* (2nd ed.). Brussels: EORTC, 1998.

Tripp-Reimer, T. Research in cultural diversity. *West J Nurs Res*, 1984, *6*(4):457-458.

West, E.A. The cultural bridge model. *Nurs Outlook*, 1993, *41*(4):229-234.

White, E.H. Giving health care to minority patients. *Nurs Clin North Am*, 1977, *12*(1):27-39.

Acculturation

Cuellar, I., Harris, L.C., & Jasso, R. An acculturation scale for Mexican American normal and clinical populations. *Hisp J Behav Sci*, 1980, *2*(3):199-217.

Mendoza, R.H. An empirical scale to measure type and degree of acculturation in Mexican-American adolescents and adults. *J Cross-Cultural Psychol*, 1989, *20*(4):372-385.

Olmedo, E.L., & Padilla, A.M. Empirical and construct validation of a measure of acculturation for Mexican Americans. *J Soc Psychol*, 1978, *105*:179-187.

Methodologic Issues

Aaronson, N.K., Acquadro, C., Alonso, J., et al. International quality of life assessment (IQOLA) project. *Qual Life Res*, 1992, *1*:349-351.

Aday, L.A., Chiu, G.Y., & Andersen, R. Methodological issues in health care surveys of the Spanish heritage population. *Am J Pub Health*, 1980, *70*(4):367-374.

Berkanovic, E. The effect of inadequate language translation on Hispanics' responses to health surveys. *Am J Pub Health*,1980, *70*(12):1273-1281.

Berzon, R., Hays, R.D., & Shumaker, S.A. International use, application and performance of health-related quality of life instruments. *Qual Life Res*, 1993, *2*(6):367-368.

Bullinger, M., Anderson, R., Cella D., & Aaronson, N.K. Developing and evaluating cross-cultural instruments from minimum requirements to optimal models. *Qual Life Res*, 1993, *2*(6):451-459.

Canales, S., Ganz, P.A., & Schag, C.A.C. Translation and validation of a quality of life instrument for Hispanic American cancer patients: Methodological considerations. *Qual Life Res*, 1995, *4*(1):3-11.

Cella, D.F., Wiklund, S.A., & Aaronson, N.K. Integrating health-related quality of life into cross-national clinical trials. *Qual Life Res*, 1993, *2*(6):433-440.

Cella, D.F., Lloyd, S.R., & Wright, B.D. Cross-cultural instrument equating: Current research and future directions. In B. Spilker (Ed.), *Quality of life and pharmacoeconomics in clinical trials (2nd ed.)*. Philadelphia: Lippincott-Raven, 1996.

Cull. A., Sprangers, M., & Aaronson, N., on behalf of the EORTC Quality of Life Study Group. *EORTC Quality of Life Study Group translation procedures*. Internal report. Edinburgh/Amsterdam: 1994.

Domino, G., Fragoso, A., & Moreno, H. Cross-cultural investigations of the imagery of cancer in Mexican nationals. *Hisp J Behav Sci*, 1991, 13(4):422-435.

Guyatt, G.H. The philosophy of health-related quality of life translation. *Qual Life Res*, 1993, 2(6):461-465.

Hayes-Bautista, D.E. Identifying "Hispanic" populations: The influence of research methodology upon public health. *Am J Pub Health*, 1980, 70(4):353-356.

Hayes-Bautista, D.E., & Chapa, J. Latino terminology: Conceptual bases for standardized terminology. *Am J Pub Health*, 1987, 77(1):61-68.

Herdman, M., Fox-Rushby, J., & Badia, X. A model of equivalence in cultural adaptation of HRQoL instruments: The universal approach. *Qual Life Res*, 1998, 7:323-335.

Howard, C.A., Samet, J.M., Buechley, R.W., et al. Survey research in New Mexico Hispanics: Some methodological issues. *Am J Epidemiol*, 1983, 117(1):27-34.

Kroeger, A. Health interview surveys in developing countries: A review of the methods and results. *Int J Epidemiol*, 1983, 12(4):465-481.

Marin, G., & Marin, B.V. Methodological fallacies when studying Hispanics. *Appl Soc Psychol Ann*, 1982, 3:99-117.

Marin, G., & Marin, B.V. A comparison of three interviewing approaches for studying sensitive topics with Hispanics. *Hisp J Behav Sci*, 1989, 11(4):330-340.

Marin, G., Marin, B.V., Perez-Stable, E.J., & Otero-Sabogal, R. Cultural differences in attitudes and expectancies between Hispanic and non-Hispanic white smokers. *Hisp J Behav Sci*, 1990, 12(4):422-436.

McArt, E.W., & Brown, J.K. The challenge of research on international populations: Theoretical and methodological issues. *Oncol Nurs Forum*, 1990, 17(2):283-286.

Montero, D. Research among racial and cultural minorities: An overview. *J Soc Sci*, 1977, 33(4):1-10.

Munet-Vilaro, F., & Egan, M. Reliability issues of the family environment scale for cross-cultural research. *Nurs Res*, 1990, 39(4):244-247.

Park, K.B., Upshaw, H.S., & Koh, S.D. East Asians: Responses to western health items. *Int J Cross-Cult Psychol*, 1988, 19(1):51-63.

Schur, C.L., Berstein, A.B., & Berk, M.L. The importance of distinguishing Hispanic subpopulations in the use of medical care. *Med Care*, 1987, 25(7):627-641.

Velasquez, R.J., & Callahan, W.J. Psychological testing of Hispanic Americans in clinical settings: Overview and issues. In K.F. Gesinger (Ed.), *Psychological testing of Hispanics*. Washington, DC: American Psychological Association, 1992.

Other Information

Anderson, R. T., Aaronson, N. K., & Wilkin, D. Critical review of the international assessments of health-related quality of life. *Qual Life Res*, 1993, 2(6):369-395.

Antle, A. Cultural and ethnic dimensions of cancer care. The American Indian. *Oncol Nurs Forum*, 1987, 14(3):70-73.

Becker, D.M., Hill, D.R., Jackson, J.S., et al. (Eds.). *Health behavior research in minority populations: Access, design, and implementation*. NIH PUB. No. 92-2965. Washington, DC: DHHS, PHS, NIH, The National Heart, Lung and Blood Institute, 1992.

Brisbane, F.L., & Womble, M. *Working with African Americans. The professional's handbook*. Needham, MA: Ginn Press, 1992. Copies are available from HRDI International Press, 222 S. Jefferson St., Suite 200, Chicago, IL, 60611.

Bureau of the Census. *Hispanic Americans today*. Washington, DC: U.S. Department of Commerce, Economics and Statistics Administration, Bureau of the Census, 1993, pp. 23-183.

COSSMHO. *Delivering preventive health care to Hispanics: A manual for providers*. Washington, DC: Author, 1990. Copies are available from Provider Education Project, 1501 16th St., NW, Washington, DC, 20036.

Guillory, J. Ethnic perspectives of cancer nursing: The Black American. *Oncol Nurs Forum*, 1987, 14(3):66-69.

Health and psychosocial instruments (HaPI). Behavioral measurement database services. PO Box 110287, Pittsburgh, PA 15232-0787. Tel.: (412) 687-6850. The HaPI database also is available online through BRS Search Services at your campus/organization library.

The Fall 1993 HaPI-CD includes an update of more than 3000 records that describe the following kinds of measurement instruments: questionnaires, rating scales, interview forms, checklists, vignettes/scenarios, indexes, coding schemes/manuals, projective techniques, tests. The database can be queried for instruments in foreign languages. The HaPI database provides information on first published sources of new instruments to access health practices and outcomes. It does not review validity data. The author and address may be provided. The *Behavioral Measurements Letter*, a companion information source, is available from Linda Perloff, PhD, editor. The Behavioral Measurements Letter, PO Box 110287, Pittsburgh, PA 15232-0787.

Kagawa-Singer, M. Ethnic perspectives of cancer nursing: Hispanics and Japanese-Americans. *Oncol Nurs Forum*, 1987, 14(3):59-65.

Naughton, M.J., & Wiklund, I. A critical review of dimension-specific measures of health-related quality of life in cross-cultural research. *Qual Life Res*, 1993, 2(6):397-432.

National Coalition of Hispanic Health and Human Services Organizations. 1501 Sixteenth St., NW, Washington, DC, 20036. Tel.: (202) 797-4335. E. Richardson is a source of information about measurement tools that have been translated into Spanish.

Office of Research on Women's Health, National Institutes of Health, 9000 Rockville Pike, Bethesda, MD, 20892. Tel.: (301) 402-1770. Coordinates the effort to include women and minorities in clinical research.

Special Populations Studies Branch, National Cancer Institute, Division of Cancer Prevention and Control. George Alexander, MD, Chief. 9000 Rockville Pike, EPN 240, Bethesda, MD 20892. Tel.: (301) 496-8589. This branch has special programs and direct interaction with investigators working with African Americans, Hispanics, Native Americans, Hawaiians, Alaskan Native residents, and underserved groups. Specific resources are the National Hispanic Cancer Control Research Network, the Native Hawaiian and American Samoan Cancer Control Research Network, and the National Outreach Initiatives Project, which includes the National Black Leadership Initiative on Cancer, the National Hispanic Leadership Initiative on Cancer, and the Appalachia Leadership Initiative on Cancer.

Surgeon General's National Hispanic/Latino Health Initiative. *Recommendations to the Surgeon General to improve Hispanic/Latino health.* Washington, DC: U.S. Department of Health and Human Services, 1993. Office of the Assistant Secretary for Health, Office of

Minority Health. This is a summary of the Executive Planning Committee meeting held on April 22 and 23,1993, and the implementation strategies identified at the meeting as crucial for prompt action. Office of Minority Health Resource Center, 1-(800)-414-6472. DHHS, PHS, Office of the Assistant Secretary for Health, Office of Minority Health. Health information and education materials and other directories are available for Asian and Pacific Islander Populations, African Americans, Native Americans, and sources of Spanish-language health materials.

The Language Assistants. Software programs to translate English- and foreign-language documents automatically or interactively. Has the capability of bidirectional translation in English, Spanish, French, German, and Italian. Information available by calling 1-(800)-851-2917, or 24-hour fax 1-(415)-345-5575.

Varricchio, C. Cultural and ethnic dimensions of cancer nursing care: Introduction. *Oncol Nurs Forum*, 1987, *14*(3):57-58.

Internet Sites for Questionnaires and Translations of Questionnaires

CDC Health-Related Quality of Life. Spanish translation of CDC's Healthy Days Measures. www.cdc.gov/hrqol/spanish.htm.

ERIC Clearinghouse on Assessment and Evaluation. Includes a search engine for searching selected assessment and evaluation sites on the Web, a "test locator," and numerous links to other Internet sources related to assessment and evaluation. www.ericae.net/.

Evaluacion Clinica y Economica de Medicamentos. Spanish-language site with pages on quality of life that include a list of instruments, databases, and bibliography. www.farmacoeconomia.com/default.htm.

FACIT Functional Assessment of Chronic Illness Therapy. Functional Assessment of Chronic Illness Therapy Measurement System. www.facit.org. www.facct.org.

Google. Useful for finding instruments available on the Internet; use keywords to search. www.google.com.

Health and Psychosocial Instruments (HAPI). A database of health and psychosocial instruments, including questionnaires, rating scales, index measures, scenarios, vignettes, observations, checklists, manuals, coding schemes, and projective techniques. www.medsearch.lib.umich.edu/. Start a UM-Medsearch session and then choose HAPI.

MAPI Research Institute. The institute has particular expertise in cultural adaptation and linguistic validation of questionnaires, helpful instrument pages, and more. www.mapi-research-inst.com.

The Mental Measurement Yearbook. Information on tests in psychology, education, and business, including availability of non-English language versions of the test. www.unl.edu/buros, or www.ericae.net/testcol.htm#trev.

QOLID. The Quality of Life Instruments Database. A comprehensive database in the field of patient-reported outcomes. QOLID lists more than 1000 questionnaires; provides detailed information on some 400; and copies of more than 240 original questionnaires, 160 translations, 70 user manuals, and descriptions of 60 databases for these questionnaires. This database is updated twice a year in collaboration with the authors of each instrument. www.qolid.org.

RAND Health. Survey section includes instruments and scoring for several important instruments. www.rand.org/health.

Search Engines such as Google, AltaVista, and Northern Light may be useful for finding a particular test.

Self-Report Measures. A collection of self-report instruments from Charles S. Carver of the University of Miami Psychology Department, including the Spanish translations of these instruments. www.psy.miami.edu/faculty/ccarver/CCscales.htm.

Sociologic Abstracts (SocioFile). Contains citations to instruments used in various sociologic studies. www.ed.ugl.lib.umich.edu:8590/?.

Taubman Medical Library. Guide to Tests and Measurement Instruments. www.lib.umich.edu/taubman/info/testsandmeasurement.htm.

Web of Science. A site that enables traces of literature and studies that employ specific tests/instruments. www.webofscience.com/.

6

Physiologic Measurement Issues

Freda DeKeyser Ganz and Linda C. Pugh

Clinical practice involves assessment and intervention in response to both psychologic and physiologic alterations. Those working in clinical practice must be familiar with techniques used to quantify psychologic as well as physiologic parameters. There is also an increasing awareness that education[1] and research[2,3] in the biologic sciences must be enhanced and encouraged within health-related disciplines such as nursing. Therefore, clinicians, educators, and researchers need knowledge of the principles of measurement related to physiologic variables.

Sources of Measurement Error

The most common tools used by clinicians to measure physiologic variables are the five senses. For example, we *see* cyanosis, we *hear* crying, and we *smell* infectious exudate. Instruments such as microscopes or stethoscopes aid and directly enhance the performance of the senses. Possibly because many physiologic variables are directly observable and are so commonly performed, they are perceived as "hard data" or as being objective and without error. However, as stated in classic measurement theory, no measurement is without error.

In fact, several sources of potential error relative to physiologic variables have been identified.[4] The first source of error stems from biologic variability. When a researcher measures a physiologic parameter at a certain time, it is probable that the value will change seconds later. The researcher does not know whether that change is due to physiologic changes within the individual or to instrument error. There also are differences among individuals. For example, in Western society there is a trend for blood pressure to increase with advancing age. A second source of error is found in specimen collection and handling. For example, the wrong name could be put on a collection tube, or a sample could evaporate. Analytical methods also can contribute to error. A technician might not add enough reagent to a step in the analysis or a transducer might not be calibrated correctly. Errors can be made after the analysis because of mistakes in transcription. Therefore, error variability leads to measurement error and so decreases the reliability and validity of measurements.

Reliability and Validity of Physiologic Measures

Errors associated with physiologic variables may be random or systematic, such as psychosocial variables. The evaluation of these errors also is described using the concepts of reliability and validity. However, the terms *reliability* and *validity* are rarely used in the biometric, medical, and medical technology literature, maybe because of a lack of familiarity with psychometric theory and the parallel development of other terms and methods deemed more appropriate. It is possible to combine aspects of both types of assessments so that practitioners from both backgrounds can evaluate physiologic variables more effectively.

Reliability

Reliability is a measure of the amount of random error of an instrument. Random measurement error refers to one-time, unusual, or chance mistakes made during the measurement process that lead to different scores on the measurement being taken. For example, if a nurse took a patient's blood pressure while the patient was speaking, the blood pressure reading would probably be higher than the patient's true blood pressure.

Within the psychosocial literature, reliability usually is determined by evaluating the internal consistency and the stability of results obtained with a tool. Internal consistency is usually calculated in psychosocial contexts with an alpha coefficient. This coefficient describes the extent to which performance on any one item or question in the instrument is a good indicator of performance on the entire tool.[5] In biomedical research this type of reliability evaluation is not common because the number of items in a measurement technique is usually very small. For some physiologic variables, investigators take a specified number of readings and report the average or mean. Grip strength has been measured in two selected studies.[6,7] These researchers reported the average of three scores. McCloy and associates[8] measured cardiac output and then averaged the next three measures as long as the three were within 10% of each other.

Test–retest, intrarater, and interrater reliability methods measure the repeatability or stability of psychosocial instruments. *Test–retest reliability* is evaluated by administering an instrument such as a questionnaire at two different times and then determining the correlation between them. This concept is similar to the duplicate measurements taken in clinical laboratories. In this context, the same specimen is divided into several parts, and then readings are taken and correlated.

Precision is a term not often seen in the psychosocial literature, but it is often used in the biometric and medical literature to describe reliability. The standard error is used to describe the variability and precision of measurements in physiologic research. The specimen is divided into several parts, and the standard error is calculated. The higher the standard error, the greater the variability and, therefore, the lower the reliability of the measurement for that sample. Theoretically, the same value should be obtained every time the test is performed.

Intrarater reliability can be evaluated by having the same technician analyze separately two halves of specimens and then determine the correlation between the two readings. *Interrater reliability* is evaluated in a similar manner, except that two people instead of one perform the analyses. Topf and Davis[9] reported interrater reliability in the assessment of sleep stage scoring. Two scorers independently rated one out of every six sleep records in their sample. Sommers, Woods, and Courtade[10] reported that investigators need to attend to interrater reliability and injectate reliability when studying cardiac output.

One method of calculating precision is the coefficient of variation. It is a common measure used by many clinical laboratories. The coefficient of variation is calculated by dividing the standard deviation by the mean (where coefficient of variation = (standard deviation/mean) * 100).[11]

Many clinical laboratories use the Levy-Jennings control chart as another method for quality control that gives the laboratory a visual depiction of precision. A standardized or control sample is divided into at least 20 parts and is then analyzed for a specific metabolite by a specific technique on subsequent days. A chart is made with the day on the x axis and the laboratory value on the y axis. The mean and standard deviations are calculated for all the days being studied. Lines are drawn through the value of the mean, as well as 2 standard deviations above and below the mean. It is expected that only 1 in 22 points will be greater than 2 standard deviations above or below the mean.[11] If more than this number of points are found to be greater than 2 standard deviations away from the mean, then that method is said to be imprecise or unreliable for that laboratory.

Validity

Validity refers to an instrument's ability to measure the true score. Validity can be seen as a measure of the amount of systematic error of a measurement. Calibration is one method commonly used with biomedical instruments to decrease the amount of systematic measurement error. Calibration is the procedure by which an instrument is adjusted to make its readings correspond as closely as possible to the true values of a known substance. For example, Derrico[12] calibrated blood pressure readings from a Dinamap monitor with a mercury gravity manometer before collecting data.

Accuracy, the term used instead of validity in biomedical literature, is said to reflect the amount of bias or difference between obtained results and the known or assumed truth.[13] Accuracy also can refer to the ability of the instrument to indicate the true value of the variable being measured. Ko[14] has defined accuracy as

$$accuracy = \frac{\text{True value} - \text{Measured value}}{\text{True value}} \times 100\%$$

Although validity has been defined as accuracy, there are several aspects related to validity that are not included in the concept of accuracy. Validity refers not only to how far empirical measurements are from true values but also to whether the instrument is measuring what it is supposed to measure. For example, a researcher who measured only white blood cell counts would be measuring only some of the many aspects of immune functioning. There are many other measures of immune function, and it would be erroneous to conclude that the entire concept was measured by white blood cell counts alone.

Accuracy is determined by three parameters: selectivity, sensitivity, and specificity. *Selectivity* refers to the ability of the instrument to identify correctly the signal under study and distinguish it from all other signals.[15] *Sensitivity*, or the true positive rate, is defined as the likelihood that a patient with a given disease will have a positive test result. *Specificity*, or the true negative rate, is the probability that a patient without the disease will have a negative test result (Figure 6.1). No test has 100% specificity and sensitivity. A test that has higher specificity usually has a lower sensitivity. Those deciding which measurement tool to use must decide whether it is more important to have a higher level of true positives or true negatives. For example, Verklan, Bickel, and Moon[16] measured the heart rate variability of neonates using energy entropy of four different domains. They found that a 100% specificity and 67% sensitivity distinguished between the neonates.

True Condition

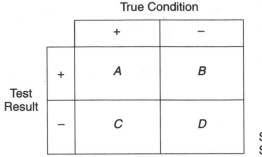

Sensitivity = $A/(A + C)$
Specificity = $D/(B + D)$

Figure 6.1   Sensitivity and Specificity

In more recent years, an alternative approach to describing accuracy has been gaining favor in the medical literature. In receiver operating characteristic (ROC) analysis, a curve is constructed in which the level of sensitivity of the test is plotted along the y axis and (1-specificity) along the x axis (Figure 6.2). The area under the resulting curve, often called a c-index or c-statistic, is used as a summary statistic to describe the accuracy of the test. A test with equal levels of sensitivity and specificity would have a value of 0.5. Often this method is described as the ability of the test to correctly discriminate between normal and abnormal.[17,18] For example, Goodwin and coworkers[19] found a 0.72 area under the curve associated with seven demographic variables that predicted premature births.

Construct Validity

Several approaches to validity can be tested and determined. *Construct validity* provides evidence of the instrument's ability to accurately measure the concept for which it was designed. It can be tested by using contrasted groups or experimental methods. When contrasted groups are used, two groups that are known to be very high and very low on the concept being studied are measured and compared by the instrument. If the groups are found to be significantly different, then the tool has adequately measured the concept. For example, Smatlak and Knebel[20] hypothesized that patients with a lowered cardiac index would have inaccurate measurements of oxygen saturation as measured by pulse oximetry. This hypothesis was supported when the investigators found that pulse oximeter measurements were up to 7% higher than actual oxygen saturation measurements measured by a co-oximeter. Therefore, this study casts some doubt on the construct validity of pulse oximetry as a measurement of oxygen saturation for patients with a low cardiac index.

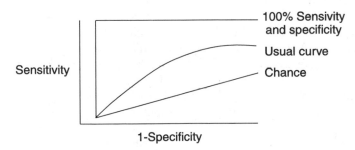

Figure 6.2   Example of ROC Curves

If a hypothesis is tested and supported with an instrument, the instrument is said to possess construct validity via experimental methods. One example of this type of construct validity is a study by McCarthy et al.[21] They hypothesized that meperidine affects temperature regulation. They found that injection of meperidine blocked the onset of fever in rats using a computerized telemetry system for body temperature monitoring. Therefore, their study demonstrated construct validity for their monitoring system.

Criterion Validity

Criterion validity is assessed when one method of analysis is compared to a known definitive method. Specimens are analyzed using this new method as well as an older, known method that has been shown to be reliable and valid. For example, a group of investigators[22] compared the spirometry readings of lung transplant patients taken at home to measurements taken in the pulmonary function laboratory. Hwu, Coates, and Lin[23] evaluated the validity of measuring heart rate by various counting methods of the radial pulse compared to that of an ECG.

Correlation coefficients are often used to compare the results of known methods with those obtained by newer ones. Bland and Altman[24] discourage this practice. They state that correlation coefficients measure relationships, not agreement between variables. Correlations also are affected by the range of true values in the sample. Tests of significance also are thought to be irrelevant because both instruments are designed to measure the same thing. Therefore, it would be unlikely *not* to find a significant relationship. Bland and Altman prefer the use of the mean absolute difference and the standard deviation of the difference as more appropriate statistics for this type of analysis. deMonterice and associates[25] report a mean absolute difference between two instruments that measure preterm infant sucking.

ROC curves also are used to compare newer technologies with known standard methods of measurement. For each method, the specificity and sensitivity are determined for various test criteria. For example, the blood pressures of known hypertensives were compared to those of normal controls with two types of automatic blood pressure machines. The blood pressures were taken using both machines on each patient. Several criteria for the definition of hypertension were then decided (e.g., systolic blood pressure: >130, >140, >150, >160). The number of true positives and true negatives were then computed for both types of measures, and the values converted into sensitivity and specificity values and plotted on a curve. The curve closest to the perfect test curve is the test with the higher validity.

Recovery experiments also are used as a type of criterion validity evaluation. A known amount of substance is added to a sample. The sample with the added substance and the sample without the added substance are then analyzed for that substance in a routine manner. The percentage of the substance found by the analysis is then calculated:[11]

$$\text{Percent recovery} = \frac{\text{Amount recovered}}{\text{Amount added}} \times 100$$

Groups of laboratories analyze the same control material and compare their results, another means of evaluating criterion validity. The results of the analysis by many labs are used to compute a mean and standard deviation. A standard deviation interval (SDI) for each lab can then be calculated as follows:

$$\text{SDI} = \frac{\text{Specific laboratory's value} - \text{Mean of all laboratories using the same method}}{\text{Standard deviation of all laboratories using the same method}}$$

A specific laboratory's results are said to be accurate if the absolute value of the SDI is less than or equal to 1, acceptable if the absolute value is less than 2 but greater than 1, and not acceptable if the absolute value is greater than 2.[11]

Content Validity

Content validity is said to exist when a tool or instrument contains most aspects of the concept being measured and is considered complete when it does not contain extraneous information. This type of validity can be evaluated in psychosocial and physiologic measures in a similar manner. Experts in the field are contacted and asked to evaluate whether the method being used in the analysis is appropriate.

The use of continuous monitoring can be seen as another step toward increasing the content validity of monitoring equipment. As technology improves, more physiologic parameters are being measured continuously in more natural settings. For example, 24-hour monitors are now available that can measure activity levels, blood pressure, ECG, and gastric motility. Although problems exist as to what data to use in the data analysis, it is thought that information gained from monitoring a person over a longer time in more natural settings has higher validity than a one-time reading taken in a doctor's office or hospital bed.

Biomedical Instrumentation

Many physiologic variables are measured with some form of biomedical instrumentation. These tools may be used in connection with clinical practice and research. They often are electrically powered[26] Every biomedical instrument is made up of three basic parts: a transducer, signal-conditioning equipment, and a display mode. Transducers convert one form of energy into another. In biomedical instruments, the transducer senses the physiologic event and converts it into an electrical signal usually measured in volts. For example, the voltage in an arterial blood pressure monitor increases as the arterial pressure increases. The transducer usually is separated from the rest of the instrument and often is applied to the body. For example, ECG electrodes are transducers that are placed on the chest.

The signal produced by the transducer is then sent to the signal-conditioning equipment. This component modifies the electrical signal so that it can be understood by other pieces of equipment, for example, by amplifying the signal or dampening extraneous noise. Noise or artifacts are unwanted signals that are not produced by the variable being measured. For example, when a patient moves in bed, noise or artifact often appears on the ECG monitor that is unrelated to electrical conduction in the heart.

The display converts the electrical signals sent by the signal-conditioning equipment into a form that can be understood by practitioners and/or stored in a computer. A strip recorder and an oscilloscope are two types of displays.

Several common properties of biomedical instruments can be used to evaluate their worth as measurement tools. These are the range, sensitivity, stability, and reliability of the instrument. The *range* of an instrument is "the complete set of values over which the instrument is designed to operate properly."[26] For example, Hanneman[27] reports that cardiac output readings are accurate within 5% for values between 0.5 and 1.0 liters/minute. If one expects values to be higher or lower than that range, one should choose another instrument.

An instrument's *sensitivity* refers to the ability of the machine to detect small differences. The higher the sensitivity, the smaller the differences that can be detected. Resolution, one aspect of sensitivity, is the smallest measurable input increment.[14] For

Table 6.1 Measurement Techniques Used in Psychosocial versus Physiologic Disciplines

	Psychosocial	Physiologic
Reliability/precision		
a) Internal consistency	Alpha coefficient	If >1 measure taken, average measurements together
b) Stability	Test–retest	Duplicate measurements
	Intrarater	Coefficient of variation
	Interrater	Standard error
Validity/accuracy		
a) Construct	Contrasted groups	Control groups
	Experimental methods	Experimental methods
b) Criterion	Correlations with	Recovery experiments
	known tools	Standard deviation interval
		Correlations with known tools
		Receiver operating characteristic curves
c) Content	Content experts	Content experts

example, a thermometer that measures in 0.1^0 differences is less sensitive than one that can detect differences of 0.01^0.[26] Ko[14] defines sensitivity as the ratio of output to input (output–input). Therefore, the larger the level of artifact or noise (or a larger input), the lower the sensitivity of the instrument.

Stability indicates the ability of a machine to maintain accurate values over repeated testings and time. A machine that has unstable readings will be subject to drift. *Drift* is a change in the sensitivity of the machine with time, temperature, or other interfering factors.[14] For example, Hanneman[27] calibrated arterial and pulmonary catheter equipment every 8 hours to control for a drift of 0.3 mm Hg per hour.

Table 6.1 compares the methods used to determine the reliability, precision, and validity or accuracy of measurement tools between the psychosocial and physiologic disciplines. Measures of internal consistency and stability can be replaced with duplicate measurements, coefficient of variation, and standard error measurements to assess the reliability and precision of a physiologic instrument. The accuracy or validity of instruments can be assessed with control groups, experimental methods, and recovery experiments, as well as less well-known methods in the psychosocial disciplines, such as ROC curves and the SDI. The use of these means to evaluate measurement issues should prove useful to researchers interested in studying complex, multidimensional concepts that include physiologic and psychosocial components.

References

1. Trnobranski, P.H. Biological sciences and the nursing curriculum: A challenge for educationalists. *J Adv Nurs*, 1993, *18*(5):493-499.
2. Sigmon, H. Answering critical care nursing questions by interfacing nursing research training, career development, and research with biologic and molecular science. *Heart Lung*, 1993, *22*(4):285-288.
3. Cowan, M.J., Heinrich, J., Lucas, M., et al. Integration of biological and nursing sciences: A 10-year plan to enhance research and training. *Res Nurs Health*, 1993, *16*(1):3-9.
4. Kringle, R.O. Statistical procedures. In C. Burtis & E. Ashwood (Eds.), *Tietz textbook of clinical chemistry* (2nd ed.). Philadelphia: Saunders, 1999.
5. Waltz, C.S., Strickland, O.L., & Lenz, E.R. *Measurement in nursing research* (2nd ed.). Philadelphia: Davis, 1991.
6. Maloni, J.A., Chance, B., Zhang, C., et al. Physical and psychosocial side effects of antepartum bed rest. *Nurs Res*, 1993, *42*(4):197-203.
7. Pugh, L.C. Childbirth and the measurement of fatigue. *J Nurs Meas*, 1993, *1*(1):57-66.

8. McCloy, K., Leung, S., Belden, J., et al. Effects of injectate volume on thermodilution measurements of cardiac output in patients with low ventricular ejection fraction. *Am J Crit Care*, 1999, *8*(2):86-92.

9. Topf, M., & Davis, J. Critical care unit noise and rapid eye movement (REM) sleep. *Heart Lung*, 1993, *22*(3):252-258.

10. Sommers, M.S., Woods, S.L., & Courtade, M.A. Issues in methods and measurement of thermodilution cardiac output. *Nurs Res*, 1993, *42*(4):228-233.

11. Ravel, R. *Clinical laboratory medicine* (6th ed.). St. Louis: Mosby, 1995.

12. Derrico, D.L. Comparison of blood pressure measurement methods in critically ill children. *Dimensions Crit Care Nurs*, 1993, *12*(1):31-39.

13. Howanitz, P.J., & Howanitz, J.H. *Laboratory quality assurance*. New York: McGraw-Hill, 1987.

14. Ko, W. Biomedical transducers. In J. Kline (Ed.), *Handbook of biomedical engineering*. New York: Academic Press, 1988, pp. 3-71.

15. Rubin, S.A. Measurement theory and instrument errors. In S.A. Rubin (Ed.), *The principles of biomedical instrumentation*. Chicago: Year Book, 1987, pp. 50-74.

16. Verklan, M.T., Bickel, D.R., & Moon, J. Heart rate variability of preterm neonates quantified by energy entropy. *Nurs Health Sci*, 1999, *1*:103-111.

17. Grunkemeier, G.L., & Ruyun, J. Receiver operating characteristic curve analysis in clinical risk models. *Ann Thoracic Surg*, 2001, *72*:323-326.

18. Schisterman, E.F., Faraggi, D., Reiser, B., & Trevisan, M. Statistical inference for the area under the receiver operating characteristic curve in the presence of random measurement error. *Am J Epidemiol*, 2001, *154*(2):174-179.

19. Goodwin, L.K., Iannaccione, M.A., Hammond, W.E., et al. Data mining methods find demographic predictors of preterm birth. *Nurs Res*, 2001, *50*(6): 340-345.

20. Smatlak, P., & Knebel, A.R. Clinical evaluation of noninvasive monitoring of oxygen saturation in critically ill patients. *Am J Crit Care*, 1998, *7*(5):370-373.

21. McCarthy, D.O., Daun, J.M., & Hutson, P.R. Meperidine attenuates the febrile response to endotoxin and interleukin-1 alpha in rats. *Nurs Res*, 1993, *42*(6):363-367.

22. Lindgren, B.R., Finkelstein, S.M., Prasad, B., et al. Determination of reliability and validity in home monitoring data of pulmonary function tests following lung transplantation. *Res Nurs Health*, 1997, *20*:539-550.

23. Hwu, Y.J., Coates, V.E., & Lin, F.U. A study of the effectiveness of different measuring times and counting methods of human radial pulse rates. *J Clin Nurs*, 2000, *9*(1):146-152.

24 Bland, J.M., & Altman, D.G. Statistical methods for assessing agreement between two methods of clinical measurement. *Lancet*, 1986, *1*:307-310.

25 deMonterice, D., Meier, P.P., Engstrom, J.L., et al. Concurrent validity of a new instrument for measuring nutritive sucking in preterm infants. *Nurs Res*, 1992, *41*(6):342-346.

26. Cromwell, L., Arditti, M., Weibell, F.J., et al. *Medical instrumentation for health care*. Englewood Cliffs, NJ: Prentice-Hall, 1976.

27 Hanneman, S.K.G. Multidimensional predictors of success or failure with early weaning from mechanical ventilation after cardiac surgery. *Nurs Res*, 1994, *43*(1):4-10.

7

Cultural Considerations in Research Instrumentation Development

Miyong T. Kim and Hae-Ra Han

Although the use of Western instruments translated from English into other languages has been a frequent feature of cross-cultural studies, many researchers have chosen to develop new instruments to measure constructs in various cultural groups while avoiding Western cultural bias. In particular, in order to study certain ethnic minorities who do not subscribe to the Western notion of health, developing new instruments might be useful and somewhat justified. This approach, however, presents some fundamental questions regarding the scientific utility of cross-cultural studies. By definition, cross-cultural studies are designed to permit valid and scientifically rigorous comparisons, and it is very difficult to make a fair comparison using an instrument that is culturally sensitive to certain cultures. The main paradox in this issue lies in the apparently difficult task of balancing sensitivity to certain cultures with the need to eliminate particular cultural biases that can influence the comparability of the measure, which ultimately compromises the conclusion validity of such studies. Ideal cross-cultural measures allow investigators to separate variance attributable to true differences in the measured phenomena from variance attributable to cultural differences or to random effects. In addition, ideal cross-cultural measures are robust with regard to within-group heterogeneity. Most measures used cross-culturally, however, are far from ideal and, in the strictest sense, absolute comparability in cross-cultural instruments is probably unattainable, and all we can do is "arrive at a reasonable compromise (p. 118)."[1]

The purpose of this chapter is to review some key steps for developing a quantitative cross-cultural instrument and for determining whether the compromise we can reach at each step is reasonable. We believe that the validity, reliability, and comparability of cross-cultural instruments can be greatly enhanced by systematic integration of substantive, conceptual, and methodologic issues. The decision-making process in cross-cultural instrumentation is presented in Figure 7.1.

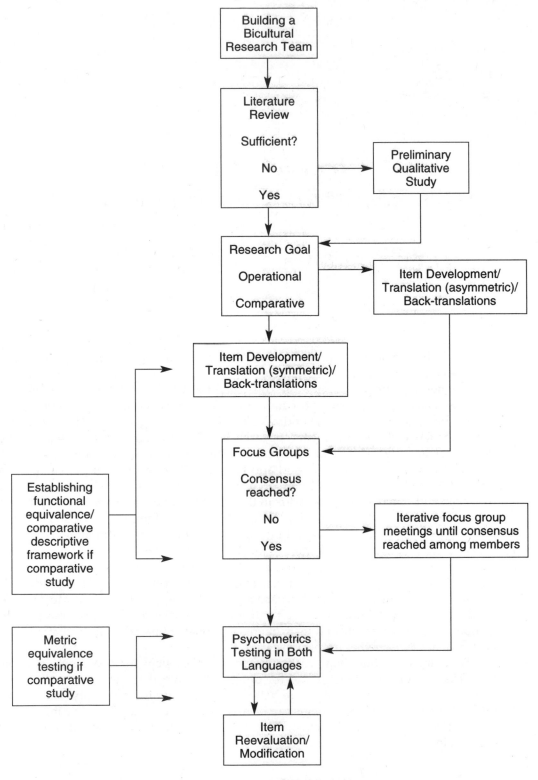

Figure 7.1   Decision tree in developing a cross-cultural instrument.

Essential Steps in Developing Instruments for Cross-Cultural Research

(1) Building a Bicultural Research Team and Conducting a Field Study as Necessary

The first step in developing a cross-cultural instrument is to develop a bicultural research team. Erkut and colleagues[2] have stressed the importance of a bilingual/bicultural research team (including indigenous researchers from the cultures being studied) as a critical component of cross-cultural instrument development. By virtue of their familiarity with the language and cultures being studied, the team, including indigenous researchers, can define concepts that provide equally valid definitions of the constructs in both cultures and determine how they can be explored. If the team decides that a review of the literature is not sufficient, a preliminary qualitative study is recommended to explore the meanings and language used by the target population to describe the phenomenon. For example, to study depression in first-generation Korean American immigrants, it was necessary to learn the words that the immigrants themselves used. The Korean immigrants were interviewed in Korean, and the interviews were transcribed verbatim. Many expressions used by the Koreans were associated with somatic symptoms (e.g., "My chest feels heavy, as if a rock is sitting on it"). The words that described emotional and somatic symptoms associated with depression and their emic concepts were drawn from the transcripts and used to design depression scales.[3]

(2) Identifying Research Goals and Matching Translation Method

The next step involves identifying the research goals as operational or comparative, and matching the translation method to the goals of the research.[4] Cross-cultural studies with operational goals consider the construct culture-specific and use one of the cultures as the criterion. When this type of study is designed, loyalty to the original language is important, even though the resulting translation into the second language can be unnatural. In contrast, if the construct is considered universal, the construct is referenced across the cultures, and a comparative study is designed. In this case, symmetric (decentered) translation is used, and loyalty of meaning is emphasized. Whichever method of translation is chosen, back-translation is the most common and highly recommended procedure for verifying the quality of a translation by independently translating back into the original language.[5]

When preparing items and translating them as necessary, Marin and Marin[6] suggest keeping the language simple, avoiding metaphors and colloquialisms, keeping the length of items short, and avoiding vague terms. Various types of response tendencies found in different cultural or linguistic groups also must be considered. For example, blacks are more likely than whites to use the extreme response categories on Likert scales.[7] Likewise, Hispanics have been found to exhibit a stronger tendency for extreme response than non-Hispanics, but only when 5-point scales were used.[8] Hui and Triandis[8] found that the use of 10-point scales reduced the extreme responses to the level of non-Hispanics, but the extreme responses of non-Hispanics were not affected by the scales. In contrast, Asians tend to endorse milder or subtler forms of expression than the stronger forms of expression used by Westerners.[9-11] Spanish speakers tend to respond "good" to items more frequently than do English speakers.[12] A specific item format can be an issue in a certain cultural group. For example, Han and coworkers[13] found that negatively worded items can be a source of measurement error, as manifested by the poor item-total correlations of the items among an Asian group.

Getting external input from members of the communities for whom the instrument is intended is a critical component in developing and translating items. Focus groups are especially useful because they allow for discussion and consensus building among a group of individuals who have common knowledge and beliefs.[14] Whenever the research team finds the feedback useful, items are modified and evaluated in successive focus groups until everyone involved is satisfied with the wording. Erkut and coworkers[2] have recognized the importance of adding monolinguals' input into the process, because their speech is not influenced by the mastery of a second language, and hence, they may be better than bilinguals at detecting awkward constructions.

(3) Testing Psychometric Properties

The measure is ready to be evaluated for its psychometric properties when the last focus group members and the research team are satisfied that the language versions are conceptually and linguistically equivalent. When the instrument is tested for its psychometric properties, additional attention should be paid to special issues of formatting and administration of the instrument. For example, by printing two language versions (i.e., Spanish and English) side by side, Ferketich and coworkers[15] made it easy for respondents to go back and forth between the two versions, in the event that the Mexican participants preferred to use Spanish vocabulary when answering certain questions. Also, social desirability is a well-known trait among certain cultural groups (i.e., Asians),[9–11] a bias which is more likely to occur when the questions relate to sensitive or culturally unacceptable behaviors (e.g., smoking among women). In such instances, self-report may be a better approach to collecting sensitive data than are face-to-face interviews; guaranteed anonymity and confidentiality could also minimize this bias.

Assessing and comparing the psychometric properties (i.e., reliability and validity) of two language versions is intended to quantify and confirm the appropriateness of the two forms. Reliability, in the form of internal consistency in most cases, is assessed by Cronbach's alpha. The target language version is treated like a new instrument,[16] with an alpha of 0.70 considered adequate. Item analysis is an additional means of finding weakness in the measure and assessing how well each item contributes to the overall measure. Item-total correlation is a correlation of each item with the total score obtained for each item. This parameter is measured using the Pearson correlation coefficient. Item-total correlation coefficients should be greater than 0.3.[16] Any item that falls below this threshold signals a potential problem and must be reviewed and reevaluated. It is then the research team's decision whether or not to retain the item to allow further analysis with a larger sample before a final deletion is made. Inter-item correlations should be less than 0.7 to indicate a lack of multicollinearity.[16] Having detailed information at the item level, the researchers can then reevaluate the non-conforming items' conceptual base and language and make the necessary revisions until adequate reliability and validity is obtained.

Once the reliability of the instrument is established, validity is addressed. The validity of the instrument is determined by whether the scale measures what it intends to measure. Validity can be assessed in a variety of ways, including content- and construct-based measures. Content validity is established by using a team of experts who agree that the items on the instrument provide adequate coverage of the concepts. Construct validity can be evaluated by testing the theoretical relationships of the construct with other relevant constructs to see if there is a significant association between the constructs, as hypothesized. Convergent and discriminant validity assessments are useful for construct validation. Convergent validity refers to substantial correlations between an instrument and other measures to which it should theoretically relate. Discriminant validity refers to the degree to which the instrument is different from other measures to which it theoretically should not be similar. If there are sufficient numbers of subjects, factor structure can be assessed. See Chapter 1, "Evaluating Instruments for Use in Clinical Nursing Research" for a more in-depth discussion of validity. Erkut and coworkers[2] recommend evaluating instruments intended for use with bilingual populations using mixed groups of bilinguals and monolinguals. To evaluate instruments intended for use with monolinguals, they recommend using groups of bilinguals and then separate groups of monolinguals in each language. The total scores of the bilingual subjects on the two versions of the instrument should demonstrate a high correlation. Erkut's group[2] has minimized potential response bias by administering two versions to bilinguals in a counterbalanced random order.

(4) Reevaluation

The final step involves turning back to the conceptual level and finalizing conceptual definitions by integrating the results from the psychometric testing, input received from subjects, and the experience and cultural knowledge of research team members. This reevaluation is an important step in allowing the cross-cultural researcher to improve the instrument and decide the future direction of instrument testing in another sample.

Achieving Equivalence in Cross-Cultural Research

Assuring cultural equivalence in conceptualizations and instrumentation between two language versions is an especially important and relevant issue when the purpose of the study is to compare a certain phenomenon across cultures, looking for similarities in the experience of two cultural groups with the phenomenon. Valid and replicable research findings across different cultures are made possible only by ascertaining equivalence across languages and cultures. This need for equivalence has significant implications for any type of instrument, regardless of its origin (i.e., translated from an existing instrument or newly developed).

According to Berry,[17] legitimate cross-cultural comparisons can be achieved through the medium of what he calls the *derived etic*, which incorporates three essential components: (1) establishing functional equivalence, (2) developing a comparative descriptive framework, and (3) establishing metric equivalence. Functional equivalence refers to the cross-cultural similarity of the function of specific behaviors (or phenomena). The critical test for functional equivalence is whether the phenomenon being studied is a naturally occurring response to the same situational context in both cultures. Developing a comparative descriptive framework involves identifying the similarities in the experience for members of both cultural groups. Identifying the boundaries that made the groups different is not the goal, but some attention to differences is necessary to provide a frame for interpreting the results fairly.

The first two activities should be completed before metric equivalence is tested. For example, after developing a bicultural research team, Phillips and coworkers[18] analyzed the experience of caregiving for elderly family members in Anglo and Mexican families through literature review and input from team members. The team concluded that there were sufficient commonalities to allow for the development of cross-culturally meaningful conceptualizations and operations. Once caregiving was defined as a functionally equivalent concept between cultures, the team adopted the decentered model to guide the research, in which the translation process is symmetric and iterative and involves changes in conceptualizations and operations for both primary and target population. As necessary, the team added more concepts (e.g., familism in Mexican culture) to the model to make the conceptualization more comparable for the two groups.

Metric equivalence refers to the psychometric properties of the instrument and indicates that the scales measure the same constructs in different cultures. Metric equivalence exists "when the psychometric properties of two (or more) cultural groups exhibit essentially the same coherence or structure" (p. 10).[17] In order for test scores from two groups to be unbiased, "they must be equally accurate" (p. 29).[19] As the final step in assessing cross-cultural comparability, metric equivalence tests seek to determine whether the identified group differences are coming from true group differences or from noncomparability of the instruments used in the study. These tests are useful for refining cross-cultural instruments and are also effective in checking an instrument's construct validity; as such, they help prevent erroneous inferences or conclusions. Several strategies can be used to test metric equivalence, at item as well as scale levels.

(1) Item-Level Analysis

Each item must be considered as a separate measurement[20] and checked for adequacy of translation, systematic item response bias, and fairness within each cultural group. The comparability of an item is then evaluated in relation to other items. Reliability coefficients and item analysis are commonly employed strategies at this level. An item is an unbiased measure of a theoretical construct if individuals from different cultural groups with the same standing on the underlying construct have the same mean score on the item.[21] In the developmental stage of the instrument, it is helpful to check differences in item means in bilinguals before administering it to monolinguals in each language. For example, Phillips et al.[18] compared item means and standard deviations for 38 bilingual subjects who answered in both English and Spanish, using t-tests and f-tests, respectively. For items with significant differences either in item means or standard deviations, the team changed the wording (accompanied by a new back-translation and reevaluation of the results) or deleted the items.

When ability tests or knowledge questionnaires are being assessed, an item difficulty test or preference index can be used. Chi-square test is another analysis technique. To use this approach, researchers devise explicitly defined test scores as common standards. The range of all test scores is then divided into a number of intervals, usually three to five.[22,23] Subjects whose scores fall within a particular interval are assumed to have the same ability level, independent of group membership. For each item, intergroup differences in the distributions of the item scores over the various intervals are then tested using chi-square analysis. An item is considered biased when a significant value is found in the test.

(2) Scale-Level Analysis

Scale-level analysis focuses on determining whether the constructs being studied perform similarly in both cultural groups. Whereas item-level analysis is especially useful in the beginning stage of instrumentation, the comparability assessment of an item is made within the context of the instrument, and the construct itself may be biased.[21] Factor analysis is the most popular approach to testing construct equivalence. Exploratory factor analysis (EFA) is a classic approach to examining the replicability of factors. The most common method of factor structure comparison using EFA is the coefficient of congruence, also known as Tucker's phi.[24] The congruence coefficient represents the degree of similarity of extracted factors across cultural groups. The coefficient is derived by summing the cross products of the loadings for two factors under consideration and dividing that amount by the square root of the product of the sums of the squared loadings.[21] The formula is as follows:

$$\sum (FaFb) \Bigg/ \sqrt{\sum (Fd^2)\sum (Fb^2)}$$

Fa and *Fb* are factor loadings of factors a and b that are derived from corresponding cultural groups a and b. In this test, all loadings are included and utilized regardless of magnitude. The value of the congruence coefficient can range from +1 (perfect agreement) to −1 (perfect inverse agreement). There are no established guidelines for minimally acceptable values for the coefficient, but the literature suggests that a coefficient greater than 0.90 is indicative of a good level of correspondence among factors.[25]

Confirmatory factor analysis (CFA) is a more advanced approach that is becoming popular. CFA tests the structural identity of a construct intended to be measured across cultures. The measurement model, including the relations between latent variables (subscales or dimensions) and observed variables (items), has to be defined first, as driven by the substantive theory underlying the relations. CFA is done with equality constraints that impose identical estimates (e.g., factor loadings) for the same parameters across the different data sets (e.g., Byrne and Campbell[26]).

Conclusion

The primary purpose of many nursing cross-cultural studies is to gain understanding about human health behaviors in both culture-specific and universal dimensions. Despite the steadily growing body of literature on cross-cultural differences and similarities, it is impossible to find an instrument that is completely free from any cultural bias. Although cultural sensitivity is the vital quality of a cross-cultural instrument, an instrument developed in one culture and used in another culture presents some potential for bias and misinterpretation. In our opinion, a good number of these newly developed instruments that accommodate certain ethnic minority cultures may lack the basic qualities of scientifically sound cross-cultural instruments. We encourage researchers to conduct thorough literature reviews and identify some strategies to modify or adopt an established instrument before they decide to develop a new instrument. When there is a justifiable need for development, the systematic approach presented in this chapter of integrating substantive, conceptual, and methodologic aspects of cross-cultural instrumentation can be taken. First, researchers need to define their research goal, determine whether they are planning operational or comparative studies, and be encouraged to develop a multicultural research team. Second, qualitative studies may be used in both instrument development and validation processes. Third, one of several empirical methods of assessing and validating the cross-cultural equivalence of instruments are chosen. Finally, the issues of response tendencies, instrument format, and administration across different cultures are essential to making a valid cross-cultural instrument for obtaining useful information about human health behaviors in a given cultural context.

References

1. Frijda, N., & Jahoda, G. On the scope and methods of cross-cultural research. *Int J Psychol*, 1966, *1*:109-127.
2. Erkut, S., Alarcon, O., Coll, C.G., et al. The dual-focus approach to creating bilingual measures. *J Cross-Cult Psychol*, 1999, *30*:206-218.
3. Kim, M.T. Measuring depression in Korean Americans: Development of Kim Depression Scale for Korean Americans. *J Transcult Nurs*, 2002, *13*:110-118.
4. Jones, E.G., & Kay, M. Instrumentation in cross-cultural research. *Nurs Res*, 1992, *41*:186-188.
5. Brislin, R. *Translation: Application and research*. New York: Wiley, 1976.
6. Marin, G., & Marin, B. *Research with Hispanic populations*. Newbury Park, CA: Sage, 1991.
7. Bachman, J.G., & O'Malley, P.M. Yea-saying, nay-saying, and going to extremes: Black-white differences in response styles. *Public Opinion Quarterly*, 1984, *48*:491-509.
8. Hui, C.H., & Triandis, H.C. Effects of culture and response format on extreme response style. *J Cross-Cult Psychol*, 1989, *20*:296-309.
9. Cheung, C.K., & Bagley, C. Validating an American scale in Hong Kong: The Center for Epidemiological Studies Depression Scale (CES-D). *J Psychol*, 1998, *13*:169-186.
10. Devins, G.M., Beiser, M., Dion, R., et al. Cross-cultural measurements of psychological well-being: The psychometric equivalence of Cantonese, Vietnamese, and Laotian translations of the Affect Balance Scale. *Am J Pub Health*, 1997, *87*: 794-799.
11. Iwata, N., Umesue, M., Egashira, K., et al. Can positive affect items be used to assess depressive disorders in the Japanese population? *Psychol Med*, 1998, *28*:153-158.
12. Hayes, R.P., & Baker, D.W. Methodological problems in comparing English-speaking and Spanish-speaking patients' satisfaction with interpersonal aspects of care. *Med Care*, 1998, *36*:230-236.
13. Han, H.R., Kim, M.T., Weinert, C. The psychometric evaluation of Korean translation of the Personal Resource Questionnaire 85-Part 2. *Nurs Res*, 2002, *15*:309-316.
14. Hughes, D., & Dumont, K. Using focus groups to facilitate culturally anchored research. *Am J Comm Psychol*, 1993, *21*:775-806.
15. Ferketich, S., Phillips, L., & Verran, J. Development and administration of a survey instrument for cross-cultural research. *Res Nurs Health*, 1993, *16*:227-230.
16. Nunnally, J.C., & Bernstein, I.H. *Psychometric theory* (3rd ed.). New York: McGraw-Hill, 1994.
17. Berry, J. Introduction to methodology. In H. Triandis & J. Berry (Eds.), *Handbook of cross-cultural psychology: Volume 2* (pp. 1-28). Boston, MA: Allyn & Bacon, 1981.
18. Phillips, L.R., de Hernandez, I.L., & de Ardon, E.T. Strategies for achieving cultural equivalence. *Res Nurs Health*, 1994, *17*:149-154.
19. Geisenger, K.F. Fairness and selected psychometric issues in the psychological testing of Hispanics. In K.F. Geisinger (ed.), *Psychological testing of Hispanics* (pp. 17-42). Washington, D.C.: American Psychological Association, 1992.
20. Bijnen, E.J., van der Net, T.Z.J., & Poortinga, Y.H. On cross-cultural comparative studies with the Eysenck Personality Questionnaire. *J Cross-Cultural Psychol*, 1986, *17*:3-16.
21. van de Vijver, F.J.R., & Leung, K. *Methods and data analysis for cross-cultural research*. Thousand Oaks, CA: Sage, 1997.
22. Scheuneman, J. A method of assessing bias in test items. *J Educ Meas*, 1979, *16*:143-152.
23. Mellenbergh, G. Conditional item bias methods. In S.H. Irvine & J. Berry (Eds.), *Human assessment and cultural factors* (pp. 293-302). New York: Plenum Press, 1982.
24. Tucker, L.R. *A method for synthesis of factor analysis studies—Personnel Research Section Report No. 984*. Washington, D.C.: Department of the Army, 1951.
25. Caprara, G.V., Barbaranelli, C., Bermúdez, J., et al. Multivariate methods for the comparison of factor structures in cross-cultural research: An illustration with the big five questionnaire. *J Cross-Cult Psychol*, 2000, *31*:437-464.
26. Byrne, B.M., & Campbell, T.L. Cross-cultural comparisons and the presumption of equivalent measurement and theoretical structure: A look beneath the surface. *J Cross-Cult Psychol*, 1999, *30*:555-574.

II

Instruments for Assessing Health and Function

8

Measuring Function

Therese Richmond, Siew Tzah Tang, Lorraine Tulman, Jacqueline Fawcett, and Ruth McCorkle

Function, which has been used as a proxy for health status and as an outcome measure for clinical research, has been receiving increasing attention since the mid-1970s from the members of many health-care disciplines. A major goal of health care is to assist individuals to maintain or regain their pre-illness level of function or to attain the maximal functional level possible given their current health status. The purposes of this chapter are to discuss the significance of measuring function, analyze the concept of function and the methodologic issues in the measurement of function, and review instruments that have been developed or used by health professionals to assess function in seriously ill adults.

Instruments that measure function can assist health professionals in both the research and the clinical arenas. In research, the use of valid and reliable instruments to measure function is critical for the development of an empirically based body of knowledge concerning the outcomes of interventions. Clinically, valid and reliable measures can assist clinicians in assessing baseline function and changes over the course of an illness, as well as in identifying the requirements for care during hospitalization and following discharge to home. Systematic identification of functioning that may be disrupted by disease or treatment can subsequently allow for planning and implementing appropriate clinical interventions at crucial times to assist patients to adjust to the changes in the performance of their usual activities, to facilitate their performance of new disease- or treatment-related activities, and to promote their optimal functioning during the entire trajectory of a disease. The ability to determine baseline function and changes over time also provides a mechanism for meaningful evaluation of the efficacy of interventions and the quality of care.

The Concept of Function

The concept of function has been defined in various ways both within the discipline of nursing and by other health-care disciplines. The terms *function, functioning, functional ability, functional status, physical function, impairment, disability, handicap,* and *health status* are frequently used interchangeably. Lack of clarity concerning the concept of function and its definition has resulted in studies that use the same term with different definitions and different measures, making comparisons across studies and integration of findings difficult, if not impossible. Moreover, different terms used to measure the same concept add to the confusion.

In general, the term *function* refers to "how people perform activities that are relevant to personal expectations and social norms."[1] Nagi[2] explained that the concept of function incorporates both the ability to perform activities or tasks that are important for independent living and the actual performance of activities and tasks crucial to the fulfillment of roles within one's current life circumstances. Although the actual terms are different, the dual approach to the concept, as proposed by Nagi, is used in this chapter. Function is viewed as a concept with two dimensions: functional ability and functional status.

Functional ability refers to the actual or potential capacity to perform the activities and tasks normally expected of an adult.[2] The inability to perform activities within the range considered normal may be temporary or permanent, static or dynamic. Instruments that measure functional ability focus on either basic activities of daily living (BADL)[3] (e.g., bathing, dressing, continence, and feeding) or a combination of BADL and instrumental activities of daily living (IADL)[4] (e.g., housekeeping, food preparation, use of transportation, and shopping).

In contrast, *functional status* refers to individuals' actual performance of activities and tasks associated with their current life roles. Limitations in functional status are said to occur when there is "a discrepancy between individual performance and average expectable role performance."[5] Emphasis is on BADL, IADL, and advanced activities of daily living (AADL) (e.g., working, traveling, engaging in hobbies, or participating in social and religious groups). Instruments designed to measure functional status differ in the breadth of measurement (the number of roles included) and the depth of measurement (the numbers and types of activities included for each role). Furthermore, measurement of functional status assumes functional ability. In order words, the assumption is made that the person has the ability to perform the roles and associated activities of interest.

Issues in the Measurement of Function

Several issues surround the selection of an instrument to measure function. Issues to consider include the primary purpose of measurement, the match between the theoretical dimension of function (functional ability, functional status), the focus of the instrument, the unique requirements of the population of interest, and methodologic concerns.

When the primary purpose of measuring function is clinical assessment, practical considerations such as the time required to administer the instrument, the ease of use by multiple care providers, the setting in which the measurement is obtained, and the clinical usefulness of the data obtained are particularly important. If the primary purpose of measuring function is research, the time required to administer the instrument continues to be a consideration. Furthermore, when functional assessment is only one of several instruments used, the degree of burden to subjects also must be considered in the choice of the instrument.

The choice of an instrument to measure function in research must be consistent with the *conceptual definition* and scope of function for that particular study. For example, if the purpose is to determine the rate and completeness with which individuals resume job responsibilities after an illness (functional status), then an instrument that yields data only on the extent to which assistance is needed with BADL (functional ability, not including ability to perform job responsibilities) is not appropriate for that study.

The unique aspects of the *population of interest* are an important consideration in choosing a measure of function. In the hospitalized adult, the clinician or researcher may be more interested in the individual's functional ability than functional status. Indeed, measurement of functional status of hospitalized persons usually is not possible because they are in a situation where IADL and AADL cannot be performed. In other situations, such as chronically ill people living in the community, measurement of functional status may be of primary interest.

The needs of the population and the purpose of measuring function may dictate whether functional assessment measures are self-report, based on clinical assessment, or reported by a proxy, also known as a surrogate. Whenever, possible, data should be collected from the patients themselves when they are able and available; otherwise, data may be provided (either totally or partially) by a proxy respondent.

Physicians and other health care providers often depend on data provided by family members (proxy respondents) in evaluating the health status of elderly and seriously ill patients and deciding on the appropriate treatment. Data provided by proxy respondents are helpful for logistical, economic, and scientific reasons.[6] Proxy respondents are asked to provide information when the study subject is unable to respond either because of functional impairments or disabilities, a language barrier, or inability of the interviewer to locate the study subject. The use of proxy-reported data increases sample size, improves representativeness of the study sample, and reduces the need for and the cost of phone or home callbacks. Without proxy data, the rate of nonresponse may be high. Researchers need, however, to weigh the advantages and disadvantages of proxy data. The use of proxy-reported data carries with it the potential for introducing a bias that may result in misclassification of respondents or in misestimated data. Respondents may under- or overestimate the true values of the data provided. Accordingly, the basic methodologic concern associated with using proxy-reported data is related to the extent of agreement between self- and proxy-reported data. When analyzing data that contain both self- and proxy-reported responses, it is important to investigate the role of proxy-reported data as both a potential confounder and an effect modifier.[7]

Flooring and ceiling effects must be considered. Specifically, patients may be at the highest level of the measure, resulting in little to no variability. Conversely, if patients have reduced function, they may be at the lowest range of the instrument and have little ability to discriminate between lower levels of function. Examining the original purpose and population for whom the instrument was developed can minimize the risk of floor and ceiling effects. For example, the Barthel Index was designed to assess the progress of patients with chronic diseases during rehabilitation. Instrument developers specifically state that the highest score does not imply the ability to live alone, cook, or keep house.[8] Consequently, use of the Barthel Index to assess function in an independent, community-based sample would predictably result in a ceiling effect.

The degree to which subtle changes in function are of interest to the investigator or clinician should be determined at the outset, as this dimension also influences the choice of an instrument. One reason why changes in function may not be seen is that the rating scale lacks the sensitivity to capture differences. Another reason why changes in function may not be detected is that the instrument uses an aggregate score that reflects overall level of function.[9] Use of subscale scores that provide a profile of the patient's level of function in various dimensions (e.g., the subscales of the Sickness Impact Profile) may be more informative.[10]

Another issue is the extent to which the *assumption of existing functional ability* is valid when measuring functional status. For example, illness may compromise one's functional ability. It is therefore recommended that both functional ability and functional status be measured. Still another consideration is the selection of an instrument that includes culturally and developmentally relevant roles and associated activities.

Instruments

A plethora of instruments have been developed to measure function. The instruments included in Appendix 8A have the following qualities: (1) They were developed, are currently used by, or have potential value for health professionals for clinical or research purposes in adult populations; (2) they have established validity and reliability; and (3) they are consistent with the definitions of function as used in this chapter. Appendix 8A presents selected instruments and a concise overview of their properties and uses are presented. Key properties of the instruments also are provided, emphasizing the dimensions of function measured, the target population for whom the instrument was developed, the number of items, and methods of administration. Concise descriptions of reliability and validity data also are included. As can be seen, several instruments contain items or discrete subscales that measure functional ability and other items or subscales that measure functional status. Clinicians and investigators who use such instruments are cautioned to be aware of the distinctions, so that appropriate interpretations of data can be made.

Summary

This chapter highlights the significance for health professionals of measuring function. The concept of function is found to consist of the dimensions of functional ability and functional status. Specific issues in the measurement of function have been explored, such as the purpose of measurement, the match between the conceptual definition and instrument, the unique requirements of the population of interest, and methodologic considerations.

Exemplar Study

McCorkle, R., Benoliel, J.Q., Donaldson, G., et al. A randomized clinical trial of home nursing care for lung cancer patients. *Cancer*, 1989, *64*:1375.

This study exemplifies the measurement of function in a prospective clinical trial designed to assess the effects of home nursing care for patients with progressive lung cancer. The three-group experimental design is described in detail, and the methods are rigorous. The study uses several instruments with established validity and reliability. The primary measure of function and level of dependency was the Enforced Social Dependency Scale. Significant differences in social dependency were found among the groups, and the results suggest that home nursing care assists in maintaining cancer patients' levels of function longer than for those who do not live in a home with nursing care.

References

1. Granger, C.V. A conceptual model for functional assessment. In C.V. Granger & G.E. Gresham (Eds.), *Functional assessment in rehabilitation medicine.* Baltimore: Williams & Wilkins, 1984, p.14.
2. Nagi, S. Disability concepts revisited: Implications for prevention. In A.M. Pope & A.R. Tarlov (Eds.), *Disability in America: Toward a national agenda for prevention.* Washington, D.C.: National Academy Press, 1991, p. 309.
3. Katz, D., Ford, A.S., & Moskowitz, R.W. The index of ADL: A standardized measure of biological and psychosocial function. *JAMA*, 1963, *185*(12):914.

4. Lawton, M.P., & Brody, E.M. Assessment of older people. Self maintaining and instrumental activities of daily living. *Gerontologist, 1969, 9*:17.

5. Moriarty, J.B. Disability concepts: Implications for research. In E.B. Whitten (Ed.), *Pathology, impairment, functional limitations, and disability—Implications for practice, research, program and policy development and service delivery.* Washington, D.C.: National Rehabilitation Association, 1975, p. 15.

6. Tang, S.T., McCorkle, R. Use of family proxies in quality of life research for cancer patients at the end of life: A literature review. *Cancer Invest, 2002, 20*(7-8):1086-104.

7. Walker, A.M., Velema, J.P., & Robins, J.M. Analysis of case-control data derived from proxy respondents. *Am J Epidemiol, 1988, 127*:905-914.

8. Mahoney, F.I., & Barthel, D.W. Functional evaluation: The Barthel Index. *Rehab Notes, 1965, 14*(2):61.

9. Feinstein, A.R., & Josephy, B.R., & Wells, C.K. Scientific and clinical problems in indexes of functional disability. *Ann Intern Med, 1986, 105*:413-420.

10. Bergner, M., Bobbitt, R.A., Carter, W.B., & Gilson, B.S. The Sickness Impact Profile: Development and final revision of a health status measure. *Med Care, 1981, 19*:787-805.

11. Frederiks, C.M., te Wierik, M., Visser, A., & Sturmans, F. The functional status and utilization of care of elderly people living at home. *J Commun Health, 1990, 15*, 307-317.

12. Frederiks, C.M., te Wierik, M., Visser, A., & Sturmans, F. A scale for the functional status of the elderly living at home. *J Adv Nurs, 1991, 16*:287-292.

13. Frederiks, C.M., te Wierik, M.J., van Rossum, H.J., et al. Why do elderly people seek professional home care? Methodologies compared. *J Commun Health, 1992, 17*:131.

14. Gulick, E.E. Parsimony and model confirmation of the ADL self-care scale for multiple sclerosis persons. *Nurs Res, 1987, 36*:278-283.

15. Gulick, E.E. The self-administered ADL scale for persons with multiple sclerosis. In C.F. Waltz & O.L. Strickland (Eds.), *Measurement of nursing outcomes: Measuring client outcomes* (vol. I). New York: Springer, 1988, p. 128.

16. Gulick, E.E. Self-assessment of health and use of health services. *West J Nurs Res, 1991, 13*:195-211.

17. Gulick, E.E. Symptom and activities of daily living trajectory in multiple sclerosis: a 10-year study. *Nurs Res, 1998, 47*:137-146.

18. Hamrin, E.K., & Lindmark, B. The effect of systematic care planning after acute stroke in general hospital medical wards. *J Adv Nurs, 1990, 15*:1146-1153.

19. Hamrin, E., & Wohlin, A. Evaluation of the functional capacity of stroke patients through an Activity Index. *Scand J Rehab, 1982, 14*:93-100.

20. Meenan, R.F., Gertman, P.M., & Mason, J.H. Measuring health status in arthritis: The Arthritis Impact Measurement Scale. *Arthritis Rheumatol, 1980, 23*:146-152.

21. Meenan, R.F. The AIMS approach to health status measurement: Conceptual background and measurement properties. *J Rheumatol, 1982, 9*:785-788.

22. Meenan, R.F., Anderson, J.J., Kazis, L.E., et al. Outcome assessment in clinical trials: Evidence for the sensitivity of a health status measure. *Arthritis Rheumatol, 1984, 27*:1344-1352.

23. Mason, J.H., Anderson, J.J., & Meenan, R.F. A model for health status for rheumatoid arthritis: A factor analysis of the Arthritis Impact Measure. *Arthritis Rheumatol, 1988, 31*:714-720.

24. Brown, J.H., Kazis, L.E., Spitz, P.W., et al. The dimensions of health outcomes: A cross-validated examination of health status measurement. *Am J Pub Health, 1984, 74*:159-161.

25. Granger, C.V., Albrecht, G.L., & Hamilton, B.B. Outcome of comprehensive medical rehabilitation: Measurement by PULSES profile and Barthel Index. *Arch Phys Med Rehab, 1979, 60*:145-154.

26. Granger, C.V., Cotter, A.C., Hamilton, B.B., et al. Functional assessment scales: A study of persons with multiple sclerosis. *Arch Phys Med Rehab, 1990, 71*:870-875.

27. Rameizl, P. CADET, a self-care assessment tool. *Geriatr Nurs, 1983, 4*:377-378.

28. Huber, M., & Kennard, A. Functional and mental status outcomes of clients discharged from acute gerontological versus medical/surgical units. *Geront ol Nurs, 1991, 17*(7):20-24.

29. Schag, C.C., Heinrich, R.L., & Aadland, R.L. Assessing problems of cancer patients: Psychometric properties of the Cancer Inventory of Problem Situations. *Health Psychol, 1990, 9*:83-102.

30. Schag, C.A., Ganz, P.A., & Heinrich, R.L. Cancer Rehabilitation Evaluation System—Short Form (CARES-SF): A cancer specific rehabilitation and quality of life instrument. *Cancer, 1991, 68*:1406-1413.

31. Fang, C.Y, Manne, S.L., & Pape, S.J. Functional impairment, marital quality, and patient psychological distress as predictors of psychological distress among cancer patients' spouses. *Health Psychol, 2001, 20*:452-457.

32. Benoliel, J.Q., McCorkle, R., & Young, K. The development of a social dependency scale. *Res Nurs Health, 1980, 3*:3-10.

33. McCorkle, R., & Benoliel, J.Q. Symptom distress, current concerns, and mood disturbance after diagnosis of life threatening disease. *Soc Sci Med, 1983, 17*:431-438.

34. Jepson, C., Schultz, D., Lusk, E., & McCorkle, R. Enforced social dependency and its relationship to cancer survival. *Cancer Practice, 1997, 5*:155-161.

35. Keith, R.A., Granger, C.V., Hamilton, B.B., & Sherwin, F.S. The Functional Independence Measure: A new tool for rehabilitation. In M.G. Eisenberg & R.C. Grzesiak (Eds.), *Advances in clinical rehabilitation.* New York: Springer, 1987, p. 6.

36. Fricke, J., Unsworth, C., & Worrell, D. Reliability of the Functional Independence Measure with occupational therapist. *Austral Occup Ther J, 1993, 40*:7-15.

37. Schipper, H., Clinch, J., McMurray, A., Levitt, M. Measuring the quality of life of cancer patients: The Functional Living Index-cancer: Development and validation. *J Clin Oncol, 1984, 2*:472-483.

38. Morrow, G.R., Lindke, J., & Black, P. Measurement of quality of life in patients: psychometric analyses of the Functional Living Index-Cancer (FLIC). *Qual Life Res, 1992, 1*:287-296.

39. Leidy, N.K. Psychometric properties of the Functional Performance Inventory in patients with chronic

obstructive pulmonary disease. *Nurs Res*, 1999, *48*, 20-28.

40. Leidy, N.K., & Haase, J.E. Functional performance in people with chronic obstructive pulmonary disease: A qualitative analysis. *Adv Nurs Sci*, 1996, *18*:77-89.

41. Jette, A.M. Functional Status Index: Reliability of a chronic disease evaluation instrument. *Arch Phys Med Rehab*, 1980, *61*:395-401.

42. Liang, M.H., Fossel, A.H., & Larson, M.G. Comparisons of five health status instruments for orthopedic evaluation. *Med Care*, 1990, *28*:632-642.

43. Calkins, D.R., Rubenstein, L.V., Cleary, P.D., et al. The Functional Status Questionnaire: Initial results of a controlled trial. *Clin Res*, 1985, *33*:244A.

44. Jette, A.M., Davies, A.R., Cleary, P.D., et al. The Functional Status Questionnaire: Reliability and validity when used in primary care. *J Gen Int Med*, 1986, *1*:143-149.

45. Jette, A.M., & Cleary, P.D. Functional disability assessment. *Phys Ther*, 1987, *12*:1854-1859.

46. Rubenstein, L.M., Voelker, M.D., Chrischilles, E.A., et al. The usefulness of the Functional Status Questionnaire and Medical Outcomes Study Short Form in Parkinson's disease research. *Qual Life Res*, 1998, *7*:279-290.

47. Fries, J.G., Spitz, P., Kraines, R.G., & Holman, H.R. Measurement of patient outcome in arthritis. *Arthritis Rheumatol*, 1980, *23*:137-145.

48. Sharpe, L., Sensky, T., & Allard, S. The course of depression in recent onset rheumatoid arthritis: The predictive role of disability, illness perceptions, pain and coping. *J Psychosomatic Res*, 2001, *51*:713-719.

49. Tulman, L., Fawcett, J., & McEvoy, M.D. Development of the Inventory of Functional Status-Cancer. *Cancer Nurs*, 1991, *14*:254-260.

50. Tulman, L., & Fawcett, J. Lessons learned from a pilot study of biobehavioral correlates of functional status in women with breast cancer. *Nurs Res*, 1996, *45*:356-358.

51. Katz, S., Ford, A.B., Moskowitz, R.W. Studies of illness in the aged: The Index of ADL, a standardized measure of biological and psychosocial function. *JAMA*, 1963, *185*:914.

52. Katz, S., Downs, T.D., Cash, H.R., & Grotz, R.C. Progress in development of the Index of ADL. *Gerontologist*, 1970, *10*(1, part I):20-30.

53. Katz, S. Assessing self-maintenance: Activities of daily living, mobility, and instrumental activities of daily living. *J Am Geriatr Soc*, 1983, *31*:721-727.

54. Aske, D. The correlation between mini-mental state examination scores and Katz ADL status among dementia patients. *Rehab Nurs*, 1990, *15*:140-142.

55. Karnofsky, D., Buchenal, J. The clinical evaluation of chemotherapeutic agents in cancer. In C.M. MacLeod (Ed.). *Evaluation of chemotherapeutic agents*. New York: Columbia University Press, 1949, p. 191.

56. Mor, V., Laliberte, L., Morris, J. N., & Weimann, M. The Karnofsky Performance Status Scale: An examination of its reliability and validity in a research setting. *Cancer*, 1984, *53*:2002-2007.

57. Schag, C.C., Ganz, P.A., Wing, D.S., et al. Quality of life in adult survivors of lung, colon and prostate cancer. *Qual Life Res*, 1994, *3*:127-141.

58. Klein, R.M., & Bell, B. Self-care skills: Behavioral measurement with Klein-Bell ADL Scale. *Arch Phys Med Rehab*, 1982, *63*:335.

59. Venable, S.D., & Mitchell, M.M. Temporal adaptation and performance of daily living activities in persons with Alzheimer's disease. *Phys Occup Ther Geriatr*, 1991, *9*(3/4):31.

60. Longman, A.J., Atwood, J.R., Sherman, J.B., et al. Care needs of home-based cancer patients and their caregivers. *Cancer Nurs*, 1992, *15*:182-190.

61. Chambers, L.W., MacDonald, L.A., Tugwell, P., et al. The McMaster Health Index Questionnaire as a measure of quality of life for patients with rheumatoid disease. *J Rheumatol*, 1982, *9*:780-784.

62. O'Boyle, C.A., McGee, H., Hickey, A., et al. Individual quality of life in patients undergoing hip replacement. *Lancet*, 1992, *339*:1088-1091.

63. Fillenbaum, G.G., & Smyer, M.A. The development, validity, and reliability of the OARS multidisciplinary functional assessment questionnaire. *J Gerontol*, 1981, *36*:428-434.

64. Rubin, C.D., Sizemore, M.T., Loftis, P.A., de Mola, N.L. A randomized controlled trial of outpatient geriatric evaluation and management in a large public hospital. *J Am Geriatr Soc*, 1993, *41*:1023-1028.

65. Weaver, T.E., & Narsavage, G.L. Reliability and validity of the Pulmonary Impact Profile Scale. *Am Rev Resp Dis*, 1989, *139*(suppl):A244.

66. Weaver, T.E., Narsavage, G.L., & Guilfoyle, M.J. The development and psychometric evaluation of the Pulmonary Functional Status Scale: An instrument to assess functional status in pulmonary disease. *J Cardiopulm Rehab*, 1998, *18*:105-111.

67. Pollard, W.E., Bobbitt, R.A., Bergner, M., et al. The Sickness Impact Profile: Reliability of a health status measure. *Med Care*, 1976, *14*:146-155.

68. Damiano, A.M. *The Sickness Impact Profile: User's manual and interpretation guide*. Baltimore, MD: Johns Hopkins University. 1996.

69. Bellamy, N., Buchanan, W.W., Goldsmith, C.H., et al. Validation study of WOMAC: A health status instrument for measuring clinically important patient relevant outcomes to antirheumatic drug therapy in patients with osteoarthritis of the hip and knee. *J Rheumatol*, 1988, *15*:1833-1840.

70. Bellamy, N., Buchanan, W.W., Goldsmith, C.H., et al. Validation study of WOMAC: A health status instrument for measuring clinically important patient relevant outcomes following total hip or knee arthroplasy in osteoarthritis. *J Orthop RheResmatol*, 1988, *1*:95.

71. Gulick, E.E. Reliability and validity of the work assessment scale for persons with multiple sclerosis. *Nurs Res*, 1991, *40*:107-112.

72. Gulick, E.E. Model for predicting work performance among persons with multiple sclerosis. *Nurs Res*, 1992, *41*:266-272.

73. Gulick, E.E., Yam, M., & Touw, M.M. Work performance by persons with multiple sclerosis: Conditions that impede or enable the performance of work. *Int J Nurs Studies*, 1989, *26*:301-311.

Appendix 8A. Instruments Used to Measure Function

Name (references)	Dimensions Measured	Dimensions of Function	Items	Administration	Reliability	Validity
Activities of Daily Living—Household Activities Scale (ADL-HAA) (11–13)	1. ADL (6 items) 2. Household activities (7 items)	Ability, status Target: elderly	13	Self-administered or structured interview Time required: a few minutes	Internal consistency: 0.86 Test-retest: ADL: 93%, HHA: 43% (81% if 1-point difference allowed) Interrater reliability: Cohen's kappas: 0.49–0.79	Discriminant: higher scores related to increased age and those receiving home care Correlation between ADL and HHA subscales: $\gamma = 0.50$
Activities of Daily Living—Multiple Sclerosis (ADL-MS) (14–17)	1. Lower body 2. Upper body 3. Recreational/ Social 4. Sensory communication 5. Intimacy 6. Urine elimination 7. Bowel elimination	Ability, status Target: patients with multiple sclerosis	1. 55 2. Short form: 15	Self-administered	Internal consistency: Entire scale: 0.96 Bowel elimination: 0.63 Other subscales: 0.75–0.97 Test-retest: 0.73–0.93 (over 2–4 weeks)	Factor analysis: 6 factors accounting for 71% of variance (lower body, upper body, intimacy, sensory/communication, recreation/socializing, bowel elimination) Convergent: correlations with Kurtze Disability Scale and Incapacity Status Scale Discriminant: discriminates patients with different length of MS in terms of decline in ADL
Activity Index (18–19)	1. Mental capacity 2. Motor activity 3. ADL functions	Ability Target: patients with CVA*	16	Clinician assessed (with familiarity with patient)	Internal consistency: Entire scale: 0.94 Mental capacity: 0.83 Motor activity: 0.79 ADL functions: 0.94	Concurrent: correlation between Activity Index and Rankin Disability Scale: $\gamma = 0.94$ Predictive: baseline scores predict scores of 3 and 12 months after stroke; predicts survival during acute hospitalization phase

*CVA = cerebral vascular accident

Appendix 8A. Instruments Used to Measure Function (*cont.*)

Name (references)	Dimensions Measured	Dimensions of Function	Items	Administration	Reliability	Validity
Arthritis Impact Measurement Scale (AIMS) (20–24)	1. Mobility 2. Physical activity 3. Dexterity 4. Household activity 5. ADL 6. Social activity 7. Anxiety 8. Depression 9. Pain 10. General health	Ability, Status Target: patients with rheumatoid arthritis (RA), other chronic illness	67	Self-administered Time required: 20 minutes	Internal consistency: Patients with RA: 0.61–0.92 Patients with other chronic illness: 0.40–0.92 Test-retest: 0.84–0.92 (6 months)	Factor analysis: 5 factors (upper- and lower-extremity function, affect, symptoms, social interaction) Convergent: high correlations within and across instruments on physical scales, lower, on psychological scales Discriminant: discriminates between diabetic and arthritis, and osteoarthritis, and rheumatoid arthritis Concurrent: correlate with functional class and disease activity (overall health)
Barthel Index of ADL Scale (8,25,26)	1. Physical disability 2. ADL 3. Mobility (7 subscales: feeding, grooming, bathing, toileting, walking or climbing stairs, propelling a wheelchair, control bowel and bladder)	Ability Target: patients with chronic disease	16	Clinician assessed (with familiarity with patient) Time required: 2 minutes	Internal consistency: 0.94–0.97 Interrater reliability: 0.99 Correlation between telephone interview and performance assessment >0.97	Concurrent: established Predictive: score <60 inversely related to subsequent morality (CVA)

Instrument	Subscales	Type/Target	Items	Administration	Reliability	Validity
CADET (27,28)	1. Communication 2. Ambulation 3. ADL 4. Elimination 5. Transfer	Ability Target: geriatric, inpatient setting	5	Clinician assessed (with familiarity with patient)	Internal consistency: 0.98 Interrater reliability: 0.94	Not specific
Cancer Rehabilitation Evaluation System (CARES) and CARES-SF (short form) (29–31)	1. Physical 2. Psychosocial 3. Medical interaction 4. Marital 5. Sexual 6. Miscellaneous	Ability, Status Target: patients with cancer	139 SF-59	Self-administered	Internal consistency: CARES: 0.82–0.94 CARES-SF: 0.60–0.85 Test-retest: CARES: 84–86% CARES-SF: 81–86%	Content: Literature, patient and professional interview Factor analysis: construct validity supported Concurrent: correlation between CARES and CARES-SF with FLIC*, symptom-checklist-90, Karnofsky, Dydadic Adjustment Scale Predictive: quality of life and psychological distress
Enforced Social Dependency Scale (ESDS) (32–34)	1. Personal competence (eating, dressing, walking, traveling, bathing and toileting) 2. Social competence (home, work, recreation, and communication)	Ability, Status Target: individuals with cancer or other life-threatening illness	10	Semistructured interview Time required: 10–20 minutes ability to distinguish	Internal consistency: 0.73–0.96 Test-retest 0.36–0.62 (over 30 days elapse)	Content: extensive interviews with patients with life-threatening illness Factor analysis: two factors (personal and social competency) Concurrent: correlation with Sickness Impact Profile: $\gamma = 0.89$ Discriminant: between situations in which recovery is likely versus not likely

*FLIC = Functional Living Index—Cancer

Appendix 8A. Instruments Used to Measure Function (*cont.*)

Name (references)	Dimensions Measured	Dimensions of Function	Items	Administration	Reliability	Validity
Functional Independence Measure (FIM) (26,35,36)	1. Self-care 2. Sphincter control 3. Mobility 4. Locomotion 5. Communication 6. Social adjustment/cooperation 7. Cognition/problem solving	Ability, selected aspects of Status Target: patients with CVA, spinal cord injury	18	Clinician assessed (with familiarity with patient) Time required: 10 minutes	Interrater reliability: 0.86–0.87 Intraclass correlations: (eating, bathing, dressing, grooming, toilet and tub transfer): 0.88	Content: interview with expert clinician Predictive: help needed by patients with MS
Functional Living Index-Cancer (FLIC) (37,38)	Functional quality of life 1. Physical well-being 2. Psychological state 3. Family/situational interaction 4. Nausea	Status Target: patients with cancer	22	Self-administered Time required: <10 minutes	Internal consistency: 0.65–0.87	Factor analysis: construct validity supported Current: validated against Karnofsky, Katz, ADL, and others Convergent-discriminant: demonstrated by a positive association with symptoms and a negative association with anxiety in the State-Trait Anxiety Inventory
Functional Performance Inventory (FPI) (39,40)	1. Body care 2. Household maintenance 3. Physical exercise 4. Recreation 5. Spiritual activities 6. Social activities	Ability, Status Target: patients with chronic obstructive pulmonary disease (COPD)	65	Self-administered	Internal consistency: subscales: 0.75–0.93 with a total scale alpha of 0.96 Test-retest: Intraclass correlation coefficient: 0.85 (2-week interval)	Content: extensive literature review and qualitative interviews with 12 men and women with COPD, content validity index of the FPI at a criterion of 86% (6 of 7 experts) was 95% and at a criterion of 71% was 100%.

						Concurrent: significant correlations between the FPI total score and the FSQ* (ADL: $\gamma = 0.68$; IADL: $\gamma = 0.68$), Duke Activity Status Index ($\gamma = 0.61$), and Kate Adjustment Scale for Relatives (socially expected activities, $\gamma = 0.53$; free-time activities, $\gamma = 0.49$) Construct: significant correlations between the FPI total score and Bronchitis-Emphysema Symptom Checklist ($\gamma = -0.59$), Basic Need Satisfaction Inventory ($\gamma = 0.61$), and Cantril's Ladder of Life Satisfaction ($\gamma = 0.63$) Discrimant: FPI discriminated between patients with severe and moderate levels of perceived severity and activity limitation and patients with $FEV^+_1 >$ and < 1.0 liter.
Functional Status Indices (FSI) (41,42)	1. Basic ADL 2. Instrumental ADL 3. Social/role function	Ability, Status Target: rheumatology patients	17	Self-administered or structured interview Time required: <15 minutes	Internal consistency: 0.93–0.96 Test-retest: 0.69–0.77 Interrater reliability: 0.61–0.78	Factor analysis: construct validity supported Criterion: agreement for basic and instrumental ADL: 0.71–0.95 when comparing self-report and direct observation

†FEV$_1$ = forced expiratory volume in 1 second

*FSQ = Functional Status Questionnaire

Appendix 8A. Instruments Used to Measure Function (*cont.*)

Name (references)	Dimensions Measured	Dimensions of Function	Items	Administration	Reliability	Validity
Functional Status Questionnaire (FSQ) (43–46)	1. Physical role function 2. Psychosocial role function 3. ADL 4. Mental health 5. Work performance 6. Social activity 7. Quality of interaction	Ability, Status Target: ambulatory patients	34	Self-administered Time required: 15 minutes	Internal consistency: 0.62–0.82	Content: established through selection of items from existing instruments Concurrent: established based on correlations with each FSQ scale and 7 variables related to function Predictive: early outcome after valvuloplasty
Health Assessment Questionnaire (HAQ) Disability Index (24,47,48)	Disability Scale: 1. Dressing/grooming 2. Arising 3. Eating 4. Walking 5. Reaching personal hygiene 6. Gripping activities	Ability Target: patients with rheumatoid and osteoarthritis primarily lived in community	21	Self-administered Time required: 5–8 minutes	Internal consistency: 0.46–0.63 Test-retest: 0.93–0.95 (1 week); 0.98 (6 months) Interrater reliability: 0.85, weighted kappa: 0.52	Factor analysis: 2 factors (gross motor and fine motor movement) Convergent: high intercorrelations within dimensions and across instruments Discriminant: discriminates between diabetics and arthritis Predictive: greater or less disability

Instrument	Components	Target	Number of Items	Administration	Reliability	Validity
Inventory of Functional Status—Cancer (IFS-CA) (49,50)	1. Personal care 2. Household and family 3. Occupational 4. Social 5. Community	Status Target: women with cancer during and after adjuvant phase of treatment	39	Self-administered or structured interview Time required: <10 minutes	Internal consistency: 1. Subscale item to subscale total scores using Fisher's z transformation: Household and Family Activities: 0.74; Social and Community Activities: 0.82; Personal Care Activities: 0.56; Occupational Activities: 0.72 2. Subscale to total IFS-CA score correlations range: Household and family activities: 0.92, Occupational activities: 0.73 Test-retest: 0.91 (over 4–7 days)	Content: Popham's average congruency established at 98.5% Construct: subscale correlations from 0.33 to 0.62 Discriminant: total functional status higher for women who completed treatment than for those still in treatment
Katz-Index of Activities of Daily Living (3,51–54)	1. Bathing 2. Dressing 3. Toileting 4. Transfer 5. Continence 6. Feeding	Ability Target: patients with hip fracture, chronic illness, and elderly	6	Clinician assessed (with familiarity with patient) Time required: A few minutes	Test-retest: Guttman characteristics-coefficient of reproducibility of 0.95–0.98 (without impairment: 0.73)	Construct: correlates highly with Mini-Mental ($\gamma = 0.76$) Concurrent: correlates with the degree of actual assistance by the patient Predictive: the longitudinal course of function, measured by mobility and house confinement
Karnofsky Performance Index (KPS) (55–57)	1. Ability to do work 2. Perform normal activities 3. Need for assistance	Ability, Status Target: patients with cancer	11	Observer, shot time	Internal consistency: 0.97 Test-retest: 0.66 (1 week, home vs clinic) Interrater reliability: 0.98, kappa: 0.53	Convergent: significant correlations with cancer inventory of problem situations, Katz ADL scale, and others Predictive: survival in days, quality of life

Appendix 8A. Instruments Used to Measure Function (*cont.*)

Name (references)	Dimensions Measured	Dimensions of Function	Items	Administration	Reliability	Validity
Klein Bell Scale (58)	1. Dressing 2. Elimination 3. Mobility 4. Bathing 5. Emergency 6. Telephone 7. Communication	Ability Target: long-term care patients	170	Clinician assessed Time required: 15 minutes	Interrater reliability: 0.92	Predictive: ADL scores correlated at discharge with assistance needed ($\gamma = -0.86$)
Lawton Instrumental Activities of Daily Living—Physical Self Maintenance Scale (IADL-PSMS) (4,59,60)	1. Instrumental ADL 2. Physical self-maintenance scale	Ability, Status Target: elderly persons living in the community	IADL: 8 items for women; 5 items for men PSMS = 6 items	Clinician assessed (with familiarity with subject) Time required: 10–15 minutes	Internal consistency: IADL: 0.92, standardized: 0.93; PSMS: 0.87, standardized: 0.90 Interrater reliability: IADL: 0.85, PSMS: 0.87–0.91	Construct: significant correlations between severity of Alzheimer's disease and IADL and PSMS Concurrent: significant correlations with physical classification, mental status questionnaire, Adjustment Rating Scale Discriminant: discriminate between groups for cancer patient-caregiver dyads; discriminate patients with and without dementia
McMaster Health Index Questionnaire (MHIQ) (61,62)	1. Physical 2. Social 3. Emotional	Ability, Status Target: rehabilitation outpatient, patients with chronic disease	59	Self-administered or structured interview Time required: 20 minutes	Test-retest: Physical (0.53–0.95), emotional (0.70–0.77), social (0.48–0.66) (1-week range)	Construct: established (better functioning for younger vs older adults)

Instrument	Dimensions	Ability/Status; Target	Administration	Reliability	Validity
OARS Multidimensional Functional Assessment Questionnaire (OMFAQ) (63,64)	A: OMFAQ (personal functioning) B: Services utilization	Ability, Status — 101; Target: community-based population	Trained interviewer Time required: 45–75 minutes	Part A Interrater reliability: social (0.82), economic (0.78), mental health (0.80), physical health (0.66) Interclass: correlation coefficients: 0.66–0.87	Part A Construct: Kendell's tau, Spearman's rank-order correlations: economic ($\gamma = 0.68$, tau = -0.62), health ($\gamma = 0.67$, tau = 0.75), self-care ($\gamma = 0.89$, tau = 0.83) Discriminant: discriminate subjects with excellent functioning from those with totally impaired functioning
Pulmonary Functional Status Scale (PFSS) (65,66)	1. Daily Activities/ Social Functioning 2. Psychological Functioning 3. Sexual Functioning	Ability, Status — 56; Target: patients with chronic pulmonary disease	Self-administered Time required: 15 minutes	Internal consistency: 0.81–0.93 Test-retest: 0.67–0.75	Content: evaluated by a panel of experts Factor analysis: construct validity supported Concurrent: correlates with the SIP ($\gamma = -0.54$); highly correlated with 12-minute walk test ($\gamma = 0.62$)
Sickness Impact Profile (SIP) (10,67,68)	1. Physical 2. Psychosocial 3. 5 additional subscales	Ability, Status — 136; Target: patients with acute and chronic illness	Self-administered or structured interview Time required: 20–30 minutes	Internal consistency: 0.81–0.97 Test-retest: 0.88 (24 hours); 0.79–0.97 (2-week)	Convergent: AIMS and SIP ($g = 0.97$) Discriminant: higher correlation between SIP and levels of dysfunction and different groups of patients

Appendix 8A. Instruments Used to Measure Function (*cont.*)

Name (references)	Dimensions Measured	Dimensions of Function	Items	Administration	Reliability	Validity
Western Ontario and McMaster Universities Osteoarthritis Index (WOMAC) (69,70)	1. Pain 2. Stiffness 3. Physical function	Ability, Status Target: patients with osteoarthritis	24	Self-administered	Internal consistency: Pain: 0.86–0.89 Stiffness: 0.90–0.91 Physical function: 0.95 Test-retest: (1 week) Pain: 0.68 Stiffness: 0.48 Physical function: 0.68	Construct: Pain: the highest levels of correlation were noted between the subscale items and the Lequesne pain and physical function components and the Doyle Index Stiffness: the highest levels of correlation were between the test items and the Doyle Index, the Lequesne pain, physical function, and stiffness components Physical function: higher levels of correlation were noted between the test items and the physical component of the Lequesne Index than with the Doyle Index, the Lequesne pain and stiffness components, the Bradburn Index and the MHIQ

Work Assessment Scale (WAS) (71–73)	WAS Impediments (WAS-I):	Status Target: patients with MS	52	Self-administered	WAS-I: Internal consistency: 0.79–0.91 Test-retest: 0.76–0.91	Content: content analysis Factor analysis: construct validity supported
	1. Mobility					Concurrent: correlates with ADL-MS subscales
	2. Hand function				WAS-E: Internal consistency: 0.77–0.89	and MS-symptom-related checklist
	3. Cognition				Test-retest: 0.67–0.81 (2–3 weeks)	
	4. Body state					
	5. Pain					
	6. Environment					
	WAS enhancers (WAS-E)					
	1. Job adjustment					
	2. Personal attributes					
	3. Social support					
	4. Environmental adjustment					
	5. Health practices					

*MHIQ = McMaster Health Index Questionnaire

9

Measuring Cognitive Status

Marquis D. Foreman and Patricia E.H. Vermeersch

Cognition comprises perception, memory, and thinking—the recognition/registration, storage, and use of information. Cognition can be affected, both positively and negatively, by illness and its treatment. The evaluation of an individual's cognitive status can be instrumental in identifying the presence of specific pathophysiologic states (e.g., delirium, dementia, or depression), a person's readiness to learn, or the effectiveness of a treatment regimen. To evaluate cognitive status, numerous instruments have been developed. These instruments range from comprehensive, full-scale batteries that require a skilled examiner and place intensive pressure on the examinee, to bedside variants that place little demand on the examiner and examinee. The bedside variants are addressed in this chapter.

The measures of cognitive status reviewed in this chapter are representative of those most frequently used in research and practice and are either considered the standard for each aspect of cognition or have been recently developed and show great promise. For each measure of cognition described, the available psychometric information is reviewed, strengths and limitations presented, and recommendations provided. The content is organized according to (1) measures of specific areas of cognition, (2) measures of global aspects of cognition, (3) measures for common disorders of cognition, (4) criteria for selecting a measure of cognitive status, and (5) conditions for using a measure of cognition. The two approaches of examination are (1) assessment of *specific* dimensions of cognition, and (2) *global* assessment of cognitive function.[1] Each has advantages and disadvantages:

Testing	Advantages	Disadvantages
Specific dimensions of cognition	Easy to administer to individuals requiring it most (e.g., fatigued, distressed, or with language or sensory limitations)	Not a comprehensive examination and may overlook an important deficit
Global assessment of cognition	All components of cognition systematically assessed	Time-consuming; may be less sensitive to some aspects of cognition; may overlook important deficits

Measures of Specific Areas of Cognition

Albert[2] identified five specific, or individual, components of cognition that should be evaluated: attention, visuospatial abilities, language, memory, and conceptualization. Each component, along with its major measures, is presented. The psychometric properties, advantages, and disadvantages of each instrument are detailed in Appendix 9A.

Attention

Attention is the ability to focus on a specific stimulus without being distracted by extraneous environmental stimuli. An individual's ability to sustain attention over time must be established before more complex cognitive functions, such as memory, can be evaluated.[2,3] According to Albert,[2] if the individual has difficulty focusing on a task for 1 to 3 minutes at a time, it will not be possible to assess other areas of cognitive function.

Evaluation of an individual's attentional abilities also is important in determining the nature of the cognitive impairment. Attentional abilities are preserved in some forms of cognitive impairment but deficient in others. For example, attentional ability is preserved in dementia, whereas an attentional deficit is a major feature of acute confusion or delirium.[4-8]

Historically, the attentional abilities of an individual have been assessed using tasks such as serial subtraction; however, these tasks are known to be biased by the individual's premorbid intellectual capability, calculating ability, and socioeconomic status.[3] Hence, in people in whom these factors could confound the interpretation of results, other tests of attention, such as digit span or repetition, the vigilance or A-test, or trail-making tests, should be substituted. However, these measures are not without limitations. The attentional abilities of individuals who have a significant language disorder, such as aphasia, cannot be assessed validly with the digit span or repetition test or test of vigilance.[3] Similarly, individuals with physical and sensory impairment may not be capable of completing the trail-making tests.[7]

Digit Span

The digit span or repetition task consists of a series of numbers that are read to the individual who repeats them in the same sequence. This task is easy to administer and interpret and requires approximately 5 minutes. In administering this task, it is important that the digits not be presented in pairs or sequences, but randomly in a normal tone of voice at the rate of one digit per second. A second attempt by the examinee is permissible; however, if both attempts fail, the task is terminated. The score on the digit span or repetition task is the number of digits correctly repeated by the examinee.

Adequate performance on this task demonstrates that the individual can attend to a verbal stimulus and sustain attention for the period of time required to repeat the digits. Persons of average intelligence can repeat five to seven digits without difficulty. According to Strub and Black,[3] repetition of less than five digits by a nonretarded patient without obvious aphasia indicates defective attention.

Test of Vigilance

The test of vigilance, also referred to as the A-test,[3] is a test that is easy to administer and interpret, requiring approximately 2 to 3 minutes. It consists of a series of random letters among which the target letter *a* appears with greater frequency. The examinee is required to indicate whenever the target letter is spoken by the examiner, who reads the list of letters to the examinee at the rate of one letter per second. Normally, an examinee should make no errors; any error is indicative of an attentional deficit. Common are (1) errors of omission, (2) errors of commission, and (3) perseverative errors. The type of error can assist in determining the nature of the cognitive impairment (e.g., perseverative errors are common with dementia). The score on this test is the absolute number of errors irrespective of their type.

Trail-Making Tests

The trail-making test (TMT) is a standardized timed test to assess visual-motor tracking skills, counting ability, spatial skills, and cognitive flexibility.[6,9] The test has two parts: Part A consists of 25 numbered circles randomly scattered on a sheet of paper. The examinee is instructed to connect these numbered circles in ascending numeric order as rapidly as possible without lifting the pencil from the paper. Part B is approximately 2.5 times more difficult than Part A[10] and consists of 13 numbered circles and 12 lettered circles randomly scattered on a sheet of paper that the examinee is to connect alternately in the proper sequence (e.g., 1-A, 2-B, 3-C, . . . 13). Practice is provided on a brief example. During the task, if a circle is connected out of sequence, the examinee is stopped, corrected, and begun again from that point. Both parts are scored according to the total time in seconds required by the examinee to compete the task. For Part B, times greater than 200 seconds are considered abnormal.[9,11–13]

The TMT has been used with various samples: individuals with organic brain damage,[9] neuropsychiatric patients,[12,14] normal adults,[9] and candidates for liver transplantation.[13,15] Delirious, elderly demented, and chronic schizophrenic patients were found to be severely impaired on the TMT;[12] however, only nine of the 20 patients with delirium could perform the test. Given these characteristics of the TMT (see Appendix 9A), the TMT may be useful in identifying an attentional deficit but not in determining the exact nature of the cognitive impairment.[7] Other measures of attention include the Mental Control and the Attention Concentration Index subsections of the Wechsler Memory Scale (discussed later in the memory section) and digit or letter cancellation.[11]

Visuospatial Ability

Because of the prevalence of visual-sensory deficits that accompany aging, the assessment of visuospatial ability is more difficult in the elderly than in the young. Many of the cognitive domains discussed in this chapter can be evaluated either orally or visually. However, this is not possible for visuospatial ability, and alternative means of testing have proven more difficult.

Constructional ability can be evaluated using two methods: figure copying or drawing on command. Albert,[16] however, warns against using drawing on command as a measure of visuospatial ability because it is confounded by conceptual impairments. Figure copying can be assessed simply by asking the examinee to copy a single line drawing, for example, copying the intersecting pentagons item of Folstein's Mini-Mental State Examination (MMSE).[17] Figure copying is useful in the diagnosis and localization of cerebral lesion; for example, patients with dementia omit essential features, whereas others oversimplify their drawings.[18] In copying a design, demented individuals also fail to preserve accurate spatial relationships.[18]

In addition to constructional ability, one should assess perceptual capacity. Figure-matching tasks are a good analogue for figure copying. They have the added advantage that they can be administered to patients with severe cognitive deficits, in whom it is otherwise difficult to meaningfully assess spatial function. However, these measures of perceptual capacity require good visual acuity of the examinee.[1] Single measures of perceptual capacity are not reviewed here, but are found as component elements of the global measures of cognition discussed later in this chapter.

The Clock-Drawing Test

The Clock-Drawing Test (CDT) is an examination of visuospatial abilities considered useful in screening for global cognitive impairment and dementia.[19-23] More recently, the CDT has been shown to test abstract conceptualization, numerical and verbal memory, and executive function.[24,25] There are three components to this test: (1) clock drawing, (2) clock setting, and (3) clock reading. Two versions exist for the clock-drawing component. In the first, the examinee is instructed to draw a clock on a blank sheet of paper, to number the face of the clock, but to omit placing the hands. In the second version, the examinee is given a sheet of paper with a predrawn circle and is instructed to draw and number the clock face, again omitting the hands on the clock. There are also two versions of the clock-setting component. The examinee is requested to place the hands on the clock depicting one to five specific times in the first version; in the second, the examinee is allowed to select the time periods. The last component of the test is clock reading. For this component, the examinee is shown one to five clocks depicting different times and is asked to read the times. The method for scoring and interpreting the results of the CDT also varies.

Language

Language is crucial for assessing most cognitive abilities. Therefore, its integrity must be established early in the evaluation.[3] If deficits in language are identified, subsequent evaluation of higher aspects of cognition are difficult, if not impossible. Assessment of language should include an evaluation of comprehension, repetition, reading, writing, and naming.[4] Several standard batteries are available for this purpose, including the Boston Diagnostic Aphasia Examination,[26] the Western Aphasia Battery (WAB),[27] and the Boston Naming Test.[28] Some of these batteries include brief aphasia screening tests that are useful for identifying the existence of a problem without giving a detailed analysis (e.g., the Halstead-Wepman Aphasia Screening Test).[29] Even if aphasia has been ruled out or is not suspected, language abilities should be a part of the assessment of an older individual, because decreases in naming ability occur with age and also are a prominent symptom of a number of disorders among the elderly (e.g., Alzheimer's disease). A variety of these measures of language abilities are presented.

Modified Halstead-Wepman

The Modified Halstead-Wepman[29] is a brief screening test of language and visuographic skills.[1,11] According to Lezak,[11] the Modified Halstead-Wepman is the most widely used of all aphasia tests because it or its variants have been incorporated into many formally organized neuropsychological test batteries, such as the Halstead-Reitan Neuropsychological Test Battery. Various modifications of the Halstead-Wepman exist. As originally devised, this test had 51 items covering all the elements of aphasic disabilities, as well as the most commonly associated communication problems. Reitan[30] pared down the list to 32 items, but still handled the data descriptively in much the same manner as the original. The emphasis of scoring is on determining the nature of the linguistic problem, once its presence has been established. Errors are coded into a diagnostic profile to describe the pattern of the patient's language disabilities. The severity of the language impairment is by breadth (the more errors in more aspects of language abilities, the more severe the impairment) and by depth (the more errors generally, the more severe the impairment). However, no provisions are made to grade test performance or classify patients on the basis of severity.

A second revision contains 37 items, the same as Reitan's with the addition of four easy arithmetic problems and the task of naming a key. A simple error-counting scoring system was established for use with a computerized diagnostic classification system that converts to a 6-point rating scale—an attempt to overcome the previous scoring limitations. However, this scoring strategy indicates the severity of an aphasic disorder, but not its nature.

Last, a short version consists of four tasks:[31] (1) copy a square, Greek cross, and triangle without lifting the pencil from the paper; (2) name each copied figure; (3) spell each name; and (4) repeat, "he shouted the warning" and then explain and write it. This version is reputed to aid in discriminating between patients with left- and right-hemisphere lesions, for many of the former can copy the designs but cannot write, whereas the latter have little trouble writing but many cannot reproduce the designs.[11]

Boston Naming Test

The Boston Naming Test[28] examines single-word expressive vocabulary or naming ability by requiring the examinee to name 60 pictured objects ordered in increasing difficulty from bed to abacus. There are various starting points for different groups of examinees: (1) children under 10 and aphasic patients start with object 1; (2) older examinees start with item 30 and continue forward unless errors are committed before item 38; if so, they return to item 29 and work backward. The pictures are presented by the examiner to the examinee in order. The examinee is allowed up to 20 seconds to respond, unless the examinee says he does not know the word before the 20 seconds. If the answer is correct, the time in seconds required for the response is noted. For other than correct responses, the verbatim response is recorded. If the examinee is unable to name an object spontaneously, the examiner provides a categoric cue, such as "It's something to eat," that is printed in brackets under the response line for each item. Again, the examinee is allowed up to 20 seconds to name the picture. If the subject still does not recognize the picture after receiving the categoric cue or misnames it, the examiner should note the response and proceed to phonemic cuing. Phonemic cues assist the examinee by providing the opening sound of the target word. It is recommended that a phonemic cue be given after every failure to respond or after any incorrect response. The scoring scheme reflects these administration procedures: (1) object correct without assistance, (2) number of categoric cues given, (3) number of objects correct after categorical cues, (4) number of phonemic cues given, (5) objects correct after phonemic cues. Provisional norms are provided in the manual for children, normal adults, and aphasic adults. However, minimal psychometric information is available.

Western Aphasia Battery (WAB)

The WAB grew out of efforts to develop an instrument from the Boston Diagnostic Aphasia Examination that would generate diagnostic classifications and be suitable for both clinical and research purposes.[11,32] Seven areas of language abilities are examined: spontaneous speech, auditory comprehension, repetition, naming, reading and writing, praxis, and construction. Some training is required for administration. Shewan and Kertesz[32] report that it takes most aphasics approximately 60 minutes to complete and less time with the more impaired patients. For individuals unable to withstand such lengthy testing, the WAB can be administered in two parts.

Memory

Memory, an essential component of cognition, consists of the mental processes for receiving, storing, and retrieving information. It should be evaluated in detail. Memory dysfunction occurs in almost all the cognitive disorders.[2] To distinguish the type and degree of memory deficit, anatomic localization, etiologic nature of the pathology, and the impact of the deficit on the individual's ability to function, various aspects of memory should be assessed in some detail.[2,3,10] Albert[2] warns that the assessment of memory in the elderly is complicated further by the fact that changes in the capacity of memory occur as people age. Therefore, careful testing often is necessary to differentiate normal from pathologic memory performance. In evaluating memory, Strub and Black[3] suggest that the following be considered: (1) the examiner must be able to verify the answers from a source other than the examinee; (2) performance on memory tasks requires sustained attention, therefore, examinees with attentional deficits will not perform optimally; (3) the examinee must be capable of relating to and cooperating with the examiner; and (4) the examinee must have no defect that impairs the comprehension or expression of language. According to Albert,[2] the most common measures of memory in use today are the Wechsler Memory Scale (WMS),[7,33] the Benton Visual Retention Test (BVRT),[34] the Randt Memory Test (RMT),[35] and Story Recall. We discuss each.

Wechsler Memory Scale

The WMS was developed to evaluate rapidly, simply, and practically a rather disparate group of memory functions.[7,36] The objective of the test battery was to create a measure that correlated well with intelligence tests without duplicating them. Seven subtests comprise the WMS and include (1) personal and current information, (2) orientation, (3) mental control (backward counting, alphabet, and counting by 30), (4) logical memory (two passages read and subject scored on average number of items retained when repeating), (5) digit span (forward and backward), (6) visual reproduction (draw geometric figures from memory), and (7) associate learning (learning 10 pairs in three trials). Performance on the subtests is summed and statistically age corrected to provide a memory quotient (MQ), which in some ways is analogous to a full-scale IQ (mean 100, SD 15). The scoring is most useful on three factors: memory, attention, and concentration. Scoring instructions published by Wechsler[7] and Klonoff and Kennedy[37] show norms for people in their eighties and nineties. For many years, the WMS was the only widely available and standardized objective test of memory for clinical use. Indices of reliability and validity[37-39] are shown in Appendix 9A.

Benton Visual Retention Test

The BVRT[34] consists of several series of simple and complex line drawings designed to assess short-term or immediate memory. Visual motor construction, visual spatial perception, and visual conceptualization also are reportedly assessed by the BVRT.[3] This series of line drawings is presented to the examinee for varying periods of time (5 to 10 seconds), depending on the administration form, in which the examinee either reproduces the designs directly or after a variable delay (immediate recall or a 15-second delay). The BVRT requires approximately 5 minutes to administer. It is recommended that the BVRT be administered by a trained psychologist, that is, one who knows the test.[40]

The BVRT exists in four alternate forms: C, D, E, and I. Form I was an attempt to remove the motor component of the BVRT to assess a more purely visual skill. In this form the examinee is asked to select the original form from a series of four alternatives.[41,42] In addition, there are three forms of administration, A through C. In administration A, the subject is shown the stimuli for 10 seconds and then is asked to reproduce them. In administration B, the subject is shown the stimuli for 10 seconds and asked to reproduce them after a delay of 5 seconds. In administration C, the subject is allowed to copy the stimuli directly.

The BVRT has explicit scoring instructions and robust normative data. Performance on the BVRT is positively correlated with IQ and negatively correlated with age.

Therefore, the norms are for the expected correct responses and the expected number of errors for each alternate form and administration for six IQ groups crossed with multiple age groups from 8 to 64 years. These norms, created with schoolchildren of various IQs and with medically ill adult patients with no history of brain disease, are available in the BVRT manual.[34]

Performance on the BVRT also is influenced by the anatomic location of the neurologic involvement. Individuals with bilateral damage average 4 to 6 errors, individuals with right-sided damage 3.5 errors, and persons with left-sided damage 1 error.[43] Other studies tend to support a right–left differential in defective copying of these designs and find that right-hemisphere patients are two or three times more likely to have difficulties.[44] However, in one study that included aphasic patients in the comparisons between groups with lateralized lesions, no differences were found in the frequency with which constructional impairment was present in the drawings of right- and left-hemisphere–damaged patients.[45] Psychometric indices[46] are shown in Appendix 9A. Form 1 may be solved by a logical strategy unrelated to the visual stimulus and requires a posttesting interview of the subject.[47]

Randt Memory Test

The RMT[35] is a set of seven subtests specifically designed to quantify mild to moderate memory loss in longitudinal studies of patients with organic brain disease. Five alternate forms were developed for repeated examination of everyday memory. The first and last subtests (General Information and Incidental Learning) are identical in all alternate forms. The other five subtests are reported to be equivalent on the basis of such relevant characteristics as word length, frequency, and imagery levels. The middle five subtests are of recall, digits forward and backward, word pairs, and a paragraph. Recognition of line drawings of common objects also is included.

There is a set order of presentation in which acquisition and retrieval from storage are differentiated by separating immediate recall and recall after fixed tasks (a subsequent subtest serves as the distractor task for each of the four subtests that have delayed recall trials). In addition, the RMT is constructed to use telephone interviews to obtain 24-hour recall data.[11]

Story Recall

Story Recall[3,11] begins with the instructions to the examinee, "I am going to read you a short story. Listen carefully, because when I finish reading, I want you to tell me as much of the story as you can remember." After reading the story, the examinee is instructed, "Now tell me everything that you can remember of that story. Start at the beginning of the story and tell me what happened." The separate items of the story are indicated by slash (/) marks. As the patient retells the story, indicate the number of ideas recalled. When an examinee reports only a few items, the examiner should encourage the examinee to try and recall more. If the examinee still does not produce much, the examiner can provide some structure for the recall through directive questioning, such as "What happened?" "Where did it happen?" "Who was involved?" In this instance, the examiner should note where the directive questioning began to keep track of spontaneous versus directed recall.

After the first recall, the examiner instructs the examinee, "In a little while, I'm going to ask you to tell me how much of the story you can still remember. I'm going to read the story to you again now so that you'll have it fresh in your memory for the next time." Recall after the second reading follows approximately 20 minutes of testing involving verbal material. Once again, the examiner asks the examinee, "Tell me everything you can remember of that story." Directed questioning should proceed as appropriate. Several versions of Story Recall can be located in Strub and Black[3] and Lezak.[11]

Conceptualization

According to Albert,[16] conceptualization is the most complex and difficult aspect of cognition to assess. Furthermore, an individual's conceptual abilities are easily confounded by general intelligence. As a result, when evaluating conceptualization, general intelligence also must be evaluated. Tasks that examine conceptualization include tests of concept formation, abstraction, set shifting, and set maintenance. These measures are thought to underestimate an individual's practical coping and problem-solving abilities.[1] Therefore, it is recommended that these formal tests be supplemented with observations of an individual's everyday decision making.[1] Other measures of conceptualization include Raven's Progressive, the Similarities subtest of the Wechsler Adult Intelligence Scale-Revised (WAIS-R), and the Verbal-Visual Test.

Proverbs Test

The Proverbs Test[48–50] is a standardized test of proverbs with regard to familiarity and difficulty. There are three alternate forms of the Proverbs Test, each containing 12 proverbs of equivalent difficulty. It is administered as a written test in which the examinee is instructed that the intent of the test is to explain what the proverb means, rather than just telling the examiner more about the proverb. The responses are scored on a 5-point rating scale that objectifies the degree of abstraction. One form is a multiple-choice version of 40 items, each with four possible answers (the best answer form). Only one choice is appropriate and abstract, the other three are either concrete interpretations or common misinterpretations.[11]

Modified Card Sorting Test

The Modified Card Sorting Test (MCST)[51] is a widely used test devised to study abstract behavior. The examinee is given a pack of 48 cards on which are printed one to four symbols (triangle, star, cross, or circle), in red, green, yellow, or blue. No two cards are identical; cards do not share more than one attribute with a stimulus card. The examinee is instructed to sort the cards according to a rule or category. Whatever category the examinee chooses first is designated "correct" by the examiner, who proceeds to inform the examinee whether or not each choice is correct until the examinee has achieved a run of six correct responses. At that point, the examinee is told that the rule has changed and is instructed to find another rule. This procedure is continued until six categories are achieved or the pack of 48 cards is used up.

Besides a score for the number of categories obtained, Nelson[51] derived a score from the total number of errors and scored as perseverative errors only those of the same category as the immediately preceding response. Results obtained from testing with the MCST readily separate examinees with unilateral neurologic lesions from control examinees. There is a tendency for patients with posterior lesions to perform better than patients whose lesions involved the frontal lobes and for patients with frontal lobe lesions to make more perseverative errors than control patients. Nelson's[51] data also suggest that this method is sensitive to aging effects. Older people perform more poorly, women outperform men, and people with higher education perform better.

Judgment: Real-Life Hypothetical Situations

Judgment is not generally evaluated in isolation from other cognitive functions, but rather as component elements in the global measures[52,53] of cognition.

Global Measures of Cognition

Global measures are used to survey multiple aspects of cognition. As a result, global measures are useful screening tools for cognitive impairment. In addition, global measures tend not to be comprehensive measures of cognition but to consist of elements that increase the sensitivity and specificity for detecting impairment. Diagnosis for cognition other than impairment is problematic using global measures. Psychometric indices, as well as advantages and disadvantages of important measures, are shown in Appendix 9B.

Mental Status Questionnaires
Mini-Mental State Examination

The MMSE,[17] is a simplified, scored form that consists of 11 questions requiring 5 to 10 minutes to complete. Each question is scored as either correct or incorrect; the total score ranges from 0 to 30 and reflects the number of correct responses. A score less than 24 is considered evidence of impaired cognition.[17,54,55] The MMSE is a reliable and valid measure. In a comprehensive review of the information about the MMSE accumulated since the mid-1960s, Tombaugh and McIntyre[56] reported that the MMSE remains psychometrically robust across settings and despite gender, race, ethnicity, and social class. Other studies document this as well.[57-61] The MMSE also is known to discriminate well among normal, depressed, demented, and depressed and demented individuals.[17] In recent reviews of cognitive screening instruments,[55-57] the MMSE was identified as the preferred instrument for use with demented elders and remains the most frequently used bedside test of cognition.

Cognitive Capacity Screening Examination

The Cognitive Capacity Screening Examination (CCSE)[62] was developed to be a sufficiently sensitive and relevant instrument for the detection of a diffuse organic mental syndrome, particularly delirium, in nonpsychiatric patients. The CCSE consists of 30 items requiring 5 to 10 minutes to administer. The test measures a variety of cognitive functions: orientation, digit span, concentration, serial sevens, repetition, verbal concept formation, and short-term verbal recall. According to the researchers, patients who score less than 20 points should be considered cognitively impaired.

Neurobehavioral Cognitive Status Examination

The Neurobehavioral Cognitive Status Examination (NCSE)[52,53] is a relatively newly developed, complete, neurologic mental status screening examination. The NCSE was designed to detect and characterize the nature of cognitive dysfunction in hospitalized adults. The NCSE is reported to provide more detailed and sensitive information about cognitive status while remaining clinically practical, that is, brief, and easy to administer (10 to 20 minutes) and score for the clinician and not fatiguing to the patient. The NCSE consists of a test and an administration and scoring manual. The instrument assesses the level of consciousness, orientation, and attention, as well as five major ability areas: language, constructions, memory, calculations, and reasoning.[52,53] With the exception of the memory and orientation categories, the other tests begin with a screen item. The screen item is a demanding test of the skill involved, and 10% to 30% of the normal population fail the screen.[52] If the screen is answered correctly, the particular skill is considered intact, and no further testing of that skill is required. If the screen is failed, the metric, a series of test items of increasing complexity, is administered. Within each cognitive ability area, the number of correct responses is totaled and recorded on the front of the test booklet, resulting in independent scores for specific cognitive ability areas rather than a single overall score. Scores below a predetermined criterion are interpreted as reflecting impairment within that particular area of cognitive functioning.[52,53]

The NCSE's clinical utility has been demonstrated in psychiatry and neurology clinics and psychiatry and neurology inpatient services and for neuropsychologic and neurosurgery patients. The NCSE occupies a middle ground between very brief instruments, which provide a global estimation of cognitive functioning, and exhaustive neuropsychologic test batteries, which offer a more thorough assessment.[52,53] It can be administered at the bedside in approximately 15 to 30 minutes.

Measures for Common Disorders of Cognition

Common disorders of cognition to be detected and evaluated relative to their nature and severity include acute confusion or delirium, dementia, and depression. Instruments for each disorder are presented and discussed. See Appendix 9C for a comparison of clinical features of these disorders.[63]

Acute Confusion/Delirium

Acute confusion, or delirium, is characterized by a disturbance in consciousness and a change in cognition that develop over a short period of time.[64] Symptoms of delirium that fluctuate diurnally include reduced ability to focus, shift, or sustain attention; memory deficits, disorientation, language disturbance; misinterpretation; and variable psychomotor behavior[4] (see Appendix 9C). Various methods have been developed to detect the presence of acute confusion accurately and promptly and to predict its occurrence.[65] Measures in addition to those discussed are shown in Appendix 9B.

Clinical Assessment of Confusion—Form A

The Clinical Assessment of Confusion—Form A (CAC-A)[66] was developed to determine the presence, pattern, and severity of confusion as perceived by nurses. The CAC-A is a checklist of 25 psychomotor behaviors, representing five dimensions of confusion: (1) cognition, (2) general behavior, (3) motor activity, (4) orientation, and (5) psychotic/neurotic behaviors. The patient is evaluated on the basis of the presence or absence of each behavior. The score is the total of the weights for each of the observed behaviors. Four or more behaviors and weighted scores greater than 8 indicates the presence of confusion. The CAC-A also implies that the more behaviors observed, the more severe the confusion. Vermeersch[66,67] provides the following recommendations for interpreting test results: 4 to 6 behaviors with a weighted score ranging from 9 to 14 indicates mild confusion; 7 to 9 behaviors with a weighted score ranging from 15 to 24, moderate confusion; more than 9 behaviors and weighted scores greater than 28, severe confusion. Psychometric indices[66–69] are shown in Appendix 9B.

NEECHAM Confusion Scale

The NEECHAM Confusion Scale[70] was designed to evaluate rapidly and nonintrusively a patient's cognitive function and behavioral performance to detect early cues to the development of acute confusion and to monitor recovery. NEECHAM places a minimal response burden on the patient by making maximal use of existing data such as the patient's performance in the environment (self-care, feeding, and use of information) and the patient's physiologic stability (vital signs, oxygen saturation, and urinary incontinence). Ratings can be repeated at frequent intervals to monitor changes in the patient's status.[70] The scale is sensitive to early changes in information processing and documents confused behavior, including delirium.[70]

The instrument consists of nine scaled items divided into three subscales of assessment: responsiveness, performance, and physiologic control. The score ranges from 0 (minimal responsiveness) to 30 (normal function) and is completed by the nurse in a manner similar to other vital function measurements conducted during routine or required nursing assessments. The authors reported that NEECHAM scores lower than 20 were strongly associated with DSM-IV criteria for delirium, whereas scores of 20 to 24 seemed to indicate borderline confusion.[71]

Delirium Rating Scale

The Delirium Rating Scale (DRS)[12] is a 10-item scale. Each of the 10 items is rated by the clinician using information obtained from an interview and mental status examination of the patient. Information from the patient's hospital record (e.g., medical history, laboratory tests, nursing observations) and family reports are also necessary.[12] The clinician-rater is instructed to complete the DRS using information obtained from at least a 24-hour period of patient observation because of the fluctuating course of the symptoms of delirium. Operationalizing the DSM-III criteria for delirium, the DRS includes items measuring the temporal onset of symptoms, perceptual disturbances, hallucinations, delusions, psychomotor behavior, cognitive status during formal testing, physical disorder, sleep–wake disturbance, lability of mood, and variability of symptoms. The total score on the DRS is the sum of the items ranging from a minimum of 0 to a maximum of 32 and is intended to reflect the severity of the delirium (the higher the score, the more severe the delirium).

The DRS is considered to represent a significant advance over earlier symptom-rating scales used to detect delirium. The criteria for delirium have been operationalized, thereby providing information on both cognitive and behavioral symptoms.

Confusion Assessment Method

Confusion Assessment Method (CAM)[5] is a four-item instrument developed to assist clinicians who have no formal psychiatric training to identify patients with delirium quickly and accurately. It has four features that are determined by information obtained by interviews of the patient, nurse, and family: (1) an acute onset of mental status changes or a fluctuating course, (2) inattention, (3) disorganized thinking, and (4) an altered level of consciousness. Delirium is diagnosed if the patient has both features 1 and 2 and either feature 3 or 4.[5] The CAM has been compared with other instruments by external reviewers and found to have the best combination of ease of use, speed of use, data acquisition, reliability, and validity.[72–76] The CAM is suitable for use at the bedside to identify patients with delirium. An Italian version shows promise.[73]

Confusion Assessment Method for the Intensive Care Unit

Confusion Assessment Method for the Intensive Care Unit (CAM-ICU)[72,76] is a modification of the CAM for use with patients who are nonverbal. The standard CAM instrument was supplemented with a picture recognition tool[77,78] and the Vigilance Test. Initial psychometric testing with critically ill, nonverbal patients has demonstrated excellent reliability and validity. The developers have concluded that the CAM-ICU may be a useful instrument for both clinical and research purposes to monitor delirium in a critically ill, nonverbal patient population.

Delirium Symptom Interview

The Delirium Symptom Interview (DSI)[79] was developed in response to previous criticism that the measurement of the symptoms of delirium was too subjective and, therefore, unreliable. Development of the DSI also was predicated on the belief that it was necessary to have structured assessments that could be administered by trained, lay interviewers so that data would be reliably collected and could be replicated by other research groups. To improve reliability and avoid the observation bias introduced by subjective opinions from clinical interviews, the DSI was constructed to structure the assessments of all the symptoms of delirium, not just the cognitive symptoms, as is typically the case. These structured assessments consist of 17 questions and 45 observations of the examinee. The symptoms assessed by the DSI are the DSM-IV diagnostic criteria for delirium: clouding of consciousness, disorientation, disturbance of sleep, perceptual disturbance, incoherent speech, increased or decreased psychomotor activity, and fluctuating behavior.

The authors report that 10 to 15 minutes are required to complete the DSI. A symptom was identified as having a rapid onset, or as new, if (1) it was not present at the patient's initial evaluation and developed subsequently in the hospital or (2) if present when the patient was first seen in the hospital, it had not been observed before the patient's hospitalization, as documented through a structured interview with a relative or caretaker. Fluctuating behavior is rated, and an etiology is sought, but not required.

Delirium Index

The Delirium Index (DI)[80] was developed to provide a standardized measure of the changes in the severity of the symptoms of delirium in delirious patients. The DI was designed to be used in conjunction with the MMSE, with each symptom of delirium rated solely on observations of patient behavior; information from family members, nursing staff, or hospital record is not necessary. The DI consists of 7 of the 9 items of the CAM, each item/symptom is rated on a scale of 0 (symptom absent) to 3 (severe impairment). The total score ranges from 0 (no symptoms) to 21 (maximum severity). The DI is reported to take 5 to 10 minutes to complete.[80–83]

Memorial Delirium Assessment Scale

Memorial Delirium Assessment Scale (MDAS)[84] was developed specifically for frequent repeated use to quantify the severity of delirium symptoms for use in clinical intervention trials. The utility of the MDAS for screening, and diagnosing delirium also has been supported.[84–89]

The MDAS is a 10-item instrument requiring 10 minutes to complete. Each item is a feature of delirium and is scored on a 4-point scale depending on its intensity and frequency, with 0 representing none and 3 representing severe; the total score ranges from 0 to 30. The first 6 items are rated on the basis of a clinical interview; the remaining 4 items are rated on the basis of a clinical interview and also from standardized nursing observations during the previous 24 hours.[80] Initial validity was established with a small sample against a clinical diagnosis of delirium as made by a psychiatrist.[84] However, mild cases of delirium were poorly detected (with cutpoint of 13), and there was substantial overlap in the scores of those rated as moderately or severely delirious.[84,89]

Dementia

Dementia is a chronic, insidious, progressive, and permanent form of cognitive impairment. It is an impairment of higher cortical functions, including memory, that is manifested by difficulties in day-to-day functioning, problem solving, and the control of emotions.[90] There are several types of dementia, based on the etiologic agent, such as primary degenerative dementia of the Alzheimer type, multi-infarct dementia, and AIDS-related dementia. A comparison of clinical features of delirium (acute confusion), dementia, and depression is found in Appendix 9A.

Mattis Dementia Rating Scale

The Mattis Dementia Rating Scale (MDRS)[91] examines five areas that are particularly sensitive to the behavioral changes that characterize Alzheimer's dementia: (1) attention, (2) initiation and perseveration, (3) construction, (4) conceptual, and (5) memory.

An interesting feature of the MDRS is that, instead of giving the items in the usual ascending order of difficulty, the most difficult item is given first. Because the most difficult items are within the capacity of most intact older persons, this feature can be a time-saver. An intact patient would only have to have three abstract answers on the first subtest, and the remaining items could be skipped. On the other hand, Mattis reports that the examination of demented patients can take 30 to 45 minutes. A motivation behind the development of the MDRS was to minimize the floor effect frequently observed when testing such persons. Scores range from 0 (poorest performance) to 144 (perfect performance).

Consortium to Establish a Registry for Alzheimer's Disease

The Consortium to Establish a Registry for Alzheimer's Disease (CERAD)[92] was organized to establish a brief and accurate method for assessing the presenting clinical manifestations and cognitive alterations in individuals with Alzheimer's disease.[93] A uniform, reliable, simple, yet accurate means of evaluation to obtain information about the clinical, neuropsychologic, and neuropathologic aspects of the disease was essential to provide appropriate health services and for research purposes. The CERAD is an extensive, comprehensive composite of other tests separated into two batteries. The first is the neuropsychological battery, which consists of tests of (1) verbal fluency, (2) modified Boston Naming Test, (3) MMSE, (4) word list memory, (5) constructional praxis, (6) word list recall, and (7) word list recognition. The second is a clinical battery, consisting of (1) demographic information, (2) drug inventory, (3) history of patient by the patient and an informant, (4) a physical examination, (5) laboratory studies, and (6) a diagnostic impression.

Depression

Depression is a disturbance of mood, consisting of dysphoria, feelings of sadness, pessimism, hopelessness, and loss of interest or pleasure in most activities.[94] It is a term used to refer to a range of disorders from a subclinical problem—a "blue" mood state and general feelings of hopelessness and demoralization—to a major depressive disorder. Most of the scales used to measure depression were developed to detect the presence of depression and to determine its level of severity.[95] Most scales, however, do not facilitate the identification of the underlying etiologic mechanisms of depression (e.g., endogenous versus nonendogenous depression).

Some problems should be considered with any of the following measures of depression:[12,96] (1) the elderly often deny feelings of depression; (2) there is a higher prevalence of somatic complaints in the elderly caused by genuine physical problems and their treatment, thereby making what are generally accepted as common somatic complaints of depression nonspecific in the elderly; and (3) it is difficult to differentiate depression from other cognitive problems, such as dementia and acute confusion. We present some measures in order of development.

Beck Depression Inventory

Beck Depression Inventory (BDI) was constructed to screen for the presence and severity of depression in adults[97] and is considered reliable and valid even with the elderly.[98]

The BDI contains 21 items, each concerned with a particular aspect of the experience and symptomatology of depression, that are rated on a four-point intensity, rather than frequency, dimension. A rating of three indicates the most severe, and zero indicates an absence of a problem in that area. As a result, the greater the score, the more depressed the individual. The ratings are made by the examinee or by an observer, who should be either a psychologist or psychiatrist. With brief training, administration takes 5 minutes.[40] Because the BDI requires a severity rating for each symptom, a finer-grained picture of the patient's distress can be obtained with the BDI than with other measures of depression. Furthermore, the BDI contains a suicide item that can be highly relevant in the assessment of older adults. Numerous validation studies[96-98] with psychiatric in- and outpatients have generated indices of reliability and validity, shown in Appendix 9B.

Hamilton Depression Rating Scale

The Hamilton Depression Rating Scale (HDRS)[99] was designed to assess the level of depression. As a result of the comprehensive coverage of depressive symptomatology, related psychopathology, and its strong psychometric properties, HDRS has remained the most commonly used rating scale of the level of depression in clinical research settings since the 1960s.[79] The HDRS relies heavily on the skill of the examiner to elicit the information required to make the ratings of depression, and therefore it is recommended that the HDRS be administered by a psychiatrist or an adequately trained individual. Training requires background knowledge of psychiatry and experience with about 10 patients.[40] The scale often is administered by two examiners, and the score is the average of both ratings. Comprising 21 items, 17 of which relate to depression, the HDRS can be completed in about 30 minutes.

Geriatric Depression Scale-Short Form

The Geriatric Depression Scale-Short Form (GDS-SF)[100] was developed for measuring depression in the elderly, for whom traditional depression scales may not be appropriate.[101,102] The GDS-SF has proven valid and reliable for measuring depression in the elderly, both those institutionalized[102] and demented.[103] None of its items focuses on the typical somatic complaints, but instead tap psychologic distress (e.g., helplessness, hopelessness, and lack of satisfaction with life).[96] It requires 5 to 7 minutes to administer; all items are answered in a yes or no format for ease of comprehension even by cognitively impaired elders. The brevity and ease of administration of the GDS-SF are important considerations with individuals who are physically frail and among whom depression may coexist with other forms of cognitive impairment (e.g., dementia and acute confusion). Sensitivity and specificity remain acceptable with MMSE scores greater than or equal to 15.

Cornell Depression Scale

The Cornell Depression Scale[104,105] is a 19-item clinician-administered scale developed to evaluate the full spectrum of depressive symptomatology with both cognitively intact and impaired patients. The examiner rates the individual on each of the 19 items using a four-point grading system: a, unable to evaluate; 0, symptom is absent; 1, symptom is present in mild or intermittent form; 2, symptom is present in severe form. The score is the total of all points assigned and can range from 0 to 38. The higher the score, the more severe the individual's depression. In a recent study by Camus et al.,[106] various parameters of reliability among three measures of depression were compared, and the Cornell Scale was found more reliable than the Sunderland or Hamilton measures.

Using a Measure of Cognition

In using an instrument to measure cognition, the following aspects should be considered:

1. Characteristics of the testing environment
   a. Maximize the comfort and privacy of both examiner and examinee.
   b. Make sure the room is well lit and of a comfortable ambient temperature (prevent glare when using laminated materials with elderly examinees).
   c. Check that the area is free from distractions (noise, test material scattered on the examination table, brightly colored or patterned clothing, jewelry; if a timer is needed, keep one that is quiet and out of the examinee's sight, as its presence, visual and auditory, could be a source of distraction).
   d. Avoid testing in the presence of others, and keep the testing emotionally nonthreatening (e.g., older adults are especially sensitive to having any difficulty thinking; therefore, stress the importance of the testing while taking care not to increase the examinee's anxiety about testing so that an environment is created in which the examinee is motivated to perform well. The order of presentation of items also can be altered so that the examinee experiences success,[11] but care should be taken not to alter the psychometric properties).
2. Characteristics of the examinee and examiner
   a. Use 15 to 20 minutes to establish rapport with the examinee and to determine the examinee's capacity to be tested. Establish whether the examinee has any special problems that could influence testing or its interpretation and implement measures to minimize disturbance. For example, for the elder with hearing impairment, take a position across from the examinee so that he or she can readily use the examiner's nonverbal language as well as read the examiner's lips.
   b. Be alert for signs of fatigue, observing for physical evidence of being tired, slurring of speech, motor slowing, or restlessness,[11] and temporarily terminate testing if necessary. If the examination must be terminated in the middle of a section, it would probably be wise to repeat the entire section when testing is resumed. Dividing of testing should consider the purpose of testing, characteristics of the examinee, and amount and type of information desired.
3. Timing of the measurement. Avoid inappropriate times of the day, such as immediately on awakening from sleep, immediately before and after meals, right before and after medical diagnostic and therapeutic procedures, or in the presence of discomfort or pain.

Interpreting Results

Interpreting results from cognitive testing is not simple and should consist of more than just the score obtained on testing. Consider the nature and pattern of the examinee's responses to testing; the examinee's behavior during testing; the context of testing; the examinee's health history, physical examination, and results of various laboratory and other tests; educational level; occupation; family history; current living situation; level of social functioning; and presence of sensory or motor deficits.[11]

The nature and pattern of the responses to testing can provide valuable information about an individual's cognitive status. Noting the examinee's verbatim responses on testing often is valuable in differential diagnosis. For example, was the examinee not motivated to respond? Did the examinee appear to be capable of performing at a higher level than was attempted? Were "I don't know" responses frequent? If such responses were typical for a given examinee, a likely conclusion would be that the individual is depressed (see Appendix 9C).

Anecdotal notes of the context of testing, the testing environment, and the appearance of the examinee during testing are also important for a better understanding of the performance on testing. Supplementary information from the examinee's health history, physical examination, and laboratory and other tests can provide valuable insight into the individual's performance on testing.

Summary

The available psychometric information, the strengths and limitations of global measures of cognition, measures of specific aspects of cognition, and measures for common disorders of cognition were reviewed in this chapter. Points to consider in selecting and using a measure of cognition and interpretations of test results were discussed. Clearly, the determination of an individual's cognitive status is important in the process and outcomes of illness and its treatment. However, additional testing and refinement of these measures of cognitive status is warranted.

Exemplar Studies

Vermeersch, P.E.H., & Henly, S.J. Validation of the structure for the Clinical Assessment of Confusion-A. *Nurs Res*, 1997, *46*(6):208-213.

This study exemplifies the need to continue debate of the theoretical properties of the concept of confusion and the accompanying measurement issues. This is a replication study to further evaluate the structure of confusion as measured by the Clinical Assessment of Confusion-A (CAC-A). In the development study, dimensions of confusion were identified: cognition, general behavior, motor activity, orientation, psychotic/neurotic behavior, and two uninterpretable factors. In this study, data from 556 nurses were analyzed to evaluate and compare three competing models of confusion: a single-factor unidimensional model, an orthogonal six-factor model, and an oblique six-factor model similar to the structure suggested in the development study. The oblique six-factor model provided the best fit in the predictive sense, and was the most satisfactory from a theoretical sense. Implications for the clinical use of these data were discussed.

Pompei, P., Foreman, M.D., Cassel, C.K., et al. Detecting delirium among hospitalized older patients. *Arch Int Med*, 1995, *155*:301-307.

This study exemplifies many of the inherent dilemmas in the measurement of delirium in older hospitalized patients. The study was a prospective cohort design of 432 elderly patients to examine the diagnostic characteristics of four instruments commonly used clinically to detect delirium: digit span, vigilance A-test, the CAC-A, and the Confusion Assessment Method. The analysis of the diagnostic characteristics of the tests was novel. Diagnostic properties were examined for each instrument; for worst, best, and median scores on each instrument; and for various combinations of the four instruments. In addition to determining sensitivity and specificity, positive and negative likelihood ratios were examined—information clinically useful for determining a specific individual's probability, or likelihood, of being delirious given their performance on the test(s). Results consistently showed that the CAC-A had the best diagnostic characteristics.

Websites for Delirium, Dementia, and Depression

The Iowa Index of Geriatric Assessment Tools (IIGAT) fmp.its.uiowa.edu/iigat

Merck Institute of Aging Health professionals toolkits
www.miahonline.org/tools/index.html

A FilemakerPro database for clinicians www.contexio.com/englishversion.htm
or www.hnet.at/gaw/GAW13E.zip

National Library of Medicine Health Services/Technology Assessment Text
hstat.nlm.gov/hq/Hquest/

"Try This," a publication of the Hartford Institute for Geriatric Nursing, is a series of assessment tools where each issues focuses on a topic specific to older adults
www.hartfordign.org/publications/trythis/

References

1. La Rue, A. *Aging and neuropsychological assessment.* New York: Plenum, 1992.
2. Albert, M.S. Assessment of cognitive dysfunction. In M.S. Albert & M.B. Moss (Eds.), *Geriatric neuropsychology.* New York: Guilford, 1988, pp. 57-81.
3. Strub, R.L., & Black, F.W. *The mental status examination in neurology* (2nd ed.). Philadelphia: Davis, 1985.
4. Foreman, M.D. Acute confusion in the elderly. *Ann Rev Nurs Res,* 1993, 11:1-30.
5. Inouye, S.K., van Dyke, C.H., Alessi, C.A., et al. Clarifying confusion: The Confusion Assessment Method. A new method for detection of delirium. *Ann Intern Med,* 1990, 113(12):941-948.
6. Levkoff, S., Liptzin, B., Cleary, P., et al. Review of research instruments and techniques used to detect delirium. *Int Psychogeriatr,* 1991, 3(2):251-268.
7. Wechsler, D. A standardized memory scale for clinical use. *J Psychol,* 1945, 19:87-95.
8. Pompei, P., Foreman, M.D., Cassel, C.K., et al. Detecting delirium among hospitalized older patients. *Arch Int Med,* 1995, 155:301-307.
9. Reitan, R.M. Validity of the Trail Making Test as an indicator of organic brain damage. *Percept Motor Skill,* 1958, 8(4):271-276.
10. Khan, A.U. *Clinical disorders of memory.* New York: Plenum, 1986.
11. Lezak, M.D. *Neuropsychological assessment* (2nd ed.). New York: Oxford University Press, 1983.
12. Trzepacz, P.T., Baker, R.W., & Greenhouse, J. A symptom rating scale for delirium. *Psychiatr Res,* 1988, 23(1):89-97.
13. Trzepacz, P.T., Brenner, R.P., Coffman, G., & van Thiel, D.H. Delirium in liver transplantation candidates: Discriminant analysis of multiple test variables. *Biol Psychiatr,* 1988, 24(1):3-14.
14. Smith, T.E., & Boyce, E.M. The relationship of the Trail Making Test to psychiatric symptomatology. *J Clin Psychol,* 1962, 18(4):450-454.
15. Trzepacz, P.T., Maue, F.R., Coffman, G., & van Thiel, D.H. Neuropsychiatric assessment of liver transplantation candidates: Delirium and other psychiatric disorders. *Int J Psychiatr Med,* 1986–1987, 16(2):101-111.
16. Albert, M.S. Assessment of cognitive function in the elderly. *Psychosomatics,* 1984, 25(4):310-313, 316-317.
17. Folstein, M., Folstein, S., & McHugh, P. Mini-Mental State Examination: A practical guide for grading the cognitive state of patients for clinicians. *J Psychiatr Res,* 1975, 12(3):189-198.
18. Moore, V., & Wyke, M. Drawing disability in patients with senile dementia. *Psychol Med,* 1984, 14(1):97-105.
19. Ainslie, N.K., & Murden, R.A. Effect of education on the Clock-Drawing Dementia Screen in nondemented elderly persons. *J Am Geriatr Soc,* 1993, 41(3):249-252.
20. Mendez, M.F., Ala, T., & Underwood, K.L. Development of scoring criteria for the Clock Drawing Task in Alzheimer's Disease. *J Am Geriatr Soc,* 1992, 40(11):1095-1099.
21. Sunderland, T., Hill, J.L., Mellow, A.M., et. al. Clock Drawing in Alzheimer's Disease: A novel measure of dementia severity. *J Am Geriatr Soc,* 1989, 37(8):725-729.
22. Tuokko, H., Hadjistavropoulos, T., Miller, J.A., & Beattie, B.L. The clock test: A sensitivity measure to differentiate normal elderly from those with Alzheimer Disease. *J Am Geriatr Soc,* 1992, 40(6):579-584.
23. Watson, Y.I., Arfken, C.L., & Birge, S.J. Clock completion: An objective screening test for dementia. *J Am Geriatr Soc,* 1993, 41(11):1235-1240.
24. Barrie, M.A. (2002). Objective screening tools to assess cognitive impairment and depression. *Top Geriatr Rehab,* 18(2):28-46.
25. Richardson, H.E., & Glass, J.N. A comparison of scoring protocols on the Clock Drawing Test in relation to ease of use, diagnostic group, and correlations with Mini-Mental State Examination. *J Am Geriatri Soc,* 2002, 50,169-173.
26. Goodglass, H., & Kaplan, E. *The assessment of aphasia and related disorders.* Philadelphia: Lea & Febiger, 1972.
27. Kertesz, A. *The Western Aphasia Battery.* New York: Grune & Stratton, 1982.
28. Kaplan, E., Goodglass, H., & Weintraub, S. (Eds.) *Boston Naming Test.* Philadelphia: Lea & Febiger, 1983.
29. Halstead, W.C., & Wepman, J.M. The Halstead-Wepman Aphasia Screening Test. *J Speech Hear Dis,* 1949, 14(1):9-15.
30. Reitan, R., & Davison, L.A. *Clinical neuropsychology: Current status and applications.* New York: Hemisphere, 1974.
31. Heimburger, R.F., & Reitan, R.M. Easily administered written test for lateralizing brain lesions. *J Neurosurg,* 1961, 18(3):301-312.
32. Shewan, C.M., & Kertesz, A. Reliability and validity characteristics of the Western Aphasia Battery (WAB). *J Speech Hear Dis,* 1980, 45(3):308-324.
33. Horner, J., Dawson, D.V., Heyman, A., & Fish, A.M. The usefulness of the Western Aphasia Battery for differential diagnosis of Alzheimer's dementia and focal stroke syndromes: preliminary evidence. *Brain Lang,* 1992, 42(1):77-88.
34. Benton, A.L. *The Revised Visual Retention Test.* Iowa City: University of Iowa Press, 1955.
35. Randt, C.T., Brown, E.R., & Osborne, D.P., Jr. A memory test for longitudinal measurement of mild to moderate deficits. *Clin Neuropsychol,* 1980, 2(4):184-194.
36. Kane, R.A., & Kane, R.L. *Assessing the elderly: A practical guide to measurement.* Lexington, MA: Lexington Books, 1984.
37. Klonoff, H., & Kennedy, M. Memory and perceptual functioning in octogenarians and nonoctogenarians in the community. *J Gerontol,* 1965, 20(3):328-333.
38. Baker, E.L., Feldman, R.G., White, R.F., et al. Monitoring neurotoxins in industry: Development of a

neurobehavioral test battery. *J Occup Med*, 1983, *25*(2):125-130.

39. Erickson, R.C., & Howieson, D. The clinician's perspective: Measuring change and treatment effectiveness. In L.W. Poon (Ed.), *Handbook for clinical memory assessment of older adults*. Hyattsville, MD: American Psychological Association, 1986, pp. 69-80.

40. Israel, L., Kozarevic, D., Sartorius, N. *Source book of geriatric assessment* (vol. 1). Geneva: World Health Organization, 1984.

41. Benton, A.L. A multiple choice type of visual retention test. *Arch Neurol*, 1950, *64*:699-707.

42. Benton, A.L., Hamsher, K. de S., & Stone, F.B. *Visual retention test: Multiple choice I*. Iowa City, IA: University of Iowa Hospital and Clinics, 1977.

43. Benton, A.L. Differential behavioral effects in frontal lobe disease. *Neuropsychologia*, 1968, *6*(1):53-60.

44. Benton, A.L. *Contributions to clinical neuropsychology*. New York: Aldine, 1969.

45. Arena, R., & Gainotti, G. Constructional apraxia and visuopractic disabilities in relation to laterality of cerebral lesions. *Cortex*, 1978, *14*(4):463-473.

46. Crookes, T.G., & McDonald, K.G. Benton's Visual Retention Test in the differentiation of depression and early dementia. *Br J Soc Clin Psychol*, 1972, *11*(1):66-69.

47. Blanton, P.D., & Gouvier, W.D. A systematic solution to the Benton Visual Retention Test: A caveat to examiners. *Int J Clin Neuropsychol*, 1985, *7*(2):95-96.

48. Gorham, D.R. A proverbs test for clinical and experimental use. *Psychol Rep*, 1956, *2*(monograph suppl. 1): 1-12.

49. Fogel, M.L. The Proverbs Test in appraisal of cerebral disease. *J Gen Psychol*, 1965, *72*(2):269-275.

50. Bromley, D.B. Some effects of age on the quality of intellectual output. *J Gerontol*, 1957, *12*(3):318-323.

51. Nelson, H.E. A modified card sorting test sensitive to frontal lobe defects. *Cortex*, 1976, *12*(4):313-324.

52. Kiernan, R.L., Mueller, J., Langston, J.W., & Van Dyke, C. The Neurobehavioral Cognitive Screening Examination: A brief but differentiated approach to cognitive assessment. *Ann Intern Med*, 1987, *107*(4):481-485.

53. Schwamm, L.H., Van Dyke, C., Kiernan, R.J., et al. The Neurobehavioral Cognitive Status Examination: Comparison with the Cognitive Capacity Screening Examination and the Mini-Mental State Examination in a neurological population. *Ann Intern Med*, 1987, *107*(4):486-491.

54. Anthony, J.C., LeResche, L., Niaz, U., et al. Limits of the "Mini-Mental State" as a screening test for dementia and delirium among hospital patients. *Psychol Med*, 1982, *12*(2):397-408.

55. Kaufman, D.M., Weinberger, M., Strain, J.J., & Jacobs, J.W. Detection of cognitive deficits by a brief mental status examination: The Cognitive Capacity Screening Examination, a reappraisal and a review. *Gen Hosp Psychiatr*, 1979, *1*(3):247-255.

56. Tombaugh, T.N., & McIntyre, N.J. The Mini-Mental State Examination: A comprehensive review. *J Am Geriatr Soc*, 1992, *40*(9):922-935.

57. Omer, H., Foldes, J., Toby, M., & Menczel, J. Screening for cognitive deficits in a sample of hospitalized geriatric patients: A re-evaluation of a brief mental status questionnaire. *J Am Geriatr Soc*, 1983, *31*(5):266-268.

58. Bird, H.R., Canino, G., Stipec, M.R., & Shrout, P. Use of the Mini-Mental State Examination in a probability sample of a Hispanic population. *J Nerv Ment Dis*, 1987, *175*(12):731-737.

59. Bleecker, M.L., Bolla-Wilson, K., Kawas, C., & Agnew, J. Age-specific norms for the Mini-Mental State Exam. *Neurology*, 1988, *38*(10):1565-1568.

60. Escobar, J.I., Burnam, A., Karno, M., et al. Use of the Mini-Mental State Examination (MMSE) in a community population of mixed ethnicity: Cultural and linguistic artifacts. *J Nerv Ment Dis*, 1986, *174*(10):607-614.

61. Magaziner, J., Bassett, S.S., & Hebel, J.R. Predicting performance on the Mini-Mental State Examination: Use of age- and education-specific equations. *J Am Geriatr Soc*, 1987, *35*(11):996-1000.

62. Jacobs, J.W., Bernard, M.R., Delgado, A., & Strain, J.J. Screening for organic mental syndromes in the medically ill. *Ann Intern Med*, 1977, *86*(1):40-46.

63. Marcantonio, E.R., Goldman, L., Mangione, C.M., et al. A clinical prediction rule for delirium after elective noncardiac surgery. *JAMA*, 1994, *271*(2):134-139.

64. American Psychiatric Association. *The diagnostic and statistical manual for mental disorders* (4th ed., text revision). Washington, DC: APA, 2000.

65. Foreman, M.D. Acute confusion in the hospitalized elderly: A research dilemma. *Nurs Res*, 1986, *35*(1):34-38.

66. Vermeersch, P.E.H. The Clinical Assessment of Confusion-A. *Appl Nurs Res*, 1990, *3*(3):128-133.

67. Vermeersch, P.E.H., & Henly, S.J. Validation of the structure for the Clinical Assessment of Confusion-A. *Nurs Res*, 1997, *46*(6):208-213.

68. Mion, L.C., & Nagley, S.J. Clinical assessment of confusion in long-term care. *Appl Nurs Res*, 1992, *5*(2):100-104.

69. Foreman, M.D. Confusion in the hospitalized elderly: incidence, onset and associated factors. *Res Nurs Health*, 1989, *12*:21-29.

70. Neelon, V.J., Champagne, M.T., Carlson, J.R., & Funk, S.G. The NEECHAM Confusion Scale: Construction, validation, and clinical testing. *Nurs Res*, 1996, *45*(6):324-330.

71. Johansson, I.S., Hamrin, E.K.F., & Larsson, G. Psychometric testing of the NEECHAM Confusion Scale among patients with hip fracture. *Res Nurs Health*, 2002, *25*:203-211.

72. Ely, E.W., Margolin, R., Francis, J., et al. Evaluation of delirium in critically ill patients:Validation of the Confusion Assessment Method for the intensive care unit (CAM-ICU). *Crit Care Med*, 2001, *29*:1370-1379.

73. Grassi, L., Caraceni, A., Beltrami, E., et al. Assessing delirium in cancer patients: The Italian versions of the Delirium Rating Scale and the Memorial Delirium Assessment Scale. *J Pain Symptom Manage*, 2001, *21*(1):59-68.

74. Rolfson, D.B., McElhaney, J.E., Jhangri, G.S., & Rockwood, K. Validity of the Confusion Assessment Method in detecting postoperative delirium in the elderly. *Int Psychogeriatr*, 2001, *11*(4):431-438.

75. Monette, J., du Fort, G., Fung, S.H., et al. Evaluation of the Confusion Assessment Method (CAM) as a

screening tool for delirium in the emergency room. *Gen Hosp Psychiatr*, 2001, *23*:20-25.

76. Ely, E.W., Inouye, S.K., Bernard, G.R., et al. Delirium in mechanically ventilated patients. Validity and reliability of the Confusion Assessment Method for the intensive care unit (CAM-ICU). *JAMA*, 2001, *286*:2701-2710.

77. Hart, R.P., Levenson, J.L., Sessler, C.N., et al. Validation of a cognitive test for delirium in medical ICU patients. *Psychosomatics*, 1996, *37*:533-546.

78. Hart, R.P., Best, A.M., Sessler, C.N., & Levenson, J.L. Abbreviated cognitive test for delirium. *J Psychosomatic Res*, 1997, *43*:417-423.

79. Albert, M.S., Levkoff, S.E., Reilly, C., et al. The Delirium Symptom Interview: An interview for the detection of delirium symptoms in hospitalized patients. *J Geriatr Psychiatr Neurol*, 1992, *5*(1):1421.

80. McCusker, J., Cole, M., Bellavance, F., & Primeau, F. Delirium: Reliability and validity of a new measure of severity of delirium. *Int Psychogeriatrics*, 1998, *10*(4):421-433.

81. McCusker, J., Cole, M., Abrahamowicz, M., et al. Delirium predicts 12-month mortality. *Arch Inter Med*, 2002, *162*:457-463.

82. McCusker, J., Cole, M., Abrahamowicz, M., et al. Environmental risk factors for delirium in hospitalized older people. *J Am Geriatr Soc*, 2001, *49*:1327-1334.

83. Han, L., McCusker, J., Cole, M., et al. Use of medications with anticholinergic effect predicts clinical severity of delirium symptoms in older medical inpatients. *Arch Intern Med*, 2001, *161*(8),1099-1105.

84. Brietbart, W., Rosenfeld, B., Roth, A., et al. The Memorial Delirium Assessment Scale. *J Pain Symptom Manage*, 1997, *13*:128-137.

85. Brietbart, W. Author's response. Re: Memorial Delirium Assessment Scale and commentary [letter]. *J Pain Symptom Manage*, 1998, *15*:74-75.

86. Lawlor, P.G., Watanabe, S., Walker, P., & Bruera, E.D. Re: Memorial Delirium Assessment Scale and commentary [letter]. *J Pain Symptom Manage*, 1998, *15*:73-74.

87. Lawlor, P.G., Nekolaichuk, C., Gagnon, B., et al. Clinical utility, factor analysis, and further validation of the Memorial Delirium Assessment Scale in patients with advanced cancer. *Cancer*, 2000, *88*:2859-2867.

88. Lawlor, P.G., Gagnon, B., Mancini, I.L., et al. Occurrence, causes, and outcome of delirium in patients with advanced cancer: A prospective study. *Arch Intern Med*, 2000, *160*:786-794.

89. Roth-Roemer, S., Fann, J., & Syrjala, K. The importance of recognizing and measuring delirium. *J Pain Symptom Manage*, 1997, *13*:125-127.

90. Bondareff, W. Biomedical perspective of Alzheimer's disease and dementia in the elderly. In M.L.M. Gilhooly, S.H. Zarit, & J.E. Birren (Eds.), *The dementias: Policy and management*. Englewood Cliffs, NJ: Prentice-Hall, 1986, pp. 13-37.

91. Mattis, S. Mental status examination for organic mental syndrome in the elderly patient. In L. Bellak

& T.B. Karasu (Eds.), *Geriatric psychiatry: A handbook for psychiatrists and primary care physicians*. New York: Grune & Stratton, 1976, pp. 77-121.

92. Morris, J., LaBarge, E., Clark, C., et al. CERAD clinical and neuropsychological assessment of Alzheimer's disease: A preliminary report of standardized procedures and reliability [abstract]. *Neurology*, 1988, *38*(suppl 1):287.

93. Welsh, K., Butters, N., Hughes, J., et al. Detection of abnormal memory decline in mild cases of Alzheimer's disease using CERAD neuropsychological measures. *Arch Neurol*, 1991, *48*(3):278-281.

94. Stabb, A., & Lyles, M. *Manual of geriatric nursing*. Glenview, IL: Scott-Foresman, 1990, pp. 528-529.

95. Thompson, L.W., Futterman, A., & Gallagher, D. Assessment of late-life depression. *Psychopharmacol Bull*, 1988, *24*(4):577-586.

96. Thompson, L.W., Gong, V., Haskins, E., & Gallagher, D. Assessment of depression and dementia during the late years. *Ann Rev Gerontol Geriatr*, 1987, *7*:295-324.

97. Beck, A.T., Ward, C.H., Mendelson, M., et al. An inventory for measuring depression. *Arch Gen Psychiatr*, 1961, *4*(6):53-63.

98. Gallagher, D., Breckenridge, J., Steinmetz, J., & Thompson, L. The Beck Depression Inventory and Research Diagnostic Criteria: Congruence in an older population. *J Consult Clin Psychol*, 1983, *51*(6):945-946.

99. Hamilton, M. Development of a rating scale for primary depressive illness. *Br J Soc Clin Psychol*, 1967, *6*(4):278-296.

100. Brink, T.L., Yesavage, J.A., Lum, O., et al. Screening tests for geriatric depression. *Clin Gerontol*, 1982, *1*(1):37-43.

101. Burke, W.J., Nitcher, R.L., Roccaforte, W.H., & Wengel, S.P. A prospective evaluation of the Geriatric Depression Scale in an outpatient geriatric assessment center. *J Am Geriatr Soc*, *40*(12):1227-1230.

102. Parmalee, P.A., Lawton, M.P., & Katz, I.R. Psychometric properties of the Geriatric Depression Scale among the institutionalized aged. *Psychol Assessment*, 1989, *1*(4):331-338.

103. Yesavage, J.A., Brink, T.L., Rose, T.L., & Adey, M. The Geriatric Depression Rating Scale: Comparison with other self-report and psychiatric rating scales. In T. Crook, S. Ferris, & R. Bartus (Eds.), *Assessment in geriatric psychopharmacology*. New Canaan, CT: Mark Powley, 1983, pp. 153-167.

104. Alexopoulos, G.S., Abrams, R.C., Young, R.C., & Shamoian, C.A. Use of the Cornell Scale in nondemented patients. *J Am Geriatr Soc*, 1988, *36*(3):230-236.

105. Alexopoulos, G.S., Abrams, R.C., Young, R.C., & Shamoian, C.A. Cornell Scale for depression in dementia. *Biol Psychiatr*, 1988, *23*(3):271-284.

106. Camus, V., Schmitt, L., Ousset, P.J., et. al. A comparative study of Hamilton, Cornell, and Sunderland depression rating scales [abstract]. *J Am Geriatr Soc*, 1993, *41*:SA42.

Appendix 9A. Advantages and Disadvantages of Specific Measures

Dimension Tested	Psychometric Properties (references)	Advantages (references)	Disadvantages (references)
Attention			
Digit Span	Sensitivity: 0.34 (8), specificity: 0.90 (8)	Brief norms available (7)	Insensitive to mild inattentiveness; confounds attention with primary memory
Vigilance Test	Sensitivity: 0.722 (7), specificity: 0.564 (7) (when used with moderately demented elderly examinees)	Can test nonverbal patients with predetermined method (eye blink); does not have educational, intellectual, or socioeconomic bias	Cannot be used with hearing-impaired persons
Trail-making test (TMT)	Sensitivity: Part A: 0.75; Part B: 0.917 Specificity: Part A: 0.821; Part B: 0.731	Useful in identifying attentional deficit but not in determining exact nature of impairment	Reliability altered by variability in examiner's reaction time and time for patient to make correction (11) High false-positive rates Practice effects; age bias; poor tolerance by older hospitalized patients (8) Cannot be used with people who are visually impaired
Visuospatial ability			
Clock-Drawing test	Internal consistency: 0.95 (20) Test–retest reliability: 0.70 (20,22) Interrater reliability: 0.48–0.95 Concurrent validity varies (correlation with MMSE 0.4; Rey Complex Figure 0.66) (17,19) Sensitivity: 0.47–0.90 Specificity: 0.48–1.00 Clock setting has greatest sensitivity (87%), specificity (82%), test–retest reliability (0.82), Kappa (0.63) and interrater reliability (0.90–0.93)	Brief and easy administration Variable methods of scoring and interpreting results	Lack of standardized performance instructions between versions preventing direct comparisons Biased against poorly educated persons May measure more complex and higher aspects cognition (abstraction, reasoning)
Language			
Halstead-Wepman Aphasia Screening Test	Not available	Brief (<30 minutes) Covers essential language abilities Discriminates among various types of aphasia	No guidelines for clinical applications so must be used by experienced examiners; no standardized scoring procedure

Appendix 9A. Advantages and Disadvantages of Specific Measures (*cont.*)

Dimension Tested	Psychometric Properties (references)	Advantages (references)	Disadvantages (references)
Boston-Naming Test	Internal consistency reliability: 0.68–0.96 (26)	Relieves examinee's frustration of failure by providing possibility of success Differentiates among types of aphasic individuals Provides evidence that a word is in examinee's potential vocabulary	Requires visual abilities
Western Aphasia Battery	Cronbach's alpha: 0.905 Bentler's coefficient theta: 0.975 Correlations among subtests: >0.60 Test–retest reliability: >0.88 Overall interrater reliability: >0.90 Construct validity Face and content validity	Discriminates aphasia from other brain damage language problems	Least able to classify patients with hemisphere strokes (33)
Memory			
Wechsler Memory Scale (WMS)	Validity questioned as to whether test measures motivation, cooperation, willingness to memorize material of little value (29) Test–retest for subscales: 0.41–0.60 (recall), 0.75–0.89 (total score) Cronbach's alpha: 0.686 (figural; 0.44; digit 0.88 Construct validity (3 factors) (7,37–39)	Easy to use, short (15–30 minutes) Allowance made for memory variances with age Memory quotient directly comparable to other intellectual functions Useful in the detection of special memory defects with specific brain injuries	Highly verbal test Overemphasis on very basic processes Combining widely variable tests to make "memory quotient" Age correction may invalidate data (3) Reliance on mental quotient when memory is multidimensional
Benton Visual Retention Test	Difficult to interpret as may use alternate form and administration Test–retest reliability (Adm A): 0.85 (43); Form C 0.58–0.60, with interrater reliability 0.95 (11) Discriminant validity for depression and dementia (standard admin, A) (46)	Three alternative forms allow use of one for a copy trial (11)	Alternative forms may not be equivalent (11,34)

Test			
Randt Memory Test	Validity of incidental learning questioned (1) Traditional indices not reported	Short (20 minutes) Accuracy in evaluating conditions associated with aging and diffuse brain diseases (11)	Highly verbal so penalizes patients with language disorders Insensitive to memory impairments involving nonverbal material (11) Requires skilled examiner so patient not questioned to point of discomfort but can push when low-level responses occur
Story Recall	Sensitive for short-term verbal recall (3,11) Traditional indices of reliability and validity not reported Equivalence among versions not done		
Conceptualization			
Proverbs Test	Not reported	Objective scores of abstractness and concreteness and can be compared with norms Decreased variation in administration and scoring (decreased bias) (11) Marginal discrimination	Scores vary by level of individual's education Concrete responses increase with age
Modified Card Sorting Test	Not reported		No scoring norms but may be rarely needed

Appendix 9B. Advantages and Disadvantages of Global Measures

Testing Dimension	Psychometric Properties (references)	Advantages (references)	Disadvantages (references)
Mental Status			
Mini-Mental State Examination	Reliable and valid Test-retest reliability: 0.82–0.98 Interrater reliability 0.88 (52) Internal consistency: 0.96 Criterion-related validity (confusion), Spearman's rho = 0.76 Discriminant validity (depression), $r = 0.38$ Concurrent validity (confusion), c, $r = 0.80$; vas-c, $r = 0.83$	Robust measurement across settings Discriminates among normal, depressed, demented, and demented depressed individuals	Total scores do not reveal precise neuropsychiatric diagnosis May be ecologically invalid
Cognitive Capacity Screening Examination	Validation studies (62) Interrater reliability: 100% Sensitivity: 0.71–0.79; specificity: 0.45 (57) Internal consistency reliability: 0.97 Concurrent validity (MMSE) is 0.78, (SPMSQ) is 0.71	Brief (5–10 minutes)	Performance influenced by age, education level, ethnicity, language (17,56–59) Cannot distinguish between acute and chronic impairment All aspects of cognition not assessed Verbal, so cannot be used with nonverbal persons
Neurobehavioral Cognitive Status Examination	More sensitive for detecting cognitive impairment than MMSE, CCSE (53) because it scores each cognitive area separately, uses graded series of test items, and assesses a larger number of areas of cognitive function	Brief (10–20 minutes) Easy to administer Provides differential profile of patient's cognitive status	
Delirium			
Clinical Assessment of Confusion-A	In hospitalized adults (8, 65, 66, 69): interrater reliability 0.88–0.89 (66, 69), concurrent validity with SPMSQ 0.71, VAS-C 0.81–0.82 (69) Test-retest: 0.85 (69) Internal consistency: 0.80 (69) Cohen's kappa: 0.79 (69) Sensitivity: 0.36, Specificity: 0.95 (8).	Checklist of 25 psychomotor behaviors Easy scoring, brief admin –5 minutes, no training needed, no response burden	Recent studies show different psychometric indices (68) Nurses in acute care may perceive confused behavior differently from nurses in intermediate care (66)

Instrument	Reliability and validity	Advantages	Disadvantages
NEECHAM Confusion Scale	In nursing home residents (68) Internal consistency KR20 0.69 Correlation with MMSE −0.51, VAS 0.81 Hospitalized and institutionalized elders (70) Interrater reliability: 0.96 Test–retest reliability: 0.98 Internal consistency (Cronbach's alpha = 0.90) Correlations to MMSE 0.25–0.64 Sensitivity (70): NEECHAM Score ≤24 = 0.95 Specificity 0.78	Reflects clinical reality low response burden	Subjective Immature scale requires training
Delirium Rating Scale (DRS)	Correlations (15) with MMSE −0.43, and TMT-B 0.66 (15) Interrater reliability 0.97 (15)	Differentiates delirious patients from normal and from those with schizophrenia and dementia Superior over earlier symptom rating scales	Scoring relies on subjective clinical judgements from unstructured clinical assessments Expensive
Confusion Assessment Method (CAM)	Face and content validity Sensitivity: 0.86–1.0 Specificity: 0.90–1.00 Positive predictive accuracy 0.91–0.94; negative predictive accuracy 0.90–1.0 Convergent validity: (MMSE) $k = 0.64$, (story recall) $k = 0.59$, (VAS-C) $k = 0.82$, (Digit Scan) $k = 0.66$ Item analysis: inattention and disorganization of thought most diagnostic for delirium Interobserver reliability: high Cohen's kappa 0.81–1.0 ($k = 0.90$)	Suitable for use at bedside to assist in identifying patients with delirium (8)	Visual and auditory ability required
Confusion Assessment Method for the Intensive Care Unit (CAM-ICU)	Interrater reliability: 0.84–0.96 (72, 76) Sensitivity: 0.93–1.0 (72, 76) Specificity: 0.89–1.0 (72, 76)	Brief and easy administration 2 minutes on average	Insufficient testing

Appendix 9B. Advantages and Disadvantages of Global Measures (*cont.*)

Testing Dimension	Psychometric Properties (references)	Advantages (references)	Disadvantages (references)
Delirium Index (DI)	Interrater reliability, between RAs, 0.78 Between RA and geropsychiatrists, 0.88 Criterion validity with DRS, r = 0.84 Convergent validity with MMSE, r = 0.60, and with Barthel Index, r = –060 Discriminant validity with IADLs, 0.42, and with the IQCODE, 0.26	Brief, easy administration Low response burden	Insufficient testing
Memorial Delirium Assessment Scale (MDAS)	Internal consistency reliability Cronbach's alpha = 0.91 (84) Concurrent validity with the DRS r = 0.88 (84); with the MMSE, r = –0.91; with a clinician's global rating of the severity of delirium, r = 0.89 Sensitivity analysis with cutpoint = 13; Sensitivity = 0.706 Specificity = 0.938 Positive predictive value = 0.923 Negative predictive value = 0.75 with cutpoint of 7, sensitivity = 0.98; specificity = 0.96 Interrater reliability, intraclass correlation coefficients, 0.69–1.00	Able to prorate ratings when information about a feature of delirium absent (84, 88) Format allows for easy, brief administration (89) Items based on current diagnostic standards (89) Potential for frequent administration (84, 89)	Low reliability in assessing severity of delirium (89) Insufficient reliability and validity testing in limited samples of small numbers (89)
Delirium Symptom Interview (DSI)	(Sample: 50 elders in acute care) Sensitivity 0.90 Specificity 0.80 Positive predictive value 0.87 Negative predictive value 0.84 Interrater reliability-Cohen's kappa 0.90 Interrater agreement on symptom domains 0.46 (fluctuating behavior) to 1.0 (disorientation, sleep disturbance) Internal consistency reliability: Cronbach's alpha, disturbance	Can be used with any population (i.e., sensory, communication deficits; very ill) Lay individuals can reliably use the DSI Less subjective rating of symptoms All domains evaluated DSI can be administered daily without burden or a learning effect	Constructed in outdated diagnostic criteria (DSM-III vs. DSM-IV) Indices of internal consistency are marginally acceptable DSI has not been used by other teams

of consciousness 0.80;
disorientation 0.75;
incoherent speech 0.61;
psychomotor behavior 0.56;
sleep disturbance 0.45

Dementia

Mattis Dementia Rating Scale (MDRS)	High test–retest reliability (1 week interval correlation was >0.90) Internal consistency reliability 0.90 Concurrent validation with other similar measures >0.67 (91)	Correlation of scores with cerebral blood flow >0.80 while scores <100 associated with death	Can take 30–45 minutes
Consortium to Establish a Registry for Alzheimer's Disease (CERAD)	(Sample: 354 patients with AD, 278 nondemented subjects) Interrater agreement: 0.092 (constructional praxis) to 1.0 (word list recall) Test–retest reliability: 0.44–0.90 (1-month interval) Discriminant validity: distinguishes AD from nondemented individual Construct validity: factor analysis: 3 factors accounting for 73% variance	More recent testing of sensitivity (93) (Sample 549 with AD and 390 controls): 0.86–0.96 Classification ability 0.91	Classification ability decreases to 0.84 when attempting to discriminate mildly from moderately impaired individuals

Depression

Beck Depression Inventory (BDI)	Split half reliability: 0.86–0.93 Test–retest reliability 0.74 (3-month interval); with elderly, depressed subjects, Excellent congruence with Research Diagnostic Criteria Specificity 0.82 (cutpoint 10) vs. 0.96 (cutpoint 17) Sensitivity 0.89 (cutpoint 10) vs. 0.57 (cutpoint 17) DSM-II criteria for depression (cutpoint 10): sensitivity 0.89, specificity 0.82; (cutpoint 17): sensitivity 0.50, specificity 0.92 Predictive validity 0.85, 0.88–0.91 Correct classification of patients, interrater reliability 0.73	Can identify major > minor depressive disorders (98) Internal consistency 0.91	Self-rating nature of scale susceptible to manipulation or socially desirable answers

Appendix 9B. Advantages and Disadvantages of Global Measures (*cont.*)

Testing Dimension	Psychometric Properties (references)	Advantages (references)	Disadvantages (references)
Hamilton Depression Rating Scale (HDRS)	Sensitive to change in elderly depressives Psychometric problems, but most laboratories report high reliability Interrater reliability: 0.80–0.90 (95) Construct validity-factor analysis up to 3 factors: (1) general factor of depression, (2) anxious depression factor, (3) index of instability subjects older adults	Provides common denominator for communicating information about level of depression across samples	Weighting shifts from frequency to intensity factor depending on dimension tested Heavily weighted toward somatic symptomatology so in elderly may result in false positives
Geriatric Depression Short-Scale Form (GDS-SF)	(Cutpoint 10): sensitivity: 0.84–0.89; specificity: 0.73–0.095 (compared to RDC and DSM-II criteria) Discriminant validity with clinical diagnosis: 0.84 Concurrent validity with HDRS and SDS High correlation with RDC definition of depression	Simple yes/no response format for symptom evaluation so may be more appropriate with cognitively impaired elders or low educational level Sensitivity and specificity acceptable when MMSE scores > 15	
Cornell Depression Scale	High sensitivity, correlates significantly with RDC diagnoses Concurrent validation with independent psychiatric diagnoses if depression R(s) = 0.81 Interrater reliability: 0.82–0.93, Cohen's kappa = 0.74 Internal consistency = 0.98	Equally sensitive in cognitively intact and impaired individuals Easy to administer and score Cornell scale most reliable compared to Hamilton and Sutherland (106)	

Appendix 9C. Comparison of the Clinical Features of Delirium, Dementia, and Depression

Feature	Delirium	Dementia	Depression
Onset	Acute/subacute; depends on cause	Chronic, generally insidious; depends on cause	Coincides with life changes; often abrupt
Course	Short, diurnal fluctuations in symptoms; worse at night, in the dark, and on awakening	Long, no diurnal effects; symptoms progressive yet relatively stable over time	Diurnal effects; typically worse in morning; situational fluctuations, but less than with delirium
Progression	Abrupt	Slow but even	Variable, rapid to slow but uneven
Duration	Hours to less than 1 month, seldom longer	Months to years	At least 2 weeks, but can be several months to years
Awareness	Reduced	Clear	Clear
Alertness	Fluctuates, lethargic, or hypervigilant	Generally normal	Normal
Attention	Impaired, fluctuates	Generally normal	Minimal impairment, distractibility
Orientation	Fluctuates in severity, generally impaired	May be impaired	Selective disorientation
Memory	Recent and immediate impaired	Recent and remote impaired	Selective or patchy impairment; "islands" of intact memory
Thinking	Disorganized, distorted, fragmented, slow, or accelerated incoherent speech	Difficulty with abstraction; thoughts impoverished; judgment impaired; words difficult to find	Intact but with themes of hopelessness, helplessness, or self-deprecation
Perception	Distorted; illusions, delusions, and hallucinations; difficulty distinguishing between reality and misperceptions	Misperceptions often absent	Intact; delusions and hallucinations absent, except in severe cases
Psychomotor behavior	Variable, hypokinetic, hyperkinetic, or mixed cycle reversed	Normal, may have apraxia	Variable; psychomotor disturbed; often early morning awakening
Associated features	Variable affective changes; symptoms of autonomic hyperarousal; exaggeration of personality type; associated with physical illness	Affect tends to be superficial, inappropriate, and labile; attempts to conceal deficits in intellect, personality changes, aphasia, agnosia may be present; lacks insight	Affect depressed; dysphoric mood; exaggerated and detailed complaints; preoccupied with personal thoughts; insight present; verbal elaboration
Mental status testing	Distracted from task	Failings highlighted by family; frequent "near-miss" answers; struggles with test; great effort to find an appropriate reply	Failings highlighted by the examinee; frequent "don't know" answers; little effort; frequently gives up, indifferent; does not care or attempt to find an answer

Adapted from Foreman, M.D. Acute confusion in the hospitalized elderly: A research dilemma. *Nurs Res*, 1986, *35*(1):34.

10

Single Instruments for Measuring Quality of Life

Geraldine V. Padilla, Marilyn Frank-Stromborg, and Setsuko Koresawa

The proliferation of health-related quality of life (HQOL) instruments since the mid-1970s makes it necessary to narrow this chapter's focus to general measures of HQOL. Many of these general measures have been adapted for use with specific diseases, such as cancer, heart failure, or arthritis; different types of cancers, such as prostate; or different types of treatments, such as bone marrow transplantation. A number of measures have been translated into a variety of languages, indicating that, despite cultural differences, some aspects of quality of life resonate across cultures. Also included in this chapter are instruments specifically designed for people with cancer. Some cancer-related quality-of-life (QOL) measures have several versions for different types of cancers or treatments. This chapter focuses on quantitative measures of HQOL and highlights four of the most commonly used quantitative instruments in the public domain. The chapter includes single instruments that yield numeric scores for the total scale or subscales and maintains older references if the references are relevant.

Definitions of Quality of Life

In 1993 an international group of investigators led by Drs. Orley, Kuyken, and Sartorius and working under the auspices of the Division of Mental Health of the World Health Organization (WHO) defined quality of life as "an individual's perception of their position in life in the context of the culture and value systems in which they live and in relation to their goals, expectations, standards and concerns." These investigators define six broad domains of quality of life: physical health, psychologic state, levels of independence, social relationships, environmental features, and spiritual concerns, including personal beliefs. This definition reflects the view that quality of life refers to a subjective evaluation, which is embedded in a cultural, social, and environmental context. As such, quality of life cannot be equated simply with the terms *health status, lifestyle, life satisfaction, mental state,* or *well-being*. Rather, it is a multidimensional concept incorporating the "individual's perception of these and other aspects of life."[1]

At a United States Public Health Service (USPHS) National Institutes of Health (NIH) workshop on QOL assessment led by Drs. Furberg and Schuttinga, a group of scientists agreed that a concise, clearly stated operational definition of HQOL was preferable to a global definition. Workshop participants adopted this working definition: "Health-related quality of life is the value assigned to duration of life as modified by the impairments, functional states, perceptions and social opportunities influenced by disease, injury, treatment or policy."[2] Both definitions of QOL and HQOL are relevant a decade later.

The WHO definition emphasizes the subjective nature of QOL evaluations, the importance of the cultural and value context in which judgments are made, and the relevance of goals, expectations, and standards.[1] The NIH QOL workshop definition reflects the scientific need for specificity and objectivity.[2] Quality is based on a value that may be assigned to the duration of life by the patient, family, health care provider, policymaker, or other person. HQOL is limited to the aspects of life that are important to the evaluator in the context of health and illness. This chapter does not adhere to a specific conceptual or operational definition of QOL except to focus on HQOL measures. It should be noted, however, that current publications use the terms *quality of life* and *health-related quality of life* interchangeably to refer to the same or different outcomes. The different HQOL definitions and measurements used across studies make it difficult to compare QOL outcomes.

Bard's 1984 views are endorsed by current investigators. He held that the term *quality of life* is too broad and inclusive to be meaningful. It is operationally defined in very different ways by different investigators, leading to measures of different aspects of QOL.[3] Representative HQOL domain frameworks are offered in Appendix 10A. Strickland points out that some QOL conceptualizations have included not only dimensions of the concept but also covariates.[4] For example, Strickland questions the inclusion of coping ability or self-esteem in QOL definitions because these variables may be covariates, not dimensions. Investigators need to be aware of these definitional differences that translate into differences in measures of QOL/HQOL.

Dimensions of Quality of Life

Flanagan's study represents an early attempt to define the dimensions that constitute QOL. He studied 3000 Americans of varying age and health status in terms of their perceptions of what constitutes QOL.[5] Using the critical incident technique, he identified the factors a healthy population would consider important for quality of life. A sample question is "Think of the last time you did something very important to you or had an experience that was especially satisfying to you. What did you do or what happened that was so satisfying to you?"[5] Flanagan asked two critical incident questions and obtained 6500 critical incidents. Categorization by independent judges resulted in 15 factors that included all of the 6500 critical incidents. A sample of 3000 people (age 30 to 70 years) was then asked one question about each of these 15 factors: "At this time in your life, how important is _____?" Flanagan found that six dimensions were extremely important to overall QOL: health, having and raising children, material comforts, work, close relationship with a spouse, and understanding oneself.

Subsequent research has clearly implicated health in determining life satisfaction and overall HQOL.[6,7] Health indices have been developed to define QOL as it applies to the state of wellness of the individual. Earlier health indices tended to concentrate on the physical functions of patients and to rely on cross-sectional (one-time) analyses of their health status. The literature indicates that this narrow, functional definition of health status has changed. A meta-analysis of 12 studies showed that patients perceive QOL as distinct from health status, thereby indicating that a measure of health status should not be used as a measure of QOL.[8] Mental health is more important than physical functioning in ratings of QOL. The reverse is true for ratings of health status, and social functioning is less important than either construct.

Many advocate the use of multidimensional measures of HQOL.[9–11] These measures include self/subjective ratings of health status; physical and psychosomatic symptoms; side effects of treatment; and physical, functional, social, emotional, and spiritual well-being. The domain frameworks in Appendix 10A provide examples of investigators who have espoused a multidimensional model of HQOL. This model consists of physical and functional well-being that includes symptom distress and nutritional status; environmental and economic well-being; social functioning and well-being; psychological, emotional, and spiritual well-being; and subjective health perceptions.

The measurement of HQOL is endorsed by many health professional associations, such as the American Society of Clinical Oncology and the Oncology Nursing Society, and by government agencies concerned with the health of their citizens. For example, in the United States, the Centers for Disease Control and Prevention's Behavioral Risk Factor Surveillance System (BRFSS) added four questions about HQOL to its 1993 survey.[12] These questions asked about subjective perceptions of general health, physical health, mental health, and impact of poor physical or mental health on usual activities (self-care, work, recreation). A module of the 2002 BRFSS survey includes QOL questions about activity limitations due to physical, mental, or emotional problems; about emotional states; and about feeling healthy and full of energy.[13] The BRFSS represents one of the most important surveillance systems used by the U.S. federal government to monitor the health behavior of its citizens.

What emerges from a review of the literature about health indices for determining QOL is the general consensus that attributes of mind, body, and spirit must all be included in any comprehensive QOL measure. This approach is recommended because of the hypothesized integration of mind, body, and spirit. Berg and colleagues constructed a values scale that included cognitive, emotional, social, and physical functions. Berg's results indicate that any attempt to define health operationally, as it relates to QOL, must include more than just aspects of physical function.[14] Mytko and Knight go further, concluding that QOL studies need to include religiosity and spirituality measures to understand the integration of mind, body, and spirit in cancer care.[15]

Subjective and objective dimensions of QOL measures are not always complementary. For instance, the study by Evans et al. of QOL in patients with end-stage renal disease found that "patients on dialysis were clearly not functioning like people who were well, despite the fact that they were enjoying life."[16] Kaasa and Loge report that important aspects of end-of-life care are spirituality and existential issues, such as patients' perceptions of purpose and meaning of life.[17] These existential dimensions are more significant than objective aspects of QOL, such as physical functioning.

Measurement of Quality of Life

Wellisch emphasizes that the optimal measurement approach to QOL is the prospective design in which the same group of patients is interviewed sequentially.[6] Evans et al. believe that subjective QOL (i.e., the individual's attitudes) is a state rather than a trait and is thus subject to variation over time.[16] If measurement takes place at only one point in the patient's experience, the true QOL picture may not emerge. Wellisch's recommended methodologic strategies for QOL research are shown in Appendices 10B and 10C.[6]

Guyatt et al. have recognized the value of both cross-sectional and longitudinal studies.[18] The former allows comparisons between people at one point in time and the latter allows evaluations of QOL changes in a person. The authors state that HQOL measures should be interpretable in a clinical sense. Differences in scores should represent the range of clinical changes from trivial or small to moderate or large. Hays and Woolley warn that defining the smallest difference in HQOL that is clinically significant (the minimal clinically meaningful difference) is problematic.[19] It is important to consider the cost of obtaining the minimal difference, the impact of the baseline value on the meaning of the change, the effect of the direction of change on the amount of change, and the influence of the distributional index and external standard or anchor on variation in the estimated magnitude.

Measures of HQOL can be generic, such as the SF-36[20] or the Nottingham Health Profile.[21,22] Instruments can address specific illnesses, such as the Functional Assessment of Cancer Therapy—Breast measure.[23] HQOL measures can combine generic and illness-specific attributes of HQOL, for example, the European Organization for Research and Treatment of Cancer Quality of Life Questionnaire Core 30[24] and the Functional Assessment of Chronic Illness Therapy.[25]

In summarizing the uses of HQOL in clinical assessments of cancer patients, Cella et al. reason that QOL changes can provide information about the impact of new drug treatments, the willingness of patients to continue treatment, and other outcomes of value to a patient besides cure or remission.[10] Naturally, any instruments used to measure QOL must be reliable and accurate. Because international collaboration in clinical trials is increasing, measurement reliability and validity needs to hold true across languages and cultures. Cella and colleagues recommend the use of item response theory to maintain QOL item banks with validated questions for different dimensions of HQOL.[10]

Osoba's review of the HQOL measurement literature in cancer includes these observations: good compliance with self-reports of HQOL is possible; HQOL can be improved with aggressive therapy; symptoms are associated with disruptions in HQOL; and pretreatment HQOL scores can predict QOL outcomes during treatment as well as survival. Osoba also reported that health care providers are poor judges of how patients feel about their QOL.[26] Studies show that proxy ratings by health care providers and family members tend to underestimate QOL, particularly for more subjective domains.[27,28]

Selecting a Quality-of-Life Instrument

The researcher who wants to measure HQOL must consider multiple issues and choose from numerous instruments. Recent books provide information on HQOL conceptual,[29] and measurement issues.[30] Older and more current general reviews, as well as this chapter, are available to assist the researcher in making a selection. The reviews include those by Cella and Tulsky,[31] Anderson and colleagues,[32] Naughton and Wiklund,[33] Coons et al.,[34] oncology-specific reviews by Cella et al.,[10] Soni and Cella;[7] and pediatric oncology reviews by Connolly and Johnson.[35] Other HQOL disease-related measures focus on stroke, such as that by Buck et al.[36] Books include those by Spilker,[37] McDowell and Newell,[38] Wenger et al.,[39] Walker,[40] Bowling,[41] and Bowling.[42] Of particular help in identifying instruments are the Websites that offer collections of QOL/HQOL measures. These collections usually include the title of the instrument, author, description of scales, and reliability and validity data. Some examples include the American Thoracic Society list of instruments www.atsqol.org/qinst.asp,[43] the MAPI Research Institute's Quality of Life Instruments Database www.qolid.org/,[44] the Quality of Life Compendium www.uib.no/isf/people/doc/qol/httoc.htm,[45] the list of QOL instruments from the toolkit of instruments to measure end-of-life care from the Center for Gerontology and Health Care Research, Brown University www.chcr.brown.edu/pcoc/Quality.htm,[46] and the Ethics Tool Database www.bc.edu/bc_org/avp/son/ethics/database.html.[47]

Multiple versus Single Instruments

The following must be considered when selecting QOL instruments:

1. Single or multiple measures: consideration of specificity, feasibility, design, cost, type of staff needed to administer the scale(s), and subject burden.
2. Generic and disease-specific measures
   a. Generic: consideration of aspects of QOL that are common across diverse samples, regardless of disease, gender, culture, and so on.
   b. Disease-specific: consideration of aspects of QOL that are unique to a group of people with the same disease.
3. Quantitative and qualitative measures
   a. Quantitative instruments: subscale scores capture multiple dimensions of the construct.
   b. Qualitative instruments: descriptive, qualitative self-reports of facets of life affected by illness.
4. Objective and subjective reports
   a. Objective instruments: observable data.
   b. Subjective instruments: patient self-evaluation or proxy evaluation of the target person's QOL.[48]
5. Objective versus subjective QOL dimensions
   a. Objective dimensions: housing, work, education, environment, socioeconomic status.
   b. Subjective dimensions: psychosocial and spiritual well-being.
   c. Combination of objective and subjective dimensions.[49,50]
6. Conceptual and linguistic translations
   a. Conceptual congruity in addition to linguistic accuracy preferred in translations.
   b. Diversity within minority groups means that direct translations may not be conceptually accurate.
   c. Interactive translations likely to achieve both conceptual and linguistic equivalence.[51]

In summary, the choice of instrument will depend on scientific and pragmatic considerations (e.g., conceptual definition of QOL, resources available to do content analysis of qualitative data, cost of interviews, literacy of sample, burdensomeness of instrument(s) selected). Sugarbaker and colleagues' study is a comprehensive approach to the measurement of QOL.[52] This cooperative, multidisciplinary effort uses multiple QOL assessment methodologies, such as objective and subjective dimensions, an interview, and self-reports. This all-inclusive approach may not always be possible or practical (see Appendix 10C). Thus, single HQOL instruments represent a realistic option for the researcher.

Measures of Quality of Life

Functional Assessment of Chronic Illness Therapy (FACIT) System

The FACIT system is composed of numerous QOL self-report measures that can be used by persons with cancer or other chronic illnesses who have at least a sixth-grade reading level. Previously, this system was called the Functional Assessment of Cancer Therapy and focused on the impact of cancer.[53] FACIT questionnaires are multidimensional QOL measures for use in clinical studies of QOL in people with chronic health conditions.[54] Cella and Nowinski administered FACIT questionnaires to a representative sample in the United States and derived FACIT population norms. These normative data can be used as reference points against which to compare the scores of people with chronic illnesses.[54]

The scales are made available for free to researchers in academic institutions, as long as the user fills out a Collaborators' Project Information Form (www.facit.org/),[55] agrees to document and share methods of data collection and analysis, and specifies the subscale(s) and translation(s) to be used. Industry users, such as pharmaceutical companies, may use FACIT questionnaires for a fee. Instructions for questionnaire use may be found on the FACIT Website.

The FACT-G questionnaire, version 4—the core of the FACIT—is a 27-item generic measure of QOL that includes subscale measures of physical well-being (7 items), emotional well-being (6 items), functional well-being (7 items), and social/family well-being (7 items). At the end of each subscale is an item that asks about QOL effects. Version 4 excludes the Relationship with Doctor (RWD) subscale, which had a ceiling effect. The questionnaire uses a 5-point Likert scale (0 = not at all, 4 = very much) and an 11-point scale (0 = not at all, 10 = very much) for the optional weighting items. The higher the score, the better the QOL. The FACT-G requires about 5 minutes to complete without assistance. A disease- or treatment-specific group of questions is added to the core FACT items for use with specific groups. For details about scoring version 4, see the Website (www.facit.org/).[55]

The FACT-G has satisfactory reliability and validity, as reported by Cella et al.,[53] and by subsequent studies, including international investigations, such as the study by Ratanatharathorn et al.[56] Initially, Cella and colleagues reported internal consistency alpha coefficients of 0.65–0.82 across subscales and 0.89 for the total instrument (version 2) in a sample of 630 patients, and test-retest reliability of 0.82–0.92 (version 2) with a sample of 60 patients.[53] Subsequent uses of the FACT-G have supported its reliability. The FACT-G is a valid and sensitive instrument that discriminates between groups with different stages of disease, levels of function, and hospitalization status. It also differentiates between groups along the dimensions of physical, functional, social, and emotional well-being. Within groups it is responsive to change over time.[23,57]

The FACIT questionnaires include disease- and treatment-specific scales, which are listed on the Website www.facit.org/.[55] A few examples of disease/treatment-specific scales include FACT-B for patients with breast cancer,[23] FACT-BR for patients with brain cancer,[58] FACT-H&N for patients with head and neck cancer,[59] FACT-L for patients with lung cancer,[60] FACT-BMT for patients undergoing bone marrow transplant,[61] FAACT for functional assessment of anorexia and cachexia,[62] FACT-An for patients with anemia,[63] and FAHI for people with HIV.[64] The FACIT system has developed scales for other areas of interest: FACT-Sp for assessment of the spiritual dimension of QOL, FAMS for the functional assessment of multiple sclerosis, and FANLT for the functional assessment of non-life-threatening conditions. The FACIT system questionnaires have been translated into other languages.[65] Currently, questionnaires are available in 38 languages. Psychometric results with the translated versions maintain good reliability and validity.

European Organization for Research and Treatment of Cancer (EORTC): Core Questionnaire, QLQ-C30

The EORTC developed the copyrighted QLQ-C30 as a generic, multidimensional measure of QOL for cancer patients. According to the Website, www.eortc.be/home/qol,[66] the

QLQ-C30 has been translated into and validated in 43 languages. Translations are also listed on the Website.

The EORTC QLQ-C30 may be used free of charge by investigators in academic settings. An agreement form must be filled out prior to its use by academics. Use by nonacademics, such as pharmaceutical companies, includes a royalty fee for each separate clinical study. Instructions for use and scoring and copies of the QLQ-C30 v3.0 questionnaire and manual may be found on the Website.[66]

The QLQ-C30 Version 2 consists of a core of 30 + 3 items representing five functional domain scales: physical (5 items), role (4 items), social (2 items), emotional (4 items), and cognitive functioning (2 items); 9 symptom scales (three, 2-item scales and six, 1-item scales); financial impact; and 3 global QOL items. The first 30 items are 4-point scales (1 = not at all, 4 = very much), and the 3 global QOL scales are 7-point scales. The time frame is the past week. Version 2 was further revised to improve the internal consistency of the role function scale and the conceptual integrity of the global QOL scale.[67] The QLQ-C30, a self-report measure, may be administered as an interview. Completion time averages between 11 and 12 minutes.[68]

In the Aaronson group study of the QLQ-C30, all internal consistency alphas were greater than 0.70, except for the role functioning scale.[68] Validity was supported in several ways. The scale structure held up as expected, except for role functioning. Interscale correlations were moderate, indicating distinct measures of QOL. Function and symptom measures generally discriminated between respondents at different performance status levels per the Eastern Cooperative Oncology Group scale. As expected, significant changes in physical and role functioning, global QOL, fatigue, and nausea and vomiting occurred with improvement or worsening of performance status. A study of the revised QLQ-C30 Version 2 carried out in Canada (n = 696) and the Netherlands (n = 485) yielded improved internal consistency alphas ranging from 0.78 to 0.88.[67] Subsequent studies further support the reliability, validity and feasibility of version 2, including translations.[69,70]

The current version, 3.0, has the same 5 functional domain scales; similar symptom scales of pain, fatigue, nausea/vomiting (2 items each scale); appetite loss, diarrhea, constipation, dyspnea, sleep disturbance (1 item each); a global health status/QOL scale; and financial impact. Changes were made in the global health status/QOL scale, the physical functioning scale, and the role functioning scale. Reliability and validity of version 3.0 have been supported in studies such as those of Arraras et al.[71] and Kyriaki et al.[72]

The core instrument QLQ-C30 is supplemented by several cancer-specific modules listed in the Website.[66] These are some examples: QLQ-BR23 for patients with breast cancer,[73] QLQ-H&N35 for patients with head and neck cancer,[74] and the QLQ-LC13 for patients with lung cancer.[75]

World Health Organization Quality of Life (WHOQOL) Group: WHOQOL-100, WHOQOL-BREF

The WHO, Programme on Mental Health launched the WHOQOL Project in 1991 with 15 centers around the world (Australia, Croatia, France, India (two centres), Israel, Japan, The Netherlands, Panama, Russian Federation, Spain, Thailand, United Kingdom, United States of America, and Zimbabwe) to develop an internationally applicable and cross-culturally comparable QOL measure.[76-78] Today, 30 centers participate in the project.

WHOQOL instruments may be used free of charge. Forms and information may be obtained at www.who.int/msa/qol/.[79] For details on computing facet and domain scores, and for syntax files for checking and cleaning data, manuals are available from The WHOQOL Group, Programme on Mental Health, World Health Organisation, CH-1211 Geneva 27, Switzerland. The Australian WHOQOL Website is very helpful: www.acpmh.

unimelb.edu.au/whoqol/.[80] The WHO Website, dosei.who.int/uhtbin/cgisirsi/Mon+Mar+31+03:37:54+MEST+2003/0/49, makes available some key reports about the development of the WHOQOL measures.[81] At the Website, enter the word WHOQOL in the "Words and phrases" box, click "Search catalogue," and a list of documents will appear. These can be viewed and printed.

The WHOQOL Group developed two instruments for measuring quality of life—the WHOQOL-100,[82] and WHOQOL-BREF.[83] The instruments are self- or interviewer-administered; may be used for medical practice, audit, policy making, and research; can be used in a variety of cultural or linguistic settings; and can be used to compare QOL in different populations and countries. The WHOQOL-100 consists of 100 items, compared to the WHOQOL-BREF with 26 items. For both questionnaires, items are rated on a 5-point scale (1 = not at all, 5 = an extreme amount). A scoring manual is available from the address above.

The WHOQOL-100 consists of 24 subscales within six domains: physical (energy and fatigue, pain and discomfort, and sleep and rest); psychologic (body image and appearance, negative feelings, positive feelings, self-esteem, thinking, learning, memory and concentration); independence (mobility, activities of daily living, dependence on medical substances and medical aids, and work capacity); social (personal relationships, social support, and sexual activity); environment (financial resources, freedom, physical safety and security, health and social care accessibility and quality, home environment, opportunities for acquiring new information and skills, participation in and opportunities for recreation/leisure, physical environment—pollution/noise/traffic/climate, and transportation); and spiritual (religion/spirituality/personal beliefs). It also measures overall QOL and health with four additional items.[82]

The WHOQOL-100 has demonstrated good validity and reliability across domains.[82] A study with a U.S. sample of 443 adults (128 healthy, 251 chronically ill, and 64 childbearing) further confirmed the internal consistency (0.82–0.95), test-retest reliability for a 2-week interval (0.83–0.96), responsiveness to change in women after childbirth, and construct validity (correlation with SF-36, ability to discriminate between groups as expected, and confirmation of conceptual structure).[84]

The WHOQOL-BREF measures four domains of the WHOQOL-100: physical health, psychologic health, social relationships and environment, and overall QOL and general health.[83] The WHOQOL-BREF correlated at 0.89 or above with relevant domain scores of the WHOQOL-100. WHOQOL-BREF domain scores also had good validity (discriminant and content) and reliability (internal consistency and test-retest).[83]

The WHOQOL-100 and WHOQOL-BREF are used to assess a variety of pathologic conditions or diseases; they are not disease specific. A recent MedLine search indicated that these instruments have been used to assess a number of conditions, including psychiatric disorders such as schizophrenia,[85] HIV infection,[86,87] chronic pain,[88] and liver transplantation.[89] Another application of these instruments focuses on community-based health issues such as post-earthquake QOL.[90] Many studies relate to cross-cultural health assessment in various countries.[91,92] Currently, 29 different language versions are available, according to the Australian Centre WHOQOL Website.[80]

Medical Outcomes Study Health Survey Based on 36 Items: RAND 36-Item Health Survey 1.0 and MOS 36-Item Short Form Health Survey (SF-36)

The Medical Outcomes Study (MOS) was a 4-year investigation conducted by RAND, Santa Monica, California to determine predictors of patient outcomes. From the battery of MOS instruments, Ware and Sherbourne published a short-form health survey called the SF-36, an easy to use, generic measure of QOL.[93,94] RAND has placed in the public domain the same 36 items in the SF-36 in an instrument called the RAND 36-item Health Survey (Version 1). Here it is referred to as the RAND 36.[95]

The SF-36 items and scoring rules are distributed by Medical Outcomes Trust, Inc. (MOT). To use the SF-36 Health Survey, researchers are required to adhere to the wording and scoring rules of the SF-36 MOT manual. MOT states that it is committed to ". . . making [our] surveys available royalty free to individuals and organizations for unfunded scholarly research." The Website for the SF-36, www.sf-36.org/, hosted by QualityMetric Inc., provides extensive information about the SF-36, and two shorter versions, the SF-12 and SF-8.[94] RAND provides a Website at which a copy of the RAND 36-item Health Survey (Version 1) can be downloaded and used by anyone free of charge. Permission to use the instrument and scoring instructions can also be downloaded at www.rand.org/health/surveys/sf36item/.[95]

The SF-36/RAND 36 consist of eight health concept subscales representing two broad dimensions of QOL: physical health and mental health. Physical health includes the constructs of physical functioning (10 items), role limitations due to physical health (4 items), bodily pain (2 items), and general health (5 items). Mental health includes energy/fatigue (4 items), social functioning (2 items), role limitations due to emotional problems (3 items), and emotional well-being (5 items). Although the SF-36 was developed as a self-administered questionnaire, it may also be administered via interview and can be completed in 5 to 15 minutes. Yes/no and Likert-type response options are used.[93,96]

The SF-36 and the RAND 36 are identical in wording but have slightly different scoring systems. For the RAND 36 instrument, instructions in the RAND manual state that precoded numeric values are recoded according to the scoring key. A high score means a more favorable health state. Each item is then scored from 0 (lowest score) to 100 (highest score). Next, items within a scale are averaged together to create a subscale score, one for each of the 8 subscales. The manual identifies the items to average together to create a subscale score.[96,97] This scoring procedure is the same for the SF-36 except in the case of the pain and general health scales. The SF-36 makes scoring of the second pain item (interference with normal work), conditional on the response to the first item (pain severity), whereas the RAND 36 scoring system is not conditional. The RAND system generally reflects less pain, although the correlation between the RAND 36 and the SF-36 pain scales is 0.99.[97] With regard to the general health scale, the RAND 36 instructions call for scoring the five general health scales in an identical manner, whereas the SF-36 instructions require that one item be scored differently. The item, "In general, would you say your health is excellent, very good, good, fair, poor?" is scored 100, 85, 60, 25, 0 for the SF-36, and the RAND 36 uses 100, 75, 50, 25, 0.[97]

The SF-36 is one of the most widely used health care survey instrument for measuring QOL. It has received rigorous evaluation.[98] More than 25 studies reported internal consistency alphas at 0.70 or greater across the eight subscales.[99] A review of 24 patient groups differing in sociodemographic and diagnostic characteristics demonstrated consistent satisfactory reliability, even for disadvantaged respondent groups, for whom reliabilities were slightly lower.[100] In summarizing findings from more than 30 studies, Ware reports that test–retest and one-year stability studies show that confidence intervals around the two summary scores for physical and mental health are smaller (± 6–7) than they are for each of the eight subscales (± 13–32).[98] With regard to validity, numerous studies across a variety of patient groups support the content, concurrent, criterion, construct,[101] and predictive validity of the SF-36.[98] It is important to note that the bodily pain score has weak convergent validity in relation to severity of medical illness,[102] and that there is a floor effect for the role functioning scales.[103] The SF-36 has been translated and tested for reliability and validity in over 40 languages. For more extensive information about the SF-36, researchers are directed to www.sf-36.org/.[94]

Summary and Future Direction

Early QOL measures (e.g., Karnofsky and Burchenal) focused on one dimension: functional status. Instruments developed later are based on a multidimensional conceptualization of QOL and a broader definition of health within the QOL construct. Health includes physical and mental health and function, health perception, physical and psychosomatic symptoms and side effects of disease and treatment, and diagnostic indicators. As the definition of QOL is broadening, investigators are insisting on more precise definitions and recommend that QOL be considered in relation to health concerns. Thus, the HQOL conceptual frameworks espouse a multidimensional model consisting of physical and functional well-being, including symptom distress and nutritional status; environmental and economic well-being; social functioning and well-being; psychologic, emotional, and spiritual well-being; and subjective health perceptions. Whether these dimensions hold true over time, disease state, and cultures awaits further research. McHorney believes that many generic measures of health lack precision. For the twenty-first century McHorney calls for equiprecise tests that would yield equally precise measures for all aspects of a construct, that is, all items and domains of health-related QOL. Equiprecise tests could be achieved with the use of computerized survey methods and item response theory such as the measurement theory.[105] The larger question is whether a computerized survey platform would be applicable for all segments of the world's population.

Exemplar Studies

Stewart, A.L., & Ware, J.E. *Measuring functioning and well-being: The medical outcomes study approach.* Durham, NC: Duke University Press, 1992.[101]

Stewart, A.L., Greenfield, S., Hays, R.D., et al. Functional status and well-being of patients with chronic conditions. Results from the Medical Outcomes Study. *JAMA*, 1989, 262(7):907-13.[106]

The Medical Outcomes Study (MOS) is a landmark observational study of over 20,000 English-speaking adult patients from Boston, Chicago, and Los Angeles and 526 physicians, clinical psychologists, social workers' and other care providers. In each city, patients and physicians were sampled from five practice settings that differed in structural characteristics. Cross-sectional and longitudinal data (over 4 years) were collected. The chronic diseases of interest were hypertension, type 2 diabetes, advanced coronary artery disease, and depression. People over 60 were overrepresented in the sample.

Part of the MOS included the measurement of HQOL in 9385 adults at the time of office visits to 362 physicians in the three target cities using the original Rand MOS Functioning and Well-Being Profile Questionnaires. The authors found that those with chronic medical conditions reported poorer functioning and well-being than those without the chronic conditions and that people with multiple chronic conditions reported poorer functioning and well-being than those with only one condition.

The Rand 36-item Health Survey, Version 1.0, and the SF-36 Health Survey (developed from the larger, original Rand MOS Functioning and Well-Being Profile Questionnaires), reflect physical, mental, and social functioning and well-being, as well as health perceptions. The MOS supported the theoretical basis, reliability, and validity of the

36-item questionnaire. The MOS led to numerous publications and hundreds of additional reports of research that used the SF-36 or Rand 36 questionnaires to measure QOL.

References

1. WHOQOL Group. Study protocol for the World Health Organization project to develop a quality of life assessment instrument (WHOQOL). *Qual Life Res*, 1993, *2*(2):153-159.
2. Patrick, D.L., & Erickson, P. *Health status and health policy: Quality of life in health care evaluation and resource allocation.* New York: Oxford University Press, 1993.
3. Bard, M. Summary of the informal discussion of functional states: Quality of life. *Cancer*, 1984, *53*(10):2327.
4. Strickland, O. Measures and instruments. *Patient outcomes research: Examining the effectiveness of nursing practice.* Proceedings of the state of the science conference sponsored by the National Center for Nursing Research, September 1991. NIH Publication No. 93-3411, 1992.
5. Flanagan, J. Measurement of quality of life: Current state of the art. *Arch Phys Med Rehabil*, 1982, *63*(2):56-59.
6. Wellisch, D. Work, social, recreation, family, and physical status. *Cancer*, 1984, *53*(10):2290-2302.
7. Soni, M.K., Cella, D. Quality of life and symptom measures in oncology: An overview. *Am J Manag Care*, 2002, *8*(18 Suppl):S560.
8. Smith, K.W., Avis, N.E., Assmann, S.F. Distinguishing between quality of life and health status in quality of life research: A meta-analysis. *Qual Life Res*, 1999, *8*(5):447.
9. Ware, J. Conceptualizing disease impact and treatment outcomes. *Cancer*, 1984, *53*(10):2316-2326.
10. Cella, D., Chang, C.H., Lai, J.S., Webster, K. Advances in quality of life measurements in oncology patients. *Semin Oncol*, 2002, *29*(3 Suppl 8):60.
11. Padilla, G.V., Grant M.M., Ferrell, B.R., & Presant, C. Quality of Life—Cancer. In Spilker, B. (Ed.) *Quality of life and pharmacoeconomics in clinical trials* (2nd ed.). New York: Lippincott-Raven, 1996, pp. 301-308.
12. Centers for Disease Control and Prevention. Current Trends: Quality of life as a new public health measure—Behavioral risk factor surveillance system, 1993. *MMWR*, 1994, *43*(20):375-380.
13. National Center for Chronic Disease Prevention and Health Promotion. 2002 Behavioral Risk Factor Surveillance System, Module 6: Quality of Life, Dec 2001. Access date 13 Mar 2003. www.cdc.gov/brfss/pdf-ques/2002brfss.pdf.
14. Berg, R., Hallauer, D., & Berk, S. Neglected aspects of the quality of life. *Health Serv Res*, 1976, *11*(4):391.
15. Mytko, J.J., Knight, S.J. Body, mind and spirit: Towards the integration of religiosity and spirituality in cancer quality of life research. *Psychooncology*, 1999, *8*(5):439.
16. Evans, R., Manninen, D.L., Garrison, L.P., Jr., et al. The quality of life with end-stage renal disease. *N Engl J Med*, 1985, *312*(9):553-559.
17. Kaasa, S., Loge, J.H. Quality of life in palliative care: principles and practice. *Palliat Med*, 2003, *17*(1):11-20.
18. Guyatt, G.H., Feeny, D.H., & Patrick, D.L. Measuring health-related quality of life. *Ann Intern Med*, 1993, *118*(8):622-629.
19. Hays, R.D., Woolley, J.M. The concept of clinically meaningful difference in health-related quality-of-life research. How meaningful is it? *Pharmacoeconomics*, 2000, *18*(5):419.
20. Ware, J.E., Kosinski, M. Interpreting SF-36 summary health measures: A response. *Qual Life Res*, 2001, *10*(5):405-413; discussion 415-420.
21. Hunt, S.M., McKenna, S.P., McEwan, J., et al. The Nottingham Health Profile: Subjective health status and medical consultations. *Soc Sci Med*, 1981, 15A:221-229.
22. Hunt, S.M., McEwen, J., McKenna, S.P. Measuring health stats: A new tool for clinicians and epidemiologists. *J Royal Coll Gen Pract*, 1985, *35*:185.
23. Brady, M.J., Cella, D.F., Mo, F., et al. Reliability and validity of the Functional Assessment of Cancer Therapy—Breast quality-of-life instrument. *J Clin Oncol*, 1997, *15*(3):974-986.
24. Fayers, P., Bottomley, A., EORTC Quality of Life Group, Quality of Life Unit. Quality of life research within the EORTC-the EORTC QLQ-C30. European Organisation for Research and Treatment of Cancer. *Eur J Cancer*, 2002, *38*(Suppl 4):S125.
25. Cella, D. Assessment methods for quality of life in cancer patients: The FACIT measurement system. *Int J Pharm Med*, *14*(2):78-81.
26. Osoba, D. Lessons learned from measuring health-related quality of life in oncology. *J Clin Oncol*, 1994, *12*(3):608-616.
27. Andresen, E.M., Vahle, V.J., Lollar, D. Proxy reliability: Health-related quality of life (HRQoL) measures for people with disability. *Qual Life Res*, 2001, *10*(7):609.
28. Novella, J.L., Jochum, C., Jolly, D., et al. Agreement between patients' and proxies' reports of quality of life in Alzheimer's disease. *Qual Life Res*, 2001, *10*(5):443.
29. King, C.R., Hinds, P.S. *Quality of life: From nursing and patient perspectives.* (2nd ed). Sudbury, MA: Jones and Bartlett, 2003.
30. Fayers, P.M., Machin, D. *Quality of life: Assessment, analysis, and interpretation.* West Sussex, England: John Wiley, 2000.
31. Cella, D.F., & Tulsky, D.S. Measuring quality of life today: Methodological aspects. *Oncology*, 1990, *4*(5):29-38.
32. Anderson, R.T., Aaronson, N.K., & Wilkin, D. Critical review of international assessments of health-related quality of life. *Qual Life Res*, 1993, *2*(6):369-395.
33. Naughton, M.J., & Wiklund, I. A critical review of dimension-specific measures of health-related quality of life in cross-cultural research. *Qual Life Res*, 1993, *2*(6):397-432.
34. Coons, S.J., Rao, S., Keininger, D.L., Hays, R.D. A comparative review of generic quality-of-life instruments. *Pharmacoeconomics*, 2000, *17*(1):13-35.

35. Connolly, M.A., Johnson, J.A. Measuring quality of life in paediatric patients. *Pharmacoeconomics*, 1999, 16(6):605.

36. Buck, D., Jacoby, A., Massey, A., Ford, G. Evaluation of measures used to assess quality of life after stroke. *Stroke*, 2000, 31(8):2004.

37. Spilker, B. *Quality of life and pharmacoeconomics in clinical trials* (2nd ed.). Philadelphia: Lippincott-Raven, 1996, pp. 301-308.

38. McDowell, I., & Newell, C. *Measuring health: A guide to rating scales and questionnaires.* New York: Oxford University Press, 1987.

39. Wenger, N.K., Mattson, M.E., Furberg, C.D., & Elinson, J. (Eds.). *Assessment of quality of life in clinical trials of cardiovascular therapies.* New York: LeJacq Publishing, 1984.

40. Walker, S.R. *Quality of life assessment: Key issues in the 1990's.* CMR Workshops Series. Boston: Kluwer, 1992.

41. Bowling, A. *Measuring health: A review of quality of life measurement scales* (2nd ed.). Maidenhead, Berkshire, UK: Open University Press, McGraw-Hill, 1997.

42. Bowling, A. *Measuring disease: A review of disease-specific quality of life measurement scales* (2nd ed.). Maidenhead, Berkshire, UK: Open University Press, McGraw-Hill, 2001.

43. Instruments, American Thoracic Society, 2003. Access date March 15, 2003. www.atsqol.org/qinst.asp.

44. Quality of Life Instruments Database (QOLID), Version 1.8, MAPI Research Institute, Lyon, France. Jan 2003. Access date Mar 15, 2003. www.qolid.org/.

45. Quality of Life Compendium. Center for Quality of Life Research in Nursing Science, University of Bergen, Norway, Sept 5, 2002. www.uib.no/isf/people/doc/qol/httoc.htm.

46. Toolkit of instruments to measure end-of-life care: Quality of life, Center for Gerontology and Health Care Research, Brown University. Aug 30, 2000. Access date Mar 15, 2003. www.chcr.brown.edu/pcoc/Quality.htm.

47. Ethics Tool Database: Boston College School of Nursing. The Trustees of Boston College, 2000. Dec 7, 2000. Access date April 2, 2003. www.bc.edu/bc_org/avp/son/ethics/database.html.

48. Sneeuw, K.C., Sprangers, M.A., Aaronson, N.K. The role of health care providers and significant others in evaluating the quality of life of patients with chronic disease. *J Clin Epidemiol*, 2002, 55(11):1130.

49. Brady, M.J., Peterman, A.H., Fitchett, G., et al. A case for including spirituality in quality of life measurement in oncology. *Psychooncology*, 1999, 8(5):417.

50. Sulmasy, D.P. A biopsychosocial-spiritual model for the care of patients at the end of life. *Gerontologist*, 2002, 42(Spec No 3):24-33.

51. Guyatt, G.H. The philosophy of health-related quality of life translation. *Qual Life Res*, 1993, 2(6):461-465.

52. Sugarbaker, P., Barofsky, I., Rosenberg, S., & Gianola, F. Quality of life assessment of patients in extremity sarcoma clinical trials. *Surgery*, 1982, 91(1):17-23.

53. Cella, D.F., Tulsky, D.S., Gray, G., et al. The Functional Assessment of Cancer Therapy Scale: Development and validation of the general measure. *J Clin Oncol*, 1993, 11:570-579.

54. Cella, D., Nowinski, C.J. Measuring quality of life in chronic illness: The functional assessment of chronic illness therapy measurement system. *Arch Phys Med Rehabil*, 2002, 83(12 Suppl 2):S10.

55. Cella, D. Center on Outcomes, Research and Education, Evanston Northwestern Healthcare. FACIT: Functional Assessment of Chronic Illness Therapy. Updated June 2002. Access date 29 March 2003. www.facit.org/.

56. Ratanatharathorn, V., Sirilerttrakul, S., Jirajarus, M., et al. Quality of life, Functional Assessment of Cancer Therapy—General. *J Med Assoc Thai*, 2001, 84(10):1430.

57. Esper, P., Mo, F., Chodak, G., et al. Measuring quality of life in men with prostate cancer using the Functional Assessment of Cancer Therapy Prostate instrument. *Urology*, 1997, 50(6):920-928.

58. Weitzner, M.A., Meyers, C. A., Gelke, C.K., et al. The Functional Assessment of Cancer Therapy (FACT) scale. Development of a brain subscale and revalidation of the general version (FACT-G) in patients with primary brain tumors. *Cancer*, 1995, 75(5):1151-1161.

59. List, M.A., D'Antonio, L.L., Cella, D.F., et al. The performance Status Scale for Head and Neck Cancer Patients and the Functional Assessment of Cancer Therapy-Head and Neck Scale. A study of utility and validity. *Cancer*, 1996, 77(11):2294-2301.

60. Cella, D.F., Bonomi, A.E., Lloyd, S.R., et al. Reliability and validity of the Functional Assessment of Cancer Therapy—Lung (FACT-L) quality of life instrument. *Lung Cancer*, 1995, 12(3):199-220.

61. McQuellon, R.P., Russell, G.B., Cella, D.F., et al. Quality of life measurement in bone marrow transplantation: Development of the Functional Assessment of Cancer Therapy—Bone Marrow Transplant (FACT-BMT) scale. *Bone Marrow Transplant*, 1997, 19(4):357-368.

62. Cella, D.F., VonRoenn, J., Lloyd, S., & Browder, H.P. The Bristol-Myers Anorexia/Cachexia Recovery Instrument (BACRI): A brief assessment of patients' subjective response to treatment for anorexia/cachexia. *Qual Life Res*, 1995, 4(3):221-231.

63. Yellen, S.B., Cella, D.F., Webster, K., et al. Measuring fatigue and other anemia-related symptoms with the Functional Assessment of Cancer Therapy (FACT) measurement system. *J Pain Symptom Manage*, 1997, 13(2):63-74.

64. Cella, D.F., McCain, N. L., Peterman, A.H., et al. Development and validation of the Functional Assessment of Human Immunodeficiency Virus Infection (FAHI) quality of life instrument. *Qual Life Res*, 1996, 5(4):450-463.

65. Bonomi, A.E., Cella, D.F., Hahn, E.A., et al. Multilingual translation of the Functional Assessment of Cancer Therapy (FACT) quality of life measurement system. *Qual Life Res*, 1996, 5(3):309-320.

66. EORTC Quality of Life web site, February 2003. Access date 2 April 2003. www.eortc.be/home/qol.

67. Osoba, D., Aaronson, N., Zee, B., et al. Modification of the EORTC QLQ-C30 (Version 2.0) based on content validity and reliability testing in large samples of patients with cancer. The study Group on Quality of Life of the EORTC and the Symptom Control and Quality of Life Committees of the NCI of Canada

Clinical Trial Group. *Qual Life Res*, 1997, 6(2):103-108.

68. Aaronson, N.K., Ahmedzai, S., Bergman, B., et al. The European Organization for Research and Treatment of Cancer QLQ-C30: A quality-of-life instrument for use in international clinical trials in oncology. *J Natl Cancer Inst*, 1993, 85(5):365-376.

69. Kemmler, G., Holzner, B., Kopp, M., et al. Comparison of two quality-of-life instruments for cancer patients: The functional assessment of cancer therapy-general and the European Organization for Research and Treatment of Cancer Quality of Life Questionnaire-C30. *J Clin Oncol*, 1999, 17(9):2932.

70. Zhao, H., Kanda, K. Translation and validation of the standard Chinese version of the EORTC QLQ-C30. *Qual Life Res*, 2000, 9(2):129.

71. Arraras, J.I., Arias, F., Tejedor, M., et al. The EORTC QLQ-C30 (version 3.0) Quality of Life questionnaire: Validation study for Spain with head and neck cancer patients. *Psychooncology*, 2002, 11(3):249.

72. Kyriaki, M., Eleni, T., Efi, P., et al. The EORTC core quality of life questionnaire (QLQ-C30, version 3.0) in terminally ill cancer patients under palliative care: Validity and reliability in a Hellenic sample. *Int J Cancer*, 2001, 94(1):135.

73. Holzner, B., Kemmler, G., Kopp, M., et al. Quality of life in breast cancer patients—not enough attention for long-term survivors? *Psychosomatics*, 2001, 42(2):117-123.

74. De Graeff, A., de Leeuw, J.R., Ros, W.J., et al. Sociodemographic factors and quality of life as prognostic indicators in head and neck cancer. *Eur J Cancer*, 2001, 37(3):332-339.

75. Jassem, J., Krzakowski, M., Roszkowski, K., et al. A phase II study of gemcitabine plus cisplatin in patients with advanced non-small cell lung cancer: Clinical outcome and quality of life. *Lung Cancer*, 2002, 35(1):73-79.

76. WHOQOL Group [Orley, J., Kuyken, W., Satorius, N., Power, M.J., et al.] Development of the WHOQOL: Rationale and current status. *Int J Mental Health*, 1994, 23:24-56.

77. WHOQOL Group. The World Health Organization Quality of Life Assessment (WHOQOL): Position paper from the World Health Organization. *Soc Sci Med*, 1995, 41:1403.

78. WHOQOL Group. The World Health Organization Quality of Life (WHOQOL) Assessment Instrument. In Spilker, B. (Ed.), *Quality of life and pharmacoeconomics in clinical trials* (2nd ed.). Hagerstown, MD: Lippincott-Raven, 1996.

79. WHOQOL Measuring quality of life: The World Health Organization Quality of Life Instruments. Access date April 2, 2003. www.who.int/msa/qol/.

80. WHOQOL Project: World Health Organization Quality of Life Project, Graeme Hawthorne, Australian WHOQOL Centre, Australian Centre for Posttraumatic Mental Health, University of Melbourne. Jan 23, 2003. Access date Mar 30, 2003. www.acpmh.unimelb.edu.au/whoqol/.

81. World Health Organization—WHOLIS webcat, Sirsi Corporation 2002. Access date April 2, 2003. dosei.who.int/uhtbin/cgisirsi/Mon+Mar+31+03:37:54+MEST+2003/0/49.

82. WHOQOL Group. The World Health Organization Quality of Life Assessment (WHOQOL): Development and general psychometric properties. *Soc Sci Med*, 1998, 46(12):1569-1585.

83. WHOQOL Group. Development of the World Health Organization WHOQOL-BREF Quality of Life Assessment. *Psychol Med*, 1998, 28(3):551-558.

84. Bonomi, A.E., Patrick, D.L., Bushnell, D.M., & Martin, M. Validation of the United States' version of the World Health Organization Quality of Life (WHOQOL) instrument. *J Clin Epidemiol*, 2000, 53(1):1-12.

85. Hasanah, C.I., & Razali, M.S. Quality of life: An assessment of the state of psychosocial rehabilitation of patients with schizophrenia in the community. *J R Soc Health*, 2002, 122(4):251-255.

86. Fang, C.T., Hsing, P.C., Yu, C.F., et al. Validation of the World Health Organization quality of life instrument in patients with HIV infection. *Qual Life Res*, 2002, 11(8):753-762.

87. Starace, F., Cafaro, L., Abrescia, N., et al. Quality of life assessment in HIV-positive persons: Application and validation of the WHOQOL-HIV, Italian version. *AIDS Care*, 2002, 14(3):405-415.

88. Skevington, S.M., Carse, M.S., & Williams, A.C. Validation of the WHOQOL-100: Pain management improves quality of life for chronic pain patients. *Clin J Pain*, 2001, 17(3):264-275.

89. O'Carroll, R.E., Smith, K., Couston, M., et al. A comparison of the WHOQOL-100 and the WHOQOL-BREF in detecting change in quality of life following liver transplantation. *Qual Life Res*, 2000, 9(1):121-124.

90. Wang, X., Gao, L., Zhang, H., et al. Post-earthquake quality of life and psychosocial well-being: Longitudinal evaluation in a rural community sample in northern China. *Psychiatry Clin Neurosci*, 2000, 55(4):427-433.

91. Skevington, S.M. Advancing cross-cultural research on quality of life: Observations drawn from the WHOQOL development. World Health Organization Quality of Life Assessment. *Qual Life Res*, 2002, 11(2):135-144.

92. Saxena, S., Carlson, D., Billington, R., WHOQOL Group. The WHO quality of life assessment instrument (WHOQOL-Bref): The importance of its items for cross-cultural research. *Qual Life Res*, 2001, 10(8):711-721.

93. Ware, J.E., & Sherbourne, C.D. The MOS 36-item short-form health survey (SF-36): I. Conceptual framework and item selection. *Med Care*, 1992, 30(6):473-483.

94. SF-36.ORG: A community for measuring health outcomes using SF tools, October 2002. Access date April 2, 2003. www.sf-36.org/.

95. RAND Health: RAND 36-Item Health Survey 1.0. Access date April 2, 2003. www.rand.org/health/surveys/sf36item/.

96. RAND. *RAND 36-Item Health Survey 1.0: RAND Health Sciences Program (Scoring manual)*. Santa Monica, CA: RAND, 1992.

97. Hays, R.D., Sherbourne, C.D., & Mazel, R.M. The RAND 36-item Health Survey 1.0. *Health Econ*, 1993, 2(3):217-227.

98. Ware, J.E., Jr. SF-36 health survey update. *Spine*, 2000, 25(24):3130-3139.

99. Tsai. C., Bayliss, M.S., Ware, JE. *SF-36 Health Survey annotated bibliography* (2nd ed., 1988-1996). Boston: Health Assessment Lab, New England Medical Center, 1997.

100. McHorney, C.A., Ware, J.E., Jr., Lu, J.F., Sherbourne, C.D. The MOS 36-item Short-Form Health Survey (SF-36): III. Tests of data quality, scaling assumptions, and reliability across diverse patient groups. *Med Care*, 1994, *32*(1):40-66.

101. Stewart, A.L., & Ware, J.E. *Measuring functioning and well-being: The medical outcomes study approach.* Durham, NC: Duke University Press, 1992.

102. McHorney, C.A., Ware, J.E., & Raczek, A.E. The MOS 36-item short form health survey (SF-36): II. Psychometric and clinical tests of validity in measuring physical and mental health constructs. *Med Care*, 1993, *31*(3):247-263.

103. Kurtin, P.S., Davies, A.R., Meyer, K.B., et al. Patient-based health status measurements in developing an outcomes assessment program. *Med Care*, 1992, *30*(Suppl 5):MS136-MS149.

104. Karnofsky, D., & Burchenal, J. *The clinical evaluation of chemotherapeutic agents in cancer.* New York: Columbia University Press, 1949.

105. McHorney CA. Generic health measurement: past accomplishments and a measurement paradigm for the 21st century. *Ann Intern Med*, Part 2, 1997, *127*:743-750.

106. Stewart, A.L., Greenfield, S., Hays, R.D., et al. Functional status and well-being of patients with chronic conditions. Results from the Medical Outcomes Study. *JAMA*, 1989, *262*(7):907.

107. Ferrans, C.E. Development of a quality of life index for patients with cancer. *Oncol Nurs Forum*, 1990, *17*(3)suppl:15-19.

108. Ferrans, C., & Powers, M. Psychometric assessment of the quality of life index. *Res Nurs Health*, 1992, *15*(1):29-38.

109. Grant, M., Ferrell, B., Schmidt, G.M., et al. Measurement of quality of life in bone marrow transplant survivors. *Qual Life Res*, 1992, *1*(6):375-384.

110. Ferrell, B.R., Dow, K.H., Grant, M. Measurement of the quality of life in cancer survivors. *Qual Life Res*, 1995, *4*(6):523.

111. Padilla, G.V., Ferrell, B.R., Grant, M.M., & Rhiner, M. Defining the content domain of quality of life for cancer patients with pain. *Cancer Nurs*, 1990, *13*(2):108-115.

112. Wellisch, D.K. Methodology in behavioral and psychosocial cancer research. Work, social, recreation, family, and physical status. *Cancer*, 1984, *53*(10 Suppl):2290-2302.

113. Grieco, A., & Long, C.J. Investigation of the Karnofsky Performance Status as a measure of quality of life. *Health Psychol*, 1984, *3*(2):129-142.

114. Zubrod, C.G., Schneiderman, M., Frei, E., et al. Appraisal of methods for the study of chemotherapy of cancer in man: Comparative therapeutic trial of nitrogen mustard and triethylene thiophosphoramide. *J Chron Dis*, 1960, *11*(1):7-33.

115. Spitzer, W.O., Dobson, A.J., Hall, J., et al. Measuring the quality of life of cancer patients: A concise QL-Index for use by physicians. *J Chron Dis*, 1981, *34*(12):585.

116. Nelson, E.C., Landgraf, J.M., Hays, R.D., et al. The functional status of patients: How can it be measured in physicians' offices? *Med Care*, 1990, *28*(12):1111-1126.

117. Nelson, E.C., Landgraf, J.M., Hays, R.D., et al. The Coop function charts: A system to measure patient function in physician's offices. In M. Lipkin, Jr. (Ed.), *Functional status measurement in primary care.* New York: Springer-Verlag, 1990, pp. 97-131.

118. van Weel, C., & Scholten, J.H.G. Report of an international workshop of the WONCA Research and Classification Committee. In J.H.G. Scholten (Ed.), *Functional status assessment in family practice.* Meditekst: Lelystad, 1992, pp. 5-51.

119. Kaplan, R.M., & Anderson, J.P. The general health policy model: An integrated approach. In B. Spilker (Ed.), *Quality of life and pharmacoeconomics in clinical trials* (2nd ed.). Philadelphia: Lippincott-Raven, 1996, pp. 309-322.

120. Bergner, M., Bobbitt, R., Pollard, W., et al. The Sickness Impact Profile: Validation of a health status measure. *Med Care*, 1976, *14*(1):57-67.

121. Johnson, J.E., King, K.B., & Murray, R.A. Measuring the impact of sickness on usual functions of radiation therapy patients. *Oncol Nurs Forum*, 1983, *10*(4):36-39.

122. Pollard, W.E., Bobbitt, R.A., Bergner, M., et al. The Sickness Impact Profile: Reliability of a health status measure. *Med Care*, 1976, *14*(2):146-55.

123. Ott, C.R., Sivarajan, E.S., Newton, K.M., et al. A controlled randomized study of early cardiac rehabilitation: The Sickness Impact Profile as an assessment tool. *Heart Lung*, 1983, *12*(2):162-170.

124. Deyo, R. Measuring functional outcomes in therapeutic trials in chronic disease. *Cont Clin Trials*, 1984, *5*(3):223-240.

125. Schag, C.A.C., & Heinrich, R.L. *Cancer Rehabilitation Evaluation System CARES Manual.* Santa Monica, CA: CARES Consultants, 1988.

126. Schag, C.A.C., Ganz, P.A., & Heinrich, R.L. Cancer Rehabilitation Evaluation System-Short Form (CARES-SF). *Cancer*, 1991, *68*(6):1406-1413.

127. Schag, C.A., Heinrich, R.L., Aadland, R., & Ganz, P.A. Assessing problems of cancer patients: Psychometric properties of the Cancer Inventory of Problem Situations. *Health Psychol*, 1990, *9*(1):83-102.

128. Schipper, H., Clinch, J., McMurray, A., & Levitt, M. Measuring the quality of life on cancer patients: The Functional Living Index-Cancer: Development and validation. *J Clin Oncol*, 1984, *2*(5):472-483.

129. Morrow, G.R., Lindke, J., & Black, P. Measurement of quality of life in patients: Psychometric analysis of the Functional Living Index—Cancer (FLIC). *Qual Life Res*, 1992, *1*(5):287-296.

Appendix 10A. HQOL Domain Frameworks

Cella et al. (53), Cella (55)	WHOQOL Group (77,79)	Ware and Sherbourne (93), Stewart and Ware (101)	Ferrans (107), Ferrans and Powers (108)	Grant, Ferrell et al. (109,110)	Padilla et al. (111)
<u>Physical dimension</u> **Physical well-being:** energy, unwellness, distress from side effects (i.e., nausea, pain), meeting family needs, cancer/HIV disease- and treatment-specific concerns	<u>Physical dimension</u> **Physical well-being:** energy and fatigue, pain and discomfort, sleep and rest	<u>Physical dimension</u> **Physical functioning and well-being:** physical functioning, energy/fatigue, pain, psycho-physiological symptoms, sleep problems	<u>Physical dimension</u> **Satisfaction and importance of health and functioning domain:** usefulness, physical independence, responsibilities, health, stress, sex life, health care and treatment, leisure activities, retirement, travel, long life	<u>Physical dimension</u> **Physical well-being and symptoms:** strength/stamina/fatigue, functional activities/ability, disease-specific symptoms (e.g., visual disturbance), coping with chronic symptoms (e.g., GVHD,* fertility), nutrition/appetite, sleep and rest, aches and pains, constipation, nausea	<u>Physical dimension</u> **Physical well-being and general functioning:** feeling healthy/sick, feeling independent/dependent, able to work/not work, feeling strong/weak, eating, sleep, rest **Disease- and treatment-specific attributes:** pain, nausea, vomiting, being hospitalized, cancer treatments
Functional well-being: able to work, accept illness, sleep well, enjoy life, enjoy leisure, enjoy quality of life.	**Independence:** mobility, activities of daily living, dependence on medical substances and aids, work capacity				
<u>Interpersonal dimension</u> **Social/family well-being:** support or communication from friends, family, and neighbors; sexual intimacy	<u>Interpersonal dimension</u> **Social:** personal relationships, social support, sexual activity	<u>Interpersonal dimension</u> **Social functioning and well-being:** social activity limitations from health, role limitations from physical health, role limitations from emotional problems	<u>Interpersonal dimension</u> **Satisfaction and importance of family domain:** family's, happiness, children, relationship with spouse/significant other, family's health	<u>Interpersonal dimension</u> **Social well-being:** appearance, roles and relationships, affection/caregiver burden, leisure activities, return to work financial burden, employment, isolation	<u>Interpersonal dimension</u> **Social support:** supportive relations, interpersonal support, relationships, marriage, friends **Social/role functioning:** making others happy, satisfying others, giving self, helping others
Relationship with doctor: confidence, communication, (deleted from Version 4)					**Fulfilling one's role:** good parent, good neighbor

142

Economic/environmental dimension
Environment: financial resources, freedom, physical safety and security, health/social care accessibility and quality, home environment, new information and skills, recreation and leisure, physical environment: pollution, noise, traffic, climate, transportation

Economic/environmental dimension
Satisfaction and importance of socioeconomic domain: standard of living, financial independence, home, job, neighborhood, overall USA conditions, friends, emotional support, education

Psychologic/spiritual dimension
Psychologic well-being: Affective/cognitive: enjoyment, happiness, spiritual support, inner peace, able to concentrate, communicate

Coping ability: feeling secure financially, housing, insurance, life style, positive mental attitude, hope, optimism, goals

Meaning pain/cancer: pain, positive/negative force, fear of disease, uncertainty, lack of control

Accomplishments: successful, satisfied, achieve goals, improve surroundings

Psychologic/spiritual dimension
Psychologic well-being: anxiety, depression, fear recurrence/diagnosis/treatment, changed priorities, cognitive/attention, normalcy, second chance, happiness, coping with survival, control, pain, distress

Spiritual well-being: strengthened belief, hope, despair, religiosity inner strength

Psychologic/spiritual dimension
Mental functioning and well-being: cognitive functioning, psychological distress, psychological well-being

Psychologic/spiritual dimension
Satisfaction and importance of psychologic/spiritual domain: satisfaction with life, happiness, satisfaction with self, achievement of goals, peace of mind, personal appearance, faith in God

Psychologic/spiritual dimension
Psychologic: body image and appearance, negative feelings, self-esteem, thinking, learning, memory, concentration

Spiritual: religion spirituality, personal beliefs

Psychologic/spiritual dimension
Emotional well-being: feeling sad, nervous, hopeless, worry about coping with illness

Health perception dimension
Health perceptions: Overall physical health

Health perception dimensions
Health perceptions: current health perceptions, health outlook

*GVHD = graft - versus - host disease.

Appendix 10B. Methodologic Approaches to Quality-of-Life Research

	Data Collection Period	Benefits	Limitations
Most optimal	**Prospective longitudinal:** For each patient, data is collected at the same time point throughout the course of treatment, usually from diagnosis through post-treatment period, and ideally continuing beyond the post-treatment period, e.g., pre, mid, end, 1-month, and 6-month follow-ups.	Offers true process evaluation of same group of patients. Offers baseline to follow-up comparisons and higher reliability estimate of quality of life.	Expensive; data takes long time to obtain; patient attrition a problem.
	Prospective single time point: For each patient, data is collected once at the same time point in the illness/ treatment trajectory, e.g. each patient is interviewed one week post treatment.	Offers uniformity of post-treatment patient evaluation.	Limited view of quality of life; possible low reliability.
	Prospective cross-sectional: Data is collected once for different groups of patients with the same illness but representing different phases of illness or treatment, e.g., three groups of breast cancer patients at diagnosis, recurrence, and near death.	Offers some view of changes in quality of life in relation to the disease trajectory; is less expensive than prospective longitudinal designs; and may increase reliability.	Patients may not be well matched other than on the disease variable, therefore, true phase comparisons are risky.
Less optimal	**Prospective single data collection, variable time points:** Data is collected once, but patients represent variable times in the illness/treatment trajectory, e.g., patients range from 1 to 10 years postmastectomy.	Offers ability to assess maximal number of patients; least expensive method of data collection.	Severe limit to comparability of patient responses due to history effects in the variability of time since diagnosis and treatment.

Based on Wellisch, D.K. Methodology in behavioral and psychosocial cancer research. Work, social, recreation, family, and physical status. *Cancer,* 1984, *53*(10 Suppl):2292.

Appendix 10C. Strategies and Technologies for Quality-of-Life Research

	Instruments	Administrator	Advantages	Disadvantages
Most optimal	Combination of structured interviewing, analogue scales, behavioral functioning/activities	Some self-administered; some administered by project staff (not the treating physician/ health care provider)	Very comprehensive; can be both general and tailored to specific illness/treatment; better content and construct validity	Expensive to implement; can be lengthy to administer; convergent validity (between measures) can suffer
Less optimal	Unstructured clinical interview	Treating physician/health care provider	Low cost, easy, and plentiful patient access	Physician bias severe; patient often skews response set to please doctor; no objective measures; low reliability
	Semistructured interview	Usually treating physician/health care provider	Low cost, easy, and plentiful patient access	Less biased than unstructured interview, but provider bias still a problem; low validity; questionable reliability
	Analogue rating scales	Can be physician/health care provider	Very brief; can be closely tailored to specific tumor types, sites, and regimens	Overly restrictive view of patient life; validity problems
	Psychologic tests	Self-administered	In-depth look at emotional status of patient	Often very poorly standardized for cancer patients; confounded with pre-illness issues; only covers emotional issues

Based on Wellisch. D.K. Methodology in behavioral and psychosocial cancer research. Work, social, recreation, family, and physical status. *Cancer*, 1984, *53*(10 Suppl):2293.

Appendix 10D. Objective Instruments That Yield Quantitative Data

Name/Description	Psychometric Testing/Comments

Karnofsky Performance Index (104)
Scale is designed to measure one dimension of a patient's life, the ability to perform activities of daily living. Karnofsky ratings:
    100—Normal, no complaints, no evidence of disease.
    60—Requires occasional assistance, able to care for most needs,
    20—Very sick, hospitalized, active supportive treatment necessary, 0—Dead
 	
Instrument is in the public domain and can be downloaded: www.hospicepatients.org/karnofsky.html.
	Tests of interrater reliability, concurrent validity, and discriminant validity indicate that, with standardized observational procedures based on a mental status exam, the Karnofsky scale is acceptably reliable and valid as a global measure, but it does not adequately capture the conceptual domain of quality of life (113, p129). One of the oldest measures of performance status (104). Measures QOL as only one dimension—physical function.

Zubrod Scale (114) The Zubrod Scale, a 0-to-5 scale in increments of 1, evaluates the patient's ability to remain ambulatory and to perform ADL (114). Instrument is in the public domain and can be viewed at (item 9) www.sts.org/file/GTSDBDefinitions.pdf.	Both the Karnofsky and Zubrod scales have been used extensively by cooperative cancer research groups because they show a correlation with tumor response to treatment and survival.
QL-Index (115) An objective scale developed by Spitzer et al. (115) A brief measure (1 minute) of health, family support, ADL, and outlook completed by a health professional. The range of scores is 0 to 10. An example from one category on the QL-Index is "During the last week the patient: has been appearing to feel well or reporting feeling 'great' most of the time (+2); has been lacking energy or not feeling entirely up to par more than just occasionally (+1); has been feeling very ill or 'lousy,' seeming weak and washed out most of the time or was unconscious (0)." Instrument can be viewed at rtog.org/members/forms/p0126/p-0126sp.html.	Discriminant construct validity, content validity, high internal consistency (Cronbach's coefficient alpha 0.775), and statistically significant interrater Spearman rank correlation ($r = 0.81$, $p < 0.001$). Cella and Tulsky report that the QL-Index is the most widely used observer-rated QOL scale (31). However, the ability of the instrument to stand alone is questionable because correlations between observer and patient ratings are modest. Grieco and Long state that the QL-Index has the advantage of brevity, but, like the Karnofsky scale, lacks standardized observational procedures (113).
Dartmouth Cooperative (COOP) (116, 117, 118) Word-picture assessment charts to measure patient function in busy clinical practices. Measure: social/role functioning; pain and emotional condition; perceptions of changes in health, overall health, quality of life; social support. Simple drawing of picture to illustrate word scale. The 1992 version is called the COOP/WONCA charts (118). Information about the Dartmouth COOP Project can be found at www.dartmouth.edu/~coopproj/index.html.	2000 patients, 4 settings (116,117) Test-retest: 0.78-0.98 elderly, 1 hour apart: 0.73-0.98 low-income, after 2 weeks: 0.42-0.88. Validity: correlations between scores on RAND scales of same dimension indicate acceptable convergent validity (0.62); average discriminant validity correlation 0.39 at one site; significant correlations between symptoms and chart scores for overall health (0.51). Useful measures of function in busy practices (36). Instrument may "detect moderate effects in physical and emotional functioning secondary to changes in health status" (17). Weaknesses: lacks disability and major daily activities.

Appendix 10D. Objective Instruments That Yield Quantitative Data *(cont.)*

Name/Description	Psychometric Testing/Comments
Quality of Well-Being (QWB) Scale (119) Utility/preference measure of HQOL outcomes. Summarizes HQOL by well years (WY) = quality adjusted life years (QALY).	Reliability and validity supported in a number of studies.
Scores: 0 (death) to 1.0 (optimal function) by combining preference-weighted measures of symptoms and functions at a specific point in time.	Applies utility analyses to treatment and policy decision
	Function scales: mobility, physical activity, social activity.
Challenge: selection of values that determine the weights. Available in many languages. To obtain information about the QWB Scale contact:	Advantages: can compare very different treatment programs and disease outcomes, sensitive to changes in health outcomes, reflects relative importance of HQOL dimensions.
Robert M Kaplan, PhD, 241 Stein Clinical Science Department of Family and Preventive Medicine University of California San Diego, La Jolla, CA 92093-0628 USA Phone: (858) 534-6058; Fax: (858) 534-7517; rkaplan@ucsd.edu	
Copyright agreement Website: medicine.ucsd.edu/fpm/hoap/images/ QWB_SAcopyrtagmnt2002.pdf.	

Numbers in parentheses correspond to studies cited in the References.

Appendix 10E. Subjective Instruments That Yield Quantitative Data

Name/Description	Psychometric Testing/Comments
Quality of Life Scale for Cancer (QOL-CA) (11) The multidimensional Quality of Life Scale for Cancer (QOL-CA), a.k.a. QLI and MQOLS-CA, is a 30-item measure that uses 100-mm linear analogue scales as the response format (0 = poorest QOL, 100 = best QOL). Subscales include psychosocial-existential well-being, physical-functional, symptom distress-nutrition, symptom distress-pain/fatigue, and attitude of worry. All versions of the instruments are in the public domain. For a copy of the questionnaire and instructions contact: Geraldine.Padilla@nursing.ucsf.edu.	Internal consistency alphas range from 0.77 to 0.91 for the subscales and total scale with the exception of pain/bowel pattern (0.68) and worry (0.52). Content validity, factor analytic construct validity, multitrait-multimethod construct validity supported (11). A revised QOL-CA2 scale consists of 33 items. It is used in a number of nursing studies with persons with cancer.
Ferrans and Powers Quality of Life Index (QLI) (107,108) The 66-item QLI produces five scores: quality of life overall and four domains (health and functioning, psychologic/spiritual, social and economic, and family). Items are rated first for satisfaction and importance. Importance ratings are used to weight satisfaction responses. Scores reflect satisfaction with QLI attributes that are important to the individual. For a copy of the most current version, scoring instructions, and permission, go to www.uic.edu/orgs/qli/index.htm.	Internal consistency alphas, across numerous studies, are consistently ≥ 0.70 for three subscales, the exception being the family subscale, which yielded a coefficient of 0.63 in one study. Test–retest reliability was demonstrated at ≥ 0.69. Content and construct validity were supported in a number of studies. The QLI is available in a number of languages and for a number of diagnoses. It is a frequently used instrument in nursing studies. All versions of the QLI are in the public domain.
Sickness Impact Profile (SIP) (120,121) The SIP provides a descriptive profile of changes in a person's behavior due to sickness. It consists of 136 items grouped into 12 categories of life activities, for example, physical, psychosocial, sleep and rest, nutrition, usual daily work, household management, leisure, and recreation (120). Typical statements on the SIP are "I laugh or cry suddenly" or "I just pick or nibble at my food." The instrument takes between 20 and 30 minutes to administer. Scores range from zero to one hundred percent disruption for a scale category or each dimension of the scale or for a total disruption score (121). Information can be found on the Ethics Tool database: www.bc.edu/bc_org/avp/son/ethics/database/3.07.07.html.	The SIP was demonstrated to be a reliable (test–retest) (122) and valid measure (120). The SIP has been used with patients with a variety of illnesses such as coronary artery disease (123). Johnson et al. used the SIP with radiation oncology patients and believe that this instrument is an acceptable QOL measure (121). The criticism has been made that, because the SIP assesses a fairly broad functional state, it may not discriminate among more subtle changes produced by the disease state or treatment (124). The lack of ability to detect change becomes important in studies attempting to show "before" and "after" QOL changes.
Cancer Rehabilitation Evaluation System (CARES) and Short Form (CARES-SF) (125,126) The CARES long form consists of 139 potential problems experienced by persons with cancer. The first 88 items pertain to all patients; the next 51 are different for each person depending on the course of treatment. The minimum number of items completed is 93, and the maximum is 132. Each item is answered on a 5-point scale from not at all (0 = no problem) to very much (4 = severe problem). If used for clinical purposes, a form is available wherein patients indicate whether they want help with the problem (yes) or not (no). The CARES consists of a global HQOL scale, five summary	Psychometric information for the CARES long form supports the reliability and validity of the instrument (127). Test-retest reliability correlations are all highly satisfactory. Alpha coefficients for three samples of 479, 1047, and 114 cancer patients ranged from 0.82 to 0.94 (126). Validity information is provided by Schag et al. (82). Studies confirm the construct validity of the five major scales; convergent and discriminant validity was supported by the patterns of correlations with other measures such as the Karnofsky Performance Scale, SCL-90, a visual analogue scale of current functioning (127).

Appendix 10E. Subjective Instruments That Yield Quantitative Data (*cont.*)

Name/Description	Psychometric Testing/Comments
scales (physical, psychosocial, marital, medical interaction, and sexual), and 31 subscales measuring everyday functioning (ambulation, weight loss, pain, difficulty working, body image, sexual and psychosocial distress, etc.). The CARES-SF (short form) contains 59 items: a minimum of 38 and a maximum of 57. Scoring is similar to the CARES long form (125,126).	
The instrument and instructions can be purchased from: Anne Coscarelli, PhD, Ted Mann Family Resource Center, 200 UCLA Medical Plaza, Ste 502, Los Angeles, CA 90095-6934. phone: (310) 794-6644, fax: (310) 794-9615.	
Functional Living Index—Cancer (FLIC) (128,129) 22-item questionnaire, Likert format (1–7 range). FLIC measures a composite of distinct factors contributing to overall functional living (physical well-being, psychologic state, family situational interaction, social ability, somatic sensation).	Validity and reliability are supported by two studies (128,129). Studies supported concurrent, discriminant, and convergent validity as well as construct validity. A similar 5-factor structure was described in both studies (128,129). Internal consistency coefficients ranged from 0.64 to 0.88.
For information about the FLIC contact: Harvey Schipper, MD World Health Org., Collaborating Centre for Quality of Life in Cancer Care St. Boniface General Hosp. Res. Centre, 351 Tache Avenue Winnipeg, Manitoba, Canada R2H 2A6, Fax: (204) 235-1231	Designed for easy, repeated patient self-administration. Popular measure of quality of life in studies of persons with cancer.
Nottingham Health Profile (NHP) (21,22) 38-item questionnaire with 6 domains: Physical mobility (8 items), pain (8 items), social isolation (5 items), emotional reactions (9 items), energy (3 items), sleep (5 items). Each item has a yes/no response format. Items are weighted. Each domain can have a score from 0 to 100. A domain score is the mean of all items within the domain. A score of 100 means the respondent believes he/she has all the problems in that domain, while a score of zero means no perceived problems. Domain scores are presented as a profile, no overall score is calculated for the whole scale.	Test–retest reliability and validity have been reported. Validity: Criterion validity established by association between consulting a doctor and subjective health status. NHP differentiated between consulters and nonconsulters of general health practitioners, after controlling for age and sex; and in the overall self-rated health between those with few versus many absences from work.
A description of the NHP can be found at www.atsqol.org/nott.asp.	
A copy of the instrument can be found at www.ildannoallapersona.com/allegati/ Nottingham%20Health%20Profile.pdf.	

11

Multiple Instruments for Measuring Quality of Life

Anna K. Omery and Hannah Dean

The continuing drive to offer cost-effective, quality care accessible to all leads to the demand for efficient and appropriate use of resources. Allocating or rationing of resources is a current and future reality. Quality of life is proposed as a goal of health care,[1,2] as an endpoint,[3–6] as an outcome of treatment,[7,8] and as a means of rank-ordering treatments for allocating resources.[9,10] Kaplan and Coons[11] assert that "health care concerns can be reduced to just two categories: life duration and quality of life." Callahan[1,2] advocates redirecting the goals of health care from extending life to favoring interventions and therapies that improve quality of life.

Padilla et al.[12] identified five purposes for examining quality of life in research. Researchers use quality of life measures to describe patient responses to disease, patient responses to symptom management, patient and family responses to cancer treatment, patient responses to rehabilitation efforts, and distress trajectories in the course of patients' disease experiences. Osaba[13] suggests that these purposes for examining quality of life are not only relevant to or for the individual or micro-level of care, they are also relevant to groups (meso-level) and care of populations (macro-level).

The proposed uses for quality-of-life measurements demand that policymakers, researchers, and clinicians be rigorous in their approach to choosing instruments and measurement schemes. The inclusion of two chapters on quality of life in this book reflects a recognition of this need for rigor. This chapter discusses using multiple instruments for measuring quality of life. Investigators will find related instruments in several other chapters of this book, including functional status, mental status, social support, coping, hope, spirituality, sexuality, anxiety, depression, loneliness, pain, and dyspnea.

Importance of Measuring Quality of Life

The conceptualization and measurement of quality of life are vital to health policy, evaluation research, and clinical decision making. References to the importance of health-related quality of life for health policy and evaluation research abound.[10,14–18] A review using citation databases (PubMed and OVID) found that more than 1000 new articles per year are being indexed under *quality of life*. They indicate the need for a means to compare the outcomes across different interventions, disease groups, and populations.[13] Some advocate a means of rank-ordering interventions by their cost-effectiveness, with quality of life as one of the factors in making the determinations.[9,10,18]

Working groups at a National Cancer Institute (NCI) sponsored workshop recommend quality-of-life assessment as an endpoint measure in Phase III clinical trial protocols, along with tumor response, survival, and toxicities of therapy.[6] Hayden et al.[3] emphasize the Southwest Oncology Group's[3] recommendation of commitment to gathering quality-of-life data because sometimes quality of life is *the* endpoint of interest when comparing one intervention against another. Caution must be exercised, however, when using quality of life as an outcome measure. For example, in the early 1980s, two evaluation studies startled the hospice community when their results failed to indicate significant differences in the quality of life for persons dying in hospice versus nonhospice settings.[19,20] Some interventions might prove to extend life at the cost of quality of life. Vaisrub alludes to the importance of quality of life as a measure of the usefulness of cardiac revascularization when he says, "The attained 'quality of life' [after cardiac revascularization] is apt to be void of social usefulness."[21] Research findings, if considered valid and replicable, could lead to limitations in funding for programs. Researchers must ensure that the measures of quality of life used are valid and sufficiently sensitive to detect differences in quality of life of populations.

Practitioners are admonished to incorporate assessment of quality of life into their clinical practices.[11,22–24] Schipper et al.[25] suggest that patients should be informed about quality of life and survival statistics as part of informed consent regarding the management of their cancers. Lynch[26] moderated grand rounds in critical care in which Engelhardt discussed the "quality of life" versus the "quality of morbidity." Engelhardt makes a strong case for the importance of providing patients with a clear picture of the impact of treatment. Informed consent requires that patients have information from which to decide whether increased lifespan is worth the morbidity associated with their conditions or their treatment or both. For example, Sugarbaker et al.[27] report evidence that suggests that amputation for sarcoma is less disruptive to quality of life than is a limb-sparing procedure involving surgery and radiation.

Issues to Consider in Measuring Quality of Life

Several significant problems related to measurement of quality of life have been raised by scholars. Yancik and Yates[28] express concern about the indiscriminate and superficial use of quality of life in clinical trials. They identify as a problem the use of a single instrument to discern differences in quality of life in patients across cancer diagnoses. Sprangers, et al.[29] note issues in addition to those across diagnoses. There can be measurement issues with multiple uses of the same instrument in the same person. That is, for a person with a very poor health status, a small increase in a quality-of-life score may be meaningful. At an earlier time, when that same person had a higher quality of life score, the same increase may have been meaningless.

In a related argument, Braden et al.[30] point to the difficulty of using quality of life as an outcome measure because the factors that affect it are so complex. They suggest that specific components of quality of life be measured that are consistent with the theoretical framework of the study and the specific expected effects or outcomes of the disease, treatment, or intervention. Smith et al.[31] conclude from their meta-analysis that quality of life and health status are separate constructs. When rating quality of life, patients give greater emphasis to mental health as opposed to physical functioning. The pattern is reversed for appraisal of health status. They reason that current health status instruments that have been used in the past to measure quality of life may no longer be appropriate measures. Furthermore, quality of life researchers increasingly propose disease-specific as opposed to generic measurement of quality of life.[32]

Investigators also question the conceptual and psychometric adequacy of Euro-American quality-of-life instruments applied to non-Euro-American populations. Kagawa-Singer[33] asserts that the Japanese, for example, hold values opposite to those of Euro-Americans. According to Kagawa-Singer, in Japanese culture life is not sacred, the individual is not autonomous, suffering is a part of life, and verbal language is viewed as a negative quality. She warns that measurements of items that have no conceptual equivalency in another culture are invalid. Kagawa-Singer recommends a framework including security, integrity, and belonging as basic needs essential to quality of life, the means of achieving which vary depending on culturally based values. Wan et al.[34] noted that in multinational clinical trials, language-adapted quality-of-life instruments focus mainly on translation issues and less on psychometric equivalency across versions.

Rosser[35] advocates a single instrument and a unitary index for ease of use for planning purposes; however, he points out that the conceptualization of quality of life has shifted, making it difficult to compare data over time. Stewart[36, p. 13] indicates that variations in conceptualizations also occur depending on the frame of reference of the observer. She concludes that "only one category, functioning or behavior, is included in all schemes." Carr and Higinson[32] identify four different definitions of quality of life:

- The extent to which hopes and ambitions are matched by experience.
- Individuals' perceptions of their position in life taken in the context of culture and value systems where they live and in relation to their goals, expectations, standards, and concerns.
- Appraisal of one's current state against some ideal.
- The things people regard as important in their lives.

Clearly, use of different definitions or reformulations of existing definitions in a study would require different instruments.

Approaches to Measuring Quality of Life

Multiple instruments are advocated because of the need for reliable, comparable, valid, and sensitive scales to measure the multidimensional concept of quality of life. Gotay et al.[5, p. 576] urge researchers to choose instruments based on a careful definition of quality of life; they say, "in a particular study, there may not be a single instrument available to carry out such a collection [of both functional and satisfaction data]." Use of multiple instruments allows flexibility in the conceptualization of quality of life while permitting comparability of specific dimensions across studies. Use of multiple instruments not only allows for comparability, it also allows for responsiveness. Employing increasingly sensitive measures for specific domains may be more feasible with the use of multiple instruments. Such an approach permits the investigator to avoid either a ceiling or a floor effect.[17] Jalowiec[37] concludes that, after a thorough examination, the advantages of the multiple-instrument approach outweigh the disadvantages.

Three general approaches to the use of multiple measures have emerged in the quality-of-life literature in the past several years: a core instrument and specific modules to be used for particular situations or conditions,[38,39] a battery of instruments, and composite instruments constructed using parts of existing instruments. The core and module approach stems from work in Europe.

The studies cited later in this chapter are examples of the battery approach to measuring the multiple dimensions of quality of life. In the early 1980s, Ware[40] suggested the wisdom of selecting a battery of health status measures because of the lack of consensus about the dimensions of the concept. Stewart[41] reiterated the breadth of the concept and indicated that there continues to be fairly wide diversity, depending on the frame of reference of the researcher. Moinpour et al.[4] recommend separate measures of physical functioning, emotional functioning, symptoms, and global quality of life; they further recommend including measures of social functioning and other "protocol-specific" variables when appropriate. Schumaker et al.[42] and Guyatt and Jaeschke[43] identify a range of problems with using a battery approach, including difficulty analyzing across time and interpreting the results of the multiple measure when they point in different directions, the complexity of study design, and the burden on the patient and staff. Nevertheless, Schumaker et al.[42] advocate a battery approach with instruments that "correspond to the dimensions of quality of life most likely to be either positively or negatively affected by treatment, and to use the best instruments to assess each of these dimensions." Spilker,[44] Spilker et al.,[45] and McDowell and Newell[46] provide valuable resources for identifying measures to be included in a battery. Many discussions and examples of the battery approach are reflected in the literature.[6,7,47–54]

The third approach to using multiple measures involves constructing composite instruments from existing measures. Cleary et al.[55] developed an instrument for examining health-related quality of life in persons with AIDS by combining specific subscales from several instruments, including the Functional Status Questionnaire, a fatigue scale from the Medical Outcomes Study short form, several questions from the Health Interview Survey, and two questions from the Memory Assessment Clinic Self-Rating Scale. DeLeo et al.[56] constructed a 31-item instrument to assess quality of life in the elderly by selecting items from eight other scales. Other examples of this approach can be found in works by Lubeck and Fries,[57] Sherbourne et al.,[58] Tuchler et al.,[59] and Wiklund et al.[60] Such an approach carries the same potential problems found in the use of a battery, with the added question of reliability and validity when previously validated instruments are cannibalized and reconstructed in new forms.

Use of multiple instruments follows from evaluation of single instruments or scales. Frank-Stromborg[61] reports on selecting a single instrument to measure quality of life. She emphasizes four decisions a researcher must make in choosing an instrument: qualitative versus quantitative measures, subjective versus objective reporters of data, subjective versus objective dimensions, and single versus multiple instruments. Other choices emerge from the literature, such as global versus domain-specific measures, societal versus individual perspectives, cognitive versus affective evaluations, global versus disease-specific measures, and population-specific measures.

As Spitzer et al. point out:

Global measures of quality of life include those that seek responses, such as the following: Please mark with an X the appropriate place within the bar to indicate your rating of this person's quality of life during the past week. (100-mm bar with "lowest quality" on the left and "highest quality" on the right).[62]

This approach assumes that the respondent can provide a valid overall assessment of quality of life. A global approach also implies unidimensionality. Domain-specific approaches seek assessments of variables related to a multidimensional concept. Domain-specific data may be achieved by either single or multiple instruments. The use of both unidimensional and multidimensional instruments in the same study may reflect the investigator's lack of conceptual clarity. Even if the investigator has a grasp of the concept and still wishes to include both global and domain kinds of quality-of-life measures, the confounding statistical issues are significant.

Societal versus individual perspectives on the quality of life may vary considerably. The researcher should clarify which approach is being used. Conclusions should reflect limitations to generalizations based on the approach used. Campbell[63] alludes to this distinction when he argues that the individual's experience of quality of life may not relate directly to societal indicators, such as education, mortality, and employment.

George[64] distinguishes between cognitive and affective evaluations of life quality. Cognitive evaluations are those based on the facts of a person's circumstances. Affective evaluations reflect how respondents feel about their quality of life irrespective of the objective facts. Both approaches have value in measuring quality of life.

Increasingly, investigators recognize the need to examine quality of life from a disease-specific perspective. The specific effects of one disease compared to another can be expected to have consequences for quality of life in different dimensions. Quality of life has been investigated in patients with rheumatoid arthritis,[48] acquired immune deficiency syndrome[5] and HIV infection,[57] stroke,[49] cardiovascular disease,[60] chronic lung disease,[65] hypertension,[11] physical disabilities,[66,69] coronary artery surgery,[68,69] heart transplants,[53] depression,[52] and cognitive impairments.[70] In addition, the range of specific cancer diagnoses and treatments addressed in the quality-of-life literature is broad, including breast cancer,[3,31] bone marrow transplant,[71,72] head and neck cancer,[73] and endometrial cancer.[74]

Gotay and Moore[73] illustrate the issue of choosing population-specific methods of measuring quality of life in their examination of studies of quality of life in head and neck cancer patients. The problem goes beyond disease-specific to population-specific issues with this patient population, for whom the comorbidities of alcohol and nicotine abuse complicate quality-of-life assessment. Other population-specific considerations include culture,[1,34,38] age,[22,54,56,70,75] and gender.[76]

Given all these possibilities when selecting multiple instruments, is there any direction for an investigator? Higginson and Carr[77] identify 10 questions for assessing quality-of-life measures for clinical practice. These questions are also applicable for researchers as they choose multiple instruments for their study. The 10 questions follow:

1. Are the domains covered relevant?
2. In what populations and settings was it developed and tested, and are these similar to the situations in which it is to be used?
3. Is the measure valid, reliable, responsive, and appropriate?
4. What were the assumptions of the assessors when determining validity?
5. Are there floor and ceiling effects? That is, does the measure fail to identify deterioration in patients who already have poor quality of life or improvement in patients who already have good quality of life?
6. Will it measure differences between patients or over time, and at what power?
7. Who completes the measure: patients, their family, or a professional? What effect will this have—that is, will they complete it?
8. How long does it take to complete the measure?

9. Do staff and patients find it easy to use?
10. Who will need to be trained and informed about the measure?

Conceptualizing Quality of Life

In spite of frequent references to quality of life in health care issues in the professional and public press, the definition of the concept remains elusive. A review of the literature reveals a variety of terms equated with quality of life, such as life satisfaction,[67,78,79] self-esteem,[80] well-being,[70,81,84] health status,[16,22,23,27,40,85,86] happiness,[87] adjustment,[88] value of life,[89] meaning of life,[90,91] and functional status.[65,92]

In addition, the dimensions of the concept of quality of life vary from study to study. Hutchinson et al.[93] identify physical, social, and emotional dimensions. Flanagan[94] describes 15 aspects in five categories, including physical and material well-being; relations with other people; social, community, and civic activities; personal development and fulfillment; and recreation. McSweeney et al.[95] define quality of life as emotional functioning, social role functioning, and participation in activities of daily living (ADL) and recreational pastimes. Linn and Linn[96] operationalize quality of life as scores on scales of depression, self-esteem, life satisfaction, alienation, and locus of control. Levy and Wynbrandt[97] report on quality of life in terms of income, sexual activity, and lifestyle. Aaronson et al.[98] point out that "research on single dimensions of quality of life, such as pain, nausea and vomiting, insomnia and psychologic distress, have led to improvements in symptom control." Guyatt et al.[65] specified dyspnea as a measure of quality of life in patients with chronic airflow limitations. City of Hope researchers expanded their quality-of-life framework to include spiritual well-being, based on extensive research with bone marrow transplant survivors.[71,72]

Acceptance of the premise that quality of life is a multidimensional concept demands a conceptual framework identifying the elements that constitute it. Three authors present specific frameworks that may prove useful in clinical nursing research.

The Ware Framework

Ware[99] proposes five elements to be used as guides in selecting instruments to measure quality of life: (1) disease; (2) personal functioning; (3) psychologic distress, or well-being; (4) general health perceptions; and (5) social or role functioning. Disease is central because it is the focus of our interest, the reason we are interested in a particular population for study. Ware recommends disease-specific measures because of the heterogeneity of the concept. *Personal functioning* is defined as the performance of or capacity to perform ADL, such as self-care, mobility, and physical activities.

Ware insists that the third element, psychologic distress and well-being, be measured using specific measures of psychologic status. *General health perceptions* refers to self-rated measures of general health and well-being. Finally, role functioning is distinguished from personal functioning and refers to the performance of or capacity to perform activities associated with an individual's usual role, such as father, mother, companion, or helpmate.

The George and Bearon Framework

George and Bearon[100] selected four dimensions to define quality of life, including both subjective evaluations and objective conditions. Their subjective evaluations include life satisfaction and self-esteem; their objective conditions include general health/ functional status and socioeconomic status. They present detailed accounts of 21 instruments for and methods of measuring the proposed dimensions, with descriptions, measurement properties, and recommendations for use of each.

The Cella Framework

Based on a review of factor analytic and aggregate index studies, Cella[101] presents four dimensions of health-related quality of life: physical, functional, emotional, and social. Cella's model is particularly apt for the purpose of this chapter because of subordinate domains linking the larger dimensions and additional areas for which the linkages are less well established. The physical dimension includes symptoms and side effects; the functional dimension, role performance, and ADL; the emotional dimension includes distress and well-being; and the social dimension comprises sociability and intimacy. Additional areas for consideration are work, sexuality, leisure, spirituality, family functioning, and treatment satisfaction.

Instruments Used to Measure Quality-of-Life Elements

The instruments described in this section are organized according to the major studies in which they were used as measures of quality of life. This arrangement illustrates conceptual frameworks and multiple instruments in quality-of-life research.

Burckhardt Study

Burckhardt[102] studied the impact of physical, psychologic, and social factors on the perception of quality of life among 94 people with arthritis in a community. She created a quality-of-life index using a single question rating the subject's overall quality of life, the Life Satisfaction Index (LSI-Z), and the Domain Satisfaction Scale.

Life Satisfaction Index (LSI-Z)

Wood et al.[103] developed the LSI-Z as a short form of the Life Satisfaction Rating (LSR). The LSI-Z consists of 13 items to which the subject is asked to respond with "agree," "disagree," or "?" An example of an item is: "This is the dreariest time of my life." "Agree" answers score 2 points, and "?" answers score 1 point. All items must be answered. The validity and reliability coefficients between the original LSR and the LSI-Z were 0.57 and 0.79, respectively.

Domain Satisfaction Scale

Burckhardt describes the Domain Satisfaction Scale as developed from empirical data by Flanagan[94] using a 7-point rating scale developed by Andrews and Withey.[104] She refers to Campbell et al.[105] when describing the reliability and validity of the tool.

Index of Domain Satisfactions

The Index of Domain Satisfactions was developed by Campbell et al.[105] Respondents rate their satisfaction with each domain on the seven-point rating scale ranging from "completely satisfied" to "completely dissatisfied." The domains explored include marriage; family life; health; neighborhood; friendships; housework; job; life in the United States, city, or county; nonwork; housing; usefulness of education; standard of living; amount of education; and savings. The nonwork item follows several questions about leisure time and are scored as 1, completely satisfied, to 7, completely dissatisfied. An example of an item is "Overall, how satisfied are you with the ways you spend your spare time?" Results are reported with overall distribution of responses on each scale and average score values. Campbell et al. report stability correlations ranging from 0.42 to 0.67 for the individual domains and 0.76 for the sum of the 14 domain satisfactions.[105] Validity is not addressed explicitly. However, the domains selected relate to everyday life and are similar to those identified by Flanagan[94] and Andrews and Withey.[104]

The Evans et al. Study

Evans et al.[106] report a study of quality of life of 859 patients with end-stage renal disease. Objective measures of functional ability were obtained using the Karnovsky Index and the patient's response to the question: "Are you *now able* to work for pay full time, part time, or not at all?" Subjective indicators were drawn from the work of Campbell et al.,[105] including the Index of Psychological Affect, the Index of Overall Life Satisfaction, and the Index of Well-Being.

Index of Psychologic Affect

The Index of Psychologic Affect (called the Index of General Affect by Campbell et al.[105]) consists of eight semantic differential items: (1) boring/interesting; (2) miserable/enjoyable; (3) useless/worthwhile; (4) lonely/friendly; (5) empty/full; (6) discouraging/hopeful; (7) rewarding/disappointing; and (8) brings out the best in me/doesn't give me much of a chance.[106] Respondents place an X in one of seven boxes between the bipolar items indicating their feelings about their present lives. Campbell et al. report a reliability coefficient of 0.89 on the Index of General Affect.[105] Correlations with the overall life satisfaction item ($r = 0.55$) and the happiness item ($r = 0.52$) provide indications of validity.

Index of Overall Life Satisfaction

Evans et al. are unclear about their use of the Index of Overall Life Satisfaction.[106] Campbell et al.[105] measure the Index of Domain Satisfactions, and they include an overall life satisfaction item:

> "We have talked about various parts of your life, now I want to ask you about your life as a whole. How satisfied are you with your life as a whole these days? Which number on the card comes the closest to how satisfied or dissatisfied you are with your life as a whole?" (1 completely satisfied; 7 completely dissatisfied.)

In a repeat interview with 285 subjects 8 months after the initial data collection, the stability correlation for the Index of Overall Life Satisfaction was 0.43.[105] Campbell et al. do not address validity explicitly.

Index of Well-Being

The Index of Well-Being[105] is a composite of the Index of Overall Life Satisfaction and the Index of General Affect. The estimated reliability coefficient is reported to be 0.89. Validity is not addressed.

The Lewis Study

Lewis's study of late-stage cancer patients is the third major study from which instrument examples are drawn.[107] Lewis chose the Rosenberg Self-Esteem Scale, the Crumbaugh Purpose-in-Life Test, and the Lewis et al. Anxiety Scale as indicators of the psychosocial aspects of quality of life.

Rosenberg Self-Esteem Scale

The Rosenberg Self-Esteem Scale[108] purports to measure a basic feeling of self-worth. It consists of 10 items to which the subject responds on a four-point scale from "strongly agree" to "strongly disagree." Lewis reports reliability coefficients from 0.85 to 0.92 and validity correlations ranging from 0.56 to 0.83 with similar measures.

Crumbaugh Purpose-in-Life Test (PIL)

The Crumbaugh PIL Test[109] is a 20-item instrument to which subjects respond on a seven-point scale. Sample items: "In life I have no goals or aims at all" (1) to "very clear goals and aims" (7) or "I am a very irresponsible person" (1) to "a very responsible person" (7).

The PIL Test is designed to measure the degree to which the subject experiences a sense of meaning and purpose in life. Split-half correlations are reported to be 0.85 in a sample of church parishioners. PIL scores correlated with therapist ratings (0.38, $n = 50$) and minister ratings (0.47, $n = 120$).

Lewis et al. Anxiety Scale

The Lewis et al. Anxiety Scale[110] was developed for cancer patients. Subjects respond to nine items on a five-point scale (1, none of the time; 5, all the time). An example is "I feel more nervous than usual." Lewis[107] reports stability reliability at 0.90 and split-half reliability at 0.79. According to Lewis, validity was established by its inverse relations with an attitude scale measuring perceived functional effectiveness.

The King et al. Study

King et al.[68] examined patient perceptions of quality of life after coronary artery surgery in a sample of 155 men and women 1 year post coronary artery bypass grafting. Their conceptual framework for quality of life encompassed life satisfaction, affect, functional disruption, and relief of angina. Data for the four elements of quality of life were collected by means of a self-administered instrument that included the Satisfaction with Life Scale, the Bi-polar Profile of Mood States, the Sickness Impact Profile, and an Angina Severity Index they developed.[68] The Angina Severity Index is not included in this chapter because King et al. fail to report validity or reliability for it.

Satisfaction with Life Scale

The Satisfaction with Life Scale (SWLS) is a five-item scale with a response set of 1 to 7 (higher score indicates greater satisfaction). The items include "In most ways my life is close to my ideal; the conditions of my life are excellent; I am satisfied with my life; so far I have gotten the important things I want in life; if I could live my live over, I would change almost nothing."[110] In the original report of the study, Diener et al.[111] report correlations from 0.58 to 0.75 with eight measures of subjective well-being. King et al.[68] report pre- and postoperative reliability coefficients of 0.82 and 0.87.

Bi-polar Profile of Mood States

The Bi-polar Profile of Mood States[112] is a 72-item instrument on which subjects indicate how they have been feeling during the past week with a response set of 0 to 4. A response of 0 indicates not at all, a response of 4 indicates extremely. Half of the items represent six positive mood states (six items for each of six positive mood states: composed, elated, agreeable, energetic, clear-headed, confident), the other half represent six negative mood states (six items for each of six negative mood states: anxious, depressed, hostile, tired, confused, unsure). High scores indicate more of the mood state, whether positive or negative. Subscale score for positive and negative mood states are calculated separately. The publisher indicates that only college norms are available for the Bi-polar Profile of Mood States.

Sickness Impact Profile (SIP)

King et al.[68] used only six of the 12 SIP scales: sleep and rest, home management, ambulation, social interaction, intellectual function, and recreation and pastimes. Other scales in the SIP include mobility, body care and movement, communications, alertness behaviors, emotional behavior, eating, and work.[113] Subjects identify which items in each scale apply to them. A sample item is[113] "I sit during much of the day." Weighted scores for each item are identified by the subject and summed, divided by the total possible score, and multiplied by 100. The result is a percentage disruption score. The widely used SIP is sometimes referred to as the "gold standard."[113] King et al.[68] report an alpha coefficient of 0.86 for the combination of the six scales in their study.

The Kinney and Coyle Study

Kinney and Coyle[66] analyzed data from structured interviews of 344 adults with physical disabilities. This study illustrates the need to design studies based on a conceptual framework appropriate to the study population. The instruments chosen afford the opportunity to examine results across populations. The interviews included four instruments aimed at measuring quality of life: the Center for Epidemiological Studies Depression Scale, Rosenberg's Self-esteem Scale, the Life 3 Scale, and 35 related life domain items from Andrews and Withey[104] and Campbell et al.[105] The authors offer clear descriptions of the first three instruments, the fourth is unclear and, therefore, omitted from our discussion.

The Center for Epidemiological Studies Depression Scale (CES-D)

The CES-D is a 20-item instrument devised using items from five sources, all previously validated depression scales. A sample item is[114] "I was bothered by things that usually don't bother me." The response set for each symptom indicates how often in the past week the subject has experienced the symptom: not at all to 1 day in the week; 1 to 2 days in the week; 3 to 4 days in the week; or 5 to 7 days in the week. Scores range from 0 (not at all to 1 day in the week for all 20 symptoms) to 60 (5 to 7 days in the week for all 20 symptoms). Kinney and Coyle[66] report a Cronbach alpha value of 0.83 on this scale for their study. They indicate that previous validity and reliability studies resulted in Cronbach alphas of 0.84 to 0.90.

Rosenberg Self-Esteem Scale

This scale was described previously in this chapter among the instruments used in the Lewis et al. study. Kinney and Coyle[66] report a Cronbach alpha of 0.83 for their study. This instrument consistently produces highly reliable values.

Life 3 Scale

Kinney and Coyle[66] use the Life 3 Scale as a criterion variable of life satisfaction, a subjective assessment of quality of life. They interjected the question "How do you feel about your life in general?" into their interviews at two separate points. Subjects were offered a response set from 1 (terrible) to 7 (delighted). The two responses were averaged for the Life 3 Scale score. Kinney and Coyle[66] report a test-retest correlation of 0.44 at 6 months. Kinney and Coyle cite Andrews and Withey[104] and Diener[115] in their discussion of the validity of the Life 3 Scale, claiming convergent validity with other measures of life satisfaction of 0.39 to 0.73.

Summary

The use of multiple instruments has the potential for solving problems of comparability and sensitivity. The researcher must, however, consider the problems that may result from this strategy such as conceptual and measurement issues, as well as administration, time requirements, and directions. Administration of instruments varies. Instruments may require completion by the researcher, a health care professional, the subject, or a significant other. When choosing multiple instruments to measure quality-of-life elements, the research must attend to variations in administration. The time required of respondents affects willingness to participate in research.[28,37] The cumulative time required to complete multiple instruments is a prime consideration. Flanagan[116] cautions about ensuring that directions to respondents are clear. The use of multiple instruments may increase the possibility of confusion.

Choosing multiple instruments for measuring quality of life has the advantage of allowing flexibility in the conceptualization of quality of life. As the concept is refined and clarified, researchers using multiple instruments can compare specific dimensions. As more sensitive instruments are developed, substitutions may be made without having to change all instruments in a battery.

Internet Resources

National Center for Chronic Disease Prevention and Health Promotion, Centers for Disease Control, Washington, DC. www.cdc.gov/hrqol.

International Society for Quality of Life Research, McLean, Virginia. www.isoqol.org.

Exemplar Studies

de Haan, R., Aaronson, N., Limburg, M., Hewer, R.L., & van Crevel, H. Measuring quality of life in stroke. *Stroke*, 1993, 24(2):320–327.

This study examines quality of life conceptually, outlines methodologic problems in measuring quality of life, reviews quality-of-life instruments, identifies criteria for selecting instruments, and proposes future directions for quality-of-life studies in stroke patients. The authors review 10 quality-of-life instruments to report their length, time needed for administration, content, scoring, and psychometric evaluation. They point out that choice of instruments depends on the specific questions addressed and on the characteristics of the patients studied. Patient and staff burden affect the feasibility of using long, comprehensive instruments; shorter instruments targeted at the specific questions of the research and compatible with patient characteristics are likely to result in a higher yield of data. The authors strongly recommend refining existing instruments rather than generating new instruments.

Bendtsen, P., & Hörnquist, J.O. Change and status in quality of life in patients with rheumatoid arthritis. *Qual Life Res*, 1992, 1(5): 297–305.

This study exemplifies an assessment package approach to measuring quality of life. The mailed package included measures of six life domains: somatic, psychologic, social, behavioral/activity, structural, and material. Subjects were asked to rate their quality of life in the various domains, statically (current performance) and dynamically (change in status related to the disease). In addition, significant others were asked to rate the patients' lives in shortened versions of the assessment package. This study is one in a series of studies published by a Swedish team anchored by J.O. Hörnquist since 1982. The team has addressed quality of life in diabetes mellitus, alcohol abuse, cancer, and rheumatoid arthritis.

References

1. Callahan, D. *Setting limits: Medical goals in an aging society.* New York: Simon & Schuster, 1987.
2. Callahan, D. *What kind of life: The limits of medical progress.* New York: Simon & Schuster, 1990.
3. Hayden, L.A., Moinpour, C.M., Metch, B., et al. Pitfalls in quality of life assessment: Lessons from a Southwest Oncology Group breast cancer clinical trial. *Oncol Nurs Forum*, 1993, 20(9):415-419.
4. Moinpour, C.M., Feigl, P., Metch, B., et al. Quality of life end points in cancer clinical trials: Review and recommendations. *J Nat Cancer Inst*, 1989, 81(7):485-495.
5. Gotay, C.C., Korn, E.L., McCabe, M.S., et al. Quality of life assessment in cancer treatment protocols: Research issues in protocol development. *J Nat Cancer Inst*, 1992, 84(8):575-579.

6. Nayfield., S.G., Ganz, P.A., Moinpour, C.M., et al. Report from a National Cancer Institute (USA) workshop on quality of life assessment in cancer clinical trials. *Qual Life Res*, 1992, 1(3):203-210.

7. Schron, E.B., & Shumaker, S.A. The integration of health quality of life in clinical research: Experiences from cardiovascular clinical trials. *Progr Cardiovasc Nurs*, 1992, 7(2):21-36.

8. Morreim, E.H. Medical ethics and the future of quality of life research. *Progr Cardiovasc Nurs*, 1992, 7(2):12-17.

9. Menzel, P.T. Oregon's denial: Disabilities and quality of life. *Hastings Center Report*, 1992, 22(6):21-25.

10. Capron, A.M. Oregon's disability: Principle or politics? *Hastings Center Report*, 1992, 22(6):18-20.

11. Kaplan, R.M., & Coons, S.J. Relative importance of dimension in the assessment of health-related quality of life for patients with hypertension. *Progr Cardiovasc Nurs*, 1992, 7(2):29-36.

12. Padilla, G.V., Grant, M.M., & Ferrell, B. Nursing research into quality of life. *Qual Life Res*, 1992, 1(5):341-348.

13. Osaba, D. A taxonomy of the uses of health-related quality of life instruments in cancer care and the clinical meaingfulness of the results. *Med Care*, 2002, 40(6, Supp. III):31-38.

14. Kaplan, R., & Bush, J. Health-related quality of life measurement for evaluation research and policy analysis. *Health Psychol*, 1981, 1(1):61-76.

15. Faden, R., & Leplege, A. Assessing quality of life. *Med Care*, 1992, 30(5) suppl:MS166-175.

16. Goldberg, H.I., Pantell, R.H., & Weber, J.R. Final panel. Reactions, reflections and predictions. *Med Care*, 1992, 30(5) suppl:MS283-293.

17. Guyatt, G.H., Feeny, D.H., & Patrick, D.L. Measuring health-related quality of life. *Ann Intern Med*, 1993, 118(8):622-629.

18. Scientific Advisory Committee of the Medical Outcomes Trust. Assessing health status and quality of life instruments: Attributes and review criteria. *Qual Life Res*, 2002, 11:193-204.

19. Wales, J., Kane, R., Robbins, S., et al. UCLA hospice evaluation study. *Med Care*, 1983, 21(7):734-744.

20. Greer, D., & Mor, V. *A preliminary report of the National Hospice Study*. Washington, DC: Department of Health and Human Services, 1984.

21. Vaisrub, S. Quality of life manqué. *JAMA*, 1976, 236(4):387.

22. Rubenstein, L.V., Calkins, D.R., Greenfield, S., et al. Health status assessment for elderly patients: Report of the Society of General Internal Medicine Task Force on Health Assessment. *J Am Geriatr Soc*, 1989, 37(6):562-569.

23. Lohr, K.N. Applications of health status assessment in clinical practice: Overview of the third conference on advances in health status assessment. *Med Care*, 1992, 30(5) suppl MS1-14.

24. Hopwood, P. Progress, problems, and priorities in quality of life research. *Eur J Cancer*, 1992, 28A(10):1748-1752.

25. Schipper, H., Clinch, J., McMurray, A., & Leavitt, M. Measuring the quality of life of cancer patients: The Functional Living Index-Cancer: Development and validation. *J Clin Oncol*, 1984, 2(5):472-483.

26. Lynch, E. To treat or not to treat—The dilemma. *Heart Lung*, 1978, 7(3):499.

27. Sugarbaker, P.H., Barofsky, I., Rosenberg, S.A., & Gianola, F.J. Quality of life assessment of patient in extremity sarcoma clinical trials. *Surgery*, 1982, 9(1):17-23.

28. Yancik, R., & Yates, J.W. Quality of life assessment of cancer patients: Conceptual and methodologic challenges and constraints. *Cancer Bull*, 1986, 38(5):217-222.

29. Sprangers, M.A.G., Moinpour, C.M., Moynihan, R.J., et al. Assessing meaningful change in quality of life over time: A users' guide for clinicians. *Mayo Clinic Proc*, 2002, 77(6):561-571.

30. Braden, C.J., Mishel, M.H., Longman, A., et al. Symposium: Quality of life in treatment for breast cancer. Presented at the 1993 Scientific Session of the American Nurses Association Council of Nurse Researchers, Washington, DC, November 1993.

31. Smith, K.W., Avis, N.E., & Assmann, S.F. Distinguishing between quality of life and health status in quality of life research: A meta-analysis. *Qual Life Res*, 1991, 8:447-459.

32. Carr, A.J., & Higginson, I.J. Measuring quality of life: Are quality of life measures patient centered? *BMJ*, 2002, 322:1357-1360.

33. Kagawa-Singer, M. Quality of life: Cross-cultural differences. Draft manuscript from the author, 1994.

34. Wan, G.J., Counte, M.A., Cella, et al. An analysis of the impact of demographic, clinical, and social factors on health-related quality of life. *Values in Health*, 1999, 2(4):308-318.

35. Rosser, R. Quality of life: Consensus, controversy and concern. In S.R. Walker & R.M. Rosser (Eds.), *Quality of life: Assessment and application*. Boston: MIT Press, 1988, pp. 297-304.

36. Stewart, A.L. The medical outcomes study framework of health indicators. In A.L. Stewart & J.E. Ware, Jr. (Eds.), *Measuring functioning and well-being: The medical outcomes study*. Durham, NC: Duke University Press, 1992, pp. 12-24.

37. Jalowiec, A. Issues in using multiple measures of quality of life. *Sem Oncol Nurs*, 1990, 6(4):271-277.

38. Orley, J. News from World Health Organization. *Qual Life Res*, 1992, 1(4):277-279.

39. Aaronson, N.K. Quality of life research in cancer clinical trials: A need for common rules and language. *Oncology*, 1990, 4(5):59-66.

40. Ware, J.E., Jr. Methodological considerations in the selection of health status measures. In N.K. Wenger, M.E. Mattson, C.D. Furberg, & J. Elinson (Eds.), *Assessment of quality of life in clinical trials*. New York: LeJacq, 1984, pp. 87-117.

41. Stewart, A.L. Conceptual and methodologic issues in defining quality of life: State of the art. *Progr Cardiovasc Nurs*, 1992, 7(1):3-11.

42. Schumaker, S.A., Anderson, R.T., & Czajkowski, S.M. Psychological tests and scales. In B. Spilker (Ed.), *Quality of life assessments in clinical trials*. New York: Raven, 1990, pp. 95-113.

43. Guyatt, G.H., & Jaeschke, R. Measurements in clinical trials: Choosing the appropriate approach. In B. Spilker (Ed.), *Quality of life assessments in clinical trials*. New York: Raven, 1990, pp. 37-46.

44. Spilker, B. (Ed.). *Quality of life assessments in clinical trials*. New York: Raven, 1990.
45. Spilker, B., Molinek, F.R., Jr., Johnston, K.A., et al. Quality of life bibliography and indexes. *Med Care*, 1990. *28*(12) suppl:S1-S45.
46. McDowell, I., & Newell, C. *Measuring health: A guide to rating scales and questionnaires*. New York: Oxford University Press, 1987.
47. Hyland, M.E. A reformulation of quality of life for medical science. *Qual Life Res*, 1992, *1*(4):267-272.
48. Bendtsen, P., & Hornquist, J.O. Change and status in quality of life patients with rheumatoid arthritis. *Qual Life Res*, 1992, *1*(5):297-305.
49. deHaan, R., Aaronson, N., Limburg, M., et al., Measuring quality of life in stroke. *Stroke*, 1993, *24*(2):320-327.
50. Ferrans, C.E. Conceptualizations of quality of life in cardiovascular research. *Progr Cardiovasc Nurs*, 1992, *7*(2):2-7.
51. Hornquist, J.O., Hansson, B., Akerlind, I., & Larsson, J. Severity of disease and quality of life: A comparison in patients with cancer and benign disease. *Qual Life Res*, 1992, *1*(2):135-141.
52. Revicki, D.A., Turner, R., Brown, R., & Martindale, J.J. Reliability and validity of a health-related quality of life battery for evaluating outpatient antidepressant treatment. *Qual Life Res*, 1992, *1*(4):257-266.
53. Strauss, B., Thormann, T., Strenge, H., et al. Psychosocial, neuropsychological and neurological status in a sample of heart transplant recipients. *Qual Life Res*, 1992, *1*(2):119-128.
54. Wray, J., Radley-Smith, R., & Yacoub, M. Effect of cardiac or heart-lung transplantation on the quality of life of the paediatric patient. *Qual Life Res*, 1992, *1*(1):41-46.
55. Cleary, P.D., Fowler, F.J., Weissman, J., et al. Health-related quality of life in persons with acquired immune deficiency syndrome. *Med Care*, 1993, *31*(7):569-580.
56. DeLeo, D., Rozzini, R., Bernardini, M., et al. Assessment of quality of life in the elderly assisted at home through a Tele-Check service. *Qual Life Res*, 1992, *1*(6):367-374.
57. Lubeck, D.P., & Fries, J.F. Changes in quality of life among persons with HIV infection. *Qual Life Res*, 1992, *1*(6):359-366.
58. Sherbourne, C.D., Meredith, L.S., Rogers, W., & Ware, J.E., Jr. Social support and stressful life events: Age differences in their effects on health-related quality of life among the chronically ill. *Qual Life Res*, 1992, *1*(4):235-246.
59. Tuchler, H., Hofmann, S., Bernhart, M., et al. A short multilingual quality of life questionnaire-practicability, reliability and interlingual homogeneity. *Qual Life Res*, 1992, *1*(2):107-117.
60. Wicklund, I., Gorkin, L., Pawitan, Y., et al., for the CAST Investigators. Methods for assessing quality of life in the Cardiac Arrhythmia Suppression Trial (CAST). *Qual Life Res*, 1992, *1*(3):187-201.
61. Frank-Stromborg, M. Selecting an instrument to measure quality of life. *Oncol Nurs Forum*, 1984, *11*(5):88-91.
62. Spitzer, W., Dobson, A., Hall, J., et al. Measuring the quality of life of cancer patients. *J Chronic Dis*, 1981, *34*(12):585-597.
63. Campbell, A. Subjective measures of well-being. *Am Psychologist*, 1976, *31*(2):117-124.
64. George, L. Subjective well-being. Conceptual and methodological issues. In C. Eisdorfer (Ed.), *Annual review of gerontology and geriatrics* (vol. 2). New York: Springer, 1981, p. 345.
65. Guyatt, G.H., Townsend, M., Keller, J., et al. Measuring functional status in chronic lung disease: Conclusions from a randomized control trial. *Respir Med*, 1991, *85*(suppl B):17-21.
66. Kinney, W.B., & Coyle, C.P. Predicting life satisfaction among adults with physical disabilities. *Arch Phys Med Rehabil*, 1992, *73*(9):863-869.
67. Evans, R.L., Dingus, C.M., & Haselkorn, J.K. Living with a disability: A synthesis and critique of the literature on quality of life, 1985-1989. *Psychol Rep*, 1993, *72*(3, part 1):771-777.
68. King, K.B., Porter, L.A., Norsen, L.H., & Reis, H.T. Patient perceptions of quality of life after coronary artery surgery: Was it worth it? *Res Nurs Health*, 1992, *15*(5):327-334.
69. Prevost, S., & Deshotels, A. Quality of life after cardiac surgery. *AACN Clin Issues Crit Care Nurs*, 1993, *4*(2):320-328.
70. Burgener, S.C., & Chiverton, P. Conceptualizing psychological well-being in cognitively-impaired older persons. *Image*, 1992, *24*(3):209-213.
71. Ferrell, B., Grant, M., Schmidt, G.M., et al. The meaning of quality of life for bone marrow transplant survivors. Part 2. Improving quality of life for bone marrow transplant survivors. *Cancer Nurs*, 1992, *15*(4):247-253.
72. Grant, M., Ferrell, B., Schmidt, G.M., et al. Measurement of quality of life in bone marrow transplantation survivors. *Qual Life Res*, 1992, *1*(6):375-384.
73. Gotay, C.C., & Moore, T.D. Assessing quality of life in head and neck cancer. *Qual Life Res*, 1992, *1*(1):5-17.
74. Lamb, M.A. The influence of endometrial cancer on intimate relationships. Part II. *Qual Life Nurs Chall*, 1993, *2*(2):32-38.
75. Stearns, D.M., Wehdon, M. Social well being and quality of life: Analysis of a journey of cancer survivorship. *Qual Life Nurs Chall*, 1993, *2*(2):23-31.
76. Omery, A., Gravell., C., & Karz, M. Gender differences in the quality of life of person with HIV/AIDS in a HMO Setting. *Communicating Nurs Res*, 2000, *33*:227.
77. Higginson, I.J., & Carr, A.J. Measuring quality of life: Using quality of life measures in the clinical setting. *BMJ*, 2001, *322*:1297-1300.
78. Brown, J., Rawlinson, M., & Hilles, N. Life satisfaction and chronic disease: Exploration of a theoretical model. *Med Care*, 1981, *19*(11):1136-1146.
79. Ferrans, C.E., & Powers, M.J. Quality of life index: Development and psychometric properties. *Adv Nurs Sci*, 1985, *8*(1):15-24.
80. Ziller, R. Self-other orientations and quality of life. *Social Indic Res*, 1974, *1*:301-306.
81. Fletcher, A., & Bulpitt, C. The treatment of hypertension and quality of life. *Qual Life Cardiovasc Care*, 1985, *1*(3):140-144.
82. House, P., Livingston, R., & Swinburn, C. Monitoring mankind: The search for quality. *Behav Sci*, 1975, *20*:57.

83. Carstensen, L., & Cone, J. Social desirability and the measurement of psychological well-being in elderly persons. *J Gerontol*, 1983, *38*(6):713-745.

84. Dow, K.H. Introduction: Social well-being and quality of life: Part II. *Qual Life Nurs Chall*, 2(2):21-22.

85. Bergner, M., Bobbitt, R., Pollard, W., et al. The Sickness Impact Profile: Validation of a health status measure. *Med Care*, 1976, *14*(1):57-67.

86. Lerner, M. Conceptualization of health and social well-being. *Health Serv Res*, 1973, *8*(1):6-12.

87. Shinn, D., & Johnson, D. Avowed happiness as an overall assessment of quality of life. *Soc Indic Res*, 1978, *5*:475-479.

88. Crewe, N. Quality of life: The ultimate goal in rehabilitation. *Minn Med*, 1980, *63*(8):586-589.

89. Bayles, M. The value of life-By what standard? *Am J Nurs*, 1980, *80*(12):2226-2230.

90. Berg, R., Hallauer, D., & Berk, S. Neglected aspects of quality of life. *Health Serv Res*, 1976, *11*(4):391-395.

91. Mount, B., & Scott, J. Whither hospice evaluation? *J Chronic Dis*, 1983, *36*(11):731-736.

92. Hochberg, F., Linggood, R., Wolfson, L., et al. Quality and duration of survival in glioblastoma multiforme. *JAMA*, 1979, *24*(10):1016-1018.

93. Hutchinson, A., Farndon, J., & Wilson, R. Quality of survival of patients following mastectomy. *Clin Oncol*, 1979, *5*:391-395.

94. Flanagan, J. A research approach to improving our quality of life. *Am Psychologist*, 1978, *33*(2):138-142.

95. McSweeney, A., Grant, I., Heaton, R., et al. Life quality of patients with chronic obstructive pulmonary disease. *Arch Intern Med*, 1982, *142*(3):473-483.

96. Linn, B., & Linn, M. Late stage cancer patients: Age differences in their psychophysical status and response to counseling. *J Gerontol*, 1981, *36*(6):689-692.

97. Levy, N., & Wynbrandt, G. The quality of life on maintenance hemodialysis. *Lancet*, 1975, *1*(7920):1328.

98. Aaronson, N.K, Meyerowitz, B.E., Bard, M., et al. Quality of life research in oncology: Past achievements and future priorities. *Cancer*, 1992, *67*(3)suppl: 839-843.

99. Ware, J. Conceptualizing disease impact and treatment outcomes. *Cancer*, 1984, *53*(10):2316-2326.

100. George, L., & Bearon, L. *Quality of life in older persons: Meaning and measurement.* New York: Human Sciences Press, 1980.

101. Cella, D.F. Functional status and quality of life: Current views on measurement and intervention. In *Functional status and quality of life in persons with cancer.* Atlanta, GA: American Cancer Society, 1991, pp. 1-12.

102. Burckhardt, C. The impact of arthritis on quality of life. *Nurs Res*, 1985, *34*(1):11-16.

103. Wood, V., Wylie, M., & Sheafor, B. An analysis of a short self-report measure of life satisfaction: Correlation with rater judgments. *J Gerontol*, 1969, *24*(4):465-469.

104. Andrews, F., & Withey, S. *Social indicators of well-being: Americans' perceptions of life quality.* New York: Plenum, 1976.

105. Campbell, A., Converse, P., & Rodgers, W. *The quality of American life: Perceptions, evaluations, and satisfactions.* New York: Russell Sage, 1976.

106. Evans, R., Manninen, D., Garrison, L., et al. The quality of life of patients with end stage renal disease. *N Engl J Med*, 1985, *312*(9):553-559.

107. Lewis, F. Experienced personal control and quality of life in late-stage cancer patients. *Nurs Res*, 1982, *31*(2):113–119.

108. Rosenberg, M. *Society and the adolescent self image.* Princeton, NJ: Princeton University Press, 1965.

109. Crumbaugh, J. Cross validation of purpose-in-life test based on Frankl's concepts. *J Individ Psychol*, 1968, *24*(1):74-81.

110. Lewis, F., Firisch, S., & Parsell, S. Clinical tool development for adult chemotherapy patients: Process and content. *Cancer Nurs*, 1979, *2*(2):99.

111. Diener, E., Emmons, R.A., Larsen, R.J., & Griffin, S. The satisfaction with life scale. *J Pers Assess*, 1985, *49*(1):71-75.

112. Lorr, M., & McNair, D. *Profile of mood states: Bi-polar form (POMS-BI).* San Diego, CA: Educational and Industrial Testing Service, 1982.

113. Bergner, M. The sickness impact profile. In N.K. Wenger, M.E. Mattson, C.D. Furburg, & J. Elinson (Eds.), *Assessment of quality of life in clinical trials of cardiovascular therapies.* New York: LeJacq, 1984, pp. 152-159.

114. Radloff, L.S. The CES-D scale: A self report depression scale for research in the general population. *Applied Psychol Meas*, 1977, *1*(3):385-401.

115. Diener, E. Subjective well-being. *Psychol Bulletin*, 1984, *95*(3):542-575.

116. Flanagan, J. Measurement of quality of life: Current state of the art. *Arch Phys Med Rehab*, 1982, *63*(2):56-59.

12

Social Support: Conceptualization and Measurement Instruments

Ada M. Lindsey and Bernice C. Yates

Some people at risk for illness become ill, whereas others with similar risk do not, and people diagnosed with the same condition vary considerably in recovery patterns and in adaptation to living with the condition. These observations have led clinicians and investigators to consider the possible contribution of other variables in influencing the onset of and the responses to illness. Social support is one variable that has received increased attention as a possible contributing factor to the observed variances in health outcomes.

There continues to be considerable literature to illustrate this burgeoning interest. There are reviews of social support,[1–13] descriptions of the properties of social support,[1,2,6,10,13,14] studies including social support as a variable,[15–19] or enhancing support through an intervention,[20–25] and reports of instrument development to measure social support.[26–80]

Current theories suggest that social support may have a protective function, serve a stress-buffering or moderating role in health maintenance, and be related to positive health outcomes.[81–85] The quality and availability of social support may have an important role in preventing illness or in recovery after illness. Loss or lack of social support has been linked with a variety of conditions and illnesses.[86–90]

Cassel,[91] one of the few investigators who has proposed a mechanism for the role of social environment in disease etiology, suggests that social environmental stressors alter the neuroendocrine balance and thus increase susceptibility to disease. People deprived of meaningful social contact do not receive adequate information or feedback. Cassel speculates that this is a key property of those with inadequate social environments. In contrast, people with adequate social support are helped in coping with crisis and adapting to change.

Socially competent individuals are likely to have well-developed social networks and, as a result, may be more resistant to stressors.[92] Persons considered to be well integrated and who function well receive more assistance from others.[93] Cobb[94] suggests there is evidence that high levels of social support influence recovery from illness, and this facilitation may occur through increased compliance with the prescribed medical regimen. Caplan[95] proposed that having social support implies that the person has an enduring pattern of relationships over time. A social support network provides "psychosocial supplies" for the individual, and these "supplies" provide for the maintenance of health of the individual. "A common impression of social support is that it provides armor to individuals who need it, can find it and use it."[3]

The quality and availability of social support may have an important role in an individual's recovery from or adaptation to an illness or surgery or in preventing illness. For example, social support perceived to be adequate may facilitate the ability to cope with stressful life events or a major crisis, to maintain health, or to adapt to changes.

Conceptualizations of Social Support

Further study is necessary to determine how social support influences health, what types of support are more important under what specific circumstances, and the mechanisms by which social support exerts an influence. Because of the heightened interest in social support interventions, definitions, conceptualizations, identification of distinguishing characteristics, and the creation of instruments to measure social support continues to evolve. The major conceptualizations of social support are reviewed in detail elsewhere.[1-4,10,13,96,97] They are briefly summarized here to provide a context for the selection of an instrument to measure social support.

The Evolution of Social Support

The development of the concept of social support has evolved steadily over the past four decades. Almost 30 years ago, Cobb[81] defined social support as the provision of information that leads people to believe they are cared for, loved, esteemed, valued, and a member of a network of communication and mutual obligation. Caplan[98] recognized that support comes from continuing, enduring relationships. From its initial treatment as a unidimensional concept meaning essentially warmth, kindness, or encouragement,[91,94] most conceptualizations[99-101] now include three or four dimensions or types of functional support. The conceptualization of social support proposed by House[99] identifies four functional dimensions of social support: emotional, instrumental, informational, and appraisal. Emotional support behaviors (closest to the original conceptualization) provide empathy and demonstration of love, trust, and caring.[99] Significant others help to mobilize psychologic resources and master emotional burdens; they are a refuge or sanctuary for stability and comfort. They share tasks and provide material supplies, skills, and cognitive guidance to improve the individual's ability to handle situations.

The perception of having a confidant or at least one close, confiding relationship is a strong indicator of social support.[102] Weiss[103] and Kahn[104] expressed social relationships as the major construct and identified six multiple functions: (1) social integration, (2) reliable alliance, (3) guidance, (4) opportunity for nurturance, (5) reassurance of worth, and (6) attachment/intimacy. Social integration is provided through a network of relationships in which participants share concerns, information, and ideas. A sense of reliable alliance is provided primarily through relationships with kin in which the person is assured of continuing assistance. Obtaining guidance occurs during stressful situations when the individual seeks emotional support and cognitive guidance from a trusted and authoritative figure. Opportunity for nurturance refers to an adult taking responsibility for the well-being of another. Reassurance of worth occurs through recognition of a person's competence in a social role. Attachment or intimacy refers to gaining a sense of security and place.

Transactions

In addition to emotional support, in the early to mid 1970s the conceptualizations of social support began to include dimensions representing behaviors inclusive of transactions such as instrumental and informational support. *Instrumental support* behaviors directly help in time of need, and *informational support* behaviors provide information that can be used in coping with personal and environmental problems. Another dimension is *appraisal support*, which reflects behaviors that transmit information relevant to self-evaluation.[99] Kahn[104] conceptualized social support as interpersonal transactions that express positive affect of one person toward another, affirm another's behaviors, perceptions, or expressed views, and provide symbolic or material aid to another person. The term *convoy* denotes the set of significant people through whom support is given or received. The characteristic of reciprocity is included in the conceptualization of social support by both Kahn[104] and Caplan.[98]

More recently, Lakey and Cohen[97] delineated the three most important theoretical perspectives of social support research as stress and coping, social constructionist, and qualities of social relationships. In describing these theoretical perspectives, they discuss the type of support that is typically measured within each perspective, how social support functions, and whether it has stress-buffering or direct effects on health outcomes. For example, within the stress and coping perspective, one way that social support is viewed is as supportive actions. It is measured as the actual support provided by others and functions by promoting coping through a stress-buffering mechanism. In contrast, the aspect of support that is emphasized within a social constructionist perspective is that people have stable beliefs about the supportiveness of others, and these beliefs are what determine how they perceive their social context, not the actual support that is provided. It is measured via global assessments of support quality or availability and functions by influencing how one evaluates oneself and others. This perspective proposes that support has a direct effect on health and well-being, regardless of stress levels, by enhancing self-esteem and self-regulation. Within the relationship perspective, the aspect of support that is emphasized and measured is companionship, intimacy, and so on—social skills that often go together with and cannot be separated from social support. From this perspective, social support would directly impact well-being. In sum, it is the theoretical perspective of the study that guides the aspects of social support that are examined and the selection of the social support measure(s); the two need to match if the research is truly going to contribute to the knowledge base of how social support functions in promoting health outcomes.

Two studies conducted in elderly persons provide examples of differences in conceptualization of social support. Rundall and Evashwick[105] make a distinction between social network and support network in their study of social network and help-seeking among 883 elderly persons. A typology of four categories was developed: engaged, abandoned, trapped, and disengaged. The typology includes the level of interaction with the network and the satisfaction with the level of interaction. The use of health and social services was found to vary with the behavior category (e.g., engaged versus abandoned). Blazer[106] measured the adequacy of social support in 33 older adults (≥65 years) living in a community. Social support was conceptualized as three parameters: (1) roles and available attachments, (2) perceived support, and (3) frequency of social interaction. In this study, all three components of social support predicted mortality.

The social support system is a composite of interpersonal relationships that satisfy specific personal social needs.[4] Social support is a component of human relationships, and these relationships are the formal and informal social support systems. An individual's social support system is comprised of multiple networks. These include the kinship network (spouse or partner, family members, and other relatives), social and role networks (friends, neighbors, and work associates), professional networks (health care providers and other professionals), and community networks (church and community groups and agencies).[4]

Family and Support Network

Social support also has been examined in the context of family functioning. Caplan[107] acknowledges that support system functions depend on stability, intactness, and integration of the family. Eight family support system functions of the contemporary U.S. family were identified; examples of these functions are family as collector and disseminator of information, as source of practical service and concrete aid, as source and validation of identity, and as haven for rest and recuperation.[98]

There are distinctions between the support network and perceived or actual social supportive behaviors. A network is the group of people with whom a person has social connections; these formal or informal relationships are described by size, density, and complexity. The network serves such functions as the provision of information and aid. The perceived impact that these network functions have on the person is social support.[30] The extent to which a person believes or feels that the supportive behaviors provided by the network meet his or her needs is the perceived level of social support. Quantitative descriptions of the social network and network analysis are beyond the scope of this chapter and are available elsewhere.[108]

Some authors suggest that the functional aspects of social support are stronger predictors of health-related outcomes than are the structural aspects, such as network size.[2,37] They make a case for the importance of focusing on the measurement of functional properties of social support, particularly in relationship to health outcomes.

The perception of support and the actual support provided may be incongruent. Individual traits, attitudes, and moods can influence both the perceived and the actual support available and provided. In stressful circumstances, a person may include available social support in the appraisal process, and the subsequent seeking of support may be a response to obtain information or other support to deal with the stressful event.[30] The social support available may thus influence the individual's subsequent coping or adaptation to the circumstance.

Distinguishing Characteristics

Social support has both qualitative and quantitative dimensions and includes both subjective and objective perceptions. Social support varies according to age and life situation.[89] Social support varies with availability of sources of support, accessibility to those sources, nature and intensity of the relationship, and changes in level of functioning. Thus, measuring social support at one point in time will not reflect this variability. In a study describing social relationships in the Danish population, Due et al.[109] found that the social network, as measured by weekly contacts, declines with age, as does the receipt of tangible aid. In contrast, emotional support is unrelated to this decline in frequency of contact. Similar levels of emotional support appear to be important for younger and older individuals.[109] Relational strain or conflict also declines with age across all types or kinds of social relations. Past experiences, perceived need, and other demands may influence provision and perception of social support available.

Social support is derived from people, places, and activities. Factors influencing the giving or receiving of social support include interpersonal, cultural, environmental, and physical; for example, the geographic proximity of support network members may facilitate or constrain the provision of supportive behaviors. In their review of the relationships between social support and diabetic management in African Americans, Ford et al.[5] found that social support is significantly linked with better diabetes management in this population. They concluded that, compared to Whites, African Americans have a tendency to depend more on their informal social networks to help with their disease-management needs. It is critical that larger numbers of African Americans and other minority groups be included in studies examining social support to increase our understanding of the associations among social support and age, gender, socioeconomic status, and other variables. This knowledge, in turn, will facilitate the development of culturally appropriate measures and interventions that are sufficiently sensitive.

Norbeck[14] developed a model that includes elements of social support and nursing practice and proposed relationships between the two that need to be studied. Properties of the individual and of the situation and the influences of these on the need for social support and on the availability of support are described.

Nonsupportive Dimensions

Much of the research and the conceptualization underlying the development of social support measures have emphasized the positive aspects of social support; a few instruments have included the negative dimensions of social support. Tilden and colleagues[45-47] describe a "darker side" of social support. Others[32,37,99] have noted there may be a "cost" in social relationships; for example, the need for reciprocal exchanges, interpersonal interchanges that are not benevolent, and the stresses of maintaining relationships.

Others argue that it is a separate dimension and should not be conceptualized as part of social support. The barrier theory, a more recent conceptualization of nonsupportive behaviors, posits that there are obstacles to accessing social support. These obstacles may include lack of access to family, lack of acceptance, lack of intimacy, feeling smothered,[110] not wanting to be a burden on family, and feeling isolated or stigmatized.[111] In a sample of HIV-positive gay men, partial support for this theory was found in that a decrease in the barriers to disclosure within the family accounted for 57% of the variance in family support.[112] The barrier theory has also explained why family members were perceived as less helpful than friends for HIV-positive gay men.[110] When measuring support, it seems appropriate to use instruments that tap not only the supportive aspects but also the cost or conflict aspects involved in the perceptions of social support and their effects on health outcomes, as these negative aspects of relationships may have adverse effects that are stronger than the positive aspects.

Gaps and Further Work

More studies need to examine the factor structure of existing social support instruments in medically ill populations. There is a need to examine the cost or conflict dimensions of supportive relationships. There is a need to determine levels of social support in healthy people to use as normative data for comparison with levels of social support in people who are ill and the satisfaction with the support available and/or provided. There is a need to study the reciprocity of social support, not just the receiving aspect. Both general and specific support scales must be included in studies to understand the processes by which support may influence behavior change and adherence.[37,59] Some unresolved questions include identification of the critical supportive behaviors and determining how they differ relative to different stressful life events and relative to specific health outcomes. What types and sources of support are most important in which circumstances? What are the most important structural properties of social support networks that allow the individual to evaluate the support as being adequate? What is the nature of the support relationships that leads to improved coping or that facilitates adjustment? Are the same elements of social support perceived to be important in all cultures? It is apparent that many very important questions about social support remain unanswered.

If, in fact, social support is a moderator variable influencing health maintenance and health outcomes, determining the level of perceived social support, the availability of support, the support received, the costs of support, and the changes in support over time become important clinical considerations. Enhancing or facilitating the quality or quantity of support may be a crucial intervention strategy. If this is the case, there is a need for a measure of social support to document baseline support in health, as well as at the time of diagnosis, and throughout the illness and treatment trajectory.[113]

Reviews of Social Support Measurement

Social support is a multidimensional construct. As yet, there is no universally accepted definition or conceptualization of social support. Efforts to create instruments to measure social support also reflect this range of diversity. For example, Vaux[114] categorized social support instruments into several categories: measures of support network resources, measures of supportive behavior, measures of support appraisals, help-seeking and support mobilization, support incidents, and support participation. Several instruments are included in more than one category, indicating that they tap more than one dimension of support.

Murawski et al.[13] suggest that measurement of social support should determine the individual's interpersonal support system, characteristics of his or her social roles in the primary support group, beliefs about sources of support that would be available during an illness, patterns of social affiliation, and need for social affiliation. The authors perceive these aspects to be critical elements of social support.

A variety of approaches to measure social support have been used. For example, questions were embedded in studies to assess social support resources, such as marital status; frequency of contacts with parents, children, and friends; living arrangements; and other indicators of social ties. Other measurement approaches included assessment of the respondent's perceptions of the supportive aspects of their social environments,[115] of receiving supportive behaviors,[51] of satisfaction with support available,[61] and of the potential availability of affect, affirmation, and aid.[57,58]

In 1977, Dean and Lin[83] were unable to locate any social support instruments with known or acceptable reliability or validity data. In 1985, Tardy[116] reviewed seven instruments designed to measure social support. He published brief descriptions and the reported validity and reliability estimates. He suggested that lack of measurement precision in the field precluded theory development and the application of findings to practice. Wood[117] reviewed 11 social support instruments in 1985 and reported similar constraints.

Stewart[118,119] reviewed studies conducted by nurse researchers and identified 21 instruments developed by nurses to measure social support. She examined these instruments according to eight dimensions she considered important in the social support literature: type (positive/negative); direction (received/given); disposition (available/enacted); description/evaluation; content (e.g., emotional, instrumental, appraisal); network/source (e.g., family, friends); duration of relationship; and level of support (e.g., satisfaction with, perceived amount of, frequency of interaction). Stewart concluded that the emphasis of most of the nurse-developed measures was emotional (available and enacted) and instrumental support from family and friends. Validity and reliability testing was reported for 7 of the 21 instruments; only six instruments had been used in more than one study. These results are comparable to Norbeck's[120] earlier finding that only 28% of the 40 social support studies used instruments with established validity and reliability.

O'Reilly[121] examined 24 measures of social support on several dimensions; one was the conceptual dimension used for the development of the instrument. Only 14 of the 24 measures were based on some conceptual definition. Problems with operational definitions of social support also were identified. Examples of issues addressed includes: whether the support measure was to be used with a general or a specific population, whether it focused on everyday support or support at critical times, and whether the questions addressed who provided the support or what support was provided. Only 11 investigators reported validity and reliability data, and several reported one or the other. O'Reilly also examined nine social network measures. Like others, he clearly distinguishes between measurement of social support and social networks.

Comparing the list of 21 nurse researcher–developed social support instruments[119] with the 24 instruments reviewed by O'Reilly,[121] only one nurse-developed instrument, the Norbeck Social Support Questionnaire,[57,58] was included in the latter list. This suggests that nurse researcher–developed instruments were not being accessed by researchers in disciplines other than nursing at that time.

Vrabec[11] reviewed the social support and caregiver burden studies and analyzed the findings in relation to clarification of the constructs, relationships among the constructs, statistical conclusion validity, and generalizability. Of the 50 studies reviewed, only 14% (n = 7) measured all three dimensions of structure, function, and nature of support (i.e., satisfaction with received support); dimensions that she advocates need to be measured to clarify the relationship between social support and burden. For example, informal sources of support, such as family and friends, generally decreased the amount of caregiving burden, but formal sources of support, such as paid providers, were not linked with reduced burden. Similarly, in relation to functional dimensions, the care recipient's level of functioning played a role in whether support was positively or negatively associated with social support. If only one or two aspects of support are measured in a study, it may not increase our understanding of the associations between variables. Similarly, she suggests measuring variables that might confound the relationship between social support and burden. In a study by Baillie, Norbeck, and Barnes,[122] social support did not mediate the relationship between stress and health but rather the years of caregiving and mental impairment of the elder. If the researchers had not measured these potentially confounding variables, they might have arrived at incorrect conclusions. It is also important to avoid using measures that confound the measurement of stress and support, which frequently occurs when the care recipient is part of the support system. To increase the statistical conclusion validity of the study, Vrabac[11] suggests using comprehensive, valid, and reliable measures of social support, with an adequate sample size. In relation to generalizability, further research using diverse groups, settings, multiple measures of support, and multiple times of measurement will increase the generalizability of this literature.

Wills and Shinar[101] reviewed social support instruments and categorized them into perceived availability of support (22 measures) and received support (5 measures). They specifically reviewed measures that were used more commonly in support research; thus, most of the measures were based on a theoretical framework and had acceptable reliability and validity evidence. Other factors to consider when choosing a tool were discussed, such as relevance, length of tool, generality versus specificity, and negative interactions. In addition, they generated a list of questions to aid intervention researchers in selecting the right tool to match the purpose of the study (e.g., "What sources of support, indigenous or grafted, does the intervention aim to influence so as to change levels of available support?").[101] They also recommend that intervention researchers include measures of both availability of support and satisfaction with support to detect any support deficiencies or support that might be underestimated because of negative perceptions of the supporter.

Now, more than 25 years after the Dean and Lin[83] 1977 report, this chapter contains 33 measures of social support with some validity and reliability data published. There now are numerous published studies in which social support has been measured in many diverse and clinical samples. The reviews cited suggest that there are a number of investigator-developed instruments that purport to measure social support. However, many of these instruments need considerable conceptual and operational development as well as psychometric testing. Others[10,97,120] also have addressed conceptual and methodologic issues in the measurement of social support.

The instruments included in this chapter purport to measure social support or some aspect of it, and represent the instruments for which there is more evidence of validity and reliability estimates. Appendix 12A alphabetically highlights important points as well as psychometric indices of each instrument.

Instruments to Measure Social Support

Arizona Social Support Interview Schedule (ASSIS)

The ASSIS[26,27] is a 30-item interview designed to tap judgments about structural components of the social network as well as adequacy of support. It measures support in the following categories: material aid, physical assistance, intimate interaction, guidance, feedback, and social participation. For each of the six categories, respondents are first asked to list the names or initials of the people who provide support (available network size). Respondents are then asked who the people were who actually provided support in the past month (utilized network size). Then they are asked if they would have liked more support (support satisfaction) and whether they received the support they needed (support need). In addition, there are two questions about interpersonal conflicts or unpleasant interactions (conflicted network size and unconflicted network size) and four questions about the personal characteristics of network members (e.g., age, ethnicity). Barrera[27] found a correlation of 0.92 between available network size and utilized network size, and thus utilized network size was analyzed in testing the instrument.

Close Persons Questionnaire (CPQ)

The CPQ was developed to assess both social network and quality and types of social support for up to four close persons identified by the respondent.[28] The support questions included assessment of the type of support needed, whether it was received in the last 12 months, and whether more support was desired. The CPQ contains three subscales: confiding/emotional support (7 items), instrumental support (4 items), and negative aspects of close relationships (4 items). Each item is rated on a 4-point Likert scale, with higher scores indicating more support (both positive and negative). The reliability and content, construct, and criterion validity of the CPQ were described.[28]

Duke Social Support and Stress Scale (DUSOCS)

The DUSOCS measures family and nonfamily social support and stress.[29-31] It is a self-reported, 24-item questionnaire. Six categories of family are used (spouse or significant other, children/grandchildren, parents/grandparents, brothers/sisters, other blood relatives, and relatives by marriage); four categories of nonfamily members are included (neighbors, coworkers, church members, and other friends). Each support source category is rated as providing no support, some support, or a lot of support. Separate scores are derived for total family support and total nonfamily support and family stress and nonfamily stress. This instrument is somewhat unique in that it assesses social support from the family separate from support provided by nonfamily members and also stress from each category. This is a strength if separation of social support from family and nonfamily is of interest.

Duke-UNC Functional Social Support Questionnaire (DUFSS)

The DUFSS is a two-scale, eight-item instrument designed for self-administration.[32] Five items assess confidant support, and three items assess affective support. The confidant support items reflect a relationship in which important life matters are discussed and shared; affective support items reflect emotional or caring support. Responses are rated on a five-point Likert scale, ranging from "as much as I would like" to "much less than I would like." An example of an item is: "I get . . . love and affection." The authors describe the development and evaluation of the DUFSS. However, this instrument measures only two dimensions of social support (confidant support and affective support).

Duke Social Support Index (DSSI)

The DSSI is a 35-item, 4-subscale instrument that measures multiple dimensions of social support.[33] Four items comprise the social network subscale; 4 items assess social interaction; 7 items reflect subjective support; 13 items measure availability of instrumental support; 4 items measure satisfaction with support; and 3 items are independent, not associated with a subscale. They are used to assess satisfaction with frequency of contact with friends and relatives, marital status, and living arrangement, and whether there is at least one close, long-term relationship. Others have developed two abbreviated scales from the DSSI; one is 23 items and the other 11 items.[34,35] The 23-item instrument includes three subscales: social interaction (4 items), subjective support (7 items), and instrumental support (11-items). The 11-item scale consists of all items on the two subscales of social interaction and subjective support.

ENRICHD Social Support Instrument (ESSI)

The ENRICHD Social Support Instrument[36] is a brief 5-item scale that was developed from other scales and items with documented predictive validity of poor outcomes in cardiac patients (e.g., low emotional support). Response options ranged from 1, none of the time, to 5, all of the time, with low scores denoting limited social support. Participants were only included in the ENRICHD trial, a social support intervention trial targeting survival and reinfarction, if they were at high risk for low social support. Preliminary reliability and validity evidence of the measure is established.

Family and Friend Support for Eating and Exercise Habits

Sallis and colleagues[37] developed four different questionnaires to measure social support from family and friends for changing dietary and exercise health habits. The Friend Support for Eating Habits Scale contains two subscales: positive comments (6 items) and negative (4 items). An example of an item from the positive subscale is "Reminded me not to eat high-salt, high-fat foods." An example of an item from the negative subscale is "Refused to eat the same foods I eat." The Family Support for Eating Habits Scale also contains two subscales: encouragement (6-items) and sabotage (7-items). An example item from the encouragement subscale is "Offer me low-salt, low-fat snacks when I visit in their homes." An example item from the sabotage subscale is "Ate high-salt or high-fat foods in front of me." The Friend Support for Exercise Habits Scale is a single subscale named "exercising together" (5 items); an example item is "Offered to exercise with me."

The Family Support for Exercise Habits Scale contains two subscales: participation and involvement (12 items) and rewards and punishments (3 items). An example item from the participation and involvement subscale is "Changed their schedule so we could exercise together." An example item from the rewards and punishments subscale is "Got angry at me for exercising." All four scales were rated on a 5-point scale ranging from 1, none, to 5, very often. These measures may capture components of supportive behavior that are context-specific for dietary or exercise changes to determine which types of supportive activities are most effective. They have been used in over 250 studies.

Family Stress and Support Inventory (FSSI)

The Family Stress and Support Inventory is a self-report instrument designed to assess intrafamilial stress and support provided by each family member, as perceived by the respondent.[38] For each family member, the respondent rates the amount of stress and the amount of support they feel they receive on a continuum of 1 to 10. The scores can be tabulated by generation (e.g., by grandparent, parent, or children generation), for the whole family, for individual family members, or some other grouping of family members. Arithmetic means of stress and support for each grouping can be determined, and a ratio of stress to support also can be calculated. Development and testing of this instrument with a sample of 382 people are described.

Interpersonal Support Evaluation List (ISEL)

The ISEL[39,40] measures perceived availability of four dimensions of support: tangible, appraisal (informational), belonging (emotional), and self-esteem. There are three forms of the ISEL: one is designed for college students, one is for use with a general population, and a third is a shortened 12-item version of the general population scale. All three are available along with scoring instructions and a 40-item Spanish version at the following Website: www.psy.cmu.edu/~scohen. The student version of the instrument has 48 statements related to perceived availability of potential social resources and respondents indicate whether each statement is probably true or probably false for them. The general population version has 40 items, 10 items for each subscale, and each item is rated on a 4-point scale: 0, definitely false; 1, probably false; 2, probably true; and 3, definitely true. The 12-item ISEL consists of 3 subscales (appraisal, belonging, and tangible) with 4 items in each. For all three versions of the ISEL, half of the statements reflect a positive direction, and half are negatively stated. Items for the college-student version are based on the elements of social relationships expected for college students. Examples of items for this version are "I know someone who would loan me $100 to help pay my tuition" or "I hang out in a friend's room or apartment quite a lot." Examples of items from the general population form are "If I needed an emergency loan of $100, there is someone (friend, relative, or acquaintance) I could get it from" and "There are several people that I trust to help solve my problems." Descriptions of instrument development and testing are well detailed.[39,40] The ISEL has been used extensively in many healthy and ill populations.

Interview Schedule for Social Interaction

The Interview Schedule for Social Interaction assesses via four subscales the perceived availability and adequacy of social relationships.[41-43] One subscale assesses the availability of confiding and emotionally intimate relationships, a second subscale assesses the availability of more diffuse relationships (e.g., friends, work associates, neighbors), and the other two subscales assess the adequacy and satisfaction with each of the two types of relationships (intimate or more diffuse). The authors describe pilot development of the instrument with various groups of subjects. The final 52-item measure was tested in a general population survey of 151 individuals and in other samples.

The instrument is designed to be administered as an interview. Four scores are derived: (1) the availability of attachment, (2) the perceived adequacy of attachment, (3) the availability of social integration, and (4) the adequacy of social integration. Scoring variations are provided in the report.

The instrument has been found useful to tap the dimensions of social support that reflect interest in specific clinical populations, such as poststroke hospitalized patients.[123] In addition, Unden and Orth-Gomer[44] shortened and adapted the ISSI for use in population surveys. They tested the original and the shortened versions in middle-aged Swedish men and demonstrated the reliability (internal consistency and split-half) and validity of the shorter version. They concluded that the shortened version had no major disadvantages.

IPR Inventory (IPRI)

The IPRI is a 39-item instrument developed to measure interpersonal relationships; it extends the measurement of social support to include reciprocity and conflict.[45] Based on evidence that conflict does occur in social relationships and that it may be deleterious to health, this instrument, by including assessment of conflict, extends beyond the more support-focused aspects of social support measures. Instrument development was based on social exchange and equity theories; thus consideration was given to the cost–benefit ratios of relationships and of reciprocation in relationships. The IPRI was refined from a previous version of a 74-item Interpersonal Relationship Index.[46] The current IPRI has three subscales: (1) social support (13 items), (2) reciprocity (13 items), and (3) conflict (13 items).

About half the items ($n = 22$) measure perceived sentiment on a five-point Likert-type scale (strongly agree to strongly disagree), and the remaining items ($n = 17$) measure perceived frequency of behavior on a five-point continuum (very often to never). Three additional items assess the structural aspects of the support network. Respondents list their network members, indicate household size, and provide information on the proximity of their relatives. The brief descriptions of the underlying theory for conceptualization and construction of this instrument, the type of testing, and the completeness of descriptions of this testing make this a particularly useful reference for instrument development in general as well as providing data on the reliability and validity of the IPRI. Description of the beginning development of this instrument also is available.[47,48] Additional psychometric evaluation has been reported, including information about the use of this instrument in 19 other studies.[49] This instrument has been translated into French and Spanish.[49,50]

Inventory of Socially Supportive Behaviors (ISSB)

Barrerra et al.[51] developed a 40-item instrument that measures the frequency with which respondents were the recipients of supportive actions. The inventory assesses help received from natural support systems. Psychometric evaluations of the ISSB[124] using exploratory[125] and confirmatory factor analysis (CFA)[124] yielded four subscales: directive guidance (12 items), nondirective support (5 items), positive social exchange (6 items), and tangible assistance (7 items). When scoring the ISSB, four pairs of items are added together to form four composite variables and, based on the CFA, 6 items were omitted from the final measurement model.[124] Each item is rated on a five-point scale according to the frequency (ranging from 0, not at all, to 4, about every day) with which it occurred during the preceding month. Examples of items are "How often has someone assisted you in setting a goal for yourself?" and "How often has someone listened to you talk about your private feelings?" The subjects for the initial and later testings of the ISSB were college students. In contrast, Krause and Markides[126] evaluated the ISSB in older adults, adding a dimension to measure social integration to the scale (13 items). This was intended to determine whether older adults provide support to persons in their social situation. The time frame was lengthened to one year and a 4-point response option was used, ranging from 1, never, to 4, very often. Before testing, 12 of the 40 items were deleted because the authors did not feel they were pertinent for assistance with stressful situations. They tested their revised tool with CFA and identified a four-factor structure: emotional, tangible, integration, and informational support. They also added a section to measure satisfaction with each of the four types of support.

MOS Social Support Survey (MOS SSS)

A good example of instrument development and evaluation is provided for the MOS SSS.[52] This instrument was tested on almost 3000 adult patients in three different geographic locations. It was developed for chronically ill patients in a medical outcomes study. The MOS SSS is a 19-item self-administered questionnaire comprising four subscales to assess functional dimensions of social support. Eighteen items are used to form the subscales: emotional/informational (8 items), affectionate (3 items), tangible (4 items), and positive social interaction (3 items). Subscale scores or the total index score can be used. Emphasis is on the perceived availability of support if needed. This instrument assesses the types of support, but not the sources of support. Respondents are asked to indicate on a Likert-type scale from 1 (none of the time) to 5 (all of the time) how often the type of support is available if needed. Examples of items are "Someone you can count on to listen to you when you need to talk" and "Someone to help with daily chores if you were sick." The instrument also includes one item to measure a structural support dimension, that is, the number of close friends and relatives. Psychometric testing supports the view that social support is multidimensional. This tool continues to be used frequently.

Multidimensional Scale of Perceived Social Support (MSPSS)

The MSPSS is a 12-item self-report measure that assesses perceived social support from family, friends, and a significant other.[53-55] Respondents rate the 12 items on a seven-point Likert-type scale, ranging from very strongly agree to very strongly disagree. An example of an item is "There is a special person with whom I can share my joys and sorrows." The beginning psychometric testing used college student samples, but it has since been used with other populations.

My Family and Friends (MFF)

My Family and Friends (MFF) is a three-part instrument developed to assess the perceptions of social support of children (6–12 years old).[56] The instrument uses 12 dialogues and props to engage children and obtain information about the availability of individuals to provide social support and the child's level of satisfaction with the type of support received. In developing and testing the instrument, the authors provide evidence that children understand and can differentiate among types of support, such as informational, emotional, companionship, and instrumental. They also claim that the instrument is sensitive to variations in perceived social support by the children when there is "family upheaval." Development of the instrument was based on cognitive developmental theory and on the social support work that has been done with adults to differentiate types of social support (emotional, instrumental, affiliative, informational, and conflictual). The addition of a dialogue that indicates conflict recognizes there may be some negative interactions in supportive relationships.

The MFF has three parts. The first part orients the child, and the child identifies support network members. Props are included in the orientation and consist of the following: (1) cards with the names of the people in the child's network (they also may be drawings or pictures of these network members), (2) a board to insert the cards in a ranked order, and (3) a large barometer with a movable indicator with points at intervals of 10 ranging from 0 to 50. The second part engages the child in the 12 dialogues.

There are five dialogues for emotional support, two each for informational, instrumental, and companionship support, and one that focuses on conflict. For each dialogue, using the cards and the board, the child ranks the network members in the order in which the child goes to the individual for the type of support indicated in the dialogue. After all network members are ranked, using the barometer movable indicator, the child is then asked how satisfied she or he is with the support provided by the individual. The authors recommend administering the 12 dialogues in two 12- to 15-minute sessions to keep the child engaged. The third part is designed to identify other persons who are important to the child. In testing and using this instrument, the examiners were carefully selected and trained to conduct the interviews with the children. The training was structured and fairly extensive; it occurred in four 3-hour sessions. An example of the dialogue stem for emotional support is "When you want to share your feelings (like feeling happy, sad, or mad) . . ." For each item, the child is asked which person they go to most often. Then, if that person is not available, whom they go to next. For the level of satisfaction for the dialogue stem, the questions are (1) "When you talk to (name of person ranked) about your feelings, how much better do you feel?" and (2) "How good does (name of person ranked) make you feel about yourself or about being you?"

An example of a dialogue stem for instrumental support is "When you need help doing something around the house, such as making or fixing something, finding something you lost, or moving something, who do you go to most often?" The satisfaction level with the instrumental support provided is assessed by the answer to the question "When you go to (name of person ranked) for help, how helpful is she/he?"

The authors note that it is possible to add other dialogues to the MFF, if there are specific areas for which information is desired. For example, constructing dialogue about social support during illness or a specific clinical situation may be of interest.

The MFF scale represents significant work in the development of an instrument to measure the perceptions of types of social support in children 6 to 12 years of age and to assess their level of satisfaction with the type of support received. It also allows the addition of dialogues that can be created to be specific for a given situation.

Norbeck Social Support Questionnaire (NSSQ)

The NSSQ[57,58] is another instrument that has been developed by nurse researchers to measure the multidimensional construct of social support. It is a short, self-administered questionnaire that taps three major components: functional aspects, network, and loss. Affect, affirmation, and aid are the functional aspects assessed, and number in the network, duration of relationships, and frequency of contact are the network properties measured. Total loss includes the number of "source of support" categories in which a loss occurred and the perceived amount of support lost.

Conceptual definitions of social support proposed by Kahn[104] were used as the theoretical basis for the NSSQ. Social support is defined as "interpersonal transactions that include one or more of the following: the expression of positive affect of one person toward another; the affirmation or endorsement of another person's behaviors, perceptions, or expressed views; the giving of symbolic or material aid to another."[104] The term *convoy* was suggested by Kahn as representing the vehicle for provision of social support:

"An individual's convoy at any point in time thus consists of the set of persons on whom he or she relies for support and those who rely on him or her for support."[104] The NSSQ includes items to tap the three supportive transaction components (affect, affirmation, and aid) and to assess representative convoy or network properties (number in network, frequency of contact, and duration of relationships).

The first item on the NSSQ asks the respondent to list each significant person in his or her life, considering "all the persons who provide personal support for you or who are important to you." Space is provided to list up to 24 people, and the respondent indicates the source or category each listed individual represents (e.g., spouse/partner, family member, relative, friend, work/school associate, neighbor, religious person). For the next set of six questions, the respondent is asked to identify the extent of support provided by each of the individuals listed in the network. For example, one of the questions used for affect is "How much does this person make you feel liked or loved?" An item used to tap affirmation is "How much does this person agree with or support your actions or thoughts?" To assess long-term aid, the question used is "If you were confined to bed for several weeks, how much could this person help you?" The rating scale ranges from 0 (not at all) to 4 (a great deal).

Other items are included to determine the duration of individual relationships (ranging from less than 6 months to more than 5 years), the frequency of contact (ranging from daily, weekly, to once a year or less), and loss (number of persons no longer available to the individual and the amount of support lost). The NSSQ also has been used to assess social support as being adequate or low and to determine the effect of adequacy of social support from specific sources of support on clinical outcome.[127] Revised scoring instructions are available and a Website has been created.[128,129] It also has been translated into several languages, including Arabic, German, and Swedish.[130,131] The NSSQ has been used in various populations, such as the elderly,[132] cancer patients,[130,133,134] adolescents,[135] pregnant women,[127,136] or chronically ill women.[137]

Partner Interaction Questionnaire (PIQ)

The PIQ[59,138,139] is a 20-item inventory designed to measure the receipt of support from a partner specifically related to smoking cessation. It includes 10 positively worded items and 10 negatively worded items that a partner might engage in during the course of a smoking cessation attempt. Responses are measured on a 4-point Likert scale from 1, never occurred, to 4, occurred more than four times. Total scores on both the positive and negative subscales are summed. An example of a positively worded item is "My spouse/ partner rewarded my quitting efforts, expressed confidence in my ability to quit smoking and maintain the program." and of a negatively worded item is "My spouse/partner expressed doubt about my ability to quit or stay quit." It did not correlate with the ISEL indicating that they assess different forms of social support.[59] This tool may be useful to tap the specific supportive and nonsupportive assistance of a partner that, in turn, may help explain the differential effects of partner support for behavior change efforts.

Perceived Social Support from Friends (PSS-Fr) and from Family (PSS-Fa)

Procidano and Heller[60] developed PSS-Fr and PSS-Fa. The authors report that these were separate valid constructs distinct from network. These represent two different sources of support categories and tap different dimensions of social relationships. Each of the measures has 20 items; a "yes," "no," or "don't know" response is given for each item. The items include receiving of supportive behaviors and a few that tap the notion of reciprocity, that is, the individual provides support to network members. An example of an item from the PSS-Fr is "Most other people are closer to their friends than I am." An example of an item from the PSS-Fa is "I get good ideas about how to do things or make things from my family." The response format of the PSS-Fr and PSS-Fa was adapted and tested using a 4-point response option (generally false, more false than true, more true than false, and generally true)[140] and a 5-point Likert scale from 1, strongly disagree, to 5, strongly agree.[112]

Personal Resource Questionnaire (PRQ) (PRQ85) (PRQ2000)

The PRQ was developed as a measure of the multidimensional characteristics of social support.[61,62] The two most recent and widely used versions of the tool are the PRQ85 and the PRQ2000.[63,141] The instrument has two parts. Information about the person's resources and satisfaction with these resources is obtained from part one and was designed to provide descriptive information about the person's social network. Part two is based on the social relationship dimensions described by Weiss[103] (intimacy, social integration, nurturance, worth, and assistance) and measures the amount of perceived social support.

Ten life situations were created for part one of the PRQ85.[141] The situations include circumstances in which the person may need assistance (e.g., urgent needs, extended care), and the respondent is asked to whom they could turn to for help (e.g., no one, spouse, child, relative, friend, spiritual advisor, professional person). Following identification of the sources of support, the individual is asked whether he or she has actually experienced the situation recently and, if so, rates the extent of satisfaction with the assistance obtained. Part two has five items for each of Weiss's[103] five social relationship dimensions. A seven-point Likert scale is used for the respondent to rate each of 25 items from 1, strongly disagree, to 7, strongly agree. A sample item is "I can't count on my relatives and friends to help me with problems." The PRQ85 has been translated into Thai, Japanese, Chinese, Dutch, Spanish,[142] and Korean.[143]

The most recent psychometric evaluation of the PRQ is part of a nationwide study of families managing multiple sclerosis (www.montana.edu/cweinert), resulting in the PRQ2000.[144] Part two of the PRQ85 was revised to clarify the underlying factor structure of the scale. Results of the factor analysis and item analysis yielded a 3-factor structure with each of the 3 factors containing 5 items. The 15 items are summed to obtain a total social support score.

Quality of Relationships Inventory (QRI)

The QRI assesses relationship-based perceptions of social support and conflict.[64] This instrument is unique in that it provides for examination of relationship-specific perceptions on three subscales (support, conflict, and depth of relationship) rather than generalized perception of social support. Respondents complete the 29-item instrument for mother, father, and up to four other relationships they consider important, such as a friend. The focus of the support subscale is perception of availability of support from the specific relationship; the focus of the conflict subscale is the conflict and ambivalence in the relationship; and the focus of the depth subscale is the significance of the relationship. Examples of items include "To what extent can you turn to this person for advice about problems?" and "How often does this person make you feel angry?" The QRI uses a 4-point Likert type scale with responses to items ranging from 1, not at all, to 4, very much. Results from instrument development testing support the underlying hypothesis that perceptions of relationship-specific support are distinct from the perceptions of general support. Additional psychometric properties and construct validity have been reported.[65]

Sense of Support Scale (SSS)

The SSS[66] is a 21-item scale designed to measure an individual's general perceived availability of the quantity and quality of social support. The items form a composite indicator of the person's sense of support rather than distinguishing among the various functions of social support. Items are rated on a 4-point Likert scale, from 0, not at all true, to 3, completely true. Six of the items are negatively worded to control for response bias. Example items include "I have a mentor(s) in my life I can go to for support/advice" and "I seldom get invited to do things with others." The authors created the scale to tap a person's sense of support that "reflects a general outlook on social life" and that affects the person's understanding of social interactions and expectations about self and others.[66]

Social Support Appraisals Scale (SSAS)

The 23-item SSAS examines the extent to which a person feels loved, respected, and involved with family, friends, or others.[67,68] The instrument development was based on Cobb's[81] conceptualization of social support. The scale can be scored as a total measure, or scores can be determined for family (8 items) and for friends (7 items). The respondents rate the items on a four-point scale from 1 (strongly agree) to 4 (strongly disagree). Examples of items are "My friends respect me" and "Members of my family don't rely on me." Descriptions of the testing of this instrument are quite helpful for those interested in instrument development. This instrument has been used with a variety of samples.

Social Support Behaviors (SSB)

The SSB is a 45-item instrument developed to assess five types of support: emotional, assistance, financial, guidance, and socializing.[69] Respondents indicate how likely a family member or a friend would be to provide the type of supportive behavior characterized in the items if needed. Perceptions of the supportive behaviors of family members and of friends are assessed separately. Examples of items are "Would visit with me or would invite me over" and "Would give me a ride if I needed it." Respondents rate, on a scale of 1 to 5, how likely either family or friends would provide the support identified in each item: 1, no one would do this, to 5, most (family/friends) would do this.

Social Support Questionnaire (SSQ)

Another measure of social support, the SSQ, has been developed and tested by Sarason et al.[70] Scores for the perceived number of social supports and satisfaction with the social support available are obtained using the SSQ. The SSQ consists of 27 items, each of which asks the respondent to list the people on whom he or she can rely for the set of circumstances described and to indicate the degree of satisfaction they have with the support provided. An example of an item is "Whom do you really count on to be dependable when you need help?" One of the options allows the respondent to answer "no one," but then the degree of satisfaction with the support is still rated (ranging 1 to 6 points from "very satisfied" to "very dissatisfied"). Two scores are calculated; the SSQ-N is the average number of network individuals available and the SSQ-S is the satisfaction with available support.

Although the instrument was developed with undergraduate college students, it has been used and found to be reliable and valid in many other populations, including adolescents[19] and adults with cancer[145] and patients with HIV.[146] It has been translated into Dutch, Polish, Japanese, German, Spanish,[147] and French.[148]

Social Support Questionnaire (SSQ)

Schaefer et al.[71] developed and used another instrument called the Social Support Questionnaire. Schaefer's SSQ is a two-part questionnaire. Nine situations are presented in part one as a measure of tangible support. An example of an item from part one is "Often people rely on the judgment of someone they know in making important decisions about their lives. Is there anyone whose opinion you consider seriously in making important decisions about your family?" Respondents list the individual(s) by initials and check the appropriate relational category. The number of situations (1–9) in which the subject could count on tangible support from another person is the person's tangible support score. In part two, respondents are provided with a list of 16 network members (i.e., mate, three closest friends, four closest relatives, four work associates, four neighbors). They then rate each person on four questions about emotional support (64-item scale) and one question about informational support (16-point scale). One of the emotional items is "How much does this person boost your spirits when you feel low?" The informational question is "How much did this person give you information, suggestions, and guidance over the last month that you found helpful?" For part two questions, the ratings range from 1, not at all, 2, slightly, to 5, extremely. The conceptualization and health-related functions of social support are described by Schaefer et al.[71] The Schaefer SSQ and the Brandt and Weinert[61] PRQ have been administered concurrently with the NSSQ and the findings are reported.[57,58]

Social Support Questionnaire

The third Social Support Questionnaire, by Revenson and Schiaffino,[72,149] is a 20-item self-administered questionnaire that was developed for use with arthritis populations. It measures the actual receipt of positive (helpful) and problematic (unhelpful) support from network members in relation to a stressor (e.g., pain or disability episode). The Positive Support Scale (16 items) can be further divided into subscales of informational (5 items), tangible (3 items), and emotional/esteem support (8 items). The respondent is asked to recall a stressor (pain or disability) episode within the past week and then rate support, also in the past week, from each of six individuals closest to them, with reference to the stress episode. Items are rated for frequency of occurrence on a 5-point Likert type scale from 1, never, to 5, always. Example items from the positive (tangible) support and problematic support scales, respectively, are "Does small favors for you, e.g., picks up a few groceries or watches the children" and "Becomes annoyed when you don't accept their advice." Although the measure was developed for arthritis populations, it can be utilized in other illness populations.

Social Support Rating Scale (SSRS)

The SSRS developed by Cauce and colleagues[73] is one of the few instruments created for use with adolescents; it was adapted from an earlier study of high school students. Respondents indicate on a three-point Likert scale the extent to which different individuals are perceived to be helpful to them: 1, not at all, to 3, great deal. The SSRS has 10 items. In addition to a total score, factor analysis of the 10 items yielded three structural support dimensions: family support, formal support, and informal support.

Social Support Scale (SSS)

Funch and colleagues[74] describe the development and use of a short scale to measure social support that can be modified for specific situations, such as support when goal is weight loss/dieting. This is a somewhat unique approach in terms of examining the specificity of social support relative to some particular desired health outcome. An example of an item they used with subjects in a health maintenance organization who were involved in a weight loss program is "When people try to diet, the people around them can sometimes help and sometimes make things harder, even if they don't realize it." The respondent is asked to indicate on a Likert-type scale, ranging from 1 (not at all helpful) to 5 (completely helpful), how helpful each person (spouse, children, other relatives, friends, coworkers) acts relative to the specific situation described. The authors provide several methods of scoring (e.g., to obtain an estimate of size of support network available) and calculations for obtaining perceived support. These two scores represent different dimensions of support. More work is required in establishing the psychometric properties of the SSS, but the idea of measuring social support specifically in relationship to an identified health outcome is very important.

Social Support Instruments for Special Populations

A few social support instruments have been designed to be used with specific populations. Several instruments that focused on social support in specific circumstances, such as eating and exercise habits,[37] weight loss/dieting,[74] or cessation,[59] were included in the previous section. Several instruments used with specific clinical populations, such as arthritis,[72] also were included above. Investigators are devoting effort to developing measures that are more sensitive to the particular social support needs of specific groups, such as mothers and stroke survivors. Specific situation examination of social support may be more helpful in some cases than is a global assessment. Selected instruments are presented and their psychometric properties are highlighted in Appendix 12B.

Hughes Breastfeeding Support Scale (HBSS)

An example of beginning development of an instrument for a specific population is the HBSS.[75] The 30-item instrument is designed to assess emotional (10 items), instrumental (10 items), and informational (10 items) support as perceived by breastfeeding mothers. It is a self-administered questionnaire using a 1-to-4 Likert-type scale format. Although the HBSS is designed to measure support in a specific population, some of the 30 items also tap the global dimensions of social support. Examples of specific and more global items are "Answered my questions about breastfeeding" and "Showed concern when I felt blue." This instrument has received some additional psychometric testing.[150,151]

Maternal Social Support Index (MSSI)

The MSSI was developed to assess a mother's perception of the amount of social support (emotional and tangible) and her satisfaction with the support provided.[76] It is a 21-question tool that can be self-administered and obtains information in seven areas: (1) help with daily tasks, (2) satisfaction with visits from kin, (3) help with crises, (4) emergency child care, (5) satisfaction with communication from male partner and (6) from another support person, and (7) community involvement. An example of one of the 10 questions related to help with daily tasks is "Who does the grocery shopping?"

Whether the social support measured by the MSSI specific to mothers would be similar to that measured by the more global measures of social support remains unknown. However, it may be useful to think of social support in more specific contexts, such as in relationship to the role of a mother. This specific examination of social support may be more helpful in some cases than a global assessment.

Nurse-Sibling Social Support Questionnaire

Murray[77] developed two tools measuring social support for school-aged siblings of children with cancer: the Nurse-Sibling Social Support Questionnaire (NSSSQ). One tool is for the siblings and one is for the parents; both measure perceptions of social support for the siblings. The author conceptualized social support using House's dimensions of emotional, informational, instrumental, and appraisal support.[99] The sibling version asks them to rate the extent to which they believe each of 30 nursing interventions helps them with the childhood cancer experience (1, not helpful, to 5, extremely helpful) and how frequently the interventions are made available to them by pediatric oncology nurses (1, never, to 5, always). The parent version of the instrument asks parents to report how helpful these same 30 nursing interventions are to their well child and how frequently the interventions are made available to the sibling. In addition, the 30-items can be separated into four subscales of emotional (12 items), informational (6 items), instrumental (6 items), and appraisal support (6 items).

Support Behaviors Inventory (SBI)

The SBI was developed to use with expectant couples.[78] It is a 45-item instrument where half of the items specifically reference pregnancy and the other half are generally applicable. The items were developed from the generation of a list of supportive behaviors identified in interviews with expectant parents. The author used House's[99] typology as the basis for the four categories of support: emotional, material, informational, and appraisal. On a six-point scale, respondents are asked to indicate the degree of satisfaction (1, very dissatisfied, to 6, very satisfied) they experience with each supportive behavior, first with their partner relationship and then with other people. Two scores are derived: One is satisfaction with partner support score, and the other is satisfaction with other people support. Conceptually, most instruments have been developed on the theory that social support is multidimensional; however, discriminant validity and factor analytic testing of the SBI suggest a broad, single dimension. Obviously, further study of this issue is required. Other studies with other instruments do support the multidimensionality of social support. A brief 11-item version of the scale (two separate scales that measure partner and other support) was created using interitem correlations and an analysis of the theoretical domain of social support.[78] Curry et al. found the 11-item scale to be reliable and valid,[152] as well as culturally appropriate for traditional Hispanic and African American Women.[153] The 45-item tool has been translated into French.[154]

Social Support in Chronic Illness Inventory (SSCII)

Development of the SSCII[79] was based on Kahn's[104] concept of convoy and a model of stress, coping, and health. It is designed for use with people with chronic illnesses, such as diabetes, hypertension, end-stage renal disease, or cardiac disease. The instrument can be completed by the chronically ill individual or the provider of support. Respondents are asked to identify the one individual who at present is most important to them and to indicate the degree of satisfaction they feel with the specified supportive behaviors. The SSCI is designed to examine perceived satisfaction with each supportive behavior relative to a specific situation, chronic illness, and the analysis is from an individual support perspective rather than from a support network perspective.

The SSCII is a 38-item measure (9 are chronic illness specific) using a six-point Likert scale that ranges from 1 (dissatisfied) to 6 (very satisfied). It has five subscales: (1) intimate interaction, (2) guidance, (3) feedback, (4) tangible assistance, and (5) positive social interaction. The respondents rate each item for one individual they identify as being the most important to them at the present time. Examples of these items are "Provided transportation for me" and "Helped me understand about my disease."

Social Support Inventory for Stroke Survivors (SSISS)

The Social Support Inventory for Stroke Survivors (SSISS)is a measure that can be administered by an interviewer or self-administered.[80,155] It consists of 75 questions, 15 for each of the following five sources of social support: personal/intimate relationship, family and close friends, community individuals, community groups, and professionals. For each of the five sources, support is measured by the three dimensions of quality, quantity, and satisfaction. Some inventory items are specific to stroke (e.g., change in available support since the stroke). The inventory is scored by the three dimensions for each of the five sources of support and by each of the dimensions across all five support sources, resulting in eight scores. The inventory was tested in stroke survivors[80] and in undergraduate college students.[155]

Selection of a Measure of Social Support

There are several major considerations in selecting an instrument to measure social support. The first is whether or not the instrument captures the dimensions of social support that you want to measure. For example, is social interaction or the availability of tangible assistance of most importance to your study or are both dimensions important for the measure you select? Whether or not the instrument assesses support perceived to be available or support that has actually been received and whether the instrument includes the costs of social support are aspects to consider in selecting a measure of social support. The populations in which the instrument has been developed, tested, and refined are important to consider and to identify other populations in which investigators have used the instrument to measure social support. A few social support instruments have been developed for children, adolescents, or elderly or for individuals with a specific illness. Some instruments include network properties as well as the support and some allow specification of the categories or specific sources of support (e.g., family, friend, coworker). Your research questions will determine which of these factors must be incorporated in the measure you select. The theoretical or conceptual basis used for the social support instrument development may be of major importance in your selection, as it should be congruent with the conceptualization of your study variables. If it is of interest to measure a variable, such as social support, over time, it is important to determine whether the instrument is a sufficiently sensitive measure for changes to be detected.

Providing a full description of every social support measure, the theoretical basis (when available) for the construction of the instrument, a full description and critique of the validity and reliability and other psychometric testing, and descriptions of samples used in the instrument development phases are beyond the scope of this chapter. Those that have been included generally have been used in more than one current study or have been newly developed with reported psychometric testing. In all cases, when selecting an instrument, it is necessary to review the original information given about the conceptual basis used to develop the measure, the samples for which it was designed, and the psychometric properties. As indicated throughout this chapter, although there are many choices of instruments designed to measure social support or some dimensions of it, not all are at the same level of development. For additional information about selecting an instrument, refer to Chapter 1.

Summary

Social support is one component of the human context of the individual's social environment. Early work has suggested that social support plays a role in mediating the effects of stressful life events, in protecting health, and in buffering against stressful circumstances or crises. Conceptualizations and measurement of social support remain varied, and several instruments designed to measure one or more dimension of social support are available and have published validity and reliability data. Many instruments require further psychometric testing. The final selection of an instrument must be based on the congruency between the variables you want to measure and what dimensions an instrument has been designed to assess.

As reflected in the diverse dimensions of social support assessed by the various instruments, there is as yet no universally accepted definition of social support. Most authors have viewed social support as multidimensional, and most instruments have been developed to tap one or more dimensions of social support. However, a few investigators have found that the subscales of the instruments they have used are very highly intercorrelated and that factor analytic techniques yield one dominant factor, suggesting that social support be viewed as one major construct. Many other investigators have found some dimensions or subscales to be separate, thus lending support to the contention that social support is a multidimensional construct. Obviously, much more work is required.

Beyond instrument development and selection, the future emphasis must be to determine more specifically how social support, or how various social support functions, affects situation- and population-specific health outcomes.

Exemplar Study: A Social Support Intervention and Assessing Adequacy of Social Support

Norbeck, J.S., DeJoseph, J.F., & Smith, R.T. A randomized trial of an empirically derived social support intervention to prevent low birthweight among African American women. *Soc Sci Med*, 1996, 43(6):947–954.[156]

This was a randomized clinical trial designed to determine if an empirically derived social support intervention would be effective in decreasing number of low-birthweight (LBW) babies in a sample of 114 African American women assessed to have low support provided by the woman's mother or the male partner. The culturally relevant social support intervention was delivered every two weeks in four face-to-face sessions and in telephone calls on each of the intervening weeks. This empirically derived and culturally appropriate social support intervention was determined to be effective in reducing the rate of LBW infants (9.1% LBW infants in intervention group [$n = 56$] compared to 22.4% LBW infants in the control groups [$n = 58$]).

This study was selected as an exemplar for several reasons. By measuring social support, the authors first identified a sample with low social support to randomly assign to an intervention or a control group. Having a sample with measured low support, the likelihood of being able to demonstrate the effectiveness of a social support intervention would be more plausible in an at-risk population. They used a standardized instrument, the NSSQ, to determine the perceived adequacy of social support. This aspect of the study was described elsewhere.[127] They selected an important clinical outcome, that of decreasing the rate of LBW infants for a population in which the rate is higher than among Caucasians. They built on previous work, in which the only two sources of social support that were important for pregnancy outcomes in this ethnic population were the woman's mother or the male partner.[127] In addition, they based their hypothesis on a model linking social support with health outcomes and on work suggesting that specific sources of support are more important then the total amount of available support.

The discussion section in this report provides critical analysis of other studies in which social support–type interventions have been found to be effective and those in which effectiveness was not found. The insights shared in this report move the social support field forward in important ways. In addition to this exemplar clinical study, many of the instrument development reports cited in this chapter provide other excellent examples of conceptualization, measurement and research incorporating social support.

Websites

In addition to the two Websites cited in the text above, there are several other sites in which social support is approached from different or a more broad perspective (e.g., the use of the Internet in social support research or the promotion of social integration). The following sites are examples.

Cornell Gerontology Research Institute, Access date April 1, 2003. www.blcc.cornell.edu/cagri/.

Social Support on the Internet. Access date April 1, 2003. homenet.hcii.cs.cmu.edu/progress/research.html.

Testing the Validity and Reliability of the Computer-mediated Social Support Measures. Access date April 1, 2003. medschool.umaryland.edu/womenshealth/whrg/nahm08.html.

The University of Alberta Social Support Research Project. Access date April 1, 2003. www.ssrp.ualberta.ca/.

References

1. Wortman, C.B. Social support and the cancer patient. Conceptual and methodological issues. *Cancer*, 1984, 53(10 suppl):2339-2362.
2. House, J.S., Kahn, R.L., McLeod, J.D., & Williams, D. Measures and concepts of social support. In S. Cohen and S.L. Syme (Eds.), *Social support and health*. New York: Academic, 1985, pp. 83-108.
3. Bruhn, J.G., & Philips, B.U. Measuring social support: A synthesis of current approaches. *J Behav Med*, 1994, 7(2):151-169.
4. Lindsey, A.M., Norbeck, J.S., Carrieri, V.L., & Perry, E. Social support and health outcomes in postmastectomy women: A review. *Cancer Nurs*, 1981, 4(5):377-384.
5. Ford, M.E., Tilley, B.C., & McDonald, P.E. Social support among African-American adults with diabetes, Part 2: a review. *J Natl Med Assoc*, 1998; 90(7):425-432.
6. Helgeson, V.S., Cohen, S., Schulz, R., & Yasko, J. Group support interventions for people with cancer: Who benefits from what? *Health Psychol*, 2000, 19:107-114.
7. Kelsey, K., Earp, J.A.L., & Kirkley, B.G. Is social support beneficial for dietary change? A review of the literature. *Fam Community Health*, 1997, 20(3):70-82.
8. May, S., & West, R. Do social support interventions ('buddy systems') aid smoking cessation? A review. *Tob Control*, 2000, 9(4):415-422.
9. Perrin, K.M., & McDermott, R.J. Instruments to measure social support and related constructs in pregnant adolescents: A review. *Adolescence*, 1997, 32(127):533-557.
10. Underwood, P.W. Social support: The promise and the reality. In V.H. Rice (Ed.), *Handbook of stress, coping, and health: Implications for nursing research, theory, and practice*. Thousand Oaks, CA: Sage Publications, 2000, pp. 367-391.
11. Vrabec, N.J. Literature review of social support and caregiver burden, 1980 to 1995. *Image J Nurs Sch*, 1997, 29(4):383-388.
12. Woodgate, R.L. Social support in children with cancer: A review of the literature. *J Pediatr Oncol Nurs*, 1999, 16(4):201-213.
13. Murawski, B.J., Penman, D., & Schmitt, M. Social support in health and illness: The concept and its measurement. *Cancer Nurs*, 1978, 1(5):365-371.
14. Norbeck, J.S. Social support: A model for clinical research and application. *Adv Nurs Sci*, 1981, 3(4):43-59.
15. Bosworth, H.B., Steffens, D.C., Kuchibhatla, M.N., et al. The relationship of social support, social networks and negative events with depression in patients with coronary artery disease. *Aging Mental Health*, 2000, 4(3):253-259.
16. Yarcheski, A., Mahon, N.E., & Yarcheski, T.J. Social support and well-being in early adolescents: The role of mediating variables. *Clin Nurs Res*, 2001, 10(2):163-181.
17. Murray, J.S. Social support for school-aged siblings of children with cancer: A comparison between parent and sibling perceptions. *J Pediatr Oncol Nurs*, 2001, 18(3): 90-104.
18. Friedman, M.M. Social support sources among older women with heart failure: Continuity versus loss over time. *Res Nurs Health*, 1997, 20(4):319-327.
19. Haluska, H.B., Jessee, P.O., & Nagy, M.C. Sources of social support: Adolescents with cancer. *Oncol Nurs Forum*, 2002, 29(9):1317-1324.

20. Smith, L., & Weinert, C. Telecommunication support for rural women with diabetes. *Diabetes Educ*, 2000, 26(4):645-655.

21. Hansell, P.S., Hughes, C.B., Caliandro, G., et al. The effect of a social support boosting intervention on stress, coping, and social support in caregivers of children with HIV/AIDS. *Nurs Res*, 1998, 47(2):79-86.

22. Keyserling, T.C., Samuel-Hodge, C.D., Ammerman, A.S., et al. A randomized trial of an intervention to improve self-care behaviors of African-American women with type 2 diabetes: Impact of physical activity. *Diabetes Care*, 2002, 25(9):1576-1583.

23. ENRICHD Investigators. Enhancing recovery in coronary heart disease (ENRICHD) study intervention: Rationale and design. *Psychosomatic Med*, 2001, 63:747-755.

24. Stewart, M., Davidson, K., Meade, D., et al. Group support for couples coping with a cardiac condition. *J Adv Nurs*, 2001, 33(2):190-199.

25. Stewart, M., Craig, D., MacPherson, K., & Alexander, S. Promoting positive affect and diminishing loneliness of widowed seniors through a support intervention. *Public Health Nurs*, 2001, 18(1):54-63.

26. Barrera, M. A method for the assessment of social support networks in community survey research. *Connections*, 1980, 3(3):8-13.

27. Barrera, M. Jr. Social support in the adjustment of pregnant adolescents: assessment issues. In B.H. Gottlieb (Ed.), *Social networks and social support*. Beverly Hills: Sage, 1981, pp. 69-96.

28. Stansfeld, S., & Marmot, M. Deriving a survey measure of social support: The reliability and validity of the Close Persons Questionnaire. *Soc Sci Med*, 1992, 35(8):1027-1035.

29. Parkerson, G.R., Michener, J.L., Wu, L.R., et al. Associations among family support, family stress, and personal functional health status. *J Clin Epidemiol*, 1989, 42(3):217-229.

30. Parkerson, G.R. Jr., Broadhead, W.E., & Tse, C.K. Validation of the Duke Social Support and Stress Scale. *Fam Med*, 1991, 23(5):357-60.

31. Parkerson, G.R., Jr., Broadhead, W.E. & Tse, C.K. Quality of life and functional health of primary care patients. *J Clin Epidemiol*, 1992, 45:1303-1313.

32. Broadhead, W.E., Gehlbach, S.H., deGruy, E.V., & Kaplan, B.H. The Duke-UNC Functional Social Support Questionnaire: A measurement of social support in family medicine patients. *Med Care*, 1988, 26(7):709-723.

33. Landerman, R., George, L.K., Campbell, R.T., & Blazer, D.G. Social support, stress, and depression: Alternative models of the stress buffering hypothesis. *Am J Community Psychology*, 1989, 17:625-642.

34. Koenig, H.G., Westlund, R.E., George, L.K. et al. Abbreviating the Duke Social Support Index for use in chronically ill elderly individuals. *Psychosomatics*, 1993, 34:61-69.

35. Goodger, B., Byles, J., Higganbotham, N., & Mishra, G. Assessment of a short scale to measure social support among older people. *Aust NZ J Public Health*, 1999, 23(3):260-265.

36. ENRICHD Investigators. Enhancing recovery in coronary heart disease patients (ENRICHD): Study design and methods. *Am Heart J*, 2000, 139(1):1-9.

37. Sallis, J.F., Grossman, R.M., Pinski, R.B., et al. The development of scales to measure social support for diet and exercise behaviors. *Preventive Med*, 1987, 16:825-836.

38. Halvorsen, J.G. The Family Stress and Support Inventory. *Fam Prac Res J*, 1991, 11(3):255-277.

39. Cohen, S., & Hoberman, H. Positive events and social supports as buffers of life change stress. *J App Soc Psychol*, 1983, 13(2):99-125.

40. Cohen, S.C., Mermelstein, R., Kamarck, T., & Hoberman, H. Measuring the functional components of social support. In I. Sarason and B. Sarason (Eds.), *Social support: Theory, research, and application*. The Hague, Holland: Martinus Nijhoff, 1985, pp. 73-94.

41. Henderson, S., Duncan-Jones, P., Byrne, D., & Scott, R. Measuring social relationships: The Interview Schedule for Social Interaction. *Psychol Med*, 1980, 10(4):723-734.

42. Duncan-Jones, P. The structure of social relationships: Analysis of a survey instrument, Part I. *Soc Psychiatry*, 1981, 16(2):55-61.

43. Duncan-Jones, P. The structure of social relationships: Analysis of a survey instrument, Part II. *Soc Psychiatry*, 1981, 16(3):143-149.

44. Unden, A-L, & Orth-Gomer, K. Development of a social support instrument for use in population surveys. *Soc Sci Med*, 1989, 29(12):1387-1392.

45. Tilden, V.P., Nelson, C.A., & May, B.A. The IPR Inventory: Development and psychometric characteristics. *Nurs Res*, 1990, 39(6):337-343.

46. Tilden, V.P., Nelson, C.A., & May, B.A. Using qualitative methods to enhance the content validity of a measure. *Nurs Res*, 1990, 39(3):172-175.

47. Tilden, V.P., & Galyen, R.D. Cost and conflict. The darker side of social support. *West J Nurs Res*, 1987, 9(1):9-18.

48. Weinert, C., & Tilden, V.P. Measures of social support: Assessment of validity. *Nurs Res*, 1990, 39(4):212-216.

49. Tilden, V.P., Hirsch, A.M., & Nelson, C.A. The Interpersonal Relationship Inventory: Continued psychometric evaluation. *J Nurs Meas*, 1994, 2(1):63-78.

50. Gauvin, M.D., Vandal, S., Mercier, P., & Bradet, R. Perception of the social support for adolescents who undergo corrective back surgery for scoliosis. *Issues Compr Pediatr Nurs*, 2002, 25(3):207-216.

51. Barrera, N., Sandler, I.N., & Ramsay, T.B. Preliminary development of a scale of social support: Studies on college students. *Am J Comm Psychol*, 1981, 9(4):435-447.

52. Sherbourne, C.D., & Stewart, A.L. The MOS Social Support Survey. *Soc Sci Med*, 1991, 32(6):705-714.

53. Zimet, G.D., Dahlem, N.W., Zimet, S.G., & Farley, G.K. The Multidimensional Scale of Perceived Social Support. *J Pers Assess*, 1988, 52(1):30-41.

54. Zimet, G.D., Powell, S.S., Farley, G.K., et al. Psychometric characteristics of the Multidimensional Scale of Perceived Social Support. *J Pers Assess*, 1990, 55(3-4), 610-617.

55. Dahlem, N.W., Zimet, G.D., & Walker, R.R. The Multidimensional Scale of Perceived Social Support: A confirmation study. *J Clin Psychol*, 1991, 47(6):756-761.

56. Reid, N., Landesman, S., Treder, R., & Jaccard, J. "My Family and Friends": Six- to twelve-year-old children's perceptions of social support. *Child Dev*, 1989, 60(4):896-910.

57. Norbeck, J.S., Lindsey, A.M., & Carrieri, V.L. The de-

velopment of an instrument to measure social support. *Nurs Res*, 1981, *30*(5):264-269.

58. Norbeck, J.S., Lindsey, A.M., & Carrieri, V.L. Further development of the Norbeck social support questionnaire: Normative data and validity testing. *Nurs Res*, 1983, *32*(1):4-9.

59. Mermelstein, R., Cohen, S., Lichtenstein, E., et al. Social support and smoking cessation and maintenance. *J Consult Clin Psychol*, 1986, *54*(4):447-453.

60. Procidano, M.E., & Heller, K. Measures of perceived social support from friends and from family: Three validations studies. *Am J Community Psychol*, 1983, *11*(1):1-14.

61. Brandt, P.A., & Weinert, C. The PRQ: A social support measure. *Nurs Res*, 1981, *30*(5):277-280.

62. Weinert, C., & Brandt, P.A. Measuring social support with the Personal Resource Questionnaire. *West J Nurs Res*, 1987, *9*(4):589-602.

63. Yarcheski, A., Mahon, N.E., & Yarcheski, T.J. Validation of the PRQ85 social support measure for adolescents. *Nurs Res*, 1992, *41*(6):332-337.

64. Pierce, G.R., Sarason, I.G., & Sarason, B.R. General and relationship-based perceptions of social support: Are two constructs better than one? *J Pers Soc Psychol*, 1991, *61*(6):1028-1039.

65. Pierce, G.R., Sarason, I.G., Sarason, B.R., et al. Assessing the quality of personal relationships. *J Soc & Pers Relationships*, 1997, *14*(3):339-356.

66. Dolbier, C.L., & Steinhardt, M.A. The development and validation of the sense of support scale. *Behav Med*, 2000, *25*(4):169-180.

67. Vaux, A., Phillips, J., Holly, L., et al. The Social Support Appraisals (SS-A) Scale: Studies of reliability and validity. *Am J Commun Psychol*, 1986, *14*(2):195-219.

68. Vaux, A. Appraisals of social support: Love, respect, and involvement. *J Commun Psychol*, 1987, *15*(October):493-502.

69. Vaux, A., Riedel, S., & Stewart, D. Models of social support: The Social Support Behaviors (SS-B) Scale. *Am J Commun Psychol*, 1987, *15*(2):209-237.

70. Sarason, I.G., Levine, H.M., Basham, R.B., & Sarason, R. Assessing social support: The social support questionnaire. *J Pers Soc Psychol*, 1983, *44*(1):127-139.

71. Schaefer, C., Coyne, J.C., & Lazarus, R. The health-related functions of social support. *J Behav Med*, 1981, *4*(4):381-406.

72. Revenson, T.A., & Schiaffino, K.M. Development of a contextual social support measure for use with arthritis populations. Paper presented at the 1990 Convention of the Arthritis Health Professionals Association, 1990.

73. Cauce, A., Felner, R., & Primavera, J. Social support in high risk adolescents: Structural components and adaptive impact. *Am J Commun Psychol*, 1982, *10*(4):417-428.

74. Funch, D.P., Marshall, J.R., & Gebhardt, G.P. Assessment of a short scale to measure social support. *Soc Sci Med*, 1986, *23*(3):337-344.

75. Hughes, R.B. The development of an instrument to measure perceived emotional, instrumental, and informational support in breastfeeding mothers. *Issues Comp Pediatr Nurs*, 1984, *7*(6):357-362.

76. Pascoe, J.M., Ialongo, N.S., Horn, W.F., et al. The reliability and validity of the Maternal Social Support Index. *Fam Med*, 1988, *20*(4):271-276.

77. Murray, J.S. Development of two instruments measuring social support for siblings of children with cancer. *J Pediatr Oncol Nurs*, 2000, *17*(4), 229-238.

78. Brown, M.A. Social support during pregnancy: A unidimensional or multidimensional construct? *Nurs Res*, 1986, *35*(1):4-9.

79. Hilbert, G. Measuring social support in chronic illness. In O. Strickland & C. Waltz (Eds.), *Measurement of nursing outcomes. Vol. 4. Measuring clients self care and coping skills.* New York: Springer, 1990, pp. 79-91.

80. Friedland, J., & McColl, M.A. Social support and psychosocial dysfunction after stroke: Buffering effects in a community sample. *Arch Phys Med Rehab*, 1987, *68*(8):475-480.

81. Cobb, S. Social support as a moderator of life stress. *Psychosom Med*, 1976, *38*(5):300-314.

82. Kaplan, B.H., Cassel, J.C., & Gore, S. Social support and health. *Med Care*, 1977, *15*(suppl 5):47-58.

83. Dean, A., & Lin, N. The stress buffering role of social support. *J Nerv Ment Dis*, 1977, *165*(6):403-417.

84. Kahn, R., & Antonucci, T. Convoys over the life course: Attachment, roles and social support. In P.B. Baltes & O. Brim (Eds.), *Life-span development and behavior*, Vol. 3. New York: Academic, 1981, pp. 253-286.

85. Broadhead, W.E., Kaplan, B.H., James, S.A., et al. The epidemiologic evidence for a relationship between social support and health. *Am J Epidemiol*, 1983, *117*(5):521-537.

86. Berkman, L.F., & Syme, S.L. Social networks, host resistance and mortality: A year follow-up study of Alameda County residents. *Am J Epidemiol*, 1979, *109*(2):186-204.

87. Nuckolls, J.B., Cassel, J., & Kaplan, B.H. Psychosocial assets, life crisis and the prognosis of pregnancy. *Am J Epidemiol*, 1972, *95*(5):431-441.

88. Lin, N., Simeone, R., Ensel, W., & Kuo, W. Social support, stressful life events and illness: A model and an empirical test. *J Health Soc Behav*, 1979, *20*(2):108-119.

89. Pilisuk, M., & Froland, C. Kinship, social networks, social support and health. *Soc Sci Med*, 1978, *12*(B):273-280.

90. Cohen, S., Doyle, W.J., Skoner, D.P., et al. Social ties and susceptibility to the common cold. *JAMA*, 1997, *277*:1940-1944.

91. Cassel, J. The contribution of the social environment to host resistance. *Am J Epidemiol*, 1976, *104*(2):107-123.

92. Heller, K. The effects of social support: Prevention and treatment implications. In A.P. Goldstein & F.H. Kanfer (Eds.), *Maximizing treatment gains: Transfer enhancement in psychotherapy*. New York: Academic, 1979, pp. 353-382.

93. Croog, S.H., Lipson, A., & Levine, S. Help patterns in severe illness: The roles of kin network, non-family resources and institutions. *J Marriage Fam*, 1972, *34*:32-41.

94. Cobb, S. Social support and health through the life course. In H.I. McCubbin, A.E. Cauble, & J.M. Patterson (Eds.), *Family stress, coping and social support*. Springfield, IL: Charles C. Thomas, 1982, pp. 189-200.

95. Caplan, G. *Support systems and community mental health*. New York: Behavioral Publications, 1974.

96. Cohen, S., Gottlieb, B.J., & Underwood, L.G. Social relationships and health. In S. Cohen, L.G. Under-

wood, & B.H. Gottlieb (Eds.), *Social support measurement and intervention*. New York: Oxford University Press, 2000, pp. 3-25.

97. Lakey, B., & Cohen, S. Social support theory and measurement. In S. Cohen, L.G. Underwood, & B.H. Gottlieb (Eds.), *Social support measurement and intervention*. New York: Oxford University Press, 2000, pp. 29-52.

98. Caplan, G. The family as a support system. In G. Caplan & M. Killilea (Eds.), *Support systems and mutual help: Multidisciplinary explorations*. New York: Grune & Stratton, 1976, pp. 19-37.

99. House, J.S. *Work stress and social support*. Reading, MA: Addison-Wesley, 1981.

100. Landmark, B.T., Strandmark, M., & Wahl, A. Breast cancer and experiences of social support. In-depth interviews of 10 women with newly diagnosed breast cancer. *Scand J Caring Sci*, 2002, 16(3):216-223.

101. Wills, T.A., & Shinar, O. Measuring perceived and received social support. In S. Cohen, L.G. Underwood, & B.H. Gottlieb (Eds.), *Social support measurement and intervention*. New York: Oxford University Press, 2000, pp. 86-135.

102. Conner, K.A., Powers, E.A., & Bultera, G.L. Social interaction and life satisfaction: An empirical assessment of late-life patterns. *J Gerontol*, 1979, 34(1):116-121.

103. Weiss, R. The provision of social relationships. In Z. Rubin (Ed.), *Doing unto others*. Englewood Cliffs, NJ: Prentice-Hall, 1974, pp. 17-26.

104. Kahn, R.L. Aging and social support. In M.W. Riley (Ed.), *Aging from birth to death: Interdisciplinary perspectives*. Boulder, CO: Westview Press for American Association for the Advancement of Science, 1979, pp. 77-91.

105. Rundall, T.G., & Evashwick, C. Social networks and help-seeking among the elderly. *Res Aging*, 1982, 4(2):205-226.

106. Blazer, D.G. Social support and mortality in an elderly community population. *Am J Epidemiol*, 1982, 115(5):684-694.

107. Caplan, G. The family as a support system. In H.I. McCubbin, A.E. Cauble, & J.M. Patterson (Eds.), *Family stress, coping and social support*. Springfield, IL: Charles C. Thomas, 1982, pp. 200-221.

108. Mitchell, R.E., & Trickett, E.J. Social networks as mediators of social support: An analysis of the effects and determinants of social networks. *Comm Ment Health J*, 1980, 16(1):27-44.

109. Due, P., Holstein, B., Lund, R., et al. Social relations: Network, support and relational strain. *Soc Sci Med*, 1999, 48(5):661-673.

110. Smith, M.Y., & Rapkin, B.D. Social support and barriers to family involvement in caregiving for persons with AIDS: Implications for patient education. *Patient Educ Couns*, 1996, 27(1):85-94.

111. Johnston, D., Stall, R., & Smith, K. Reliance by gay men and intravenous drug users on friends and family for AIDS-related care. *AIDS Care*, 1995, 7(3):307-319.

112. Serovich, J.M., Brucker, P.S., & Kimberly, J.A. Barriers to social support for persons living with HIV/AIDS. *Aids Care*, 2000, 12(5):651-662.

113. Lindsey, A.M. Social support: Selection of a mea-

surement instrument. *Oncol Nurs Forum*, 1984, 11(2):88-89.

114. Vaux, A. *Social support theory, research and intervention*. New York: Praeger, 1988.

115. Moos, R.H. *Evaluating educational environments: Procedures, measures, findings, and policy implications*. San Francisco: Jossey-Bass, 1979.

116. Tardy, C.H. Social support measurement. *Am J Comm Psychol*, 1985, 13(2):187-202.

117. Wood, Y.R. Social support and social networks: Nature and measurement. In P. McReynolds & G.J. Chelune (Eds.), *Advances in Psychological Assessment*. San Francisco: Jossey-Bass, 1985, pp. 312-353.

118. Stewart, M.J. Social support intervention studies: A review and prospectus of nursing contributions. *Int J Nurs Stud*, 1989, 26(2):93-114.

119. Stewart, M.J. Social support instruments created by nurse investigators. *Nurs Res*, 1989, 38(5):268-275.

120. Norbeck, J.S. Social support. *Ann Rev Nurs Res*, 1988, 6:85-109.

121. O'Reilly, P. Methodological issues in social support and social network research. *Soc Sci Med*, 1988, 26(8):863-873.

122. Baillie, V.S., Norbeck, J.S., & Barnes, L.E. Stress, social support, and psychological distress of family caregivers of the elderly. *Nurs Res*, 1988, 37(4):217-222.

123. Morris, P.L.P., Robinson, R.G., Raphael, B., & Bishop, D. The relationship between the perception of social support and post-stroke depression in hospitalized patients. *Psychiatry*, 1991, 54(August):306-315.

124. Finch, J.F., Barrera, M., Jr., Okun, M.A. et al. The factor structure of received social support: Dimensionality and the prediction of depression and life satisfaction. *J Soc Clin Psychol*, 1997, 16(3):323-342.

125. Barrera, M., Jr., & Ainley, S.L. The structure of social support: a conceptual and empirical analysis. *J Commun Psychol*, 1983, 11:133-143.

126. Krause, N., & Markides, K. Measuring social support among older adults. *Int J Aging Hum Dev*, 1990, 30(1):37-53.

127. Norbeck, J.S., & Anderson, N.J. Psychosocial predictors of pregnancy outcomes in low-income black, Hispanic and white women. *Nurs Res*, 1989, 38(4):204-209.

128. Norbeck, J. *Revised scoring instructions for the Norbeck Social Support Questionnaire (NSSQ)*. San Francisco: University of California, 1995.

129. Norbeck Social Support Website. Access date March 13, 2003. nurseweb.ucsf.edu/www/ffnorb.htm.

130. Lindsey, A.M., Ahmed, N., & Dodd, M. Social support network and quality as perceived by Egyptian cancer patients. *Cancer Nurs*, 1985, 8(1):37-42.

131. Berterö, C.M. Types and sources of social support for people afflicted with cancer. *Nurs Health Sci*, 2000, 2:93-101.

132. Nelson, P.B. Social support, self-esteem, and depression in the institutionalized elderly. *Issues Ment Health Nurs*, 1989, 10(1):55-68.

133. Larson, P.J., Lindsey, A.M., Dodd, M.J., et al. Influence of age on problems experienced by patients with lung cancer undergoing radiation therapy. *Oncol Nurs Forum*, 1993, 20(3):473-480.

134. Lindsey, A.M., Larson, P., Dodd, M., et al. Co-morbidity, nutritional intake, social support, weight,

and functional status over time in older cancer patients receiving radiation therapy. *Cancer Nurs*, 1994, 17(2):113-124.

135. Kang, D-H, Coe, C.L., Karaszewski, J., & McCarthy, D.O. Relationship of social support to stress responses and immune function in healthy and asthmatic adolescents. *Res Nurs Health*, 1998, 21:117-128.

136. Norbeck, J.S., & Anderson, N.J. Life stress, social support, and anxiety in mid- and late-pregnancy among low income women. *Res Nurs Health*, 1989, 12(5):281-287.

137. Primomo, J., Yates, B.C., & Woods, N.F. Social support for women during chronic illness: The relationship among sources and types to adjustment. *Res Nurs Health*, 1990, 13(3):153-161.

138. Mermelstein, R., Lichtenstein, E., & McIntyre, K. Partner support and relapse in smoking cessation programs. *J Consult Clin Psychol*, 1983, 51(3):465-466.

139. Cohen, S., & Lichtenstein, E. Partner behaviors that support quitting smoking. *J Consult Clin Psychol*, 1990, 58(3):304-309.

140. Windle, M., & Miller-Tutzauer, C. Confirmatory factor analysis and concurrent validity of the perceived social support-family measure among adolescents. *J Marriage Fam*, 1992, 54(4):777-787.

141. Weinert, C. A social support measure: PRQ85. *Nurs Res*, 1987, 36(5):273-277.

142. Orshan, S.A. Acculturation, perceived social support, self-esteem, and pregnancy status among Dominican adolescents. *Health Care Women Int*, 1999, 20(3):245-257.

143. Han, H., Kim, M.T., & Weinert, C. The psychometric evaluation of Korean translation of the Personal Resource Questionnaire 85-part 2. *Nurs Res*, 2002, 51(5):309-316.

144. Weinert, C. Measuring social support: PRQ2000. In O. Strickland & C. DiIorio (Eds.), *Measurement of nursing outcomes: Vol 3. self-care and coping*. New York: Springer, 2003, pp. 161-172.

145. Poole, G.J. Social support for patients with prostate cancer: The effect of support groups. *Psychosoc Oncol*, 2001, 19(2):1-16.

146. Feaster, D.J., & Szapocznik, J. Interdependence of stress processes among African American family members: Influence of HIV serostatus and a new infant. *Psychol Health*, 2002, 17(3):339-363.

147. Acuna, L., & Bruner, C.A. Estructura factorial del cuestionario de apoyo social de Sarason, Levine, Basham, y Sarason en Mexico [Factorial structure of the social support questionnaire of Sarason, Levine, Basham, and Sarason in Mexico]. *Rev Mex de Psicologia*, 1999, 16(2):267-279.

148. Rascle, N., Aguerre, C., & Bruchon-Schweitzer, M. Soutien social et sante: Adaptation francaise du questionnaire de soutien social de Sarason, le S.S.Q. [Social support and health: A French adaptation of Sarason's S.S.Q.]. *Cahiers Internationaux de Psychologie Sociale*, 1997, 33:35-51.

149. Revenson, T.A., Schiaffino, K.M., Majerovitz, S.D., & Gibofsky, A. Social support as a double-edged sword: The relation of positive and problematic support to depression among rheumatoid arthritis patients. *Soc Sci Med*, 1991, 33(7):807-813.

150. McNatt, M.H., & Freston, M.S. Social support and lactation outcomes in postpartum women. *J Hum Lact*, 1992, 8(2):73-77.

151. Wambach, K.A. Breastfeeding intention and outcome: A test of the theory of planned behavior. *Res Nurs Health*, 1997, 20(1):51-59.

152. Curry, M.A., Campbell, R.A., & Christian, M. Validity and reliability testing of the prenatal psychosocial profile. *Res Nurs Health*, 1994, 17:127-135.

153. Curry, M.A., Burton, D., & Fields, J. The prenatal psychosocial profile: A reseach and clinical tool. *Res Nurs Health*, 1998, 21(3):211-219.

154. Goulet, C., Gevry, H., Gauthier, R.J., et al. A controlled clinical trial of home care management versus hospital care management for preterm labour. *Int J Nurs Stud*, 2001, 38(3):259-269.

155. McColl, M.A., & Friedland, J. Development of a multidimensional index for assessing social support in rehabilitation. *Occup Ther J Res*, 1989, 9(4):218-234.

156. Norbeck, J.S., DeJoseph, J.F., & Smith, R.T. A randomized trial of an empirically-derived social support intervention to prevent low birthweight among African American women. *Soc Sci Med*, 1996, 43(6):947-954.

157. Fuhrer, R., Stansfeld, S.A., Chemali, J., & Shipley, M.J. Gender, social relations and mental health: Prospective findings from an occupational cohort (Whitehall II study). *Soc Sci Med*, 1999, 48(1):77-87.

158. Blumenthal, J.A., Burg, M.M., Barefoot, J., et al. Social support, type A behavior, and coronary artery disease. *Psychosom Med*, 1987, 49:331-40.

159. Uphold, C.R., Lenz, E.R., & Soeken, K.L. Social support transactions between professional and nonprofessional women and their mothers. *Res Nurs Health*, 2000, 23(6):447-460.

160. McCall, W.V., Reboussin, B.A., & Rapp, S.R. Social support increases in the year after inpatient treatment of depression. *J Psychiatr Res*, 2001, 35(2):105-110.

161. Gigliotti, E. A confirmation of the factor structure of the Norbeck Social Support Questionnaire. *Nurs Res*, 2002, 51(5):276-284.

162. Lyons, J.S., Perrotta, P., & Hancher-Kvam, S. Perceived social support from family and friends: Measurement across disparate samples. *J Pers Assess*, 1988, 52(1):42-47.

163. Swanson, K.M. Predicting depressive symptoms after miscarriage: A path analysis based on the Lazarus paradigm. *J Women's Health Gender-based Medicine*, 2000, 9(2):191-206.

164. Corbeil, R.R., Quayhagen, M.P., & Quayhagen, M. Intervention effects on dementia caregiving interaction: A stress-adaptation modeling approach. *J Aging Health*, 1999, 11(1):79-95.

Appendix 12A. Measures of Social Support

Instrument	Description	Psychometric Indices
Arizona Social Support Interview Schedule (ASSIS)[26,27]	5 indicators are constructed: (1) total network size, (2) conflicted network size, (3) unconflicted network size, (4) support satisfaction, and 5) support need Scores are calculated across the following categories of support: material aid, physical assistance, intimate interaction, guidance, feedback, social participation, and interpersonal conflicts	Test-retest reliabilities in college students: total network size (0.88), conflicted network size (0.54), support satisfaction (0.69), support need (0.80) In ethnically diverse sample, alpha reliabilities: support satisfaction (0.50), support need (0.70) Evidence for predictive validity in that support satisfaction and need were the strongest predictors of depression; conflicted network size was positively correlated with several symptom dimensions[27]
Close Persons Questionnaire (CPQ)[28]	Assesses both social network and quality and types of social support (emotional, instrumental, negative aspects) of up to 4 persons close to respondent A cumulative weighted total score for each type of support can be calculated to include the responses for all close persons nominated (most weight [score of 1] given to the 1st close person, 0.25 given to 2nd person, 0.15 to 3rd and 0.10 given to 4th person)[157]	May have utility for large population/epidemiologic surveys Internal consistency (Cronbach's alpha): 0.85 (confiding/emotional), 0.82 (instrumental), 0.63 (negative aspects) Test-retest reliabilities (Spearman correlations): 0.88 (confiding/emotional), 0.71 (instrumental), 0.72 (negative aspects) Evidence for content, construct, and criterion validity provided[28]
Duke Social Support and Stress Scale (DUSOCS)[29-31]	Self-report measure of family and nonfamily social support and stress 24-item questionnaire 6 categories of family (spouse/significant other, children/grandchildren, parents/grandparents, brothers/sisters, other blood relatives, relatives by marriage) 4 categories of nonfamily (neighbors, coworkers, church members, other friends) Each support category rated as to degree of support provided (none to a lot) Separate total scores for family and nonfamily support	Pearson correlation for test-retest (range 7- to 39-day interval): 0.76 (family support), 0.67 (nonfamily support) 0.40 (family stress), 0.68 (nonfamily stress) Validity: Spearman rank order correlation family support with family strength 0.43, $p = 0.0001$; family stress with FILE I & II 0.45, $p = 0.0001$ Internal consistency reliability of 4 subscales range from 0.53 to 0.71
Duke-UNC Functional Social Support Questionnaire (DUFSS)[32]	2-scale, 8-item self-administered measure of 2 dimensions of social support 5 items assess *confidant* support (reflect relationship in which important life matters discussed and shared) 3 items assess *affective* support (reflect emotional or caring support) Responses rated on 5-point Likert scale ranging from "as much as I would like" to "much less than I would like"	Test-retest reliability: 0.66 (1- to 4-week interval, for 22 of 40 married, young females in a primary care clinic) Internal consistency for the two subscales was 0.62 and 0.64 Construct and concurrent validity reported with significant correlations with other measures Further testing in other populations necessary

Instrument	Description	Reliability and Validity
Duke Social Support Index (DSSI)[33-35]	Original instrument, 35-item, 4-subscale measure of multiple dimensions of social support: network, social interaction, subjective support, instrumental support, and items measuring satisfaction with support[33] Two shorter versions of this instrument have been developed: One is 23 items with 3 subscales (social interaction, subjective support and instrumental support) and the other includes 11 of those 23 items using just 2 subscales (social interaction and subjective support)[34]	Additional psychometric testing on the long and shorter versions will be necessary for use in specific populations Factor analysis supported Shorter version of instrument[34] Acceptable validity and reliability reported for the 11-item instrument[35] used in elderly community-dwelling sample
ENRICHD Social Support Instrument (ESSI) (ENRICHD, 2000)[36]	Brief 5-point scale with response options ranging from 1 (none of the time) to 5 (all of the time) Subjects were included in the ENRICHD trial if they scored ≤ 3 on 2 or more items and have a total score ≤ 18	Cronbach alpha reliability of the ESSI: 0.86 Validity evidence: ESSI correlated with the Perceived Social Support Scale (0.62)[158] ISSB (0.35), and the Beck Depression Inventory (−0.39)[36,158]
Family and Friend Support for Eating and Exercise Habits (FFSEEH)[37]	Friend support (eating)—2 subscales: positive comments (6 items), negative comments (4 items) Family support (eating)—2 subscales: encouragement (6 items), sabotage (7 items) Friend support (exercise)—one scale: exercising together (5 items) Family support (exercise)—2 subscales: participation and involvement (12 items), rewards and punishment (3 items) Amount of support rated on a 5-point Likert scale ranging from 1 (none) to 5 (very often)	Test-retest and alpha reliabilities (respectively): positive comments 0.81, 0.87 negative comments 0.78, 0.80 encouragement 0.86, 0.87 sabotage 0.57, 0.83 exercising together 0.79, 0.84 participation 0.77, 0.91 rewards 0.55, 0.61 Subscales were validated with factor analysis; only factors with eigen values > 2.0 were retained for further analysis
Family Stress and Support Inventory (FSSI)[38]	Self-report measure of intrafamilial stress and support provided by each family member as perceived by the respondent For each family member, respondent rates amounts of stress and support received on 1-to-10 continuum Scores can be tabulated by generation, whole family, or individual family members Arithmetic means of stress and support for each grouping determined; ratio of stress to support can be calculated	Test-retest reliability: 0.78 (support), 0.68 (stress) Concurrent validity correlation of 0.50 found between the Family Inventory of Life Events and the FSSI-Stress score; Halvorsen[38] used Marlowe-Crown Social Desirability Scale to determine whether respondents had a social desirability bias in their responses or based responses on true perception of support or stress; scores did not correlate with social desirability

Appendix 12A. Measures of Social Support (*cont.*)

Instrument	Description	Psychometric Indices
Interpersonal Support Evaluation List (ISEL)[39,40]	Measures of perceived availability of support for 4 dimensions of support: tangible, appraisal (informational), belonging (emotional), self-esteem 3 versions: one for college students (48 statements, 12 items per subscale), respondents indicate whether statement is probably true or false for them; one for general population (40 items, 10 items per subscale), respondents indicate whether statement is definitely or probably true or definitely or probably false for them; shorter version of general population (12 items, 4 items per subscale), 4-point scale 50% of items positively worded 50% negatively worded	Validity evidence was provided by correlations between ISEL and other social support measures[40] Internal reliabilities (alpha coefficients): *Total student* (0.77–0.86), *Total general* (0.88–0.90), *Subscales* Student General Appraisal (0.77–0.92) 0.70–0.82 Tangible (0.71–0.74) 0.73–0.81 Belonging (0.75–0.78) 0.73–0.78 Self-esteem (0.62–0.73) 0.62–0.73 Test-retest (total student, 4-week interval): 0.87, subscales: 0.80–0.87 Test-retest (general): (2-day interval) 0.87, (6-week interval) 0.70; (subscales): (2-day) 0.67–0.84, (6-week interval) 0.63–0.69 Validity testing reported
Interview Schedule for Social Interaction (ISSI)[41-43]	Measures the perceived availability and adequacy of attachment and social integration in social relationships (4 subscales) Interview (52-item) or self-report (33-item) measure	Cronbach's alpha: coefficients 0.79–0.90 Test-retest reliability (Pearson product moment correlations): 0.63–0.80 Construct validity correlation of 0.31 between extraversion subscale and the availability of social integration subscale[41]
IPR Inventory (IPRI)[45,49]	39-item measure of interpersonal relationships (includes reciprocity and conflict) Based on theories of social exchange and equity, and refined from a previous 74-item Interpersonal Relationship Index[46] 3 subscales: social support (13 items), reciprocity (13), conflict (13) Items either measure perceived sentiment on 5-point Likert-type scale (agree to disagree) or measure perceived frequency of behavior on a 5-point continuum (very often to never) 3 additional items assess structural aspects of support network	Internal consistency reliability coefficients: (Cronbach's alpha), 0.92 (support), 0.83 (reciprocity), 0.91 (conflict) Factor analysis determined (detailed description) Criterion-related validity determined for support and conflict Normative scores developed for 3 subscales is an important contribution

Instrument	Description	Reliability/Validity
Inventory of Socially Supportive Behavior (ISSB)[51]	40-item measure of the frequency with which respondents receive support from natural support systems Items rated on 5-point scale as to frequency during preceding month (0, not at all, to 4, about every day) 4 subscales identified in college students: directive guidance (12 items), nondirective support (5 items), positive social exchange (6 items), and tangible assistance (7 items)[124] 4 different subscales developed and tested in older adults: emotional, tangible, integration, and informational support[126] Another modification of the ISSB was to measure only frequency of exchange of supportive behaviors (not quality or availability); subjects were asked to rate support on an 8-point scale over the past year[159]	In college students, confirmatory factor analysis (CFA): appropriate to use 4 dimensions of ISSB separately Evidence for predictive validity in that 4 dimensions were differentially related to depression and life satisfaction[124] In older adults, alpha reliabilities: emotional (0.83), tangible (0.67), integration (0.81), and informational support (0.81) CFA indicated four dimensions Evidence for predictive validity in that all 4 subscales of support buffered impact of bereavement on depressive symptoms In the modified ISSB, alpha coefficients ranged from 0.86 to 0.92[159]
MOS Social Support Survey (MOS SSS)[52]	Developed for use with chronically ill patients in a medical outcomes study 19-item, self-administered questionnaire measuring functional dimensions of social support 4 subscales (emotional/informational, affectionate, tangible, positive social interaction) Can use subscale scores (recommended) or total index score One item measures the number of close friends and relatives Respondents indicate how often the type of support is available if needed on Likert-type scale (1, none of the time, to 5, all of the time) 1 item measures structural support dimension Good example of instrument development and evaluation	Tested on approximately 3000 adult patients in 3 sites Internal consistency reliability (Cronbach's alpha): all above 0.91 (each subscale, total scale) Alpha reliabilities for subscales ranged from 0.79 to 0.93 in depressed inpatients[160] Validity tested with multitrait and factor analysis methods resulted in strong convergent and discriminant validity Findings support view that social support is multidimensional
Multidimensional Scale of Perceived Social Support (MSPSS)[53–55]	Self-report measure of 3 subscales: perceived social support from family, friends, and a significant other 12 items rated on a 7-point Likert-type scale (very strongly agree to very strongly disagree)	Testing performed on college students Internal reliabilities (Cronbach's alpha) for subscales: 0.85–0.91, and total score: 0.88 Test-retest reliability 0.72–0.85 for the subscales and 0.85 for total scale Factor analysis showed factors loading on each of subscales; significant low to moderate correlation

Appendix 12A. Measures of Social Support (*cont.*)

Instrument	Description	Psychometric Indices
My Family and Friends (MFF)[56]	3-part measure of perceptions of social support of children aged 6–12 years old 12 dialogues (5, emotional support; 2 each, informational, instrumental, and companionship support; 1, conflict), and props used to engage children and gather data about availability of individuals to provide social support and child's level of satisfaction with type of support received Based on cognitive developmental theory and social support work Significant contribution and allows the addition of dialogues created for specific situations	Sensitive to variations in perceived social support during "family upheaval" Test-retest reliability: 0.68 (network member rankings), 0.69 (satisfaction with support) Overall internal consistency (Cronbach's alpha): dialogues: 0.72, emotional support: > 0.75, instrumental support: teacher 0.28, sibling 0.83 (range attributed to stems: 1 focused on help with schoolwork, other on help around the house)
Norbeck Social Support Questionnaire (NSSQ)[57,58,128,129]	Developed by nurse researchers to measure multidimensional construct of social support Short, self-administered questionnaire tapping 3 areas: functional aspects (affect, affirmation, aid); network (number in network, duration of relationships, frequency of contact); loss (number of support categories in which loss occurred and perceived amount of support lost) Theoretical bases are Kahn's conceptual definitions of social support[104] Ratings scale ranges from 0 (not at all) to 4 (a great deal) Has been used in diverse populations (low-income pregnant women[127,136]; elderly[132]; patients with cancer[130,133,134]; chronically ill women[137]; adolescents[135]	Test-retest reliability: functional and network property items: 0.85–0.92 Internal consistency (each of 3 functional aspects of social support): 0.89 or higher Correlations: among 3 network property items (0.88–0.96), 3 loss items (0.54–0.68) Concurrent validity with Social Support Questionnaire: moderate (0.31–0.56 for subscales) Construct validity demonstrated Normative database (working adults) reported[58] Confirmation of factor structure has been reported[161]
Partner Interaction Questionnaire (PIQ)[59,138,139]	20-item measure of behaviors specific to smoking cessation: 10 positive statements and 10 negative statements Items are measured on a 4-point Likert scale from 0, never, to 3, often Two subscales are created: one indicating positive actions and one indicating negative actions	Respondents who were successful abstainers reported receiving more support from their partners during treatment than either those who never quit or quit and relapsed[138]

Perceived Social Support from Friends (PSS-Fr) and from Family (PSS-Fa)[60]	Measure of valid constructs distinct from network 20-item, yes, no, or don't know response for each instrument (friends, family) Items include receiving supportive behaviors and reciprocity (providing support to network members) Response format changed to a 5-point Likert scale from 1, strongly disagree to 5, strongly agree[112] or a 4-point scale (generally false, more false than true, more true than false, and generally true)[140]	In undergraduate college students: Internal consistency (Cronbach's alpha): PSS-Fr (0.88); PSS-Fa (0.90) Factor analysis: single factor for each scale Subjects with high PSS-Fr scores had significantly lower scores on trait anxiety In diabetic and chronic psychiatric patients: alpha reliabilities: PSS-Fa 0.89, 0.91; PSS-Fr 0.84, 0.92 Construct validity correlation between PSS-Fa and PSS-Fr was 0.40 (16% shared variance) indicating two distinct subscales Criterion-related validity: college student and diabetic patient samples perceived significantly higher levels of family support than the chronic psychiatric sample; the college sample perceived significantly higher friend support than chronic psychiatric patients[162] In HIV-positive gay men: alpha reliabilities of 5-point Likert scale: PSS-Fa were 0.89; PSS-Fr was 0.90[112] In a middle adolescent sample using 4-point scale (PSS-Fa only), a 3-factor model was found using confirmatory factor analysis: Support received (alpha = 0.93) Support provided (alpha = 0.87) Family intimacy (alpha = 0.62) Composite score (alpha = 0.94) Test-retest correlations (6-month interval) were 0.77, 0.71, 0.55, and 0.78, respectively Convergent validity correlations between the PSS-Fa subscales and several characteristics of adolescents and their parents (e.g., maternal support) were significant[140]
Personal Resource Questionnaire[61,62] PRQ85[141] PRQ2000[144]	Measure of multidimensional characteristics of social support—theoretical basis is Weiss[103] dimensions of social relationships PRQ85—2 parts: (I) subject's resources and satisfaction with social network in 10 life situations, (II) social relationship dimensions (5 subscales) measured on a 25-item, 7-point Likert scale PRQ2000: Part II revised to clarify the underlying factor structure of the scale; yielded a 3-factor solution with 15 items	PRQ85—High internal consistency reliabilities for part II (total scale): 0.87 to 0.93[144] Moderate intercorrelations (0.52 to 0.73) for intimacy, social integration, worth, assistance, nurturance subscale independent[141] Established reliability and validity in multiple populations and across cultures[62,63,141-143,163] PRQ2000—Internal consistency reliabilities for 3 factors ranged from 0.82 to 0.86; for total scale, 0.87 to 0.93 Intercorrelations among the three factors ranged from 0.60 to 0.70 Construct validity correlations between the PRQ2000 and the CES-D ranged from −0.44 to −0.51[144] PRQ2000 warrants further evaluation

Appendix 12A. Measures of Social Support (*cont.*)

Instrument	Description	Psychometric Indices
Quality of Relationships Inventory (QRI)[64,65]	Measure of relationship-based perceptions of social support and conflict, using 3 subscales (support, conflict, depth of relationship), not generalized perception 29-item questionnaire completed for mother, father, and up to 4 other important relationships (parent and college student participants) Additional psychometric testing has been reported	Alpha coefficients: support subscale for (M) mother (0.83), (F) father (0.88), (Fr) friend (0.85); conflict subscale M (0.88), F (0.88), Fr (0.91); depth subscale M (0.83), F (0.86), Fr (0.84) Moderate to strong associations of 3 subscales for each relationship category Reliability and construct validity of QRI reported: quality of specific relationships
Sense of Support Scale (SSS)[66]	21-item composite measure of global perceived availability of support Tested in corporate employees (mean age = 38.7 yrs) and undergraduate students (mean age = 20.9 yrs)	Alpha reliability of scale was 0.86 Test-retest reliability was 0.91 Concurrent validity: Correlations between SSS and Social Provisions Scale (0.72) and ISEL (0.78) Convergent validity: SSS was positively related to hardiness and approach-coping Divergent validity: SSS was negatively related to illness symptoms, stress, and avoidance-coping
Social Support Appraisals Scale (SSAS)[67,68]	23-item measure of extent to which person feels loved, respected, and involved with friends, family, others Based on Cobb's conceptualization of social support[81] Scale scored as total measure or subscales (family, 8 items; friend, 7 items) or total, 23 items Items rated on a 4-point scale (1, strongly agree, to 4, strongly disagree) Instrument testing helpful to researchers interested in instrument development	Convergent and divergent validity studied using 5 college and 5 community samples Internal consistency (Cronbach's alpha): 3 scales (0.80–0.90) Attempts to derive subscales to tap love, respect, and involvement resulted in 3 factors, but difficulty with third factor[68]
Social Support Behaviors (SSB)[69]	45-item measure of 5 types of support: emotional, assistance, financial, guidance, socializing Respondents indicate how likely a family member or friend would provide identified support	High internal consistency reliabilities reported for subscales Subscale validity, content validity, and subscale sensitivity demonstrated
Social Support Questionnaire (SSQ)[70]	27-item measure of perceived number of social supports, and satisfaction with them Respondent asked to list people on whom they can rely for the set of circumstances described in each item and degree of satisfaction with support Can also calculate the number of supporters for each role (e.g., family, friend)	Correlations of SSQ with personality, adjustment, life change measures reported Correlations of items with total score (0.48–0.72); satisfaction scores (coefficient alpha) was 0.94 Test-retest (4-week interval) correlations for satisfaction (0.83) and for the number listed (0.90) Stability and high internal consistency among items reported Alpha coefficients for family support was 0.81 and for all other supports was 0.88[146]

Instrument	Description	Psychometric Properties
Social Support Questionnaire (SSQ)[71]	2-part questionnaire: (1) measure of tangible support—9 situations; (2) respondents are provided with a list of 16 network members (i.e., mate, three closest friends, four closest relatives, four work associates, four neighbors) and rate each person on four questions about emotional support (64-item scale) and one question about informational support (16-point scale) Has been used in combination with other measures[57,58]	Test-retest (9-month interval) reliability: tangible support (0.56), emotional support (0.66), informational support (0.58) Internal consistency: information (0.81), emotional support (0.95); tangible support (0.31)[71] In Alzheimer's caregivers, reliabilities of the emotional scale was 0.80 (test-retest) and 0.96 (internal consistency)[164]
Social Support Questionnaire (SSQ)[72,149]	Consists of two scales: positive support scale (16-item) and problematic support scale (4-item) Positive support scale can be analyzed as subscales of emotional/esteem (8 items), tangible (3 items), and informational (5 items) support Developed for use with arthritis populations but can be used in other illness populations	Alpha coefficients for pain episode: positive support (0.90), emotional (0.86), tangible (0.79), informational (0.75), problematic support (0.64) Alpha coefficients for disability episode: positive support (0.95), emotional (0.91), tangible (0.76), informational (0.89), problematic support (0.70) Four-factor structure emerged for all network members except the spouse, where a two-factor structure emerged (positive and problematic)
Social Support Rating Scale (SSRS)[73]	One of few instruments developed for use with adolescents 10-item scale, uses 3-point Likert scale to measure extent to, which different classes of available individuals are perceived to be helpful Allows examination of separate sources of support: formal, informal, and family support in addition to total support scale	Factor Analysis: 3 factors (formal, informal, and family support) Additional psychometric testing is necessary
Social Support Scale (SSS)[74]	Short scale used to measure social support; unique in that tool can be modified for use with specific situations (desired health outcome, e.g., weight loss) Likert-type scale used to measure how helpful each person (spouse, children, other relatives, friends, and coworkers) is relative to specific situation (1, not at all helpful, to 5, completely helpful)	Requires more work in establishing psychometric properties of scale

Key: Superscript numbers correspond to references.

Appendix 12B. Social Support Instruments for Special Populations

Instrument	Description	Psychometric Indices
Hughes Breast feeding Support Scale (HBSS)[75]	30-item measure of support: emotional (10 items), instrumental (10 items), and informational (10 items) as perceived by breastfeeding mothers Self-administered questionnaire using 1–4 Likert-scale format Measures specific and global dimensions	Corrected split-half reliability scores for 3 subscales 0.85–0.89 Internal consistency alpha coefficients: 0.84–0.88 Internal consistency (alpha coefficients) ranged from 0.91–0.95 for the 3 subscales and total scale Convergent validity supported by a correlation of 0.60 ($p < 0001$) between HBSS and a single item measuring overall support[151]
Maternal Social Support Index (MSSI)[76]	Measure of mother's perception of amount of social support (emotional and tangible) and her satisfaction with provided support 21-item, self-administered measure directed to 7 areas: help with daily tasks, satisfaction with visits from kin, help with crises, emergency child care, satisfaction with communication from male partner, other support person, community involvement	Test–retest reliability: 0.72 (6- to 8-week interval), correlations for individual items 0.58–0.81 Internal consistency (coefficient alphas): 0.60–0.63, If clustered child care and non-child care items into 2 groups, was 0.72 (child care) and 0.78 (non-child care) Concurrent validity supported by correlations of the MSSI and Family Relations Scale ($r = 0.50$) and the CES-D scale ($r = 0.30$)[76]
Nurse-Sibling Social Support Questionnaire (NSSSQ)[77]	Sibling version—measures the extent to which 30 nursing interventions help them with the childhood cancer experience (1, not helpful, to 5, extremely helpful) and how frequently the interventions are made available to them by pediatric oncology nurses (1, never, to 5, always) Parent version—measures how helpful these same 30 nursing interventions are to their well child, and how frequently the interventions are made available to the sibling The 30 items can be separated into four subscales of emotional (12 items), informational (6 items), instrumental (6 items), and appraisal support (6 items)	Internal consistencies (alpha coefficients): sibling helpfulness scale: 0.92; sibling frequency scale: 0.90; parent helpfulness scale: 0.94; parent frequency scale: 0.90 All 4 subscales demonstrated acceptable internal consistency reliabilities (alphas > 0.82)[17] Content validity index of 100% agreement was found among 5 expert pediatric oncology nurses that items measured appraisal support (6 items) the concept of social support Warrants further testing
Support Behaviors Inventory (SBI)[78]	45-item instrument Brief 11-item version of the scale is also available (for both partner and other support) Uses 6-point scale to derive two satisfaction scores: satisfaction with partner support and satisfaction with other people support (for both the 45-item and 11-item scales)	Internal reliability (Cronbach's alpha): scores (1) partner support (0.97), (2) other people support (0.98), (3) subscales very highly intercorrelated (0.86–0.93) Discriminant validity and factor analytic techniques support broad single dimension not 4 separate dimensions Warrants further study French version (45-item) internal consistency reliabilities: 0.97–0.98[154] Cronbach alphas of 11-item scales were (1) partner support (0.90–0.95), (2) other people support (0.94–0.95)[152]

Instrument	Description	Psychometric Properties
		Test-retest reliabilities (10-week interval): 0.54–0.68[153]
		Construct validity supported by correlations between stress and partner support ($r = 0.42$) and other people support ($r = 0.57$)[152]
		Factor structure of 45-item scale warrants further study
Social Support in Chronic Illness Inventory (SSCII)[79]	38-item measure of perceived satisfaction with specified supportive behaviors, relative to a specific situation (chronic illness)	Internal consistency (alpha coefficients): total scale (0.98), subscales (0.84–0.94)
	Can be completed by provider of support or chronically ill individual	Test-retest reliability (2-week interval): 0.48
	Based on Kahn's[104] concept of convoy, and a model of stress, coping, and health	Factor analysis did not confirm separate subscales but one main factor (intimate interaction)
	Designed for use with persons with chronic illness, e.g., diabetes, hypertension, end-stage renal, cardiac disease	Further refinement may be necessary
	Uses 6-point Likert scale (1, dissatisfied, to 6, very satisfied)	
	5 subscales: intimate interaction, guidance, feedback, tangible assistance, and positive social interaction	
Social Support Inventory for Stroke Survivors (SSISS)[80]	Self-report inventory of 8 aspects of social support, administered in a structured interview format	Internal consistency (Cronbach's alpha): 0.84
	Source of social support: personal, friend, community, groups, profession	Test-retest reliability (2-week interval): 0.76 in stroke survivors[80]
	Support measured by 3 dimensions (quality, quantity, satisfaction)	In undergraduate students, test-retest reliability (1-week interval): 0.91[55]
	Inventory items specific to stroke	Concurrent validity supported by a correlation of 0.484 between personal and friend support and an attachment subscale of the Interview of Socially Supportive Interactions[155]
	8 scores, scored by 3 dimensions for (1) each of 5 sources of support and by (2) each of 3 dimensions across all 5 support sources	Construct validity supported by correlations among depression and satisfaction with support ($r = -0.295$), quantity of support ($r = -0.262$), and personal/intimate support ($r = -0.240$)[155]
		Warrants further testing

Key: Superscript numbers correspond to references.

Acknowledgment: We want to recognize the contributions of Catherine de Flores and Majeda El-Banna, graduate research assistants, in obtaining the new references and of LaDonna Tworek, administrative assistant, in the preparation of this revised chapter.

13

Measuring Coping

Jo Ann Wegmann and Kimberly McClane

Coping as a concept has received much attention in the literature and has been investigated by various disciplines and avenues of study. Early, classic work concerning coping as a stress response includes empirical studies by Angell,[1] Koos,[2] and Hill.[3] These works are now viewed as classics in the field. Interest in family stress has continued to develop systematically, which has resulted in many examples of research strategies, methods, and reliable and valid instruments to study coping.[4]

Multiple, often overlapping, definitions of coping exist. In this chapter, *coping* is defined as the cognitive and behavioral strategies used to master conditions of harm, threat, or challenge when a normal or routine response is not available.[1,5] As such, coping involves two separate frameworks, psychologic and sociologic. According to Lazarus, the psychologic taxonomy of coping includes direct action and palliative modes. Direct actions are associated with (related to) physiologic responses to stress and become evident with threats of change in a person's social or physical environment. Palliative coping encompasses thoughts or actions designed to relieve the emotional impact of stress. Unlike direct actions, palliative coping does not alter threatening or damaging events but serves to make the person feel better. This has also been referred to as active versus avoidant coping. Sociologic coping behaviors rely on the resources of individuals or groups, such as families. Early research into families recognized the importance of family resources, such as cohesion and adaptability, to maintain family organization and functioning during stressful events.[3] Such coping tendencies are closely related to aspects of social support discussed elsewhere in this book.

Instruments to Measure Coping

A comprehensive list of data-collection techniques or instruments used to measure coping would be extensive, and there would be much duplication among tools. The purpose of this chapter is to identify instruments used for research into coping. Resources include family sociology, psychology, psychiatry, and nursing. All the instruments described are designed to measure the effect of adequate coping behaviors on some outcomes and they appear to be suitable for clinical studies.

Typically, coping processes have been investigated for two reasons: validation or confirmation of a particular theory and evaluation of a patient with a diagnostic clinical instrument.[6] It also is valuable to investigate individual and family coping strategies to identify inappropriate or inadequate coping patterns that can affect health outcomes.

When identifying instruments for the study of coping, it is valuable first to explore broader issues of research into this phenomenon. Because coping represents responses to stressors, the astute investigator must be aware of the sensitive nature of such research, as well as the ethical issues inherent in such exploration. Brailey[7] identifies three research issues in the study of coping strategies: (1) obtaining an accurate picture of routine personal coping strategies, (2) delineating the functions of coping in order to determine the effectiveness of coping, and (3) determining appropriate measurements of coping efficacy. Brailey describes four methods of data collection or types of instrumentation used in the study of coping: (1) direct observation during normal events, (2) use of vignettes to elicit personal responses to stressful events, (3) use of structured instrumentation to obtain usual responses to general sources of stress, and (4) personal accounts of coping responses to actual stressful events.[7]

Direct observation of the subject while he or she is coping with normal events is the first method Brailey describes. This strategy typically involves a longitudinal study, with the risk of observer effect on responses. Another means of data collection involves the use of vignettes of stressful situations, from which subject responses are obtained. This may provide information about coping strategies, but Brailey cautions that vignettes may not represent realistic situations. A third data-collection technique seeks responses to how subjects usually cope with general stressors. Structured instruments typically provide a list of coping responses, rated by the subject on a Likert-type scale. Many instruments that measure coping are designed in this format, yet discrepancies may exist between what subjects say they do and what they actually do in specific situations. The fourth data-collection method involves the use of real events from subjects' own lives and asks them to describe the coping strategies they used. Although this use of real-life events appears advantageous, a potential problem with self-report is selective distortion; this method of data collection is used infrequently.

Singer[6] elaborates somewhat on Brailey's descriptions. This psychologist identifies two types of coping studies. One strategy assumes a theoretical position on how people function. From such a position, the researcher identifies categories or descriptors for coping behaviors. Scales and other measurement instruments can then be developed based on the identified categories. Examples of studies that arise from a theoretical position include comparisons of the relative successes of people employing one category of coping style with those in another.

The second type of coping study Singer describes examines a particular stress or stresses, such as illness or bereavement. Examples include inferential studies about patterns of reactions and functional adaptation to common stressors.

Jalowiec Coping Scale

In beginning discussion of various coping instruments, it is valuable to describe one such tool in detail. The Jalowiec Coping Scale (JCS) is presented here as an exemplar of an instrument developed by a nurse. The JCS is a 60-item, self-report psychometric instrument developed in 1977 by a registered nurse master's student and colleagues at the University of Illinois, Chicago Medical Center. The respondent rates how often each of the coping strategies is used on a four-point (0–3) rating scale (ranging from "never used" to "often used"). Additionally, there is space at the beginning of the questionnaire to list which stressor or stressful event is under investigation. This permits the examination and comparison of situation-specific coping.[8]

Eight coping styles are identified: confrontive, evasive, optimistic, fatalistic, emotive, palliative, supportant, and self-reliant. The subscales were rationally derived by the authors via thematic clustering.

Confrontive	Constructive problem-solving, facing up to and confronting the problem or situation
Evasive	Doing things to avoid confronting the problem
Optimistic	Positive thinking or positive attitudes about the problem or situation
Fatalistic	Pessimistic thinking or pessimistic attitudes toward the problem or situation
Emotive	Expressing or releasing emotions
Palliative	Doing things to make yourself feel better
Supportant	Using support systems (including religious support systems)
Self-Reliant	Depending on yourself to deal with the situation, rather than on others

The JCS consists of two parts. Part A (use) is scored according to the targeted stressor. The subject rates the use of each coping strategy on the four-point Likert-type rating scale. Part B (effectiveness) has the subject rating the effectiveness of each item used. The scale for Part B is 0, not helpful; 1, slightly helpful; 2, fairly helpful; and 3, very helpful. If the subject did not use a particular coping strategy, then he or she should not rate the effectiveness of the item. Ratings for the coping strategies are summed separately for use and effectiveness.

The authors also addressed the validity of the JCS. Content validity is reported as 0.85 for the eight subscales. Empirical construct validity is reported as 75% for all eight subscales, following agreement of 25 nurse researchers. Criterion validity indicates that subjects with a larger social support network used more supportant coping strategies, as reported by the lead author (A. Jalowiec, personal communication, February 4, 2003).

This instrument is widely used and has undergone substantial revision since 1987. It is useful for adults of all ages, including adolescents and the elderly, in both clinical and well population settings. It has been used with patient populations and family members of patients. It is available in English and 22 known foreign languages, with a reading level at the sixth grade (A. Jalowiec, personal communication, February 4, 2003).

The instruments designed to measure coping described here are organized into six broad categories: those derived from studies of disease and health-care outcomes; those related to family sociology research, work, and employment issues; issues in the elderly; coping issues in today's world and terrorism; and global issues. In discussing specific instruments, methods of data collection and analysis are addressed. Issues of reliability and validity also are addressed for each instrument. The specific instruments discussed are summarized in Appendix 13A.

Disease and Health Care Outcomes

Disease, illness, and alterations in overall health present loss experiences that frequently result in the activation of coping mechanisms to regain or compensate for such losses. The list of disease-specific and age-specific coping strategies is extensive. Several instruments to measure coping in generalized illness situations are presented here.

Coping Strategy Questionnaire

The Coping Strategy Questionnaire[9] assesses cognitive and behavioral pain coping mechanisms in a sample of patients with chronic low back pain. This self-report questionnaire consists of six cognitive coping strategies (e.g., thinking of things that serve to distract one away from the pain) and two behavioral coping strategies (e.g., engaging in active behaviors that divert one's attention away from the pain) when the subject feels pain. Items are scored on a seven-point scale, and the respondent indicates how often he or she uses that particular strategy when feeling pain (0, never; 3, sometimes; and 6, always).

This questionnaire is internally reliable, with an alpha coefficient of 0.71. The authors discuss the predictive value of this questionnaire when working with people experiencing chronic pain. The value of an instrument such as this one to nursing research in a variety of settings is evident.

Coping Health Inventory for Parents

The Coping Health Inventory for Parents assesses the relationship between parental attitudes toward a child's chronic illness and parental coping patterns. Eighty items of coping behavior are operationally defined. Parents are asked to record how helpful (scale of 0 to 3) each behavior is in their family situation.[10] Three subscales are measured. McCubbin et al.[11] report Cronbach's alphas of 0.97, 0.79, and 0.71 for the three subscales. Coefficient alphas also are reported and range between 0.84 and 0.89 for the three subscales.[12]

Chronicity Impact and Coping Instrument: Parent Questionnaire (CIC:PQ)

Hymovich reports on the CIC:PQ.[13] This instrument was developed to determine the impact of a child's chronic illness on parents and to understand how parents cope. The author describes the results of three tests and the three phases of the instrument.

The current format of the CIC:PQ contains 167 items divided into six sections, including your child, yourself, your spouse, brothers and sisters, hospitalization, and other. This self-report instrument is completed by parents. There are 60 stressor items, 61 coping items, and nine value/attitude/belief items. Other items seek demographic information.

Hymovich reports that internal consistency was determined for each of the three revisions of this instrument. The current version of the CIC:PQ has a Hoyt reliability coefficient of 0.95, which the author cautions may be artificially inflated. She states further that the test-retest reliability still needs to be determined. Although this is a relatively new instrument for measuring family coping, its value lies in its ability to determine the impact of chronic disease on parents and their coping practices with chronically ill children and predict the outcome of intervention with these families.

Goldstein Cooper-Avoider Sentence Completion Test (SCT)

Cohen and Lazarus investigated the relationship between the mode of coping with preoperative stress and recovery from surgery.[14] Among the instruments used to gather information was the Goldstein Cooper-Avoider SCT. This test consists of a series of sentence-completion items; responses are scored by the investigator for either avoidance or coping. An example of one item is "My greatest fear is . . ." The authors acknowledge that there may be gender differences in responses. No information is offered on the reliability or validity of this instrument. Nevertheless, this test appears to be easily administered and elicits predictive information about individuals' coping styles before a threatening event. As such, it offers potential value to nursing research.

Preoperative Coping Scale

Another study of surgical patients used a preoperative coping scale to assess the extent to which patients desired and sought information about impending surgery.[15] The preoperative coping scale consists of 15 items that address location and size of incision, length of the operation, expected level of pain, and type of postoperative treatment. Sime reports that quantitative data were derived by assigning a plus or minus to each item and summing across items. The possible range of scores is –15 to 15, with extreme minus scores representing limited information seeking and extreme positive scores indicating extensive information seeking. Very little other information is available about the preoperative coping scale. Validity and reliability are not addressed in Sime's paper. This scale, too, appears to be a likely instrument for future development in nursing research.

Response to Illness Questionnaire (RIQ)

Pritchard reports on the development of the RIQ, a 34-item, self-report survey designed to measure aspects of illness behavior.[16] This instrument was administered to two groups of patients undergoing long-term hemodialysis. The actual instrument is not fully described in this brief report, but temporal reliability was tested. Weighted kappa values ranged from 0.22 to 0.89. Pritchard concludes that the RIQ has a substantial level of temporal reliability and suggests that it is a valuable instrument for studies of illness behavior.

Bedsworth and Molen's Semistructured Interview

To measure the psychologic stress of spouses of myocardial infarction patients immediately after admission to a coronary care unit, Bedsworth and Molen[17] developed a semistructured interview. Four open-ended questions identify perceived threats and perceived coping strategies. These authors identified 45 actual coping strategies and the total actions taken against the perceived threats by a specific group of spouses.

Little information about this semistructured interview is available, yet it appears to be congruent with the second method of data collection described by Brailey,[7] that is, obtaining subjects' responses to vignettes of stressful situations. Bedsworth and Molen[17] do not address issues of validity or reliability, and indeed, one problem with this type of data collection is the potential for selective distortion by the respondent. Nevertheless, identification of actual coping behaviors used by spouses provides valuable information and suggests possible directions for future research.

Ways of Coping Checklist

The Ways of Coping Checklist (WCC) was developed by Folkman and Lazarus.[18] This 66-item, four-point Likert-type response category checklist assesses behavioral and cognitive coping strategies in eight subscales. This instrument has been widely used in assessing coping in such areas as bereavement, chronic illness, and functional disability. Cronbach's alphas in three studies range from 0.56 to 0.79.[19]

Cancer Inventory of Problem Situations

Heinrich and Schag[20] developed an instrument to document day-to-day physical and psychosocial problems confronted by cancer patients. The Cancer Inventory of Problem Situations is a self-report test that takes approximately 20 minutes to complete. It consists of 131 problem statements with a five-point rating scale, with responses ranging from "not at all" to "very much." The problem statements are grouped into 27 categories. The instrument evaluates the patient's previous month and how each statement applied to him or her during that time. The content and face validity of this instrument have been established.

Pain Experience Inventory

The Pain Experience Inventory is composed of 37 questions answered on a four-point Likert-type scale ("not at all" to "very much"). It was designed to measure cognitive factors perceived to influence the pain experience. Content analysis by a panel of experts revealed a content validity index of 0.92.[21]

Pain Coping Tool

The Pain Coping Tool measures 14 coping elements, 4 behaviors, and 10 strategies. It is a 28-item tool in which subjects respond to a four-point Likert-type scale ("not at all" to "very much"). Content analysis by a panel of experts revealed a content validity index of 0.94. Cronbach's alpha is reported at 0.71.[21]

Family Inventories

Early attempts at defining and measuring coping arose from research into families and family stress management. Much of the recent literature on coping is grounded in sociology. McCubbin et al. explore recent investigations into family stress and coping in a decade review of these topics.[10] These authors note that the study of family coping depends on multiple cognitive psychologic theories and sociologic sources. Coping strategies are described in terms of both the individual and the family by Olson et al.[22]

Olson et al., at the University of Minnesota Department of Family Social Science, have developed a series of instruments called Family Inventories.[23] These inventories consist of nine instruments that measure various aspects of family life, adaptability, cohesion, and coping. Three instruments in particular were developed as part of the Family Stress and Coping Project, and are identified in the following sections.

Ongoing research into families, resiliency, and the passage of time has utilized the following instruments. Recent work by McCubbin et al. has examined cross-cultural and ethnic group differences in family functioning and coping.[24]

Family Inventory of Life Events and Changes (FILE)

The FILE scale was developed as an index of family stress and records both normative and nonnormative life events and changes experienced by the family unit.[11] FILE consists of 72 items grouped into nine subscales. A high raw score indicates low stress, and a low raw score indicates high stress. One subscale is labeled "losses" and includes the following item: "A parent/spouse died." Responses to each statement are recorded as yes or no, and a total scale score is obtained. The authors suggest that the total scale score be calculated rather than the subscales separately, as the subscale scores are not empirically stable.

Reliability for the overall scale is 0.81 (Cronbach's alpha), with subscale scores varying from 0.30 to 0.73. These scores support use of the total scale score, rather than scoring by individual subscales. Instrument validity was determined by discriminant analyses between low-conflict and high-conflict families ($p < 0.01$).

Adolescent-Family Inventory of Life Events and Changes (A-FILE)

The A-FILE[25] is a 50-item self-report instrument designed to record normative and nonnormative life events and changes as perceived by an adolescent during the immediately preceding 12 months of family life. This instrument measures adolescent–family life changes and records events experienced by any member of the family. The instrument is comprised of six conceptual dimensions, including life transitions. One statement from this dimension is "Parent started school." Subjects respond yes (coded as 0) or no (coded as 1) to each statement. A high score implies low stress.

The total scale alpha reliabilities for the A-FILE are 0.83 and 0.80 and were determined by two different samples. Validity assessments were made by correlating the conceptual dimensions with two outcome measures—adolescent substance use and adolescent health locus of control ($p < 0.01$). A suggested future use of this instrument is in research with adolescents diagnosed with chronic or catastrophic illnesses.

Family Coping Strategies (F-COPES)

The F-COPES instrument[26] was created to identify effective problem-solving approaches and behaviors used by families in response to problems or difficulties. The F-COPES is a 30-item self-report instrument. Each item is answered on a Likert-type scale, with answers ranging from "strongly disagree" to "strongly agree." One dimension of the F-COPES is to seek spiritual support. An example of one statement from this dimension is "Attending church services."

The instrument is conceptually organized for internal family coping patterns (three scales) and external family coping patterns (five scales) (A.J. Thompson, personal communication, October 7, 1993). Because of the interval nature of the data, scores can be obtained and parametric statistical analyses can be performed on the results. Scores may be obtained for each dimension or for the total instrument. Reliability for the F-COPES was determined by Cronbach coefficient alpha (0.86 and 0.87 for two samples) and test–retest.

Family APGAR

The Family APGAR measures personal satisfaction with one's own family function in five parameters: adoption, partnership, growth, affection, and resolve. It is a five-item, Likert-type self-report questionnaire. Cronbach's alpha is reported at 0.86.[27]

Two-Part Coping Assessment Scale

Sidel et al. developed a structured, easily scored assessment scale for coping strategies.[28] Their two-part coping scale includes three problem situations for which the subject lists possible approaches or strategies, and a list of 10 strategies for coping with the situation is provided. In the second part of this scale, the subject responds, on a seven-point scale, to the likelihood of using each of the 10 strategies. The authors conclude that both free responses and ratings are important because they may elicit different sources of information about coping strategies. The validity and reliability of this scale are not addressed. This study is an early attempt to develop a pencil-and-paper measure to learn more about less socially approved ways of coping and is the groundwork for the development of more recent instruments. This tool illustrates the use of vignettes[7] for data collection.

Parental Coping Scale (1962)

In this classic work, Hurwitz et al. sought to develop a tool to assess parent–child relationship patterns in families with juvenile delinquents.[29] Five areas of parental coping are assessed via interviews with both parents, together and separately. These areas are rated immediately after the interviews using a four-point scale ranging from "very constructive" to "very destructive." This type of data collection represents Brailey's[7] fourth method of study, that is, having subjects identify coping responses used in relation to specific events or situations. Hurwitz et al. state that reliability for the scoring of the interviews was determined by chi-square analysis ($p \leq 0.05$). Validity was achieved by differentiating constructive from destructive parental coping mechanisms.

Cooperative Extension Program Evaluation Survey (CEPES)

The CEPES evaluates family life programs in parenting, communication, conflict resolution, stress management, and balancing work and family. This involves a pretest early in an educational program that includes family coping-coherence and quality-of-life subtests. CEPES posttests were mailed to participants two to five months after the educational program to determine the effectiveness of the program. Thirteen program sites were utilized for data collection, and 50 to 88% of the respondents reported making one to three positive behavioral changes. The authors recommend the use of the CEPES by agencies and programs for enhancing human relationship skills in a variety of populations.[30]

Workplace and Employment Issues

Identifying coping in the workplace and employment issues is deeply interrelated to coping with many issues in adult life. Some of the issues include the individual's personality, response to personal anxiety related to job performance and anxiety experienced on the job, family and financial issues that can affect the ability to transition to or from a position for individual satisfaction, as well as the effects of the overall economy of the country. Most scales designed to measure job satisfaction, job efficacy, and job content are offered through various private organizations and consult firms. Several scales are available to measure coping related to unemployment issues. The Canadian Mental Health Association has identified the loss of employment to be the fourth on the scale of life crises, preceded by personal injury, death of a family member, and divorce.[31]

One specific area of employment that has not been addressed in the literature is the ability to cope with reentry into the job market following retirement. Economic changes in the early twenty-first century have forced many individuals over the age of 65 to seek employment in order to maintain their daily existence. Assessments have been completed involving unemployment and retrenchment[32] and recovery following unemployment related to a plant closure.[33] However, no specific assessment instruments were derived from these works. These areas of employment and coping should be researched in the future.

Coping Inventory for Stressful Situations (CISS)

The CISS is a multidimensional scale to rate coping in a variety of situations, including the loss of employment.[34] CISS can also be useful in assessment and placement of individuals in a variety of environments, including patients in psychiatric or medical care programs, stress and wellness programs, and inmates in correctional institutions. There are two scales available, adolescent and adult, and they contain age-specific content.

The instrument consists of 48 questions on a five-point Likert scale in the domains of tasks, emotion, and avoidance. There is also a shorter 21-question version available. The administrator's manual contains 10 training case studies to promote internal consistency and test-retest reliability, factor analysis, and construct validity.[34]

Coping Scale for Adults (CSA)

The CSA is modeled from the Adolescent Coping Scale to provide a comprehensive overview of adult coping in a self-administered instrument. The entire test scale is 73 items, with two short forms containing 19 items, and two long forms ranging from 57 to 73 items. The CSA evaluates the individual coping techniques in 19 areas: social support, problem solving, work ethic, worry, personal relationships, wishful thinking, stress reduction, social responsibilities, identifying problems, self-blame, introversion, spiritual needs, positivity, the ability to seek personal or professional assistance, relation methods, physical activities, self-protection, humor, and ability or lack of ability to cope with life changes.[35,36]

The CSA can be used in a variety of settings and life situations by individuals over the age of 18 years. Reliability of 88% of the questions was measured at 0.58. The test-retest reliability was high (> 0.75). With correlations of validity 0.73 or greater, the author of the instrument identified the short form as a practical indicator of coping dimensions.[36]

The Proactive Coping Inventory (PCI)

The PCI is a multidimensional instrument dealing with coping that is particularly well suited for work stress and burnout. This scale is significant for three reasons:

1. The integration of planning and preventative approaches related to self-regulated goal attainment
2. The integration of proactive goal attainment with the association and application of available social resources
3. The facilitation of proactive coping skills for the achievement of identified personal goals.

The PCI is composed of six categories to measure the individual's proactive coping skills. These include the proactive coping scale (14 questions), the reflective coping scale (1 question), strategic planning scale (4 questions), the preventative coping scale (10 questions), the instrumental support scale (8 questions), and emotional support-seeking scale (5 questions). The validity and reliability are reported as "good," with no numeric values available.[37,38]

Issues in the Elderly

The issue of coping in the aging individual is a multifocal problem that has issues involving physical, emotional, and mental functioning, social and family support, environmental factors, and matters relating to retirement and developmental staging. The relationship between these issues makes the concept of coping in general difficult to identify. Several assessment scales related to the issue of coping in the elderly will be identified here. A Coping Strategies Questionnaire used in several areas of elder assessment has been related to specific disease pathologies and depression.[39–41]

Beck Hopelessness Scale (BHS)

The BHS is an assessment tool that focuses on an elder's negative perspective on his or her future. This can be indicative of inability to cope with current life issues expressed by hopelessness. The BHS is a 20-item, true-false scale, and it has not been translated into any other languages. The domains assessed are feelings about the future, loss of motivation and drive, and limitations of future expectations. It has a reported internal consistency of 0.93, and the alpha coefficient was 0.86 in present combined samplings.[42]

Geriatric Depression Scale Long Form (GDS-LF)

The GDS-LF is an example of several geriatric depression scales available, which can assist in evaluating the coping skills of the individual over 60 years of age. Developed in 1982, it has been translated into Chinese. The GDS-LF is a self-administered survey of 30 questions in a yes/no format, taking approximately 10 to 15 minutes to complete. The domains evaluated include depression and symptoms of depression that are free of ageism. The test-retest reliability is 0.85 and internal consistency is 0.94. The GDS-LF is a revised scale using 15 items, and it has been found reliable in the geriatric population.[43,44]

The Duke-UNC Functional Social Support
Questionnaire (DUFSS)

The DUFSS scale aims to identify social support that an elderly person has established to assist him or her to cope with the stresses and challenges of daily life. It is a short, 8-item self-administered survey. Most studies utilizing DUFSS have been related to terminal or life-threatening illnesses in a longitudinal manner. Due to the limitation of application, the current reliability and validity is questionable, which indicates that the instrument should be used with a larger sample population.[45]

The Elder Life Adjustment Interview Scale (ELAIS)

The purpose of ELAIS is to assess coping as related to depression, life satisfaction, and associated theoretical factors in an elder's life. Developed in 1996 by Dubanski, Helby, Kameoka, and Wong, the subscale domains include depression, life fulfillment, environmental factors, perceived health status, and personal behavior. The responses are measured on a five-point Likert scale with a total of 230 questions. It has been evaluated for reliability and validity and translated into Japanese.[46]

The General Perceived Self-Efficacy Scale

The General Perceived Self-Efficacy Scale was developed in the early 1980s in Germany, initially 20 questions in length. Following research and translation, it is now available in a 10-question or 13-question format. The underlying theory is that self-efficacy creates a mood of motivation and decreases depression, anxiety, and helplessness. This in turn reflects a positive attitude toward coping with life issues. The internal alpha consistencies range from 0.75 to 0.91. The validity varies with the translation (13 languages and two genders) as well as age of the sample.[47]

The Satisfaction with Life Scale (SWLS)

The SWLS is a brief five-question survey that is intended to measure overall satisfaction with an individual's life. The responses are submitted on a seven-point Likert scale, with scores ranging from 35 to 5, and are evaluated in a global manner. The test-retest correlation coefficient is reported as 0.82, with an alpha coefficient of 0.87.[48,49]

The Role of the Elder as Caregiver

Individuals often experience the role of caregiver over the age of 65 years within their spousal relationship, family, and friends. In increasing numbers, grandparents are becoming caregivers to their grandchildren. The stress of the caregiver role often negatively influences the aging individual, creating frustration and an inability to cope with daily responsibilities.[50]

The Perceived Caregiver Burden Scale (PCBS)

Developed in 1990 by Stommel, Given, and Given, the PCBS is a 31-item survey with responses based on a 4-point Likert scale. The subscales address the caregiver's perceived burdens as related to physical and emotional health, family and social relationships and activities, personal finance, and employment. It has been translated into Hindi and has reliability coefficients of 0.72 to 0.92.[50]

The Perceived Support Scale (PSS)

The PSS identifies the perceived level of support the individual has in the role of caregiver. It is an 11-item questionnaire with a 4-point Likert scale for response. The domains identified in the PSS are tangible support, informational support, and emotional support.[51]

Global and Post Terrorism Issues

In the early twenty-first century, it has become necessary and expedient to confront issues of large-scale terrorism. After the September 2001 attacks, the Office for Victims of Crime prepared the *Handbook for Coping after Terrorism*.[52] Included is a list of practical coping ideas, five of which are discussed here.

1. Simplify your life for a while. Identify your individual responsibilities; make a list. Then, determine which are absolutely necessary and which can be put aside.
2. Reestablish former routines at work, home, or school as much as possible. This helps to begin to restore order. Occupy your mind with work, and stay busy, but avoid immersing yourself in frantic activity.
3. Rely on people you trust for information, advice, and help. Avoid potentially unscrupulous individuals who may attempt to take advantage of victims in the aftermath of a disaster.
4. Help others in small ways to ease your own suffering.
5. Contemplate hope. Identify things that give you hope and make a list of these. Refer to this list as needed, especially on bad days.

Sadly, our world has changed forever. Health care professionals can employ basic, useful tactics such as those in the preceding list, to help others realize that things will get better. Despair about past and potential future terrorism can merge into hope for peace through dialogue, planning, and sharing strategies for healthy recovery and safe practice.

Summary

Both theory testing and clinical instrument development are considered important elements in measuring coping. As the concept of coping becomes better defined and as coping behaviors are more systematically studied, other properties of coping may emerge.[7]

This chapter identified 31 instruments of varying designs for use in the measurement of coping. Self-report scales using Likert-type responses usually facilitate data collection and are amenable to a variety of analytic tests. Not addressed in this chapter are other, more qualitative methods of data collection, including interviews, patient narrative reports, some forms of participant observation, and grounded theory. The reader is encouraged to consider such methods for research into coping, because it is possible to gather much rich, descriptive data through qualitative methods.

Instruments used to measure coping are varied and derive from many disciplines. As this concept is further understood and empirically measured, its value as a moderator variable in health outcomes should become better documented. Coping represents an area that is ripe for clinical research, and it is anticipated that this summary of instruments that measure coping will be expanded and refined.

For purposes of this chapter, instruments to measure coping have been discussed within six broad categories. These include studies of disease and health care outcomes, family sociology research, work and employment issues, issues in the elderly, and issues in today's world and terrorism within a global construct. It is understood that there are many more constructs in which coping can be studied. Future health care professionals are encouraged to explore these and other areas and to maintain a global focus, as we all can serve to assist others with global concerns of coping. The specific instruments discussed in this chapter are summarized in Appendix 13A.

Exemplar Studies

Bowers, S.P. Gender role identity and care giving experience of widowed men, *Sex Roles*, 2002, *41*:9–10.

The relationship between gender role identity and caregiving experience was explored in a sample of elderly widowed men. A total of 200 males (82.5% Caucasian) were interviewed 12 to 16 months after the death of their wives. Results indicated that men who had served as caregivers scored higher on the masculine dimension of the Bem Sex Role Inventory, and masculinity was a significant predictor of well-being for both caregivers and noncaregivers. Following a cognitive dissonance model, the results do not support the adoption of feminine or androgynous ideals as a way of coping with this life demand. Instead, the results add to the growing body of work in support of a masculine model of well-being.

McFarland, P.L., & Sanders, S. Male caregivers: Preparing men for nurturing roles. *Am J Alzheimer's Dis*, 1999, *14*(5):278-282.

This article reports the results of a series of focus groups conducted about males who provide care to females with Alzheimer's disease. Male caregivers' coping skills, unique needs, role development, task provision, utilization of services, and potential service gaps were explored. These men were found to focus on the provision of concrete caregiving tasks and to minimize their emotional reactions to caregiving. Obtaining education about Alzheimer's disease also proved to be important because it gave them a sense of control over their situation and thus improved their coping abilities. Through these findings, new strategies for practitioners working with male caregivers are suggested, including development of support networks and wellness programs, increased utilization of services, and the design of a male-specific support group.

Internet Resources for Coping Assessment Tools

CINHALnews.com, 1998 Fall/Winter. *Research instruments.* Retrieved January 25, 2003, from www.cinahl.com/library.

Griffith University. *Test library.* Retrieved February 22, 2003, from www.gu.edu.au/school/psy/testlibrary/index.htm.

MAPI Research Institute, September 2002. *Home page: Access to instruments.* Retrieved February 22, 2003, from 195.101.204.50:443/instruments6.html.

Mental Health Counts. (n.d.). *Resources: Diagnostic and assessment Tools.* Retrieved September 25, 2003, from www.mental-health-matters.com/resources/diagnostic.php.

Quantana Healthcare Solutions, Inc., October 2002. *The Medical Algorythms Project.* Retrieved February 22, 2003, from www.medical.org/index.html.

The Scottish Executive, July 2001. *Identifying learning and support needs: A digest of assessment tools.* Retrieved September 25, 2002, from The University of Strathclyde in Glasgow Website: www.scotland.gov.uk/library3/education/ilsn-00.asp.

University of Iowa. (n.d.). *Table of contents: Iowa Index of Geriatric Assessment Toolsl.* Retrieved September 30, 2002, from www.uiowa.edu/~centrage/docs/Geriatric%20Assessment%20Tools/TABLE_OF_CONTENTS.html.

References

1. Angell, R.C. *The family encounters the depression.* New York: Scribners, 1936.
2. Koos, E.L. *Families in trouble.* New York: King's Crown Press, 1946.
3. Hill, R. *Families under stress.* Norwalk, CT: Greenwood, 1949.
4. McCubbin, H.I., Cauble, A.E., & Patterson, J. (Eds.). *Family stress, coping, and social support.* Springfield, IL: Charles C. Thomas, 1982.
5. Lazarus, R. *Psychological stress and the coping process.* New York: McGraw-Hill, 1966.
6. Singer, J.E. Some issues in the study of coping. Proceedings of ACS Workshop on Methodologies in Behavioral Physiological Cancer Research, April 1983. *Cancer*, 1984, *53*(suppl):2303–2315.
7. Brailey, L.J. Issues in coping research. *Nurs Papers Perspect Nurs*, 1984, *16*(1):5.
8. Jalowiec, A., Murphy, S., & Powers, M. Psychometric assessment of the Jalowiec Coping Scale. *Nurs Res*, 1984, *33*(3):157–161.
9. Rosentiel, A., & Keefe, F. The use of coping strategies in chronic low back pain patients: Relationship to patient characteristics and current adjustment. *Pain*, 1983, *17*(1):33.
10. McCubbin, H.I., Joy, C.B., Cauble, A.E., et al. Family stress and coping: A decade review. *J Marriage Fam*, 1980, *42*:855–871.
11. McCubbin, H.I., Patterson, D., & Wilson, M. FILE-Family Inventory of Life Events and Changes. In D.H. Olson, H.I. McCubbin, H. Barnes, et al. (Eds.),

Family inventories. St. Paul, MN: Family Social Science, University of Minnesota, 1982, p. 69.

12. Kessner Austin, J., & McDermott, N. Parental attitude and coping behaviors in families of children with epilepsy. *J Neurosci Nurs*, 1988, 20(3):174.

13. Hymovich, D. Development of the Chronicity Impact and Coping Instrument: Parent Questionnaire (CIC:PQ) *Nurs Res*, 1984, 33(4):218.

14. Cohen, F., & Lazarus, R. Active coping processes, coping dispositions, and recovery from surgery. *Psychosom Med*, 1973, 35(5):375.

15. Sime, A.M. Relationship of preoperative fear, type of coping, and information received about surgery to recovery from surgery. *J Pers Soc Psychol*, 1976, 34(4):716–724.

16. Pritchard, M. Temporal reliability of a questionnaire measuring psychological response to illness. *J Psychosom Res*, 1981, 25:63.

17. Bedsworth, J., & Molen, M. Psychological stress in spouses of patients with myocardial infarction. *Heart Lung*, 1982, 11(4):450.

18. Folkman, S., & Lazarus, R.S. An analysis of coping in a middle-aged community sample. *J Health Soc Behav*, 1980, 21(3):219-239.

19. Gass, K.A. & Chang, A.S. Appraisals of bereavement, coping, resources, and psychosocial health dysfunction in widows and widowers. *Nurs Res*, 1989, 38(10):31–36.

20. Heinrich, R., & Schag, C. Living with cancer: The Cancer Inventory of Problem Situations. *J Clin Psychol*, 1984, 40(4):972.

21. Arathuzik, M.D. The appraisal of pain and coping in cancer patients. *West J Nurs Res*, 1991, 13(6):714–731.

22. Olson, D.H.J., McCubbin, H.I., Barnes, H., et al. *Families: What makes them work?* Beverly Hills, CA: Sage, 1983.

23. Olson, D.H., McCubbin, H.I., Barnes, H., et al. *Family inventories.* St. Paul, MN: Family Social Science, University of Minnesota, 1982.

24. McCubbin, H., Thompson, E., Thompson, A., & Futrell, J. (Eds.). *Resiliency in ethnic minority families: African-American families, Vol. 2.* Boston: Sage, 1995.

25. McCubbin, H.I., Patterson, J.M., Bauman, E., & Harris, L.H. A-FILE-Adolescent Family Inventory of Life Events and Changes. In D.H. Olson, H.I. McCubbin, H. Barnes et al. (Eds.), *Family inventories.* St. Paul, MN: Family Social Science, University of Minnesota, 1982, p. 89.

26. McCubbin, H.I., Larsen, A.S., & Olson, D.H. F-COPES-Family Coping Strategies. In D.H. Olson, H.I. McCubbin, H. Barnes, et al. (Eds.), *Family inventories.* St. Paul, MN: Family Social Science, University of Minnesota, 1982, p. 101.

27. Smith, C.E., Mayer, L.S., Parkhurst, C., et al. Adaptation in families with a member requiring mechanical ventilation at home. *Heart Lung*, 1991, 20(4):349.

28. Sidel, A., Moos, R., Adams, J., & Cady, P. Development of a coping scale. *Arch Gen Psychiatr*, 1969, 20(2):226.

29. Hurwitz, J., Kaplan, D., & Kaiser, E. Designing an instrument to assess parental coping mechanisms. *Soc Casework*, 1962, 43(1):527.

30. Fetsch, R.J., & Gebke, D. A family life program accountability tool. *Extension*, 1994, 32(1):140.

31. Canadian Mental Health Association Newfoundland and Labrador Division. Job loss stages. Retrieved February 6, 2003, from www.cmhanl.ca/education/publications/gcwu/04-joblossstages.html.

32. Endler, N.S., & Parker, J.D. CISS: Coping inventory for stressful situations. Retrieved 1999 from www.mhs.com.

33. Frydenberg, E., & Lewis, R. Coping scale for adults. Retrieved 1997 from www.getting-on.co.uk/toolkit/adult-scale.html.

34. Greenglass, E.R. Proactive coping, work, stress, and burnout. Retrieved April 2001 from www.isma.org.uk/stressnw/proactive.htm.

35. Greenglass, E., Schwarzer, R., Jakubiec, D., et al. The proactive coping inventory (PCI): A multidimensional research instrument. Retrieved July 1999 from userpage.fu-berlin.de/~health/poland.htm.

36. Gibson, J. Coping Scale for Adults, 1997. Retrieved from www.getting-on.co.uk/toolkit/adult-scale.html.

37. Waters, L.E. *Psychological reactions to unemployment following retrenchment*, 2000. Melbourne, Australia: University of Melbourne, Department of Management.

38. Castro, F.G., & Romero, G.J. Recovery from unemployment in Latina women after a plant closure. Retrieved from www.sscnet.ucla.edu/issr/paper/issr3-7.txt, 1987.

39. Lin, C. Development of cancer pain coping strategies questionnaires and the use of pain coping strategies among cancer patients. *Nurs Res*, 2000, 6:405-416.

40. Burckhardt, C.S., & Henriksson, C. The Coping Strategies Questionnaire–Swedish version: Evidence of reliability and validity in patients with fibromyalgia. *Scand J Behav Ther*, 2001, 30:97-107.

41. Tan, G., Robinson-Whelan, M.P., Thronby, J.I., & Monga, T.N. Coping with chronic pain: A comparison of two measures. *Pain*, 2001, 90:127-133.

42. Crocker, J. (n.d.) Beck Hopelessness Scale. Psychosocial measures for Asian Americans: Tools for practice and research. Retrieved from www.columbia.edu/cu/ssw/projects/pmap.

43. Mui, A.C. (n.d.) Geriatric Depression Scale Long Form (GDS-LF) and Short Form (GDS-SF). Psychosocial measures for Asian Americans: Tools for practice and research. Retrieved from www.columbia.edu/cu/ssw/projects/pmap.

44. Rapp, S.R., Parisi, S.A., Walsh, D.A., & Wallace, C.E. Detecting depression in elderly medical patients. *J Consult Clin Psychol*, 1998, 56(4):509-513.

45. Team Care: Instrument Review. (n.d.) The Duke Functional Social Support Questionnaire (DUFSS). Retrieved from the Duke scale review.doc. www.hkrdgp.org.au/pdf%20files/The%20DUKE%20scale%20review.pdf.

46. Dubanoski, J.P., Helby, E.M., Kameoka, V.A., & Wong, E. The Elder Life Adjustment Interview Schedule (ELAIS for depression). Psychosocial measures for Asian Americans: Tools for practice and research. Retrieved from www.columbia.edu/cu/ssw/projects/pmap.

47. Schwarzer, R. General perceived self-efficacy in 14 cultures. Retrieved from userpage.fu-berlin.de/~health/world14.htm.

48. Yoshioka, M.R. (n.d.) Satisfaction with Life Scale. Psychosocial measures for Asian Americans: Tools for practice and research. Retrieved from www.co-

lumbia.edu/cu/ssw/projects/pmap.

49. Diener, E. (n.d.) Satisfaction with Life Scale. Retrieved from www.psych.uiuc.edu/~ediener/hottopic/hottopic.html.

50. Gupta, R. Perceived Caregiver Burden Scale. Psychosocial measures for Asian Americans: Tools for practice and research. Retrieved from www.columbia.edu/cu/ssw/projects/pmap.

51. Gupta, R. (n.d.) Perceived Support Scale. Psychosocial measures for Asian Americans: Tools for practice ad research. Retrieved from www.columbia.edu/cu/ssw/projects/pmap.

52. *Office for Victims of Crime Handbook for coping after terrorism.* Washington, DC: U.S. Department of Justice, 2001.

Appendix 13A. Summary List of Instruments Used in Research into Coping

Tool	Reliability Information	Validity Information	Population
Two-part Coping Assessment Scale[25]	No	No	Adults
Parental Coping Scale (1962)[29]	Yes	Yes	Parents
FILE[11]	Yes	Yes	Parents
A-FILE[25]	Yes	Yes	Adolescents and parents
F-COPES [26]	Yes	Yes	Adults
Chronicity Impact and Coping Instrument[13]	Yes	No	Parents
Goldstein Cooper-Avoider Sentence Completion Test[14]	No	No	Adults
Preoperative Coping Scale[15]	No	No	Adults
Coping Strategy Questionnaire[19]	Yes	No	Adults with low back pain
Response to Illness Questionnaire[16]	Yes	No	Long-term hemodialysis adults
Bedsworth and Molen Semistructured Interview[17]	No	No	Spouses of patients with myocardial infarction
Cancer Inventory of Problem Situations[20]	No	Yes	Adults
Jalowiec Coping Scale[8]	Yes	Yes	Adults
Family APGAR[27]	Yes	No	Adults
Coping Health Inventory for Parents (CHIP)[10,11]	Yes	No	Parents
Ways of Coping Checklist (WCC)[18]	Yes	No	Adults
Pain Experience Inventory[21]	No	Yes	Adults
Pain Coping Tool[21]	No	Yes	Adults
Cooperative Extension Program Evaluation Survey (CEPES)[30]	No	No	Families
Coping Inventory for Successful Situations (CISS)[34]	No	No	Adolescents, adults
Coping Scale for Adults (CSA)[35,36]	Yes	Yes	Adults
Proactive Coping Inventory (PCI)[37,38]	No	No	Adults
Beck Hopelessness Scale (BHS)[42]	No	No	Adults
Geriatric Depression Scale Long Form (GDS-LF)[43,44]	Yes	Yes	Adults
Duke-UNC Functional Social Support Questionnaire (DUFSS)[45]	Yes	Yes	Adults
Elder Life Adjustment Interview Scale (ELAIS)[46]	Yes	Yes	Adults
General Perceived Self-Efficacy Scale[47]	Yes	Yes	Adults
Satisfaction of Life Scale (SWLS)[48,49]	Yes	Yes	Adults
Role of Elder as Caregiver[50]	No	No	Adults
Perceived Caregiver Burden Scale (PCBS)	Yes	Yes	Adults
Perceived Support Scale (PSS)[51]	No	No	Adults

14

Measuring Hope

Martha H. Stoner

Hope, a subtle, if not unconscious, expectation regarding an abstract but positive aspect of the future, is an important factor influencing the quality and quantity of life for people who have life-threatening or chronic illnesses. Health care professionals have recognized an empirical relationship between the apparent loss of hope and eventual deterioration and death of patients with serious illnesses.[1-5] Practitioners working with people who have a life-threatening diagnosis have become interested in the influence of hope and hopelessness on patients' abilities to cope with the uncertainty associated with their diagnosis.[6-15] Interventions designed to maintain and instill hope in patients are described[7,16-21] Health professionals continue to try to understand the meaning of hope for themselves as well as for the patients and families for whom they provide care.[22-28] Research studies on hope, including the development of instruments to measure this concept, continue to be reported.[29-60] Hopelessness, frequently considered the polar opposite of hope, also has been measured and researched.[61-65] Because hope is such a complex, abstract phenomenon, a review of the theoretical foundation of the concept, including concept analyses and qualitative studies of hope, is presented. Instruments that measure hope are described.

Theoretical Description of Hope

Hope, thought of as wishful thinking or desire, frequently has been discredited as an impure mode of thought. An exception to this rejection of hope as unworthy of consideration is found in the works of philosopher Gabriel Marcel.[66-68] Marcel described hope as something very real that transcends all particular objects and is more concerned with a person as a being. Central to Marcel's view of hope is the association between hope and captivity and despair with the need to be delivered from some present condition or state. Although described as an inner sense, Marcel believed that there must be an interaction between one who gives and one who receives hope. This intersubjectivity (or bond of love) between self and others is essential to hope as a mysterious, but important, inner force for human survival.

Lynch also rejected the commonly held view of hope as something vague or nega-tive.[69] Hope was described as something very definite and positive. Hope is an interior sense that needs a response from the outside and has meaning only as it relates to oth-ers, that is, as an act of collaboration or mutuality. Another similarity Lynch shared with Marcel was the placement of hope in a framework of captivity; the need to imagine a way out of difficulty was central.

Stotland[70] defined hope as the perceived probability of success in obtaining a goal. The person is convinced that the desired goal is truly obtainable. Much of Stotland's analysis was devoted to understanding hope as a psychodynamic force in relation to other factors, such as motivation, achievement, and goal attainment. These philosophic and behavioral science perspectives of hope have contributed to a greater understanding of this abstract phenomenon. In addition, they provide conceptual frameworks for the de-velopment of measures of hope.

Measurement of Hope

Behavioral scientists and health professionals other than nurses have an interest in hope and have developed instruments to measure the concept. These instruments are described in the following section.

Gottschalk-Gleser Hope Scale

Gottschalk measured hope as a set of predetermined weighted categories indicating positive or negative levels of hope.[31-33] This method of quantifying hope, one of several scales within the Gottschalk-Gleser scales, used typescripts of 5-minute tape-recorded speech samples elicited from subjects in response to purposely ambiguous instructions to talk about any interesting or dramatic personal life experience.[31] One positive cate-gory consists of reference to self or others' getting or receiving help, advice, support, sus-tenance, confidence, or esteem from others or self. Negative categories reference not being, not wanting, or not seeking to be the recipient of good fortune, good luck, or God's favor or blessing. Gottschalk reported acceptable construct validity for his Hope Scale and used it in a number of studies.[31,33]

Erickson, Post, and Paige Hope Scale

Erickson, Post, and Paige[30] developed a 20-item, self-report instrument based on Stot-land's theoretical constructs of hope,[70] that is, the importance of future-oriented goals and the probability of attaining those goals. The goals were focused but not situation-specific in an attempt to reflect goals common to American society. Examples of goals in-cluded "To have enough money for basic needs," "To see my children turn out well," and "To have good bodily health."

Subjects rate each goal on a seven-point scale of importance and then indicate the 0 to 100% probability of attaining those same goals. Erickson and associates reported test-retest reliabilities of 0.79 and 0.78 ($p = 0.001$) for importance and probability scales, re-spectively, when administered one week apart to undergraduate students.

Hope Index Scale (HIS)

The HIS defines hope as "a state of mind which results from the positive outcome of ego strength, perceived human family support, religion, education, and economic assets."[71] Obayuwana and associates[71] analyzed Kübler-Ross's five stages of dying and Engel's five characteristics of the giving-up–given-up complex and discovered what they judged to be very similar determinants of hope. They then conducted a telephone survey of ran-domly selected people ($n = 500$) to learn the meaning of hope. Interviewees were asked to give one-word descriptions of hope, and these words were clustered into themes. The HIS was constructed with 60 yes/no items representing those themes and the resultant definition of hope.[71] Ten of the 60 items test for social desirability and are not included in the scoring. Desirable responses are assigned 10 points for a maximum of 500 points. The HIS was tested with more than 3000 people in a series of studies evaluating the concurrent and predictive validity of the instrument. A significant and high negative correlation (Pearson's $r = -0.88$, $p < 0.001$) was found between the HIS and the Beck Hopelessness Scale. The HIS discriminated between and among normal controls, psychiatric patients, depressed patients without suicide ideation, and suicide attempters. Obayuwana and associates[71] indicate that the HIS is suitable for both clinical and research evaluation of hope.

The Hope Index

Staats, a psychologist, developed the Hope Index based on Beck's self-other-world depressive triad and a definition of hope as the "interactions between wishes and expectations."[72] The Hope Index stresses the cognitive rather than the affective aspect of hope and focuses on specific events rather than general optimism. Half of the items ($n = 8$) are self-references such as "To be more competent" and "To have good health." The other eight items focus on others or on global circumstances such as "Other people to be more helpful" and "Understanding by my family." Multiplying each "wish score" by each "expect" score and summing them is the method of scoring the Hope Index. Scores for Hope-self, Hope-other, Wish, and Expect subscales can be derived. Staats does not reference Stotland's[70] theoretical description of hope as the importance and probability of goal attainment, but the Hope Index seems to reflect a similar theoretical perspective.

The Hope Scale

The Hope Scale developed by Snyder and colleagues[73] is based on a two-factor construct. One factor, agency, is goal-directed determination; a sample item is "I energetically pursue my goals." The second factor, pathways, is illustrated by the item "There are lots of ways around any problem," and involves the planning of ways to meet goals. The wording of items can be modified to address different goals, such as work goals versus school goals. The number of items ranges from 6 to 12, and the total hope score is the sum of the items for agency and pathways. The instrument has been used in business and schools with reports of acceptable psychometric properties.

Nursing Investigations of Hope: Qualitative Approaches

Nurses continue to investigate hope in an attempt to increase their understanding of this concept for use in research and in clinical practice. These inquiries range from clinicians' recognition of the importance of hope for their patients, a practical need for nursing interventions to support hope, to highly sophisticated research studies of hope using a variety of instruments and methods.

In one of the earliest efforts by a nurse to explicate the concept of hope, Stanley[36] used an existential, phenomenologic method. Her purpose was to isolate discrete, descriptive elements common to the experience of hope in healthy young adults, not to measure levels of hope. Junior and senior college students ($n = 100$) were asked to describe how they felt when they experienced hope in a situation. The phenomenologic analysis identified the following seven elements common to experiencing hope: (1) expectation of a significant future outcome, (2) being confident of outcome, (3) taking action to effect outcome, (4) experiencing comfortable feelings, (5) experiencing uncomfortable feelings, (6) having interpersonal relatedness, and (7) having a quality of transcendence. These common elements were synthesized into a general structure of hope as follows: "The lived experience of hope is a confident expectation of a significant future outcome, accompanied by a quality of transcendence and interpersonal relatedness and in which action to effect the outcome is initiated."[36]

Thompson[40] investigated hope-related variables identified from the literature as they correlated to the perception of hope in 10 cancer patients. Field study methods with in-depth interviews, responses to scale items, and observation of behavior were used. Scaled items included patient and investigator ratings of hope on a four-point continuum, from lacking hope to hopeful. Findings incorporated a description of hope as "a complex phenomenon involving the variables of love, mutuality, freedom, and newness communicated through a positive orientation."[40] Hope was manifested by a positive orientation and expectations for the future.

In a study of hope in elderly persons with cancer, Dufault used participant observation with 22 women and 13 men between the ages of 65 and 89.[28,29] She reported that her findings support hope as multidimensional and process oriented. Dufault defined hope as "a multi-dimensional dynamic life force characterized by confident yet uncertain anticipation of realistically possible and personally significant desirable future good having implications for action and for interpersonal relatedness."[28] Dufault identified two related, but distinct, spheres of hope. Generalized hope included a general sense that future nonspecific developments would be beneficial. The second sphere, particularized hope, concerned the confident expectation of a specific future goal or personally significant future good for self. All subjects spoke of the behavior of significant others as a source of hope. Dufault's conceptualization of hope has influenced the work of other nurse researchers, including serving as a framework to develop instruments to measure hope.[22,26,56]

McGee developed a model of hope in which hope and hopelessness represent opposite ends of a continuum.[34] At one extreme is the unjustifiably or totally hopeful person who may be immobilized by feelings of invulnerability. At the other extreme is the unrealistically hopeless person who gives in to what is perceived as inevitable. The desirable balance in this model is achieved by what McGee labels the realistic copers: people who have a positive outlook on life while accepting areas of actual hopelessness in life.

Most investigations of hope have been conducted with adults facing a life-threatening illness. Adolescents, some well ($n = 17$) and some being treated for substance abuse ($n = 8$), participated in a grounded theory study of hope by Hinds.[52] Analysis of the data revealed a construct definition of hope for adolescents: ". . . the degree to which an adolescent believes that a personal tomorrow exists; this belief spans four hierarchical levels proceeding from lower to higher levels of believing."[52] In another grounded theory investigation of hope, Hinds and Martin[53] learned from adolescents with a variety of cancer diagnoses how they achieve hopefulness and what nursing strategies influenced their hopefulness. Adolescents described four sequential phases to sustain their hopefulness: cognitive discomfort, distraction, cognitive comfort, and personal competence.[53] Nursing strategies positively influencing adolescent hopefulness were embedded in the involvement of the nurse in a personal and committed relationship with the adolescent.[74] The specific strategies identified were as follows: Truthful explanations do something; nursing knowledge of survivors; caring behaviors; cognitive clutter; careful competence; and future focus.

Hall explored the concept of hope as experienced by 11 men with HIV disease.[23] From her own experience of being given a terminal diagnosis and the data from study participants, Hall defined hope as "something all people need until they take their last breath."[23] She further explains "that life is hope, and that hope, in our culture, is an orientation toward the future that must be maintained in every stage of life, regardless of one's degree of frailty or the potential hazards of an uncertain future."[23] Hall offers a compelling argument that it is just as important to have hope immediately before death as it is at other times in life. She supports her position with the knowledge that we will all die, and simply having more certain knowledge of the timing of one's death does not alter one's need to maintain hope. Hall urges health professionals not to label the hope expressed by terminally ill people as denial and thus deprive them of the comfort that hope brings to them.

Saleh and Brockopp[9] conducted a phenomenologic study to learn about the experience of hope from hospitalized patients with cancer who were awaiting a bone marrow transplant. Analysis of data from semistructured interviews with nine participants revealed that religious practices and family members were the most frequently identified sources of hope.

Qualitative inquiries about hope have supported extant theoretical and philosophic conceptualizations of hope. These studies of hope contribute to the understanding of hope and provide further foundation for instrument development and for nursing interventions.

Nursing Investigations of Hope: Quantitative Approaches

Evidence of the importance of the concept of hope to nurses is apparent in the number of research reports that continue to be published. Measurement of hope remains a challenge, but some of the instruments to measure hope have been used in multiple studies with consistently acceptable psychometric properties. Some of the instruments and their use in research are summarized in the following sections.

Time Opinion Survey

Raleigh investigated hope as it was manifested in physically ill adults within the theoretical framework of Rogers' unitary man.[35] She interviewed 45 individuals with chronic illnesses and 45 with a life-threatening form of cancer. The purposes of the study were to identify and describe attributes of hope as exhibited in the physically ill adult, to describe what these individuals believed to be factors that influenced their hope, and to explore possible relationships among types of illness, degree of hope, personal control, and length of illness. To accomplish her purposes, Raleigh designed a Time Opinion Survey as the measure of hope.

In a subsequent study,[60] Raleigh developed and used a 23-item interview guide, the Sources of Support Interview Schedule, to learn whether oncology patients differed from patients with other chronic illnesses in their sources of hope and their extensions of hope into the future. Respondents indicated how hopeful they were on a 1-to-10 scale. Both types of patients were generally optimistic and able to think positively about their illnesses. Patients used the strategies of (1) getting busy, (2) praying or participating in religious activities, (3) thinking about something else, and (4) talking to others to ease feelings of hopelessness.

Stoner Hope Scale (SHS)

One of the earliest attempts by a nurse researcher to meet the need for a valid and reliable measure of hope was the Stoner Hope Scale.[37,38] A preliminary form of the SHS adhered closely in both form and content to the scale based on Stotland's theory of hope[70] developed by Erickson and associates.[30] Problems in the use of this form of the scale encountered in a pilot study with 10 cancer patients resulted in modifications. Stotland's[70] conceptualization of hope as the importance and probability of attainment of future-oriented goals was retained. However, the theoretical frameworks of Lynch[69] and Marcel,[66–68] which recognize hope as an interior sense requiring interaction with external resources, had not been adequately reflected. To strengthen this aspect of the scale, three domains of hope representing spheres of involvement replaced generic and specific categories of hope. Intrapersonal, interpersonal, and global hope were designated as the three domains of hope. The domains and the goals within them were identified in consultation with nurse clinicians in oncology and psychiatry. Each domain has 10 goals, and subjects are asked to respond to each of the 30 goals on a four-point Likert-type response set, first for the importance of the goal and then for the probability of attainment of each goal. In addition, some items incorporate the conceptualization of hope as a need to escape from some difficulty. An example of this can be seen in the item "to be free from pain."

Intrapersonal hope is defined as the domain of hope grounded on interior resources and beliefs. Although it may be influenced by external stimuli, intrapersonal hope arises from within the person and is not dependent on transaction with another being. One item within the intrapersonal domain is to overcome fears.

Interpersonal hope is the domain of hope in which the sphere of involvement extends beyond the self and is definitely dependent on transactions with external resources. Thus, interpersonal hope occurs or exists because of the connection between individuals. An example of a goal in this domain is to have people seek me out as a friend.

Global hope refers to the broad scope of issues and concerns important to people in a general sense. Global hope goes beyond the person and interpersonal relationships to the sphere of involvement, including hope for the human race, the world, and beyond. One goal in the global hope domain is to see an end to the threat of nuclear war.

Scoring of the SHS was based on Stotland's conceptualization of hope and included both importance and probability as parameters. For each item, the importance score was multiplied by the probability score. These products were then summed to yield subscale scores (intrapersonal, interpersonal, and global) as well as a total hope score, for a maximum total score of 480.

To estimate content validity, three expert judges, all with postgraduate nursing education, independently placed goals into domains, with nearly 100% agreement.[37] Concurrent validity of the SHS was assessed through the use of the Beck Hopelessness Scale (BHS) as a criterion measure.[61,62] The BHS was designed to measure hopelessness and provides a measure of the construct hope in the opposite direction. The BHS has a high degree of internal consistency with a KR-20 reliability coefficient of 0.93 reported by Beck et al.[61] for a sample of 294 suicide attempters. The demonstrated negative relationship ($r = -0.47$, $p = 0.001$) between the SHS and the BHS indicates moderate concurrent validity for the SHS.

With a sample of 58 cancer patients, the SHS had a high degree of internal consistency, as evidenced by a Cronbach alpha coefficient[75] of 0.93. Item-to-total correlations ranged from 0.37 to 0.65, with a mean interitem correlation of 0.53. When the SHS was subjected to canonical factor analysis,[76] in which the number of factors was limited to one, all 30 of the items loaded positively on the first factor and only four items weighted more heavily on another factor. This suggests that all the items were measuring a single construct, presumed to be hope. The computed reliability coefficient omega for the SHS was 0.94.

In a descriptive, correlational study of hope with 58 people with cancer, Stoner found positive associations between hope and religiosity ($r = 0.37$, $p = 0.01$), social support ($r = 0.34$, $p = 0.01$), and having close contact with other people with cancer ($r = 0.23$, $p = 0.05$).[37] In a further analysis of data from 55 subjects in this study, Stoner and Kaempfer[38] found no significant difference in the level of hope between subjects grouped by phase of illness: (1) no evidence of disease, (2) in active treatment, and (3) terminally ill. People who recalled being given information about their prognosis at the time of diagnosis had significantly lower hope scores than did those who had no recall of being told about their prognosis.

The SHS has been used in a number of studies by nurses, particularly graduate students, and by investigators from other disciplines. In a series of articles, Farran and associates[42–44] report on a study of 126 community-living older adults, in which a modified version of the SHS and multiple instruments were used. The modified SHS used only the intra- and interpersonal subscales and only the probability responses were scored. In a report involving 72 of the subjects, a predictive model in which hope was the outcome variable was used. The researchers found that the model was stable over time.[42] Another report describes the association between hope and social support and interpersonal control.[43] The authors suggest that practitioners can influence hope in older people not by denying the losses associated with aging, but by focusing on reality-based hope. They identify the SHS as an appropriate measure for interactive attributes of hope. However, they noted that some items may not represent realistic hope for older adults.[44]

Nowotny Hope Scale (NHS)

The original NHS was composed of 47 items within six dimensions of hope identified from the literature.[39,58] The dimensions were (1) orients to future, (2) includes active involvement, (3) comes from within, (4) is possible, (5) relates to or involves others or a higher being, and (6) relates to meaningful outcomes to individuals. Sample items are "In the future I plan to accomplish many things" and "I have difficulty in setting goals."

In a methodologic study, Nowotny asked 306 adults, both well and having a cancer diagnosis, to think of a significant life event that they considered stressful. Subjects then responded to the objective statements using a four-point, scaled response of "strongly agree," "agree," "disagree," and "strongly disagree."

Internal consistency reliability was demonstrated by a Cronbach coefficient alpha of 0.897. A negative correlation coefficient of –0.471 ($p = 0.001$) between the NHS and the BHS indicates moderate concurrent validity. The final NHS consisted of 29 items within six factors: (1) confidence, (2) relating to others, (3) the feeling that the future is possible, (4) religious faith, (5) active involvement, and (6) the feeling that hope comes from within. The 29-item NHS has a reliability of 0.90, and the subscale alphas and item-to-item correlations were stronger. The mean for NHS was 82.7 (SD = 9.8), with a range of scores of 49 to 104.

Nowotny applies her research in measuring hope to clinical practice by stating that nurses should record their assessment of patients' hope in the medical record.[59] She advocates the use of the NHS as a clinical assessment instrument and suggests nursing interventions to facilitate hope within each of the dimensions measured.

The NHS was used in a study of spiritual well-being, religiousness, and hope in women with breast cancer.[77] In this study of 175 women the coefficient alpha was again 0.90. These women had higher mean hope scores, 95.4 (SD = 9.7), than subjects in Nowotny's study. Hope was positively associated with spiritual well-being.

Herth Hope Scale (HHS)

The HHS and an abbreviated version of the scale, the Herth Hope Index, have been used extensively in research with a variety of subjects.[45-51] The original HHS was developed from Lazarus and Folkman's Stress Appraisal and Coping theoretical perspective and Stotland's theory of hope. Hope was defined as "an energized mental state characterized by an action-oriented, positive expectation that goals or needs for self and future are obtainable, and that the present state or situation is temporary."[45] This original 32-item scale used a categoric response set, in which respondents were asked to indicate "applies to me" or "does not apply to me" to items. The HHS was used in a descriptive study to determine the existence and nature of the relationship between hope and coping (Jalowiec Coping Scale) in 120 people with a variety of types of cancer who were receiving chemotherapy. A significant positive association between level of hope and level of coping response was found ($r = 0.80$, $p = 0.001$).

In a later report,[48] Herth described modifications of the HHS in which she incorporates the model of hope by Dufault and Martocchio.[29] Items were conceptualized within the spheres of generalized and particularized hope. Six dimensions of hope were combined into three: (1) cognitive-temporal, (2) affective-behavioral, and (3) affiliative-contextual. An example of a positively worded item is "I believe a favorable outcome is possible." "My life has little meaning and value" is representative of negatively worded items. Each of the three dimensions had 10 items for a total of 30 items. The response set was modified to a four-point summated rating scale (0, never applies, to 3, often applies).[48]

The HHS was used in a study of well adults ($n = 185$) to establish normative data on well adults.[49] The mean hope score was 80 (range 60 to 90). A 3-week test-retest with 20 subjects yielded a correlation coefficient of 0.90. The HHS was negatively correlated ($r = -0.74$) with the BHS.[61] In a similar study to obtain normative data with an elderly population, the HHS was given to 40 randomly selected elderly people.[50] The Cronbach's alpha was 0.94, and a 3-week test-retest reliability coefficient with 20 subjects was 0.89. The mean hope score was 72 (SD = 6.31) and a range of 52 to 88. The HHS and BHS correlation was $r = -0.69$, $p = 0.01$. In a third study of 75 bereaved elderly people,[51] the Cronbach's alpha for the HHS was 0.95, and a 3-week test-retest reliability of 0.91 was obtained with a sample of 20.[51] The mean hope scores were lower at 54 (SD = 5.6), with a range of 29 to 83.[46,51]

Data from these three studies were pooled ($n = 300$) and subjected to factor analysis. Three factors consistent with the theoretical conceptualization of the HHS were supported: (1) temporality and future (cognitive-temporal dimension), (2) positive readiness and expectancy (affective-behavioral dimension), and (3) interconnectedness (affiliative-contextual dimension). The alpha coefficients for the subscales were 0.91, 0.90, and 0.87, respectively.

Herth Hope Index (HHI)

Herth developed and evaluated an abbreviated instrument to measure hope, the HHI, to meet the need for an instrument to measure hope that is concise, simple, and has acceptable psychometric properties.[49] Because the HHI is intended for clinical application as well as research, the 12 items focus on adults who have an alteration in their health status. Four items in each of the three subscales parallel the conceptual foundation of the

HHS. Example items of the HHI are "I have specific possible short-, intermediate-, or long-range goals," "I see a light in the tunnel," and "I have faith that gives me comfort." The Likert-type response set is retained and each item is scored on an ordinal scale from 1 (strongly disagree) to 4 (strongly agree), with a total range of scores from 12 to 48.

A study to evaluate the psychometric properties of the HHI involved 172 adults from diverse settings, illness status, and backgrounds.[49] Validating instruments included the HHS, the Existential Well-Being Scale (EWS), the NHS for concurrent criterion-related validity, and the Hopelessness Scale (HS) to assess divergent validity. Factor analysis confirmed the original conceptualization represented by the three subscales. High correlations were obtained between the HHI and all of the criterion measures, HHI and the HHS ($r = 0.92$), the EWS ($r = 0.84$), and the NHS ($r = 0.81$). The correlation between the HHI and the HS was inverse ($r = -0.73$). All the instruments attained acceptable Cronbach's alphas, including a 0.97 for the HHI. The respondents used the full range of scores (12 to 48) with a mean HHI score of 32.39 (SD = 9.61). The HHI takes only minutes to administer and is useful for both clinical assessment to facilitate nursing interventions and for research purposes.[49]

Herth has continued to use and evaluate the HHI with other populations.[47,50,51] In a study of terminally ill adults, all of whom were receiving hospice care, the range of scores on the HHI was 16 to 45. The mean score was 39 (SD = 4.34).[47] The mean HHI score of 38 (SD = 3.12), with a range of scores from 12 to 46, was found in a study of 60 older adults residing in one of three settings.[50] Using a similar research protocol, Herth studied family caregivers of terminally ill people ($n = 25$).[51] With this sample the mean HHI score was 37 (SD = 4.11), with a range of scores from 15 to 46. In these three studies, Herth used methodologic triangulation by adding a qualitative interview to enrich her data and validate her findings. The semistructured interviews explored subjects' perception of hope and identified strategies they believed fostered their hope based on their personal experience. Analysis of the interviews increases the understanding of the meaning of hope to diverse segments of the population and provides a framework for nursing interventions based on the categories of hope-fostering strategies. Herth's focused research efforts in developing and evaluating instruments to measure hope have made a significant contribution to the understanding of hope and to its use in both clinical practice and research.

The Miller Hope Scale (MHS)

The MHS is a 40-item instrument with a five-point Likert-type response set (5 representing strong agreement, 1 strong disagreement). The range of possible scores is 40 to 200, with a high score indicating high levels of hope. An example of a positively worded item is "I look forward to an enjoyable future"; "I feel trapped, pinned down" is a sample negatively worded item. Hope is described as a state of being characterized by anticipation of a continued good state, an improved state, or a release from a perceived entrapment. The conceptualization of the MHS was based on the works of Dufault,[28,29] Lynch,[69] and Marcel.[66–68] Critical elements of hope identified are (1) mutuality-affiliation, (2) sense of the possible, (3) avoidance of absolutizing, (4) anticipation, (5) achieving goals, (6) psychologic well-being and coping, (7) purpose and meaning in life, (8) freedom, (9) reality surveillance-optimism, and (10) mental and physical activity.

In a study to evaluate the psychometric properties of the MHS, 522 college students completed the MHS and construct validation instruments.[56] The Psychological Well-Being Scale (PWBS), the Existential Well-Being Scale (EWBS), and a single-item 10-point self-assessed Hope Scale were used to evaluate criterion-related validity. The Hopelessness Scale (HS) was used to assess discriminant validity. The mean score for the MHS was 164.46 (SD = 16.31), with a range of scores from 105 to 198. Cronbach's alpha on the MHS was 0.93 and with a subsample of 308 students, a 2-week test-retest reliability of 0.82 was obtained. Construct validity was supported by correlation coefficients of 0.71 with the PWBS, 0.82 with the EWBS, and 0.69 with the single-item self-assessment of hope. A negative correlation of 0.67 was found between the MHS and the HS. Factor analysis produced three factors: (1) satisfaction with self, others, and life; (2) avoidance of hope threats; and (3) anticipation of the future. Hope was considered a complex, multidimensional construct, that is, a state of being that is more than goal attainment.

Miller[57] conducted a qualitative descriptive study of hope with a sample of 60 people, aged 38 to 83, who had been critically ill. The purpose of the study was to learn from patients what strategies they used to maintain or increase hope when they felt their existence was threatened. A 20-item structured interview guide was used to generate data analyzed to identify nine categories of hope-inspiring themes. The categories are (1) cognitive strategies, (2) determinism, (3) world view, (4) spiritual strategies, (5) relationship with caregivers, (6) family bonds, (7) control, (8) goals, and (9) other. Subjects were less able to identify threats to their hope, perhaps since they felt good because they had survived a recent health crisis. Although, as in other studies, nurses were not specifically identified as a source of hope, Miller identified some strategies for maintaining hope that could guide nursing interventions related to hope.

The MHS was used in a study of hope, self-esteem, and social support in people with multiple sclerosis.[78] Data were gathered on 40 participants, aged 32 to 70 years, with a mean age of 48.2. The mean MHS score was 157.9, and scores ranged from 108 to 200. Hope was correlated with both self-esteem ($r = 0.74$, $p = 0.001$) and social support ($r = 0.68$, $p = 0.001$). These findings suggest that nursing interventions targeting increasing self-esteem and social support also may increase the level of hope in people with multiple sclerosis.

In a similar study,[79] the MHS was used to evaluate hope in patients with spinal cord injuries. Participants ($n = 77$) were 18 to 73 years of age (mean = 34.79) and had numerous physical impairments. The range of scores on the MHS was 54 to 197 with a mean of 153.51 out of a possible range of 40 to 200. Correlations of 0.908 ($p = 0.001$) between hope and self-esteem and 0.891 ($p = 0.001$) between hope and social support were detected. The authors concluded that nursing care to promote hope in those with spinal cord injuries is appropriate.

Assessment of hope in psychiatric ($n = 48$) and chemically dependent ($n = 144$) patients was the focus of another research report[80] in which the MHS was used with a convenience sample with a mean age of 38.35. The mean MHS score of 135.73 (SD = 25.17) with this population was statistically significantly lower than Miller and Powers' findings with healthy adults.[56] These findings add to the construct validity of the MHS because hope scores were lower at time of admission than just before discharge. In addition, this population's hope scores were lower than those of healthy adults.

The MHS was used in a study[81] of functional status and hope in elderly people with ($n = 86$) and without cancer ($n = 88$). The Philadelphia Geriatric Center's Multilevel Assessment Instrument was used to measure functional status. Having cancer was not a threat to hope, but declining physical health and lower socioeconomic status were significantly associated with lower levels of hope.

The growing number of research reports about hope provides the foundation for evidence-based practice related to interventions designed to support hope in people with diagnoses that might result in a change in or loss of hope.[9,16,77-87] The body of knowledge of hope is being strengthened by the findings from studies that focus on specific populations such as the elderly,[88-90] adolescents,[91] people with mental health diagnoses,[7,92] and homeless people.[94] A particularly informative series of articles by Herth and Cutcliffe[6,94-98] addresses the concept of hope beginning with a discussion of the meaning of hope.[6] Subsequent articles explicate hope as an issue for specific areas of nursing practice: mental health nursing,[94] palliative care nursing,[95] gerontologic nursing,[96] and critical care nursing.[97] In the final article Herth and Cutcliffe[98] discuss policy, practice, and education issues related to hope and make recommendations for further research.

Summary

Because hope is a complex, abstract phenomenon, this review of instruments to measure hope includes a discussion of the theoretical analysis from the perspective of philosophy and the behavioral sciences. Themes common to most of the discussion of hope, including theoretical, clinical, and measurement issues are (1) a future orientation, (2) an expectation of attainment of important goals, (3) recognition of hope as an interior sense that is dependent on interaction with others, and (4) a need to escape from some feeling of captivity or despair. Additional research to refine and evaluate the existing instruments for research purposes is ongoing. Progress in developing instruments to be used in collecting data on hope and to direct interventions to maintain hope have been made. The Miller Hope Scale[54,57,91] and the Nowotny Hope Scale[39,58,59] continue to be used in nursing research studies. The Herth Hope Scale[48] and especially, the Herth Hope Index,[49] have been used most extensively, including translation and use in international studies. The exemplar study presented in the following section illustrates the use of the Herth Hope Index to evaluate a nursing intervention based on the Hope Process Framework[20] designed to influence levels of hope in patients confronting a life-threatening diagnosis. Additional research investigating hope and therapeutic nursing interventions with other patient groups have and will continue to contribute to nursing science.

Exemplar Study

Herth, K. Enhancing hope in people with a first recurrence of cancer. *J Adv Nurs*, 2000, 32(6):1431.

In this quasi-experimental study Dr. Herth investigated the impact of an intervention program designed to enhance hope in 115 people experiencing a first recurrence of cancer. Subjects were randomly assigned to one of three groups: a treatment group in which hope interventions were implemented, a control group given information, and a control group given the usual treatment. Based on findings from prior research, Herth used a Hope Process Framework to guide the hope intervention group sessions.[P1434] The first two sessions were devoted to an experiential process of searching for hope. In the third session participants recognized and investigated ways to achieve a sense of connectedness with family, friends, and support groups. Creative expressions of hope and other life-awareness activities were used to help participants identify sources of strength during the fourth session. Two sessions were devoted to assisting participants with cognitive and practical strategies for sustaining hope. A final session included identification of methods for participants to continue to work together as desired via e-mail, phone, and a chat room.

Data were gathered on variables recognized as possible correlates of hope using a self-report Background Data Form. Measures of hope using the Herth Hope Index and Quality of Life using the Cancer Rehabilitation and Evaluation Systems, Short Form were obtained at baseline; two weeks; and three, six, and nine months after intervention. Data analysis included evaluation of the psychometric properties of the instruments, description of the sample, and one-way analysis of variance to test for group differences at each of the time points using baseline scores as covariates.

Participants in the hope program had a significantly higher mean score on hope than participants in either of the control groups at all the time points post intervention. The quality of life of participants in the hope program was also significantly higher than that in the two control groups across time. Although the intervention was designed to engender hope, the higher quality-of-life scores were expected because hope is assumed to be a coping strategy for enhancing quality of life. This study provides a basis for a theoretically based intervention to engender hope that could serve as a model for other interventions and for the continued evaluation of the impact of those interventions.

Website Resources

Herth Hope Scale. sourcebook.fsc.edu/nursing/wellbe/wbm4/Herth%20Hope%20Index.pdf

Hope Research—The role of hope in managing chronic physical pain. www.ualberta.ca/HOPE/studies/pain.htm

C.R. Snyder, Professor, University of Kansas—Hope Research. www.ku.edu/~crsnyder/

References

1. Engel, G.A life setting conducive to illness: The giving-up given-up complex. *Bull Menninger Clin*, 1968, 32(6):355-365.
2. Hyland, J. Death by giving up. *Bull Menninger Clin*, 1978, 42(4):339-349.
3. Richter, C.P. On the phenomenon of sudden death in animals and man. *Psychosom Med*, 1957, 19(3):191-198.
4. Stewart, W.K. Hopelessness following illness in middle age. *Psychosomatics*, 1977, 18(2):29-32.
5. Vaux, K.L. *Will to live, will to die*. Minneapolis, MN: Augsburg Publishing House, 1978.
6. Cutcliffe, J.R., Herth, K. The concept of hope in nursing 1: Its origins, background and nature. *Br J Nurs*, 2000, 11(12):832-840.
7. Landeen, J., Seeman M.V. Exploring hope in individuals with schizophrenia. *Int J Psychosocial Rehab*, 2000, 5:45-52.
8. Rustoen T., Wiklund I. Hope in newly diagnosed patients with cancer. *Cancer Nursing*, 2000, 23(3):214–219.
9. Saleh, U.S., Brockopp, D.Y. Hope among patients with cancer hospitalized for bone marrow transplantation. *Cancer Nurs*, 2001, 24(4):308-314.
10. Srivastava, R. Beyond hope? *JAMA*, 2002, 288(10):1203–1204.
11. Wonghongkul, T., Moore, S.M., Musil, C., et al. The influence of uncertainty in illness, stress appraisal, and hope in coping in survivors of breast cancer. *Cancer Nurs*, 2000, 23(6):422–429.
12. Ersek, M. The process of maintaining hope in adults undergoing bone marrow transplantation for leukemia. *Oncol Nurs Forum*, 1992, 19(6):883–889.
13. Chen, M-L., Pain and hope in patients with cancer: A role for cognition. *Cancer Nurs*, 2003, 26(1):61–67.
14. O'Connor, A.P., Wicker, C.A., & Germino, B.B. Understanding the cancer patients' search for meaning. *Cancer Nurs*, 1990, 13(3):167-175.
15. Scanlon, C. Creating a vision of hope: The challenge of palliative care. *Oncol Nurs Forum*, 1989, 16(4):491–496.
16. Bays, C.L. Older adults' descriptions of hope after a stroke. *Rehab Nurs*, 2001, 26(1):23–27.
17. Duggleby, W. Hope at the end of life. *J Hospice Palliative Nurs*, 2001, 3(2):51-57.
18. Glynn, S. Multiple sclerosis: The Treetops model of residential care. *Br J Nurs*, 2002, 11(9):9-22.
19. Herth, K. Enhancing hope in people with a first recurrence of cancer. *J Adv Nurs*, 2000, 32(6):1431-1441.
20. Herth, K.A. Development and implementation of a hope intervention program. *Oncol Nurs Forum*, 2001, 28(6):1009–1017.
21. Wall, L.M. Changes in hope and power in lung cancer patients who exercise. *Nurs Sci Q*, 2000, 13(3):234-242.
22. Haase, J.E., Britt, T., Coward, D.D., et al. Simultaneous concept analysis of spiritual perspective, hope, acceptance and self-transcendence. *IMAGE: J Nurs Scholar*, 1992, 24(2):141–147.
23. Hall, B.A. The struggle of the diagnosed terminally ill person to maintain hope. *Nurs Sci Q*, 1990, 4(3):177-184.
24. Begley, A., Blackwood, B. Truth-telling versus hope: A dilemma in practice. *Int J Nurs Pract*, 2000, 6:26-31.
25. Stephenson, C. The concept of hope revisited for nursing. *J Adv Nurs*, 1991, 16(12):1456-1461.
26. Yates, P. Towards a reconceptualization of hope for patients with a diagnosis of cancer. *J Adv Nurs*, 1993, 18(5):701–706.
27. Van Ness, P.H., Larson, D.B. Religion, senescence, and mental health: The end of life is not the end of hope. *J Ger Psychiatr*, 2002, 10(4):386-397.
28. Dufault, K.J. *Hope of elderly persons with cancer* (doctoral dissertation, Case Western Reserve University). *Dissertation Abstracts International*, 1981, 42(05):1820B (University Microfilms No. 8118642).
29. Dufault, K.J., & Martocchio, B. Hope: Its spheres and dimensions. *Nurs Clin North Am*, 1985, 20(2):379-391.
30. Erickson, R.C., Post, R.D., & Paige, A.B. Hope as a psychiatric variable. *J Clin Psychol*, 1975, 31(a):324-330.
31. Gottschalk, L.A. A hope scale applicable to verbal samples. *Arch Gen Psychiatr*, 1974, 30(6):779-785.

32. Gottschalk, L.A., Lolas, F., & Viney, L.L. (Eds.). *Content analysis of verbal behavior: Significance in clinical medicine and psychiatry.* New York: Springer-Verlag, 1986.

33. Gottschalk, L.A., & Hoigaard, J. Emotional impact of mastectomy. In L.A. Gottschalk, F. Lolas, & L.L. Viney (Eds.), *Content analysis of verbal behavior: Significance in clinical medicine and psychiatry.* New York: Springer-Verlag, 1986, p. 171–187.

34. McGee, R.F. Hope: A factor influencing crisis resolution. *Adv Nurs Sci,* 1984, 6(4):34-44.

35. Raleigh, E.D. *An investigation of hope as manifested in the physically ill adult* (doctoral dissertation, Wayne State University). *Dissertation Abstracts International,* 1980, 41(04):1313B (University Microfilms No. 8022786).

36. Stanley, A.T. "The lived experience of hope: The isolation of discrete descriptive elements common to the experience of hope in healthy young adults" (doctoral dissertation, The Catholic University of America). *Dissertation Abstracts International,* 1978, 39(03):1212B (University Microfilms No. 7816899).

37. Stoner, M.J.H. "Hope and cancer patients" (doctoral dissertation, The University of Colorado). *Dissertation Abstracts International,* 1982, 44(1):115B (University Microfilms No. 8312243).

38. Stoner, M.H., & Kaempfer, S.H. Recalled life expectancy information, phase of illness and hope in cancer patients. *Res Nurs Health,* 1985, 8(3):269-274.

39. Nowotny, M.L. *Measurement of hope as exhibited by a general adult population after a stressful event.* Doctoral dissertation, Texas Woman's University, Denton, TX, 1986.

40. Thompson, M. *An investigation of the relationship of love, mutuality, freedom, and newness with the perception of hope in patients with the diagnosis of cancer.* Unpublished thesis, California State University, 1980.

41. Grimm, P.M. "Hope, affect, psychological status and the cancer experience" (doctoral dissertation, University of Maryland at Baltimore). *Dissertation Abstracts International,* 1989 (University Microfilms No. PUZ8924458).

42. Farran, C.J., & McCann, J. Longitudinal analysis of hope in community-based older adults. *Arch Psychiatr Nurs,* 1989, 3(5):272–276.

43. Farran, C.J., & Popovich, J.M. Hope: A relevant concept for geriatric psychiatry. *Arch Psychiatr Nurs,* 1990, 4(2):124-130.

44. Farran, C.J., Salloway, J.C., & Clark, D.C. Measurement of hope in a community-based older population. *West J Nurs Res,* 1990, 12(1):42-59.

45. Herth, K.A. The relationship between level of hope and level of coping response and other variables in patients with cancer. *Oncol Nurs Forum,* 1989, 16(1):67-72.

46. Herth, K. Relationship of hope, coping styles, concurrent losses, and setting to grief resolution in the elderly widow(er). *Res Nurs Health,* 1990, 13(1):109-117.

47. Herth, K. Fostering hope in terminally-ill people. *J Adv Nurs,* 1990, 15(11):1250–1259.

48. Herth, K. Development and refinement of an instrument to measure hope. *Scholar Inquiry Nurs Pract Int J,* 1991, 5(1):39-51.

49. Herth, K. Abbreviated instrument to measure hope: Development and psychometric evaluation. *J Adv Nurs,* 1992, 17(10):1251–1259.

50. Herth, K. Hope in older adults in community and institutional settings. *Issues Ment Health Nurs,* 1993, 14(2):139-156.

51. Herth, K. Hope in the family caregiver of terminally ill people. *J Adv Nurs,* 1993, 18(4):538-548.

52. Hinds, P.S. Inducing a definition of "hope" through the use of grounded theory methodology. *J Adv Nurs,* 1984, 9(4):357-362.

53. Hinds, P.S., & Martin, J. Hopefulness and the self-sustaining process in adolescents with cancer. *Nurs Res,* 1988, 37(6):336-340.

54. Fehring, R.J., Miller, J.F., & Shaw, C. Spiritual well-being, religiosity, hope, depression, and other mood states in elderly people coping with cancer. *Oncol Nurs Forum,* 1997, 24(4):663-671.

55. Farran, C.J., Wilken, C., & Popovich, J.M. Clinical assessment of hope. *Issues Ment Health Nurs,* 1992, 13(2):129-138.

56. Miller, J.F., & Powers, M.J. Development of an instrument to measure hope. *Nurs Res,* 1988, 37(1):6-10.

57. Miller, J.F. Hope-inspiring strategies of the critically ill. *Appl Nurs Res,* 1989, 2(1):23-29.

58. Nowotny, M.L. Assessment of hope in patients with cancer: Development of an instrument. *Oncol Nurs Forum,* 1989, 16(1):57-61.

59. Nowotny, M.L. Every tomorrow, a vision of hope. *J Psychosoc Oncol,* 1991, 9(3):117-125.

60. Raleigh, E.D.H. Sources of hope in chronic illness. *Oncol Nurs Forum,* 1992, 19(3):443–447.

61. Beck, A.T., Lester, D., Trexler, L., & Weisman, A. The measurement of pessimism: The hopelessness scale. *J Consult Clin Psychol,* 1974, 42(6):861–865.

62. Durham, T.W. Norms, reliability, and item analysis of the hopelessness scale in general psychiatric, forensic psychiatric, and college populations. *J Clin Psychol,* 1982, 38(3):597-600.

63. Carson, V., Soeken, K.L., Shanty, J., & Terry, L. Hope and spiritual well-being: Essentials for living with AIDS. *Perspect Psychiatr Care,* 1990, 26(2):28-34.

64. Campbell, L. Hopelessness: A concept analysis. *J Psychosoc Nurs,* 1987, 25(2):18-22.

65. Rideout, E., & Montemuro, M. Hope, morale and adaptation in patients with chronic heart failure. *J Adv Nurs,* 1986, 11(4):429-438.

66. Marcel, G. *Homo viator* (E. Crawford, trans.). San Francisco, CA: Harper & Row, 1962.

67. Marcel, G. *The mystery of being. Vol. 11: Faith and reality. Death and hope.* South Bend, IN: Regnery/Gateway, 1951, pp. 146-165.

68. Marcel, G. *Desire and hope.* In N. Lawrence & D. O'Connor (Eds.), Readings in existential phenomenology. Englewood Cliffs, NJ: Prentice-Hall, 1967, p. 277.

69. Lynch, W.F. *Images of hope.* Baltimore, MD: Helicon, 1965.

70. Stotland, E. *The psychology of hope.* San Francisco: Jossey-Bass, 1969.

71. Obayuwana, A.O., Collins, J.L., Carter, A.L., et al. Hope index scale: An instrument for the objective assessment of hope. *JAMA,* 1982, 74(6):761–765.

72. Staats, S. Hope: A comparison of two self-report measures for adults. *J Person Assess,* 1989, 53(2):366-375.

73. Snyder, C.R., Harris, C., Anderson, J.R., et al. The will and the ways: Development and validation of an individual-differences measure of hope. *J Personality Soc Psychology,* 1991, 60:570-585.

74. Hinds, P.S., Martin, J., & Vogel, R.J. Nursing strategies to influence adolescent hopefulness during oncologic illness. *J Assoc Pediatr Oncol*, 1987, *4*(1&2): 14-22.

75. Mitchell, S.K. Interobserver agreement, reliability, and generalizability of data collected in observational studies. *Psychol Bull*, 1979, *86*(2):376.

76. Anastasi, A. *Psychological testing* (4th ed.). New York: Macmillan, 1970.

77. Mickley, J.R., Soeken, K., & Belcher, A. Spiritual well-being, religiousness and hope among women with breast cancer. *IMAGE: J Nurs Scholar*, 1992, *24*(4):267-272.

78. Foote, A.W., Piazza, D., Holcome, J., et al. Hope, self-esteem and social support in persons with multiple sclerosis. *J Neurosci Nurs*, 1990, *22*(3):155–159.

79. Piazza, D., Holcombe, J., Foote, A., et al. Hope, social support and self-esteem of patients with spinal cord injuries. *J Neurosci Nurs*, 1991, *23*(4):224-230.

80. Holdcraft, C., & Williamson, C. Assessment of hope in psychiatric and chemically dependent patients. *Appl Nurs Res*, 1991, *4*(3):129-134.

81. McGill, J.S., & Paul, P.B. Functional status and hope in elderly people with and without cancer. *Oncol Nurs Forum*, 1993, *20*(8):1207–1213.

82. Phillips, K.D., & Sowell, R.L. Hope and coping in HIV-infected African-American women of reproductive age. *J Nat Black Nurs Assoc*, 2000, *11*(2):18-24.

83. Kylma, J., Vehvilainen-Julkunen, K., & Lahdevirta, J. Hope, despair and hopelessness in living with HIV/AIDS: A grounded theory study. *J Adv Nurs*, 2001, *33*(6):764-775.

84. Stanton, A.L., Danoff-Burg, S., & Huggins, M.E. The first year after breast cancer diagnosis: Hope and coping strategies as predictors of adjustment. *Psycho-Oncology*, 2002, *11*(2):93-102.

85. Ebright, P.R., & Lyon, B. Understanding hope and factors that enhance hope in women with breast cancer. *Oncol Nurs Forum*, 29(3):561-568.

86. Lin, C.C., Lai, Y.L., & Ward, S.E. Effect of cancer pain on performance status, mood states, and level of

87. hope among Taiwanese cancer patients. *J Pain Symptom Manage*, 2003, *25*(1):29-37.

87. Lohne, V. Hope in patients with spinal cord injury: A literature review related to nursing. *J Neurosci Nurs*, 2001, *33*(6):317-325.

88. Touhy, T.A. Nurturing hope and spirituality in the nursing home. *Holistic Nurs Pract*, 2001, *15*(4):45-56.

89. Cutcliffe, J.R., & Grant, G. What are the principles and processes of inspiring hope in cognitively impaired older adults within a continuing care environment? *J Psychiatr Ment Health Nurs*, 2001, *8*(5):427-436.

90. Westburg, N.G. Hope, laughter, and humor in residents and staff at an assisted living facility. *J Ment Health Couns*, 2003, *25*(1):16-32.

91. Canty-Mitchell, J. Life change events, hope, and self-care agency in inner-city adolescents. *J Child Adolesc Psychiatr Nurs*, 2001, *14*(1):18-31.

92. Bland, R., & Darlington Y. The nature and sources of hope: Perspectives of family caregivers of people with serious mental illness. *Perspect Psychiatr Care*, 2002, *38*(2):61-68.

93. Partis, M. Hope in the homeless people: A phenomenological study. *Prim Health Care Res Devel*, 2003. *4*:9-19.

94. Cutcliffe, J.R., & Herth, K. The concept of hope in nursing 2: Hope and mental health nursing. *Br J Nurs*, 2002, *11*(13):885-889, 891-893.

95. Herth, K.A., & Cutcliffe, J.R. The concept of hope in nursing 3: Hope and palliative care nursing. *Br J Nurs*, 2002, *11*(14):977-983.

96. Herth, K.A., & Cutcliffe, J.R. The concept of hope in nursing 4: Hope and gerontological nursing. *Br J Nurs*, 2002, *11*(17):1148-1156.

97. Cutcliffe, J.R., & Herth, KA. The concept of hope in nursing 5: Hope and critical care nursing. *Br J Nurs*, 2002, *11*(18):1190-1195.

98. Herth, K.A., & Cutcliffe, J.R. The concept of hope in nursing 6: Research/education/policy/practice. *Br J Nurs*, 2002, *11*(21):1401-1411.

15

Instruments to Measure Aspects of Spirituality

Jan M. Ellerhorst-Ryan and Sharon Fish Mooney

Commitment to viewing people in need of health care in a holistic manner must include their spiritual concerns. Burkhardt and Nagai Jacobson have noted that spirituality, derived from the Latin *spiritus* and the Greek *pneuma*, meaning breath, is "the essence of who we are and how we are in the world."[1] Highfield and Cason stated, "We cannot abdicate our responsibility for treating a person's spiritual needs to the chaplain, any more than we can abdicate our responsibility for man's physical needs to the physician, or his psychosocial needs to the psychologist and social worker."[2]

Historically, research on spirituality has focused on religiosity and more organized systems of belief shared by groups.[3] Moberg and Brusek,[4] in comparing religiosity and spiritual well-being, associate the former with institutional goals and behaviors. Measures of religious practice, however, are not always reliable indicators of spirituality.[3,5]

Spirituality, a concept common to nursing, is more than the sum of the client's religious beliefs and practices. Moberg has written that spirituality is "the totality of man's inner resources, the ultimate concerns around which all other values are focused, the central philosophy of life that guides conduct, and the meaning-giving center of human life which influences all individual and social behavior."[6] It also encompasses the need to find satisfactory answers to questions about the meaning of life, illness, suffering, and death.

The Third National Conference on Classification of Nursing Diagnoses recognized the importance of spirituality by including spiritual concerns, spiritual distress, and spiritual despair in the list of approved nursing diagnoses. At the Fourth National Conference in 1980, only the diagnosis of spiritual distress was retained. It is currently defined as "a disruption in the life principle that pervades a person's entire being and that integrates and transcends one's biological and psychosocial nature."[7] This is still the most common definition used in nursing. Spiritual needs, often the focus of research, generally arise out of situations of spiritual distress.

Spiritual concepts apply to persons who are religious in both the traditional and nontraditional sense, but also to atheists and agnostics, based on a broader definition of spirituality that includes a search for meaning. Given that both a religious component and a psychosocial component are involved in spiritual concerns, both should be and have been incorporated in tools designed to assess aspects of spirituality.

The concept and understanding of "God" does not easily conform to a universal definition. It is, therefore, important to consider ways of eliciting information about the subject's perception of God. People who hold traditional views generally characterize God as personal and transcendent and as Ultimate Deity. People of more Eastern or metaphysical orientations may believe in many gods (polytheism) or conceive of God or divinity in more impersonal terms or as an energy force. Proponents of a "New Age" or "New Consciousness" world view often have a pantheistic belief, in which the divine is thought to exist in everything and everyone. For others, God may be whatever that person values most, the focal point of life: work, family, or community service.[8]

In view of the significant influence the Judeo-Christian world view has had on the development of Western culture, the formal instruments reviewed most often reflect that perspective. They are especially relevant for use with an older adult population. Information on their applicability to people of other religious orientations is included when available. Increasingly, qualitative researchers are addressing the spiritual concerns of people with varying medical conditions and religious or spiritual orientations. See, for example, Hall's study on patterns of spirituality in persons with advanced HIV disease based on qualitative methodologic assumptions derived from interpretive interactionism[9] and the narratives of Kahn and Steeves[10,11] on critical experiences with the terminally ill.

Instruments

Before selecting a measurement tool, the researcher must first decide which aspect of spirituality is to be investigated. Spiritual needs in general may be studied, or the focus may be limited to a specific spiritual need or aspect of spirituality. Commonly identified spiritual needs include hope, forgiveness, love and relatedness, and meaning and purpose in life. Other related concepts for which measurement tools are available include spiritual well-being, spiritual coping, spiritual maturity, religious motivation, and spiritual transcendence.

Consideration also must be given to the population under study (e.g., adults versus children, nurses versus patients) to ensure appropriate measurement tool selection.

Spiritual Needs: Quantitative Tools
Spiritual Health Inventory (SHI)
The SHI[12] is a 31-item self-report instrument worded in the first person. Respondents rank how often they have experienced the feeling or behavior described on a 1-to-5 Likert scale. SHI content is consistent with the author's definition of spiritual health; that is, having satisfactorily met spiritual needs for self-acceptance; a trusting relationship with self based on a sense of meaning and purpose in life (e.g., "I feel valuable as a person even when I cannot do as much as before"); relationships with others and/or a supreme other characterized by unconditional love, trust, and forgiveness (e.g., "I believe my nurses and doctors care about me," "I feel a need to be forgiven for some of my thoughts and feelings"); and hope (e.g., "I worry about life after death").[12] A ranking of 5 indicates frequent occurrence, and a ranking of 1 indicates infrequent occurrence. Scores are determined by reversing subject-recorded ratings of each negative indicator of spiritual health, then summing ratings for all items. Higher scores are associated with higher levels of spiritual health.

Content and construct validity for the SHI are based on a review of the literature, input from an expert panel, and factor analysis. Three factors, representing the spiritual needs for self-acceptance, relationships, and hope, account for 71.5% of variance. Analysis using 23 subjects produced a Cronbach's alpha of 0.77.[12]

Spiritual Perspective Scale (SPS)

Formerly titled the Religious Perspective Scale, the SPS contains 10 items that measure the subjects' "perspectives on the extent to which spirituality permeates their lives and (their degree of engagement) in spiritually-related interactions."[13] The SPS can be administered either as a structured interview or questionnaire. Responses are ranked on a 1-to-6 scale. Scores are determined by calculating the arithmetic mean across all items, with higher scores indicating greater spiritual perspective. An example of an item is "In talking with your family or friends, how often do you mention spiritual matters?" with response options ranging from 1, not at all, to 5, about once a day.

Reliability and validity for the SPS have been demonstrated in both healthy and terminally ill adult populations. Internal consistency was measured by Cronbach's alpha, with alpha coefficients ranging from 0.93 to 0.95. Interitem analysis revealed average correlations between 0.57 and 0.68. The fact that subjects who reported having a religious background scored higher on the SPS provided evidence for construct validity.[13,14]

Serenity Scale

The 40-item Serenity Scale is designed to measure serenity, "a spiritual experience of inner peace that is independent of external events."[15] Although related to peace of mind, serenity goes further, bringing comfort to those confronted by harsh circumstances that are difficult and sometimes impossible to change. Attributes of serenity, as defined by the authors of the scale, include hope, forgiveness, love and relatedness, and meaning and purpose in life.[15]

Items are scored using a Likert scale, with subjects rating frequencies of personal experiences from 1, never, to 6, always. Thirteen of the 40 items are negatively stated and require reverse scoring. Higher scores indicate greater levels of serenity. Examples of test items include "I experience an inner calm even when under pressure" and "I experience an inner quiet that does not depend on events."

Content validity of the Serenity Scale was established by an expert panel analysis during instrument development. Internal consistency was established by Cronbach's alpha, reported as 0.92. Factor analysis revealed nine factors that explained 58.2% of the variance: inner haven, acceptance, belonging, trust, perspective, contentment, present centered, beneficence, and cognitive restructuring.[15] The authors acknowledge questionable validity with low-literacy subjects.

Serenity transcends formal religious dogma; therefore, the Serenity Scale can be used with subjects holding a variety of religious views, including atheism. Participants in field studies represent a wide range of age and economic status from both rural and urban areas. The authors note, however, that the scale has been tested on primarily white and well-educated adults.

Spiritual Needs: Qualitative Tools

Interview schedules using open-ended questions may be more useful for qualitative spiritual research. The interview tools described here can be utilized in populations of individuals with diverse religious beliefs and orientations.

Stallwood (a.k.a. Hess)[16,17] and Stoll[18] are well known for their interest in spiritual concerns of patients. They have defined spiritual needs as "any factors necessary to establish and/or maintain a dynamic personal relationship with God (as defined by the individual) and out of that relationship to experience forgiveness, love and relatedness, hope, trust, and meaning and purpose in life."[16] Both authors have developed assessment tools useful for interviewing and data collection. Two more recent assessment tools used in nursing have been developed by Reed[19] and Burkhardt.[1]

Hess's Spiritual Needs Survey

Hess's Spiritual Needs Survey was designed for use in hospitals or extended care facilities but could easily be modified for use in other settings.[17] Five questions focus on the patient's awareness of his or her spiritual needs and efforts to address them:

- Were you aware of having a spiritual need at any time during your hospitalization?
- Are you able to describe it? Can you tell me about it?
- With whom did you discuss this need?
- How did you feel about the assistance you received?
- Has your need been met to any degree, or is it still present?[17]

Stoll's Guidelines for Spiritual Assessment

Although Stoll's Guidelines for Spiritual Assessment were not designed for use as a research tool, they have been used in conjunction with other measurement scales to evaluate the ability of hospitalized patients to meet their spiritual needs.[18,21,22] Stoll's Guidelines include 13 questions addressing the person's concept of God, sources of hope and strength, religious practices, and relationship between spiritual beliefs and health. A sample item is "To whom do you turn when you need help?"

Fish and Shelly[23] modified Stoll's Guidelines to organize the questions into four categories: understanding a person's beliefs about and involvement with God and religious practice, determining the extent to which a person's religious practices serve as a resource for faith and life, assessing whether resources for hope and strength are founded in reality, and extending an opportunity to accept spiritual help. Excluding the fourth category, which is an invitation for intervention by the interviewer, the remaining three categories make up 11 open-ended questions.

The Reed Interview Schedule

The Reed Interview Schedule is designed to elicit information on patient preferences for spiritually related nursing interventions.[19] The schedule consists of one structured item and one open-ended item. The first question, "In what ways could hospital nurses help you in your spiritual needs?" is followed by descriptions of seven spiritually related interventions identified in a review of current nursing literature. Interventions included reading to or with the patient; allowing time for personal prayer or meditation; talking with the patient about beliefs and concerns; providing time for the patient to talk or pray with family members; arranging a visit with a minister, priest, or rabbi; and helping the patient to attend the hospital chapel. Participants may select more than one intervention in response to the question. The second open-ended item invites participants to describe other interventions important to them but not listed in the first item.

Burkhardt's Spiritual Assessment Tool

The Spiritual Assessment Tool was developed by Burkhardt, based on a conceptual analysis of spirituality from a critical review of the literature. Major categories are meaning and purpose, inner strengths, and interconnectedness. Open-ended questions allow for more exploration of personal perceptions and understanding of spirituality, varying concepts of God, and spiritual care practices such as prayer and meditation.[1,3,20]

Singular Concepts of Spiritual Need

An alternative to investigating spiritual needs is to limit the scope of the study to one or more specific spiritual needs. The concepts of hope, meaning and purpose in life, forgiveness and love, and relatedness are briefly reviewed and a measurement tool for each is highlighted.

Hope

Dufault and Martocchio have defined hope as a "multidimensional life force characterized by a confident yet uncertain expectation of achieving a future good which . . . is realistically possible and personally significant."[24] These characteristics are clearly demonstrated in the Nowotony Hope Scale (NHS).[25]

The NHS is a 29-item questionnaire that assesses six components of hope: (1) confidence in outcome, (2) relationships with others, (3) belief in the possibility of a future, (4) spiritual beliefs, (5) active involvement, and (6) inner readiness. Responses are recorded using a four-point scale (strongly agree, agree, disagree, strongly disagree). An example of an NHS item is "Sometimes I feel I am all alone."[25]

Reliability analysis of the NHS using Cronbach's alpha yielded a coefficient of 0.90. Concurrent validity was established by comparing participant scores on NHS with scores on the Beck Hopelessness Scale. Pearson's product moment correlation produced $r = -0.47$ ($p < 0.001$).[25]

Meaning and Purpose in Life

Crumbaugh Purpose in Life Test (PIL) is designed to measure the degree to which a person experiences a sense of meaning and purpose in life.[26] The tool was developed based on Frankl's concepts of noogenic neurosis that occurs in response to an absence of purpose in life, manifested by "existential frustration" and boredom.[26,27]

The PIL consists of 20 items to which respondents reply on a seven-point scale. Construct validity was established by comparing scores of healthy subjects with those of clients undergoing psychiatric therapy. Differences reported were significant and in the direction predicted. Concurrent validity was demonstrated by correlating PIL scores with therapists' ratings for psychiatric clients and ministers' ratings of healthy subjects. Correlations were 0.37 ($n = 50$) and 0.47 ($n = 120$), respectively. Reliability testing, using split-half correlation ($n = 120$), yielded a coefficient of 0.85, corrected to 0.92 by the Spearman-Brown formula.[28]

Love and Relatedness

Although the definitions of social support vary, factors consistently identified include the perception that one is cared about, loved, esteemed, and valued, and the perception that support is readily available when needed. These elements of love and relatedness are not only essential components of relationships with other people but also present to varying degrees in a person's relationship with God.[29]

Maton's Spiritual Support Scale employs three items to assess perceived support from God. Responses are recorded using a five-point scale, ranging from "not at all accurate" to "completely accurate." The first two items, "I experience God's love and caring on a regular basis" and "I experience a close personal relationship with God," were found in a prior study to predict well-being in a congregational sample and to correlate positively with other measures of intrinsic religion.[30] A third item, "My religious faith helps me cope during times of difficulty," elicits faith aspects of perceived spiritual support.

Cronbach's alpha produced a reliability coefficient of 0.92, with test–retest reliability yielding $r = 0.81$ ($n = 66$).[29]

The Spiritual Support Scale has been used to evaluate the relationship between perceived levels of spiritual support and well-being among two groups of high-stress and low-stress individuals.[29] Among recently bereaved parents and adolescents experiencing three or more uncontrollable life events, perceived spiritual support correlated significantly with multiple measures of well-being in the direction predicted. No significant relationships were found between spiritual support and well-being in low-stress populations. Limitations acknowledged by the author in testing the Spiritual Support Scale include small sample size and inadequate minority representation.[29]

Forgiveness

Studzinski has defined forgiveness as a "response to suffering which an individual has incurred at the hands of someone else. . . . the choice presented to the sufferer is between harbouring resentment or allowing the healing of forgiveness to take place."[31] Two scales measuring forgiveness were developed by Mauger et al.[32] as part of a project to produce an objective personality inventory that would examine multiple dimensions of behavior related to personality disorders. The scales, Forgiveness of Self (FS) and Forgiveness of Others (FO), are actually subscales of the Behavior Assessment System I (BAS), an inventory consisting of 301 true-false items.[33,34] Each of the forgiveness scales is composed of 15 statements. Items on the FO scale focus on taking revenge, justifying retaliation, and holding grudges: "I would secretly enjoy hearing that someone I dislike had gotten into trouble" and "It is not right to take revenge on a person who tries to take advantage of you." The FS scale assesses feelings of guilt over past mistakes, perceptions of oneself as sinful, and having a variety of negative attitudes toward self: "I am often angry at myself for the stupid things I do" and "It is easy for me to admit that I am wrong."[32]

Test–retest reliability was calculated with 21 graduate students who completed the scales with a 2-week interval between administrations. Reliability for the FO was reported at 0.94, for FS, 0.67. In reviewing these differences, the authors suggest that "forgiveness of others is a stable characteristic across time, but our attitude toward ourselves, as reflected in feelings of guilt, anger at ourselves, and having a negative evaluation of ourselves, fluctuates over time."[32]

Further testing of validity and reliability on the FS and FO was performed using data from 237 outpatient counseling clients from Christian counseling centers. Clients completed both the BAS and the Minnesota Multiphasic Personality Inventory (MMPI) as part of the initial intake process. The authors noted a correlation of 0.37 between scores on the FO and FS, indicating that the scales measure two related, but different, phenomena. In addition, factor analysis revealed different loading patterns for the FO and FS scales. The FO scale loads significantly on a factor labeled Alienation from Others, which includes other scales such as cynicism, negative attitudes toward others, and passive aggressive behavior. The FS scale loads primarily on the factor neurotic immaturity, along with negative self-image, self-control deficit, and motivation deficit scales. Correlations between the forgiveness scales and scales of the MMPI indicate an association between problems with forgiveness and other types of psychopathology, including depression, anxiety, anger, distrust, and negative self-esteem.[32]

Information on demographics of subjects involved in validity and reliability testing for the FS and FO is limited to age, sex, and education, with gender being the only variable with clinical significance. Women tended to report slightly more difficulty in forgiving themselves than did men. There are no references in either scale to religious beliefs, which would appear to make the FS and FO useful regardless of religious orientation.

Spiritual Well-Being

An alternative approach to assessing spiritual needs is the evaluation of spiritual well-being (SWB), which has been defined by the National Interfaith Coalition on Aging as "the affirmation of life in a relationship with God, self, community and environment that nurtures and celebrates wholeness."[35]

Moberg summarized the universality of SWB:

> A central concern of the Christian faith, if not also of Islam, Judaism, Hinduism, and Buddhism, is to enhance the SWB of people. Although the semantics and theology of this concern vary from one group to another, it is located at the very core of many religious goals. It also is central to the ultimate values of Soviet Marxism, which hopes to shape "the new man" who combines "spiritual richness" with "moral purity."[36]

The Spiritual Well-Being Scale (SWB Scale)

The SWB scale, a 20-item Likert-type tool, was developed in conjunction with the social indicators movement in the 1960s and 1970s by Paloutzian and Ellison.[35,37] The scale reflects the belief that SWB involves a vertical and a horizontal dimension. The vertical dimension refers to the sense of well-being in the relationship with God, and the horizontal refers to sense of purpose in and satisfaction with life. These two subjective dimensions can be addressed separately using one of the two subscales comprising the SWB scale. The Religious Well-Being (RWB) subscale measures the vertical component, and the Existential Well-Being (EWB) subscale focuses on the horizontal. For example, the statement, "I have a personally meaningful relationship with God" refers to RWB, and "I believe that there is some purpose for my life" refers to EWB.[35] Responses to each item range from "strongly agree" to "strongly disagree."

Factor analysis of the SWB scale using varimax rotation was performed on data obtained from 206 students at three colleges having a religious orientation. The items clustered together as expected, with existential items loading into two subfactors, life direction and life satisfaction.[35,37]

The scale was then administered to 100 student volunteers at the University of Idaho. Test–retest reliability coefficients were 0.93 (SWB), 0.96 (RWB), and 0.86 (EWB). Internal consistency was evaluated using coefficient alpha, yielding 0.89 (SWB), 0.87 (RWB), and 0.78 (EWB).[35]

Examination of item content supports the face validity of the scale. In addition, the SWB scale scores have correlated in predicted ways with other theoretically related measures, including the PIL and Intrinsic Religious Orientation.[35]

The authors of the SWB scale acknowledge that the tool arises from the Judeo-Christian perception of religious well-being in which God is viewed in personal terms. However, they note that "it is possible that those from eastern religions such as Hinduism and Buddhism may be able to use the scale if they can meaningfully interpret the statements about relationship with God."[35]

The SWB scale continues to be one of the most widely used scales in all disciplines[38] and is particularly relevant for an older population as some questions presume the subject holds a traditional view of God. A recent study using the scale also compared ethnic differences between Caucasians and African Americans.[39] One criticism of the scale over the years has been the problem of ceiling effects that appear to affect scores of subjects from certain religious traditions; evangelical Protestants, for example, generally score very high on the scale. Scott, Agresti, and Fitchett[40] conducted research to determine if significant ceiling effects would be evidenced when the scale was used with a psychiatric inpatient sample, based on the theory that the scale might prove to be more useful with people who are struggling with issues of faith. They also conducted an exploratory factor analysis using oblique rather than orthogonal rotation. The three factors that emerged were affiliation (positive connection with God and self), alienation (sense of disconnection from God and self), and dissatisfaction with life. No significant ceiling effects were found with this population.[40]

Moberg's Indexes of SWB

Moberg's Indexes of SWB, a 45-item questionnaire, include a variety of factors that may influence SWB: social attitudes; self-perceptions; theologic and religious contexts; and religious beliefs, opinions, experiences, preferences, and affiliations.[36] Seven indices identified through factor analysis include Christian faith, self-satisfaction, personal piety, subjective SWB, optimism, religious cynicism, and elitism.

Response categories for most items range from "strongly agree" to "strongly disagree." Items in the personal piety index differ in that they require a response that indicates how frequently the subject participates in a particular activity. An example from this tool is "How often do you pray privately?" (personal piety).[36]

The instrument indexes of SWB are believed to have face validity, as the items were based on information gained through multiple earlier studies performed by the tool's author.[36] Preliminary data support criterion validity of the indices. When scores for evangelical Christians were compared with those of other Christians, differences were in the expected direction. Likewise, scores for Christians were higher than scores for people professing to be agnostic or atheist.[36] Additional testing with other criterion groups is needed to establish the tool's validity further. Further analysis of the validity of the indices has demonstrated coefficients ranging from 0.60 to 0.86 when scores were correlated with the SWB scale.

Moberg's indexes of SWB represent a major attempt to demonstrate the multifaceted nature of SWB. However, two characteristics may limit its usefulness in clinical research. The tool in its present form is somewhat lengthy and may not be practical to use with populations with extensive disease, who would tire easily. The indexes also are specific to Christianity and could not be used in their present form with patients of Jewish or Eastern orientations.

JAREL Spiritual Well-Being Scale

A spiritual well-being scale developed by nurses to assess spiritual well-being in older adults is the JAREL Spiritual Well-Being Scale, a 24-item Likert-type scale.[41] The name is based on the initials of the first names of the four principal investigators. The scale was developed in a two-phase study using factor analysis. Three factors identified were: (1) faith/belief dimension, (2) life/self-responsibility, and (3) life-satisfaction/self-actualization. Items that loaded 0.05 and above in factor 1 related to spiritual beliefs, belief in a supreme power, purpose in life, prayer, and life after death. The authors also identified four primary areas of nursing interventions related to the scale: affirmation, therapeutic communication, reminiscence, and referral.[42]

Phase 1 of the study consisted of data collection over an 18-month period from 31 in-depth interviews and approximately 150 hours of participant observation of older adults (aged 65–85) with varying belief systems and in a variety of settings. Validity of the categories of data that emerged was determined by consensus of the four investigators.

One of the core categories was relationship, subdivided into Ultimate other, other/nature, and self. The other core category that emerged was time (past, present, future).[41,42]

Spiritual Coping

Nurses often overlook the importance of religious faith when routinely assessing how a person responds to disease and copes with illness. Investigating spiritual coping may appear, on the surface, to document the performance of religious activities. In reality, spiritual coping looks beyond the actual behavior to the meaning or significance the behavior holds for the individual. In many research studies incorporating open-ended questions when subjects are given an opportunity to express what helped them most to cope with a crisis situation, prayer and faith are the variables mentioned most frequently.[43]

Patient Spiritual Coping Interview

The Patient Spiritual Coping Interview was developed by McCorkle and Benoliel[44] and adapted for use in a one-time interview format by Sodestrom and Martinson.[45] This semistructured interview contains 30 items that investigate relationship with God or a higher being, use of spiritual behaviors or resource persons, expressions of spiritual needs, and perception of the nurse's role in spiritual care.[45] Questions include "Do you ever watch religious TV or listen to religious radio?" "Have you spoken about your spiritual thoughts or concerns to someone?" and "How do you think nurses can assist you with your spiritual needs?"

The content validity of the interview was established by its consistency with the current literature and an expert panel of judges, three in oncology nursing research and two in theology. All agreed the items included were adequate and appropriate. Reliability was inferred by the assumption that subjects are reliable sources of information pertaining to the use of spiritual coping strategies.[45]

Spiritual Maturity

Spiritual maturity is another concept that has been studied, specifically from a Judeo-Christian perspective for use by pastoral counselors, clinical researchers, and psychotherapists. The growing specialty of parish nursing has also created more of a demand for spiritual assessment tools of this nature for use in congregations.[46]

Spiritual Assessment Inventory (SAI)

The SAI is based on a model of spiritual maturity that integrates relational maturity with God and experiential God-awareness.[47] Relational maturity is viewed from an object relations perspective. God-awareness is based on New Testament teaching and principles drawn from the literature of contemplative spirituality. Following the development of a pool of 54 self-report items to measure these two hypothesized dimensions of spiritual maturity, two factor analytic construct validity studies were conducted. In the second study, after revision and expansion of the SAI, five factors were identified: awareness of God, instability, grandiosity, realistic acceptance, and defensiveness/disappointment. Each subscale demonstrated good internal consistency reliability (0.73–0.95). Factors in the second study correlated with the Bell Object Relations Inventory, thereby supporting the underlying theory and validity of the SAI. The five-factor structure was corroborated by a 1999 study by Hall and Edwards.[48]

The authors of this study have also noted the theoretical and psychometric weaknesses of other spirituality assessment instruments, including the widely used SWB scale, noting that factor analysis had not supported the two-scale scoring of the two items of EWB and SWB, thus raising questions about that scale's validity for clinical use.[49,50]

Faith Maturity Scale

The Faith Maturity Scale is a 38-item self-report scale developed by the Search Institute; it was originally used in a national study of six Protestant mainline denominations.[51] It was designed to function as the primary criterion variable to evaluate the effectiveness of religious education. Development of the scale was based on the theory that religious education should help faith to mature and that mature faith would be evidenced by both a vertical and a horizontal dimension that included faith in God and service (obligation and action) to other people. Reliability coefficients (Cronbach alpha) ranged from 0.84 to 0.89. A fourfold faith typology was supported by the data: undeveloped faith (low vertical and horizontal), vertical faith (high vertical, low horizontal), horizontal faith (low vertical, high horizontal), and integrated faith (high vertical and horizontal). The scale holds promise for the measurement of spiritual maturity with other subjects in a variety of disciplines.[51]

Religious Motivation

Religious motivation, both internal and external, has also been a subject for measurement.

Intrinsic Religious Motivation Scale

The importance of spirituality in a person's life was evaluated by the Intrinsic Religious Motivation Scale developed by Hoge.[52] An intrinsically motivated person is one whose most central and ultimate motive in life can be found in his or her religious faith. The extrinsically motivated person views his or her religion as subservient to other aspects of life, such as economic or social status.[53] The scale consists of 10 statements to which the participant answers yes or no. "One should seek God's guidance when making every important decision" indicates intrinsic motivation. "It doesn't matter what I believe as long as I lead a moral life" is consistent with extrinsic motivation.[52]

The Intrinsic Religious Motivation Scale was administered to 42 adult Protestants, 21 of whom were judged by their ministers as intrinsically motivated and 21 judged as extrinsically motivated. The initial scale included 30 items. The final scale is composed of the 10 items having highest validity, reliability, item-to-item correlations, and item-to-scale correlations.

All 10 items correlated with the ministers' judgments in the direction predicted beyond 0.03 level of significance. The reliability of the scale, measured by Kuder-Richardson formula 20, was 0.901. Item-to-item correlations ranged from 0.132 to 0.716, with 22 of 45 item-to-item correlations greater than 0.5.[52]

The shorter version of the scale may be easier to use than the Patient Spiritual Coping Interview. However, the Intrinsic Religious Motivation Scale fails to identify specific behaviors that provide a source of comfort or strength to the subject. Another potential problem with the scale lies in the classification of items. Seven of the items are indicative of intrinsic motivation, but only three reflect external motivation. The author has acknowledged this limitation and suggests deletion of the intrinsic item "My faith sometimes restricts my actions." With this change, the Kuder-Richardson score becomes 0.902.[52]

Spiritual Transcendence

Transcendence and interconnectedness have been more recent recurring themes in spirituality research in nursing as well as in other disciplines.

Spirituality Assessment Scale (SAS)

Howden's SAS is a 28-item scale with seven response categories ranging from strongly agree to strongly disagree.[54] The SAS operationalizes spirituality in relation to four critical dimensions: unifying interconnectedness, innerness or inner resources, transcendence, and purpose and meaning in life. Howland's scale, especially the nine items related to interconnectedness, might be more suitable for people with a basic underlying world view that is Eastern metaphysical or New Age/New Consciousness. Items in this category include a feeling of harmony with self and others and a feeling of oneness with the universe or Universal Being. Transcendence is also interpreted by Howden as related to self-healing, rising above or beyond usual experiences as opposed to the concept of reaching outside oneself to a transcendent God or higher power. Psychometrics yielded a high internal consistency for the SAS (alpha = 0.9164).

Spiritual Transcendence Scale (STS)

Piedmont's STS is based on the theory that spirituality is an expression of an innate need for spiritual transcendence.[55] Spiritual transcendence is viewed as an independent dimension of personality. Piedmont defines spiritual transcendence as "the capacity of individuals to stand outside of their immediate sense of time and place to view life from a larger, more objective perspective."[55] In developing the STS, 65 items were originally formulated based on a review of Christian, Jewish, and Hindu texts and consultation with religious leaders from these faiths. Factor analysis and confirmatory factor analysis were conducted. The three subscales operationalizing spiritual transcendence are C, Connectedness (relationships with others); P-F, Prayer Fulfillment (prayer and meditation); and U, Universality (meaning and purpose of life). Subscale P-F appears to measure more traditional religion or spirituality. Scales C and P-F appear to be more consistent with measurements of nontraditional humanistic spiritualities, atheism, or agnosticism.

Spiritual Needs of Children

The potential difficulties in obtaining spiritual data from children are summarized by Shelly:

> If sound assessment is crucial to caring for adults, it is even more important in the pediatric setting. Children, especially young children, have a limited ability to communicate, particularly about abstract concepts.[56]

A study of adolescents reported by Elkind and Elkind[57] used only two questions: "When do you feel closest to God?" and "Have you ever had a particular experience when you felt especially close to God?" Responses from 144 ninth-grade students to these items indicated differences between males and females and between honor students and "average" students ($p < 0.05$). Differences also were noted between Protestants, Catholics, and Jews; however, the uncertainty about exact numbers represented in each denomination precluded statistical analysis.

A Nurses Christian Fellowship task force developed a seven-question assessment tool to obtain information about the spiritual needs of children: "How do you feel when you're in trouble?" or "Do you know who God is? What is He like?"[56]

Additional information can be obtained from young children by asking them to draw pictures of God and themselves or significant others. Using this technique requires special skill in interpretation to obtain meaningful data.

Nurse Recognition of Spiritual Needs of Patients

Several tools measure nurses' awareness of and appropriate interventions for spiritual needs. Chadwick devised a seven-item multiple-choice questionnaire to investigate "awareness and preparedness of nurses to meet spiritual needs."[58] Sample questions include "How long has it been since you last recognized a spiritual need in your patients?" and "Have you ever read the Bible or prayed with a patient?"

Sodestrom and Martinson developed a nurse interview schedule to correspond to the one discussed above for patients. Seventeen items were selected from the patient interview and modified to evaluate nurses' awareness of the spiritual strategies patients use in coping with disease.[45] Nurse participants answer yes, no, or don't know to questions such as "Do you know if your patient has spoken to a clergyman?" "Do you know if s/he has read the Bible?" and "Does your patient make reference to guilt feelings related to God?" Reliability and validity for the nurse interview are based on the same data as the Patient Spiritual Coping Interview.

Highfield and Cason developed a 49-item questionnaire for their study of nurses' ability to identify behaviors and conditions expressive of spiritual health or spiritual need.[2] Nurse participants are instructed to note whether the behavior or condition described is related to either the spiritual or psychosocial dimension. They also are to rate on a scale of 1 to 5 how frequently each behavior or condition is seen in their patients. Finally, participants are to note each item considered a patient problem.

The items contained in the Highfield-Cason questionnaire were identified from the nursing and pastoral care literature and were submitted to a review panel of theology and psychology experts. Although many items in the questionnaire are legitimately a part of the spiritual domain (e.g., "expresses fear of tests and diagnosis," "is unable to pursue creative outlets"), the less specific items could easily represent a psychosocial problem rather than or in addition to a spiritual problem. This ambiguity must be addressed by researchers who choose to use the Highfield-Cason questionnaire.

Summary

Clinical research related to spiritual issues in the past had been hampered by a variety of factors, including discomfort among health professionals who believe that spirituality and spiritual needs are a private matter, difficulty in distinguishing psychosocial needs from spiritual needs, lack of valid and reliable measurement tools that address spiritual concerns, and confusion about differences between spiritual concerns and religiosity. Some of these issues remain, especially the conceptual fuzziness between psychosocial and spiritual needs and definitions of spirituality that tend to be focused exclusively on one's relationship with self, other people, and the environment rather than any acknowledgment of the transcendent. The tools described here represent a heightened awareness of different aspects of spirituality. The development of new measures and further refinement of tools currently available will enable us to expand our understanding of this underresearched but important area.

Exemplar Study

Carson, V., Loeken, K.L., Shanty, J., & Terry, L. Hope and spiritual well-being: Essentials for living with AIDS. *Perspect Psychiatr Care*, 1990, 26:28–34.

The purpose of the study was to evaluate levels of hope and SWB among HIV-positive homosexual men. Sixty-five subjects were recruited, 25 of whom had been diagnosed with AIDS. Participants completed the Beck Hopelessness Scale and the SWB Scale (SWBS) while waiting in an outpatient clinic to see a physician. Only four subjects had scores consistent with hopelessness, with half scoring in the range of no or minimal pessimism. People with AIDS were found to be significantly more hopeful than those with AIDS-related complex (ARC; $p < 0.05$). SWBS scores were determined for overall SWB, existential well-being (EWB), and religious well-being (RWB). Participants were found to have positive levels of SWB; those with higher SWB scores tended to be more hopeful. A similar pattern was seen with EWB and RWB scores; however, the relationship between hope and EWB was significantly stronger than that between hope and RWB.

The authors note that EWB enables individuals to respond to a crisis as a challenge and as an opportunity for personal growth. They suggest that EWB's greater contribution to overall SWB reflects feelings of alienation and abandonment experienced from society and from organized religion.

The study is important in that it examines the spiritual health of a group of gay men who are HIV-infected. The findings support those of other studies demonstrating a direct relationship between SWB and hope.[59,60] Moreover, the results are consistent with subjective observations that homosexual men often are poorly accepted in organized religion. Denying homosexual men access to religious participation (e.g., opportunities to experience RWB) may compromise overall SWB for some, although the population studied may have offset their RWB losses to some degree through EWB enhancement.

References

1. Burkhardt, M.A., & Nagai Jacobson, M.G. Spirituality and health. In B.M. Dossey, Keegan, L., & Guzzetta, C.E. (Eds.), *Holistic nursing: A handbook for practice* (3rd ed.). Gaithersburg, MD: Aspen, 2000, p. 92-108.
2. Highfield, M., & Cason, C. Spiritual needs of patients: Are they being recognized? *Cancer Nurs*, 1983, 6(3):187-191.
3. Larson, D.B., Swyers, J.P., & McCullough, M.E. (Eds.). *Scientific research on spirituality and health: A consensus report*. Rockville, MD: National Institute for Healthcare Research, 1998.
4. Moberg, D., & Brusek, P. Spiritual well-being: A neglected subject in quality of life research. *Soc Indicators Res*, 1978, 5(3):303.
5. Emblen, J. Religion and spirituality defined according to current use in nursing literature. *J Prof Nurs*, 1992, 8:41-47.
6. Moberg, D.O. Development of social indicators of spiritual well-being for quality of life research. In D.O. Moberg (Ed.), *Spiritual well-being: Sociological perspectives*. Washington, DC: University Press of America, 1979.
7. McFarland, G.K., & McFarlane, E.A. *Nursing diagnosis and intervention: Planning for patient care* (3rd ed.). St. Louis: Mosby, 1997
8. Sire, J. *The universe next door* (3rd ed.). Downers Grove, IL: InterVarsity Press, 1988.
9. Hall, B.A. Patterns of spirituality in persons with advanced HIV disease. *Res Nurs Health*, 1998, 21:143-153.
10. Kahn, D.L., & Steeves, R.H. Spiritual well-being: A review of the research literature. *Qual Life: A Nursing Challenge*, 1993, 2(3):60-64.
11. Steeves, R.H., & Kahn, D.L. Experience of meaning in suffering. *IMAGE: J Nurs Scholar*, 1987, 19:114-116.
12. Highfield, M.F. Spiritual health of oncology patients. *Cancer Nurs*, 1992, 15(1):1-8.
13. Reed, P.G. Spirituality and well-being in terminally ill hospitalized adults. *Res Nurs Health*, 1987, 10:335-344.
14. Reed P.G. Religiousness among terminally ill and healthy adults. *Res Nurs Health*, 1986, 9:35-42.
15. Roberts, K.T., & Aspy, C. Development of the serenity scale. *J Nurs Meas*, 1993, 1(2):145-164.
16. Stallwood, J. Spiritual dimensions of nursing practice. In I. Beland & J. Passos (Eds.), *Clinical nursing*. New York: Macmillan, 1975.
17. Hess, J.S. Spiritual needs survey. In S. Fish & J.A. Shelly, *Spiritual care: The nurse's role*. Downers Grove, IL: Intervarsity Press, 1983, p. 157.
18. Stoll, R. Guidelines for spiritual assessment. *Am J Nurs*, 1979, 79:1574.
19. Reed, P.G. Preferences for spiritually-related nursing interventions among terminally ill and nonterminally ill hospitalized adults and well adults. *Appl Nurs Res*, 1991, 4(3):122-128.
20. Dossey, B.M. *AHNA Core curriculum for holistic nursing*. Gaithersburg, MD: Aspen, 1987, pp. 46-47.
21. Stoll, R. *Spiritual assessment: A nursing perspective*. Presented at the Spirituality in Nursing workshop, Marquette University, Milwaukee, WI, August 1984.
22. Fordyce, E. *An investigation of television's potential for meeting the spiritual needs of hospitalized persons*. Doctoral dissertation, Catholic University of America, 1981. *Dissertation Abstracts International*, 1982.
23. Fish, S., & Shelly, J.A. *Spiritual care: The nurse's role*. Downers Grove, IL: Intervarsity Press, 1983
24. Dufault, K., & Martocchio, B.C. Hope: Its spheres and dimensions. *Nurs Clin North Am*, 1986, 20(2): 379.
25. Nowotony, M.L. Assessment of hope in patients with cancer: Development of an instrument. *Oncol Nurs Forum*, 1989, 16(1):57
26. Crumbaugh, J.C., & Maholick, L.T. An experimental study in existentialism: The psychometric approach to Frankl's concept of noogenic neurosis. *J Clinical Psychol*, 1964, 20:200.
27. Frankl, V. *Man's search for meaning*. New York: Washington Square Press, 1984.

28. Crumbaugh, J.C. Cross-validation of purpose in life test based on Frankl's concepts. *J Indiv Psychol*, 1968, *24*:74.

29. Maton, K.I. Stress-buffering role of spiritual support: Cross-sectional and prospective investigations. *J Sci Study Rel*, 1989, *28*(3):310-323.

30. Maton, K.I. Empowerment in a religious setting: An exploratory study. [Unpublished Master's Thesis, University of Illinois at Urbana-Champaign, IL, 1984.]

31. Studzinski, R. Remember and forgive: Psychological dimensions of forgiveness. In C. Floristan & C. Duquoc (Eds.), *Forgiveness*. Edinburgh: T & T Clark, 1986, p. 12.

32. Mauger, P.A., Perry, J.E., Freeman, T., et al. Measurement of forgiveness: Preliminary research. *J Psychol Christian*, 1992, *11*(2):170.

33. Mauger, P.A., Webb, J.H., Davis, R., et al. Development of a multi-dimensional inventory for the diagnosis of personality disorders. Paper presented at the annual meeting of the Southeastern Psychological Association, Atlanta, GA, 1985.

34. Mauger, P.A. *Behavior assessment system I, preliminary manual, version 2.1*. Atlanta, GA: Automated Assessment, 1991.

35. Ellison, C.W. Spiritual well-being: Conceptualization and measurement. *J Psychol Theol*, 1983, *11*(4):330-340.

36. Moberg, D. Subjective measures of spiritual well-being. *Rev Relig Res*, 1984, *25*(4):351.

37. Paloutzian, R., & Ellison, C.W. Loneliness, spiritual well-being, and the quality of life. In A. Peplau & D. Perlman (Eds.), *Loneliness: A sourcebook of current theory, research, and therapy*. New York: Wiley, 1982, p. 224.

38. Bufford, R.K., Paloutzian, R.F., & Ellison, C.W. Norms for the Spiritual Well-Being Scale. *J Psychol Theol*, 1991, *19*:56-70.

39. Miller, G., Fleming, W., & Brown-Anderson, F. Spiritual well-being scale ethnic differences between Caucasians and African-Americans. *J Psychol Theol*, 1998, *26*(4):358-364.

40. Scott, E.L., Agresti, A.A., & Fitchett, G. Factor analysis of the 'Spiritual Well-Being Scale' and its clinical utility with psychiatric inpatients. *J Sci Study Rel*, 1998, *37*(2):314-321.

41. Hungelmann, J.A., Kenkel-Rossi, E., Klassen, L., & Stollenwerk, R.M. Development of the JAREL spiritual well-being scale. In R.M. Carrol-Johnson (Ed.), *Classification of nursing diagnoses: Proceedings of the eighth conference, North American Nursing Diagnosis Association*. Philadelphia: Lippincott, 1998, p. 393.

42. Hungelmann, J.A., Kenkel-Rossi, E., Klassen, L., & Stollenwerk, R.M. Focus on spiritual well-being: Harmonious interconnectedness of mind-body-spirit—Use of the JAREL Spiritual Well-Being Scale. *Geriatr Nurse*, 1996, *17*(6):262-266.

43. McCullough, M.E. Prayer and health: Conceptual issues, research review, and research agenda. *J Psych Theol*, 1995, *23*(1):15-29.

44. McCorkle, R., & Benoliel, J.Q. *Manual of data collection instruments*. [Unpublished manual.] Seattle: University of Washington, 1981.

45. Sodestrom, K.E., & Martinson, I. Patient's spiritual coping strategies: A study of nurse and patient perspectives. *Oncol Nurs Forum*, 1987, *14*(2):41-46.

46. Wilson, R.P. What does a parish nurse do? *J Christian Nurs*, 1997, *14*(1):13-16.

47. Hall, T.W., & Edwards, K.J. The initial development and factor analysis of the spiritual assessment inventory. *J Psychol Theol*, 1996, *24*(3):233-246.

48. Slater, W., Hall, T.W., & Edwards, K.J. Measuring religion and spirituality: Where are we and where are we going? *J Psychol Theol*, 2001, *29*(1):4-21.

49. Ledbetter, M.F., Smith, L.A., Fischer, J.D., et al. An evaluation of the construct validity of the Spiritual Well-Being Scale: A confirmatory factor analytic approach. *J Psychol Theol*, 1991, *19*:94-102.

50. Ledbetter, M.F., Smith, L.A., Vosler-Hunter, W.L., & Fischer, J.D. An evaluation of the research and clinical usefulness of the Spiritual Well-Being Scale. *J Psychol Theol*, 1991, *19*:49-55.

51. Benson, P.L., Donahue, M.J., & Erickson, J.A. The Faith Maturity Scale: Conceptualization, measurement, and empirical validation. *Res Soc Sci Study Religion*, 1993, *5*:1-26.

52. Hoge, D.R. Validated Intrinsic Religious Motivation Scale. *J Sci Study Rel*, 1972, *11*:369.

53. Soderstrom, D., & Wright, E.W. Religious orientation and meaning in life. *J Clin Psychol*, 1977, *33*(1):65-68.

54. Howden, S.W. "Developmental and psychometric characteristics of the spirituality assessment scale." [Unpublished doctoral dissertation.] Denton, TX: Texas Women's University College of Nursing, 1992.

55. Piedmont, R.L. Does spirituality represent the sixth factor of personality? Spiritual transcendence and the five-factor model. *J Personality*, 1999, *67*(6):986-1013.

56. Shelly, J.A. *Spiritual needs of children*. Downers Grove, IL: Intervarsity Press, 1982.

57. Elkind, D., & Elkind, S. Varieties of religious experience in young adolescents. *J Sci Study Rel*, 1962, *2*(1):102.

58. Chadwick, R. Awareness and preparedness of nurses to meet spiritual needs. In S. Fish & J.A. Shelly, *Spiritual care: The nurse's role*. Downers Grove, IL: Intervarsity Press, 1983.

59. Carson, V., Soeken, K.L., & Grimm, P.M. Hope and its relationship to spiritual well-being. *J Psychol Theol*, 1988, *16*(2):159-167.

60. Mickley, J.R., Soeken, K., & Belcher, A. Spiritual well-being, religiousness, and hope among women with breast cancer. *IMAGE: J Nurs Scholar*, 1992, *24*(2):267.

16

Measuring Body Image

Julie F. Robertson

The concept of body image has application in a wide range of disciplines, including medicine, nursing, psychology, physical therapy, dentistry, and dietetics. The importance of body image in our culture is significant: One has only to note the tremendous expenditure of time, effort, and money by people seeking to alter their appearance to resemble an ideal image.

Life events that alter one's body can profoundly affect how one perceives oneself and functions in society. Such alterations can be very disrupting and anxiety provoking. Physical alterations caused by trauma, surgery, or treatment can lead to depression and lowered self-esteem. Health care professionals encounter patients experiencing a variety of alterations in body image, including changes in body structure and function, deformities, loss of body boundaries, and depersonalization. Whether the change is the consequence of surgery, drugs, sensory deprivation, fatigue, stress, immobility, or anesthesia, adequate assessment of body image change is key to effective intervention that will promote, reestablish, or maintain self-esteem. Health care that successfully assists patients to integrate physical changes can significantly influence adaptation and survival. Quality of life is inextricably linked with body image.

The Concept of Body Image

The concept of body image has been well researched by multiple authors, who have produced several classic articles on the subject.[1,2] Schilder defined *body image* as "the picture of our own body which we form in our mind . . . the way in which the body appears to ourselves."[1] Body image in this instance refers to a psychologic experience and focuses on individuals' feelings and attitudes toward their bodies.[2] Norris believes that body image is a "social creation . . . basic to identity and it has been referred to as the somatic ego."[3] Body image in this case is subjective and is grounded in life experiences.

Acknowledgment: The author wishes to thank Judy M. Diekmann for her invaluable contributions in writing this chapter in the first edition of the book.

The concept of body image has been researched from different perspectives, including neurologic, somatic, and psychologic characterizations and has been found to be a multidimensional construct.[4] Definitions have included both direct perceptions of the body through visual, tactile, and proprioceptive senses and indirect perceptions via attitudes, emotions, and reactions.[5,6]

Body image also has been defined as an adaptive mechanism that perpetuates balance among the physiologic, psychologic, and sociocultural components of the body.[7] Certain behavioral aspects of body image disturbance, such as avoiding social situations that might be associated with food or appearance, also have garnered the attention of researchers.[8] Body image differs from self-concept. *Body image* refers to perception, whereas *self-concept* denotes feelings about oneself. These terms have been used interchangeably despite the fact that they are distinct concepts.

Neurologists have observed that patients with selective brain lesions demonstrate a wide range of distorted body images.[5] Such patients were unable to distinguish one side of the body from the other, denied the existence of various body parts, denied the incapacitation of various parts, or falsely attributed new body parts to themselves. It is believed that body image disturbances can occur with brain lesions at any level. However, the parietal region of the minor hemisphere is commonly regarded as a site of special significance because of the relationship that exists between right parietal disease and body image disorders.[2,9]

In the field of psychiatry, investigators reported that numerous schizophrenic patients demonstrate almost the same range in distortions of body image as that observed in neurologic patients.[10] In a classic study, Fisher and Cleveland[2] reviewed and classified the bizarre body perceptions reported by schizophrenics. They grouped these distortions into several categories The first centers around issues of masculinity and femininity and includes such distortions as feeling that one has the body parts of the opposite sex or that one is half-man, half-woman. A second group of distortions involves feelings of body disintegration and deterioration. The third category refers to feelings of depersonalization, in which schizophrenics lose a sense of reality about the existence of body parts or the total body. The fourth category of distortions is a sense of body boundary loss. Schizophrenics with this disorder feel that things happening elsewhere and to other people are happening to them.

The relationship between psychiatric disorders and body image is multiplex. Early research focused on the emotional distress that results from disfigurement. However, this changed when Freud[5] hypothesized that concerns about appearance resulted from psychologic conflict. A growing body of evidence indicates that poor body image has a detrimental affect on a person's mental health.[11]

Much research has been conducted on the relationship between eating disorders and body image. Studies of patients with the syndrome of anorexia nervosa support a relationship between body image distortions and feelings of inadequacy.[12] This syndrome is characterized by a negative evaluation of body appearance and the tendency to overestimate body size. Studies also have found a relationship between distorted body image and obesity[13,14] or bulimia.[15] In 1980, the *Diagnostic and Statistical Manual of Mental Disorders* included body image disturbance as a diagnostic criteria for bulimia and anorexia nervosa.[16]

Research in the area of body image is proliferating. Many investigators have turned from clinical analysis to the analysis of body perception as a psychologic phenomenon in healthy populations. They postulate that the normal person's attitude toward his or her body influences behavior in the same way as attitudes do. Feelings about the body appear to affect decisions at all levels; even decisions relating to survival may be biased by one's prevailing body image. Findings of recent studies demonstrate a strong correlation between body image disturbance and feelings of low self-worth and depression in normal populations.[11,17]

A growing body of evidence indicates that a person's developmental stage and gender influence body image. In the past, body image studies focused primarily on adolescent and young adult females.[18] However, recent studies show that children as young as 8 or 9 may engage in dieting because of poor body image and concerns about being overweight.[19] Recent findings also suggest that body image disturbances among adolescent and adult males is an increasing problem in Western societies.[18] More research is needed on body image changes across the lifespan, with a focus on children and older adult populations.

Sociocultural and cross-cultural research on body image has increased worldwide in the past decade. The preponderance of evidence indicates that there are important differences in body image related to race and ethnicity. Social and cultural influences are now believed to significantly affect body image and closely tie body parts and appearance to personality development and socialization.[20,21]

Researchers have increasingly focused on the role that media plays in the development of body image. Growing evidence indicates that sociocultural messages portrayed in the media are powerful forces contributing to body image disturbances among adolescent girls. This association has not been adequately explored for males and other age groups.[21] Experts predict that body image disturbance will continue to increase, especially among women, as a result of the emphasis that Western societies place on beauty, youth, and slimness.[22] These powerful cultural messages have been shown to produce body dissatisfaction among non-eating disordered women.[12,23] Some researchers claim that body dissatisfaction is now normative in Western societies in females beginning as early as age eight.[4]

Measuring the Body Image Concept

Despite the proliferation of body image research, there is little consensus about the best procedure to measure body image. In recent years, many techniques were developed to measure body image, and many of these focus on body size estimation. The diversity of instruments and procedures has led to methodologic concerns that study results cannot truly be compared.[6,24] In addition, many of these methods have not been psychometrically validated.[6]

The most popular measurement techniques used for the major dimensions of body image include questionnaires, scales (see Appendix 16A), body image boundary determinations, direct measurement of perceived body size, distortion techniques, silhouettes, and videotape feedback (see Appendix 16B). The assistance of a psychologist or psychiatrist may be helpful in interpreting results of these instruments.

Three body measurement techniques used by investigators with increasing frequency are (1) mirror images and other self-representations that measure a subject's internalized picture of his or her body's physical appearance, (2) videotape recordings that give people an opportunity to scrutinize how they appear to others, and (3) direct video monitoring using a TV screen to assess body image. Examples of these measurement tools are listed in Appendix 16B.

In several studies employing direct video monitoring, Gardner et al. found that the use of the TV video was "quite accurate" in determining body size.[13,25] These researchers advocate the use of this methodology because it "allows a direct, simultaneous, and exact assessment of body image"[13] and is a viable technique to use with a variety of populations, including eating-disordered individuals and children.[25] Gardner et al. reported that several researchers have found that TV video methodology has acceptable reliability and validity as a measure of body image.[25] In the 1990s, Gardner et al. further perfected the TV video methodology.[26]

Since the late 1970s, nurses have shown increasing interest in studying the phenomenon of body image in a variety of populations, resulting in the development of a number of measures of body image. Populations studied include pregnant women and their spouses,[27] multiple sclerosis patients,[28] cancer patients,[29,30] ill children,[31] patients with halo braces,[32] immobilized patients,[33] older adults,[34] overweight women,[35] and patients who have undergone head and neck surgery,[36] cerebral bypass surgery,[37] and mastectomy.[38] Nurse researchers also have examined adaptation to body image distortion[39] and nurses' perceptions of what constitutes acceptable female body size.[40] Nurse-developed instruments are shown in Appendix 16A[33,36] and 16B.[35]

Summary

Many techniques are available to measure the different aspects of body image. It is important to note that body image is a complex construct that cannot be measured with any single method. Most likely, multiple instruments and methods will be necessary. Nurse researchers are in an excellent position to expand the knowledge about body image across the lifespan in both healthy and ill populations. It is evident that continuing work is needed to determine the usefulness, reliability, and validity of each of the instruments and techniques described in this chapter.

Exemplar Studies

Grant, K., Lyons, A., Landis, D., et al. Gender, body image, and depressive symptoms among low-income African American adolescents. *J Soc Issues*, 1999, *55*(2):299.

This study investigated gender differences in body image and depression among a sample of sixth–eighth grade African American adolescents from low-income families. Methods are well described and rigorous. Data collection instruments have excellent documented reliability and validity.

Stice, E., & Bearman, S.K. Body-image and eating disturbances prospectively predict increases in depressive symptoms in adolescent girls: A growth curve analysis. *Dev Psychol*, 2001, *37*(5):597.

This study was a longitudinal investigation that tested whether body image and eating disorder disturbances predicted depression in adolescent girls. Methods are well described and rigorous. Nine instruments were used to collect the data, all of which possess acceptable psychometric properties.

Websites

Alliance for Eating Disorders. Access date 5 March 2003. www.eatingdisorderinfo.org. Body Image Task Force. Access date 5 March 2003. home.earthlink.net/~dawn_atkins/bitf.htm.

Eating Disorders Coalition for Research Policy and Action. Access date 5 March 2003. www.eatingdisorderscoalition.com.

Body Positive: Boosting Body Image At Any Weight. Access date 5 March 2003. www.bodypositive.com.

National Eating Disorders Screening Program. Access date 5 March 2003. www.mentalhealthscreening.org/eat.htm.

References

1. Schilder, P. *Image and appearance of the human body*. New York: International Universities Press, 1950 (originally published in 1935).
2. Fisher, S., & Cleveland, S. *Body image and personality*. New York: Dover, 1968.
3. Norris, C. The professional nurse and body image. In C. Carlson & B. Blackwell (Eds.), *Behavioral concepts and nursing intervention* (2nd ed.). Philadelphia: Lippincott, 1978, p. 5-36.
4. Grogan, S. *Body image: Understanding body dissatisfaction in men, women, and children*. London: Routledge, 1999.
5. Lacey, J.H., & Birtchnell, S.A. Body image and its disturbances. *J Psychosom Res*, 1986, 30(6):623-631.
6. Gardner, R.M. Methodological issues in assessment of the perceptual component of body image disturbance. *Br J Psychol*, 1996, 87:327-337.
7. Dropkin, M.J. Change in body image associated with head and neck cancer. In L.B. Marino (Ed.), *Cancer Nursing*. St. Louis: Mosby, 1981, p. 560-581.
8. Rosen, J.C., Srebnik, D., Saltzberg, E., & Wendt, S. Development of a body image avoidance questionnaire. *Psychol Assess J Consult Clin Psychol*, 1991, 3(1):32-37.
9. Van Deusen, J. *Body image and perceptual dysfunction in adults*. Philadelphia: Saunders, 1993.
10. Cash, T.F., & Pruzinsky, T. *Body image: Development, deviance, and change*. New York: Guilford Press, 1990.
11. Grant, K., Lyons, A., Landis, D. et al. Gender, body image, and depressive symptoms among low-income African American adolescents. *J Soc Issues*, 1999, 55(2):299-315.
12. Haworth-Hoeppner, S. The critical shapes of body image: The role of culture and family in the production of eating disorders. *J Marriage Fam*, 2000, 62(1):212-227.
13. Gardner, R.M., Martinez, R., & Espinoza, T. Psychological measurement of body image of self and others in obese subjects. *J Soc Behav Person*, 1987, 2(2):205-217.
14. Friedman, M.A., & Brownell, K.D. Psychological correlates of obesity: Moving to the next research generation. *Psychol Bull*, 1995, 117(1):3-20.
15. Showers, C.J., & Larson, B.E. Looking at body image: The organization of self-knowledge about physical appearance and its relation to disordered eating. *J Personality*, 1999, 67(4):659-700.
16. American Psychiatric Association. *Diagnostic and statistical manual of mental disorders* (3rd ed.). Washington, DC: American Psychiatric Association, 1980.
17. Stice, E., & Bearman, S.K. Body-image and eating disturbances prospectively predict increases in depressive symptoms in adolescent girls: A growth curve analysis. *Dev Psychol*, 2001, 37(5):597-607.
18. Hayslip, B., Cooper, C.C., Dougherty, L.M. et al. Body image in adulthood: A projective approach. *J Personality Assess*, 1997, 68(3):628-649.
19. Kostanski, M., & Gullone, E. Dieting and body image in the child's world: Conceptualization and behavior. *J Genet Psychol*, 1999, 160(4):488-499.
20. Monteath, S., & McCabe, M.P. The influence of societal factors on female body image. *J Soc Psychol*, 1997, 137:708-727.
21. Ricciardelli, L., & McCabe, L.A. (2001). Self-esteem and negative affect as moderators of sociocultural influences on body dissatisfaction, strategies to decrease weight, and strategies to increase muscles among adolescent boys and girls. *Sex Roles*, 2001, 44(3):189-207.
22. Wolszon, L.R. Women's body image theory and research: A hermeneutic critique. *Am Behav Sci*, 1998, 41(4):542-557.
23. Stevens, C., & Tiggemann, M. Women's body figure preferences across the life span. *J Genet Psychol*, 1998, 159:94-102.
24. Smeets, M.A.M., Smit, F., Panhuysen, G.E.M., et al. The influence of methodological differences on the outcome of body size estimation studies in anorexia nervosa. *Br J Clin Psychol*, 1997, 36:263-277.
25. Gardner, R.M., Morrell, J., Urrutia, R., & Espinoza, T. Judgments of body size following weight loss. *J Soc Behav Person*, 1989, 4(5):603-613.
26. Gardner, R.M., Friedman, B.N., & Jackson, N.A. Body size estimations, body dissatisfaction and ideal size preferences in children six through thirteen. *J Youth Adolesc*, 1999, 28(5):603-618.
27. Fawcett, J., & Frye, S. An exploratory study of body image dimensionality. *Nurs Res*, 1980, 29(5):324-327.
28. Sammonds, R.J., & Cammermeyer, M. Perceptions of body image in subjects with multiple sclerosis: A pilot study. *J Neurosci Nurs*, 1989, 21(3):190-194.
29. Padilla, G.V., & Grant, M.M. Quality of life as a cancer nursing outcome variable. *Adv Nurs Sci*, 1985, 8(1):45.
30. Ramer, L. Self-image changes with time in the cancer patient with a colostomy after operation. *J ET Nurs*, 1992, 19(6):195-203.
31. Beardslee, C., & Neff, J.A. Body-related concerns of children with cancer as compared with the concerns of other children. *Mat Child Nurs J*, 1982, 11:121.
32. Olson, B., Ustanko, L., & Warner, S. The patient in a halo brace: Striving for normalcy in body image and self concept. *Orthopaed Nurs*, 1991, 10(1):44-50.
33. Baird, S.E. Development of a nursing assessment tool to diagnose altered body image in immobilized patients. *Orthopaed Nurs*, 1985, 4(1):47-54.
34. Janelli, L.M. The realities of body image. *J Gerontol Nurs*, 1986, 12(10):23-27.
35. Popkess-Vawter, S., & Banks, N. Body image measurement in overweight females. *Clin Nurs Res*, 1992, 1(4):402-417.
36. Droughton, M.L., & Verbic, M. Body image reintegration after head and neck surgery: Application and evaluation of three nursing interventions. *J Off Pub Soc Otorhinolaryngol Head-Neck Nurs*, 1988, 6(1):19-22.

37. Stewart-Amidei, C., & Penckofer, S. Quality of life following cerebral bypass surgery. *J Neurosci Nurs,* 1988, 20(1):50-57.

38. Bredin, M. Mastectomy, body image and therapeutic massage: A qualitative study of women's experience. *J Adv Nurs,* 1999, 29(5):1113-1120.

39. Norris, J., Kunes-Connell, M., & Spelic, S.S. A grounded theory of reimaging. *Adv Nurs Sci,* 1998, 20(3):1-12.

40. Wright, J. Female nurses' perceptions of acceptable female body size: An exploratory study. *J Clin Nurs,* 1998, 7:307-315.

41. Fisher, S. *Body experience in fantasy and behavior.* New York: Appleton-Century-Crofts, 1970.

42. Gleghorn, A.A., Penner, L.A., Powers, P.S., & Schulman, R. The psychometric properties of several measures of body image. *J Psychopathol Behav Assess,* 1987, 9(2):203-218.

43. Ben-Tovim, D.I., & Walker, M.K. Women's body attitudes: A review of measurement techniques. *Int J Eating Dis,* 1991, 10(2):155-167.

44. Secord, P., & Jourard, S. The appraisal of body cathexis: Body cathexis and self. *J Consult Clin Psychol,* 1953, 17:343-347.

45. Jourard, S.M., & Secord, P.F. Body-cathexis and the ideal female figure. *J Abnorm Soc Psychol,* 1955, 50:243.

46. Mayer, J.D., & Eisenberg, M.G. Body concept: A conceptualization and review of paper-and-pencil measures. *Rehabil Psychol,* 1982, 27(2):97.

47. Franzoi, S.L., & Shields, S.A. The Body Esteem Scale: Multidimensional structure and sex differences in a college population. *J Person Assess,* 1984, 48(2):173-178.

48. Thomas, C.D., & Freeman, R.J. The Body Esteem Scale: Construct validity of the female subscales. *J Person Assess,* 1990, 54(1&2):204-212.

49. Secord, P. Objectification of word-association procedures by the use of homonyms: A measure of body cathexis. *J Person,* 1953, 21:479-495.

50. Jupp, J.J., & Collins, J.K. Instruments for the measurement of unconscious and conscious aspects of body image. *Aust J Clin Exp Hypnosis,* 1983, 11(2):89-110.

51. Winston, B.A., & Case, T.F. Reliability and validity of the Body-Self Relations Questionnaire: A new measure of body image, March 1984. Paper presented at the meeting of the Southeastern Psychological Association, New Orleans.

52. Brown, T.A., Cash, T.F., & Mikuka, P.J. Attitudinal body-image assessment: Factor analysis of the Body–Self Relations Questionnaire. *J Person Assess,* 1990, 55(1&2):135-144.

53. Cash, T.F., & Green, G.K. Body weight and body image among college women: Perception, cognition, and affect. *J Person Assess,* 1986, 50(2):290-301.

54. Cooper, P.J., Taylor, M.J., Cooper, Z., & Fairburn, C.G. The development and validation of the Body Shape Questionnaire. *Int J Eating Dis,* 1987, 6(4):485-494.

55. Hadigan, C.M., & Walsh, B.T. Body shape concerns in bulimia nervosa. *Int J Eating Dis,* 1991, 10(3):323-331.

56. Bunnell, D.W., Cooper, P.J., Hertz, S., & Shenker, I.R. Body shape concerns among adolescents. *Int J Eating Dis,* 1992, 11(1):79-83.

57. Thompson, J.K., Fabian, L.J., Moulton, D.O., et al. Development and validation of the Physical Appearance Related Teasing Scale. *J Person Assess,* 1991, 56(3):513-521.

58. Ben-Tovim, D.I., & Walker, M.K. The development of the Ben-Tovim Walker Body Attitudes Questionnaire (BAQ), a new measure of women's attitudes towards their own bodies. *Psychol Med,* 1991, 21(3):775-784.

59. Cash, T.F., & Fleming, E.C. The impact of body image experiences: Development of the Body Image Quality of Life Inventory. *Int J Eat Dis,* 2002, 31(4):455-460.

60. Candy, C.M., & Fee, V.E. Underlying dimensions and psychometric properties of the Eating Behaviors and Body Image Test for Preadolescent Girls. *J Clin Child Psychol,* 1998, 27(1):117-127.

61. Polce-Lynch, M., Kliewer, W., & Meyers, B.J. Gender differences in early adolescent self-esteem: The mediating role of body image, Unpublished manuscript, 1994, Virginia Commonwealth University.

62. Polce-Lynch, M., Meyers, B.J., Kliewer, W., et al. Adolescent self-esteem and gender: Exploring relations to sexual harassment, body image, media influence, and emotional expression. *J Youth Adolesc,* 2001, 30(2):225-244.

63. Hopwood, P., Fletcher, I., Lee, A. et al. A body image scale for use with cancer patients. *Eur J Cancer,* 2001, 37(2):189-197.

64. Wooley, O.W., & Roll, S. The Color-a-Person Body Dissatisfaction Test: Stability, internal consistency, validity, and factor structure. *J Person Assess,* 1991, 56(3):395-413.

65. Askevold, F. Measuring body image: Preliminary report on a new method. *Psychother Psychosom,* 1975, 25:71-111.

66. Fichter, M.W., Meister, I., & Koch, H.J. The measurement of body image disturbances in anorexia nervosa: Experimental comparison of different methods. *Br J Psychiatr,* 1986, 148:453-461.

67. Ajzen, Y., & Iagolnitzer, E.R. Dimensionality of revisited body awareness. *Percept Motor Skills,* 1985, 60:455.

68. Thomas, C.D., & Freeman, R.J. Body-Image Marking: Validity of body-width estimates as operational measures of body image. *Behav Mod,* 1991, 15(2):261-270.

69. Dillon, D.J. Measurement of perceived body size. *Percept Motor Skills,* 1962, 14:191.

70. Dillon, D.J. Estimation of bodily dimensions. *Percept Motor Skills,* 1962, 14:219.

71. Slade, P.D., & Russell, G.F. Awareness of body dimension in anorexia nervosa: Cross-sectional and longitudinal studies. *Psychol Med,* 1973, 3:188-199.

72. Meerman, R., Vandereycken, W., & Napierski, C. Methodological problems of body image research in anorexia nervosa patients. *Acta Psychiatr Belgica,* 1986, 86(1):42-51.

73. Ruff, G.A., & Barrios, B.A. Realistic assessment of body image. *Behav Assess,* 1986, 8:237-251.

74. Mizes, J.S. Validity of the body image detection device. *Addict Behav,* 1991, 16:411-417.

75. Fawcett, J., & Chodil, J.J. The topographic device: Development and research. In E. Bauwens (Ed.), *Research for clinical nursing: Its strategies and findings.* Monograph Series 1979: 3. Indianapolis, IN: Sigma Theta Tau, 1980.

76. Allebeck, P., Hallberg, D., & Espmark, S. Body image—An apparatus for measuring disturbances in

estimation of size and shape. *J Psychosomat Res*, 1976, *20*:583-589.

77. Collins, J.K. The objective measurement of body image using a video technique: Reliability and validity studies. *Br J Psychol*, 1986, *77*:199-205.

78. Collins, J.K. Methodology for the objective measurement of body image. *Int J Eating Dis*, 1987, *6*(3):393-399.

79. Williamson, D.A., Davis, C.J., Bennett, S.M., et al. Development of a single procedure for assessing body image disturbances. *Behav Assess*, 1989, *11*:433-446.

80. Fitts, W. *Tennessee Self-Concept Scale*. Nashville: Counselor Recordings and Tests, 1964.

81. Sherman, D.K., Iacono, W.G., & Donnelly, J.M. Development and validation of body rating scales for adolescent females. *Int J Eat Dis*, 1995, *18*(4):327-333.

82. Stunkard, A.J., Sorenson, T., & Schlusinger, F. Use of the Danish Adoption Registry for the study of obesity and thinness. In S. Kety (Ed.), *The genetics of neurological and psychiatric disorders*. New York: Raven Press, 1983, pp. 115-129.

83. Collins, M.E. Body figure perceptions and preferences among preadolescent children. *Int J Eat Dis*, 1991, *10*(2):199-208.

Appendix 16A. Important Questionnaires and Scales Used in the Measurement of Body Image Dimensions

Instrument	Description	Psychometric Indices
Body Distortion Questionnaire (BDQ) Developed by Fisher (41)	Affective measure of body image, identifies abnormal attitudes related to body appearance and function 82-item questionnaire, offers 3-response format (yes, not, undecided)	High Kuder-Richardson reliability (0.95) High convergent correlations with other affective measures of body image (42) Discriminates well between normals and bulimics (42), and anorexics (43)
Body Parts Satisfaction Questionnaire (BPSQ) Developed by Berscheid et al. and modified by Gleghorn et al., 1987 (42)	Modified version has 25 items, uses 7-point Likert scale	High internal consistency (Cronbach's alpha): 0.92 Good convergent correlations with other affective measure of body image Construct validity: known groups technique showed statistically significant differences between normal and bulimic individuals: $F(1,108) = 91.06$, $p < 0.001$ (42)
Body Cathexis Scales Developed by Secord and Jourard (44)	Measures body cathexis (45) (degree of self-reported satisfaction with one's own body) 2 scales: body cathexis scale (46 items); self-cathexis (general self-satisfaction); sum of scores indicates body esteem Use expanded to include patients with multiple sclerosis (28), older adults (34), and others	Split-half reliability ($r = 0.81$) (46) Unidimensional, "tight internal structure" when 51-item version used; recommended use in researching role of body feelings in self-concept and personality Moderately good test–retest reliability; contains 3–4 factors (43)
Secord and Jourard Modified Body Cathexis Questionnaire (45)	Modified to include 12 body parts, each rated on a 7-point scale (1 "strong, positive feeling" to 7 "strong negative feeling") Scoring: total score divided by 12 to give final score (1–7)	Internal consistency (all subscales), Cronbach's alpha: 0.74 (27)
Body Esteem Scale (BES) Developed by Franzoi and Shields (47)	36 items (23 original Body Cathexis scale items plus 12 new) Body esteem shown to be multidimensional construct differing for males and females Female subscales sound and meaningful, offer potentially useful method for assessing body image in high-risk populations (48)	Factor analysis: Clusters of variables (men: physical attractiveness, upper body strength, physical condition; females: sexual attractiveness, weight concern, physical condition) Cronbach's alpha: 0.78–0.87 Convergent validity: moderate correlation between self-esteem on Rosenberg Self-Esteem Scale and each of 3 body esteem subscales of BES Discriminant validity established: Wilkes lambda stepwise selection method: "weight concern subscale" discriminates anorexic females from nonanorexic (lambda = 0.86, $p < 0.001$, canonical correlation = 0.37); same means of analysis for male

Instrument	Description	Psychometric Properties
Secord Homonym Test (49)	Word-association technique eliciting associations to a recited list of 100 homonyms, each with meanings pertaining to body parts/processes or nonbody meanings Also includes stimulus words Score is number of body reference responses given Taps changes in unconscious body involvement (50)	data: upper-body subscale differentiated male weightlifters from nonweightlifters (lambda = 0.90, $p < 0.01$, canonical correlation = 0.34) (47, 48) Interrater reliability: 0.95 Test–retest reliability: 0.94 Split-half reliability: 0.85 (48)
Body–Self Relations Questionnaire (BSRQ) (51, 52)	Subscale of Multidimensional Body–Self Relations Questionnaire (MBSRQ) (51) 54-item scale using 5-point Likert format ("definitely agree" to "definitely disagree") Measures attitude toward body image related to physical appearance, fitness, health 3 dimensions of attitude: cognitive, affective, behavioral	Cronbach's alpha: 0.83–0.92 Test–retest reliabilities (over 1 month): 0.85–0.91 (53) Convergent and discriminant validity established Factor analysis: 7-factor, stable structure consistent for males and females (52)
Body Shape Questionnaire (BSQ) Developed by Cooper et al. (54)	Measures concerns about body shape, especially "feeling fat" (features of body image distortion) in both bulimia and anorexia nervosa 34-item scale, using a 6-point format ("never" to "always") Subjects asked to respond about feelings toward their appearance over last 4 weeks Valid measure of body shape concerns (55, 56)	Validated using 4 samples of women (bulimics, attending family planning clinic, occupational therapy students, undergraduate students) Concurrent validity: moderate to high correlations between BSQ, Eating Disorder Inventory (EDI), and Eating Attitudes Test (EAT) among bulimic patients and students Discriminant validity established (54)
Physical Appearance Related Teasing Scale (PARTS) Developed by Thompson et al. (57)	Measures role teasing plays in development of negative body image and eating disorders 18-item scale, using a 5-point format ("never" to "frequently") 2 subscales: Weight/Size Teasing Scale (W/ST), General Appearance Teasing Scale (GAT)	Internal consistency reliability (coefficient alpha): 0.91 (W/ST) and 0.71 (GAT) Test–retest reliability: 0.86 (W/ST), 0.87 (GAT) Convergent and discriminant validity established: (1) strong relationship between teasing about weight/size and adult eating disturbances and body image dysfunction, (2) GAT statistically significant predictor of bulimic behavior (57)
Ben-Tovim Body Attitudes Questionnaire (BAQ) Developed by Ben-Tovim and Walker (58)	Measures broad range of body-related attitudes held by women 44-item questionnaire 6-factors: feelings of fatness, feelings of disgust with body, perceived physical strength/fitness, importance of weight and shape in one's life, perceived physical attractiveness, feeling of lower-body fatness	Normed with large sample of community women ($n = 504$) Factor analysis: 6 factors Kuder-Richardson reliability: 0.92 Test–retest reliability (4-week period): 0.83 Good convergent validity with existing instruments (58)

Appendix 16A. Important Questionnaires and Scales Used in the Measurement of Body Image Dimensions (*cont.*)

Instrument	Description	Psychometric Indices
Body Image Avoidance Questionnaire (BIAQ) Developed by Rosen et al. (8)	Body image viewed as multidimensional construct where negative body image expressed by dysfunctional behaviors related to grooming, dressing, socialization 19-item questionnaire, using 6-point scale Instrument may yield information "above and beyond typical attitudinal measures of body image" (8)	Internal consistency reliability (Cronbach's alpha): 0.89 Test–retest reliability (2 weeks): 0.87 Concurrent validity established: self-reported behavioral avoidance strongly associated with negative attitudes towards weight and shape (Body Shape Questionnaire): $r(351) = 0.78, p < 0.001$ (8) Discriminant validity: discriminates between bulimic and normal subjects (8)
Baird Body Image Assessment Tool (BBIAT) Developed by Baird (33)	11-item assessment tool Copy of instrument found in *Orthopaedic Nursing* (33)	Interrater reliability: adequate for 6/11 items Validation: preliminary work done by comparing to standard Further testing warranted
Body Image Reintegration Tool (BIRT) Developed by Droughton and Verbic (36)	13-item tool, intended to determine whether certain nursing interventions corrected or minimized patients' alterations in body image Yes/no response to description of patient outcomes expected to occur if nursing interventions successful Intervention successful if 11 or more out of 13 responses positive 4 weeks after hospital discharge	No reliability or validity data reported.
Body Image and Body Change Inventory Developed by Ricciardelli & McCabe (21)	Consists of 3 subscales: Body dissatisfaction (7 items that assess attitudes to 7 body parts), strategies to decrease weight (6 items), and strategies to increase muscles (6 items)	Adequate internal consistency and test–retest reliability for all 3 scales. Confirmatory factor analysis; concurrent and discriminant validity demonstrated by authors (21)
Body Image Quality of Life Inventory Developed by Cash & Fleming (59)	19-item questionnaire using a 7-point bipolar scale measures positive and negative results of body image on feelings about self, life in general, sexual relations, eating, exercise, grooming, and family and work/school situations	Internal consistency reliability (Cronbach's alpha): 0.95 Test–retest reliability: 0.79 Convergent validity: significant correlation with several measures of body image evaluation (59)

Eating Behaviors and Body Image Test for Preadolescent Girls Developed by Candy & Fee (60)	Assesses the onset of problem eating and body image disturbances in preadolescent girls; 38-item, Likert-type scale indicating degree to which the subject engaged in the behaviors 2 subscales: Body Image Dissatisfaction/Restrictive Eating subscale (BID/RE) and Binge Eating Behaviors (BEB)	Internal consistency reliability (Cronbach's alpha): 0.91 (BID/RE) and 0.75 (BEB) Test–retest reliability: 0.90 (BID/RE) and 0.79 (BEB) Factor analysis: 2 factors Initial validity established by moderate to strong correlation with Body Image Silhouettes and sociodemographic variables (60)
Media Influence Scale (MIS) Developed by Polce-Lynch, et al. (61)	Assesses how adolescents' thoughts and feelings about their physical appearance is affected by movies, television, and advertisements 12-item instrument that uses a Likert-type scale (1 "never" to 4 "always"); high total score indicates that media affects perceptions of physical appearance	Internal consistency reliability (Cronbach's alpha): 0.88 (62)
Body Image Scale for Cancer Patients Developed by Hopwood et al. (63)	A short body image scale developed for use in clinical trials 10-item scale using a 4-point Likert scale, with "0" meaning "not at all" and "3" meaning "very much"	High internal consistency reliability (Cronbach's alpha): 0.93 Clinical validity: all items fulfilled the response criteria Discriminant validity: statistically significant differences between women treated with mastectomy compared with those who received conservative surgery ($p < 0.001$) (63)

Numbers in parentheses correspond to studies cited in the References.

Appendix 16B. Important Techniques to Measure Body Image

Instrument	Description	Psychometric Indices
Color-a-Person Body Dissatisfaction Test (CAPT) Developed by Wooley and Roll, 1991 (64)	2 gender-appropriate drawings (front and side views of human body) are shown to subjects Subjects asked to indicate level of satisfaction/dissatisfaction with 16 body parts by coloring the 2 drawings: red, very dissatisfied; yellow, dissatisfied; black, neutral; green, satisfied; blue, very satisfied 3 scores calculated: CAPT total (mean of all 16 parts), CAPT score I (mean of abdomen, hips, buttocks, thighs), CAPT score II (mean of remaining parts)	Test-retest reliability: 0.72–0.89 (2- to 4-week intervals, no gender differences) Cronbach's alphas (all): 0.70–0.88 (both normal and subjects with eating disorders) Validity established by correlation with Secord and Jourard's Body Cathexis Scale and Rosenberg's Self-esteem Scale Factor analysis/varimax rotation for 3 groups (female, male college students, eating disorder patients): face, extremities, torso (64)
Askevold Method for Measuring Body Image (Image Marking) (65)	Subject asked to draw specific marks: to measure accuracy of determining dimensions in general; to identify specified body parts while imagining self in mirror (body height, acromioclavicular joints, narrowest waist width, femoral trochanter bones) Investigator assists in marking as well as noting differences in position of actual body parts compared to those marked	Discriminates best between anorexics and controls as compared to video monitor procedure and movable caliper procedure (66) Reliability and validity (tested with group of bulimic and normal women): reliability 0.72–0.92; construct validity (multitrait-multimethod matrix): met 2 of 3 standards (67) Recent evidence suggests Image Marking may reflect error variance rather than meaningful assessments of body width (68)
Direct Measurement of Perceived Body Size Developed by Dillon (69)	Directly measures visually perceived body height, width, depth Device constructed of wooden beams; subject asked to adjust beams to form a doorway they can just fit through; subjects estimate dimensions during 10 sessions (vertical, then horizontal, ascending, and descending estimates)	Error of estimate (estimate minus actual measure): no systematic variation except for estimate of knee height (70) Test-retest reliability: 0.85–0.95 Validity coefficients: 0.00–0.95 (significant for full height, mouth height, shoulder height, r = 0.95) Gradual increase in reliability and validity as estimate progressed from knee to full height (70)
Slade and Russell Moving Caliper Technique (71)	Apparatus consists of 2 lights mounted on horizontal bar; subjects asked to adjust the lights to estimate the dimensions of body regions Estimates compared to actual dimensions and expressed as ratio or index (perceived × 100 divided by real): 100 corresponds to accurate, < 100 shows underestimation of physical size, > 100 shows overestimation	Variable reliability estimates (0.25–0.94) (72) Discriminates well between anorexic and normal subjects (42, 66) Correlates well with other perceptual measures of body image (42)

Instrument	Description	Reliability/Validity
Body Image Detection Device (BIDD) Developed by Ruff and Barrios (73)	Modification of Slade and Russell's technique Overhead projector, projecting a 1-cm-wide horizontal band of light used by subjects to estimate widths of 5 body parts by adjusting beam of light 2 measures: Body Perception Index (BPI): difference between actual and perceived body dimensions; Subjective Rating Index (SRI): subjective rating of weight status assigned by the subject to each body site (74)	Respectable reliability for both measures coefficient alphas: BPI, 0.83–0.93; SRI, 0.79–0.81. Test–retest: BPI, 0.75–0.92; SRI, 0.60–0.93 Validity studies inconsistent (74)
Fawcett Measure of Perceived Body Space Originally developed by Schlachter, then modified by Fawcett and Chodil (75)	54-inch square sheet of opaque yellow ochre vinyl on which are superimposed concentric circles ranging in diameter from 11 to 54 inches: each circle is 1 inch larger than the preceding one; each circle is designated by a 2-digit random number; subject asked to position self in center circle and to identify circle that represents space body occupies	Has face validity Test–retest reliability coefficients: 0.89 (3-hour interval) 0.74 (1 week) (27) Requires further testing
Allebeck et al. Apparatus for Measuring Disturbances in Size and Shape (76)	Picture of subject or external object displayed on TV monitor; subject adjusts size and height/width proportions Deviations from correct measures read directly by electrical instrumentation	Respectable reliability estimates (56): internal consistency (Cronbach's alpha): 0.87–0.97; test–retest: eating disorder subjects ($r = 0.91$), normal subjects ($r = 0.83$) Validity unclear; does not discriminate between anorexic and control groups (66)
Video Camera Developed by Collins (77)	Polaroid picture of subject distorted by videocamera to provide range of representations from thin to obese Subjects asked to change image on TV screen to match own image of their body	Test–retest reliability (67): 0.83–0.96 (5 consecutive assessments of body image 10 minutes apart); 0.63 (24 hours apart); 0.61 (8 weeks apart) Limited data on construct validity (77, 78)
Body Image Assessment (BIA) Developed by Williamson et al. (79)	Inexpensive, simple measure of body image disturbances in women Subject selects silhouette of female body frames perceived to resemble own current and ideal body size 3 scores: Current Body Size Score (CBS), Ideal Body Size (3- to 8-week interval) Score (IBS), discrepancy score	Reliability and validity data obtained from large sample ($n = 659$) of eating disorder and normal subjects Test–retest reliability: CBS, discrepancy scores: 0.72–0.93 (1- to 8-week interval); IBS: 0.60 Validity: correlates well with 2 other measures of eating disorders; discriminates between eating disorder patients and normals (79) Further studies warranted

Appendix 16B. Important Techniques to Measure Body Image (*cont.*)

Instrument	Description	Psychometric Indices
Body Image Photo Technique (BIPT) Developed by Popkess-Vawter & Banks (35)	Uses videotapes of the subject's front, back, and side views wearing a blouse and slacks. Subjects complete a semantic differential composed of 15 bipolar adjectives related to body image before and after viewing their 1-minute videotape.	Internal consistency reliability (Cronbach's alpha): 0.80 (pre) and 0.90 (post) Test–retest reliability: 0.60 (pre) and 0.81 (post) Construct validity: moderate correlation with body image Tennessee Self-Concept Scale (80, 35)
Body Rating Scales for Adolescent Females (BRS) Developed by Sherman, et al. (81)	Simple method to assess body size distortion in adolescent girls; includes 2 scales modified from the Figure Rating Scale (FRS), (82) one representing preadolescent girls (BRS11) and the other adolescent girls (BRS17); each scale includes nine figures ranging from thin to fat.	High intercorrelations among raters and scales and between body ratings and the body mass index (81)
Child Figure Drawings Developed by Collins (83)	Simple method to assess body size distortion in boys and girls [modified from the Figure Rating Scale (FRS) (82) consists of a series of seven figures; one scale for boys, one for girls. Figures progress from very thin to very obese; subjects asked to use the figure scale to make five figure selections	Test–retest reliability: range from 0.38 to 0.71 for the 5 selections Further reliability and validity testing is required (83)

Numbers in parentheses correspond to studies cited in the References.

17

Measuring Sexuality: Physiologic, Psychologic, and Relationship Dimensions

Margaret Chamberlain Wilmoth (formerly Metcalfe) with Angela D. Berry

Human sexuality is an integral aspect of quality of life, yet it is distinct enough to be studied as a separate entity. A frequently cited definition of human sexuality comes from the World Health Organization: "the integration of somatic, emotional, intellectual, and social aspects of sexual being in ways that are enriching and that enhance personality, communication, and love."[1]

Sexuality is a complex construct that has historically defied a precise theoretical definition. This lack of a theoretical definition has complicated efforts to develop measures that clearly operationalize the construct and facilitate systematic study of human sexuality. Sexuality has been of scholarly interest since the time of Hippocrates,[2] with more formal study beginning with authors such as Havelock Ellis[3] and Krafft-Ebing.[4] Measurement of the construct began in earnest with the publication of Kinsey's[5,6] work and that of Masters and Johnson.[7] Human sexuality is a complex construct, too complex to be examined in its entirety. Thus, research generally examines a subcomponent of human sexuality, such as sexual response, sexual activity, sexual functioning, sexual behaviors, or body image, level of satisfaction, and frequency of sexual activity. Regardless of what aspect of human sexuality is studied, it is critical that the theoretical definition of the component under study is linked to the way it is operationalized or measured for the study results to have any validity or applicability.

Human sexuality can be viewed as the degree of maleness or femaleness in a person's personality and physique. Our sexuality also influences how we act and react to our world, ourselves, and each other. Sexuality and resultant sexual behavior are a composite of physiologic, intrapsychic, interpersonal, and sociocultural phenomena. The physiologic

[1]*Acknowledgment:* The work of the original chapter (1986) was supported in part by National Cancer Institute predoctoral training grant 1F31 CA08000.

dimension represents the function of the organs involved in the biology of the sexual response, commonly referred to as the sexual response cycle. The intrapsychic or psychologic dimension represents the private experience of sexual functioning, including knowledge and attitudes about sexuality, level of sexual satisfaction, sexual fantasies, gender role definition, body image, sexual experience, and basically how an individual defines himself or herself as a sexual being. The interpersonal dimensions represent the nature and degree of social, interactive sexual behavior. The sociocultural dimension includes values, traditions, roles, and customs related to sexuality of ethnic groups and cultures.

Research on Human Sexuality

Current research on the construct of human sexuality includes work from the sociologic, anthropologic, and psychologic perspectives, as well as from the health care professions. Levels of study can be viewed as occurring from the macro- to the microlevel. The macrolevel includes broad social and cultural issues. Methods used by this level of study are beyond the scope of this chapter. Midlevel study, which is covered here, includes research into interpersonal and psychologic aspects of sexuality, and the micro level of study focuses on physiologic, hormonal, and anatomic aspects of sexuality. Techniques used in studying the microlevel of sexuality are also beyond the scope of this chapter.

Sociocultural Research

Sociocultural research uses anthropologic methods, such as ethnography and field studies, to describe sexual scripts in differing cultures. Surveys are also used to describe social norms of sexual behavior; those done by Kinsey and associates are well-known examples.[5,6] Examples of cultural sexual scripts are gender role behaviors, use of circumcision, and views of same-gender relationships.

Interpersonal and Psychologic Research

Psychologic research in sexuality involves psychometric documentation of affect, libido, knowledge, and attitudes toward sexual function and sexual experience. Psychologic research not only has drawn on standard and well-established psychologic testing methods but also has begun to generate valid and reliable instruments designed specifically to measure the personal or intrapsychic dimensions of sexuality.[8-10]

Research on the interpersonal aspects of sexuality addresses the sexual adjustment of couples. Measurement of sexuality as it relates to dyads is less well developed than either physiologic or psychologic methodologies. Nonpsychometric surveys of interpersonal components of sexuality abound and in general consist of tools for assessment, counseling, and discussion involving premarital, marital, and family interventions in nonresearch settings. Such tools were not intended to be used for scientific investigation, and little, if any, psychometric data are available on them.

Physiologic, Hormonal, and Anatomic Research

Physiologic research on sexuality occurs in the laboratory setting at either the cellular, hormonal, or vascular level, using techniques that are beyond the scope of this chapter.

Neurovascular Research

Neurovascular research pertains to mechanisms underlying autonomic innervation (glandular and smooth-muscle function); regulation by central nervous system structures (e.g., the limbic system) and neurotransmitters (e.g., peptides and monoamines); and hemodynamics.

Physiologic Research

Physiologic research typically uses the sexual response cycle as the paradigm for study. The sexual response cycle was first identified by Masters and Johnson[7] as comprising 4 phases: excitement, plateau, orgasm, and resolution. It has been modified by Kaplan[11] to three phases: desire, arousal, and orgasm. Physiologic research also deals with the grossly observable outcomes of neurovascular mechanisms. Traditionally, this has entailed measuring autonomically mediated effects on such parameters as heart rate, blood pressure, respiration, skin conduction, and papillary response. Such indices are generally not considered sufficiently sensitive or discriminating. Instead, genital measures seem to distinguish sexual arousal from other emotional states more reliably. For example, erectile function in males, including determination of penile tumescence, has been demonstrated to correlate with self-reports of sexual arousal. Pelvic vascular competency in male sexual arousal also has been investigated. Alternatively, psychophysiologic research on female sexual response has included measurement of vaginal lubrication and acidity, labia minora temperature, clitoral engorgement, and genital vasoconstriction during sexual arousal.[12]

Gonadal Research

Sexuality as reflected by gonadal function has been approached through endocrine studies (e.g., circulating levels of gonadal steroids, gonadotropins, prolactin, thyroid-stimulating hormone, and thyroid hormones), fertility evaluation (e.g., menstrual history, contraceptive use, gonadal biopsy, semen evaluation), physical assessment of the genitalia and secondary sexual characteristics, and clinical manipulation of the endocrine milieu (e.g., endocrine ablation or replacement therapies).[13]

A great deal of attention has been focused in recent years on the effects of menopause and aging on sexuality. These effects are physiologic, interpersonal, intrapersonal, and sociocultural in nature. The use of hormone replacement therapies continues to be controversial and of interest across the health professions. Research in this area is most comprehensively studied using a combination of physiologic and self-report measures.

Human Sexuality in Illness and Disability

Any illness involving distress, fatigue, pain, fear, anxiety, or depression may affect sexuality.[14] Pathology that impairs anatomic structures alters sexual function and may negatively affect the sexual response cycle. Sexual drive, however, may still persist in the presence of altered sexual functioning, regardless of etiology. Many individuals live full sexual lives in the context of their chronic illness, but little is known about the prevalence and type of sexual difficulties or dysfunctions experienced with many chronic illnesses. Medications are another common source of sexual functioning difficulty, and their use should be assessed with any measure of psychologic and interpersonal sexuality. Many measures developed to assess sexuality in illness and disability are specific to that particular disease state, with no "healthy" norms on which to base analysis. Thus, it is often difficult to determine the degree of sexual difficulty or disability specifically caused by the disease. Furthermore, few health professionals are prepared to assist their patients in dealing with the impact of chronic disease on sexuality.

Sexuality Education

Sexuality education remains a controversial topic in both public and higher education. Health professionals are legally obligated to provide full disclosure of the risks and benefits of any intervention; this implies disclosure related to sexuality and sexual functioning. Thus, health professionals require sexuality education as it relates to disease, treatments, and medications. Educational programs must be evaluated for their ability to positively influence knowledge and subsequent behaviors.

Classic Measures of Sexuality

Sexual Performance Evaluation Questionnaire of the Marriage Council of Philadelphia

Interviews are a commonly used method of obtaining information related to sexual issues. A particularly comprehensive interview guideline is that based on the Sexual Performance Evaluation Questionnaire of the Marriage Council of Philadelphia.[15] Useful in obtaining a sexual history, the lines of inquiry addressed are under the major topic headings of childhood sexuality; onset of adolescence; orgasmic experiences; feelings about self as masculine or feminine; sexual fantasies and dreams; dating; engagement; marriage; extramarital sex; sex after widowhood, separation, or divorce; sexual deviations; certain effects of sex activities; and use of erotic material. A related sexual performance evaluation outline covers investigation of specific characteristics of an individual's coital activities.

Participation in an interview can be a therapeutic experience for an individual. This method of data collection, however, is very time consuming, and the resulting findings are often difficult to quantify. Research conclusions obtained in this way can become extremely tenuous. However, such data can describe phenomena from which concepts can be identified that can lead to the development of more quantifiable instruments.

Derogatis Sexual Function Inventory (DSFI)

The most comprehensive and thoroughly evaluated psychometric instrument to measure sexual function is the Derogatis Sexual Function Inventory (DSFI).[16,17] On the assumption that sexuality consists of multiple behavioral domains, 10 constructs are operationalized in the subscales of the 245-item DSFI, as follows: (1) information (sexual knowledge); (2) experience (sexual behavior); (3) drives (biologically determined and subject to neuroendocrine control); (4) sexual attitudes (liberal versus conservative); (5) psychologic symptoms (such as obsessive-compulsiveness or somatization); (6) affect (such as depression, anxiety, or guilt); (7) gender role definition or identity (relative masculinity or femininity is conceived along a continuum); (8) sexual fantasy (rehearsal and vicarious fulfillment or expression of sexual drives); (9) body image (self-evaluation of physical attractiveness as well as the reflected perceptions of others); and (10) satisfaction (sexual frequency and novelty, achievement of orgasm, communication between partners).

These constructs are designed to permit valid clinical prediction of current sexual functional status and provide conceptual clarity in deliberations on the nature and breadth of human sexuality as a component of personality and biologic function.

The DSFI has been well tested in a broad variety of populations, including male and female heterosexuals, homosexuals, transsexuals, and sexually dysfunctional individuals. Test–retest reliabilities for the 10 subscales range from 0.42 to 0.96. Internal consistency reliability coefficients range from 0.56 to 0.97. Predictive validity of the DSFI has been demonstrated in populations of individuals having sexual dysfunctions and their partners and in populations consisting of male and female transsexuals. Normed scores from 200 normal and 200 sexually dysfunctional individuals also are available. Factor analysis based on a group of 380 patient and nonpatient subjects revealed seven empirical dimensions that underlie the DSFI: (1) body image, (2) psychologic distress, (3) heterosexual drive, (4) autoeroticism, (5) gender role, (6) sexual satisfaction, and (7) sexual precociousness.

The other psychometric instruments described in this chapter lack the comprehensiveness of the DSFI and instead focus more on the dimensions of human sexuality they endeavor to quantify. Except where specified by a certain technique, such as factor analysis, the dimensions measured reflect the conceptual framework of the researcher.

National Survey of Sexual Attitudes and Lifestyles

This British survey of sexual attitudes and lifestyles has been done twice—once in 1990 and again in 2000. The survey covered topics such as family and learning about sex, first sexual experiences, sources and use of contraceptives, attitudinal questions, sexual practices, sexually transmitted diseases, sexual dysfunction, cohabitation history, and demographic questions.[18]

Measuring Sexuality

The literature has been reviewed for sexual assessment measures from a broad variety of perspectives and is organized according to their originally intended use. This chapter reflects a relatively thorough treatment of human sexuality research instrumentation, with emphasis on research done at the midlevel of study (psychologic and interpersonal). However, the discipline of the study of human sexuality is developing rapidly and new instruments or adaptations of available instruments to different subject populations are continually in progress. Appendix A gives six critical reviews of sexuality literature.

Organization of Appendices

Evaluation of Sexuality Curricula

Several instruments have been developed specifically to determine the effects of sex education programs on changes in the sexual knowledge and attitudes of participants. In these settings, success is judged by an increase in sexual knowledge or a change in attitudes reflecting greater permissiveness. Five instruments are presented with psychometric indices in Appendix 17B. Other available measures are summarized in Appendix 17C.

Psychologic and Interpersonal Research

Sexual Experience, Knowledge, or Attitudes

A number of instruments that assess the different components of sexual experience, knowledge, or attitudes have reported reliability and validity information and are accessible to researchers. These tools were designed for use in clinical and research settings with normal and dysfunctional individuals. Additional measures of this component of the psychologic dimension of sexuality are summarized in Appendix 17C.

Measures of Gender Role Definition and Attitudes

Sexual orientation and sexual roles are viewed from three perspectives: gender role definition, gender identity, and sexual deviancy. Appendix 17D lists the most commonly used instruments.

Measures of Sexual Dysfunction

Sexual dysfunction is a broad concept that can encompass both physiologic and psychologic components. Approaches to the medical evaluation of infertility or sterility have been described, as well as problems with sexual performance or response. This discussion is limited to psychometric determination of the nature and extent of an individual's sexual health. Four important measures are described in Appendix 17E.

Instruments Used to Measure Body Perception

Body perception or image is an integral component of an individual's sexuality and can make a significant contribution to sexual health or dysfunction. Because of the growing recognition of and interest in body image disturbance among people with physical illness and disability, it is given separate consideration here. Major instruments are detailed in Appendix 17F.

Measures of the Interpersonal Dimension of Sexuality

Measures of the interpersonal dimensions of sexuality address marital or dyadic characteristics, including a range of parameters and indicators of adjustment and satisfaction. Measures of this dimension of sexuality are summarized in Appendix 17G.

Measures of Sexuality Used in Special Populations

Research into the demands imposed on one's sexuality by the presence of physical illness is being conducted by researchers in a wide variety of disciplines. To illustrate the form this has taken in different realms of clinical expertise, efforts to assess the psychosexual impacts in the presence of several types of chronic illness are briefly presented in Appendix 17H.

Summary

Psychometric instrumentation in the field of sexuality is becoming increasingly sophisticated and complex. The growing recognition of sexuality as a critical component of quality of life has permitted evolution in measurement of the construct. Critical to validity of research findings is the requirement for researchers to link the theoretical definition with operationalization of the subconcept of sexuality being studied. Without this linkage, it is nearly impossible to say findings have any valid clinical application.

The preceding discussion of instruments available for the measurement of issues related to sexuality is fairly extensive both in breadth and depth of inquiry. Rigor in psychometric evaluation of tools is essential before widespread use in either clinical or research application. A common concern for many instruments is that they have typically been normed on college students and have had limited validation with other populations, such as a variety of ages, genders, orientations, educational backgrounds, and socioeconomic classes. Also left out are those who are culturally divergent and those who are dealing with acute and chronic illness and its impact on their sexuality. Controlled studies using the different instruments with different populations are needed to test reliability and validity. At the same time, researchers will be able to define more clearly the issues around sexuality that are most important to those they wish to serve.

Since the 1960s the groundwork has been laid not only to question the concepts and issues of sexuality, but also to provide an atmosphere of sensitivity, awareness, and openness that allows for scientific and conscientious study of an individual's sense of his or her sexuality and what affects it in what way. However, there are possible limitations to research in the field of sexuality. First, because of the sensitive nature of sexuality, it often is quite difficult to obtain objective data from the subject or partner. Some people are unwilling to participate in research related to sexual matters because of embarrassment, denial, fear, or a desire for privacy. Similarly, people who have sexual problems and are seeking help may self-select to participate in such studies, thus creating a biased sample. Some subjects may respond to inquiries based on what they suppose to be the desirable or socially acceptable response because of reluctance to reveal unusual or unconventional sexual values and practices.

Still it is hoped that this chapter has provided enough depth to meet the interests of those who would wish to continue the work that has been started in this field. Some of the instruments, though begun as a research tool, are also quite useful as part of an assessment package designed to identify problems and help individuals with specific issues.

Exemplar Studies

Rudy, E.B., & Estok, P.J. Running addiction and dyadic adjustment. *Res Nurs Health*, 1990, *13*:219-225.

This study exemplifies the use of the Dyadic Adjustment Scale by Spainer to determine the effects of runner's addiction, as described by the Runners Addiction Scale, on the relationship of the individual and his or her spouse. The sample was 45% of a group of runners who had just completed a marathon, with an almost equal sample of males and females and an age range from 25 to 71. The study concept was well researched and led logically to this comparison. A Pearson's product moment correlation was used to determine the relationship between addiction and dyadic adjustment. Dependent *t*-tests were used to analyze the differences between spouses. This study extended the work of Spainer by using the tool with both members of a marital dyad instead of a single member, as had been done previously. The authors showed that there is no significant difference between the members, which supports the accuracy of using the instrument with only one member of a dyad.

Wilmoth, M.C., & Townsend, J. A comparison of the effects of lumpectomy versus mastectomy on sexual behaviors. *Cancer Practice*, 1995, *3*:279-285.

This study exemplifies the use of the Wilmoth Sexual Behaviors Questionnaire—Female by Wilmoth and Tingle in measuring the impact of breast cancer on sexuality and the measure's sensitivity in distinguishing between women who underwent mastectomy versus lumpectomy. The sample comprised 165 women, the majority of whom were Caucasian. Women were between 6 months and 10 years post diagnosis and had received adjuvant therapy in addition to the primary surgical treatment for their disease. Findings indicate that no significant difference existed in sexuality between women treated by lumpectomy and those treated by mastectomy. Women who had received chemotherapy as adjuvant treatment experienced a more negative impact on sexual behaviors regardless of the surgical approach. Other factors with a significant positive effect on sexuality included a history of minimal alcohol use and tamoxifen use. This study exemplifies the importance of using a validated measure with congruence between theoretical and operational definitions of the construct being studied.

References

1. World Health Organization. *Education and treatment in human sexuality: The training of health professionals.* Technical Report Series No. 572. Geneva: WHO, 1975.
2. Westheimer, R.K., & Lopater, S. *Human sexuality: A psychosocial perspective.* Philadelphia: Lippincott & Williams, 2002.
3. Ellis, H. *Studies in the psychology of sex.* Philadelphia: FA Davis, 1900.
4. Krafft-Ebing, R. Van. *Psychopathia sexualis.* Brooklyn, NY: Physicians and Surgeons Book Company, 1906.
5. Kinsey, A.C., Pomeray, W.B., & Martin, C.E. *Sexual behavior in the human male.* Philadelphia: Saunders, 1948.
6. Kinsey, A.C., et al. *Sexual behavior in the human female.* Philadelphia: Saunders, 1953.
7. Masters, W.H., & Johnson, V.E. *Human sexual functioning.* Boston: Little, Brown & Co., 1966.
8. Davis, C.M., Yarber, W.L., Schreer, G., & Davis, S.L. *Handbook of sexuality-related measures.* Thousand Oaks, CA: Sage, 2002.
9. Talmadge, L.D., & Talmadge, W.C. Sexuality assess-

ment measures for clinical use: A review. *Am J Fam Ther*, 1990, *18*(1):80-105.

10. Daker-White, G. Reliable and valid self-report outcome measures in sexual (dys)function: A systematic review. *Arch Sex Behav*, *31*(2):197-210.

11. Kaplan, H.S. *The new sex therapy: Active treatment of sexual dysfunctions*. New York: Brunner/Mazel, Publishers, 1974.

12. Whipple, B. Beyond the G spot: New research on human female sexual anatomy and physiology. *Scand J Sexology*, 2000, *3*(2):35-42.

13. Schiavi, R.C., & Schreiner-Engel, P. Physiologic aspects of sexual function and dysfunction. *Psychiatr Clin North Am*, 1980, *3*(1):81.

14. Sipski, M.L., & Alexander, C. J. *Sexual function in people with disability and chronic illness*. Gaithersburg, MD: Aspen, 1997.

15. Group for the Advancement of Psychiatry. *Assessment of sexual function: A guide to interviewing*. New York: Jason Aronson, 1974.

16. Derogatis, L.R. Psychological assessment of psychosexual function. *Psychiatr Clin North Am*, 1980, *3*(1):113.

17. Derogatis, L.R., & Melisaratos, N. The DSFI: A multi-dimensional measure of sexual functioning. *J Sex Mar Ther*, 1979, *5*(3):244-280.

18. Johnson, A.M., Mercer, C. H., Erens, B., et al. Sexual behavior in Britain: Partnerships, practices, and HIV risk behaviors. *Lancet*, 2001, *358*(9296):1835-1842.

19. Hoon, E.F., Hoon, P.W., & Wincze, J.P. An inventory for the measurement of female sexual arousability: The SAI. *Arch Sex Behav*, 1976, *5*(4):291-300.

20. Chambless, D.L., & Lifshitz, J.L. Self-reported sexual and anxiety arousal: The expanded Sexual Arousability Inventory. *J Sex Res*, 1984, *20*(3):241-254.

21. Allen, R.M., & Haupt, T.D. The Sex Inventory: Test–retest reliabilities of scale scores and items. *J Clin Psychol*, 1966, *22*(4):367-386.

22. Thorne, F.C. The Sex Inventory. *J Clin Psychol*, 1966, *22*(4):367-374.

23. Perkel, A.K. Development and testing of the AIDS Psychosocial Scale. *Psychol Rep*, 1992, *71*:767-778.

24. Quirk, F.H., Heiman, J.R., Rosen, R.C., et al. Development of a sexual function questionnaire for clinical trials of female sexual dysfunction. *J Women's Health Gender-Based Med*, 2002, *11*(3):277-290.

25. Lief, H.I., Fullard, W., & Devlin, S.J. A new measure of adolescent sexuality: SKAT-A. *J Sex Educ Ther*, 1990, *16*(2):79-91.

26. Snell, W.E., Jr., Fisher, T.D., & Miller, R.S. Development of the Sexual Awareness Questionnaire: Components, reliability, and validity. *Ann Sex Res*, 1991, *4*:65-92.

27. Snell, W.E., Jr., Belk, S.S., Papini, D.R., & Clark, S. Development and validation of the Sexual Self-Disclosure Scale. *Ann Sex Res*, 1989, *2*:307-334.

28. Miller, W.R., & Lief, H.I. The sex knowledge and attitude test (SKAT). *Arch Sex Behav*, 1979, *5*:282-287.

29. Fisher, S.G., & Levin, D. The sexual knowledge and attitudes of professional nurses caring for oncology patients. *Cancer Nurs*, 1983, *6*(1):55-61.

30. Zuckerman, M., Tushup, R., & Finner, S. Sexual attitudes and experience: Attitude and personality correlates and changes produced by a course in sexuality. *J Consult Clin Psychol*, 1976, *44*(1):7-19.

31. Carey, M.P., Morrison-Beedy, D., & Johnson, B.T. The HIV-Knowledge Questionnaire: Development and evaluation of a reliable, valid, and practical self-administered questionnaire. *AIDS Behav*, 1997, *1*(1):61-74.

32. Bem, S. The measurement of psychological androgyny. *J Consult Clin Psychol*, 1974, *42*(2):155-162.

33. Campbell, T., & James, A. The factor structure of the BEM sex-role inventory (BSRI): Confirmatory analysis of long and short forms. *Educ Psychol Meas*, 1997, *57*(1):118-125.

34. Holt, C.L., & Ellis, J.B. Assessing the current validity of the Bem Sex-Role Inventory. *Sex Roles*, 1998, *39*(11/12):929-941.

35. Sugihara, Y., & Warner, J.A. Endorsements by Mexican-Americans of the Bem sex-role inventory: Cross-ethnic comparison. *Psychol Rep*, 1999, *85*(1):201-211.

36. Hoffman, R.M., & Borders, L.D. Twenty-five years after the Bem Sex-Role Inventory: A reassessment and new issues regarding classification variability. *Meas Eval Counsel Devel*, 2001, *34*(1):39-56.

37. MacDonald, A.P., Jr. Identification and measurement of multidimensional attitudes toward equality between the sexes. *J Homosex*, 1974, *1*(2):165-182.

38. King, L.A., & King, D.W. Validity of the sex-role egalitarian scale: Two replication studies. *Sex Roles*, 1994, *31*(5/6):339-348.

39. McGhee, M.R., Johnson, N., & Liverpool, J. Assessing psychometric properties of the Sex-Role Egalitarianism Scale (SRES) with African Americans. *Sex Roles: J Res*, 2001, *45*(11-12):859-866.

40. Snell, W.E., & Finney, P.D. Interpersonal strategies associated with the discussion of AIDS. *Ann Sex Res*, 1990, *3*:425-451.

41. MacDonald, A.P., Jr., Huggins, J., Young, S., et al. Attitudes toward homosexuality: Preservation of sex morality of the double standard? *J Consult Clin Psychol*, 1973, *40*:161-164.

42. Sambrooks, J.E., & MacCullock, M.J. A modification of the sexual orientation method and an automated technique for presentation and scoring. *Br J Soc Clin Psychol*, 1973, *12*(2):163-174.

43. Berkey, B.R., Perelman-Hall, T., & Kurdek, L.A. The Multidimensional Scale of Sexuality. *J Homosex*, 1990, *19*(4):67-87.

44. Schover, L.R., Friedman, J.M., Weiler, S.J., et al. Multiaxial problem-oriented system for sexual dysfunction. *Arch Gen Psychiatry*, 1982, *39*(5):614-619.

45. Jensen, S.B., & Schover, L.R. Brief sexual counseling for medical patients: A workshop for training professionals. *J Sex Marital Ther*, 1988, *14*(1):13-28.

46. Sondhaus, E.L., Kurtz, R.M., & Strube, M.J. Body attitude, gender, and self-concept: A 30-year perspective. *J Psychol*, 2001, *135*(4):413-430.

47. Snell, W.E., Jr., & Papini, D.R. The Sexuality Scale: An instrument to measure sexual-esteem, sexual-depression, and sexual-preoccupation. *J Sex Res*, 1989, *26*(2):256-263.

48. Koleck, M., Bruchon-Schweitzer, M., Cousson-Gelie, F., Gilliard, J., & Quintard, B. The body-image questionnaire: An extension. *Percept Motor Skills*, 2002, *94*(1):189-196.

49. Freeston, M.H., & Plechaty, M. Reconsideration of the Locke-Wallace Marital Adjustment Test: Is it still

relevant for the 1990s? *Psychol Rep*, 1997, *81*(2):419-434.

50. Foster, A.L. The sexual compatibility test. *J Consult Clin Psychol*, 1977, *45*(2):332-333.

51. Spainer, G.B. Measuring dyadic adjustment: New scales for assessing the quality of marriage and similar dyads. *J Mar Fam*, 1976, *38*(1):15-28.

52. Crane, D.R., & Middleton, K.C. Establishing criterion scores for the Kansas marital satisfaction scale and the revised Dyadic Adjustment Scale. *Am J Fam Ther*, 2000, *28*(1):53-60.

53. Hunsley, J., & Pinsent, C. Construct validity of the short forms of the Dyadic Adjustment Scale. *Fam Rel*, 1995, *44*(3):231-237.

54. Hunsley, J., Best, M., Lefebvre, M., & Vito, D. The seven-item short form of the Dyadic Adjustment Scale: Further evidence for construct validity. *Am J Fam Ther*, 2001, *29*(4):325-335.

55. Reiss, I.L. *The social context of premarital sexual permissiveness*. New York: Holt, Rinehart, & Winston, 1967.

56. Barret-Lennard, G.T. The Relationship Inventory: Later developments and adaptations. *JSAS Catalog of "Selected Documents in Psychology,"* 1978, *8*:68 (MS No. 1732).

57. Gurland, B.J., Yorkston, N.J., Stone, A.R., et al. The Structured and Scaled Interview to Assess Maladjustment (SSIAM). I. Description, rationale and development. *Arch Gen Psychiatr*, 1972, *27*(2):259-263.

58. Gurland, B.J., Yorkston, N.J., Goldberg, K., et al. The Structured and Scaled Interview to Assess Maladaptation (SSIAM). II. Factor analysis, reliability and validity. *Arch Gen Psychiatr*, 1972, *27*(2):264.

59. LoPiccolo, J., & Steger, J. The Sexual Interaction Inventory: A new instrument for assessment of sexual dysfunction. *Arch Sex Behav*, 1974, *3*(6):585-595.

60. McCoy, N.N., & D'Agostino, P.A. Factor analysis of the Sexual Interaction Inventory. *Arch Sex Behav*, 1977, *6*(1):25-35.

61. Vaughn, M.J., & Baier, M.E. Reliability and validity of the Relationship Assessment Scale. *Am J Fam Ther*, 1999, *27*(2):137-147.

62. Van den Broucke, S., Vertommen, H., & Vandereycken, W. Construction and validation of a marital intimacy questionnaire. *Fam Rel*, 1995, *44*(3):285-290.

63. Noller, P. *Nonverbal communication in marital interactions*. Elmsford, NY: Pergamon, 1984.

64. Bienvenue, M.J., Sr. Measurement of marital communication. *Fam Coord*, 1970, *19*(1):26-31.

65. Schaefer, M.T., & Olson, D.H. Assessing intimacy: The PAIR Inventory. *J Mar Fam Ther*, 1981, *7*(1):47-60.

66. Waring, E.M., & Reddon, J.R. The measurement of intimacy in marriage: The Waring Intimacy Questionnaire. *J Clin Psychol*, 1983, *39*(1):53-57.

67. Hatfield, E., & Sprecher, S. Measuring passionate love in intimate relationships. *J Adolesc*, 1986, *9*:383-410.

68. Wilmoth, M.C., & Tingle, L.R. Development and psychometric testing of the Wilmoth sexual behaviors questionnaire-female. *Can J Nurs Res*, 2001, *32*(4):135-151.

69. Waterhouse, J., & Metcalfe, M. Development of the sexual adjustment questionnaire. *Oncol Nurs Forum*, 1986, *13*(3):53-59.

70. Bruner, D.W., Scott, C.B., McGowan, D., et al. The RTOG Modified sexual adjustment questionnaire: Psychometric testing in the prostate cancer population. *Int J Rad Oncol, Phys, Biol*, 1998, *42*(1):202.

71. Althof, S.E., Coffman, C.B., & Levine, S.B. The effects of coronary bypass surgery on female sexual, psychological and vocational adaptation. *J Sex Mar Ther*, 1984, *10*(3):176-184.

72. Molassiotis, A. Measuring psychosexual functioning in cancer patients: Psychometric properties and normative data of a new questionnaire, including commentary by White, I. and Robinson, L. *Eur J Oncol Nurs*, 1998, *2*(4):194-207.

73. Watts, R.J. Sexual functioning, health beliefs and compliance with high blood pressure medications. *Nurs Res*, 1982, *31*(5):278-283.

74. Pieper, B.A., et al. Perceived effect of diabetes on relationship to spouse and sexual function. *J Sex Educ Ther*, 1983, *9*(2):46.

75. Jensen, S.B., & Soren, B. Diabetic sexual dysfunction. A comprehensive study of 16 insulin-treated diabetic men and women—An age matched control group. *Arch Sex Behav*, 1981, *10*:493-504.

76. Jensen, S.B., & Soren, B. Sexual dysfunction in insulin-treated diabetics: A six year follow-up study of 101 patients. *Arch Sex Behav*, 1986, *15*(4):271-283.

77. Rubin, Z. Liking Scale Relationship quality of gay men in closed or open relationships. *Journal of homosexuality*, *12*:85-99.

78. Williams, A.M., & Miller, W.R. The design and use of assessment instruments and procedures for sexuality curricula. In N. Rosenzweig and F.P. Pearsall (Eds.), Sex Education for the health professional: A curriculum guide. New York: Grune & Stratton, 1978, p. 137.

79. Green, R., & Weiner, J. (Eds.). Methodology in sex research. Rockville, MD: DHHS, National Institute of Mental Health, 1981.

Appendix 17A. Critical Reviews of Sexuality

Author	Focus	Comments
Schiavi and Schreiner-Engel (13)	Psychometric instruments and measuring more than 1 aspect of sexual activity and marital interaction with heterosexual individuals and dyads	Early overview; provides names, authors, description of instruments, reliability and validity data
Talmadge and Talmadge (9)	Clinical instruments	Excellent reference: describes usefulness of measures of research
Williams and Miller (78)	Criteria for evaluating effectiveness of curricula on sexuality	9 questionnaires summarized
Green and Wiener (79)	Research issues in the study of human sexuality	Sex and aging, sexual dysfunction, heterosexual relationships, rape, neurobiologic components, homosexuality, psychosexual differentiation addressed
Daker-White (10)	Measures of sexual function and dysfunction	Includes discussion of psychometric properties
Davis et al. (8)	Text of sexual assessment measures with psychometric data and references	Very thorough compendium of broad range of sexual outcome and knowledge measures

Numbers in parentheses correspond to studies cited in the References.

Appendix 17B. Major Instruments Used in Evaluating Sexuality Curricula

Name	Description	Psychometric Indices
Sex Knowledge and Attitude Test (SKAT) (8, 28)	149 items, self-administered Measures sexual knowledge, attitudes, level of experience in sexual activity Attitude section: 4 subscales (sexual myths, heterosexual relations, abortion, autoeroticism) containing 35 Likert-format items Knowledge section: 1 subscale (psychologic, biologic social, psychobiologic), 71 true/false items	Used in wide range of educational settings, including nursing Standardized scores available for comparison (based on results of 850 medical students from 16 U.S. schools tested in 1971)
Sex Knowledge and Attitude Test for Adolescents (SKAT-A) (25)	Comprehensive scale with 3 main sections (knowledge, attitudes, behavior) Identifies behaviors that put adolescent at risk for acquiring/transmitting HIV or becoming parent teenager Knowledge section: 61 items (40 true/false, 21 multiple-choice, randomly placed) Attitude section: 43 statements scored on 5-point Likert scale randomly placed Behavior section: 43 items (yes/no, checklist format)	Factor analysis: 4 subscales in attitude scale (sexual myths, responsibility, sex and its consequences, sexual coercion) Test-retest reliability: 0.804 (knowledge) and 0.916 (attitude scale) Internal consistency: Cronbach's alpha (knowledge): 0.70; (attitude): 0.89 Validity: correlations with KIRBY Knowledge and Attitude scales: 0.41–0.60 (similarities in expected areas) SKAT-A explores important attitudes that other measures do not, "consequences" of behavior and "responsibility" toward others
Human Sexual Knowledge and Attitude Inventory (HSKAI) (29)	Designed for use with nurses 163 items (multiple-choice, true/false forced choice, rating scales) Measures biographic information, sexual attitudes and experience Assesses sexual knowledge	Test-retest reliability: 0.84 Construct validity: (sexual knowledge established by jury rating)
Human Sexuality Questionnaire (HSQ) (8, 30) Developed by Zuckerman et al. (can be used only with authors' permission)	Focuses on the cumulative heterosexual and homosexual experiences Guttman-type behavioral self-report questionnaire Measures sexual experiences and attitudes: 6 experience scales (heterosexual, homosexual, numbers of hetero- or homosexual partners, orgasmic experience, masturbation) Attitudes: scale of items dealing with parental attitudes about children's sexuality and adult heterosexual activities	Coefficients of reproducibility: 0.97 for both males and females Rank-order correlations for male and female items: 0.95 (confirming ordinality of scales, high reliability)
HIV-Knowledge Questionnaire (HIV-K-Q) (8, 31)	Evaluates knowledge about human immunodeficiency virus infection for use in program evaluation 45 items Requires a sixth-grade education Requires 7 minutes to complete	Internally consistent (alpha = 0.91) Test-retest reliability: 0.83–0.91

Numbers in parentheses correspond to studies cited in the References.

Appendix 17C. Instruments Measuring the Psychologic Dimension of Sexuality

Name	Description	Psychometric Indices
Sexuality Arousability Inventory (SAI) (8,19,20)	Self-report of sexual arousability in women Descriptions of 28 sexual activities and situations are rated on a 7-point Likert scale (−1 "adversely affects arousal" to +5 "always causes sexual arousal")	Discriminates between normal and sexually dysfunctional individuals (from middle and upper-middle socioeconomic class) Cross-validation with 2 different samples; coefficient alphas: 0.91, 0.92 Test–retest reliability coefficient: 0.69 (8-week interval)
Sexual Arousability Inventory-Expanded (SAI-E) (20)	Measures amount of arousal and anxiety experienced during specific sexual behaviors Behavioral self-report 28 items, answered once for arousal and once for anxiety (total 56 items) Scored on 7-point Likert scale (−1 "adversely affects arousal/extremely anxiety provoking" to +5 "extremely arousing/relaxing")	Factor analysis: 5 factors (preparation/participation in intercourse, pornography, nongenital sex play, breast stimulation, other sex play) Split-half Spearman-Brown reliability coefficient (females): 0.92 (arousal), 0.94 (anxiety) Can be used with males regardless of sexual orientation or marital status
Sex Inventory (SI) (21,22)	200 true/false items Self-report measure of sexual attitudes and behavior in adult men 9 subscales (sex drive and interest, sexual maladjustment, neurotic conflict, fixation, repression, loss of control, confidence, homosexuality, promiscuity)	Test–retest reliability: 0.40–0.50 (23) Discriminates between normal and clinical groups and among clinical groups
AIDS Psychosocial Scale (23)	Measures self-concept, defenses (denial, repression, rationalization), peer pressure, perceived empowerment (locus of control, self-efficacy) Revised to 28 items, 7 subscales Scored in a 5-point Likert format	Concurrent validity of subscales: eigen values > 1.00 Cronbach's alpha: 0.84
Sexual Function Questionnaire (SFQ) for Heterosexuals (8,24)	Comprehensive measure of sexual functioning 6 sections (biographic, present sexual experience, past experience, intrapersonal factors, interpersonal factors, medical history) 7 domains of female sexual function related to desire, physical arousal-sensation, physical arousal-lubrication, enjoyment, orgasm, pain, and partner relationship	Lacks normative, reliability, and validity data Test–retest reliability: 0.21–0.71 (Quirk) Internal consistency of 7 domains: 0.65–0.91 (Quirk) Discriminant validity and sensitivity established

Appendix 17C. Instruments Measuring the Psychologic Dimension of Sexuality (cont.)

Name	Description	Psychometric Indices
Sexual Risk Taking Scale (SERT-A) (25)	Being developed to accompany Sex Knowledge and Attitude Test for Adolescents (SKAT-A) Attempts to measure immediate/future risk of HIV infection, pregnancy, sexually transmitted diseases in teens	No data available
Sexual Awareness Questionnaire (SAQ) (26)	36-item self-report, measuring 4 personality factors (subscales) associated with sexual awareness and assertiveness Scored using a 5-point Likert scale (0–4)	Convergent and discriminant validity established Cronbach's alpha (male, female): sexual consciousness (M, 0.83; F, 0.86); sexual monitoring (M, 0.80; F, 0.82); sex appeal consciousness (M, 0.89; F, 0.92); sexual assertiveness (M, 0.83; F, 0.81)
Sexual Self-Disclosure Scale (SSDS) (27)	Measures sexual communication issues (extent to which an individual would discuss sexual topics) 12 subscales related to sexual esteem, sexual depression, and sexual preoccupation 60-items, 5-point Likert scale Revised (SSDS-R) to include 12 new subscales (sexual behaviors, values preferences, attitudes and feelings); total of 24 subscales 72 items 5-point Likert scale	Internal consistency of 12 subscales: Cronbach's alpha: female therapist: 0.83–0.93 (average 0.90); male therapist 0.84–0.94 (average 0.92) Reliability, validity established
National Survey of Sexual Attitudes and Lifestyles (NSSAL) (18)	A comprehensive survey of sexual education, sexual experiences, contraceptive use	No data available

Numbers in parentheses correspond to studies cited in the References.

269

Appendix 17D. Instruments Used to Evaluate the Success of Sex Education Curricula*

Instrument Name/Author	Number of Items	Response Format	Types of Data Elicited
Minnesota Sexual Attitudes Scales (MSAS)/Held et al.	35	Rating scale	Attitudes toward and feelings about designated groups of people (e.g., married adults) engaging in certain categories of sexual activities
Sexual Attitude and Behavior Survey (SABS)/Kilpatrick & Smith	40	Rating scale	Sexual attitudes and experience Attitudinal measures elicit reported permissibility/liberality of male, female and personal behavior and fantasy
Test for Assessing Sexual Knowledge and Attitudes (TASKA)/Hawkins	122	True/false; completion; rating scale; forced choice	Biographical information, sexual attitudes, experience, changes in personal behavior, and suggestions for sexuality course development
National Sex Forum Questionnaire/McIlvenna	26	Rating scale	Biographic information; sexual attitudes and experience
Harvard Sex Questionnaire/Nadelson & Shaw	61	True/false; forced choice	Biographic information; sexual attitudes, experience and knowledge
Obstetrics-Gynecology Sexuality Course Evaluation Questionnaire/Montgomery & Singer	6	Likert scale	Emotional discomfort experienced in response to hypothetical clinical situations
Physicians Workshop Questionnaire/Pion	40	Essays; fill-in-blanks; rating scales	Sexual attitudes and knowledge; change in professional behavior; suggestions for sexual course development

*Adapted from William, A.M., & Miller, W.R. The design and use of assessment instruments and procedures for sexuality curricula. In N. Rosenzweig and F.P. Pearsall (Eds.), *Sex education for the health professional: A curriculum guide.* New York: Grune & Stratton, 1978.

Appendix 17E. Measures of Gender Role Definitions and Attitudes

Name	Description	Psychometric Indices
BEM Sex Role Inventory (BSRI) (32–36)	60 item, self-report of gender role definition Scored on 7-point Likert scale (masculinity, femininity androgyny subscale scores, plus social desirability scale) Applicable to Mexican Americans as well as non-Hispanic European Americans	Test–retest reliability: 0.76–0.94 (4-week interval) Coefficient alpha (3 scales): 0.75–0.90 Concurrent validity with other measures of masculinity, femininity Normative data available
Sex Role Survey (SRS) (37–39)	53-item, self-report measure of attitudes toward sex roles in the home, sex role-appropriate behavior, equality in business, equal involvement in social/domestic work) 9-point scale Applicable to African Americans	Alpha coefficients: 4 factors and total score: 0.85–0.96 power (4 dimensions: Cross-validation studies have been performed; normative data available Construct validity has been evaluated
AIDS Discussion Strategy Scale (40)	Measures 6 specific types of discussion tactics to persuade a partner to discuss AIDS (rational, manipulative, withdrawal, charm, subtlety, persistence)	Unavailable
AIDS Empathy Scale (8, 40)	Measures the extent to which an individual reports feeling empathy toward a person with AIDS	Unavailable
Attitudes Towards Homosexuality Scale (ATHS) (41)	Measures attitudes towards homosexuality (general, lesbian, male) 28-item, self-report 9-point scale ("strongly agree" to "strongly disagree")	Split-half reliability: 0.93 Alpha coefficients: 0.93–0.94
Sexual Orientation Method (42)	Self-report test of relative hetero-erotic and homoerotic orientation of homosexual men 120 paired questions (half re: attitudes toward men; half re: attitudes toward women) 5-point scale of degree of sex attributes (attractive, interesting, hot, handsome, exciting, pleasurable)	Test–retest reliability: 0.80–0.94 in control subjects of adult males Homosexual scores significantly different from controls
Multidimensional Scale of Sexuality (MSS) (43)	Self-report questionnaire with 9 categories of sexuality (heterosexuality, homosexuality, asexuality plus 6 categories of bisexuality) 45 items, 5 items relating to each category 3 sets of scores for each of the 9 categories: behavior, cognitive/affective, description of oneself	Reliability: chi-square analysis (MSS compared to Kinsey scale) showed significant relationship ($p < 0.001$) Normed using college students Additional research needed to validate categories

Numbers in parentheses correspond to studies cited in the References.

271

Appendix 17F. Measures of Sexual Dysfunction

Name	Description	Psychometric Indices
Multiaxial Problem-Oriented System for Sexual Dysfunction (44)	Comprehensive measure of specific behavioral sexual problems associated with different phases of sexual cycle (e.g., desire, arousal, orgasm, coital pain) (43) Uses history format and produces a normed computerized sexual function profile May be used to classify sexual dysfunction in clinical situations and research	Not available
Sexual History Form (Derived from multiaxial problem-oriented system) (45)	28-multiple-choice item questionnaire May be used to classify sexual dysfunction in clinical situations and research	Norms available for sexually well-functioning people
Index of Sexual Satisfaction (ISS) (8)	Used to determine degree of satisfaction and dissatisfaction in a relationship 25-item self-report questionnaire reflecting common problems (12 positively worded and 13 negatively worded) Items rated on Likert scale; scoring takes 5 to 8 minutes	Normed on large Hawaiian multiethnic sample Reliability alpha coefficients: 0.906–0.925 Test-retest reliability: 0.93 Discriminant validity (compared to IMS and SAS): differed significantly from Index of Marital Satisfaction—IMS ($p < 0.001$)
Golombok Rust Inventory of Sexual Satisfaction (GRISS) (8, 10)	Brief and well-organized measure of sexual quality and present function in heterosexuals (10) 28-item self-report questionnaire (male/female versions) Responses on 5-point Likert scale (never to always) Takes 3–8 minutes to complete, 4–10 minutes to score Overall global functioning score (higher score, higher level of dysfunction) 4 subscales: 2 for males (impotence, premature ejaculation), 2 for females (anorgasmia, vaginismus) Other items: lack of sensuality, avoidance, dissatisfaction, infrequency, noncommunication Value in diagnosing potency and helpful in understanding pattern of couple's interrelatedness	Normed on group of sexual therapy clients Split-half reliabilities: 0.94 (female), 0.87 (male) for scales Internal consistencies, all scales: 0.61–0.83 (mean 0.74) Test-retest reliabilities: 0.47–0.84 (mean 0.65) Discriminant validity established

Numbers in parentheses correspond to studies cited in the References.

Appendix 17G. Instruments Used to Measure Body Perception

Name	Description	Psychometric Indices
Body Attitude Scale (BAS) (8, 46)	Self-report semantic differential rating scale of attitude toward outer body form 30 different body concepts rated on 7-point, bipolar adjective scale ("most negative" to "most positive") Constructs comprise 3 primary attitude dimensions (evaluative, potency, activity)	Generalizability coefficients (both sexes): 0.93–0.98 Individual differences in body attitude score correlate with gross variations in physique Distinguishes between normal and chronically ill subjects Reliability and validity established
Sexuality Scale (SS) (47)	Measures concepts of [1] sexual esteem, [2] sexual depression, [3] sexual preoccupation 30-item measure, scored on 5-point Likert scale (+2 agree to −2 disagree) 10 items measure each of 3 concepts Studies comparing SS with people's attitudes, empathy with persons with AIDS to determine predictability (0.68): significant gender effect only for subscale 3 (M > F) SS subscales compared to measures of locus of control, anxiety, depression, guilt, self-esteem, sexual awareness: Cronbach's alphas high for all. [1], [3] more associated with positive orientation toward sex; [2] accompanied by greater levels of anxiety, depression, and less self-esteem and sexual assertiveness	Cronbach's alpha coefficients for each concept subscale for W (women) and M (men): [1] W: 0.88, M: 0.93, all: 0.92; [2] W: 0.88, M: 0.94, all: 0.90; [3] W: 0.88, M: 0.79, all: 0.88 Test–retest reliability ($p < 0.001$): [1] 0.69–0.74; [2] 0.67–0.76; [3] 0.70–0.76 Significant correlations between subscales: negative between [1] and [2] among both men and women Correlations established in 1 study (46), but the reverse found in a later study (39): positive between [1], [3] in women; positive between [2], [3] in men (46) SS compared to Beck Depression Inventory (BDI) and Rosenberg Self-Esteem Scale (RSE): factor analysis showed inadequate fit in subscale [3]. Deleted items with reliabilities < 0.50 and created short form (SF) (5 items for each subscale). Reliabilities for SS-SF improved: reliability coefficients: [1] W: 0.92, M: 0.94; [2] W, M: 0.89; [3] W: 0.96, M: 0.92 Correlations: [1], [2] highly negatively correlated, and unrelated to [3] Question on sexual esteem too narrow, but [1] does differentiate from "self-esteem" (47)
Body Image Questionnaire (48)	Evaluates correlation of body image with sex and health	No data available

Numbers in parentheses correspond to studies cited in the References.

Appendix 17H. Measures of the Interpersonal Dimension of Sexuality

Name	Description	Psychometric Indices
Locke-Wallace Marriage Inventory (49)	Self-report measure of marital adjustment 15 items in 4 formats: multiple-choice, 6-point scale (always agree to always disagree), selection of applicable items from a checklist ("very unhappy" to "perfectly happy")	Discriminates between adjusted and maladjusted couples Split-half reliability (Kuder-Richardson): 0.90
Sexual Compatibility Test (50)	101-item self-administered measure of sexual activity, attitudes, satisfaction, responsiveness in couples Specific sexual activity rated along 6 dimensions Normative data available	Cronbach's alphas: 0.90–0.96 Product moment correlations: 0.79–0.97 Concurrent validity: omega-squared ranges from 0.08–0.48
Dyadic Adjustment Scale (marital or similar dyads) (51)	32-item self-report measure of dyadic satisfaction, dyadic consensus, dyadic cohesion, affectional expression Items rated on 6-point scale	Cronbach's alpha (total, subscales): 0.73–0.96 Criterion-related and construct validity demonstrated (differentiates between married and divorced people) Correlation coefficients: 0.86 (married) and 0.88 (divorced) Coefficient alpha: 0.80–0.92 No significant gender differences noted
Revised Dyadic Adjustment Scale (RDAS) (52)	Evaluates dyadic adjustment in distressed and nondistressed relationships 14 items consisting of 3 subscales: dyadic consensus subscale, dyadic satisfaction subscale, and dyadic cohesion subscale	Cronbach's alpha coefficient: 0.90 Spearman-Brown split-half reliability coefficient: 0.95
Short Form of Dyadic Adjustment (DAS-1, DAS-6, DAS-7, Satisfaction Subscale) (53, 54)	Evaluate and classify couples as distressed or nondistressed. Available in 4 forms: [1] one-item, [2] six-item, [3] seven-item, and [4] Satisfaction subscale.	Correlations for Males and Females for each form: [1] = data unavailable; [2] = M (0.34–0.58), F (0.51–0.67), Total (0.45–0.62); [3] = M (0.38–0.64), F (0.55–0.65), Total (0.49–0.62); [4] M (0.24–0.71), F (0.22–0.71) Cronbach alpha values for [3]: M (0.75), F (0.79), Total (0.78) Reliability and validity established for [3]
Reiss Premarital Sexuality Permissiveness (PSP) (55)	12 item self-report attitudinal scale Assesses kissing, petting, coitus, each considered under 4 conditions of affection (engagement, no affection, strong affection, love) Rating scale used to show degree of agreement or disagreement	Guttman Scale reliability criteria met with coefficient of reproducibility > 0.90 Coefficient of scalability > 0.65 and pure scale types 50%–60%
Barrett-Lennard Relationship Inventory (RI) (56)	Measures 4 dimensions of interpersonal relationships (congruence, level of regard, empathetic understanding, unconditionality) 64 items (for each dimension, 8 positively and 8 negatively worded items) Rated from +3 (strongly true) to –3 (strongly not true) Scale scores for each dimension	Split-half and test-retest reliability of each component scale averages 0.85 Correlates with other measures of marital relationship adequacy

Instrument	Description	Reliability/Validity
Structured and Scaled Interview to Assess Maladjustment (SSIAM) (57, 58)	60-item, structured interview format Measures maladjustment in 5 areas (work, family, marriage, sex, social) 11 dimensions for each area rated on a 10-point scale	Interrater reliability established Correlation coefficients of reliability of subscales: 0.78–0.97 Patient self-ratings yielded correlation coefficients 0.20–0.70 compared to ratings of close informants
Sexual Interaction Inventory (SII) (59, 60)	Self-report inventory of sexual adjustment and satisfaction of heterosexual couples Useful in determining treatment for sexual dysfunction 17 items, with 6 questions on each item, rated on 6-point scale Issues: degree of satisfaction with frequency/range of sexual behaviors, sexual pleasure, self-acceptance, partner acceptance	Test–retest reliability: 0.53–0.90 over 2-week period Cronbach's alpha: 0.85–0.93 Validity established Discriminates between sexually satisfied couples and sexually dysfunctional couples; scales correlate with global ratings of sexual satisfaction
Relationship Assessment Scale (RAS) (61)	Measures one's subjective evaluation of a close relationship Not limited to marriage relationships Has shown strong predictive validity with dating couples	Coefficient alpha: 0.35–0.80 (total scores = 0.91) No significant gender differences noted
Marital Intimacy Questionnaire (MIQ) (62)	85-item self-report questionnaire Measures 5 components of marital intimacy as well as marital satisfaction, perceived global intimacy, and communication intimacy	Validity established
Marital Communication Scales (MCS) (63)	Measure of nonverbal communication accuracy Couples participate in dyadic, face-to-face testing situation 16 hypothetical situations presented (8 where 1 member of couple is expresser, other receiver, and 8 with roles reversed)	Discriminates between satisfied and dissatisfied couples Split-half reliability using Spearman-Brown correction: coefficients 0.87 (2 groups)
Marital Communication Inventory (MCI) (64)	Self-report measure of success or failure in marital communication (emotions, feelings, economics, behaviors, communication patterns) 46 items with responses: usually, sometimes, seldom, never Separate male and female versions	Corrected odd-even split-half correlation coefficient: 0.93 (Spearman-Brown correction formula) Mann-Whitney U test: significant difference between matched groups (with and without marital problems)
Personal Assessment of Intimacy in Relationships (PAIR) (65)	75-item measure of 5 types of intimacy: social, emotional, intellectual, sexual, recreational Subjects respond to statements using a 5-point Likert scale in 2 steps: perceived, "as it is now" and expected, "how he or she would like it to be"	Factor analysis and split-half reliabilities of the PAIR have been evaluated Validity demonstrated by its correlation with measures of marital adjustment, self-disclosure, and family environments Cronbach's alpha reliability coefficient for each of 6 subscales of the PAIR: >= 0.70

Appendix 17H. Measures of the Interpersonal Dimension of Sexuality (*cont.*)

Name	Description	Psychometric Indices
Waring Intimacy Questionnaire (WIQ) (66)	160-item true–false format Assesses 8 components of marital intimacy (sexuality, cohesion, affection, conflict resolution, identity, expressiveness, autonomy, compatibility)	Test–retest reliability: 0.70–0.90 KR 20 reliabilities: 0.52–0.87 High significant correlation with PAIR Inventory
Passionate Love Scale (PLS) (67)	30-item, nonbehavioral self-report questionnaire 9-point Likert format Assesses level of longing for union with another Includes component of sexual desire and profound physiological arousal 3 components of construct: cognitive, emotional, behavioral	Internal consistency: coefficient alphas 0.94 and 0.91 (short version) Uncontaminated by social desirability Convergent validity compared to Rubin's Liking and Loving scales (77): $r = 0.86$, $p < 0.001$ PLS measures romantic, sexual component of love; may be good outcome measure for effectiveness of sexual therapy

Numbers in parentheses correspond to studies cited in the References.

Appendix 17I. Measures of Sexuality Used in Special Populations

Name	Description	Psychometric Indices
Sexual Behaviors Questionnaire-Female (SBQ-F) (68)	Assesses a broad spectrum of female behaviors 8 scales (original version) scored on Likert scale (communication, appearance, desire, arousal, activity level, techniques, orgasm, satisfaction) Originally tested on convenience sample of healthy women and women having breast cancer for at least 6 months Offers reliable measure of sexuality for both healthy women and women with cancer; can be used in quality of life research to assess effects of cancer therapy over time	Index of Content validity: 1.00 Factor analysis: 7 scales (communication, techniques, sexual response, self-touch, body scar, masturbation, relationship) MANOVA: significant differences between healthy women and women with breast cancer, but not difference between women having lumpectomy versus mastectomy Convergent validity tested using Watt's Sexual Functioning Questionnaire Internal consistency: reliability: 0.94 Alpha coefficients: 0.53–0.94 Pearson's correlation coefficients: 0.57–0.87
Sexual Adjustment Questionnaire (SAQ) (69, 70)	Measures changes in sexual expression following a cancer diagnosis Subsections: activity level, desire, relationship, arousal, orgasm, techniques	Test–retest reliability: 0.54–0.94 (mean 0.67) Construct validity: scores of patients with cancer Patients with cancer significantly lower than nonpatients (activity level, techniques, relationship subsections)
Althof et al. Semi-structured interview (71)	Developed to evaluate preoperative and longitudinal postoperative effects on sexuality of women undergoing coronary bypass surgery Female cardiac surgery patients	Unavailable
Psychosexual Functioning Questionnaire (PSFQ) (72)	Measures psychosexual functioning in cancer patients Supplies information about sexual satisfaction, sexual interest, altered body image, psychological and physical symptoms, and impotence-related difficulties	Reliability and validity established
Sexual Functioning Questionnaire Patients receiving antihypertensive medications (73)	17-item instrument 5-point Likert rating scale High score indicates positive sexual functioning Assesses major elements of sexual experience	Test–retest reliability: 0.83 (72 hours) Cronbach's alpha: 0.55–0.65
Perception of Diabetes Mellitus Questionnaire (PDM) (74–76) Patients with diabetes mellitus	Assesses perceived impact of diabetes on sexual functioning and relationships with a spouse or partner 7-item relationship score (RS), and 6-item Sexual Function Score (SF) Rated on 7-point scale (1 "minimal effect" to 7 "great effect")	Coefficient alphas: 0.79 (RS), 0.83 (SF)
Jensen Sexual History Form Male and female insulin-treated diabetics	Adaptation of the Sexual History Form (from the Multiaxial Problem-Oriented System for Sexual Dysfunction) (43)	Unavailable

Numbers in parentheses correspond to studies cited in the References.

18

Measuring Dietary Intake and Nutritional Outcomes

Nancy A. Stotts and Nancy Bergstrom

Nutrition is an important consideration in health maintenance and treatment of disease. Selecting instruments to measure dietary intake as well as nutritional outcomes is important in clinical research. This chapter addresses the measurement of nutrition, specifically measures of ingestion, clinical evaluation, energy expenditure, biochemical measures, and body composition. Within each category, various measures are presented; each measure described; and their usability, accuracy, and precision are discussed.

Measures of Ingestion

Various approaches have been used to measure the type and amount of intake. Direct observation and weighing food, diet recall, dietary records or food diary, food frequency records, and dietary scoring are frequently used approaches.

Direct Observation and Weighing Food

Direct observation of food intake and the weighing of food are methods of dietary evaluation that allow valid measurement of nutrients consumed, especially for people in institutional settings. Direct observation and weighing are done by research or dietary staff. Before food is placed on trays, dietary staff weigh and measure the food and then weigh and measure or just observe it when removing the tray after determining that the food was not saved or discarded. Menus from the dietary department provide data on food served, serving size, and variations based on special diets. Recipes are obtained to assist in computer analysis of nutrient intake.[1] To mitigate the effect of being observed, photographs of the tray can be taken before and after each meal. The photography method of nutritional assessment yielded the same information as direct observation by research staff in a study done of nutrient intake of nursing home residents.[2] In reality, it is not clear that a photograph is an improvement over a trained observer, and it requires the use of additional equipment and data interpretation.

Calorie counts used in hospitalized patients are one form of direct observation. Breslow and Sorkin[3] compared 1-day and 3-day calorie counts in hospitalized patients, in hopes that the 1-day count would provide data comparable with 3-day data. Using 30 patients, they found mean 3-day intake (952 ± 91 calories) and first-day intake were similar (918 ± 116 calories). The first day had high sensitivity (calories 96%, protein 93%) and had positive predictive value (calories 100%, protein 96%). These data suggest that the 1-day calorie count may be a valid alternative to the 3-day dietary intake record.

The major advantage of direct observation is that an accurate or valid record of intake can be accomplished. Memory and motivation are not critical to this method. Disadvantages are that having intake observed may precipitate behavior change and thus the recorded intake may not represent the usual intake. Observation is expensive because of the number of hours a trained observer is needed. Error is present, but neither the amount nor direction of error with this method can be anticipated.[4] Some data indicate that direct observation can be accurate if the observer receives adequate training. Visual estimates of food were highly correlated with measured or weighed food ($r = 0.96$) even when carried out in a field study in Nepal.[5]

Direct observation of dietary intake in patients in a free-living situation usually is too expensive if data must be collected for more than 1 day.[4] Thus direct observation is not a technique that can be used readily in outpatient or large epidemiologic studies, in which case, the subject may be asked to monitor food intake. The degree of precision requested of the subject can vary from recording dietary intake to weighing foods before eating them. Either method is more practical and frequently used in the free-living population.[4]

One approach that has been tested in an effort to enhance accuracy is the recording of intake using a computerized system. Kretsch and Fong[6] compared food intake of a small sample of research volunteers ($n = 9$) recorded on a computer with intakes recorded by the metabolic unit dietary staff. In this one small study, mean differences were less than 5% for the two methods of documenting intake, and correlations were between 0.81 and 0.92. Further testing of the system is needed with larger samples and among those who are free-living.

Another study compared weighing food with an estimate of the proportion of the family food that was ingested by pairs of adult women in the family. Data from 64 young and middle-aged women showed a high correlation ($r = 0.90 - 0.92$) between the two techniques.[7] Further work is needed to confirm the validity of this method in other populations (e.g., older persons, men).

Twenty-Four-Hour Dietary Recall

The work of Burke[8] forms the foundation for *dietary recall*, a quantitative approach to the assessment of recent diet intake. Subjects are interviewed and asked to recall all the food they consumed in the previous 24 hours, usually from the time of the last snack on the night before until bedtime.[9] The interviewer guides the subject through the day asking questions such as "What did you eat for breakfast?" Specific food items are usually not suggested by the interviewer to avoid leading the subject. The interviewer may stimulate the subject to be more complete by asking broad questions such as "Did you eat your toast dry?" The quantity of food is determined by asking the person to describe the amount. Food models and measuring cups and spoons are used to assist the subject in recalling the serving size. The interview takes 30 to 60 minutes when conducted by a trained interviewer.[4]

The advantages of this method are that it requires memory only for the past 24 hours, and most people can remember intake over that time.[10,11] Data are collected rather quickly and may be obtained by telephone interview. In addition, because this method is used only once, there is no training effect.

The disadvantages are numerous.[11,12] The method requires accurate short-term memory, which may be problematic for some elderly people. Subjects may report what they think the researcher wants to hear or may have difficulty estimating portion size. Data analysis can be tedious and difficult, requiring the calculation of nutrients ingested. This method does not have enough precision to evaluate the usual dietary intake or the adequacy of the diet to meet specific nutritional needs or to assess deficiency states. The inability to diagnose deficiencies has led some investigators to conclude that the 24-hour recall has limited utility.[12] When 24-hour recall is used to measure the intake of specific nutrients, estimates of reliability vary widely, necessitating multiple recall studies to place subjects in the same quartile for specific nutrients.[11]

Interrater reliability must be established for any investigation in which two or more interviewers collect data. The use of a standardized training manual helps investigators to become and remain reliable. The validity of the 24-hour recall technique is established by comparing observed dietary intake and a subject's recalled intake. High correlation has been found between these two measurement methods, thereby supporting concurrent validity of the recall method. For example, the 24-hour recall and 3-day food record estimate for total calories was significantly correlated ($r = 0.67$), thus establishing the validity of the measures, when used by women on a low-fat diet.[13]

The Dietary Record or Food Diary

The dietary record or food diary is used to determine what an individual has eaten for 1, 3, or 7 days.[10,14] Subjects are instructed how to keep the record. Each food or fluid ingested and a measure of quantity are recorded as close to the time of ingestion as possible to reduce memory-related inaccuracies. Subjects may or may not be asked to weigh or measure the quantity of food. When subjects are asked to weigh food, a food scale is generally made available and the subject is instructed in weighing and measuring. Subjects are told to weigh or otherwise measure food before eating or drinking.

The dietary record approach often is used as the gold standard for validating other methods, when observation or food weighing is not possible.[4] The reliability of dietary records has been evaluated over a 2-week period[15] and at 1- and 9-month intervals.[16] Intake was not significantly different when dietary intake for 1 week was compared with that of a second week.[17] Correlations were 0.70 to 0.85 for the dietary intake at 1- and 9-month intervals.[16] One year later repeated 5-day food records also yield a high correlation for energy and energy-yielding nutrients ($r = 0.66$), vitamins and minerals ($r = 0.58$), and foods ($r = 0.58$).[18] These studies provide evidence of the validity and reliability of the dietary record.

Factors that affect the accuracy of reporting diet records include the need to provide socially acceptable responses, simplifying or truncating food intake by recalling fewer food items, inaccurate perception of portion size, the type of food, personal preferences, product serving sizes, and comparison of personal servings with those of others.[19] In addition, the diversity of intake may be reduced to avoid the necessity of weighing and recording more items, thus, the diet may appear more homogeneous and less varied than might be normally expected.

Self-reported dietary assessment has been shown to underestimate energy intake, and this bias is most evident for high-fat foods.[20,21] Underreporting affects the accuracy of dietary data more among women, those categorized as overweight, minority groups, and younger adults.[22] Dietary records are most accurate when completed by a dietician[23] or patients or subjects trained by a dietician.[4]

The advantages of the diet record include limited dependence on memory; increased accuracy in serving size data if foods are weighed or measured; ability to record data over a prolonged period, thus increasing the representativeness of the data; and the need for fewer research personnel to collect data and the resulting lower costs of data collection.[4,10]

Major disadvantages of diet records are that adherence is required, those who record all food intake may differ from people who do not, and the existence of a potential training effect (i.e., intake may change because it is being recorded).[4] In addition, subjects must be highly motivated to record and measure their intake or weigh food. Memory-related errors may be replaced with recording errors, and the generation of copious data requires significant time for analysis.[10] All these factors represent potential threats to validity and reliability.

Food Frequency Records or Questionnaires

The food frequency record, questionnaire, or interview asks the individual how often a specific food is eaten in a given time frame. Food items are selected with the study purpose in mind, such as foods high in saturated fat to study heart disease risk or foods high in calcium when studying osteoporosis. Data usually are analyzed to indicate adequacy of intake in broad categories such as quartiles.[4,10,24] Advantages of this method include the low cost and representativeness of the data on usual intake.[4] Cost-saving methods can include having subjects independently complete records or complete records through brief interviews, telephone calls, or mailed questionnaires. Questionnaires may be easily formatted for computerized scanning. Disadvantages relate to the nature of the food list to be studied. These include the order of the questions, the specificity of the foods listed,[25] and cultural differences in food preferences.[4] These problems can threaten accuracy and specificity. It should be noted that no more validity is added to the food frequency record by including portion size for items that do not come in natural units.[26]

Intake estimated using self-administered semiquantitative food frequency records was compared with data obtained from five 2-day diet records in 53 elderly people. The mean intake difference for most nutrients was less than 5% between the two methods. Intake correlations between the diet records and the food frequency record were quite variable, for example, 0.34 for zinc in women to 0.75 for protein, zinc, and calcium in men. For most nutrients, the diet records classified 70% of the subjects in the same quartile as that assigned by the food frequency record. These data suggest that for individuals and groups, the food frequency record can produce data similar to that from 10 days of diet records.[27]

A cross-cultural food frequency record was developed for a major epidemiologic study of breast and colorectal cancer in Spain. Subjects completed the food frequency record before and after a 4-day food intake record. Validity varied, with reliability coefficients of 0.20 for vitamin A and 0.88 for alcohol. When measured at 1-year intervals, reliability coefficients ranged from 0.51 for saturated fat to 0.88 for alcohol.[28] These data suggest that culturally specific food frequency records can be created.

A study using a combination of the assessment methods showed that both food frequency questionnaire (FFQ) ($r = 0.91$) and the structured 72-hour recall ($r = 0.69$) provided valid estimates of nutrient intake and showed average intraclass correlation.[29] When FFQ, food records, and 24-hour direct recall were used to assess fat in 13 men, FFQ seemed to overestimate dietary intake. There were no differences in energy and nutrient intake in comparing food records and 24-hour recall.[30]

Dietary Scoring

The dietary score is a method used to evaluate whether the food consumed represents the composite of nutrients required to meet an individual's needs. It is based on the premise that various food groups contribute unique nutrients and together meet the individual's nutritional needs. The score is the sum of the points assigned for food items from each group.[31]

The validity of this method has been evaluated by Guthrie and Scheer.[31] They assigned dietary scores to the 24-hour dietary records obtained from 212 university students. Dietary scores were compared with diet records, and a nutrient ratio was calculated. The Recommended Daily Allowance (RDA), using the relevant age and gender chart, was the standard against which the adequacy of the diet was judged. This method is valid because a maximum dietary score of 16 met the RDA for 7 of 12 nutrients, and the remaining 5 nutrients met 80% (an acceptable value) of the RDA.

Data were examined to evaluate 24-hour recalls to determine variety among the 5 major food groups (dairy, meat, grain, fruit, vegetable) using a dietary diversity score.[32] Data showed that age-adjusted mortality was inversely related to the diet diversity score ($p < 0.0009$). The relative risk of death in men and women consuming two or fewer food groups was 1.5 (95%, confidence interval [CI] 1.2–1.8) for men and 1.4 (95%, CI 1.1–1.9) for women. Analysis from the same data set showed that African Americans had lower diet diversity scores than whites and that scores for both groups increased with income and educational preparation.[33]

The strengths of dietary scoring are that it can be administered and analyzed by most health care professionals and many clients and families; it can be modified to assess the needs of specific groups; and data analysis takes only minutes. Limitations are that evaluation of mixed food (e.g., casseroles, ethnic food combinations) requires judgment; it is difficult to rate fast food; and the method is not sensitive to portion size, and therefore a wide range of caloric and nutrient levels may be ingested without being accurately reflected in the score.[4]

Analysis of Dietary Intake Data

A computer program generally is used to analyze dietary intake data. Input includes both the volume of food (e.g., half cup, 8 ounces), as well as the specific food (e.g., fresh green beans, 2% milk). The program provides information on the nutrient composition of the diet. The accuracy of this method may be threatened because some dietary items do not adequately represent the composition of foods such as stir-fries, casseroles, salads, and less well-known foods. The nutrient database for foods should be appropriately selected and made known by the computer software company. A very accurate assessment of nutrients ingested can be generated by software.

Many computer programs can be used to analyze nutrient intake data. Price and program sophistication vary widely, and the user must be sure there is a fit between the planned use and the program selected. Some programs have a limited database and calculate a limited number of nutrients. Others include fast foods, convenience foods, and special diets. Some permit the user to update values, add recipes, or provide supplementary information about specific nutrients. For both research and clinical purposes, evaluation of the nature of the database used in the computer program selected is critical to ensure that the data generated are consistent with the user's purpose. The individual who enters the data must be trained adequately to maximize accuracy of the data.

Clinical Evaluation

Clinical evaluation has been the mainstay of nutritional assessment. Methods of clinical assessment include accurate history and physical examination and anthropometric measures.

History and Physical Examination

The health history and physical examination are the oldest and probably the most widely used evaluation of nutritional status. Numerous texts and journal articles address the techniques for eliciting an accurate nutritional assessment.[34,35]

The health history provides information about events that led to or have the potential for leading to changes in dietary intake or digestion with implications for nutrition. For example, difficulty swallowing or diarrhea may affect nutritional status. Useful data commonly obtained in the history include usual weight, weight change, change in the pattern or variety of food ingested, changes in appetite, and signs and symptoms of gastrointestinal problems, such as nausea, vomiting, anorexia, and diarrhea. Data from the health history provide the focus for subsequent physical examination.

The physical examination can help to identify nutritional adequacy or deviations. Because signs and symptoms of malnutrition are not often seen in the United States, skill and constant vigilance are needed to identify changes in physical findings. An adjunct to physical examination is photographic comparison.[36] When considering the diagnosis of nutritional alterations, there is a need to rule out confounding factors, such as disease process, medication side effects, metabolic abnormality, age, and the half-lives of nutrients suspected as being deficient.

The major advantage of the history and physical examination as a source of nutritional data is its ubiquitous presence in the United States health care system. The practitioner who can identify manifestations of nutritional defects is well positioned to suggest additional diagnostic tests, implement appropriate treatment, and take steps toward prevention in those at high risk.

There are disadvantages in using the health history and physical as a routine means of detecting abnormalities. They include time; money; the need for additional tests to confirm the diagnosis; variations in examiner's skills to identify, interpret, and diagnose problems; and the fact that deficiencies must be severe or persistent to produce visible symptoms.[36]

The accuracy of physical examination has been studied by documenting agreement between objective findings, usually laboratory test findings, and subjective findings, documented by physical examination and history in the clinical impression. Clinical judgments by two surgeons were compared with laboratory data. Correlations for one surgeon were 60% of cases and for another, 65% of cases.[37] In part, this may be explained by the lack of specificity of laboratory data for various nutritional states.

The reliability of physical examination data has been evaluated in several nutritional studies.[38] These studies suggest there is significant variability in the use of this fundamental measure of nutritional status. However, much of this variability can be mitigated with training and ongoing evaluation.

Anthropometric Measures

Anthropometric measures are easy to perform and have been a cornerstone in the evaluation of nutritional status. Areas addressed include weight, mid-arm muscle circumference, skinfold measures, and head circumference. Knee height and calf circumference also are used to evaluate height and weight in those who are elderly or not ambulatory.

In older adults (> 60 years), anthropometry (height, weight, skinfold thickness, and circumferences) is the most reliable and specific indicator of malnutrition.[39]

Weight has been used as a measure of nutritional status. It can be used alone or in combination with height or frame size. A loss of 5% of usual weight, weighing less than 90% of ideal body weight, or the loss of 10 pounds in 30 days or less all signal actual or potential nutritional problems. Data indicate that weighing is not performed consistently in tertiary care teaching hospitals. In examining patients ($n = 300$) in three centers 24 to 36 hours after admission, only 66% reported having been weighed. When weights recorded on the chart were compared with those obtained by research personnel, more than 25% differed by 5 or more pounds.[40]

Body mass index (BMI) is being used by increasing to evaluate weight and weight changes because BMI indexes weight to height.[41,42] The BMI is calculated by dividing weight in kilograms by height in meters squared. It is used to diagnose undernutrition and obesity, controlling for age and gender. In obesity, BMI does not characterize the distribution of fat, and increased intraabdominal fat is an independent health risk. Guidelines thus recommend measurement of waist circumference.[43] Some limited data indicate that providing tape measures to medical students during an outpatient rotation increased the percentage of medical students who used waist circumference to identify patients at risk for metabolic syndrome.[44]

Arm muscle circumference and skinfold measurement have been employed in underdeveloped countries to evaluate nutritional status.[45] More recent work has led to the establishment of age-related standards in the United States; standards also have been developed for a limited number of minority populations.[39,46]

Mid-upper-arm circumference is a measure of muscle mass, bone, and skin. It is used to calculate mid-arm muscle circumference as a measure of lean body mass and is derived by the following formula:[45]

arm muscle mass (cm) = mid-upper-arm circumference (cm) – (0.314 × triceps skinfold (mm))

Decreases in arm muscle mass can occur because of muscle disease, inactivity, or nutritional deficiencies. Severe depletion is defined as the lowest fifth percentile on established tables, and those in the sixth to twenty-fifth percentile are classified as moderately depleted.

Skinfold measures are performed to evaluate fat stores. A skinfold caliper, produced by manufacturers such as Lange, Holtain, and Harpenden, is used to measure skinfold thickness. Many sites can be measured (e.g., scapula, waist, triceps), but the most frequently used site is the triceps. In hospitalized patients for whom edema may be a consideration, the triceps site often is selected because less edema forms in the upper arm than in the more dependent body parts.

Fat is a concentrated energy store in the body. Because fat stores do not change rapidly, skinfold measures are not a sensitive measure of malnutrition. Depletion generally indicates chronic malnutrition or a severe hypermetabolic state leading to rapid fat utilization. Head circumference is used in children to evaluate growth. Using normative tables, children are classified according to percentiles. Chronic undernutrition results in delayed head growth, and its identification and treatment are important to prevent permanent damage.[47]

In nonambulatory or elderly patients who are unable to stand erect, alternative approaches to height and weight measurement are necessary.[48,49] Knee height to evaluate height and calf circumference has been suggested to evaluate weight. Knee height is the distance from the heel of the left foot to the top of the thigh. It is measured with a caliper with the subject supine, on the left leg, and at a 90-degree angle. Overall height is then calculated by using the formula:

$$\text{Height (cm)} = 105.9 \ (\pm 11.6) + 6.48 \ (\pm 1.81) \times \text{sex} + 0.988 \ (\pm 0.24) \times \text{knee height (cm)}$$

A nomogram has been constructed based on this formula.[49]

Body weight in the nonambulatory can be calculated using calf circumference. It is measured on the left leg at the widest point with the subject in the supine position. The distance measured, as well as knee height, mid-upper-arm circumference, and subscapular skinfold, are used to derive body weight for a female from the standard formula:

$$(0.98 \times \text{arm circumference}) + (1.27 \times \text{calf circumference}) + (0.4 \times \text{subscapular skinfold thickness}) + (0.87 \times \text{knee height}) - 62.35$$

Available coefficients are used to calculate weight in men with a similar formula.[48]

The validity and reliability of anthropometric measures are an important consideration. Instrument accuracy is important. The manufacturer's specifications, reports of previous studies, and personal experience are all considered in instrument evaluation. For example, the Lange calipers (Scientific Industries, Cambridge, MA) apply $10 \ \text{g}/\text{mm}^2$ of pressure to measure skinfold thickness. Accuracy is determined by using a standard calibration block provided by the manufacturer. If the caliper registers 10 mm while resting on the first step and 10 ($\pm$ 0.5) additional mm on each of the four subsequent steps, its precision is established. If the instrument is not calibrated, it needs to be returned for servicing.

Sources of error in the measurement of skinfold thickness can include the selection of different skin sites, variations in body and hand positions that affect the amount of tissue grasped, and the length of time the caliper is applied before taking a reading.[50] Standardized protocols and adequate training sessions and supervision reduce measurement variability. Planned periodic interrater reliability testing is needed to maintain the stability of measurement techniques over time and to ensure precision.

Energy Expenditure

Energy expenditure is the heat released and mechanical work performed by the body that is necessary to sustain life and lifestyle.[51] It reflects the metabolism of substrates. It is measured by direct and indirect calorimetry, doubly labeled water, and oxygen consumption derived from pulmonary artery data.

Direct and Indirect Calorimetry

Direct calorimetry is a measure of heat production. Knowing that specific substrates produce a given amount of heat allows energy expenditure to be derived. The findings are used to plan nutritional therapy. Direct calorimetry requires that a subject be placed in a chamber where heat production is measured. It is the criterion measure against which other methods are compared. There is excellent accuracy (1%) and precision ($\pm$ 2–3%).[52] The advantage of direct calorimetry is accuracy. Alternatively, it restricts activity, changes the subject's usual activity patterns, and requires expensive equipment and considerable investigator time.

Indirect calorimetry measures the gas exchange associated with the oxidation of energy substrates. The metabolic cart used for gas measurement can be taken to the subject's bedside. It is less expensive than direct calorimetry. Accuracy of indirect calorimetry is enhanced in critically ill patients who have an established steady state of at least 5 minutes in which oxygen consumption and carbon dioxide production change by less than 10%.[53] Its disadvantages are primarily that it remains an expensive technique and requires the use of a hood or a mask that the subject may find confining. McClave et al. recommend that indirect calorimetry be incorporated as an integral part of nutritional assessment in the critical care unit.[54]

Doubly Labeled Water

Energy expenditure can be measured with doubly labeled water. This method involves giving the subject a loading dose of water labeled with the stable isotope deuterium and ^{18}O. The deuterium is eliminated as water and the ^{18}O is disposed of as both carbon dioxide and water; the difference in the two elimination rates is a measure of carbon dioxide production. The rate of isotope elimination, and hence energy expenditure, is measured by collection of urine for isotope analysis. The method is accurate to 1% with precision of 4% to 7% when measured in free-living, community-dwelling persons.[55]

Comparisons were made of estimates of daily energy expenditure using energy intake from 7-day self-reported diet records, metabolizable energy intake balance, doubly labeled water, and room calorimetry.[51] Results indicated that self-reported diet records and room calorimetry underestimate daily energy expenditure. Doubly labeled water is a more direct approach to determining energy expenditure in free-living individuals than the use of intake methods of calorimetry.[51]

The advantage of the doubly labeled water technique is its accuracy. Disadvantages include the need for isotope administration, urine gathering, and sophisticated instruments and trained personnel for isotope data analysis.[52]

Oxygen Consumption Measurement via Pulmonary Artery Catheter

Another means to measure energy expenditure is with oxygen consumption measured using a pulmonary artery catheter in critically ill patients. Data show a strong correlation between energy expenditure measured by indirect calorimetry using a metabolic cart and that calculated from the Fick equation with data obtained from a pulmonary artery catheter. There is a strong correlation ($r = 0.83$, $p < 0.001$) between oxygen consumption obtained by the two methods, with a mean difference of 4%. There also is a strong correlation ($r = 0.82$, $p < 0.001$) in energy expenditure between the two methods, but the range of differences is large (-36% to $+40\%$). These differences reflect a hyperdynamic and metabolically stressed critically ill population. Cardiac output measures tend to be overestimated at higher values and therefore are a potential source of error. Thus when indirect calorimetry is not available, the Fick method can be used to estimate energy expenditure in patients with pulmonary artery line in place, if its limitations are kept in mind.[56]

Biochemical Measures

Biochemical parameters reflect the end-product of ingestion, digestion, absorption, and metabolism of nutrients. A simple approach that can be measured with minimal invasive strategies, biochemical measures often are used to evaluate nutritional status. They involve laboratory techniques and can be performed on blood, serum, plasma, hair, nails, urine, sweat, and stool. They offer an objective measure of nutritional status and in some cases provide data about subclinical deficiencies. Important considerations are selecting the appropriate test, sample collecting and handling, sample analysis, and interpretation of the findings.[57]

Selecting the Measure

Laboratory studies are performed to determine nutrient concentration; nutrient-balance studies; nutrient needs; changes in blood components related to intake; and responses to tests, doses, or loads. The investigator must be familiar with the alternative laboratory tests and determine which tests provide the most direct, valid, and reliable data. Knowing the purpose of the study thus becomes critical in selecting the outcome measure.

Sample Collecting and Handling

Serious consideration must be given to sample collection and handling. The timing of sampling may be an important consideration as food and fluid intake influence the results of some tests. Also, some tests are sensitive to circadian rhythms, and so measurement needs to be performed at a consistent time. If it is necessary to fast for the test or a special test meal is required, planning is required. For all tests, subjects will require instruction. Special equipment may be needed to collect the sample; for example, specific tubes may be needed, and some tests may require that the tubes be chilled immediately to stop metabolic processes.

Selecting a Clinical Laboratory

Most researchers are required to use a clinical laboratory for at least a portion of their assays. Labs must be state certified, because patient care decisions are based on the findings. Laboratory test accuracy, precision, and sensitivity should be evaluated. Sensitivity is important when perhaps a thousandth of a milliliter may be crucial to data.[57]

The accuracy of the assay itself can be ensured by using appropriately calibrated equipment and known standards. Results that agree with known standards across a range of values (highest to lowest expected) provide evidence to support the validity of the assay. The precision of the analysis can be evaluated by submitting samples in duplicate or triplicate for analysis and evaluating the agreement between the results generated. The decision as to the acceptable degree of variability is the investigator's. Reliability is worthless, however, if the test is not accurate. The laboratory will provide the researcher with information about accuracy, precision, and sensitivity on request; it is important to know the technique used by the laboratory when performing the test so that it can be reported as part of any publication arising from the study.

Some data from France show variability in analyses of biochemical marker of nutritional status, that is, 7% variability in albumin and prealbumin, among 30 different laboratories participating in a multisite study.[58] These data raise the question of whether a single center should be used in multicenter trials or, at least, whether the issue should be addressed prospectively in the study design.

Interpretation of Laboratory Data

Interpretation of laboratory results requires careful judgment. Clinical laboratories provide information about acceptable normal values for a specific laboratory. Data about the nature of the sample on whom the laboratory test was normed ideally should be similar to the study population. When using published norms, the rationale for cutoff points created by authors of tables should be clear and acceptable to the investigator.

Example: A Biochemical Measure of Protein Status

An example of the process of selecting a biochemical parameter is the choice of a measure of protein status. The serum proteins are biochemical indicators of malnutrition.[59] They are synthesized by the liver and vary primarily in their rate of turnover. The following are serum protein measures frequently used to evaluate protein status: albumin, transferrin, nitrogen balance, urine creatinine, prealbumin, 3-methylhistidine, and retinol-binding protein. For all of them, hydration status is important in their validity; dehydration produces falsely elevated serum levels. It should be noted that posture and circadian rhythm also can affect hydration and the accuracy of the values.

Probably the most frequently measured laboratory evaluation of protein status is serum albumin level. Albumin has a long half-life (18–20 days), is not sensitive to rapid changes in nutritional status, and falls late in malnutrition. It therefore is not appropriate to use low serum albumin to diagnose either recent or mild to moderate malnutrition. Low albumin is associated with increased morbidity and mortality in patients who are ill.[59]

Transferrin, another frequently used measure of protein status, has a shorter half-life (8–10 days) and a smaller body pool. Its major function is to transport iron. Normally, about one third of the body transferrin is bound to iron. Although initially recommended as a measure of protein malnutrition, it is affected by many factors other than protein-calorie malnutrition and so is not a meaningful measure. For example, an iron deficiency is seen with protein-calorie malnutrition, which stimulates hepatic synthesis, and elevated levels of transferrin are seen. At the other extreme, inflammatory states, liver disease, and some anemias result in depressed transferrin levels.

Prealbumin, another plasma protein, has a short half-life (2 days). It also is known as thyroxin-binding prealbumin and transthyretin. It transports a portion of thyroxine and vitamin A. Because of its short half-life, prealbumin decreases quickly when protein or calorie intake is decreased. In contrast, it responds quickly when nutrients are provided exogenously. This measure provides a better evaluation of nutritional status than intake because prealbumin reflects not only what has been ingested but also what has been able to be absorbed, digested, and metabolized. On the other hand, prealbumin is quite sensitive to inflammatory response and will decrease dramatically because of a decrease in protein synthesis.

Retinol-binding protein has a very short half-life (12 hours) and very low serum levels. It participates with prealbumin in the transport of vitamin A, and its response follows that of prealbumin. Although it has a theoretical advantage over other plasma proteins by virtue of its short half-life, its low normal values and the technical difficulties in measurement have not demonstrated its superiority over other measures of nutrient status.

Another frequently used measure of protein metabolism is urine creatinine. Creatinine is the by-product of muscle catabolism and so is a measure of lean body mass. Diurnal variations occur, but over a 24-hour period its excretion is relatively constant. Creatinine excretion is a theoretically strong measure of nutritional status but is subject to many threats to validity. It requires normal renal function and urinary output, an accurately collected 24-hour specimen, and adequate hydration. In addition, it is not accurate in patients who have been on prolonged bed rest and those who have had a recent high-protein meal.[53] Normally nutritional status with creatinine is evaluated using a 24-hour urine creatinine excretion divided by normal creatinine for height, producing a creatinine height index. Valid age-specific tables are required to accurately interpret the data that are generated.

Similarly, 3-methylhistidine is another measure of skeletal muscle breakdown. Its excretion is seen as a sensitive measure of catabolism, but because there is a large pool of 3-methylhistidine outside of skeletal muscle, it is not a specific test. It is threatened by all the measures noted for creatinine. In addition, reference tables are lacking for children.

Fundamental to any discussion of protein status is the concept that nitrogen turnover is in balance, that is, that intake and loss from the body are carefully regulated and closely approximate each other under normal nutritional circumstances. For anabolism and repair to occur, a positive nitrogen balance is needed. To measure nitrogen balance, protein intake and loss in the urine are measured for a 24-hour period. A standard formula is used to calculate nitrogen balance, and it takes into consideration nonurine nitrogen loss, such as stool and skin.

During periods of starvation and concomitant catabolism, intake of nitrogen is not as great as output, and so nitrogen balance is negative. Threats to the validity of this test are posed by liver function, renal function, hydration status, medications, and the accuracy of the 24-hour urine data. It is important to realize that this measure provides no information about nutritional status or protein stores, but rather only about the immediate intake and metabolic balance.

Selection of the measure or measures of protein status must first be addressed from a theoretical perspective, that is, what dimension of protein status is of interest and over what period of time. Is it synthesis of plasma proteins, breakdown of exiting protein stores, or nitrogen turnover? Consideration then must be given to the accuracy, precision, and sensitivity of the test. Accuracy is evaluated both through the literature and by understanding the accuracy available in the laboratory that you plan to use.

It is important when evaluating accuracy in the literature to consider whether the sample studied and the outcome evaluated reflect your situation. One example of this is a study in which the ability of anthropometric and biochemical indices to predict death among patients (n = 294) in a general medical ward was assessed.[60] Death within 3 months was predicted with a linear discriminant analysis method with a sensitivity of 83% and specificity of 84%, using the variables sex, functional ability, urea, total protein, alkaline phosphatase, and albumin-adjusted calcium. The authors report that the anthropometric and biochemical indices did little to improve the accuracy of the prediction, and they acknowledge that these data contradict findings among surgical patients. The precision of tests also should be evaluated based on the literature. Interpretation requires that the researcher consider practical issues, such as the cost, ease of data collection, and subject burden.

Measures of Body Composition

Bioelectrical impedance analysis (BIA) often is used to measure body composition. BIA is a noninvasive measure that involves passing alternating electric current over body tissues from electrodes on the extremities. Resistance is provided by various body tissues that are low in lean tissue and high in fat tissue and bone. Analysis provides a quantitative measure of fat-free mass, body fat, resistance, and reactance.

The value of BIA was demonstrated by Kyle et al., who showed that single-frequency BIA, using the FENEVA equation, was valid in pre- and post-transplant patients and permits prediction of their fat-free mass (r = 0.974).[61] Body composition from the NHANES III bioelectrical impedance data showed that males had greater fat-free mass than females, regardless of age or racial-ethnic status.[46] Fat-free mass increased in all groups up to mid-adulthood and then decreased in the elderly. Mean total body fat also increased with older groups until about age 60 and then decreased. These data provide a descriptive reference for several United States populations, including non-Hispanic whites, non-Hispanic blacks, and Mexican Americans.

To examine the validity of BIA, skinfold thickness measurement and BIA were compared with each other and with dual-energy absorptiometry (DXA) as the criterion measure to evaluate body composition in elderly women ($n = 93$).[62] BIA had better agreement with DXA in measuring fat and fat-free mass than did skinfold measurement. The authors used the BIA data to develop a predictive equation for body composition. Data showed that the equation for fat-free mass yielded a small amount of error, whereas data for fat mass was positive correlated with the degree of fat mass. However, the use of manufacturer's equations resulted in significant error. Data supporting the importance of the equation used to calculate body composition is found in a meta-analysis that explored different methods to assess percentage body fat when compared with underwater weighing. The comparison of four common BIA equations revealed large variations in over- or underestimations of body fat percentage.[63]

Nonetheless, the expanding role of BIA in health care has received recent attention. Because fat-free mass and fat mass are important determinants of basal energy expenditure, Barak et al. hypothesized they could use BIA to estimate energy requirements of patients receiving nutritional support.[64] The goal was to develop a more accurate measure of resting energy requirement than was possible using the Harris-Benedict equation. Using 40 subjects (20 men and 20 women), they used body composition data derived from BIA and took into account age and gender when they developed predictive equations with multiple regression. Equations were subsequently tested in 36 subjects. The researchers found that the BIA-derived equations were more accurate in predicting resting energy expenditure than the Harris-Benedict equation ($r^2 = 0.65$) in approximately 75% of the patients. This demonstrates an additional role for BIA.

The advantage of BIA is that it is easy to use, fast, and relatively inexpensive. Its major limitation is that error in measurement of body composition may be introduced by proprietary equations used to interpret BIA data. In addition, ingestion of meals and hydration status can affect the accuracy of the measure.[65]

Summary

Serious consideration must be given to all available measurement techniques as a study is designed. Selection and use of the most appropriate instruments for measurement are pivotal to producing data on which health care knowledge can be built.

Exemplar Studies

Braga, M., Gianotti, L., Radaelli, G., & DiCarlo, V. Nutritional approach in malnourished surgical patients: A prospective randomized study. *Arch Surg*, 2002, *137*(2):174–180.

Malnourished cancer patients ($n = 196$) scheduled for surgery were randomized to enteral feeding with a standard diet within 12 hours of surgery (control group); another group received 1 liter/day for 7 days of a liquid diet enriched with arginine, omega-3 fatty acids, and RNA (preoperative group); and a third group were given enteral feeding of the enriched liquid diet both before and after surgery (perioperative group). Malnutrition in these cancer patients was defined by weight loss. The groups were compared for homogeneity in terms of demographics, biochemical markers, comorbid factors, and surgical variables. The main outcome variables were postoperative complications and length of hospital stay.

Wouters-Wesseling, W., Wouters, A.E., Kleijer, C.N., et al. Study of the effect of a liquid nutrition supplement on the nutritional status of psycho-geriatric nursing home patients. *Eur J Clin Nutr*, 2002, *56*(3):245–251.

This study used weight, Barthel index of daily activities, bowel function, serum level albumin, C-reactive protein, homocystine, thiamine, vitamin B6 and B12, folic acid, and vitamin D to evaluate the effect of a multinutrient liquid nutrition supplement in psychogeriatric nursing home patients. The researchers used a double-blind, placebo-controlled design and assessed outcomes at baseline, 6 weeks, and 12 weeks.

References

1. Porter, C., Schell, E.S., Kayser-Jones, J., & Paul, S.M. Dynamics of nutrition care in nursing home residents who are eating poorly. *J Am Diet Assoc*, 1999, *99*(11):1444-1446.
2. Simmons, S.F., & Reuben, D. Nutritional intake monitoring for nursing home residents: A comparison of staff documentation, direct observation, and photography methods. *J Am Geriatr Soc*, 2000, *48*(2):209-213.
3. Breslow, R.A., & Sorkin, J.D. Comparison of one-day and three-day calorie counts in hospitalized patients: A pilot study. *J Am Geriatr Soc*, 1993, *41*:923-927.
4. Barrett-Connor, E. Nutrition epidemiology: How do we know what they ate? *Am J Clin Nutr*, 1991, *54*:182S-187S.
5. Gittelsohn, J., Shankar, A.V., Pokhrel, R.P., et al. Accuracy of estimating food intake by observation. *J Am Diet Assoc*, 1994, *94*(11):1273-1277.
6. Kretsch, M.J., & Fong, A.K. Validation of a new computerized technique for quantitating individual dietary intake: The Nutritional Evaluation Scale System (NESS) vs. weighed food record. *Am J Clin Nutr*, 1990, *51*(3):477-484.
7. Iwaoka, F., Yoshiike, N., Date, C., et al. A validation study on a method to estimate nutrient intake by family members through a household-based food-weighing survey. *J Nutr Sci Vitaminol*, 2001, *47*(3):222-227.
8. Burke, B.S. The dietary history as a tool in research. *J Am Diet Assoc*, 1947, *23*(12):1041.
9. Freidenreich, C.M., Slimani, N., & Riboli, E. Measurement of past diet: Review of previously proposed methods. *Epidemiol Rev*, 1992, *14*:177-196.
10. Block, G. Human dietary assessment: Methods and issues. *Prev Med*, 1989, *18*(5):653-660.
11. Beaton, G.H., Milner, J., Corey, P., et al. Sources of variance in 24 hour dietary recall data: Implications for nutrition study design and interpretation. *Am J Clin Nutr*, 1979, *32*:2456-2459.
12. Willett, W. Nutritional epidemiology: Issues and challenges. *Int J Epidemiol*, 1987, *16*(suppl):312-317.
13. Simon, M.S., Lababidi, S., Djuric, Z., et al. Comparison of dietary assessment methods in a low-fat dietary intervention program. *Nutr Cancer*, 2001, *40*(2):108-117.
14. Lee-Han, H., McGuire, V., & Boyd, N.F. A review of the methods used by studies of dietary measurement. *J Clin Epidemiol*, 1989, *42*(3):269-279.
15. Adelson, S. Some problems in collecting dietary data from individuals. *J Am Diet Assoc*, 1960, *36*(5):453-460.
16. Heady, J.A. Diets of bank clerks. Development of a method of classifying the diets of individuals for use in epidemiological studies. *J Res Stat Soc* [A], 1961, *124*:336.
17. Linusson, E.F.I., Sanjur, D., & Erikson, E.C. Validating the 24-hour recall method as a dietary survey tool. *Arch Latino Am Nutr*, 1975, *24*:277.
18. Almendingen, K., Trygg, K., Hofstad, B., et al. Results from two reseated 5 day dietary records with a 1 year interval among patients with colorectal polyps. *Eur J Clin Nutr*, 2001, *55*(5):374-379.
19. Vuckovic, N., Ritenbaugh, C., Taren, D.L., et al. A qualitative study of participants' experiences with dietary assessment. *J Am Diet Assoc*, 2000, *100*(9):1023-1028.
20. Black, A.E., & Cole, T.J. Biased over- or underreporting is characteristic of individuals whether over time or by different assessment methods. *J Am Diet Assoc*, 2001, *101*:70-80.
21. Krebs-Smith, S.M., Graubard, B., Cleveland, L., et al. Low energy reporters vs others: A comparison of reported food intakes. *Eur J Clin Nutr*, 2000, *54*:281-287.
22. Johansson, L., Solvoll, K., Bjorneboe, G.E., et al. Under- and overreporting of energy intake related to weight status in a national-wide sample. *Am J Clin Nutr*, 1998, *68*:266-274.
23. Champagne, C.M., Bray, G.A., Kurtz, A.A., et al. Energy intake and energy expenditure: a controlled study comparing dieticians and non-dieticians. *J Am Diet Assoc*, 2002, *102*(10):1428-1432.
24. Block, G., & Hartman, A.M. Issues in reproducibility and validity of dietary studies. *Am J Clin Nutr*, 1989, *50*:1133-1138.
25. Sertoli, M., Beers, T., Coates, R., et al. Assessing consumption of high-fat foods: The effect of grouping foods into single questions. *Epidemiology*, 1992, *3*(6):503-508.
26. Jonneland, A.T., Haraldsdottir, J., Overvad, K., et al. Influence of individually estimated portion size on the validity of a semiquantitative food frequency questionnaire. *Int J Epidemiol*, 1992, *21*(4):770-777.
27. Horwath, C.C. Validity of a short food frequency questionnaire for estimating nutrient intake in elderly people. *Br J Nutr*, 1993, *70*(1):3-14.
28. Martin-Moreno, J.M., Boyle, P., Gorgojo, L., et al. Development and validation of a food frequency questionnaire in Spain. *Int J Epidemiol*, 1993, *22*(3):512-519.
29. Schroder, H., Covas, M.I., Marrugat, J., et al. Use of a three-day estimated food record, a 72-hour recall and a food-frequency questionnaire for dietary assessment in a Mediterranean Spanish population. *Clin Nutr*, 2001, *20*(5):429-437.
30. Herbert, J.R., Hurley, T.G., Chiriboga, D.E., et al. A comparison of selected nutrient intakes derived from three diet assessment methods used in a low-fat maintenance trial. *Public Health Nutr*, 1998, *1*(3):207-214.

31. Guthrie, H.A., & Scheer, J.C. Validity of a dietary score for assessing nutrient adequacy. *J Am Diet Assoc*, 1981, *78*(3):240-242.

32. Kant, A.K., Schatzkin, A., Harris, T.B., et al. Dietary diversity and subsequent mortality in the First National Health and Nutrition Examination Survey Epidemiologic follow-up study. *Am J Clin Nutr*, 1993, *57*(3):434-440.

33. Kant, A.K., Block, G., Schatzkin, A., et al. Dietary diversity in the U.S. population, NHANES II, 1976-1980. *J Am Diet Assoc*, 1991, *91*(12):1526-1531.

34. Hoffer, L.J. Clinical nutrition: 1. Protein-energy malnutrition in the inpatient. *CMAJ*, 2001, *165*(10):1345-1349.

35. Bickley, L.S., Szilagyi, P.G. *Bates' guide to physical examination and history taking.* (8th ed.). Philadelphia: Lippincott Williams & Wilkins, 2003.

36. Fitzpatrick, T.B., Johnson, R.A., Polano, M.K., et al. (Eds.). *Color atlas and synopsis of clinical dermatology: Common and serious diseases.* (2nd ed.). New York, McGraw-Hill, 1992.

37. Baker, J.P., Detsky, A.S., Wesson, D.E., et al. Nutritional assessment: A comparison of clinical judgement and objective measures. *N Engl J Med*, 1982, *306*(16):969-972.

38. Pettigrew, R.A., Charlesworth P.M., Farmilo, R.W., & Hill, G.L. Assessment of nutritional depletion and immune competence: A comparison of clinical examination and objective measurements. *J Par and Ent Nutr*, 1984, *8*(1):21-24.

39. Kuczmarski, M.F., Kuczmarski, R.J., & Najjar, M. Descriptive anthropometric reference data for older Americans. *J Am Diet Assoc*, 2000, *100*(1):59-66.

40. Jensen, G.L., Friedmann, J.M., Henry, D.K., et al. Noncompliance with body weight measurement in tertiary care teaching hospitals. *J Par and Ent Nutr*, 2003, *27*(1):89-90.

41. Thomas, D.R., Ashmen, W., Morley, J.E., et al. Nutritional management in long-term care: Development of a clinical guideline. *J Gerontol* Medical Sciences, 2000, *55A*(12):M725-M734.

42. National Heart, Lung, and Blood Institute. *Clinical guidelines on the identification, evaluation and treatment of overweight and obesity in adults.* Bethesda, MD: National Institutes of Health, 2002.

43. Noel, P.H., & Pugh, J.A. Management of overweight and obese adults. *BMJ*, 2002, *325*:757-61.

44. Carson, J.A. Pocket tape measure for waist circumference: Training medical students and residents on a simple assessment of body composition. *J Nutr*, 2003, *133*(2):547S-549S.

45. Jeliffe, D.B. Direct nutritional assessment of human groups. In *The assessment of nutritional status of the community.* Monograph No. 53. Geneva: World Health Organization, 1966, pp. 238-239.

46. Chumlea, W.C., Guo, S.S., Kuczmarski, R.J., et al. Body composition estimates from NHANES III bioelectrical impedance data. *Int J Obes Rel Metab Disord*, 2002, *26*(12):1596-1609.

47. Carney, D.E., & Meguid, M.M. Current concepts in nutritional assessment. *Arch Surg*, 2002, *137*(1):142-145.

48. Chumlea, W.C., et al. Prediction of body weight for the nonambulatory elderly from anthropometry. *J Am Diet Assoc*, 1988, *88*(5):564-568.

49. Haboubi, N.Y., Hudson, P.R., & Pathy, M.S. Measurement of height in the elderly. *J Am Geriatr Soc*, 1990, *38*(9):1008-1010.

50. Burkinshaw, L., Jones, P.R., & Krupowicz, D.W. Observer error in skinfold thickness measurements. *Human Biol*, 1973, *45*(2):273-279.

51. Seale, J.L., & Rumpler, W.V. Comparison of energy expenditure measurements by diet records, energy intake balance, doubly labeled water and room calorimetry. *Eur J Clin Nutr*, 1997, *51*(12):856-863.

52. Schoeller, D.A., & Racette, S.B. A review of field techniques for the assessment of energy expenditure. *J Nutr*, 1990, *120*:1492-1495.

53. McClave, S.A., Spain, D.A., Skolnick, J.L., et al. Achievement of steady state optimizes results when performing indirect calorimetry. *J Par and Ent Nutr*, 2003, *27*(1):16-20.

54. McClave, S.A., McClain, C.J., & Snider, H.L. Should indirect calorimetry be used as part of nutritional assessment? *J Clin Gastrointerol*, 2001, *33*(1):14-19.

55. Schoeller, D.A. Measurement of energy expenditure in free-living humans by using doubly labeled water. *J Nutr*, 1988, *118*:1278-1289.

56. Corbean, R.A., Gentillo, L.M., Parker, A., et al. Nutritional assessment using a pulmonary artery catheter. *J Trauma*, 1992, *33*(3):452-456.

57. DeKeyser, F.G., & Pugh, L.C. Approaches to physiologic measurement. In C. Waltz, O. Strickland, & E. Lentz (Eds.), *Measurement in nursing.* (2nd ed.). Philadelphia: Davis, 1991, pp. 387-412.

58. Cardenas, D., Blonde-Cynober, F., Ziegler, F., et al. Should a single center for the assay of biochemical markers of nutritional status be mandatory in multicenter trials? *Clin Nutr*, (2001), *20*(6):553-558.

59. Hensrud, D.D. Nutrition screening and assessment. *Med Clin North Am*, 1999, *83*(6):1525-1546.

60. Woo, J., Mak, Y.T., Lau, J., & Swaminathan, R. Prediction of mortality in patients in acute medical wards using basic laboratory and anthropometric data. *Postgrad Med J*, 1992, *68*(806):954-960.

61. Kyle, U.G., Genton, L., Mentha, G., et al. Reliable bioelectrical impedance analysis estimate of fat-free mass in liver, lung, and heart transplant patients. *J Par and Ent Nutri*, 2001, *25*(2):45-51.

62. Haapala, I., Hirvonen, A., Niskanen, L., et al. Anthropometry, bioelectrical impedance and dual-energy x-ray absorptiometry in the assessment of body composition in elderly Finnish women. *Clin Physiol Funct Imaging*, 2002, *22*(6):383-391.

63. Fogelholm, M., Van Marken Lichtenbelt, W. Comparison of body composition methods: A liteature review. *Eur J Clin Nutr*, 1997, *51*:495-503.

64. Barak, N., Wall-Alonso, E., Cheng, A. & Sitrin, M.D. Use of bioelectrical impedance analysis to predict energy expenditure of hospitalized patients receiving nutritional support. *J Par and Ent Nutri*, 2003, *27*(1):43-46.

65. Slinde, F., & Rossander-Hulthen, L. Bio-electrical impedance: Effect of 3 identical meals on diurnal impedance variation and calculation of body composition. *Am J Clin Nutr*, 2001, *74*:474-478.

19

Measuring Sleep

Felissa R. Lashley

Sleep is an active, rather than passive, process that is part of a cyclic circadian alternation of sleep and wakefulness.[1] This sleep-wake rhythm is regulated by neural systems that include a neural pacemaker and various neurochemical systems. It is influenced by other factors and conditions, such as light and darkness.[1]

In humans, sleep consists of two major states: rapid-eye-movement (REM) sleep, and non-REM (NREM) sleep. REM sleep usually is not divided into stages, but various stages have been identified in NREM sleep. NREM sleep is subdivided in stages from 1 to 4 corresponding to an approximate continuum of depth of sleep from light to deep. Each of these stages have distinct electroencephalographic (EEG) characteristics.[2] NREM sleep is controlled by multiple neuronal groups and systems involving the hypothalamus, basal forebrain, midbrain, pons, and medulla, but REM sleep is controlled by systems located mainly in the pons.[3]

In normal adults, there is a cyclical alternation of REM and NREM sleep, with NREM sleep occurring first in the transition from wakefulness to sleep. The first sleep cycle is usually shorter, with both NREM and REM sleep normally alternating in cycles averaging approximately 90 to 110 (but ranging from 70 to 120) minutes through the night. A normal adult will have between four and six cycles per night. REM sleep occupies about 20% to 25% of total sleep, and NREM sleep accounts for 75% to 80% of total sleep in normal young adults.[1] Various factors influence sleep stages, including age, circadian rhythms, temperature, drugs, and pathologic alterations.[2]

Typically, in adults, in the first part of the night, NREM sleep predominates; and as the night wears on, REM sleep occupies an increasing proportion of the approximate 90-minute cycle. Sleep normally begins with NREM stage 1 sleep (drowsiness), which is a transitional state between wakefulness and deeper levels of sleep. It usually comprises only 5% to 10% of normal sleep time. People can be easily aroused from this stage. Stage 2 NREM sleep (light sleep) usually follows and comprises the greatest proportion (45% to 55%) of adult sleep. As stage 2 sleep continues, the EEG shows slow-wave activity that eventually meets the criteria for stage 3 sleep. Stages 3 and 4 sleep typically follow. NREM stages 3 and 4 sleep often are called slow-wave, delta, or deep sleep. NREM stage

3 sleep comprises 4% to 6% of total sleep time, usually appearing in the first third of the sleep episode.

In the first sleep cycle, NREM stage 4 sleep lasts about 20 to 40 minutes. NREM stage 4 sleep represents 12% to 15% of sleep time, and slow-wave sleep predominates. Then, usually, sleep returns to stages 3 and 2. From stage 2 sleep, REM sleep may be entered, preceded by a series of body movements. REM sleep normally appears after a full cycle of NREM sleep has occurred. The REM sleep stage has spontaneous, rapid eye movements with high brain activity and metabolism. Dreaming occurs during this stage. NREM sleep stages 3 and 4 usually predominate during the first half of the sleep period and are reduced later. REM sleep occurs more in the second half of the sleep period, usually alternating with NREM stage 2 sleep. As the night or sleep period wears on, the cycles repeat, but the REM periods become longer, and NREM sleep may reach only stages 2 or 3.[4-7]

Variation in sleep patterns are characteristically associated with age. Newborns spend about half of their sleep in the REM stage; this percentage is higher in premature infants.[8] Slow-wave sleep is at a maximum in children and decreases with age. In some older individuals, stage 4 sleep may be absent.[1,2] Other observed changes in the elderly are shorter total sleep times (although in one survey, older respondents reported more sleep than younger ones[9]), increased night awakenings, and increased fragmentation of sleep. The nighttime awakenings are sometimes due to physical problems, such as the need to urinate or pain.[10] The elderly frequently take medications to help them sleep. An inadequate amount of sleep or poor sleep quality often are reflected in daytime napping, lack of alertness, and fatigue.[11]

In the United States approximately 40 million people have chronic sleep disorders, and 20 to 30 million have intermittent sleep problems.[1] Sleep disorders affect infants (e.g., sudden infant death syndrome), children, adults (e.g., sleep apnea, insomnia, circadian rhythm disorders due to shift work), the elderly (> 50% of those 65 years and older), and individuals with medical and/or psychiatric illness.

Disorders of sleep and arousal have been variously classified. In 1990, the new International Classification of Sleep Disorders, produced by the American Sleep Disorders Association, was released and later revised.[12] This detailed classification system summarizes diagnostic and coding information. An outline of this system is shown:[12]

1. Dyssomnias
   Intrinsic sleep disorders
   Extrinsic sleep disorders
   Circadian rhythm sleep disorders
2. Parasomnias
   Arousal disorders
   Sleep-wake transition disorders
   Parasomnias usually associated with REM sleep
   Other parasomnias
3. Sleep disorders associated with medical/psychiatric disorders
   Associated with mental disorders
   Associated with neurologic disorders
   Associated with other medical disorders
4. Proposed sleep disorders

The first category, the dyssomnias, includes many of the disorders commonly associated with either insomnia (difficulty in initiating or maintaining sleep) or excessive sleepiness. Dyssomnias are a heterogeneous grouping that include the major primary sleep disorders associated with either disrupted nocturnal sleep or impaired wakefulness and excessive sleepiness.[12] Included are intrinsic sleep disorders (those in which the primary cause is an internal abnormality originating within the body, such as narcolepsy or central sleep apnea syndrome); extrinsic sleep disorders (those in which the primary cause is outside the body, such as environmental sleep disorder or hypnotic-dependent sleep disorder); and circadian rhythm disorders, in which the underlying problem is chronophysiologic, such as shift work sleep disorder.[12]

The second category, parasomnias, are undesirable physical phenomena that usually occur during, or are exacerbated by, sleep. These may occur during REM sleep, arousal, or the transition from sleep to awakening or vice-versa, and include such disorders as bruxism (teeth grinding), sleepwalking, rhythmic movement disorder, night terrors, nightmares, and sudden infant death syndrome.[12]

The third category consists of sleep disorders associated with medical/psychiatric disorders and may include alcoholism, psychoses, parkinsonism, sleep-related asthma, and peptic ulcer disease. The final category is called "proposed sleep disorders" and includes pregnancy-associated sleep disorder.[12]

Issues in the Measurement of Sleep

Selecting a measure of sleep depends on the problem being investigated and the purpose of the investigation. Is the investigator interested in the problem from a research or a clinical perspective? Is the aim of the investigation diagnostic, evaluation of management and treatment, or assessment of a given sleep parameter under different conditions? Because *sleep* is a general term, the investigator must determine in advance what parameters or variables are of interest for the particular study. Possible variables and parameters related to sleep are:

Time spent in bed
Sleep quantity or total sleep time
Time and percentage spent in various stages of sleep
Number of sleep stage shifts
Sleep onset latency (time from "lights out" to sleep)
"Lights out" time
Time of falling asleep
Difficulty/ease in falling asleep
Quality of sleep
Bedtime rituals
Use of medications to promote sleep
Sleep arousals per night (number, length, time of night, circumstance [e.g., urination], difficulty/ease in falling back to sleep)
Sleep sufficiency
Sleep efficiency
Sleep fragmentation
Soundness of sleep
Satisfaction with sleep
Time of arising
Difficulty/ease in awakening in the morning
Feeling rested or refreshed after sleep
Moods or feelings on awakening
Occurrence of parasomnias or sleep-related symptoms
Dreams
Daytime sleepiness/alertness
Napping during the day (time of day, number, duration, circumstances)

Certain aspects of sleep can be measured objectively provided that instrumentation is calibrated correctly, the results are examined by a skilled interpreter, and reliability and validity issues, including the appropriateness of the measure for the problem, are addressed. Aspects of sleep that lend themselves to measurement by instrumentation include the time spent in each stage of sleep, sleep latency, total sleep time, number of arousals or awakenings, time of awakening, amount and type of movement, and the like. However, if an investigator wishes to assess the prevalence of general sleep problems in relation to another parameter in a large population, he or she may choose survey research methodology and devise one or two questions related to sleep, as discussed later in this chapter.

Objective techniques are useful for many purposes, but it often is of interest to know how respondents perceive their sleep. In some ways, measuring sleep perception is similar to measuring pain perception in that there are important subjective perceptions to assess. These can include sleep quality, whether sleep was "good" or not, and whether the person felt rested on awakening. Other considerations that guide the choice of measurement include budget, the number of professionals participating in the project, the availability of specialized equipment or space, expertise of the investigator or consultants, the size of the sample, the anticipated cooperation of subjects and any inconvenience to them, and time constraints. The gold standard for traditional sleep studies is polysomnography, but this method may not be available to all investigators. Furthermore, it may not provide the type of information desired and may provide data not necessary to the particular study. Instrumentation also has been used to indirectly assess sleep states through activity monitoring or movement.

Another approach to assess sleep has been the use of questionnaires. These can be particularly useful for screening, triage, and assessing the effects of treatment. They are inexpensive, nonintrusive, and may subjectively assess the respondent's perceptions. Instruments with credible reliability and validity are desirable. Unfortunately, many questionnaires developed to measure sleep have not predefined the aspects of sleep they measure; the reference time of the inquiry may be unclear; psychometric information may not be available; scoring information may be absent; intentional and unintentional bias may be present;[13] data are usually retrospective, and recall bias may play a significant role; and the population on which the tool was normed may be homogeneous, leading to problems of generalization (e.g., age, sex, ethnic group). Many questionnaires have been developed by an author for a specific study and have not been tested again. Questionnaires may be administered by self-report and interview. Because few researchers, even in studies using single sleep-related questions, have used consistent wording in the question and response choices, it is difficult to make cross-study comparisons.

Instruments such as sleep diaries and sleep logs have been used as self-reports or as charts completed by observers. Sleep diaries permit comparison between sleep parameters and other events of interest over a continuous period but can be burdensome. Observational techniques, such as those by health care providers, bed partners, or parents, have been used alone or in conjunction with instrumentation and self-reports and may include the use of time-lapse photography or video/audio recording. Indirect measures of sleep have been through daytime performance testing or psychologic testing. These are discussed later in this chapter.

A brief discussion of the relationship between subjective and objective measures of sleep is warranted. Results have varied, and ultimately the relationship between objectively measured and subjectively perceived parameters, such as length of time slept, may depend on the definition of the variable; the extent and significance of the variation of the parameter; factors related to the individual subject, such as age, mood, drug use, cognition, and disease state; instrument-related factors, such as question wording; selection of the objective and subjective measures; unintentional investigator bias; and the method used to compare the objective and subjective measures. Furthermore, although an overnight sleep study may objectively indicate restlessness and arousals, a subject may report "good" sleep and indeed may feel rested. Both results are useful.

Some researchers[14] have documented that people can accurately describe at least some sleep parameters, but other researchers comparing other sleep parameters with electrophysiologic monitoring have found less reliability with estimates of depth of sleep and the number of brief awakenings.[14] Turner and Ascher reported a correlation of 0.84 between roommate report and self-report on sleep latency.[15] Researchers finding acceptable correlations between various variables measured by objective and subjective counterparts are numerous,[16,17] as are those who find questionable relationships between the two approaches.[18] Others find variation within the same experimental setting.[19] Thus, it cannot be assumed that all subjective measures are invalid and that subjective assessments do provide unique information, but caution is needed in instrument selection and interpretation.

This chapter is organized by instrumentation: questionnaires (including rating scales) and interviews, single- and few-item survey-type questions, sleep diaries and logs, observation, and performance and psychologic testing.

Instrumentation Used to Measure Sleep

Polysomnography

The gold standard for monitoring sleep is polysomnography. A sleep study is usually done overnight in a sleep laboratory and employs a standardized scoring method.[20] Monitoring may include the recording of sleep-related physiologic parameters, such as respiratory, neuromuscular, cardiac, genitourinary, gastrointestinal, and/or endocrine functions.[21] An individualized, tailored protocol may be designed for a given person based on the type of problem suspected. The EEG is the core of polysomnography, but other standard assessed measures include the continuous monitoring of (1) eye movement activity by electrooculogram (EOG), (2) cardiac rhythm monitoring by electrocardiogram (ECG), (3) muscle monitoring by electromyogram (EMG), and (4) respiratory parameters. At least one channel of EEG is monitored (e.g., C3/A2 or C4/A1). More extensive monitoring may be desirable to evaluate seizures or the parasomnias. The EOG records eye-movement activity during sleep and is particularly useful in detecting REM sleep (distinguished by bursts of rapid eye movements), sleep onset, and transition into NREM stage 1 (when slow rolling eye movements may be seen). At least two channels are recommended. For the EMG, usually the muscles beneath the chin (mentalis/submentalis muscles) are monitored. However, additional muscle monitoring specific to a particular interest may be added. For example, the anterior tibialis muscles are of particular interest in detecting periodic leg movements or restless legs syndrome. To monitor bruxism, the masseter muscle may be an EMG location. Other parameters may be added, including respiratory parameters, core temperature determinations, heart rate, blood pressure, penile tumescence, and esophageal pH. The minimal respiratory parameters necessary to evaluate breathing disorders during sleep, such as in sleep apnea, include airflow or exchange monitoring through the nose and mouth, respiratory effort, and a measure of oxygen saturation (usually oximetry). These concurrent measurements should be recorded and interpreted by certified experts, using standardized procedures and scoring.[22] Sleep-stage scoring techniques have been well developed and standardized.[20] The standard for scoring remains the visual interpretation, although computer-aided systems are expected to become the norm in the near future.

Audio and video monitoring during the overnight recording, combined with behavioral observation, are useful to characterize arousal disorders, assess seizure activity, and observe body position and movement during sleep.[22] After the person has settled in, electrodes are applied, and the mechanical apparatus is calibrated. Recording is usually done on chart paper 300 mm wide recorded at a chart speed of 10 or 15 mm/second. To begin polysomnography, the lights should be turned off as close to the person's regular bedtime as possible; testing should be concluded as close to the normal time of arising as possible. These times should be marked on the chart paper. A technologist usually observes the patient throughout the procedure. If possible, 8 hours of recording (and at least 6.5 hours) should be done. Sleep recordings are commonly scored by dividing the paper tracing into segments or epochs. The most commonly used epoch lengths are 20 or 30 seconds. A first night effect has been described for adaptation to the sleep laboratory. Some researchers believe that even after several adaptation nights, an accurate assessment of the subject's usual asleep is not possible; hence the interest in at-home measures and other ways of assessment.[23]

Multiple Sleep Latency Test (MSLT)

The MSLT consists of polygraphic monitoring with a standard recording montage that usually includes EEG, EOG, EMG, ECG, respiratory flow, and respiratory sounds. The major purposes of the MSLT are to assess readiness to fall asleep, detect daytime sleepiness, and detect sleep-onset REM episodes (SOREMPs). SOREMPs do not usually occur in normal adults, as sleep usually begins with NREM sleep. The MSLT can be used (1) to diagnose narcolepsy; (2) to assess responses to drug therapy; and (3) to evaluate the experimental effects of different drugs, the manipulation of dosages or changing nighttime sleep schedules.[24] The MSLT generally is done on the day after overnight polysomnography. The subject should have kept sleep diaries for one to two weeks before admission because values on the MSLT can be influenced by previous sleep. Drugs influencing sleep (e.g., caffeine, alcohol, hypnotics, amphetamines, sedatives, antihistamines, and others) must be withdrawn 2 weeks prior to this test. The patient is in street clothes and between tests is not in bed. To begin the test, the recording equipment is attached to the patient. Specific standardized instructions are given. The patient lies down in a dark room with a nonstimulating environment and is given the opportunity to nap at 2-hour intervals for four to five times during the day. The usual times are 10:00 A.M., noon, 2:00 P.M., 4:00 P.M., and 6:00 P.M. These nap periods are usually 20 minutes long. The time to sleep onset (sleep latency) and the types of sleep are monitored. In normal persons, sleep onset usually is 10 minutes or more. The mean sleep latency is shorter in persons with narcolepsy, usually averaging less than 5 minutes. Normal people usually begin REM sleep 75 to 90 minutes after going to sleep; sleep onset does not normally begin with REM sleep. REM sleep usually is not experienced during a short nap period. The occurrence of two or more SOREMPs during the MSLT nap period is virtually diagnostic of narcolepsy, especially if other causes of early onset of REM sleep, such as severe sleep deprivation, have been ruled out. The MSLT is said to have a sensitivity of 84% and specificity of 99% using narcoleptic diagnosis criteria of less than 5 minutes to fall asleep and at least 2 SOREMPs.[22,24,25] Studies of the use of nasal continuous positive airway pressure (CPAP) for both chronic snorers and sleep apneics showed an improvement in MSLT scores with CPAP administration,[26] suggesting validity of the MSLT. Other research has demonstrated that the MSLT scores are related to the amount of sleep on one or more previous nights, time of day, and other variables in normal subjects.[27] One study in six insomniacs demonstrated a test-retest reliability over 3 to 90 weeks of 0.65.[28] Another study demonstrated that the MSLT is highly reliable in testing daytime sleepiness in normal subjects even over periods exceeding a year. However, these researchers cautioned that at least three and preferably four MSLTs were necessary for good reliability. For four tests, the test-retest reliability in 14 normal subjects was reported as 0.97 by Zwyghuizen-Doorenbos and colleagues.[29] The MSLT has also been used to investigate sleep latency in persons undergoing smoking cessation.[30] The MSLT shows promise for use in an ambulatory setting, although its use is not yet widespread.[31] The MSLT has been called "the accepted clinical standard" for the diagnosis of daytime sleepiness.[24]

Maintenance of Wakefulness Test (MWT)

The MWT evolved from the MSLT. It also is a polysomnographic procedure in which the variables monitored include EEG, EOG, EMG, ECG, and respiratory parameters. The MWT uses a multiple-nap approach but measures the subject's ability to stay awake rather than to fall asleep. Subjects are instructed to "try to stay awake for as long as possible" while sitting in a comfortable chair in a dark room for five 20-minute trials between 10:00 A.M. and 6:00 P.M.[32] This procedure evaluates the degree of alertness and can detect sleep tendency at inappropriate times.[22]

Another test, said to be similar to the MWT, has been referred to as "lapses." It consists of a 10-minute tapping test, 5 minutes with the eyes open and 5 minutes with the eyes closed. The person is instructed to stay awake during tapping, and a lapse is scored if the time between taps is longer than 3 seconds. The number of lapses in the 10 minutes is scored and used as a measure of sleepiness. Freeman et al. found a negative correlation of 0.51 between lapses and the MSLT.[33]

Repeated Test of Sustained Wakefulness (RTSW)

The RTSW also is a polygraphic test and examines the effects of treatment on the ability to sustain wakefulness in persons who are excessively sleepy.[34] The subject lies in bed in a dimly lit room and is instructed to remain awake. Some researchers believe that the MWT and RTSW are more sensitive to nighttime changes in sleepiness and alertness than the MSLT and in one study discriminated between subjects in nap, and no-nap conditions.[34]

Modified Assessment of Sleepiness Test (MAST)

The MAST is a modification of the MSLT. Subjects are studied in alternating conditions in both a "bed nap" setting and a "chair nap" setting. The researchers[35] believe that the "chair" setting has face validity and that the MAST may provide a sensitive measure, particularly in the assessment of sleepiness in patients with some type of hypersomnia.[35]

Home or Ambulatory Monitoring

Among the disadvantages of polysomnography is the expense, including an overnight stay in the sleep laboratory and the need for all-night technologists and for specialized equipment and facilities.[36] In addition, recorded sleep may be influenced by of the unnatural environment. Technologic advances have resulted in some ambulatory and home-monitoring devices that allow the recording of sleep and associated physiologic parameters outside the sleep laboratory.[21] Advantages include allowing data collection in a more natural environment, less expense, round-the-clock data collection, and free movement. Disadvantages include the potential for the monitoring device to develop a glitch and for the patient to misunderstand the instructions; uncontrolled conditions;

and the lack of immediate medical backup if needed. Ambulatory or home monitoring may be particularly suited to document disorders occurring sporadically, such as the parasomnias or seizures.[31] Some systems allow for transmission of the home-collected sleep data by telephone lines directly to the sleep laboratory.[37] Both analogue ambulatory recorders (e.g., Medilog 9000 system, Oxford Medical Systems, Clearwater, FL) and digital systems (e.g., the Vitalog portable recorder, Vitalog Corporation, Palo Alto, CA) can be used for home monitoring. Each has certain suitabilities and advantages and disadvantages. Sewitch and Kupfer compared analogue ambulatory and laboratory recordings to monitor sleep in normal persons and found that the results were essentially the same.[38] A consensus statement issued by the American Thoracic Society has not recommended home monitoring devices for the diagnosis of sleep-related respiratory problems at this time.[39] As devices have been refined, agreement between home and laboratory studies, especially for sleep apnea, have increased.[40] Portable devices such as Embletta and the WATCH PAT 100 (a portable device based on measuring peripheral arterial tone) are being used for unattended sleep studies in obstructive sleep apnea syndrome, resulting in cost savings.[41,42]

Pupillometry

Pupillometry is a nonintrusive technique that evaluates the ability of the subject to maintain alertness by measuring pupillary constriction. The behavior of the pupil reflects autonomic activity: The sympathetic nervous system predominates in maintaining alertness, and the parasympathetic system is associated with sleep. In pupillometry an infrared pupillograph is used to measure the length of time a person maintains a large and stable pupillary diameter (characteristic of alertness) when seated in a dark room. Persons who are sleepy, such as in narcolepsy, may show progressive pupillary constriction or miosis over the 15-minute testing period and/or marked variation in pupillary diameter or oscillations, called hippus.[43]

Pupillometry has been used to follow patients under various types of treatment for insomnia. Some studies have reported that parameters such as baseline pupil diameter, pupillary light reflex, and the pupillary orienting response do not differentiate between normal individuals and those with narcolepsy.[44] Other studies have shown that pupillometry can distinguish sleep-deprived normals from controls or those with narcolepsy from normals and can accurately measure inalertness during attempts to stay awake.[45]

Pupillometry is relatively inexpensive and is not as time-consuming as polysomnography. However, standardization has not been accomplished, and the recognition of and procedure for dealing with artifacts such as involuntary eyeblinks remain an issue.[46]

Activity Measurement

An indirect method of studying sleep is by examining activity or motility. In sleep, major body movements occur mainly before and after REM sleep, long periods of immobility are associated with NREM sleep, and small body movements have been found to be associated with REM sleep.[47] The latter has been demonstrated by combining time-lapse videorecording with electrophysiologic monitoring.[47] Movement-sensing devices to measure sleep or wakefulness have been applied to studies of sleep in humans.[48] The actigraph is a small box containing a movement detector and memory storage that can be worn by subjects on the wrist or ankle. It allows continuous recording for several days during normal activities in the home. The internal piezoelectric sensor in the actigraph records movement and interpretation is based on the fact that fewer limb movements occur during sleep than during wakefulness.[49] Thus, it is used to infer sleep and wake periods. The time-based recording system uses various time periods or epochs for measurement, such as 5, 30, or 60 seconds. Various models are available, including the Motion-logger and the Actillume (both from Ambulatory Monitoring, Inc., Ardsley, NY, 10502; 914-693-9240). Scoring may be accomplished by various methods, including a hand-scoring method, a computer-scoring system called Sleepest that has several options,[49] Actigraphic Scoring Analysis, and the "Action" algorithm supplied with the actigraph. Appendix 19A presents research activities to demonstrate correlation of the actigraph with EEG.[48-64] Actigraphy is increasingly used to diagnose some sleep-wake disorders and evaluate treatment effects but seem less useful for documenting sleep apnea and long periods of wakefulness with little motion.[63]

In summary, the actigraph is useful because it can provide data over time in the home environment, is relatively inexpensive, appears more accurate than sleep logs, and for some parameters, particularly the distinction between sleep and wakefulness and total sleep time, correlates well with data from polysomnography. The method of scoring and characteristics of the population influence the accuracy of the results obtained. Other monitoring devices are highlighted in Appendix 19B.

Questionnaires and Interviews

A variety of questionnaires have been devised to measure various aspects of sleep and sleep-related behavior. As discussed, the self-report questionnaires are largely subjective and have both advantages and disadvantages. In some cases, questionnaires are wholly concerned with sleep, but in other cases, sleep is only one of several parameters investigated. A number of questionnaires will be discussed fully, and the others are detailed in Appendix 19C.

The Stanford Sleepiness Scale (SSS)

The SSS is a self-rating scale in which subjects are asked to record the number corresponding to the statement best describing their degree of sleepiness.[65] The SSS is administered every 15 minutes during waking activities and may be averaged over the hour. When averaged in this way, a decrease of approximately three scale values indicates a significant decrease in performance in those affected by sleep loss. Validity ratings of mean SSS values using the Wilkinson Addition Test and the Wilkinson Vigilance Test was reported at a correlation of 0.68; and correlation on an abridged version of the Williams Word Memory test was reported at 0.47. Reliability using alternate forms has been reported at 0.88.[65] The SSS is said to measure feelings of sleepiness or tiredness at a particular point in time. It is more often used in research protocols than in clinical evaluation and diagnosis.[24]

Two early validity studies were done. One found the SSS sensitive to total acute sleep deprivation.[66] Correlations were low and/or variable with level of performance and sleep deprivation, and therefore the elevated sleep ratings were not predictive of performance efficiency for individual subjects on the Wilkinson Auditory Vigilance test, a four-choice serial RT test, a visual simple RT test, anagrams, and the Wisconsin Card Sorting test.[67]

In another investigation using four short-duration performance tasks and the Wilkinson Auditory Vigilance task along with the SSS, Glenville and Broughton[68] found that the SSS was a reliable indicator of acute sleepiness and that there were significant (but unreported) correlations between the SSS and a decrease in performance on vigilance, choice reaction, and simple reaction time, but not with short-term memory and handwriting.[68] Reliability of the SSS in chronically sleep-deprived patients and those with cumulative partial sleep deprivation, as well as in narcoleptics, has been questioned.[69] When comparing a group of normal subjects with a group of patients with sleep apnea and excessive daytime sleepiness, Roth and colleagues did not find differences in SSS scores.[70]

The Epworth Sleepiness Scale (ESS)

The ESS measures general levels of sleep propensity, defined as the probability of falling asleep at a particular time.[71] Sleep propensity will vary by time of day and from day to day depending on activity, drugs, sleep deprivation, pathology, and cognitive and affective state. Average sleep propensity over a prolonged period, such as a week, can be calculated.[71] In terms of validity, the ESS was said to distinguish significantly between patients with disorders of excessive daytime sleepiness and those without and was significantly correlated with the MSLT and with polysomnography. The test-retest reliability of the ESS in a group of medical students in one study was 0.82. Patients with sleep apnea showed ESS scores that were statistically significantly lower after treatment than before treatment was started, as would be expected with successful treatment. Internal consistency reliability showed Cronbach's alphas of 0.88 for the patients and 0.73 for the students, showing a reasonably high consistency. A factor analysis was performed on the ESS scores of 150 patients and 104 students; one main factor was identified for each group. The ESS is reliable, internally consistent, and has one main dimension in its variance.[72] It has been used to assess sleep-disordered breathing in Hispanics and non-Hispanics.[73] An Italian-language version has been compared with the MSLT and found to be useful for preliminary screening of daytime sleepiness.[74]

For this paper-and-pencil questionnaire, the subject is asked to rate on a scale of 0 (low) to 3 (high) the chances that they would doze in certain situations. Thus, when the 8-item scores are summed, the individual's score can range from 0 (abnormally low sleepiness) to 24 (very high level of sleepiness).

The Pittsburgh Sleep Quality Index (PSQI)

The PSQI measures subjective sleep quality. This subjective, self-rated, paper-and-pencil questionnaire consists of 19 items. In addition, clinical information is assessed by the bed partner in 5 additional questions that are not used in the scoring. Responses to the 19 items are grouped into 7 component scores that are weighted equally on a 0-to-3 scale, as some components consist of one question and others have several questions. The 7 components of the PSQI are sleep quality, sleep latency, sleep duration, habitual sleep efficiency, sleep disturbances, use of sleeping medication, and daytime dysfunction. The 7 component scores also can be summed to produce a global PSQI score that can range from 0 to 21. Higher scores indicate more severe complaints and worse sleep quality.[75] A geriatric version has been used to examine sleep in older adults in various fitness programs.[76]

Internal consistency reliability for each component via Cronbach's alpha ranged from 0.35 to 0.76, with an overall reliability coefficient of 0.83. Test-retest reliability for 91 patients revealed a correlation for global scores of 0.85, and individual components ranged from 0.65 to 0.84. In regard to validity, global PSQI scores were compared across controls, depressives, and two groups of persons with sleep disorders. Patients were discriminated from controls, and concurrent polysomnographic findings supported the questionnaire findings. A global PSQI score above 5 was said to have a diagnostic sensitivity of 89.6% and specificity of 86.5% in differentiating good from poor sleepers.[75] Other instruments to measure sleep are found in Appendix 19C.[77–115]

Other Instruments

Single- or Few-Item Sleep Surveys

A number of investigators have examined various aspects of sleep, either singularly or as part of multidimensional studies of health in large populations. The latter studies usually include instruments with one or a few sleep-related items that are obtained by mailed survey or as part of large-scale telephone or face-to-face interviews.[116,117] Single-item inquiries about sleep often have less sensitivity and specificity than do composite scales.[80] Results from survey questions often can be difficult to compare because of methodologic differences, variations in the question phraseology, and differences in the type and wording of response choices.

Sleep Diaries/Sleep Logs/Charts

Polysomnographic recordings provide objective information about sleep, its stages, awakenings, and the like, but information about how individuals evaluate their sleep is not obtained in that manner. Sleep diaries are usually self-reports of sleep, are obtained daily, and, although subjective, they may be less biased than retrospective recalls obtained on an infrequent basis. Generally these day-to-day reports of sleep activities may be used not only at bedtime, but also to give a 24-hour picture of sleep-wake activities and patterns over a period of time, such as a week. Diaries are clinically relevant and over time may provide insights into patterns affecting sleep and the degree of disruption experienced by the patient. For example, in examining nocturnal enuresis in a child, the daily log may indicate that this occurred on nights when the child's daily nap was skipped, thus suggesting a possible cause-and-effect relationship and opportunity for intervention.[118]

Advantages of sleep diaries include their ease of use, convenience, low expense, reflection of the natural setting, relative nonobtrusiveness, and recording of the person's perceived sleep experience.[13] Diaries may be used independently or in conjunction with polysomnography to obtain a picture of usual behavior. They may be used to monitor adherence to therapy, such as scheduled naps; facilitate longitudinal data collection, such as in shift workers; evaluate treatment progress; monitor symptoms; and promote self-management.[119] Problems include the fact that they can be burdensome, they are subject to intentional and unintentional bias, subjects may not keep them daily and thus fill them in just before collection, and they are subjective. Sleep diaries may have a single focus, such as recording the number of minutes required to fall asleep in the previous night;[120] may combine this information with other data to judge the success of a relaxation treatment for long sleep-onset periods; or they may have multiple purposes. Depending on why the diary is being kept, daytime activities that influence sleep, as caffeine intake, alcohol or drug use, smoking, meals and snacks, medication use, and exercise may be recorded. Sometimes a sleep log may be kept by an observer, as in the case of a child.[119]

A major question regarding the use of self-reported sleep diaries or logs concerns reliability and validity. Haythornthwaite and colleagues[121] examined the use of diaries to study sleep in patients with chronic pain. The reliability of coefficients of stability was examined among subjects, as were reliability coefficients across four nights. They reported item ranges of 0.38 to 0.62 for coefficients of stability. Using the Spearman-Brown prophecy formula for reliability coefficients across four nights, they reported ranges of 0.69 to 0.87. Regarding validity they noted that subjects accurately discriminated different aspects of sleep behavior and reported adequate concurrent and convergent validity with individual items relative to sleep in other instruments. Rogers and colleagues[16] compared recordings in a sleep diary about nocturnal sleep and the time and duration of daytime naps with ambulatory polysomnographic recordings in 25 normal and 25 narcoleptic subjects. Agreement between the sleep diaries and polysomnographic data for these parameters was reportedly high (kappa = 0.87), as was the sensitivity (92.3%) and specificity (95.6%). They concluded that sleep diaries were reliable for collecting information about sleep-wake patterns in most subjects. Subjects with fluctuations in daytime vigilance were said to require greater sensitivity to detect short frequent naps.[16] In studies of sleep diaries, estimates of sleep latency were compared with observer estimates from the same night. Correlations have ranged from 0.84 to 0.99.[15,122] Other methods include daily sleep diary and spouse sleep diaries,[123] sleep card,[124] and a modified sleep card.[125]

Observation

Observation of sleep and wakefulness may occur through several methods, including direct behavioral observations by one or more observers (such as roommates, bedpartners, or nurses);[10] video,[47,126] and time-lapse photography, or motion pictures.[127] The latter is now used less frequently. Observation by a trained observer and/or by audio and video recording may accompany polysomnography. The issue of reliability is important. Direct observation often involves the use of a variety of investigator-developed protocols, descriptors, and/or forms. Often, these are developed according to what that the investigator wishes to observe. Thus, as in survey methodology, it often is difficult to make comparisons across studies.

Visual Analog and Rating Scales

Visual analog scales and adjective checklists often are used to assess subjective parameters, such as sleep, pain, fatigue, dyspnea, and moods. Detailed discussions may be found elsewhere.[128–131]

Performance and Psychologic Tests

Performance, vigilance, and psychologic tests sometimes are used as indirect measures of alertness or sleepiness. A consequence of impaired nighttime sleep and the use of certain medications, such as depressants, are decreased alertness, increased daytime sleepiness, and altered mood states.[132] As a result, daytime performance can decline.[133] Consistency has been demonstrated between objectively measured sleepiness, performance, vigilance, and certain moods.[132] Some of the most commonly used tests to measure performance or vigilance that have been used in regard to increased sleepiness and decreased alertness include the Wilkinson four-choice reaction time; Wilkinson addition test; the trailmaking test; the digit-symbol substitution test; symbol copying test; tracking tasks; auditory reaction time; complex visual reaction time; tapping rates; Serial 7 Subtraction; the Shipley-Hartford Abstraction Scale; Sentence Completion Test; card sorting; the Wechsler Memory Scale and other short- and long-term memory tests; reaction time tests; manual dexterity tests; and paired-associates tests.[133] Determining the psychologic parameters affected by sleep, such as mood, anxiety, hopelessness, and depression, also is common in conjunction with sleep-related measures. Commonly used tests in sleep-related studies have included mood-related visual analogue scales, the Profile of Mood States, the Multiple Affect Adjective Checklist, the Crown-Marlowe Social Desirability Scale, the Rotter Locus of Control, the Beck Depression Inventory, the Spielberger State/Trait Anxiety test, Minnesota Multiphasic Personality Inventory, the California Personality Inventory, and the Cornell Index. A discussion of these tests is beyond the scope of this chapter.

Summary

A variety of methods are available to measure the broad area of sleep. The choice of instrument and method depends on the purpose of the study, the aspect of sleep being studied, available resources, and the expertise of the investigator. Any choice of instrument should consider the issues of validity and reliability. Many of the more recently developed questionnaires have paid more attention to these issues. Promising advances have been made in less expensive instrumentation and in ambulatory monitoring. These approaches may offer more options for future studies.

References

1. National Commission on Sleep Disorders. *Research report. Vol. 1. Executive summary and executive report.* Bethesda, MD: National Institutes of Health, 1993.
2. Carskadon, M.A., & Dement, W.C. Normal human sleep: An overview. In M.H. Kryger, T. Roth, & W.C. Dement (Eds.). *Principles and practice of sleep medicine* (3rd ed.). Philadelphia: Saunders, 2000, pp. 15-25.
3. Siegel, J.M. Mechanisms of sleep control. *J Clin Neurophysiol*, 1990, 7(1):49-65.
4. Thorpy, M.J. (Ed.). *Handbook of sleep disorders.* New York: Marcel Dekker, 1990.
5. Thorpy, M.J., & Yager, J. *The encyclopedia of sleep and sleep disorders* (2nd ed.). New York: Facts on File, 2001.
6. Pressman, M.R., & Fry, J.M. What is normal sleep in the elderly? *Clin Geriatr Med*, 1988, 4(1):71-81.
7. Kryger, M.H., Roth, T., & Dement, W.C. (Eds.). *Principles and practice of sleep medicine* (3rd ed.). Philadelphia: Saunders, 2000.
8. Horne, J. Annotation: Sleep and its disorders in children. *J Child Psychol Psychiatr All Disc*, 1992, 33(3):473-487.
9. Kripke, D.F., Simons, R.N., Garfinkel, L., & Hammond, E.C. Short and long sleep and sleeping pills. Is increased mortality associated? *Arch Gen Psychiatr*, 1979, 36(1):103-116.
10. Webb, W.B., & Swinburne, H. An observational study of sleep of the aged. *Percept Motor Skills*, 1971, 32(3):895-898.
11. Goldstein, M.Z. Practical geriatrics: Insomnia in later life. *Psychiatr Serv*, 2001, 52:1573-1575.
12. American Sleep Disorders Association, Diagnostic Classification Steering Committee (Thorpy, M.J., Chairman). *International classification of sleep disorders: Diagnostic and coding manual.* Rochester, MN: American Sleep Disorders Association, 1997.
13. Bootzin, R.R., & Engle-Friedman, M. The assessment of insomnia. *Behav Assess*, 1981, 3:107-126.
14. Browman, C.P., & Tepas, D.I. The effects of presleep activity on all-night sleep. *Psychophysiology*, 1976, 13(6):536-540.
15. Turner, R.M., & Ascher, L.M. Controlled comparison of progressive relaxation, stimulus control and paradoxical intention therapies for insomnia. *J Consult Clin Psychol*, 1979, 47(3):500-508.

16. Rogers, A.E., Caruso, C.C., & Aldrich, M.S. Reliability of sleep diaries for assessment of sleep/wake patterns. *Nurs Res*, 1993, 42(6):368-372.
17. Edwards, G.B., & Schuring, L.M. Pilot study: Validating staff nurses' observations of sleep and wake states among critically ill patients, using polysomnography. *Am J Crit Care*, 1993, 2(2):125-131.
18. Weiss, B.L., McPartland, R.J., & Kupfer, D.J. Once more: The inaccuracy of non-EEG estimations of sleep. *Am J Psychiatr*, 1973, 130(11):1282-1285.
19. Monroe, L.J. Psychological and physiological differences between good and poor sleepers. *J Abn Psychol*, 1967, 72(3):255-264.
20. Rechtschaffen, A., & Kales, A. (Eds.). *A manual of standardized terminology, techniques and scoring system for sleep stages of human subjects.* NIH Publication No. 204. Washington, DC: Public Health Service, U.S. Government Printing Office, 1968.
21. Kayed, K. Use of home monitoring in a sleep disorders clinic. In L.E. Miles and R.J. Broughton (Eds.), *Medical monitoring in the home and work environment.* New York: Raven, 1990, pp. 245-254.
22. American Electroencephalographic Society guidelines for polygraphic assessment of sleep-related disorders (polysomnography). *J Clin Neurophysiol*, 1992, 9(1):88-96.
23. Johns, M.W., & Dore, C. Sleep at home and in the sleep laboratory: Disturbance by recording procedures. *Ergonomics*, 1978, 21(5):325-330.
24. Carskadon, M.A. Measuring daytime sleepiness. In M.H. Kryger, T. Roth, & W.C. Dement (Eds.). *Principles and practice of sleep medicine* (2nd ed.). Philadelphia: Saunders, 1994, pp. 961-962.
25. Carskadon, M.A., Dement, W.C., Mitler, M.M., et al. Guidelines for the multiple sleep latency test (MSLT): A standard measure of sleepiness. *Sleep*, 1986, 9(4):519-524.
26. DiPhillipo, M.A., Fry, J.M., & Pressman, M.R. Objective measurement of daytime sleepiness following treatment of obstructive sleep apnea with nasal CPAP. *Sleep Res*, 1988, 17:167.
27. Richardson, G.S., Carskadon, M.A., Orav, E.J., & Dement, W.C. Circadian variation of sleep tendency in elderly and young adult subjects. *Sleep*, 1982, 5(suppl 2):S82-S94.

28. Seidel, W.F., & Dement, W.C. The Multiple Sleep Latency Test: Test-retest reliability. *Sleep Res,* 1981, 10:284.

29. Zwyghuizen-Doorenbos, A., Roehrs, T., Schaefer, M., & Roth, T. Test-retest reliability of the MSLT. *Sleep,* 1988, 11(6):562-565.

30. Prosise, G.L., Bonnet, M., Berry, R.B., & Dickelj, M.J. Effects of abstinence from smoking on sleep and daytime sleepiness. *Chest,* 1994, 105(4):1136-1141.

31. Broughton, R.J. Ambulant home monitoring of sleep and its disorders. In M.H. Kryger, T. Roth, & W.C. Dement (Eds.), *Principles and practice of sleep medicine* (2nd ed.). Philadelphia: Saunders, 1994, pp. 978-983.

32. Mitler, M.M., Gujavarty, K.S., & Browman, C.P. Maintenance of wakefulness test: A polysomnographic technique for evaluating treatment efficacy in patients with excessive somnolence. *Electroencephalogr Clin Neurophysiol,* 1982, 53(6):658-661.

33. Freeman, C.R., Johnson, L.C., Spinweber, C.L., & Gomez, S.A. The relationship among four measures of sleepiness. *Sleep Res,* 1988, 17:334.

34. Sugerman, J.L., & Walsh, J.K. Physiological sleep tendency and ability to maintain alertness at night. *Sleep,* 1989, 12(2):106-112.

35. Erman, M.K., Beckham, B., Gardner, D.A., & Roffwarg, H.P. The modified assessment of sleepiness test (MAST). *Sleep Res,* 1987, 16:550.

36. Ancoli-Israel, S. Evaluating sleep apnea with a portable modified Medilog/Respitrace system. In L.E. Miles & R.J. Broughton (Eds.), *Medical monitoring in the home and work environment.* New York: Raven, 1990, pp. 275-283.

37. Sewitch, D.E. Evaluation of commercially available home recording systems for all-night sleep recordings: The telediagnostic and Oxford Medilog 9000 systems. In L.E. Miles & R.J. Broughton, *Medical monitoring in the home and work environment.* New York: Raven, 1990, pp. 231-243.

38. Sewitch, D.E., & Kupfer, D.G. Polysomnographic telemetry using Telediagnostic and Oxford Medilog 9000 systems. *Sleep,* 1985, 8(3):288-293.

39. American Thoracic Society Consensus Conference on Indications and Standards for Cardiopulmonary Sleep Studies. *Am Rev Resp Dis,* 1989, 139(2):559-568.

40. Golpe, R., Jimenez, A., & Carpizo, R. Home sleep studies in the assessment of sleep apnea/hypopnea syndrome. *Chest,* 2002, 122(4):1156-1161.

41. Bar, A., Pillar, G., Dvir, I., et al. Evaluation of a portable device based on peripheral arterial tone for unattended home sleep studies. *Chest,* 2003, 123(3):695-703.

42. Dingli, K., Coleman, E.L., Vennelle, M., et al. Evaluation of a portable device for diagnosing the sleep apnoea/hypopnoea syndrome. *Eur Respir J,* 2003, 21(2):253-259.

43. McLaren, J.W., Erie, J.C., & Brubaker, R.F. Computerized analysis of pupillograms in studies of alertness. *Invest Ophthalmol Vis Sci,* 1992, 33(3):671-676.

44. Newman, J., & Broughton, R. Pupillometric assessment of excessive daytime sleepiness in narcolepsy-cataplexy. *Sleep,* 1991, 14(2):121-129.

45. Yoss, R.E., Moyer, N.J., & Ogle, K.N. The pupillogram and narcolepsy. A method to measure decreased levels of wakefulness. *Neurology,* 1969, 19(10):921-928.

46. Eshler, B., Mercer, P., Merritt, S., & Cohen, F.L. Three methods of handling invalid pupillometry data. *Sleep Res,* 1992, 21:338.

47. Aaronson, S.T., Rashed, S., Biber, M.P., & Hobson, J.A. Brain state and body position. *Arch Gen Psychiatr,* 1982, 39(3):330-335.

48. Kripke, D.F., Mullaney, D.J., Messin, S., & Wyborney, V.G. Wrist actigraphic measures of sleep and rhythms. *Electroencephalogr Clin Neurophysiol,* 1978, 44(5):674-676.

49. Hauri, P.J., & Wisbey, J. Wrist actigraphy in insomnia. *Sleep,* 1992, 15(4):293-301.

50. Mullaney, D.J., Kripke, D.F., & Messin, S. Wrist-actigraphic estimation of sleep time. *Sleep,* 1980, 3(1):83-92.

51. Sadeh, A., Lavie, P., Scher, A., et al. Actigraphic home-monitoring sleep-disturbed and control infants and young children: A new method for pediatric assessment of sleep-wake patterns. *Pediatrics,* 1991, 87(4):494-499.

52. Pollmaecher, T., & Schulz, H. The relation between wrist-actigraphic measures and sleep stages. *Sleep Res,* 1987, 16:55.

53. Urbach, D., Lavie, P., & Alster, J. Screening for sleep disorders by actigraphic recordings. *Sleep Res,* 1988, 17:357.

54. Newman, J., Stampi, C., Dunham, D.W., & Broughton, R. Does wrist-actigraphy approximate traditional polysomnographic detection of sleep and wakefulness in narcolepsy-cataplexy? *Sleep Res,* 1988, 17:343.

55. Borbely, A.A. New techniques for the analysis of the human sleep-wake cycle. *Brain Devel,* 1986, 8(4):482-488.

56. Stampi, C., & Broughton, R. Ultrashort sleep-wake schedule: Detection of sleep state through wrist-actigraph measures. *Sleep Res,* 1988, 17:100.

57. van Hilten, J.J., Braat, E.A.M., van der Velde, E.A., et al. Ambulatory activity monitoring during sleep: An evaluation of internight and intrasubject variability in healthy persons aged 50-98 years. *Sleep,* 1993, 16(2):146-150.

58. Thoman, E.B., & Glazier, R.C. Computer scoring of motility patterns for states of sleep and wakefulness: Human infants. *Sleep,* 1987, 10(2):122-129.

59. Lichstein, K.L., Nickel, R., Hoelscher, T.J., & Kelley, J.E. Clinical validation of a sleep assessment device. *Behav Res Ther,* 1982, 20(3):292-297.

60. Keefe, M.R., Kotzer, A.M., Reuss, J.L., & Sander, L.W. Development of a system for monitoring infant state behavior. *Nurs Res,* 1989, 38(6):344-347.

61. Korner, A.F., Thoman, E.B., & Glick, J.H. A system for monitoring crying and noncrying, large, medium and small neonatal movements. *Child Dev,* 1974, 45(4):946-952.

62. Keefe, M.R. Comparison of neonatal nighttime sleep-wake patterns in nursery versus rooming-in environments. *Nurs Res,* 1987, 36(3):140-144.

63. de Souza, L., Benedito-Silva, A.A., Pirez, M.L. et al. Further of actigraphy for sleep studies. *Sleep,* 2003, 26(1):81-85.

64. Sadeh, A., & Acebo, C. The role of actigraphy in sleep medicine. *Sleep Med Rev,* 2002, 6(2):113-124.

65. Hoddes, E., Zarcone, V., & Dement, W.C. Cross-validation of the Stanford Sleepiness Scale. *Sleep Res,* 1972, 1:91.

66. Glenville, M., & Broughton, R. Reliability of the Stanford Sleepiness Scale compared to short duration performance tests and the Wilkinson auditory vigilance task. In P. Passouant & I. Oswald (Eds.), *Pharmacology of the states of alertness*. Oxford: Pergamon, 1979, pp. 235-244.

67. Herscovitch, J., & Broughton, R. Sensitivity of the Stanford Sleepiness Scale to the effects of cumulative partial sleep deprivation and recovery oversleeping. *Sleep*, 1981, 4(1):83-92.

68. Glenville, M., & Broughton, R. Reliability of the Stanford Sleepiness Scale compared to short duration performance tests and the Wilkinson auditory vigilance task. *Sleep Res*, 1982, 5:S135.

69. Broughton, R. Performance and evoked potential measures of various states of daytime sleepiness. *Sleep*, 5(suppl 2):S135-S146.

70. Roth, T., Hartse, K.M., Zorick, F., & Conway, W. Multiple naps and the evaluation of daytime sleepiness in patients with upper airway sleep apnea. *Sleep*, 1980, 3(3-4):425-439.

71. Johns, M.W. Daytime sleepiness, snoring, and obstructive sleep apnea. The Epworth Sleepiness Scale. *Chest*, 1993, 103(1):30-36.

72. Johns, M.W. Reliability and factor analysis of the Epworth Sleepiness Scale. *Sleep*, 1991, 15(4):376-381.

73. Sitton, S., & Chediak, A.D. The Epworth Sleepiness Scale correlates with indices of sleep disordered breathing in a population of Hispanics and Nonhispanics with obstructive sleep apnea. *Sleep Res*, 1994, 23:328.

74. Vignatelli, L., Plazzi, G., Barbato, A., et al. Italian version of the Epworth sleepiness scale: External validity. *Neurol Sci*, 2003, 23(6):295-300.

75. Buysse, D.J., Reynolds, C.F., III, Monk, T.H., et al. The Pittsburgh Sleep Quality Index: A new instrument for psychiatric practice and research. *Psychiatr Res*, 1989, 28(2):193-213.

76. Vitiello, M.V., Prinz, P.N., & Schwartz, R.S. The subjective sleep quality of healthy older men and women is enhanced by participation in two fitness training programs: A nonspecific effect. *Sleep Res*, 1994, 23:148.

77. Jenkins, C.D., Stanton, B.A., Savageau, J.A., et al. Physical, psychological, social and economic outcomes six months after cardiac valve surgery. *Arch Int Med*, 1983, 143(11):2107-2113.

78. Croog, S.H., Levine, S., Testa, M.A., et al. The effects of antihypertensive therapy on the quality of life. *N Engl J Med*, 1986, 314(26):1657-1664.

79. Jenkins, C.D., Stanton, B.A., Niemcryk, S.J., & Rose, R.M. A scale for the estimation of sleep problems in clinical research. *J Clin Epidemiol*, 1988, 41(4):313-321.

80. Rose, R.M., Jenkins, C.D., & Hurst, M.W. Health change in air traffic controllers: A prospective study I. Background and description. *Psychosom Med*, 1978, 40(2):142-165.

81. Zomer, J., Peled, R., Rubin, A-H.E., & Lavie, P. Mini Sleep Questionnaire (MSQ) for screening large populations for EDS complaints. In W.P. Koella, E. Ruther, & H. Schulz (Eds.), *Sleep '84*. Stuttgart: Gustav Fischer Verlag, 1985, pp. 467-470.

82. Ellis, B.W., Johns, M.W., Lancaster, R., et al. The St. Mary's Hospital Sleep Questionnaire: A study of reliability. *Sleep*, 1981, 4(1):93-97.

83. Leigh, T.J., Bird, H.A., Hindmarch, I., et al. Factor analysis of the St. Mary's Hospital Sleep Questionnaire. *Sleep*, 1988, 11(5):448-453.

84. Ellis, B.W., Harris, R.I., Hayward, S.J., et al. Factors in the sleep of preoperative patients. *Br J Surg*, 1982, 69(5):281-282.

85. Parrott, A.C., & Hindmarch, I. The Leeds Sleep Evaluation Questionnaire in psychopharmacological investigations—A review. *Psychopharmacology*, 1980, 71(2):173-179.

86. Kronholm, E., & Hyyppa, M.T. Age-related sleep habits and retirement. *Ann Clin Res*, 1985, 17(5):257-264.

87. Hyyppa, M.T., Lindholm, T., Kronholm, E., & Lehtinen, V. Functional insomnia in relation to alexithymic features and cortisol hypersecretion in a community sample. *Stress Med*, 1990, 6(2):277-283.

88. Hyyppa, M.T., & Kronholm, E. Quality of sleep and chronic illnesses. *J Clin Epidemiol*, 1989, 42(7):633-638.

89. Douglass, A.B., Bornstein, R., Nino-Murcia, G., & Keenan, S. Creation of the "ASDC Sleep Disorders Questionnaire." *Sleep Res*, 1986, 15:117.

90. Douglass, A.B., Bornstein, R., Nino-Murcia, G., et al. The Sleep Disorders Questionnaire I. Creation and multivariate structure of SDQ. *Sleep*, 1994, 17(5):160-167.

91. Douglass, A.B., Bornstein, R., Nino-Murcia, G., et al. Test-retest reliability of the Sleep Disorders Questionnaire (SDQ). *Sleep Res*, 1990, 19:215.

92. Lee, K.A. Self-reported sleep disturbances in employed women. *Sleep*, 1992, 15(6):493-498.

93. Schramm, E., Hohagen, F., Grasshoff, U., et al. Test-retest reliability and validity of the structured interview for sleep disorders according to DSM-III-R. *Am J Psychiatr*, 1993, 150(6):867-872.

94. Reynolds, C.F., III, Giles, D.E., Buysse, D.J., et al. The structured interview for sleep disorders according to DSM-III-R. *Am J Psychiatr*, 1993, 150(6):857-858.

95. Rumble, R., & Morgan, K. Hypnotics, sleep and mortality in elderly people. *J Am Geriatr Soc*, 1992, 40(8):787-791.

96. Johnson, J.E. Progressive relaxation and the sleep of older men and women. *J Comm Health Nurs*, 1993, 10(1):31-38.

97. Snyder-Halpern, R., & Verran, J.A. Instrumentation to describe subjective sleep characteristics in healthy subjects. *Res Nurs Health*, 1987, 10(3):155-163.

98. Verran, J., & Snyder-Halpern, R. Do patients sleep in the hospital? *Appl Nurs Res*, 1988, 1(2):95.

99. Verran, J. Personal correspondence, March, 1994.

100. Richards, K. Techniques for measurement of sleep in critical care. *Focus Crit Care*, 1987, 14(4):34-40.

101. McDonald, D.G., & King, E.A. Measures of sleep disturbance in psychiatric patients. *Br J Med Psychol*, 1975, 48(1):49-53.

102. Nicassio, P.M., Mendlowitz, D.R., Fussell, J.J., & Petras, L. The phenomenology of the pre-sleep state: The development of the pre-sleep arousal scale. *Behav Res Ther*, 1985, 23(3):263-271.

103. Coren, S. Prediction of insomnia from arousability predisposition scores: Scale development and cross-validation. *Behav Res Ther*, 1988, 26(5):415-420.

104. Bootzin, R.R., Shoham, V., & Kuo, T.F. Sleep anticipatory anxiety questionnaire: A measure of anxiety about sleep. *Sleep Res*, 1994, 23:188.

105. van Diest, R. Subjective sleep characteristics as coronary risk factors, their association with type A behaviour and vital exhaustion. *J Psychosom Res*, 1990, *34*(4):415-426.

106. Kapuniai, L.E., Andrew, D.J., Crowell, D.H., & Pearce, J.W. Identifying sleep apnea from self-reports. *Sleep*, 1988, *11*:430-436.

107. Webb, W.B., Bonnet, M., & Blume, G. A post-sleep inventory. *Percept Motor Skills*, 1976, *43*(3, part 1):987-993.

108. Domino, G., Blair, G., & Bridges, A. Subjective assessment of sleep by sleep questionnaire. *Percept Motor Skills*, 1984, *59*(1):163-170.

109. Hunt, S.M., et al. A quantitative approach to perceived health status. *J Epidemiol Comm Health*, 1980, *34*(4):281-286.

110. Alonso, J., Anto, J.M., Gonzalez, M., et al. Measurement of general health status of non-oxygen-dependent chronic obstructive pulmonary disease patients. *Med Care*, 1992, *30*(suppl 5):MS125-MS135.

111. McKenna, S.P., Hunt, S.M., & McEwen, J. Weighting the seriousness of perceived health problems using Thurstone's method of paired comparisons. *Int J Epidemiol*, 1981, *10*(1):93-97.

112. McKenna, S.P., McEwen, J., Hunt, S.M., & Papp, E. Changes in the perceived health of patients recovering from fractures. *Publ Health Lond*, 1984, *98*(2):97-102.

113. Hunt, S.D., McEwen, J., McKenna, S.P., et al. Subjective health status of patients with peripheral vascular disease. *Practitioner*, 1982, *226*(1363):133-136.

114. McDowell, I., & Newell, C. (Eds.). *Measuring health: A guide to rating scales and questionnaires.* New York: Oxford University Press, 1987.

115. Acebo, C., Sadeh, A., Seifer, R., et al. Mothers' assessment of sleep behaviors in young children: Scale reliability and validation during actigraphy. *Sleep Res*, 1994, *23*:96.

116. Morgan, K., Dallosso, H., Ebrahim, S., et al. Characteristics of subjective insomnia in the elderly living at home. *Age and ageing*, 1988, *17*(1):1-7.

117. Morgan, K., Dallosso, H., Ebrahim, S., et al. Prevalence, frequency, and duration of hypnotic drug use among the elderly living at home. *Br Med J*, 1988, *296*(6622):601-602.

118. Ferber, R. *Solve your childs sleep problems.* New York, Simon & Schuster, 1985.

119. Douglass, A.B., Carskadon, M., & Houser, R. Historical data base, questionnaires, sleep and life cycle diaries. In L.E. Miles & R.J. Broughton (Eds.), *Medical monitoring in the home and work environment.* New York: Raven, 1990, pp. 17-28.

120. Borkovec, T.D., & Weerts, T.C. Effects of progressive relaxation on sleep disturbance: An electroencephalographic evaluation. *Psychosom Med*, 1976, *38*(3):173-180.

121. Haythornthwaite, J.A., Hegel, M.T., & Sterns, R.D. (1991). Development of a sleep diary for chronic pain patients. *J Pain Symptom Man*, 1991, *6*(2):65-72.

122. Tokarz, T., & Lawrence, P. An analysis of temporal and stimulus factors in the treatment of insomnia. In R.R. Bootzin, & M. Engle-Friedman, The assessment of insomnia. *Behav Assess*, 1981, *3*:107-126.

123. Coates, T.J., Killen, J.D., George, J., et al. Estimating sleep parameters: A multitrait-multimethod analysis. *J Consult Clin Psychol*, 1982, *50*(3):345-352.

124. Lewis, H.E., Matthew, H., Proudfoot, A.T., et al. Nitrazepam-A safe hypnotic. *Lancet*, 1957, *2*(7008):1262-1266.

125. Tune, G.S. The influence of age and temperament on the adult human sleep-wakefulness pattern. *Br J Psychol*, 1969, *60*(4):431-441.

126. Anders, T.F., Keener, M.A., & Kraemer, H. Sleep-wake state organization, neonatal assessment and development in premature infants during the first year of life. II. *Sleep*, 1985, *8*(3):193-206.

127. Kligman, D., Smyrl, R., & Emde, R.N. A "nonintrusive" longitudinal study of infant sleep. *Psychosom Med*, 1975, *37*(5):448-453.

128. Herbert, M., Johns, M.W., & Dore, C. Factor analysis of analogue scales measuring feelings before and after sleep. *Br J Med Psychol*, 1976, *49*(4):373-379.

129. Gift, A. Visual analogue scales: Measurement of subjective phenomena. *Nurs Res*, 1989, *38*(5):286-288.

130. Cline, M.E., Herman, J., Shaw, E.R., & Morton, R.D. Standardization of the visual analogue scale. *Nurs Res*, 1992, *41*(6):378-380.

131. Wewers, M.W., & Lowe, N.K. A critical review of visual analogue scales in the measurement of clinical phenomena. *Res Nurs Health*, 1990, *13*(4):227-238.

132. Roth, T., Roehrs, T., & Zorick, F. Sleepiness: Its measurement and determinants. *Sleep*, 1982, *5*(suppl 2):S128-S134.

133. Johnson, L.C., Spinweber, C.L., Gomez, S.A., & Matteson, L.T. Daytime sleepiness, performance, mood, nocturnal sleep: The effect of benzodiazepine and caffeine on their relationship. *Sleep*, 1990, *13*(2):121-135.

134. Netzer, N.C., Stoohs, R.A., Netzer, C.M., et al. Using the Berlin Questionnaire to identify patients at risk for the sleep apnea syndrome. *Ann Intern Med*, 1999, *131*(7):485-491.

135. Harding, S.M. Prediction formulae for sleep-disordered breathing. *Curr Opin Pulm Med*, 2001, *7*(6):381-385.

Appendix 19A. Studies Illustrating the Accuracy of Actigraphy

Author	Study Description	Results
Kripke et al. (48)	Compared EEG and actigraph (24 hours; n = 5)	Positive correlation for total sleep time (0.98) Positive correlation of minutes for wake time (0.85)
Hauri and Wisbey (49)	Compared duration of sleep data in insomniacs (1 week, n = 36)	Wrist actigraphy more exact than sleep logs but less exact than polysomnography
Mullaney et al. (50)	Wrist actigraph compared to EEG (n = 85)	Positive correlation for total sleep time (0.89) Positive correlation for wakening after sleep onset (0.70) Positive correlation for mid-sleep awakenings (0.25)
Sadeh et al. (51)	Compared sleep-disturbed and normal children (leg actigraph)	Discriminated between 2 groups Correct assignment rate 79.4% (sleep-disturbed) and 91.2% (control)
Pollmaecher and Schulz (52)	Compared EEG and actigraph (n = 26)	Excellent agreement in deeper sleep stages Poor agreement in transition from wakefulness and sleep (insomniacs or supine subjects)
Urbach et al. (53) Newman et al. (54)	Efficacy of treatment for elder insomnia	Actigraph sensitive to treatment effects; reliably distinguishes sleep apnea from insomnia; distinguishes between sleep and wake states in narcolepsy
Borbely (55)	Usefulness of wrist activity to examine medication course of action	Measured motor activity and to document sleep attacks in narcolepsy patient
Stampi and Broughton (56)	Compared wrist actigraph and polysomnography (n = 1)	Excellent agreement on total sleep time (baseline 99% and recovery 96.1%) Less agreement for ultrashort sleep (78.8%)
de Souza et al. (63)	Compared actigraphy and polysomnography (n = 21)	Actigraphy sensitive for Cole's and Sadeh's algorithms but had low sensitivity
van Hilten et al. (57)	6 nights of study	Much intrasubject variability; varying results depending on subject and sleep parameter

Numbers in parentheses correspond to studies cited in the References.

Appendix 19B. Instrumentation Measuring Sleep: Other Monitoring Devices

Name/Description	Psychometrics	Comments
Static charge–sensitive bed (SCSB, Biomatt, Biorec, Inc.) Flexible, sensitive plate placed under mattress	Not widely tested or used in the United States	Used to study heart, respiratory, and body movements during sleep Can combine with other assessments Inexpensive
Home monitoring system (HMS) Uses pressure-sensitive mattress pad, signals from respiration and body movements are transmitted Patterns of signals identify sleep, wakefulness, respiratory events, leg movements	Signal scoring procedure reliable and valid (58)	Has been used with elderly and infants
Pressure-sensitive mattress with capacitance-type sensor/amplifier (electronic monitors)	Tandberg instrument recorded 5 states of sleep, computer results compared to observer (58)	Used to study infants
Holter ECG with ear oximetry and breath sound monitoring	In obstructive sleep apnea, there is progressive bradycardia associated with apnea followed by abrupt tachycardia	Used to measure cyclic variation of heart rate and snoring Inexpensive ($100)
Medilog/Respitrace recording system (Ambulatory Monitoring, Inc.)	Wrist actigraph transducer distinguishes sleep from waking (36)	Respirations recorded on Respitrace bands; combined with tibialis EMG
Sleep assessment device (SAD) (Farrall Instruments, Inc., Grand Island, Nebraska)	Compared to EEG recording and sleep questionnaire: percent agreement 83.3–100% (59)	If awake, subject verbally acknowledges soft tone played every 10 minutes (tape recorded)
Infant state bassinet monitor consists of foam cell air mattress connected via tube to stratham pressure unit (Burwin baby monitor) with output sent to digital event recorder	High correlation with standard sleep polygraph (60) Infant respiratory patterns and movements can be assessed (60)	Pressure-sensitive foot mat to detect caregiver can be added (61) Modified version used to categorize infant movements (62)

Numbers in parentheses correspond to studies cited in the References.

Appendix 19C. Other Questionnaires and Interviews to Measure Sleep

Name/Description	Psychometric Indices	Comments
Sleep Dysfunction Scale/Sleep Problems Scale 4 questions to ascertain the number of days the subject has problems: falling asleep, staying asleep, awakening early, or tired Coding is a 0–5 Likert-type scale (ATC) or 1–4 Scores may be summed: lower scores, less sleep disturbance	Cronbach's alpha: 0.79 (ATC) and 0.63 (CSRS) (77); 0.79 (78) Test–retest reliability: 0.59 (79) Concurrent validity (taking or not taking certain medications)	Developed from Air Traffic Controllers (ATC) and Cardiac Surgery Recovery Study (CSRS) (77,80) Called Sleep Problems Questionnaire by Jenkins et al. (79)
MiniSleep Questionnaire (MSQ) Contains 7 items Scaled from 1 (never) to 7 (always)	Mean scores for each item and for total MSQ can be determined "Outstanding stability" (81)	Developed to assess excessive daytime somnolence in large populations Work continues on refining selection criteria
St. Mary's Hospital Sleep Questionnaire 14 items evaluate sleep and early-morning behavior in past 24 hours 3 variables (sleep latency, sleep period time, awake onset latency) High score means "good sleep"	"Good" test–retest reliability Factor analysis showed no completely clear structure (83) 2 factors emerged: sleep latency and sleep quality	Evaluates sleep in hospitalized patients Has been used to detect changes in sleep of hospitalized surgical patients (84) and to compare the sleep of patients with arthritic diseases
Leeds Sleep Evaluation Questionnaire (SEQ) Consists of 10 questions, with responses on a visual analogue scale (10-cm line with words denoting extremes at each end) subject is asked to mark the line where it approximates his answer	Factor analysis revealed 4 factors corresponding to the 4 areas questioned Reasonable degree of reliability and validity (85)	Formerly known as Sleep Evaluation Questionnaire Used to monitor self-reported perceptions of sleep during drug treatment for sleep problems Questions explore 4 areas: getting to sleep, quality of sleep, awakening, and behavior following wakefulness
Rehabilitation Research Center Sleep Habit Questionnaire (RRC-SHQ) Originally consisted of 65 multiple-choice items Scoring has several indices (additive and dichotomous)	2 factors: depression-related insomnia and satisfaction with sleep (account for 39% of variance) (86) Good test–retest stability (87) "Acceptable validity and reliability" (88)	Questions relate to sleep environment, behavior, subjective feelings re: wakefulness, satisfaction with sleep quality, daytime sleepiness, initiating and maintaining sleep, dreams, other (88)
Sleep Questionnaire and Assessment of Wakefulness (SQAW) 863 items (multiple-choice, dichotomous, and fill-in)	No data found	Developed by Laughton Miles at Stanford University Clinical screening tool No scoring information available

311

Appendix 19C. Other Questionnaires and Interviews to Measure Sleep (*cont.*)

Name/Description	Psychometric Indices	Comments
ASDC Sleep Disorders Questionnaire 165 variables		Shortened version of SQAW Designed to predict, polysomnographic diagnosis (89)
Sleep Disorders Questionnaire Intent to develop "triage" questionnaire with diagnostic point of view 175 items plus body mass index, at 8th-grade reading level Response choices 1 to 5 on Likert-type scale Scoring manual being developed (90)	Reliability 0.7 overall correlation (2 weeks) (90) Canonical discriminant function analysis performed Criterion validity: related polysomnography and MSLT results to the specific group	Derived from SQAW May serve as a database and screening tool for referrals to sleep laboratory (89,90) Specific diagnostic scales developed were: sleep apnea, narcolepsy, psychiatric sleep disorder, and periodic leg movements
General Sleep Disturbance Scale (GSDS) 21 items Self-rated 10-point scale from 0 (never) to 9 (all the time) Can be broken down into 7 subscales Score: summed from 0 to 189 Higher score, more severely disturbed sleep (92)	Cronbach's alpha: overall 0.88 3 subscales: (1) use of sleep aids: 0.62; (2) sleep quality: 0.79; (3) sleepiness: 0.82 Validity: developed refined from SQAW and statistical difference between permanent and rotating shift nurses	Developed by Lee, a nurse investigator Items address sleep quality, quantity, initiating sleep, fatigue, alertness at work, use of drugs for sleep, others
Structured Interview for Sleep Disorders (DSM-III-R) (SIS-D) Structured clinical interview: semistructured section (e.g., health, meds), structured (sleep disorder symptoms) Takes 20–30 minutes Summary score sheet Instruction manual (93)	Validity: concordance between consensus diagnosis and polysomnographic data (90% confirmation) Test–retest reliability (Cohen's kappa: mean: 0.77) Reliability: 0.56–0.89 Interrater reliability 97%–100% (93)	Fits with forthcoming DSM-IV criteria (94) Used to screen and diagnose sleep disorders Useful screening instrument (94)
Nottingham Longitudinal Study of Activity and Aging Profiles health, well-being and assesses sleep and sleep meds	Not reported	Begun in 1985 to collect baseline data No significant relationships between mortality and subjective insomnia or sleep duration (95)
Baekland, Hoy: Unnamed Sleep Log Modified from Antrobus et al. (92) Also known as sleep pattern questionnaire 2-week log of (A) state of mind, fatigue before retiring, on awakening (3 items); and (B) 8 items completed on awakening (time fell asleep, number of awakenings, state of sleep, dreams)	No composite scoring Test–retest reliability: (A) 0.84 and (B) 0.97 only 7 items (96) Theta reliability: 0.76 (97)	Questionnaire results similar to EEG (14)

Scale	Reliability/Validity	Comments
Verran and Snyder-Halpern (VSH) Sleep Scale Uses visual analogue scale (97,98) Author-modified original scale (8 items sleep, 2 dreams)	Original scale compared to St. Mary's Hospital's Sleep Q and Baekland/Hoy log: theta reliability coefficient: 0.82; factor analysis and correlations showed validity	New scale has 15 items (disturbance, effectiveness, supplementation) Can calculate total sleep period (TSP) Ongoing testing in U.S. and Taiwanese populations (99)
Richards–Campbell Sleep Questionnaire (100) 5-item VAS (e.g., to sleep depth, quality), 0 (poorest quality) to 100 (optimal)	Content construct validity Cronbach's alpha (internal consistency reliability): 0.82	Revised instrument requires further testing (100)
Complaints of Sleep Disturbance Scale (CSD) 20 items from the MMPI (sleep, fatigue, dreams)	Correlation between sleep monitor and CSD score: 0.62 (101)	Distinguishes between subjects with high and low sleep motility
Pre-sleep Arousal Scale (PSAS) (102) 16 item, self-report 2 subscales: (A) somatic and (B) cognitive Subscale scores range from 8 to 40	Face validity 100% Somatic subscale (A) correlates significantly with CSAQ (0.36), as does cognitive subscale (B) (0.49) Construct validity Internal consistency reliability (A) 0.79–0.84 and (B) 0.67–0.88 Test–retest correlations (over 3 weeks): 0.76 (A) and 0.72 (B)	Discriminates among normal sleepers and insomniacs
Arousal Predisposition Scale (APS) Premise is that insomniacs have higher levels of autonomic activity (19,103) Initial 70 items reduced to 12 Items summed for composite score (higher scores show greater arousal)	Internal consistency reliability: 0.83–0.84 Validation studies conducted; "valid and reliable indicator of a pattern of sleep disruptions and insomnia"	Value: predicts tendency toward sleep disruption in general population (103)
Sleep Anticipatory Anxiety Questionnaire (SAAQ) (104) Assesses presleep anxiety 10 items Higher scores indicate more anxiety	Cronbach's alpha for internal consistency: 0.83 Factor analysis: (1) overall degree of presleep anxiety, (2) extent of cognitive experience as opposed to somatic arousal	Construct validity currently being evaluated
Sleep Wake Experience List (SWEL) 15 items	Screening quality: average to high (kappa: 52.3%–90.3%) (105) Diagnostic/prognostic: average (kappa = 51.1%–78.0%) (105)	Also used to assess snoring, napping, and sleep duration

Appendix 19C. Other Questionnaires and Interviews to Measure Sleep (*cont.*)

Name/Description	Psychometric Indices	Comments
Apnea Score Derived from Hawaii Sleep Questionnaire (106) 2 items	Said to be 10% effective in identifying individuals with moderate to severe sleep apnea by polysomnography	2 items refer to (1) presence of loud snoring and (2) stopping breathing during sleep
Post Sleep Inventory (107) 29 items, bipolar anchor endpoints 13-point scale	Orthogonal rotation, principal component analysis: 7 factors High construct validity Sensitive measure	3 categories of items
Sleep Questionnaire 55 items Choices are Likert-type Scoring not described	Test–retest reliability (10 weeks): 0.79 (108) Internal consistency reliability, Cronbach's alpha: 0.76 (median) Factor analysis: 7 factors (71.7% of variance)	Clinical judgment and factor scales undergoing further testing
Nottingham Health Profile (109) Self-report, 2-part questionnaire 5 sleep-related items (yes–no) Weighted score or summed score (110, 111)	Questionnaire valid, reproducible, sensitive to change (110,112) Face, content and criterion validity established (109) Test–retest reliability: 0.75–0.88 (113,114)	
Child Sleep Habits Questionnaire (SHQ) Parental assessment of child sleep habits 63 items, 5 scales	High test–retest reliability; good internal consistency for "bedtime" scale, moderate reliability for remainder (115)	Scales are bedtime problems, sleep problems, night waking, daytime sleepiness, morning problems
Berlin Questionnaire (134) Identifies people in the primary care population at risk for sleep apnea	Consists of questions on snoring, daytime sleepiness, sleepiness while driving, and hypertension as well as information on age, sex, neck circumference, ethnicity, weight, and height (the latter are used to calculate the body mass index).	Sensitivities are reported as ranging from 76% to 96%, specificities from 13% to 54%, and positive predicitive values of 69% to 77% (135)

Numbers in parentheses correspond to studies cited in the References.

20

Attitudes Toward Chronic Illness

Rebecca F. Cohen

Chronic illness is the number-one health problem in the United States. Between 1900 and 1970, a shift was seen in mortality patterns. Death from acute infections was surplanted by an increase of more than 250% in mortality rates from major chronic diseases. These changes have brought about the need for a new arrangement of values and priorities in health care policy, finance, and management.[1]

Traditionally, professionals approached chronic symptom management in terms of compliance and service utilization and attempted to engineer the patient to the health team's treatment goals. However, it has been noted that this approach fails to incorporate an appreciation of the role of personality variables in the development and outcome of chronic illness, as well as how chronic illness affects the individual emotionally and psychologically.

If health care providers are to influence the patient's adaptation to chronic illness, they must acknowledge the lay perception of illness and understand what the patient sees as relevant. A strong relationship has been shown between coping styles and attitudes and treatment results. This is important to remember because ineffective coping styles and damaging attitudes can adversely affect treatment outcomes and, therefore, need to be identified early. By studying coping styles, perception, attitudes, beliefs, and illness behavior, we may be able not only to affect treatment outcomes (including mortality rates) and adaptation to chronic illness, but also the initial development of the illness process itself.[1]

There has been a proliferation of chronic illness studies from a variety of perspectives designed to evaluate the outcome of physical illness and its treatments, as well as the patient's response to physical disease.[2] Some of the instruments used to measure a patient's attitudes toward chronic disease discussed in this chapter also appear in other chapters. In terms of function, this overlap of instruments should be considered when determining which tool to use for a research project. Chronic illness affects an individual in many ways: physically, psychologically, spiritually, and emotionally. Often, what appears simple on the surface really is quite complicated (e.g., when measuring disability). It is important not only to consider what the patient cannot do, but also what he or she *will* not do, for each may result in the same degree of confinement. As we learn more about the human mind and body, the measurement tools used grow more comprehensive in terms of approaching the patient as a whole. This chapter points out, and emphasizes, the growth that has occurred in the development of tools to measure patient attitudes.

Measures of Ability to Function

With the increasing numbers of elderly in our society, and a similar increase in the need for long-term care, many instruments have been developed to measure physical functioning to determine patient needs so that a patient can be assigned to the appropriate level of care. These instruments also assess the adequacy and composition of staff and determine how patients respond to various modes of treatment. Some scales, such as the Sickness Impact Profile (SIP)[3] and Rand Measures of Health Status,[4] measure the patient's overall health as described by diagnoses, doctor visits, days in bed, number of therapeutic drugs, self-assessed health, pain, and other variables, including the ability to perform everyday activities. Other measures, such as the Cumulative Illness Rating Scale,[5] measure impairment, that is, the extent of organic pathologic change determined by a physician. Disability, or how limitations of activities and functioning affect a person, often is measured by using the Barthel Index[6,7] and the Evaluation of Levels of Subsistence.[8]

Parts of scales that measure disability can be divided further into items that specifically measure either activities of daily living (ADL) or instrumental activities of daily living (IADL). Examples of ADL scales include the Index of ADL[9] and the Physical Self-Maintenance Scale.[10] Examples of IADL scales are the Instrumental Activities of Daily Living Scale[10] and a subscale of the OARS Multidimensional Functional Assessment Scale.[11] Some scales combine ADL and IADL items or may include other health status variables.

Linn and Linn[12] point out that in institutions most functional status tests are completed by nurses or nursing attendants according to their observations of the patients. When used in the community, rating systems are often self-report inventories. Scales vary regarding the numbers of response choices, ranging from simple dichotomous (yes/no) scales to the 11-point SIP scale. Although the purpose of the yes/no response is to allow untrained persons to rate the answers reliably, one disadvantage is that less variance in behavior can be described, and thus the scale may not be sensitive to treatment changes or to discrimination among levels of functioning. On the other hand, even trained raters find it difficult to distinguish between 11 different levels of an item such as bathing. Generally, scales that maintain the best discrimination—and are easy to administer—involve only four to seven responses. Van Hook and Berkman[11] also identified the length of the interview and the expense involved in training interviewers as limitations of tools that measure functional status, such as the OARS, when used in the primary care setting.

Van Hook and Berkman[11] and Linn and Linn[12] have identified another problem with most of the instruments available to measure physical functioning: the lack of definition specificity and frequent unrealiability. For example, does one measure whether an activity *is* or *can be* performed? A person may be physically able to dress unassisted but does not do so because of severe depression. One observer could rate the subject as able to dress without assistance, and another could rate the subject as requiring full assistance. Another source of discrepancy arises from the lack of specificity about conditions for making assessments. The scale may not indicate whether the person is to be evaluated with or without glasses, a hearing aid, or other prostheses. Van Hook and Berkman[11] state that "summated indexes of function may obscure task specific limitations and are often too imprecise to identify the specific nature of the functional deficits" (p. 232). Several other problems related to measuring functional status also were discovered during their investigations: Functional measures may not identify the disability well and are not meaningful in terms of range of tasks and activities performed; there may be a disparity between performance and capacity; and cognitive impairment and cultural variation may also cause unreliable results.

The following four instruments measure the impact of chronic illness on the patient's ability to function and offer unique, broad approaches to the concept of human health. The Rapid Disability Rating Scale-2 and Simplified Disability Assessment Scales are geared toward what the patient actually does, not what they are able to do, as well as certain psychologic functioning. The SIP measures the impact of illness in terms of dysfunction, not levels of positive functioning, and evaluates psychosocial and physical health. The Arthritis Impact Measurement Scale measures physical health and emotional well-being.

Rapid Disability Rating Scale-2

In response to the limitations of available instruments, Linn and Linn[12] revised Linn's Rapid Disability Rating Scale[13] into the Rapid Disability Rating Scale-2 (RDRS-2). Ratings in the RDRS-2 are based on what the person does, not on what he or she is able to do. There are 18 items, with four-point scales ranging from no assistance or disability to severe disability. The first group of items measures the ADL, and later items assess related disabilities and special problems of confusion, depression, and uncooperativeness to provide clues concerning the reasons for disability.

Items on the RDRS-2 are scored from 1 (none) to 4 (severe). Total scores can range from 18 (no disability) to 72 (if the responses are all chosen from the most severe disabilities). Item definitions and instructions for ratings appear on the scale, so that little training is needed in making assessments. The scale can be used by any person who knows the subject to be rated and who has observed him or her performing ADL.[12]

Intraclass reliability correlations between the findings of two nurses who independently rated the same 100 patients were found to range from 0.62 to a high of 0.98; all were statistically significant. Reliability also was shown by testing the same 50 patients twice within a 3-day period. Test-retest values ranged from 0.58 to 0.96 between the first and second ratings by Pearson's product-moment correlations.[12]

Rating scale measurements using both the RDRS-2 and the Maryland-Barthel Disability Index[7] found that the test of functional status usefully predicts outcome. Items on the RDRS-2 were used to predict mortality in a stepwise multiple regression analysis as well as by discriminant function analysis. All items together reached an r of 0.20, with the best predictors of mortality being the need for assistance with eating, incontinence, time in bed, diet, and depression. For accuracy of classification, the scale held a 72% accuracy rate in mortality prediction.[12]

Rapid Disability Assessment Scale

A simplified test for the evaluation of patients with chronic illness developed by Sett[14] is an attempt to simplify the measurement of disability in hospitalized patients. Although developed quite some time ago, it can still serve as a useful tool in caring for patients with chronic illnesses and should be expanded beyond its use with cerebrovascular accident (CVA) patients.

Sett[14] studied other disability instruments and chose among ADL three areas he considered the most essential factors for patient independence for self-care at home: ambulation, self-care, and communication. Four examiners separately performed the testing procedures on 20 patients who had had a CVA. They were instructed not to communicate their findings until each had tested the patient in the designated ADL areas. The chi-square test was applied to the data to determine the statistical significance. The p value was less than 0.01 in all three areas. This simplified disability test was conducted in the following manner:[14]

> *Ambulation.* The patient was asked to demonstrate his ability to walk or perform a transfer to or from a wheelchair. A five-point scale (0, patient is confined to bed, to 5, patient walks without assistance) was used.
>
> *Self-care.* The self-care item tested the patient's ability to carry out ADL such as eating, dressing, bathing, and toilet care. Seven questions plus observation were used to rate the patient on a five-point scale (0, patient is unable to perform any of the ADL without assistance, to 5, patient performs ADL using both upper extremities).
>
> *Communication.* Scores on nine questions ranged from 0 (patient has severe expressive-receptive [global] aphasia) to 5 (patient has neither aphasia nor dysarthria). The test was a modification of the Schuell technique.

Sickness Impact Profile (SIP)

The SIP was developed to provide a measure of perceived health status sensitive enough to detect changes or differences in health status occurring over time or between groups. The SIP is useful for a variety of illness types and severity, as well as demographic and cultural subgroups. Furthermore, the SIP, which measures the behavioral impact of illness in terms of dysfunction, not levels of positive functioning, is intended to provide a measure of the efforts or outcomes of health care that can be used for evaluation, program planning, and policy formulation.

The instrument contains 136 questions answered in a yes/no format and takes 15 to 35 minutes to complete. It can be administered by an interviewer or self-administered. In completing the SIP, the subject must check only those statements that describe him on a given day and are related to his health.[15] Each item is weighted. The instrument has 12 subscales, seven of which aggregate into two dimensions, physical (ambulation, mobility, body care, and movement) and psychosocial (alertness, emotional behaviors, social activities, and communication). A global score (the seven subscales plus eating, recreation, home maintenance, sleep, and rest) is calculated as the weighted sum of all items.[16]

The test-retest reliability of the SIP was 0.92, internal consistency was 0.94, and overall reliability in terms of score was high ($r = 0.75–0.92$) Reliability did not appear to be significantly affected by the variables examined, and results suggest that the SIP is potentially useful for measuring dysfunction under a variety of administrative conditions and with a variety of subjects.[17]

The SIP has been used widely in health services and clinical research since the 1970s. It is considered one of the most responsive instruments used to measure the impact of joint arthroplasty on quality of life[16] and it has been used with people who have a variety of chronic diseases.[18–24] In addition, Sanders and colleagues [25] tested the instrument on subjects with chronic low-back pain in six different culture groups, including Americans, Japanese, Mexicans, Colombians, Italians, and New Zealanders. Findings from their study indicate that the SIP is useful in identifying important cross-cultural differences in chronic pain patients' self-perceived level of dysfunction. American patients were found to be the most dysfunctional, and various explanations for this difference were suggested by the authors. A French version of the original U.S. version of the SIP also has been created because it was felt that a simple, direct translation of the scale was inadequate.[26]

The SIP shows good correlations with other health status and functional status measures and appears to be a reliable instrument with sufficient content validity, but a number of questions regarding its effectiveness remain unanswered. In assessing the SIP and literature related to the use of this tool, DeBruin et al.[27] and Lipsett et al.[28] found unresolved questions related to the theoretical implications of the construct of sickness, the effect of age and gender on SIP scores, the construct validity judged by factor analysis, the responsiveness of the instrument, and whether the list can be shortened and the scoring procedure simplified. At the time, they suggested that further evaluation of the methodologic and theoretical aspects of the instrument should be done if it is to be used as an international standard measure of functional status. Pollard and Johnston,[29] in their investigation of the SIP, also found that problems in scoring have often led to inconsistent and illogical scores. The method of scoring, they found, is incompatible with the underlying theoretical scaling framework, the nature of the items in the SIP, and the properties of the items. They have suggested a new method of scoring that reduces the number of items that most respondents, including people with severe limitations, would be asked and believe that the new method will resolve problems identified by many researchers.

An interesting question about the results of the SIP scale, as useful as it may be, is that of the reliability of self-ratings versus ratings by service providers when analyzing disability or dysfunction. Kivela[30] points out that there are three main methods by which disability can be measured: clinical assessment of the individual's performance, questioning the individual about the level of daily performance, and standard tests of individual performance conducted by a trained observer. This study compared a questionnaire-based measure of disability with evaluations by health care professionals. A total of 205 patients with chronic illness and elderly persons receiving home nursing or home help services or both were included in the study. A questionnaire was developed that used the activities listed in standardized measurements of ADL and IADL. Comparisons between the self-report and rater assessments of performance were then made for individual activities of self-care and domestic duties, including the following six activities: dressing, eating, daily washing, bathing or sauna, cooking, and cleaning.[30]

Results indicated that agreement between the questionnaire-based and the provider ratings was high for basic self-care activities but not high for housework. Kivela[30] points out that the extent of the observer's earlier knowledge about the patient's performance and environment may have affected the results, as may have the differences in the educational levels of the observers.

Arthritis Impact Measurement Scales (AIMS)

Meenan et al.[31] developed the AIMS to measure three areas of human health (physical, emotional, and social well-being) and to meet the need for a reliable, valid, and comprehensive measure of the health of patients with arthritis.

AIMS was built on two previously tested health status measures: Bush's Index of Well-Being and the Rand Health Insurance Study batteries. The Index of Well-Being is a behaviorally based scale that includes three function/dysfunction scales (mobility, physical activity, social activity) and a symptom-problem complex. The Rand approach combines the three behavioral components of the Index of Well-Being with psychologic scales for anxiety and depression. Both approaches have undergone extensive testing and refinement.[31] In addition, the AIMS has been translated into several languages and found to meet the goals of the World Health Organization, thus, it appears to meet the needs of its users throughout the world.[32]

AIMS consists of demographic and health status items arranged into nine scale groups as follows: mobility (5 items); physical activity (5); social activity (9); social role (7); ADL (5); pain (5); dexterity (5); anxiety (8); and depression (6). The remaining 11 items relate to health perceptions and overall estimates of functional status and arthritis severity.[31] These nine subscales can be aggregated into three health status dimensions: physical function, psychologic function, and pain. Each dimension has a range of 0 to 10, with a higher score indicating more limitation and lower health status.[33]

Shortened forms of the AIMS have been tested on patients with rheumatoid arthritis or total hip replacement.[30,34] Lorish et al.[34] and Potter and Zauszniewski[35] found that after reducing the 45-item AIMS to 22 items, alpha reliabilities and test-retest correlations indicated that the full and short scales were comparably reliable on all scales except for pain. Although the convergent validity coefficients were comparable between the short and full versions, the short mobility, pain, depression, and anxiety scales were not comparable to the full scales in detecting changes from baseline. Thus, if minimizing the number of items used with the AIMS is desired, while maximizing reliability and validity, the short versions of physical activity, household activity, dexterity, ADL, and social activity should be used with the full version of mobility, pain, depression, and anxiety. Katz et al.[16] used a shortened version of the AIMS (sAIMS), which was an 18-item questionnaire divided into 9 subscales, on 54 patients undergoing total hip replacement. Two of the five items from each subscale of the original AIMS that had the highest internal consistency and correlation with the total AIMS score were selected. Results from their study indicated that the sAIMS was sensitive to clinical change on the global dimension, but not on the physical dimension. Potter and Zauszniewski[35] used a collapsed version of the AIMS2 and combined it with Ellison's Spiritual Well-Being Scale and Rosenbaum's Self-Control Schedule in a single survey format. The impact of social, emotional, and physical factors on older adults with arthritis was measured, and the additive and mediating effects of learned resourcefulness and spirituality on general health perception were investigated.

In the initial research conducted by Meenan et al.,[31] individual health status items showed an impressive degree of disease impact in the study group. The AIMS instrument was found to be easily completed by patients; the scales had face validity and were easy to score in either Guttman or Likert format; and, after deleting some questions that led to confusion or had low item-total correlation, all the scales, with the exception of Social Activity, fulfilled a number of generally accepted criteria for reliability and scalability. The significance of the correlations held for both patient-generated and physician-generated health status proxies.

A later study of patients with osteoarthritis, conducted by Weinberger et al.,[36] found that both exposure to stressors and low self-esteem support were associated with increased disability along all AIMS dimensions. Physical disability was associated with being older and having less "tangible" support; psychologic disability with being younger, Caucasian, and having less "belonging" support; and pain with being younger, Caucasian, and having less education. Self-esteem was the most consistent social support dimension when predicting functional status. Thus, the AIMS instrument was found to be practical, simple, and dependable and should prove useful for evaluating a wide variety of interventions in the field of rheumatology.[31]

Measures of Illness Behavior

The concepts of illness behavior and sick role have tremendous implications for public health programs, estimated needs for medical care, medical economics, and our understanding of health and illness in general. For example, what is the influence of various norms, values, fears, and expected rewards and punishments on how a symptomatic person behaves? What makes one person suffer in silence, whereas another seeks immediate health care for the slightest discomfort? Are there systematic differences in illness behavior in given populations, and, if so, what effect would these differences have on the provision of educational and informational programs? All these questions have been addressed in various research investigations through three very important instruments: Dimensions of the Sick Role, the Illness Behavior Questionnaire (IBQ), the Illness Self-Concept Repertory Grid, and the Mishel Uncertainty in Illness Scale.

Dimensions of the Sick Role

The term *illness behavior* refers to the ways in which symptoms may be differentially perceived, evaluated, and acted (or not acted) on by different kinds of people. Kassebaum and Baumann[37] conducted research more than 35 years ago to study the sick role and illness behavior in patients with chronic illness.

Patients with one or more primary diagnoses of chronic illness respond to 20 statements with stipulated response alternatives ranging from "strongly disagree" to "strongly agree" on a seven-point Likert-type scale. Factor analysis was selected because it permits subjects to group items cognitively. A scale was constructed for each factor, using the factor's most highly loaded items. Each respondent was given a sum score on each factor's scale. The distribution of scores for each factor scale was trichotomized into high, medium, and low categories. Factor analysis yielded four distinct dimensions in underlying sick role expectations: dependence, reciprocity, role performance, and denial.

High scores on individual dimensions of the sick role varied with age, sex, ethnic origin, education, occupational category, and diagnosis. Chronic illness, the investigators suggested, may therefore be regarded as one subtype of sick role, having special characteristics. Patients with chronic illness are likely to perceive the structure of the sick role along dimensions that differ from those perceived by patients with acute, temporary illness. Also, within the broad classification of chronic illness, they found that different diagnoses had different consequences for people (e.g., patients with arteriosclerotic heart disease were found to have almost double the number of high scores on the dimensions of dependence, reciprocity, role performance, and denial than patients with diabetes; diabetics were distinguished from other diseases studied by their low level of denial). For this reason, the authors suggested further research into the concept of the sick role and illness behavior in terms of different types of illness, different social settings, and different segments of the population.[37] The IBQ was later developed to serve as a useful tool in such research efforts.

Illness Behavior Questionnaire (IBQ)

To better understand the concept of illness behavior in relation to a specific symptom (in this case, pain), Pilowsky and Spence[38] conducted a research study with unselected patients (48 men and 52 women with a mean age of 49.1 years) referred to either the pain clinic or the psychiatric service of a large metropolitan hospital for the management of intractable pain. They developed the 52-item IBQ to determine the patient's attitudes and feelings about illness, perception of the reactions of significant others in the environment (including doctors) to self and illness, and the patient's own view of his or her current psychosocial situation. Pain is addressed in another chapter, but this questionnaire is discussed in the section on chronic illness measurements because of its potential for a variety of medical illnesses and symptoms and its importance in trying to understand how patients feel about their illness or symptoms.

The seven subscales of the IBQ are general hypochondriasis, disease conviction, psychologic versus somatic perception of illness, affective inhibition, affective disturbance, denial of problems, and irritability.[38]

The results of data analysis showed six principal clusters of patients, each with definite illness behavior characteristics. Groups 1 to 3 had a relatively nonneurotic, reality-oriented attitude toward illness indicated by low scores on the first three scales. The symptom (pain) experience seemed to be an adaptive reaction to stress, but one that obscured all other aspects of the stress response. Groups 4 to 6 related more clearly to the syndrome of abnormal illness behavior. The symptom (pain) was interwoven with, and was symptomatic of, a personality disorder or an essentially maladaptive response to psychologic stress.[38]

Besides being used with patients with pain, the IBQ has been used to assess behavior in patients with neurologic diseases, psychiatric disorders, cancer, and a variety of other diseases, including EI, environmental illness.[39] It is interesting to note the study by Tatarelli et al.[39] of patients with gynecologic cancer. Findings suggest that illness behavior is almost totally involved in a belief dimension: Cultural stereotypes of cancer as a fatal illness influence patients' reactions to the disease as well as their delay in seeking care.

Illness Self-Concept Repertory Grid (ISCRG)

In an attempt to extend use of the IBQ, Large[40] used a repertory grid technique involving various self-concepts as "elements" and concepts drawn from the IBQ as "constructs." It was expected that, because they presumably conceived of themselves as being ill, subjects scoring high on the disease conviction scale of the IBQ would similarly rate themselves toward the ill pole of the illness construct of the grid. Because illness is considered undesirable, one might expect a considerable difference on this construct between the patient's actual self-concept and his or her ideal self-concept. The patients with the greatest discrepancy between actual self-concept and ideal self-concept were hypothesized to have the most self-dissatisfaction and, therefore, would have the most motivation toward treatment and show the greatest improvement.

The grid is constructed using *elements* ("as I am, as I would like to be, as others see me, as my doctor sees me") and bipolar constructs.[40] In the original study done by Large,[40] 18 patients with chronic musculoskeletal pain were told that the purpose of the study was to gain some insight into their views of themselves and their world and, therefore, they were being asked to complete a questionnaire. The repertory grids were then completed by each patient during an initial interview in which the subject was exposed to biofeedback. A second grid was completed at the final interview (post-trial), using identical elements and constructs.

The grids were analyzed by means of the principal component analysis devised by Slater for use with individual grids. The main focus of interest was the distance between element 1 (as I am), or self, and element 2 (as I would like to be), or ideal self, derived from the initial grid for each subject. The Spearman rank-correlation coefficient was computed between three rankings: changes in pain scores calculated pre- and post-trial; distances between element 1 (self) and 2 (ideal-self); and correlations between electromyelogram activity ratings and pain scores. The rank correlation between pain score changes and element 1 to 2 distances was 0.43, ($p < 0.05$). Thus, the greater the distance between elements 1 and 2, the greater the decline in pain scores.[40]

In another study by Large,[41] the effect of participation in a pain-management program on self-concept and attitudes toward illness was investigated. It was found that, despite the fact that no change in symptoms was seen, differences between the pre- and postrepertory grids showed a significant increase in the distance between "as I would like to be" and "like a physically ill person." This suggested that physical illness had become less desirable after participation in the pain-management program. It appeared that the program helped the patients to adopt a more balanced view of physical illness as being undesirable and as including both physical and emotional factors. He hypothesized that the findings indicate that attitudes may be more important than symptoms in determining subsequent illness behavior. Large and James,[42] investigating the use of hypnosis for pain, suggest from their results that pain relief may so powerfully alter self-concept that a shift occurs in self-view from illness to wellness. However, it also is possible that a fixed self-view of illness may neutralize treatments such as hypnosis.

The ISCRG is, therefore, a useful research tool because of its flexibility and ability to produce quantifiable data that allow comparison across individuals as well as time. The tool provides insight into the individual and can be used to guide the clinician in evaluating and planning treatment because of its ability to identify clinically meaningful changes in self-concept. The grid could be useful as an instrument to predict the optimum timing of treatment and to predict when the patient is ready to respond to treatment, but further testing is needed to determine whether some of the instability found in measurement is due to treatment effects.[42]

Mishel Uncertainty in Illness Scale (MUIS)

Uncertainty, according to Mishel and colleagues[43-48] has been defined as the inability to determine the meaning of illness related to events. It occurs as a result of ambiguity concerning the state of the illness, complexity of treatment options and system of care, lack of information about the diagnosis and seriousness of the illness, and the unpredictable course of the disease. Influencing factors in uncertainty include familiarity of symptoms and events, the individual's ability to process the information he or she is given, and resources available to the individual to assist in the interpretation of illness-related events. The degree of uncertainty experienced by an individual has been found to be strongly related to the presence of stress, emotional distress, mood disturbance, anxiety, poor quality of life, and poor psychosocial adjustment to illness. A significant relationship has not been found to exist between uncertainty, gender, marital status, age, and employment status.[49]

The MUIS is a self-administered, 5-point Likert-type scale in which respondents state the degree to which they agree with uncertainty statements. Scores range from a low of 23 to a high of 115, and higher scores indicate higher levels of uncertainty in illness. It is a tool that is available in four versions, including a 33-item adult version (MUIS-A) for use with ill, hospitalized adults; a 23-item community version (MUIS-C) for use with chronically ill individuals and their families residing in the community; and a 31-item Parent's Perception of Uncertainty in Illness (PPUS) to measure uncertainty in parents of ill children. The PPUS can also be used with a spouse, friend, or other relative by replacing the word *child* with the appropriate relationship name.[43-48]

Measures of Locus Control

Closely related to the concept of illness behavior are beliefs about internal versus external control. Through comprehensive investigation of how patients with chronic illness feel about themselves, the world around them, and the relationship between the two, techniques can be tailored to individual expectancies to increase the possibility of a successful treatment outcome. Two different reinforcement patterns lead to either the general expectancy that rewards are contingent on internal resources (such as effort) or the general expectancy that rewards are externally related to things such as luck, chance, fate, or powerful others. General expectancy is referred to as *locus of control*. The Health Locus of Control (HLC) Scale, Health Specific Locus of Control Beliefs Questionnaire, and the

Attribution Interview Schedule are three instruments related to locus of control. These measures are described in Appendix 20A.[50–58]

Although the presence of attributional thinking in everyday life has been supported in numerous studies, the assumption that it always occurs in important or unexpected life situations was not as readily evident. Lowery et al.,[59] wanting to investigate the finding that some patients search for a cause to their illness while others do not, compared a sample of chronically ill and acutely ill patients to determine differences in causal search. Chronic patients had either diabetes, arthritis, or hypertension, and acute patients were hospitalized with stable myocardial infarction.

The results of this study indicated that more than half of each sample had not thought "Why me?" These subjects, in both acute and chronic illness groups, had better affect scores and higher expectations for recovery than those who had engaged in causal thinking. The length of time an individual had had a chronic illness also was not related to their having thought about the question "Why me?"[59]

Thus, contrary to Weiner's theoretical contention that causal thinking is pervasive, differences in affect were not found between those who had and those who had not come up with a cause. Rather, it was the element of the search itself that was associated with affective and expectancy differences, not the construction of a cause.[59] These results also were verified in a study conducted by Weaver and Narsavage[60] with patients with chronic obstructive pulmonary disease. Findings from both studies suggested that causal search may not be the first step in adjustment to a problem and may, in fact, not be the best adjustment mechanism in acute and chronic illness situations. Contemplating causal questions appears to play a significant role in functional status by producing discontentment and disappointment in illness situations where answers are not well defined. Preoccupation with causal search may limit problem solving, thus interfering with the adjustment process.[59,60]

Measures Related to Children with Chronic Diseases

Although many instruments have been developed to evaluate how the patient with a chronic illness feels and thinks, few are geared specifically to assessing the perceptions of parents who have children with chronic disease. The Chronicity Impact and Coping Instrument: Parent Questionnaire is used to evaluate the effect of chronic disease on the family and to gain information related to how parents cope with the difficulties encountered as a result of their child's illness. Another tool, the Roberts Apperception Test for Children (RATC), has been used to assess the presence of serious emotional disturbances in children. Its use has been extended to help identify maladaptive coping mechanisms in children with chronic diseases. Both are described in Appendix 20B.[61–63]

Appendix 20C presents other available measures.[64–80] These tools are different from those previously discussed in that they tend to be less conceptual and more straightforward concerning attitudes toward chronic disease and characteristics of individuals with chronic disease. Some were tested only on well subjects, and others included well subjects, but they all have many implications for use with patients with chronic disease.

Summary

This chapter reviews concepts underlying the development of instruments to measure the impact of chronic illness on patients and, in the case of children, on their parents. Specific instruments are discussed, and others are presented for reference.

Exemplar Studies

Winters, C.A. Heart failure: Living with uncertainty. *Prog Cardiovasc Nurs,* 1999, *14*(3):85–93.

This study exemplifies the measurement of attitudes toward chronic illness. The purpose of the study was to describe the uncertainty experienced by men and women with heart failure and to extend the theoretical understanding of uncertainty in chronic illness. Data were collected from 22 adults living in urban and rural areas of a rural Western state and included audiotaped interviews, clinical and demographic information, and scores from the community form of the Mishel Uncertainty in Illness Scale. Three major themes of uncertainty were identified related to symptoms and treatment, attempts to stay well, and quality of life and death. The study contributed to the uncertainty in illness theory by demonstrating the influence of age-related changes on the ability to recognize and respond to symptoms and the presence of cautious trust of health care providers. The study had many implications for health care providers in terms of understanding the ability of people with heart failure to reframe their view of health and change their personal behaviors to accommodate the changes that occur as a result of their illness. The study also stresses the importance of beginning education early for patients with heart failure in order to reduce uncertainty.

Mann, W.C., Tomita, M., Hurren, D., & Charvat, B. Changes in health, functional and psychosocial status and coping strategies of home based older persons with arthritis over three years. *Occup Ther J Res,* 1999, *19*(2):126–146.

This study exemplifies the measurement of attitudes toward chronic illness and the many variables that affect the patient's attitude. The study was done at the University of Buffalo Consumer Assessments Study, where 61 cognitively intact elders, as measured by the Mini Mental Status Exam, were retrospectively selected for inclusion. Criteria for participation included having arthritis that affected activities, living at home at an initial interview, and living at home at a three-year follow-up interview. Paired *t*-tests found significant changes at the three-year follow-up in four measures of health status: number of medications, number of chronic illnesses, pain, and vision. Functional status declined significantly as measured by the SIP and the IADL section of the OARS. No significant changes were found for psychosocial status. Satisfaction with the use of assistive devices was high. A significant decline in health and functional status was found, as was clear evidence of the use of successful coping strategies. The study suggested the need for occupational therapy services to take a strong role in the care of elders with arthritis.

Internet Resources

- The RAND Corporation has included information about various research projects being conducted, the tools used, and methods and procedures. Several different chronic illnesses are included in the studies, and the interview tools utilized are offered for the reader to download. Interview tools ask many different kinds of questions, including attitudes about illness and health care.

    Research areas link: www.rand.org/health/research_areas.html.
    Additional Current Research link: www.rand.org/health_areas/healthproj.html.
    Improving Chronic Illness Care Evaluation link: www.rand.org/health/ICICE/.
    Interview tools for CHF, diabetes, depression, adult asthma, parents of adolescents who have asthma (12-17), and parents of children who have asthma (2-11).

- Center for Research on Chronic Illness: www.unc.edu/depts/crci/. University of North Carolina at Chapel Hill School of Nursing received a grant from the National Institute of Nursing Research to initiate the Center for Research on Chronic Illness. Currently funded studies are discussed, including work done on uncertainty in patients with chronic illnesses by Dr. Merle Mishel.

- The Hospital for Sick Children: www.sickkids.on.ca/. The Hospital for Sick Children is conducting research on adaptation to childhood chronic illness. This cite is reached by going into the home page, then clicking Healthcare Professionals, then Child Health Services, then Programs and Projects. Direct cite address for research is www.sickkids.on.ca/kidscancope/about.asp.
- The Agency for Health Care Policy and Research (AHCPR): www.ahcpr.gov/news/focus/chchild.htm. This cite lists a source for a Spanish-English scale for asthma in Latino children. Asthma is the most common chronic illness affecting Latino children. A new Spanish-English scale developed with Agency for Healthcare Research and Quality support will help health care workers get information from Latino parents about the level of control over their child's asthma despite language and educational barriers.
- Agency for Healthcare Research and Quality Home Page: www.ahcpr.gov/.

  Research Findings: www.ahcpr.gov/research/.
  Data and Surveys: www.ahcpr.gov/data/.

References

1. Forsyth, G.L., Delaney, K.D., & Gresham, M.L. Vying for a winning position: Management style of the chronically ill. *Res Nurs Health*, 1984, 7(3):181-188.
2. Morrow, G.R., Chiarello, R.J., & Derogatis, L.R. A new scale for assessing patient's psychosocial adjustment to medical illness. *Psychol Med*, 1978, 8:605-610.
3. Bergner, M., Bobbitt, R.A., Carter, W.B., & Gilson, B.S. The Sickness Impact Profile: Development and final revision of a health status measure. *Med Care*, 1981, 19(8):787-805.
4. Brook, R.H., Ware, J.E., Davies-Avery, A., et al. Overview of adult health status measures fielded in Rand's health insurance study. *Med Care*, Jul; 1979, 17(7):iii-x, 1-131.
5. Linn, B.S., Linn, M.W., & Gurel, L. Cumulative Illness Rating Scale. *J Am Geriatr Soc*, 1968, 16(5):622-626.
6. Mahoney, R.I., & Barthel, D.W. Functional evaluation: The Barthel Index. *Maryland State Med J*, 1965, 14:61-65.
7. Wylie, C.M., & White, B.K. A measure of disability. *Arch Environ Health*, 1964, 8:834.
8. Gauger, A.B., Brownwell, W.M., Russell, W.W., et al. Evaluation of levels of subsistence. *Arch Phys Med Rehab*, 1964, 45:286.
9. Katz, S., Ford, A.B., Moskowitz, R.W., et al. Studies of illness in the aged. The Index of ADL: A standardized measure of biological and psychosocial function. *JAMA*, 1963, 185:914.
10. Lawton, M.P., & Brody, E. Assessment of older people: Self-maintaining and instrumental activities of daily living. *Gerontologist*, 1969, 9(3):179-186.
11. Van Hook, M.P., & Berkman, R.B.D. Assessment tools for general health care settings: PRIME-MD, OARS, and SF-36. *Hlth Soc Wrk*, 1996, 21(3):230-234.
12. Linn, M.W., & Linn, B.S. The Rapid Disability Rating Scale-2. *J Am Geriatr Soc*, 1982, 30(6):378-382.
13. Linn, M.W. A rapid disability rating scale. *J Am Geriatr Soc*, 1967, 15(2):211-214.
14. Sett, R.F. Simplified tests for evaluation of patients with chronic illness (cerebrovascular accidents). *J Am Geriatr Soc*, 1963, 11:1095.
15. Carter, W.B., Bobbitt, R.A., Bergner, M., & Gilson, B.S. Validation of an interval scaling: The Sickness Impact Profile. *Health Serv Res*, 1976, 11(4):516-528.
16. Katz, J.N., Larson, M.G., Phillips, C.B., et al. Comparative measurement sensitivity of short and longer health status instruments. *Med Care*, 1992, 30(10):917-925.
17. Pollard, W.E., Bobbitt, R.A., Bergner, M., et al. The Sickness Impact Profile: Reliability of a health status measure. *Med Care*, 1976, 14(2):146-155.
18. Drossman, D.A., Leserman, J., Li, Z.M., et al. The rating form of IBD patient concerns: A new measure of health status. *Psychosom Med*, 1991, 53(6):701-712.
19. Fox, E., McDowall, J., Neale, T.J., et al. Cognitive function and quality of life in end-stage renal failure. *Ren Failure*, 1993, 15(2):211-214.
20. Juniper, E.F., Guyatt, G.H., Ferrie, P.J. & Griffith, L.E. Measuring quality of life in asthma. *Am Rev Resp Dis*, 1993, 147(4):832-838.
21. Schuling, J., Greidanus, J., & Meyboom de Jong, B. Measuring functional status of stroke patients with the Sickness Impact Profile. *Disab Rehab*, 1993, 15(1):19-23.
22. Baker, C.A. Factors associated with rehabilitation in head and neck cancer. *Cancer Nurs*, 1992, 15(6):395-400.
23. Granger, C.V., Cotter, A.C., Hamilton, B.B., & Fiedler, R.C. Functional assessment scales: A study of persons after stroke. *Arch Phys Med Rehab*, 1993, 74(2):133-138.
24. Syrjala, K.L., Chapko, M.K., Vitaliano, P.P., et al. Recovery after allogeneic marrow transplantation: Prospective study of predictors of long-term physical and psychosocial functioning. *Bone Marrow Transplant*, 1993, 11(4):319-327.
25. Sanders, S.H., Brena, S.F., Spier, C.J., et al. Chronic low back pain patients around the world: Cross-

cultural similarities and differences. *Clin J Pain,* 1992, *8*(4):317-323.

26. Chwalow, A.J., Lurie, A., Bean, K., et al. French version of the Sickness Impact Profile: Stages in the cross cultural validation of a generic quality of life scale. *Fund Clin Pharmacol,* 1992, *6*(7):319-326.

27. DeBruin, A.F., DeWitte, L.P., Stevens, F., & Diederiks, J.P. Sickness Impact Profile: The state of the art of a generic functional status measure. *Soc Sci Med,* 1992, *35*(8):1003-1014.

28. Lipsett, P.A., Swoboda, S.M., Campbell, et al. Sickness Impact Profile Score versus a modified short-form survey for functional outcome assessment: Acceptability, reliability, and validity in critically ill patients with prolonged intensive care unit stays. *J Trauma Inj Infect Crit Care,* 2000, *49*(4):737-743.

29. Pollard, B., & Johnston, M. Problems with the Sickness Impact Profile: A theoretically based analysis and a proposal for a new method of implementation and scoring. *Soc Sci Med,* 2001, *52*(6):921-934.

30. Kivela, S.L. Measuring disability—Do self-ratings and service provider ratings compare? *J Chron Dis,* 1984, *37*(2):115.

31. Meenan, R.F., Gertman, P.M., & Mason, J.H. Measuring health status in arthritis. *Arthr Rheum,* 1980, *23*(2):146-152.

32. van Kuyk-Minis, M.H., & Liu, L. Issues related to the translation of measurement scales: A comparison of versions of the Arthritis Impact Measurement Scale. *Occup Ther J Res,* 1998, *18*(4):143.

33. Burckhardt, C.S., Woods, S.L., Schultz, A.A., & Ziebarth, D.M. Quality of life of adults with chronic illness: A psychometric study. *Res Nurs Health,* 1989, *12*(6):347-354.

34. Lorish, C.D., Abraham, N., Austin, J.S., et al. A comparison of the full and short versions of the arthritis impact measurement scales. *Arthr Care Res,* 1991, *4*(4):168-173.

35. Potter, L., & Zauszniewski, J.A. Spirituality, resourcefulness, and arthritis impact on health perception of elders with rheumatoid arthritis. *J Holistic Nurs,* 2000, *18*(4):311-331. Discussions 332-336.

36. Weinberger, M., Tierney, W.M., Booher, P., & Hiner, S.L. Social support, stress and functional status in patients with osteoarthritis. *Soc Sci Med,* 1990, *30*(4):503-508.

37. Kassebaum, G.G., & Baumann, B.O. Dimensions of the sick role in chronic illness. *J Health Hum Behav,* 1965, *6*(1):16.

38. Pilowsky, I., & Spence, N.D. Illness behavior syndromes associated with intractable pain. *Pain,* 1976, *2*(1):61-71.

39. Tatarelli, R., Atlante, G., dePisa, E., et al. Illness behavior in a sample of patients with gynecological cancer compared to other benign pathologies. *New Trends Exp Clin Psychiatr,* 1991, *7*(4):187.

40. Large, R.G. Prediction of treatment response in pain patients: The Illness Self-Concept Repertory Grid and EMG Feedback. *Pain,* 1985, *21*(3):279-287.

41. Large, R. Self-concepts and illness attitudes in chronic pain: A repertory grid study of a pain management programme. *Pain,* 1985, *23*(2):113-119.

42. Large, R.G., & James, F.R. Personalized evaluation of self-hypnosis as a treatment of chronic pain: A repertory grid analysis. *Pain,* 1988, *35*(2):155-169.

43. Mishel, M.H. The measurement of uncertainty in illness. *Nurs Res,* 1981, *30*(5):258-263.

44. Mishel, M.H. Parents' perception of uncertainty concerning their hospitalized child. *Nurs Res,* 1983, *32*(6):324-330.

45. Mishel, M.H. Perceived uncertainty and stress in illness. *Res Nurs and Health,* 1984, *7*:163-171.

46. Mishel, M.H., Hostetter, T., King, B., & Graham, V. Predictors of psychosocial adjustment in patients newly diagnosed with gynecological cancer. *Cancer Nurs,* 1984, *7*:291-299.

47. Mishel, M.H., & Braden, C.J. Finding meaning: Antecedents of uncertainty in illness. *Nurs Res,* 1988, *37*(2):98-103,127.

48. Mishel, M.H. Reconceptualization of the uncertainty in illness theory. *IMAGE: J Nurs Schol,* 1990, *22*(4):256-262.

49. Winters, C.A. Heart failure: Living with uncertainty. *Prog Cardiovasc Nurs,* 1999, *14*(3):85-91.

50. Lowery, B.J. Misconceptions and limitation of locus of control and the I-E scale. *Nurs Res,* 1981, *30*(5):294-298.

51. Wallston, B.S., Wallston, H.A., Kaplan, G.D., & Maides, S.A. Development and validation of the health locus of control (HLC) scale. *J Consult Clin Psychol,* 1976, *44*(4):580-585.

52. Rock, D.L., Meyerowitz, B.E., Maisto, S.A., & Wallston, K.A. The derivation and validation of six multidimensional health locus of control scale clusters. *Res Nurs Health,* 1987, *10*(3):185-195.

53. Strickland, B.R. Internal-external expectancies and health-related behavior. *J Consult Clin Psychol,* 1978, *46*(6):1192-1211.

54. Wallston, K.A., Maides, S., & Wallston, B.S. Health-related information seeking as a function of health-related locus of control and health value. *J Res Person,* 1976, *10*(2):215.

55. Sugarek, N.J., Deyo, R.A., & Holmes, B.C. Locus of control and beliefs about cancer in a multi-ethnic clinic population. *Oncol Nurs Forum,* 1988, *15*(4):481-486.

56. Lau, R.R., & Ware, J.F. Refinements in the measurement of health-specific locus-of-control beliefs. *Med Care,* 1981, *19*(11):1147-1158.

57. Nagy, V.T., & Wolfe, G.R. Cognitive predictors of compliance in chronic disease patients. *Med Care,* 1984, *22*(10):912-921.

58. Lowery, B.J., & Jacobsen, B.S. Attibutional analysis of chronic illness outcomes. *Nurs Res,* 1985, *34*(2):82-88.

59. Lowery, B.J., Jacobsen, B.S., & Murphy, B.B. An exploratory investigation of causal thinking of arthritics. *Nurs Res,* 1983, *32*(3):157-162.

60. Weaver, T.E., & Narsavage, G.L. Physiological and psychological variables related to functional status in chronic obstructive pulmonary disease. *Nurs Res,* 1992, *41*(5):286-291.

61. Hymovich, D.P. The chronicity impact and coping instrument: Parent questionnaire. *Nurs Res,* 1983, *32*(5):275-281.

62. Humovich, D.P., & Baker, C.D. The needs, concerns and coping of parents of children with cystic fibrosis. *Family Relations: J Appl Fam Child Stud,* 1985, *34*(1):91.

63. Palomares, R.S., Crowley, S.L., Worchell, F.F., et al. The factor analytic structure of the Roberts apperception test for children: A comparison of the standard-

ization sample with a sample of chronically ill children. *J Person Assess*, 1991, *56*(3):414-425.

64. Counte, M.A., Bieliauskas, L.A., & Pavlou, M. Stress and personal attitudes in chronic illness. *Arch Phys Med Rehab*, 1983, *64*(6):272-275.

65. Pollock, S.E., & Duffy, M.E. The Health Related Hardiness Scale: Development and psychometric analysis. *Nurs Res*, 1990, *39*(4):218-222.

66. Viney, L.L., & Westbrook, M.T. Patterns of anxiety in the chronically ill. *Br J Med Psychol*, 1982 Mar; *55*(PT):87-95.

67. Rahe, R.H., & Holmes, T.H. The social readjustment rating scale. *J Psychosom Res*, 1967, *11*(2):213-218.

68. DeVon, H.A., & Powers, M.J. Health beliefs, adjustment to illness, and control of hypertension. *Res Nurs Health*, 1984, *7*(1):10-16.

69. Rodrigue, J.R., Kanasky, W.F., Jackson, S.I., & Perri, M.G. The Psychosocial Adjustment to Illness Scale—Self-Report: Factor structure and item stability. *Psycho Assess*, 2000, *12*(4):409-413.

70. Derogatis, L.R. The Psychosocial Adjustment to Illness Scale (PAIS). *J Psychosom Res*, 1986, *30*(1):77-91.

71. Stubbing, D.G., Haalboom, P., & Barr, P. Comparison of the Psychosocial Adjustment to Illness Scale—Self-Report and clinical judgment in patients with chronic lung disease. *J Cardiopulm Rehab*, 1998, *18*(1):32-36.

72. Drummond-Young, M., LeGris, J., Browne, G., et al. Interactional styles of outpatients with poor adjustment to chronic illness receiving problem-solving counseling. *Health Soc Care Comm*, 1996, *4*(6):317-329.

73. Browne, G.B., Byrne, C., Roberts, J., et al. The Meaning of Illness Questionnaire: Reliability and validity. *Nurs Res*, 1988, *37*(6):368-373.

74. Viney, L.L., & Westbrook, M.T. Coping with chronic illness: Strategy preferences, changes in preferences and associated emotional reactions. *J Chron Dis*, 1984, *37*(6):489-502.

75. Cantril, H. A study of aspirations. *Sci Am*, 1963, *8*(2):41.

76. Laborde, J.M., & Powers, M.J. Life satisfaction, health control orientation, and illness-related factors in persons with osteoarthritis. *Res Nurs Health*, 1985, *8*(2):183-190.

77. Lubin, B., Rahaim, S., Rinck, C.M., & Nickel, E.J. MMPI experimental scale correlates of the MAACL-R with male alcoholics. *Psychol Rep*, 1991, *69*(2):460-462.

78. Stevenson, J.S. Construction of a scale to measure load, power and margin in life. *Nurs Res*, 1982, *31*(4):222-225.

79. Rosenberg, S.J., Hayes, J.R., & Peterson, R.A. Revising the Seriousness of Illness Rating Scale: Modernization and re-standardization. *Int J Psychiatr Med*, 1987, *17*(1):85-92.

80. Sacks, C.R., Peterson, R.A., & Kimmel, P.L. Perception of illness and depression in chronic renal disease. *Am J Kidney Dis*, 1990, *15*(1):31-39.

81. Weir, R., Browne, G., Roberts, J., et al. The Meaning of Illness Questionnaire: Further evidence for its reliability and validity. *Pain*, 1994, *58*(3):377-386.

82. Milne, B.J., Logan, A.G., & Flanagan, P.T. Alterations in health perception and life-style in treated hypertensives. *J Chron Dis*, 1985, *38*(1):37.

Appendix 20A. Instruments Used to Determine Locus of Control

Instrument	Description	Psychometric Indices
Multidimensional Health Locus of Control Scale (MHLC) (50–53)	3 subscales of locus of control beliefs: (1) Internal Scale (IS) assesses degree to which individual believes own behavior responsible for health (H) or illness (I); (2) Chance Scale (CS): assesses belief that level of H or I is a function of luck, fate, or uncontrollable factors; (3) Powerful Others (PO): assesses belief that degree of H or I is determined by important figures (e.g., physician) Scaled on 6-point, Likert-type scale: externally worded items: 1, strongly disagree, to 6, strongly agree, and internally worded items: reverse scored; range 11 (most internal) to 66 (most external)	Alpha reliability: 0.72 Concurrent validity: 0.33 correlation ($p < 0.01$) with Rotter's Internal–External scale Wallston et al. found correlation of 0.25 (54) Tested in culturally diverse populations (55) using revised MHLC scale: test–retest reliability of Spanish locus of control scale: IS (0.68), CS (0.36), PO (0.61); Cronbach's alpha: IS (0.20–0.40), CS (0.46), PO (0.61–0.72) Suggests that poorly educated people need greater direction to take active role in health maintenance (55)
Health Specific Locus of Control Beliefs Questionnaire Developed by Lau and Ware (56)	Measures person's beliefs about self-control over health, provider control over health, chance health outcomes, general health threat, health care attitudes, health status perceptions, and value placed on health 28 items: statement of opinion about control over health with 7-point response scale (strongly agree to strongly disagree) 4 dimensions (subscales): self-care, provider control, chance, general health threat (independent of others)	Test–retest (3-week interval) performed Internal consistency reliability estimates (alpha) performed Factor analysis performed
Nagy and Wolfe's Compliance Tool (57)	Authors used health locus of control construct and Health Belief Model to predict compliance with medical regimen in chronically ill patients Reemphasizes multidimensional nature of compliance and suggests that cognitive variables in general, and health locus of control beliefs specifically, play limited role in determining compliance in chronic illness	Found lack of relationship between health locus of control scales and compliance measures
Attribution Interview Scale (58)	Uses Weiner's Attribution Model (causal explanations predict behavioral and emotional reactions to life events) Weiner found that causes fall into 3 dimensions: (1) locus (cause internal or external to person); (2) stability (whether or not cause is changeable); (3) control (whether cause is under volitional control or controlled by outside forces) Self-esteem found to be linked to locus dimension	Reliability coefficients (for 3 dimensions): (1) 0.72, (2) 0.86, (3) 0.89

Numbers in parentheses correspond to studies cited in the References.

20B. Instruments Used to Assess the Impact of Chronic Illness in Children or Their Parents

Instrument	Description	Psychometric Indices
Chronicity Impact and Coping Instrument: Parent Questionnaire (CICI:PQ) (61,62)	167-item self-administered measure of the impact of chronic childhood illness on parents; parental coping; parental perception of needs Items include: (A) demographic data; (B) parent relationships; (C) hospitalization experiences; (D) concerns of oneself (Self-concern) and spouse (Spouse concern); (E) help wanted for child and siblings (Help); (F) coping strategies of self (Self cope) and spouse (Spouse cope); (G) communication with siblings (Sib talk); (H) beliefs (Belief) Responses scaled using Likert-format	Internal reliability of subscales (Cronbach's alpha) Help, Self-Concern, Spouse concern scales combined to form Stressor scale Scale: (number of items) reliability (r): Help (23) $r = 0.95$; Self-concern (16) $r = 0.89$; Spouse concern (15) $r = 0.91$; Self cope (40) $r = 0.80$; Spouse cope (15) $r = 0.80$; Sib talk (9) $r = 0.84$; Beliefs (9) $r = 0.43$; Stressor (54) $r = 0.72$ CICI:PQ helps parents express their concerns to health professionals (62)
Roberts Apperception Test for Children (RATC) (51)	Story-telling technique combining a projective technique with a standardized scoring system Children (6–15 years old) are presented with card series depicting common childhood situations involving parents, peers, and schools 13 scales: 8 adaptive and 5 clinical scales Scored on adaptive (e.g., resolution) and clinical (e.g., depression) scales Helps in identifying children with serious emotional disturbance	Linear Structural Relations Model (LISREL) analysis Chi-square goodness of fit used to evaluate 3-factor solution Cluster analysis of chronically ill sample resulted in 2 cluster solution based on T scores for each scale

Numbers in parentheses correspond to studies cited in the References.

Appendix 20C. Selected Other Instruments Measuring Attitudes Toward Chronic Disease

Instrument	Description	Psychometric Indices
Multiple Sclerosis Adjustment Scale (64)	Used to identify the multiple sclerosis (MS) patient's capacity to maintain distress within manageable limits, to invest emotional concern and energy in non-MS areas, to reevaluate life value and priorities, and to maintain optimism and interest in the future Self-report scale Statements scored in either a positive (good adaptation) or a negative (poor adaptation) direction on a Likert-type scale Can be used to determine ability to adapt to "life with disease" and disease exacerbations in patients with other chronic illness	Testing done on 97 adult MS patients in a treatment center Reliability = –0.79
Health Related Hardiness Scale (65)	51-item, self-report measure of commitment (15 items), challenge (15), and control (21) Target population: adults with multiple sclerosis, hypertension, rheumatoid arthritis, and diabetes Items scored on 6-point Likert scale Higher scores indicate greater hardiness	High internal consistency (alpha coefficient): 0.91 Test–retest Pearson: $r = 0.90$ (2 week); $r = 0.80$ (3 months) Content and construct validity established
Total Anxiety Scale (66)	Interview format with tape-recorded responses Patient asked questions about feelings related to death (fears of dying); mutilation (fears); separation (loneliness, loss); guilt (moral disapproval, criticism); shame (self-criticism); diffuse (tension, vague fears)	Reliability and validity tested using canonical correlation to analyze relationship between each set of continuously measured variables Can be used to study relationship between anxiety patterns in chronically ill patients and indices of rehabilitation
Social Readjustment Rating Scale (SRRS) (67)	Self-report using a yes/no checklist of 43 life changes (life change assigned value based on adjustment required for each change during prior year); high stress shown by SRRS > 300 Can be used to study relationship between event and onset of medical illness	Correlation coefficients between discrete groups (Pearson's r) > 0.90, except for relationship between white and black subjects (0.82) Kendall's coefficient of concordance (W) = 0.477 ($p < 0.0005$)
Psychosocial Adjustment to Medical Illness (PAIS) and Psychosocial Adjustment to Medical Illness Self-Report Revised (PAIS-SR) (2,68,69–73)	PAIS: a multidimensional, semistructured clinical interview designed to assess the psychosocial and social adjustment of medical patients, or members of their immediate families, to the patient's illness. 7 independent domains (health-care orientation; sexual relationships; role function (*vocational and domestic environments*); social support (*extended family relationships and social environment*); and intrapsychic functioning (*psychologic distress*). Scored using 4-point Likert scale and then summed for each domain and overall adjustment score calculated. PAIS-SR: a self-report version of the PAIS. It is a structured, self-report, 46-item questionnaire and each item is rated on a 4-point scale from 0, no improvement or no change since illness, to 3, a great deal of negative change since illness. The higher score indicates less psychosocial adjustment to illness.	Reliability: interrater reliability coefficients significant (> 0.50) for all except Family domain (> 0.33) Validity established except for vocational and family domains High degree of internal consistency (Cronbach alphas 0.80 to 0.90) based on responses of subjects with cardiac, lung cancer, and renal disease. High degree of interrater reliability to rate the change in adjustment for breast cancer and Hodgkins disease (intraclass correlation coefficients, 0.61 to 0.86).

Appendix 20C. Selected Other Instruments Measuring Attitudes Toward Chronic Disease (cont.)

Instrument	Description	Psychometric Indices
Coping with Chronic Illness: A Self-Appraisal Device (74)	Subject presented with 6 clusters of coping strategies on 6 separate cards Statement given to patients indicating use of the strategy: (1) action; (2) control; (3) escape; (4) fatalism; (5) optimism; (6) interpersonal coping Asked to rank strategies from (1) the one they were most likely to use to (6) the one least likely to use Context and structure of interview schedule described as pertaining to their illness and its implications for them Administered in interview format Useful in determining the extent to which certain factors are related to preferences for different coping strategies (e.g., demographic characteristics, lifestyles, illness roles, degree of disability, perceived handicap, and achievement of rehabilitation goals)	Tested in 3 separate studies: (1) 92 ill vs. well subjects to determine differences in coping strategies (in hospital); (2) 46 chronically ill subjects to determine differences in strategy preferences among patients with different types of chronic illness in different situations (in-hospital and at home); (3) chronically ill patients to determine associations between preferences for coping strategies and emotional reactions to chronic illness (in hospital and at home) Reliability coefficient ($n = 45$, few stresses and relatively stable lives over 1 month): 0.70 (1) action: 0.43; (2) control: 0.30; (3) escape: 0.30; (4) fatalism: 0.50; (5) optimism: 0.38; (6) interpersonal: 0.54 Reliability coefficient over 1 day ($n = 10$) shows higher estimates Overall $r = 0.90$ (range 0.79–0.92 for all clusters)
Cantril's Self-Anchoring Striving Scale (75,76)	Used in variety of research exploring life satisfaction 10-step ladder to assess a person's general sense of well-being at three points in time: past, present, future Subject asked to describe the best possible life for him/her and the worst possible life Shown drawing of ladder with 10 rungs (top, best possible life; bottom, worst life) Asked to show on the ladder where they stand now, where they stood 5 years ago, where they hope to be 5 years from now Interview format Scoring: answers are coded into meaningful categories to enable comparison of different groups Further study with a variety of diseases and populations to determine the effect of chronic illness	Endpoints of scale are self-defined and numeric ratings reflect individual criteria Traditional notions of reliability may not be applicable Extremes are personal, and the meaning of endpoints remains relatively constant for a given individual over time, thereby minimizing error variance Test–retest reliability coefficient (sample of 378 community residents over 2-year period): 0.65 Face validity supported by overt relationship between the nature of the instrument and life satisfaction
Multiple Affect Adjective Check List (MAACL) and revised form (MAACL-R) (77)	Measure of an individual's mood as it varies day to day Self-report checklist of 132 adjectives best reflecting feelings that day Subscales: MAACL: 3 negative effects: anxiety, depression, hostility; MAACL-R: above 3 plus positive affect, sensation seeking, dysphoria	Reliability: MAACL: 0.65–0.92; MAACL-R: acceptable internal and test-retest reliabilities Validity: MAACL: 0.41–0.79; MAACL-R: concurrent and discriminant validity confirmed

Measure	Description	Reliability/Validity
Margin in Life Scale (MIL) (78)	94-item, self-report measure of vitality or freedom a person has to continue living (McClusky's construct of Margin of Life) Subjects rate load, power, and importance of each item 6 subscales (Self, Family, Religiosity/Spirituality, Body, Extra-Familial Relationships, Environment) Higher scores mean greater innate vitality or margin in life	Validity established through factor analysis and known-groups approach to construct validity Test–retest reliability: stability Cronbach's alpha reliability coefficients: body (0.87), self (0.84), family (0.69), religiosity (0.67), other human relationships (0.37), environment (−0.16)
Seriousness of Illness Rating Scale (revised) (SIRS-R) (79)	SIRS-R is an ordinal-level scale that reliably measures current views on the severity of illness and can be used with a variety of subjects and in psychosomatic research Examines the relationship of biologic, psychologic, and social variables to disease prevention, diagnosis, and treatment Used extensively in health psychology research to examine the link between the occurrence of stressful life events and onset of illness, mediating effects of personality on illness, and emotional factors in medical inpatients Original SIRS has 126 disease items evaluated by magnitude estimates of seriousness, ranked in quantitative order SIRS-R (revised) includes recently discovered disorders (e.g., AIDS) for final list of 137. A self-report questionnaire is used.	Geometric mean score determined ranking of each disorder Kendall's coefficient of concordance (W) signifies extent of interrater reliability in rank-ordering of disease items: Kendall's $W = 0.716$ ($p < 0.00001$); Mann-Whitney U test used to test differences in rankings of each disorder among the 3 levels of raters; homogeneity of disease item rating shown within the sample
Illness Effects Questionnaire (IEQ) (80)	20-item questionnaire measuring perception of illness-related effects on personal and social behavior 7-point Likert scale with scores ranging from 0 to 140	Internal reliability alpha: 0.93 Test–retest reliability: 0.99 Scale score correlates moderately with depression in medical patients and changes in depression among patients receiving treatment for chronic pain
Meaning of Illness Questionnaire (MIQ) (81)	MIQ measures a variety of concurrent yet divergent meanings given to an illness: its impact on life, the amount of type of stress (harm, loss, threat) and functional context (disability, disfiguring, deteriorating), the simultaneous view of illness associated with sense of hope, motivation and control, the degree of stress, change in commitment, and a secondary appraisal of more or less coping resources. Each of the 33 MIQ items is scored on a 3-point or 7-point scale from "not at all" to "a great deal." Score of factors are not summed into a local score and tests of total score internal consistency is not applicable. Two open-ended questions concern a person's previous and current life beliefs and commitments.	Test–retest reliability ranged between kappa −0.45 and 1.00, with the majority between 0.60 to 0.77. The MIQ has a strong relationship to health outcomes and greater utility than coping behaviors in explaining variance in adjustment to chronic illness in patients attending outpatient clinics.

Appendix 20C. Selected Other Instruments Measuring Attitudes Toward Chronic Disease (*cont.*)

Instrument	Description	Psychometric Indices
Hypertensive Interview Schedule (82)	Used to determine the effect of being treated for hypertension on health perception and lifestyle and the duration of any alterations after first being diagnosed 3 sections addressed: (1) Measures of Health Perception: health status: 9-point scale (1, poorest health; 9, best health); presence of symptoms: asked to identify symptoms from a list of 16, and to rate frequency (1, never, to 7, always), individual symptom scores summed to produce total score; worry about health: 9-point scale (1, no worry; 9, most worried possible) (2) Lifestyle: participation in physical and social activities; ability to participate: 9-point scale (1, no worry; 9, most worried possible); self-care behaviors (list) (3) Problems and Beliefs (list): interview format	Tested on 100 adult hypertensives and 50 normotensive controls Reliability and validity: between-group comparisons: Yate's chi square test of Fisher's exact proportions test used to assess nominal level data Mann-Whitney U test for ordinal- or interval-level data Kendall's tau used to measure strength of association between pairs of variables Analysis of variance used to test for differences between groups

Numbers in parentheses correspond to studies cited in the References.

21

Selecting a Tool for Measuring Cancer Attitudes

Nancy Burns

The word *cancer* generates in all of us a terror that we have difficulty defining. The illogical, unspoken, and often unrecognized attitudes or beliefs that lead to this intense emotion occur to some degree in everyone, regardless of rationality, sophistication, or education. These attitudes or beliefs occur in cancer patients and their family members as well as in health professionals and the community at large.

Impact of Attitudes and Beliefs on the Cancer Situation

Concern about the attitudes or beliefs about cancer comes from their impact on the cancer situation. The dictionary definition of *situation* is "a state of affairs of special or critical significance" and "the aggregate of biological, psychological, and sociocultural factors acting on an individual or group to condition behavioral patterns."[1] Experiencing the risk of having cancer or the diagnosis of cancer or living through the event of yourself or a significant other having cancer is a situation of critical significance. This situation affects in a holistic way the behavioral patterns of the individual and of those in the individual's social environment. The phrase *cancer situation* describes this phenomenon, which affects not only the person with cancer, but also family members, social support systems, and the health professionals providing care.

Attitudes and beliefs drive psychosocial responses to the threat and diagnosis of cancer. A number of basic research findings have made a compelling case for a link between psychosocial responses and cancer survival.[2] Variations in measures of natural killer (NK) cells and other dimensions of immunologic functioning have been linked to variations in psychosocial variables, such as stress,[3,4] depression,[5] interpersonal relationships,[6] marital disruption,[7] and social support.[8] When the person with cancer experiences high levels of psychosocial distress, particularly in the absence of an effective support system, the level of NK cells decreases. Longitudinally, levels of NK cells vary inversely with the level of psychosocial distress.[9] The level of NK cells is more predictive of the probability of metastasis and survival length than is any other variable, including medical treatment. This explanation of the link between psychosocial and physiologic elements in cancer is referred to as the psychoneuroimmunology model. The model explains relationships among variables that have been demonstrated through research for many years but were not understood.

Decision making also is influenced by attitudes and beliefs. Treatment decisions are made by the patient, family unit, society, and health professionals and may have a major impact on the healthiness of the response to the cancer situation.

Patient and Family Decisions

Patient and family decisions influenced by cancer beliefs may include decisions about lifestyles, self-examination, participation in cancer-screening activities, the speed with which symptoms are reported to a health professional, initiating and adhering to treatment regimens, and self-esteem, quality of life, and degree of hopefulness. Family members' plans for the future, such as job changes, purchasing of new homes or other large expenditures, sending children to college, or moving to another region of the country, are often heavily influenced by attitudes about cancer.[10,11]

Societal Decisions

The social treatment of a person with cancer by his or her family, and of the patient and family by the community, is related to beliefs about cancer. The loss of social support and the abandonment of the patient-family unit by the community, which often occur in the cancer situation, may have serious long-term consequences, not only for the person with cancer but also for the present and future mental health of family members. Negative community attitudes also influence social and political systems. The fear and horror associated with cancer have generated a demand that something be done to prevent it or cure it. These negative attitudes have been helpful in compelling Congress and private foundations to provide increased funding for cancer research. However, they also have led to problems related to rehabilitation, insurability, and employability. People who have had cancer often are labeled "cancer patients" for the rest of their lives—a stigmatizing label affecting self-esteem and social functioning.

Culture

A recent upsurge of research addresses the effect of cultural beliefs on participation in screening, prevention activities, and early detection. Failure to understand cultural views of cancer may impair communication between nurse and patient and affect patient outcomes. Educational materials must be designed in culturally sensitive language.[12–27]

Health Professionals' Decisions

The decisions of health professionals are influenced by their personal attitudes about cancer. Concern has been expressed about this repeatedly in the nursing and medical literature, and many studies have been conducted to examine the impact of cancer attitudes on practice.[28–32] Also of concern is the impact of various educational approaches on cancer attitudes and subsequent practice decisions. Although links have been established between cancer attitudes and the use of prevention and screening interventions for cancer, the impact on other areas of practice remain essentially unstudied. Given the nature of primary care, the issues of concern are difficult to measure and often require self-report strategies that, given the topic, lend themselves to a number of biases. To decrease the risk of biases, Osborn et al.[33] used a medical record audit to examine the primary care activities of physicians and medical educators. Creative strategies should be used to understand situations in which negative cancer attitudes affect clinical decisions and interventions that can improve primary care outcomes. Several primary care situations might be influenced by negative cancer attitudes. For example, a primary care provider with negative cancer attitudes may believe that a cancer diagnosis is a presage of death and might react by refusing to consider the possibility that a patient might have this "horrible" disease. Such an attitude can influence the interpretation of physical examination findings, resulting in signs and symptoms of cancer being overlooked, minimized, or discounted; lumps may be watched for months. When cancer is diagnosed or considered a possibility, negative cancer attitudes may influence the choice of referral sources and selection of appropriate treatments. The relationship between the health professional and the client may be altered by a health provider's negative attitudes about cancer because such providers have difficulty addressing the emotional reactions of the patient and family members to a cancer diagnosis and initiate avoidance strategies. If a caregiver's attitudes about cancer are unrealistically negative, he or she may provide physical care but not psychologic care, and rehabilitative strategies may not be considered. Personal closeness with the patient may be avoided. Such caregivers may remain unaware of the feelings and problems faced by the patient-family unit and thus deprive them of needed care. A number of the instruments described in this chapter were developed to address some of these concerns.

Choices about a career in the health professions can be related to cancer attitudes. Such decisions often are made early in one's professional career. In one study, beginning student nurses had more negative beliefs about cancer than any other group tested.[34] These beliefs became even more negative during the nursing school experience. Students reported avoiding the selection of cancer patients to care for and feeling helpless to make a difference in the patient's status. Nursing staff on general medical-surgical units were perceived by the students to provide only minimal care to cancer patients. Few students were assigned to oncology units for clinical experience. Nursing faculty seemed to avoid clinical contact with cancer patients and tended to limit the number of hours of classroom content related to cancer nursing. These behaviors clearly influenced career decisions by the new graduate.

Beliefs, Attitudes, and Values:
A Theoretical Perspective

Beliefs, attitudes, and values are related ideas but are not the same. Most theorists make clear distinctions among the three. According to Michael Rokeach, *beliefs* reflect an individual's perception of reality.[35] Richer and Ezer distinguish between belief and meaning in a concept analysis which suggests that meaning exists at two levels. Attributes and anticedents are identified and a model case provided for each concept.[36] Scheibe proposes that beliefs allow the person to make inferences about what expectations he or she can have in a given situation.[37] Thus, a belief reflects what a person expects to happen in the external world in a given situation. Beliefs often develop during childhood, tend to be unconscious, and cannot be directly observed. Therefore, beliefs must be measured by indirect means.[33] Carl Jung saw beliefs as part of the collective unconscious and thus as acquired from one's culture but also influencing one's culture.[38] Antonovsky considered beliefs as important factors that influence a person's sense of coherence and thus his or her state of health.[39] Caplan thinks that beliefs are important in determining whether a person responds in an effective or ineffective way to a crisis situation.[40]

Rokeach sees *attitudes* as emerging from the belief system.[35] Attitudes involve the joining together of several beliefs. Attitudes are more likely to be conscious and, therefore, can be obtained by direct measurement.

Values are defined by Rokeach as a special type of belief, an abstract idea about ideal ways of behaving and ideal goals of life.[35] For example, values would be involved in determining the beliefs a health care provider "should" have about cancer. It would be possible, then, to compare the ideal belief with the actual belief.

Ajzen and Fishbein have developed a theory of reasoned action that suggests relationships between beliefs, attitudes, intentions, and behavior.[41] They believe that humans are rational rather than driven by uncontrollable desires and that behavior is carefully reasoned as opposed to automatic. They propose that beliefs that a certain behavior will lead to a certain outcome lead to attitudes about that behavior, that attitudes about the behavior lead to intentions to perform a specific behavior, and that intentions are highly predictive of the actual behavior of an individual.

Berrenberg proposes three models that may explain the effects of attitudes toward cancer on behavior.[42] The first model, the *Familiarity Model*, is derived from research demonstrating that contact with minority group members leads to more positive attitudes toward that group.[43] These findings are explained by proposing that contact reduces fear and negative stereotyping. Berrenberg proposes that contact with a disease such as cancer may have a similar effect—more positive attitudes toward cancer.

Second, the *Vulnerability Model* suggests that attitudes toward a disease may not operate in the same way as attitudes toward minorities. Increased contact with cancer may increase the sense of aversion to it by familiarizing the individual with the ravages of the disease. Personal experience with cancer and contact with cancer patients might increase a person's sense of vulnerability. If this model is correct, one could predict that increasingly negative attitudes would occur with greater experience with cancer. Berrenberg suggests that the Familiarity Model and the Vulnerability Model can be conceptualized as linear functions between experience with cancer and cancer attitudes.

Last, the *Dual Process Model* predicts that the most positive cancer attitudes will be found among those with the highest levels of cancer experience—those with a personal history of cancer. This explanation derives from the Familiarity Model. However, the Dual Process Model goes beyond this to suggest that experience with cancer may result in the individual finding renewed meaning in life. In addition, the cancer experience may enhance a person's sense of competence as a result of achieving mastery in coping with a traumatic life event. Unlike the Familiarity and Vulnerability Models, the Dual Process Model proposes that individuals with moderate levels of cancer experience, such as family members of persons with cancer, will have the most negative cancer attitudes. This proposition is derived from Coyne's social learning theory of depression.[44] Coyne suggests that the social needs of the depressed person over time alienate others and thus elicit negative social feedback, leading ultimately to social rejection. This rejection occurs because repeated attempts to relieve the depressed person fail, producing frustration. Berrenberg suggests that there are similarities between the social interactions of cancer patients and those of depressives.[42] She supports this proposition with the research of Wortman and Dunkel-Schetter, who found that the awkward nature of interpersonal contact with cancer patients can increase negative feelings and therefore increase the tendency to derogate the patient.[45] Negative feelings generated from a single experience with a cancer patient tend to be generalized to the disease itself. Thus, the Dual Process Model proposes a curvilinear relationship between cancer attitudes and cancer experience. Those with personal cancer experience will hold the most positive attitudes, and those having the familial experience with cancer will hold the most negative attitudes. Individuals with minimal experience with cancer should have attitudes somewhere in between these two groups. Berrenberg does not address where health professionals fit in on this attitude curve. Berrenberg has developed an instrument to measure cancer attitudes and conducted studies to test the three models. These are described later in the chapter. The study findings are consistent with the predictions of the proposed Dual Process Model.

Measurement of Beliefs and Attitudes

There is not yet a generally accepted conceptual definition within the body of knowledge of the essential elements of beliefs or attitudes about cancer. Therefore, each scientist has operationalized the concept using somewhat different criteria. Various methods for measuring beliefs and attitudes about cancer have been developed, but few have been used repeatedly in studies. Many of the existing tools need further work to develop validity and reliability.

Gaps in the Literature

Research examining attitudes and beliefs about cancer has not been a focus of studies in recent years. A high priority of psychosocial oncology research has been the examination of variations in quality of life as a consequence of treatment strategies. However, attitudes and beliefs most likely influence many of the dimensions of quality of life, and this probable relationship needs to be studied. Studies also are needed to document the impact of cancer attitudes and beliefs of the patient, family members, and social support groups on the quality of life of people with cancer.

The examination of cancer attitudes and beliefs in healthy populations also is important because of the shift in today's health care delivery system from an illness orientation to the promotion of health and prevention of illness. Research is needed to understand how cancer attitudes influence health choices. It is not known whether beliefs and attitudes about cancer, which tend to be acquired early in life and thus may be entrenched, can be changed or if changes are short term or long term. It is important to identify (1) situations in which unrealistic negative beliefs occur, (2) activities that can modify beliefs, and (3) the impact of revised beliefs on responses to the cancer situation.

Studies are needed to examine the current cancer attitudes of faculty who educate health care professionals and their students and to assess the effectiveness of teaching strategies designed to promote positive attitudes. The cancer attitudes of students must be examined longitudinally and correlated with relevant clinical experiences during their education. Many studies have examined cancer attitudes before and after continuing education programs related to cancer care.[46-51] However, many of these studies have not been well designed. Attitude measurement immediately after a program in which the desired attitudes have been discussed introduces a social desirability problem in that the participants tend to respond by giving the desired response rather than their actual attitude. The lack of comparison groups in many of these studies also is problematic. The cancer attitudes of health care providers must be examined longitudinally by taking repeated measures.[46] For example, attitudes might be measured at the time of initial employment in an oncology setting, during a staff-development program about oncology, and at set intervals thereafter.

Correlational studies to examine the relationship of cancer beliefs to other variables of interest in the cancer situation are needed. Studies to specifically examine the validity and reliability of existing tools will make a valuable contribution to the current level of knowledge about such tools. The cultural sensitivity of existing instruments needs to be examined and the cultural sensitivity of new instruments developed to measure cancer attitudes should be reported.[52] Theoretical studies of cancer beliefs and attitudes are badly needed. Corner, in a review of measures of cancer attitudes, suggests that there has been little progress toward understanding the influences that create such pessimism about cancer.[53]

Selection of a Belief or Attitude Tool

Selecting a belief or attitude tool involves deciding how well the tool measures the dimensions of attitudes or beliefs about cancer, the established validity and reliability of the tool, the time required to administer the tool, ease in completing and scoring the tool, and the complexity of data analysis. It also is important to determine whether the tool fits conceptually with the researcher's perception of cancer beliefs or attitudes and the theoretical framework of the study.

Researchers have used a variety of techniques to measure cancer beliefs and attitudes. Early measurement strategies used open-ended interviews.[54] Other studies use stimulus stories followed by questions.[55] Qualitative research methods have been used to examine cancer attitudes.[56,57] Questions related to knowledge about cancer, hopelessness, and self-esteem have been used in many studies to reflect cancer attitudes indirectly.[58] However, the use of quantitative questionnaires and scales to measure cancer beliefs and attitudes is more common.

American Cancer Society Studies

The American Cancer Society initiated the measurement of cancer attitudes using questionnaires. The American Cancer Society questionnaire includes items about how likely the respondent believes a patient is to tell people he or she has cancer; the respondent's willingness to work next to someone who has cancer; his or her belief that cancer is curable, that cancer is contagious, that cancer is the worst thing that could happen to a person, or that a diagnosis of cancer is a death sentence; any tendency to read news releases about cancer; the expectation that a cure for cancer will be found; and the desire to be informed of a diagnosis of cancer. Two instruments are reviewed in depth. Additional measures are presented in Appendix 21A.

The Haley Cancer Attitude Survey

In 1968, Haley et al. developed a tool to measure the cancer attitudes of medical students.[59] The tool evolved from 600 statements that expressed attitudes toward cancer and the care of cancer patients. From these statements, a preliminary form with 33 questions was developed and given to 163 physicians, 89 medical students, and 13 laypersons. Responses were examined using factor analysis, from which three dimensions of cancer attitude were identified: "(a) attitudes toward the patient's inner resources to cope with serious illness such as cancer (CAS I); (b) attitudes toward the value of early diagnosis and aggressive treatment (CAS II); and attitudes toward personal immortality and preparation for and acceptance of death (CAS III)."[50]

A second sample of 94 physicians was used to develop the tool further. Correlational analysis of the new data led to the subdivision of CAS II into two subscales: CAS IIa, early diagnosis, and CAS IIb, aggressive treatment. The instrument used a nine-point Likert-type scale with responses ranging from "strongly disagree" to "strongly agree." Scoring used –4 for "strongly disagree," 0 for "no opinion," and +4 for "strongly agree." Completion of the instrument requires approximately 15 minutes.

Examples from the survey include:

- A physician can be so discouraged by the low cure rate of cancer that he will not feel the need to do routine "cancer tests," especially when he is so busy working with sick patients.
- Aggressive treatment of cancer frequently subjects the patient to illness, pain, and expense without much actual benefit to him.
- The dying patient has to be kept happy since he has nothing to look forward to.

Reliability data for this instrument were not reported. Face validity and content validity must be inferred from the tool-development process. Initial steps toward construct validity were obtained through factor analysis and the formation of clearly defined factors. However, no report was given of the constancy of the factors across samples.

The tool was used in a study reported by Haley et al. in 1977 as part of a battery of tests given to examine the cancer-related attitudes of medical students.[50] Findings indicated that cancer attitudes evolved throughout medical school and were unrelated to the student's intellectual ability or to personal needs associated with daily interactions with others. Cancer attitudes were associated with values in life and the degree of openness to others. Responses tended to be neutral early in medical education, but definite attitudes emerged as medical education and experience progressed. There were increases in CAS I, decreases in CAS IIa and CAS IIb, and increases in CAS III. The cancer attitudes of medical students were different from those found in a comparison group of physicians. Medical students had more positive values on CAS I (the patient's psychologic resources) and less positive values on CAS IIa (early diagnosis) and CAS IIb (aggressive treatment) than did practicing physicians. In 1981, the tool was revised by Blanchard et al.[51] Twenty-seven new items were added to address changes in medical practice and modifications in the doctor–patient relationship since the original tool had been developed. The structure of the original tool was kept intact, and the new items were added to the end of the instrument. Using only the original 33 questions, Blanchard failed to replicate the original factor structure reported by Haley. Responses demonstrated a high degree of variability, and only 50% of the variance could be explained by the eight factors. In 1982, Cohen et al. used the revised tool in a comparative study of the responses of cancer patients, medical students, medical residents, physicians, and medical cancer educators.[60] The sample was purposely selected to allow comparison with Haley's original sample. However, factor analysis apparently was not performed on the new data, and therefore no additional information on the factor structure is available from this study.

In 1986, Raina et al. reported the use of the CAS over several years to examine the cancer attitudes of medical students and found that it yielded inconsistent results and discriminated poorly.[61] They report that "a rigorous analysis of the three subscales based on the CAS showed them lacking in reliability and internal consistency." Peters et al. used the CAS in 1987 in a study of the effect of a course in cancer prevention on medical student's attitudes and clinical behavior.[47] Students and a control group were followed for 3 years after completing the course. The authors found little change in attitude scores over time as measured by the CAS. Corner and Wilson-Barnett used the CAS on a sample of newly registered nurses in London in 1992.[46] They reported that the CAS did not appear to be particularly responsive to changes in attitudes among subjects. Responses to the CAS were compared to data on attitudes collected during interviews, using questions relating to each of the factors of the CAS. In contrast to the CAS, the interview questions did provide evidence of changes in attitude.

In 1996, Annunziata et al. used the CAS to determine the influence of demographic and professional factors on the cancer attitudes of Italian physicians. Variables included emotional involvement with patients, perception of the need for aggressive treatment, and communication of diagnosis and prognosis. Most physicians (77%) indicated that they were able to deal with the needs of the cancer patient. However, 44% indicated that patient anxiety was sometimes unbearable to them.[62]

The Burns' Cancer Beliefs Scales

The Burns' Cancer Beliefs Scales were developed between 1977 and 1981 as part of a doctoral dissertation.[63] A concept analysis of cancer beliefs was performed, and the essential elements were obtained from the literature and personal experience. A semantic differential format was used to develop the instrument. Therefore, each item is considered a separate scale. The semantic differential was designed to measure meaning. It tends to capture the affective component of meaning rather than factual meaning. It uses strategies similar to the word association used by psychotherapists to reflect the unconscious. Thus, the significance of the responses goes far beyond the simple dictionary definition of the word used in the instrument—it provides a link with the unconscious belief structure of the individual. The intensity of the response and the correlation of groupings of scales reflects experience or thought that often cannot be expressed directly.

The instrument was first tested on 13 family members of cancer patients participating in a family support group. Then four groups ($n = 153$) were selected to test the instrument: American Cancer Society volunteers, high school teachers, beginning nursing students, and members of a Baptist church. It was hypothesized that the American Cancer Society volunteers would score highest, high school teachers and beginning nursing students would have moderate scores, and the Baptist church members would score lowest. American Cancer Society volunteers scored highest and beginning nursing students had the lowest scores. Using analysis of variance (ANOVA), the group scores showed a statistically significant difference at the 0.001 level. To examine further the structure of the instrument, factor analysis was performed. Three distinct factors emerged and were labeled fear of the cancer situation, hopelessness, and stigma.

Researchers using the tool were asked to send their data to Burns to allow further examination of the instrument structure, validity, and reliability. Data from the original study and from various additional sources were pooled, resulting in a diverse sample of 767 subjects. Using this sample, correlations between the factor scores and other variables of interest were examined. Factor analysis was performed on this sample with the same factors emerging. Items with a factor loading of 0.4 or greater were selected for inclusion in each factor. All the items loaded on one of the three factors; there were no secondary loadings. However, because subjects from the original sample were included in the sample, validation of the factor structure will require additional work, including a confirmatory factor analysis. Weights on the items in each factor are available, as well as normative values, such as means and other statistical data for each scale from the 767 subjects.

The Burns' Cancer Beliefs Scales contain 23 semantic differential scales consisting of bipolar adjectives or descriptive terms associated with beliefs about cancer. Each opposing set of descriptive terms is placed at opposite ends of a seven-point scale. Positive and negative responses to an item are randomly assigned to the right or left side of the scale to diminish the probability of global scoring by the respondent. Instructions for completing the scale are included on the instrument form. Individuals are instructed to respond quickly with their initial gut reaction to the descriptive terms by marking one space on each scale.

- *Factor I, fear of the cancer situation,* consists of the following scales: painless to severe, constant, untreatable pain; no fear to terror; body mutilation to no body changes; pleasant odors to foul odors; independency to dependency; no life changes to sudden, overwhelming life changes; extreme suffering to no suffering; nourished to wasting away; certain future to uncertain future; and destructive, uncontained growth to normal growth.
- *Factor II, hopelessness,* consists of the following scales: punishment to no punishment, worthlessness to worth, shame to pride, acceptance to rejection, alienation to belonging, being wanted to not being wanted, unloved to loved, and abandoned to cared for.
- *Factor III, stigma,* consists of the following scales: hopefulness to hopelessness, certain death to being cured, helplessness to control, optimism to pessimism, and unknown to known.

Instrument administration is fairly simple and should take only 5 to 10 minutes. Participants must be instructed to respond to each item quickly and spontaneously with as little thought as possible. Completion of the tool can generate emotional responses in patients and family members; therefore, it is recommended that a health professional be present when the tool is used with these groups.

Scoring is performed by rating the most negative response as 1 and increasing each space by 1 to the most positive response, which is rated as 7. The lowest possible score is 23, and the highest possible score is 161. Added insight can be obtained by calculating factor scores for each of the three factors.

Internal consistency estimates were examined using the alpha coefficient. Alpha coefficients for the three factors range from 0.76 to 0.91. These statistics indicate an acceptable level of internal consistency for the tool.

Content validity was developed through literature review and concept analysis. The instrument was reviewed by family members of cancer patients, nurses practicing oncology, and nursing doctoral students, and then it was revised based on their suggestions.

Construct validity was examined using factor analysis. The grouping of the concepts that form the scales leads to the formation of a higher construct defined by the factor. Factor structure has been further examined using a sample of 767 subjects, providing some evidence of factorial validity.

Concurrent validity was obtained by administering the tool to a sample of people concurrently with other instruments thought to measure the same concept. The Hoffmeister Cancer Attitudes Questionnaire and the Beck Hopelessness Scale[64] were administered with the Burns' Cancer Beliefs Scales to 58 subjects. Factor scores of the Beck scale and the Hoffmeister questionnaire were correlated with factor scores of the Burns scales, using Pearson's product–moment correlations. All three factors of the Burns scales correlated significantly ($p < 0.001$) with the factors of the Hoffmeister questionnaire. The pessimism factor in the Beck scale correlated beyond the 0.001 level with all factors of the Burns scales. Correlations of the other two factors in the Beck scale (factor 2, loss of motivation, and factor 3, future expectations) with the Burns factors, and the Hoffmeister clusters indicated no significant correlations. The two factors from the Beck scale apparently measure a phenomenon not related to cancer attitudes and beliefs. The results of the correlations indicate concurrent validity for both the Burns scale and the Hoffmeister questionnaire.

Divergent validity was examined by correlating the three factors on the Burns scale with the Cancer Optimism Cluster in the Hoffmeister questionnaire. The two scores were significantly negatively correlated, suggesting divergent validity.

Ash et al. used the instrument in 1988 in a cancer-prevention and -detection course for 14 nurses in developing countries.[65] They report that the mean score (83.64) compared favorably with Burns's sample of 767 subjects (99.78). Additional measures of cancer attitudes can be found in Appendix 21A.

Summary

Attitudes toward cancer influence emotional health and behavior in the cancer situation. A number of methods for measuring cancer attitudes have been developed, but few have been used repeatedly in studies. Many of the existing tools need further work to develop validity and reliability. Research examining attitudes about cancer has not been the focus of studies in recent years. A high priority in psychosocial oncology research has been the examination of variations in quality of life as a consequence of various treatment strategies. However, attitudes and beliefs influence many of the dimensions of quality of life. The examination of cancer attitudes in health populations also is important because of the shift in our health care delivery system to promotion of health and prevention of illness. Studies are needed to examine current attitudes about cancer among health professions' faculty and students and to evaluate the effectiveness of teaching strategies designed to promote more positive attitudes about cancer.

Exemplar Studies

Hailey, B.J., Carter, C.L., & Burnett, D.R. Breast cancer attitudes, knowledge, and screening behavior in women with and without a family history of breast cancer. *Health Care for Women International*, 2000, 21:701-715.

This study exemplifies a comparative descriptive design sufficient to assess differences in the breast cancer attitudes, knowledge, and screening behaviors in two groups of women: those with a family history of breast cancer and those without a family history of breast cancer. Although a framework is not expressed, the authors critically examine previous studies whose findings guide the development of hypotheses and direct the methodology. The authors propose that women with a first-degree relative (FDR) would "(1) have more negative attitudes about cancer, (2) perceive themselves as having a high risk for breast cancer, (3) be more likely to engage in appropriate screening behavior, and (4) be more interested in genetic testing" (p. 703). An improvement over previous studies addressing these questions was the inclusion of a comparison group. The Cancer Attitude Inventory (Berrenberg, 1991) was used to examine attitudes toward breast cancer by inserting the word breast before cancer in each item. The first three hypotheses were validated. Thus, women with a first-degree relative had more negative attitudes about breast cancer. The fourth hypothesis was not supported. More than 80% of the subjects indicated a desire to be tested: 88% of the FDR group and 73% of the comparison group. The difference between the groups was not statistically significant.

Taylor, K.L., Kerner, J.F., Gold, K.R., & Mandelblatt, J.S. Ever vs. never smoking among an urban, multi-ethnic sample of Haitian-, Caribbean-, and U.S.-born blacks. *Preventive Medicine*, 1997, 26:855-865.

This study exemplifies the use of a cancer attitudes measure to compare three ethnic black groups who were living in New York City: Haitian, Caribbean, and United States-born. A structured telephone interview assessed smoking status, alcohol use, cancer-related attitudes and beliefs, and demographic information. The Cancer Attitudes Scale (Schottenfeld & Kerner, 1984) was included in the interview questions. Multiple logistic regression was used to examine the research questions.[93] Caribbean- and Haitian-born participants were significantly less likely to have ever smoked than United States-born blacks. Alcohol use was strongly correlated with smoking across groups. The belief that smoking was not related to cancer was related to "an almost twofold increase of ever smoking" (p. 855). There were significant differences among the groups in the two subscales of the Cancer Attitudes Scale. However, cancer attitudes were not significantly related to smoking behavior.

Internet Resources

CANSA Research. www.cansa.co.za/facts_myths_attitudes.asp. National Breast Cancer Center. www.nbcc.org.au/pages/info/resource/nbccpubs/cultatt/contents.htm.

New York Task Force on Immigration Health. www.med.nyu.edu/cih/docs/FocusGroupRep.pdf.

References

1. Stein, J. *The Random House dictionary of the English language.* New York: Random House, 1967, p. 1333.
2. Sabbioni, M.E.E. Psychoneuroimmunological issues. *Cancer Invest,* 1993, *11*(4):440-450.
3. Levy, S.M., Herberman, R.B., Maluish, A.M., et al. Prognostic risk assessment in primary breast cancer by behavioral and immunological parameters. *Health Psychol,* 1985, *4*(2):99-113.
4. Khansari, D.N., & Murgo, Faith, R.E. Effects of stress on the immune system. *Immunol Today,* 1990, *11*(5):170-175.
5. Calabrese, J.R., Kling, M.A., & Gold, P.W. Alterations in immunocompetence during stress, bereavement, and depression: Focus on neuroendocrine regulation. *Am J Psychiatr,* 1987, *144*(9):1123-1134.
6. Kennedy, S., Kiecolt-Glaser, J.K., & Glaser, R. Immunological consequences of acute and chronic stressors: Mediating role of interpersonal relationships. *Br J Med Psychol,* 1988, *61*(1):77-85.
7. Kiecolt-Glaser, J.K., Fisher, L.D., Ogrocki, P., et al. Marital quality, marital disruption, and immune function. *Psychosom Med,* 1987, *49*(1):13-34.
8. Levy, S.M., Herberman, R.B., Whiteside, T., et al. Perceived social support and tumor estrogen/progesterone receptor status as predictors of natural killer cell activity in breast cancer patients. *Psychosom Med,* 1990, *52*(1):73-85.
9. Glaser, R., Rice, J., Sheridan, J., et al. Stress-related immune suppression: Health implications. *Brain Behav Immun,* 1987, *1*(1):7-20.
10. Foster, L.W., & McLellan, L. Cognition and the cancer experience: Clinical implications. *Cancer Pract,* 2000, *8*(1):25-31.
11. Hailey, B.J., Carter, C.L., & Burnett, D.R. Breast cancer attitudes, knowledge, and screening behavior in women with and without a family history of breast cancer. *Health Care Women Int,* 2000, *21*:701-715.
12. Ali, N.S., & Khalil, H.A. Cancer prevention and early detection among Egyptians. *Cancer Nurs Int J Cancer Care,* 1996, *19*(2):104-111.
13. Bartroso, J., McMillan, S., Casey, L., et al. Comparison between African-American and white women in

their beliefs about breast cancer and their health locus of control. *Cancer Nurs Int J Cancer Care,* 2000, *23*(4):268-276.
14. Champion, V.L., & Scott, C.R. Reliability and validity of breast cancer screening belief scales in African American women. *Nurs Res,* 1997, *46*(6):331-337.
15. Ellis, P.M., Butow, P.N., Simes, R.J., et al. Barriers to participation in randomized clinical trials for early breast cancer among Australian cancer specialists. *Austr N Z J Surg,* 1999, *69*(7):486.
16. Goldstein, D., Thewes, B., & Butow, P. Communicating in a multicultural society II: Greek community attitudes towards cancer in Australia. *Intern Med J,* 2002, *32*:289-296.
17. Granda-Cameron, C. The experience of having cancer in Latin America. *Cancer Nurs Int J Cancer Care,* 1999, *22*(1):51-57.
18. Guidry, J.J. Assessing cultural sensitivity in printed cancer materials. *Cancer Practice,* 1999, *7*(6):291-296.
19. Jennings-Dozier, K., & Lawrence, D. Sociodemographic predictors of adherence to annual cervical cancer screening in minority women. *Cancer Nurs Int J Cancer Care,* 2000, *23*(5):350-356.
20. Mitchell, J.L. Cross-cultural issues in the disclosure of cancer. *Cancer Practice,* 1998, *6*(3):153.
21. Moore, R.J. African American women and breast cancer: Notes from a study of narrative. *Cancer Nurs Int J Cancer Care,* 2001, *24*(1):35-42.
22. Ong, K.J., Back, M.F., Lu, J.J., et al. Cultural attitudes to cancer management in traditional southeast Asian patients. *Australasian Radiol,* 2002, *46*:370-374.
23. Phillips, J., Cohen, M.Z., & Tarzian, A.J. African American women's experiences with breast cancer screening. *J Nurs Scholar,* 2001, *33*(2):135-140.
24. Sadler, G.R., Dhanjal, S.K., Shah, N.B., et al. Asian Indian women: Knowledge, attitudes and behaviors toward breast cancer early detection. *Public Hlth Nurs,* 2001, *18*(5):357-363.
25. Salazar, M. K. Hispanic women's beliefs about breast cancer and mammography. *Cancer Nurs Int J Cancer Care,* 1996, *19*(6):437-446.

26. Suarez, L., Ramirez, A.G., Villarreal, R., et al. Social networks and cancer screening in four U.S. Hispanic groups. *Am J Prev Med*, 2000, *19*(1):47-52.

27. Taylor, K.L., Kerner, J.F., Gold, K.F., & Mandelblatt, J.S. Ever vs. never smoking among an urban, multi-ethnic sample of Haitian-, and U.S.-born Blacks. *Prevent Med*, 1997, *26*:855-865.

28. Liberati, A., Apolone, G., Nicolucci, A., et al. The role of attitudes, beliefs, and personal characteristics of Italian physicians in the surgical treatment of early breast cancer. *Am J Pub Health*, 1990, *81*(1):38-42.

29. Bostick, R.M., Spraffka, J.M., Virnig, B.A., et al. Knowledge, attitudes, and personal practices regarding prevention and early detection of cancer. *Prev Med*, 1993, *22*(1):65-85.

30. Chlebowski, R.T., Sayre, J., Frank-Stromborg, M., et al. Current attitudes and practice of American Society of Clinical Oncology-member clinical oncologists regarding cancer prevention and control. *J Clin Oncol*, 1992, *10*(1):164-169.

31. Flanagan, J., & Holmes, S. Social perceptions of cancer and their impacts: Implications for nursing practice arising from the literature. *J Adv Nurs*, 2000, *32*(3):740-749.

32. Roman, E.B., Sorribes, E. & Ezquerro, O. Nurses attitudes to terminally ill patients. *J Adv Nurs*, 2001, *34*(3):338-345.

33. Osborn, E.H., Bird, J.A., McPhee, S.J., et al. Cancer screening by primary care physicians. Can we explain the differences? *J Fam Pract*, 1991, *32*(5):465-471.

34. Burns, N. Development of the Burns' Cancer Beliefs Scales. *Proceedings of the American Cancer Society Third West Coast Cancer Nursing Research Conference*, August 4–5, 1983, Portland, OR.

35. Rokeach, M. *Beliefs, attitudes and values*. San Francisco: Jossey-Bass, 1968.

36. Richer, M., & Ezer, H. Understanding beliefs and meanings in the experience of cancer: A concept analysis. *J Adv Nurs*, 2000, *32*(5):1108-1115.

37. Scheibe, K.E. *Beliefs and values*. New York: Holt, Rinehart, & Winston, 1970.

38. Read, H., Fordham, M., & Adler, G. (Eds.). *The collected works of C.G. Jung*. New York: Pantheon, 1960.

39. Antonovsky, A. *Health, stress, and coping*. San Francisco: Jossey-Bass, 1979.

40. Caplan, G. *Support systems and community mental health*. New York: Grune & Stratton, 1976.

41. Ajzen, I., & Fishbein, M. *Understanding attitudes and predicting social behavior*. Englewood Cliffs, NJ: Prentice-Hall, 1980.

42. Berrenberg, J.L. Attitudes towards cancer as a function of experience with the disease: A test of three models. *Psychol Health*, 1989, *3*(4):233-243.

43. Amir, Y. The contact hypothesis in ethnic relations. *Psychol Bull*, 1969, *71*(5):319-342.

44. Coyne, J.C. Depression and the response of others. *J Abnorm Psychol*, 1976, *85*(2):186-193.

45. Wortman, C.B., & Dunkel-Schetter, C. Interpersonal relationships and cancer: A theoretical analysis. *J Soc Issues*, 1979, *35*(1):120-155.

46. Corner, J., & Wilson-Barnett, J. Newly registered nurse and the cancer patient: the educational evaluation. *Int J Nurs Studies*, 1992, *29*(2):177-190.

47. Peters, A.S., Schimpfhauser, F.T., Cheng, J., et al. Effect of a course in cancer prevention on students' attitudes and clinical behavior. *J Med Ed*, 1987, *62*(7):592-600.

48. Scott, C.S., & Neighbor, W.E. Preventive care attitudes of medical students. *Soc Sci Med*, 1985, *21*(3):299-305.

49. Schmelkin, L.P., Wachtel, A.B., Hecht, D., et al. Cancer opinionnaire: Medical students' attitudes toward psychosocial cancer care. *Cancer*, 1986, *58*(3):801-806.

50. Haley, H.B., Huynh, H., Paiva, R.E., & Juan, I.R. Students' attitudes towards cancer: Changes in medical school. *J Med Educ*, 1977, *52*(6):500-507.

51. Blanchard, C.G., Ruckdeschel, J.C., Cohen, R.E., et al. Attitudes toward cancer: The impact of a comprehensive oncology course on second-year medical students. *Cancer*, 1981, *47*(11):2756-2762.

52. Nielsen, B.B., McMillan, S., & Diaz, E. Instruments that measure beliefs about cancer from a cultural perspective. *Cancer Nurs Int J Cancer Care*, 1992, *15*(2):109-115.

53. Corner, J.L. Assessment of nurses' attitudes towards cancer: A critical review of research methods. *J Adv Nurs*, 1988, *13*(5):640-648.

54. Mitchell, G.W., & Glicksman, A.S. Cancer patients: Knowledge and attitudes. *Cancer*, 1977, *40*(1):61-66.

55. Sloan, R.P., & Gruman, J.C. Beliefs about cancer, heart disease, and their victims. *Psychol Rep*, 1983, *52*(2):415-424.

56. Dodd, M.J., Chen, S., Lindsey, A.M., et al. Attitudes of patients living in Taiwan about cancer and its treatment. *Cancer Nurs Int J Cancer Care*, 1985, *8*(4):214-220.

57. Halldorsdottir, S., & Hamrin, E. Experiencing existential changes: The lived experience of having cancer. *Cancer Nurs Int J Cancer Care*, 1996, *19*(1):29-36.

58. Blinov, N.N., Komiakov, I.P., & Shipovnikov, N.B. Cancer research in Russia, II: Patients' attitudes to the diagnosis of cancer. *Soc Work Soc Sci Rev*, 1993, *4*(1):83-87.

59. Haley, H.B., Juan, I.R., & Galen, J.F. Factor-analytic approach to attitude scale construction. *J Med Educ*, 1968, *43*(3):331-336.

60. Cohen, R.E., Ruckdeschel, J.C., Blanchard, C.G., et al. Attitudes towards cancer: A comparative analysis of cancer patients, medical students, medical residents, physicians and cancer educators. *Cancer*, 1982, *50*(6):1218-1223.

61. Raina, S., Alger, E.A., Stolman, C., et al. Limitations in testing for attitudes toward cancer. *J Cancer Educ*, 1986, *1*(3):153-160.

62. Annunziata, M.A., Talamini, R., Tumolo, S., et al. Physicians and death; comments and behavior of 605 doctors in north-east of Italy. *Support Care Cancer*, 1996, *4*(5):334-340.

63. Burns, N. *Evaluation of a supportive-expressive group for families of cancer patients*. Unpublished dissertation, Denton Texas Woman's University, 1981.

64. Beck, A., Weissman, A., Lester, D., et al. The measurement of pessimism: The hopelessness scale. *J Consult Clin Psychol*, 1974, *42*(6):861-865.

65. Ash, C.R., McCorkle, R., & Tiffany, R. Cancer prevention and detection course for nurses in developing countries. *Cancer Nurs Int J Cancer Care*, 1988, *11*(4):230-236.

66. Hocloch, F.J., & Coulson, M.E. Developing an attitude inventory. *J Nurs Ed*, 1968, 7(3):9-13.
67. Sherif, C.W., Sherif, M., & Nebergall, R.E. *Attitudes and attitude change.* Philadelphia: Saunders, 1965.
68. Craytor, J.K., Brown, J.K., & Morrow, G.R. Assessing learning needs of nurses who care for persons with cancer. *Cancer Nurs Int J Cancer Care,* 1978, 1(3):211-220.
69. Hoffmeister, J. *First year evaluation results: Test development information, oncology nursing project.* Contract #1-CN-65185. Pittsburgh: University of Pittsburgh National Cancer Institute, 1976.
70. Lebovits, A.H., Croen, L.G., & Goetzel, R.Z. Attitudes towards cancer: Development of the Cancer Attitudes Questionnaire. *Cancer,* 1984, 54(6):1124-1129.
71. Damrosch, S., Denicoff, A.M., St. Germain, D., et al. Oncology nurse and physician attitudes toward aggressive cancer treatment. *Cancer Nurs Int J Cancer Care,* 1993, 16(2):107-112.
72. Davison, R.L. Opinion of nurses on cancer, its treatment and curability—A survey among nurses in Public Health Service. *Br J Prevent Sociol Med,* 1965, 19(1):24-29.
73. Whelan, J. Oncology nurses' attitudes toward cancer treatment and survival. *Cancer Nurs Int J Cancer Care,* 1984, 7(5):375-383.
74. Fanslow, J. Attitudes of nurses toward cancer and cancer therapies. *Oncol Nurs Forum,* 1985, 12(1):43-47.
75. Donovan, M., Yasko, J., Wolpert, P., et al. *Cancer attitude survey.* Contract #1-CN-55186-07. Pittsburgh: University of Pittsburgh National Cancer Institute, 1977.
76. Gutteling, J.M., Seydel, E.R., & Wiegman, O. Perceptions of cancer. *J Psychosoc Oncol,* 1986, 4(3):77-93.
77. Becker, M.H., Haefner, D.P., Kasl, S.V., et al. Selected psychosocial models and correlates of individual health related behaviors. *Med Care,* 1977, 15(suppl 5):27-46.
78. Hailey, B.J., & Lalor, K.M. Perceptions about breast cancer patients: The effect of the type of relationship with the patient. *J Psychosoc Oncol,* 1990, 8(1):119-132.
79. Domino, G., Affonso, D.A., & Hannah, M.T. Assessing the imagery of cancer: The Cancer Metaphors Test. *J Psychosoc Oncol,* 1991, 9(4):103-121.
80. Domino, G., & Lin, J. Images of cancer: China and the United States. *J Psychosoc Oncol,* 1991, 9(3):67-78.
81. Domino, G., & Lin, W. Cancer metaphors: Taiwan and the United States. *Int J Psychol,* 1993, 28(1):45-56.
82. Domino, G., Fragoso, A., & Moreno, H. Cross-cultural investigations of the imagery of cancer in Mexican nationals. *Hisp J Behav Sci,* 1991, 13(4):422-435.
83. Berrenberg, J.L. The Cancer Attitude Inventory: Development and validation. *J Psychosoc Oncol,* 1991, 9(2):35-44.
84. Rounds, J.B., & Zevon, M.A. Cancer stereotypes: A multidimensional scaling analysis. *J Behav Med,* 1993, 16(5):485-496.
85. Berman, S.H., & Wandersman, A. Measuring knowledge of cancer. *Soc Sci Med,* 1991, 32(11):1245-1255.
86. Derogatis, I.R. *SCL-90-R.* Towson, MD: Clinical Psychometric Research, 1992.
87. Pettingale, K.W., Burgess, C., & Greer, S. Psychological response to cancer diagnosis—I. Correlations with prognostic variables. *J Psychosom Res,* 1988, 32(3):255-261.
88. Greer, S., Morris, T., Pettingale, K.W., et al. Psychological response to breast cancer and 15-year outcome. *Lancet,* 1990, 335(8680): 49-50.
89. Nelson, D.V., Friedman, L.C., Baer, P.E., et al. Attitudes to cancer: Psychometric properties of fighting spirit and denial. *J Behav Med,* 1989, 12(4):341-355.
90. Frank-Stromborg, M. Reaction to the diagnosis of cancer questionnaire: Development and psychometric evaluation. *Nurs Res,* 1989, 38(6):364-369.
91. Frank-Stromborg, M., Wright, P., Segalla, M., et al. Psychological impact of the cancer diagnosis. *Oncol Nurs Forum,* 1984, 11(3):16-22.
92. Mandelblatt, J.S., Gold, K., O'Malley, A.S., et al. Breast and cervix cancer screening among multiethnic women: Role of age, health, and source of care. *Prev Med,* 1999, 28:418-425.
93. Schottenfeld, D., Kerner, J.F. Final report: Cancer control development grant. Bethesda, MD: National Cancer Institute, 1984.

Appendix 21A. Additional Important Measures of Cancer Attitudes

Instrument	Description	Psychometric Indices
Cancer Attitude Inventory developed by Hocloch and Coulson, 1968 (66)	Measure of nursing students' attitudes toward cancer based on Sherif's conceptual framework of attitude change (67) 36-item, Likert-type scale	Content validity established Test–retest reliability: 0.96
Craytor's Oncology Nursing Questionnaire Developed by Craytor et al., 1978 (68)	Measures attitudes and learning needs of nurses caring for cancer patients Nurses asked to respond to item in 2 ways: (1) importance of cancer patient care activities, (2) how successfully activity performed Modified as cancer nursing skills have changed over time	Reliability data not given Validity: factor analyses for 2 factors: psychosocial care and physical care
The Cancer Attitudes Questionnaire developed by Hoffmeister, 1976 (69)	21-item measure of cancer attitudes using 5-point Likert-type format Cluster analysis revealed 4 clusters: fatalism, optimism, cancer phobia, stigma	Reliability: test–retest (1-week interval) performed Validity: cluster characteristics of the measure indicate clusters valid (internal consistency) Face-content validity established
Croen and Lebovits's Cancer Attitudes Questionnaire developed by Lebovits et al., 1984 (70)	28 items representing seven attitudinal dimensions (3–6 in each dimension) 50% of items in each dimension expressed negatively and 50% positively 6-point Likert forced-choice scale (no undecided or neutral responses) Instrument modified to contain 5 factors (71)	Construct validity: established by expert panel Factor analysis performed Reliability: interrater: determined by repeated measures; ANOVA internal consistency: alpha coefficient: 0.96
Nurses' Attitude Questionnaire modified from the original (72) by Whelan, 1984 (73)	14-multiple-choice-question measure used to compare cancer attitudes of nurses in the United States and England	No reliability or validity data available
Fanslow's Cancer Attitudes Instrument Developed by Fanslow, 1985 (74)	49-item measure derived from American Cancer Society Questionnaire and Craytor's Oncology Nursing Questionnaire 15 items address attitudes about skills in cancer nursing, 34 items address cancer-related myths and knowledge, 5-point Likert scale used (5 most positive, 1 most negative) Higher total score reflects more positive attitude towards cancer	Internal consistency satisfactory: alpha 0.9 (skill), 0.9 (knowledge) Face and content validity established Higher scores may relate to nurse's ability to effectively care for patients with cancer and knowledge about cancer
Yasko and Power's Cancer Attitude Survey developed by Donovan et al., 1977 (75)	38-item measure using a forced-choice 4-point Likert-type scale for responses Derived from previous questionnaires; items added	Reliability reported to be 0.80

Cancer Opinionnaire developed by Schmelkin et al., 1986 (49)	Developed to measure medical students' attitudes toward psychosocial cancer care Revised to total 50, then 38, items with 6-point Likert-type response scale 5 subscales: (1) outcome expectations (10 items); (2) candor (10); (3) interest in treating cancer (6); (4) psychosocial concerns: role of physician (7); (5) psychosocial concerns: importance to the patient (5)	Principal axis factor analysis performed and 5-factor solution selected: oblique factor rotation indicated factors not correlated; varimax rotation used for item inclusion on subscales Alpha coefficients: (1) 0.79, (2) 0.82, (3) 0.75, (4) 0.68, (5) 0.68
Perceptions of Cancer developed by Gutteling et al., 1986 (76)	Based on Health Belief Model (77) 4 subscales: (1) cancer knowledge (15 multiple-choice items); (2) health attitudes (11 statements with 5-point Likert-scaled responses); (3) behavioral intention (items ask subjects to rate probability of behaving in a particular way to 5 daily situations); (4) fear of cancer (same situations as in (3) but subjects rate reactions on a 5-point scale)	Reliability and validity of subscales tested: (1) Cronbach's alpha: 0.73, item-total correlations averaged 0.34; (2) factor analyses used, principal component analysis revealed 4 factors (eigenvalues > 1.0, accounting for 57.9% of variance); (3) Cronbach's alpha: 0.64, item-total correlation averaged 0.40; (4) Cronbach's alpha: 0.90, item-total correlation averaged 0.58
Cancer Perception Vignettes developed by Hailey and Lalor (78)	3 one-paragraph vignettes describing a breast cancer patient who recently received a mastectomy Subject asked to imagine what it would be like to visit her Relationship changes in each vignette: 1st is mother, 2nd is close family friend, and 3rd is a distant neighbor; 12-item questionnaire then completed by subject concerning perceptions of patient and reactions to her 5 possible responses for each item (5 most negative, 1 most positive); higher total score, more pessimistic attitude toward patient	Factor analysis for 4 factors with eigenvalues > 1, accounting for 59% of variance: (1) reactions and attitudes of others, (2) psychological effects, (3) noticeable effects of illness, (4) optimistic vs. pessimistic attitudes toward illness
Cancer Metaphors Test (CMT) developed in 1991 (79)	Developed to assess image of cancer Subject asked to indicate the appropriateness of 32 metaphors in giving an image of what cancer is ("very appropriate" to "very inappropriate") Factors identified in factor analysis: (1) total pessimism (33.8% variance); (2) future optimism (14.2%); (3) natural disaster (10.3%); (4) foreign intruder (8.3%) Instrument used to compare images in China (80), Taiwan (81), Mexico (82)	Test-retest reliability (10- to 12-week interval) > 0.70 Convergent and discriminant validity: factor analysis for 4 factors (25 of 32 metaphors, and 66.6% total variance); 4 factors statistically differentiated Health Locus of Control from CMT Internal consistency reliability of factors: (1) 0.85; (2) 0.88; (3) 0.79; (4) 0.73 Significant correlations with Health locus of control, Quality of life index

Appendix 21A. Additional Important Measures of Cancer Attitudes (*cont.*)

Instrument	Description	Psychometric Indices
Berrenberg's Cancer Attitude Inventory (CAI) developed in 1989 (83)	Developed to test the 3 models explaining cancer attitudes: familiarity, vulnerability, and dual process Final 41-item inventory, derived from extensive review of the literature, questionnaire survey of 54 cancer survivors, and studies examining cancer attitudes	Reliability and validity tested on 302 undergraduate students Factor analysis for 2 factors, analyzed by varimax rotation; factor structure could not be defined suggesting unidimensional scale Cronbach's alpha: 0.91 Test-retest in 2 samples: 0.90, 0.91
Measure of Cancer Stereotypes developed by Rounds and Zevon, 1993 (84)	Measures preconceptions or stereotypes of general public and cancer patients Intended to identify the attributes most salient to cancer stereotype to develop strategies to alter the public's view of the cancer patient Identified attributes important to organization of perception of a medical condition: such as severity, visibility, familiarity, and comfort in socialization with affected person Subject asked to rate each attribute on a 7-point scale and to also rate these attributes for 11 other illnesses as well as cancer, and finally, asked to make comparisons of similarity between pairs of illnesses	Sample tested: 68 physically healthy psychology students Multidimensional scaling analyses for 2-dimensional solution, I: physical-functional health; II: normality Cancer was perceived as normal but not having the most extreme physical impact Responses to cancer clearly distinct from other illnesses Further research on structure of illness stereotypes warranted
Fear of Cancer Index (FCI) developed by Berman and Wandersman, 1992 (85)	Indirect measure of fear of cancer by asking subjects to interpret meanings of various physical symptoms Can also be used to explain health-seeking behavior related to cancer prevention and screening Composite score: distress ratings of 25 items from Symptom Checklist (SCL-90-R) (86) including 7 Warning Signs of Cancer, and 25 items from the Knowledge of Cancer Warning Signs Inventory (KCWSI) (85,87) Scoring: summed cross product values between each of identical KCWSI and SCL-90-R items (max. score 300)	Reliability not addressed Validity testing (correlation and regression analysis) demonstrated construct validity Warrants further study
Cancer Adjustment Survey developed by Nelson et al., 1989 (89)	Developed to measure the concepts of denial and "fighting spirit," reported to extend cancer survival (53,88) Eight 5-point Likert-scale items used	Factor analysis for 3 factors: (1) fighting spirit, (2) information seeking, (3) denial (weak) Test-retest reliability performed in samples with breast cancer (BC), and other cancers (OC): (1) BC: 0.71, OC: 0.51; (2) BC: 0.75, OC: 0.81; (3) BC: 0.57, OC: 0.35

Reaction to the Diagnosis of Cancer Questionnaire (RDCQ) developed by Frank-Stromborg, 1989 (90)	Developed to assess initial reactions of persons diagnosed with cancer, from work begun in 1984 (91) Initial RDCQ comprised of 19 items, either distress or confronting responses, using yes/no format Revised RDCQ contains 17 items using 5-choice modified Likert format Further revised to improve internal consistency of the 2 groups of items, resulting ultimately in a 28-item instrument	Convergent and discriminant validity: suggest "fighting spirit" has 2 components (fighting back, information seeking) Denial is weak factor requiring further study Internal consistency reliability, coefficient alphas: (1) 17-item, initial revised RDCQ: 0.89 (confronting response items 0.72); (2) final 28-item RDCQ: 0.90 (confronting subscale, 0.82, distress subscale, 0.91) Factor analysis confirmed the multidimensional construct measured by the RDCQ Test-retest (2-week interval): 0.89 (distress scale 0.92; confronting scale 0.87)
Cancer Attitudes Scale developed by Schottenfeld & Kerner (1984)[93]	Developed for a cancer control development grant The scale includes an anxiety subscale (6 items) a helplessness subscale (8 items) and a denial subscale (2 items) Subscales can be combined into a single score where a higher score reflects less anxiety and hopelessness and a lower level of denial. In addition to these subscales, cancer "superstitions" beliefs (e.g., not having faith in God, not being a good person, or having another person wish bad things about you . . . increase your chances of getting cancer) and embarrassment about being examined were included (92)	Anxiety subscale (Kuder-Richardson, KR = 0.58) Hopelessness subscale (KR = 0.72) Denial subscale (KR = 0.46) The subscales have similar factor loadings and distributions. Total score (KR = 0.75)

Numbers in parentheses correspond to studies cited in the References.

22

Measuring Family Outcomes

Gloria Juarez, Betty R. Ferrell, and Michelle Rhiner

Cancer, an often chronic illness with significant physical and psychosocial consequences, has an impact on the whole family. It is estimated that two of every three individuals will have a family member who receives a cancer diagnosis.[1] Oncology nurses recognize the integral role of the family in caring for the person with cancer and have contributed significantly to the research related to cancer's impact on the family.

Any discussion on measuring family outcomes must begin with definitions of both *family* and *outcomes*. There is consensus that *family* is best defined by the individual patient, rather than interpretations of family limited to blood relations or those related by marriage. *Family* is a broad term and may include any significant relationship, such as friend, life partner, lover, relative, or spouse.

Family theorists agree that the family is more than the sum of its individuals. Family is viewed as a social system. Germino and O'Rourke, major contributors to conceptualization of family outcomes in oncology, defined *family* as a social system in which members have ties to each other, are interdependent, have some common history, and share some goals.[1]

Health care research has emphasized the need to measure outcomes of nursing and medical interventions. This focus on outcomes has been extended to family research. In a thorough review of the methodologic and conceptual issues in family research, Feetham defines *family outcomes* as "the changes or stabilization in family functioning as an endpoint of nursing practice, or the abilities/functions of the family (at the family system or family member level) as an endpoint of nursing practice."[2]

Thus, the measurement of family outcomes is best guided by a broad definition of family and by selecting outcomes that result from nursing care of the patient and family across the spectrum of illness and disease. The inclusion of family outcomes in health care research is imperative, and the theoretical and methodologic challenges of this research are significant.

Theories to Guide Research

Several authors have acknowledged the lack of family theories to guide research.[3,5] Research often is conducted on individual roles or relationships, such as family caregiving in chronic illness, but these studies seldom use a family framework.

Researchers frequently have used nursing theories that include concepts of social support, family, or social well-being to guide family research. These theories or conceptual models, however, are generally individual-specific models with reference to the interaction between patient and family. Feetham promotes the need for research that adds to our knowledge of family functioning and structure and contributes family theories to science.[2]

Methodologic Challenges

Increased attention to family outcomes is timely, particularly in light of health care reforms that have transferred both acute and chronic care to family members. The burden on family members to provide health care occurs at a time when care also has become complex-high-tech care in the living room. Decreased hospital stays and increased outpatient care have resulted in family members' assuming responsibilities that are both physically and psychologically taxing.

Nursing has historically included family members in interventions such as teaching.[8] However, family members often have been viewed only as components of the patient's environment, rather than recipients of nursing care or as critical outcomes of such care.

Historically, family members often were included in research as proxy measures of patient outcomes. Proxy measures, however, lack validity for most patient variables. More recently, nurse researchers have recognized the importance of family outcomes as distinct and valuable outcome measures of nursing care. Research has demonstrated that care that benefits patients, such as improved pain management, may occur at the risk of creating a significant burden on family caregivers.[9,10]

Feetham observes that there has been limited research expertise in family outcomes research, family research, and research involving the interaction of practitioners and families.[2] She also recognizes the need to identify predictors of family outcomes in light of diminishing health care resources to identify high- and low-risk families.[2] For example, it is important to identify families most in need of assistance after outpatient surgery to best distribute resources for home care.

A critical measurement issue in family outcomes research is the identification of the unit of analysis. Outcomes may focus on an individual family member or be applicable to several family members. Some experiences will be similar for the patient and family members, whereas other experiences will be unique or contradict other experiences. Some outcomes focus on the concept of caregiving and thus are primarily concerned with the individual(s) most involved in direct care. Other outcomes, such as family coping, require an analysis of the total family experience and involve multiple family members.

Dimensions of the Concept

Family outcomes have been explored in oncology as a multidimentional concept. Several key variables frequently surface, one of the most common being family communication. Investigators have evaluated the effect of cancer on patterns of communication, generally citing the difficulties imposed by a cancer diagnosis.[11] This variable illustrates the dynamic nature of the concept of family outcomes as family communication varies across the illness trajectory from initial diagnosis to treatment, remission, relapse, and terminal illness.

An additional variable frequently explored in family research is the need for information.[12] Descriptive and exploratory investigations have assessed the need for education, particularly in the area of home care. A closely related variable is the need for support services. Coping and social support often have been extracted from patient outcomes research and applied to family members.[1,12,13]

Several researchers have identified caregiving demands associated with cancer care.[13-16] Laizner and colleagues[17] reviewed 14 studies between 1982 and 1993 that evaluated caregiver needs. Three general areas of need were identified: (1) personal needs (bathing, self-care), (2) instrumental needs (meals, housework, transportation), and (3) administrative needs (financial and legal). The authors stressed the importance of assessing caregiving demands adequately over time to address the changing nature and intensity of caregiving.

The importance of selecting appropriate concepts for measurement resounds throughout the family research literature. The initial response of family members to a cancer diagnosis may be best measured by concepts such as anxiety or coping but may later focus on entirely different concepts, such as anticipatory grief or loss.[18] Other concepts, such as hope or the need for information, may remain relevant over time, yet take on altered meaning over the course of the illness.[19]

Despite global definitions of family, most family research has remained focused on individual members. The impact of the diagnosis on the spouse has been the predominant area of research.[19,20] The greatest methodologic challenge for the future is to broaden the scope of research to include multiple family members and measurement of the total family experience. Accomplishing this goal requires an interdisciplinary approach in which all researchers benefit from the involvement of other disciplines,[6] attention to the methodologic issues,[2] as described above, and a critical evaluation of the instruments currently used with individuals for their applicability to other family members or to family system outcomes.

Issues Involved in Selecting Instruments

Feetham[4] provides an excellent review of the methodologic issues involved in measuring family outcomes. Researchers recognize that reliability issues are important in family research, as the family system is dynamic and outcomes are expected to change significantly over time. Validity issues are a challenge in family outcome research because researchers need to evaluate the relevance of using outcomes borrowed from patient research in family outcomes analyses. The content of instruments that measure anxiety, coping, or hope may in fact be quite different in the context of the family. Likewise, issues of construct validity are challenged when applied to family caregivers because issues such as the relationship of the individual family member to the patient may have a significant impact on the validity of that concept. For example, the concepts of grief or loss vary greatly in family members caring for a child rather than a grandparent with cancer.

Germino has addressed the pragmatic issues of measuring family outcomes. She discusses issues such as respondent burden in relation to family members.[21] Family members may be both physically and psychologically exhausted, and in fact the burden on family caregivers may exceed the needs of the patient. Germino recognizes the difficulties associated with recruiting family subjects. Gaining access to family members outside of the clinic setting and arranging appropriate sites for data collection may be more difficult than in patient research.

Numerous cultural factors also must be considered in any evaluation of family outcomes. The cultural meanings associated with family, religion, family traditions, and ethnic influences are very relevant in family research.[22]

Family outcomes research is not simply a replication of the outcomes and variables in patient research to families. Many concepts and outcomes are appropriate, but recognizing the unique nature of the family requires careful analysis and selection of outcomes. A clear understanding of the meaning of family and of the family as a system requires both qualitative and quantitative approaches.[23]

Most limitations of family research concern sample selection. Most family research has been conducted on highly articulate family members with advanced education and high socioeconomic status. The inclusion of family members from diverse backgrounds and skills requires attention to the readability and the total appropriateness of evaluation methodologies. Several investigators have noted differences in family outcomes based on individual characteristics, such as gender[14,24] and age.[25,26] Further exploration of these individual characteristics should enhance our understanding of family outcomes.

Clark and Gwin[27] advocate the identification of additional variables of interest, including the health of the family caregivers, the marital relationship, and adaptation of the children of adults with cancer. Survivorship in pediatric cancer also challenges researchers to explore outcomes of interest for this population.[28-30] The diagnosis of cancer in a child has a significant impact on the entire family over time and on the child into adulthood.[28-30]

Instruments Available for Measuring Family Outcomes

Instruments that have been used in family outcomes research are described in Appendix 22A.[31-56] The concepts measured include family functioning, social support, coping, caregiving demands, caregiver reactions, marital adjustment, and quality of life. The reader should note that many other instruments and concepts presented in this text also are relevant for family outcomes research.

Summary

Changes in the health care environment continue to thrust the burden of caregiving onto the family and emphasize the need for careful evaluation of caregiver needs or burden for effective intervention. A variety of instruments can measure the impact of medical and nursing interventions on family outcomes. However, additional instrument development and refinement clearly are needed.

Exemplar Study

Endo, E., Nitta, N., Inayoshi, M., et al. Pattern recognition as a caring partnership in families with cancer. *J Adv Nurs*, 2000, 32(3):603.

This study addressed the process of a caring partnership by elaborating pattern recognition as a nursing intervention with families with cancer. It was based on Newman's theory, in which a hermeneutic, dialectic method was used to engage Japanese families. The wife-mothers were hospitalized due to cancer diagnosis. The family included at least the woman with cancer and her primary caregiver. Each of the four research nurses entered into partnership with a different family and conducted tape-recorded, semistructured interviews with each family.

The data revealed five dimensions of a transformative process: (1) the family-nurse mutual concern and evolution of family's pattern, (2) recognition of the family's pattern as a whole and their own pattern as part of the whole, (3) revelation of meaning in the family's pattern, (4) caring and action potential, and (5) transformation.

The study is exemplary because the investigator uses the patient and at least one family member to grasp the pattern of the family as a whole and experience the meaning of caring. The study contributes to an understanding of the process of pattern recognition as a caring partnership with families. It also illustrates how qualitative research can direct future research.

Most families found meaning in their patterns and made the shift from separated individuals within the family to trustful, caring relationships. The families showed increasing openness, connectedness, and trustfulness in caring relationships. The author concludes by stating that this research method was designed to meet the reality of clinical nursing practice.

Internet Resources

Promoting Excellence: Key Clinical Assessment and Research Tools: Introduction to the tools. Access date 4 Feb 2003. www.promotingexcellence.org/instruments/.

QOLID Quality of Life Instruments Database. Access date 4 Feb 2003. www.qolid.org/.

References

1. Germino, B. & O'Rourke, M.E. Cancer and the family. In R. McCorkle, M. Grant, M. Frank-Stromborg, & S.B. Baird (Eds.), *Cancer nursing: A comprehensive textbook*. (2nd ed.). Philadelphia: Saunders, 1996, pp. 81-92.
2. Feetham, S.B. *Family outcomes: Conceptual and methodological issues*. NIH Publication No. 93-3411. Washington, DC: Department of Health and Human Services, 1992, pp. 103-111.
3. Friedman, M.M. *Family nursing research, theory, and practice* (4th ed.). Stanford, CT: Appleton & Lange, 1998.
4. Feetham, S.L. Conceptual and methodological issues in research of families. In A.L. Whall & J. Fawcett (Eds.), *Family theory development in nursing: State of the science and art*. Philadelphia: Davis, 1991, pp. 43-58.
5. Astedt-Kurki, P., Paavilainen, E., & Lehti, K. Methodological issues in interviewing families in family nursing research. *J Adv Nurs*, 2001, 35(2):288-293.
6. Knafl, K. Family outcomes: Practitioner/family interface. In P. Moritz (Ed.), *Patient outcomes research: Examining the effectiveness of nursing practice*. Rockville, MD: National Center for Nursing Research, 1992.
7. Gilliss, C.L. Family nursing research, theory and practice. *IMAGE: J Nurs Scholar*, 1991, 22(4):19-22.
8. Ferrell, B., Grant, M., Borneman, T., et al. Family caregiving in cancer pain management. *J Pallia Med*, 1999, 2(2):185-195.
9. Ferrell, B.R. The family. In H.G. Doyle & N. MacDonald (Eds.). *Oxford textbook of palliative medicine* (2nd ed.). Oxford: Oxford University Press, 2002, pp. 909-917.
10. Davies, B. Supporting families in palliative care. In B. Ferrell & N. Coyle (Eds.). *Textbook of palliative nurs-*

ing (2nd ed.). Oxford: Oxford University Press, 2001, pp. 363-373.
11. Cassileth, B.R., & Hamilton, J. The family with cancer. In B.R. Cassileth (Ed.), *The cancer patient: Social and medical aspects of care*. Philadelphia: Lea & Febiger, 1979, pp. 233-247.
12. Barsevich, A.M., Much, J., Sweeney, C. Psychsocial responses to cancer. In C.H. Yarbro, M.H. Froge, M. Goodman, & S.L. Groenwald (Eds.). *Cancer nursing principles and practice* (5th Ed.). Philadelphia: Saunders, 2000, pp. 1529-1549.
13. Boland, D., & Sims, S. Family caregiving at home as a solitary journey. *IMAGE: J of Nurs Scholar*, 1996, 28(4):55-58.
14. Stetz, K. Caregiving demands during advanced cancer. *Cancer Nurs Int J Cancer Care*, 1987, 10:260-268.
15. Oberst, M.I., & Scott, D.W. Postdischarge distress in surgically treated cancer patients and their spouses. *Res Nurs Health*, 1988, 11(4):223-233.
16. Hinds, C. The needs of families who care for patients with cancer at home: Are we meeting them? *J Adv Nurs*, 1985, 10(6):575-581.
17. Laizner, A.M., Shegda Yost, L.M., Barg, F.K., & McCorkle, R. Needs of family caregivers of persons with cancer: A review. *Sem Oncol Nurs*, 1993, 9(2):114-120.
18. Frank-Stromborg, M., & Wright, P. Ambulatory cancer patients' perceptions of the physical and psychosocial changes in their lives since the diagnosis of cancer. *Cancer Nurs Int J Cancer Care*, 1984, 7(2):117-129.
19. Gotay, C. The experience of cancer during early and advanced stages: The view of patients and their mates. *Soc Sci Med*, 1984, 18(7):605-613.
20. Northouse, L.L. The impact of breast cancer on pa-

tients and husbands. *Cancer Nurs Int J Cancer Care,* 1989, *12*(5):276-284.

21. Germino, B.B. Quality of life for families with cancer: Research issues. *Meniscus Health Care Comm, Qual Life-Nurs Chall,* 1993, 2(2):39-45.

22. Kagawa-Singer, M. Cultural systems. In R. McCorkle, M. Grant, M. Frank-Stromborg, & S.B. Baird (Eds.). *Cancer nursing: A comprehensive textbook* (2nd ed.). Philadelphia: Saunders, 1996, pp. 38-52.

23. Clarke-Steffen, L. A model of the family transition to living with childhood cancer. *Cancer Pract,* 1993, *1*(4):285-292.

24. Siegel, K., Raveis, V.H., Mor V., et al. The relationship of spousal caregiver burden to patient disease and treatment-related conditions. *Ann Oncol,* 1991, *2*(7):511-516.

25. Carey, P.J., Oberst, M.T., McCubbin, M.A., & Hughes, S.H. Appraisal and caregiving burden in family members caring for patients receiving chemotherapy. *Oncol Nurs Forum,* 1991, *18*(8):1341-1348.

26. Hileman, J.W., Lackey, N.R., & Hassanein, R.S. Identifying the needs of patients with cancer. *Oncol Nurs Forum,* 1992, *19*(5):771-777.

27. Clark, J.C., & Gwin, R.R. Pschosocial responses of the family. In S.L. Groenwald, M.H. Frogge, M. Goodman, & C.H. Yarbro (Eds.). *Cancer nursing principles and practice* (3rd ed.). Sudbury, MA: Jones & Barlett, 1993, pp. 468-483.

28. Lichtman, R.R., Taylor, S.E., Wood, J.V., et al. Relations with children after breast cancer: The mother-daughter relationship at risk. *J Psychosoc Oncol,* 1984, 2:1-19.

29. Birenbaum, L.K., & Yancey, D. Children's response to parent's cancer. *Second National Conference on Cancer Nursing Research,* Baltimore, MD: American Cancer Society, 1992.

30. Baird, S.B. The effect of cancer in a parent on role relationships with the nurse/daughter. *Cancer Nurs,* 1988, *11*(1):9-17.

31. Feetham, S.L. Family research: Issues and directions for nursing. In H. Werley & J.J. Fitzpatrick (Eds.). *Annual review of nursing research* (2nd ed.). New York: Springer, 1984, pp. 3-25.

32. Roberts, C.S., & Feetham, S.L. Assessing family functioning across three areas of relationship. *Nurs Res,* 1982, *3*(4):231-235.

33. Knafl, K., Gallo, A., Breitmayer, B., et al. One approach to conceptualizing family response to illness. In S. Feetham, S. Meister, J. Bell, & K. Gilliss (Eds.), *The nursing of families.* Newbury Park, CA: Sage, 1992, pp. 70-78.

34. Norbeck, J.S., Lindsey, A.M., & Carrieri, V.L. The development of an instrument to measure social support. *Nurs Res,* 1981, *30*(5):264-269.

35. Norbeck, J.S., Lindsey, A.M., & Carrieri, V.L. Further development of the Norbeck Social Support Questionnaire: Normative data and validity testing. *Nurs Res,* 1983, *32*(1):4-9.

36. Lewis, F.M., Woods, N.F., Hough, E.E., & Bensley, L.S. The family's functioning with chronic illness in the mother: The spouse's perspective. *Soc Sci Med,* 1989, *29*(11):1261-1269.

37. Lewis, F.M., & Hammond, M. Psychosocial adjustment of the family to breast cancer: A longitudinal analysis. *JAMA,* 1992, *47*(5):194-200.

38. Lewis, F.M., Hammond, M., & Woods, N.F. The family's functioning with newly diagnosed breast cancer in the mother: The development of an explanatory model. *J Behav Med,* 1993, *16*(4):351-370.

39. Woods, N.F., Haberman, M., & Packard, N.J. Demands of illness and individual, dyadic and family adaptation in chronic illness. *Western J Nurs Res,* 1993, *15*(1):10-30.

40. Stetz, K.M. The experience of spouse caregiving during advanced cancer. Unpublished doctoral dissertation. Seattle: University of Washington, 1986.

41. Stetz, K.M. The relationship among background characteristics, purpose in life, and health in spouse caregivers. *Sch Inq Nurs Pract,* 1989, *3*(2):133-153.

42. Given, C.W., Given, B., Stommel, M., et al. The caregiver reaction assessment (CRA) for caregivers to persons with chronic physical and mental impairments. *Res Nurs Health,* 1992, *15*(4):271-283.

43. Stommel, M., Wang, S., Given, C.W., & Given, B. Focus on psychometrics confirmatory factor analysis (CFA) as a method to assess measurement equivalence. *Res Nurs Health,* 15(5):399-405.

44. Ferrell, B., Rhiner, M., & Rivera, L.M. Development and evaluation of the Family Pain Questionnaire. *J Psychosoc Oncol,* 1993, *10*(4):21-35.

45. Ferrell, B.R., Grant, G., Chan, J., et al. The impact of pain education on family caregivers of elderly patients. *Oncol Nurs Forum,* 1995, *22*(8):1211-1218.

46. Robinson, B. Validation of a caregiver strain index. *J Gerontol,* 38(3):344-348.

47. Smilkstein, G., Ashworth, C., & Montano, D. Validity and reliability of the family APGAR as a test of family function. *J Fam Pract,* 1982, *15*(2):303-311.

48. Smilkstein, G. Family APGAR analyzed. *Fam Med,* 1993, *25*(5):293-294.

49. Spanier, G.B. Measuring dyadic adjustment: New scales for assessing the quality of marriage and similar dyad. *J Marital Fam Ther,* 1976, *31*:15-28.

50. Lewis, F.M., & Deal, L.M. Balancing our lives: A study of the married couple's experience with breast cancer recurrence. *Oncol Nurs Forum,* 1995, *22*(6):943-953.

51. McCubbin, H.I., & Comeau, J. FIRM: Family inventory of resources for management. In H.I. McCubbin, & A.I. Thompson (Eds.), *Family assessment inventories for research and practice.* Madison: University of Wisconsin-Madison, Family Stress Coping and Health Project, 1987, pp. 145-160.

52. McCubbin, H., & Patterson, J. FILE: family inventory of life events and changes. In H. McCubbin & A. Thompson (Eds.), *Family assessment inventories for research and practice.* Madison: University of Wisconsin Press, 1987, pp. 81-100.

53. Olson, D.H., Portner, J., & Bell, R. Family adaptability and cohesion evaluation scales (FACES II). St. Paul: University of Minnesota, Family Social Services, 1982.

54. Olson, D.H., Sprenkle, D.H., & Russell, C.S. Circumplex model of marital and family systems. I. cohesion and adaptability dimensions, family types and clinical applications. *Fam Process,* 1979, *18*(1):3-28.

55. Weitzner, M.A., Jacobsen, P.B., Wagner, H. Jr, et al. The Caregiver Quality of Life Index—Cancer (CQOLC) scale: Development and validation of an instrument to measure quality of life of the family caregiver of patients with cancer. *Qual Life Res,* 1999, 8:55-63.

Appendix 22A. Instruments to Measure Family Outcomes

Instrument/ Target Population	Dimensions/Description	Psychometric Indices
Feetham Family Functioning Survey (FFFS) (31,32) Family's ability to function as a unit within the community and their internal system	21-item, self-report measure of 3 constructs: (1) family interactions with the community, (2) family relationship to various subsystems, (3) reciprocal relationships within the family structure Subjects answer 3 questions on each item on a 7-point Likert scale (1 little, 7 much): (1) "How much is there now?", (2) "How much should there be?" and (3) "How important is it to me?"	Cronbach's alpha for the 3 measures: 0.66–0.84 Test-retest reliability: 2-week interval: 0.93; 5-week interval: 0.83 Correlations between scores of husbands and wives: 0.72
Defining and Managing Chronic Illness Parent interviews #1, #2 Child's interviews #1, #2 Sibling's interviews #1, #2 (33) Target population: families with a child diagnosed with a chronic illness	Interview guides developed to tape-record the child with a chronic illness, the parents and siblings, covering topics of history of illness; course of illness; child's condition, medication, and treatment; how the family takes care of the illness; school situation; health care situation; family events from the parents', child's, and siblings' perspective	None described
Norbeck Social Support Questionnaire (NSSQ) (34,35) Measures social support from all sources, including family members	Respondent asked to list each significant person, and relationship (9 questions measure the perceived support with regard to functional properties of social support) Uses 5-point Likert scale (1 not at all, 5 a great deal) Self-administered to groups or by mail; takes about 10 minutes to complete Separate score for family support can be calculated; allows for cultural variation as studies show the most effective sources of support may differ among cultural groups	Tested on nursing students Test–retest reliability n = 67 with 2-week interval: 0.85–0.92 Kendall tau B correlation coefficients: number of categories of persons lost: 0.83 ($p < 0.001$); amount of support lost: 0.71 ($p < 0.001$) Internal consistency tested through intercorrelations among all items: 2 affect items: 0.97; 2 affirmation items: 0.96; 2 aid items: 0.89 3 network property items: 0.88–0.96; correlations highly related to affect and affirmation (0.88–0.97) and moderately related to aid (0.69–0.80) Validity: did not correlate with Marlowe-Crowne Test of Social Desirability-SF Concurrent validity testing: parallels between tangible support (Social Support Questionnaire) and aid and informational support and affect Construct validity: low but significant relationship with Profile of Mood States depression and confusion subscales and NSSQ total loss subscale

F-COPES (36–38) Women with breast cancer and their family	49-question measure of psychosocial adjustment of the family to breast cancer Uses 5-point Likert scale (1 never, 5 almost always) Families interviewed by a 2-person interview team; partners independently complete the self-report questionnaire	Internal consistency reliabilities (coefficient alpha): women and partner's measures: ≥ 0.83 (most 0.90); mother's measure of quality of mother–child relationship: 0.74 Stability reliability coefficients: (4-month interval): 0.58–0.83 Depression and experienced illness demands changing the most over time
Demands of Illness Inventory (DOII) (39) Families with chronic illness	125-question measure of psychosocial adjustment of the family to diabetes and breast cancer Questionnaire can identify demands associated with a recent diagnosis of a chronic illness and with long-term adaptation Questions assess 7 subscales: (1) physical symptoms, (2) personal meaning, (3) family functioning, (4) social relationships, (5) self-image, (6) monitoring symptoms, (7) treatment issues Parallel instrument for partners Employs 4-point Likert scale (1 not at all, 4 extremely) Families interviewed at home; partners complete self-report questionnaire	Internal consistency reliability (alpha coefficients) of 7 dimensions (subscales): demands experienced (0.78–0.91); intensity of demands (0.86–0.92) Cronbach's alphas (total score): number score (0.96); intensity score (0.97)

Caregiving Demands Scale (CDS) (40,41)
Caregivers of individuals with chronic illness in the home
	Self-report questionnaire
	3 dimensions measured: (1) physical care, (2) role alterations, (3) financial alterations
	All scales/dimensions have one or more subscales
	All scales have 2 conceptually different components for measuring demands: (1) caregiving actions or behaviors, (2) perceived level of difficulty on carrying out that behavior
	5-point Likert scale used (1 not at all difficult, 5 extremely difficult)
		Physical care scale
		  Alpha coefficient, total scale: 0.78
		  Internal consistency reliability: meals (0.69); intimate care (0.71); walking/transfers (0.80); meds/treatment (0.60); supervision (0.94); new skill acquisition (0.60); rest (0.45)
		  Content validity established
		Role alteration
		  Alpha coefficient (total score): 0.78
		  Internal consistency reliability coefficients: social participation (0.66); interpersonal relationships (0.83)
		Financial alterations
		  Reliability not established
		  Overall validity confirmed using sample procedures of other 2 scales

Appendix 22A. Instruments to Measure Family Outcomes (*cont.*)

Instrument/Target Population	Dimensions/Description	Psychometric Indices
Caregiver Reaction Assessment (CRA) (42,43) Caregivers of the elderly with physical impairments or dementia in the home	24-item measure of differences in the reactions of various groups of caregivers and how their reactions change over time 5 subscales: caregiver esteem, lack of family support, impact on finances, impact on schedule, impact on health 5-point Likert scale used (1 strongly agree, 5 strongly disagree) Measure completed during an in-person interview with repeat administration over time to assess change	Internal consistency of subscales calculated using Cronbach's alpha All items forming each subscale loaded within 20 points or less of one another (lowest scores 0.60) Loadings range for Impact on Health Scale: 0.91–0.52
Family Pain Questionnaire (FPQ) (44) Caregivers managing chronic cancer pain at home	14-item linear analogue measure of knowledge of a family caregiver in managing chronic cancer pain Administered by mail or in person	Established reliability (test–retest, internal consistency) and validity (content, construct, concurrent) content validity: CVI > 0.90 construct validity: ANOVA, $p < 0.05$ concurrent validity: ($r > 0.60$, $p < 0.05$) factor analysis: 2 subscales of knowledge and experience test–retest reliability ($r > 0.80$) with retest or caregivers ($n = 67$)
Quality of Life (family version) (45) Caregivers of persons with cancer in the home	20-item linear analogue measure of quality of life of a family member caring for a patient with cancer Subscales include physical, psychologic, social, and spiritual well-being Administered by mail or in person	Psychometric analysis in progress with 60 subjects, 180 observations
Caregiver Strain Index (CSI) (46) Caregivers	13-item ordinal scale that measures family caregiver's strain in providing various degrees of care to patients at home Administered by mail or in person	Internal consistency (Cronbach's alpha): 0.86 (81 cases) Evidence of construct validity obtained in 3 areas: (1) patient characteristics, (2) subjective perceptions of the caretaking relationship by caregivers, (3) emotional health of caregivers
Family APGAR (47,48) Individual's perception of family function	5-item questionnaire that measures a family member's perception of family function 5 parameters measured: adaptation, partnership, growth, affection, and resolve 3-point ordinal scale (0–2) used for each item Self-administered	Correlated with previously validated instrument, Pless-Satterwhite Family Index and with estimates made by psychotherapists of family function: APGAR/Pless-Satterwhite correlation: 0.80; APGAR/Therapist correlation: 0.64 Family APGAR scores of married graduate students (mean = 8.24) significantly higher than scores of community mental health clinic patients (mean = 5.89)

Instrument	Description	Reliability/Validity
Dyadic Adjustment Scale (DAS) (49, 50) Married or unmarried, cohabiting couples	Spanier DAS is a 32-item questionnaire measuring a family member's perception of family function 5 parameters measured: adaptation, partnership, growth, affection, and resolve Uses 5-point Likert scale (1 always disagrees, 5 always agree) Tool useful for assessing marital adjustment Self-administered or can be adapted for interview use	Cronbach coefficient alpha (total DAS and component subscales): 0.73–0.96 Criterion-related and construct validity established (tool's ability to differentiate between married and divorced people) Correlation coefficient (Locke-Wallace Marriage Inventory): 0.86 (married individuals), 0.88 (divorced individuals)
Family Inventory of Resources for Management (FIRM) (51) Patients and family members, including all adults and children	69-item questionnaire measuring family's ability to deal with stressors 4 factors evaluated: (1) family strengths (esteem and communication), (2) family strengths (mastery and health), (3) extended family social support, (4) family well-being 4-point Likert scale used (1 not at all, 4 very well) Self-report	Cronbach's alpha: 0.89 (4 primary subscales: 0.62–0.85) Total FIRM scores correlated with measures of: family cohesion (0.46), expressiveness (0.27), conflict (0.30), organization (0.25)
Family Inventory of Life Events and Changes (FILE) (52) Adult family members	71-item measure designed for adult members of the family unit Items ask family members to check all events experienced by any member of the family over a 1-year period Individual family score is compared to the norm in the appropriate stage and is a means of classifying the family into a high-stress, moderate-stress, or low-stress group Self-report	No data available at this time
Family Adaptability and Cohesion Evaluation Scales (FACES) (53,54) Family members	FACES II is a 20-item questionnaire designed to classify families into 3 general and 16 specific types on adaptability and cohesion dimensions Subjects rate the frequency of a behavior on a 5-point scale (1 almost never, 5 almost always) Family cohesion is measured as a means of evaluating family's ability to adapt/adjust during illness Self-report and should be completed independently	Cronbach's alpha (estimated): cohesion (0.77); adaptability (0.67); total scale (0.68) Scores between family members ranged from 0.30 to 0.40
Caregiver Quality of Life Index-Cancer (CQOLC) (55,56) Specific for family caregiver of cancer patients	Self-administered rating scale designed to assess QOL issues in family caregivers of patients with cancer 35-item questionnaire uses a 5-point Likert-type scale (0 not at all, 4 very much)	Test-retest reliability was 0.95 and internal consistency was 0.91

Numbers in parentheses correspond to studies cited in the References.

23

Measuring Anxiety

Margaret S. Soderstrom and Patricia M. Grimm

September 11, 2001, is forever etched in the memories of many Americans. Since that day of devastating terrorist attacks, the term *anxiety* has taken on a different dimension. The *New York Times* reported psychogenic rashes erupting in schoolchildren,[1] anxiety manifestations related to the juxtaposition of coincidence and predestination applied to the terrorist attacks,[2] and generalized anxiety and posttraumatic stress experienced by people all over the world who watched the attacks live through instant media access. Anxiety, a word that is familiar to almost everyone, has taken on a different value. Generally speaking, and depending on its application, anxiety can be considered a normal response to contemporary life stresses and strains; an exaggerated outcome to a traumatic event and, as such, a precursor to posttraumatic stress disorder (PTSD); an expected reaction to the demands of illness; an intrinsic personality characteristic; or a psychiatric diagnosis. The measurement of anxiety, therefore, depends on the researcher's perspective and purpose. This chapter reviews the conceptualizations of anxiety (both historical and contemporary), issues in the selection of a measure of anxiety, available instruments, and current trends in anxiety research. This revised chapter identifies the value of survey qualitative data in measuring anxiety and related somatic presentations, which were particularly evident in the follow-up research in the 9/11 aftermath. Eighteen months after the terrorist attacks, two-thirds of Americans polled reported anxiety related to thinking about the event several times a week.[3,4]

Definition

Anxiety can be defined as "an unpleasant subjective experience associated with the perception of real or imagined threat."[5] Or, more comprehensively, "an emotion that signifies the presence of danger that cannot be identified, or if identified, is not sufficiently threatening to justify the intensity of the emotion."[6] The word *anxiety* comes from the Greek word *agon*, from which we derive the terms *anguish* and *agony*. *Agon* also relates to the German word *Angst*, which is used in modern times by the existential philosophers Kierkegaard and Sartre to describe painful feelings of terror and dread.[6,7] In contemporary psychologic thinking, anxiety is seen as playing a central role in the functioning of personality. We all experience some degree of anxiety to foster creativity and face daily challenges; however, anxiety can also impair cognitive and intellectual functioning as well as interfere with effective problem solving.[7] Anxiety can take on a somatic presentation, making the primary cause, anxiety, easy to overlook by a primary care provider focused on the somatic complaint.[3] The origins of anxiety, and the human responses defined as anxiety, have evolved over time and within the social context of those times. Silver et al. concluded, "The psychological effects of a major national trauma are not limited to those who experience it directly, and the degree of response is not predicted simply by objective measures of exposure to or loss from the trauma."[3]

Conceptualization

Since Greco-Roman times and before, anxiety has been associated with ideas of self-awareness and individuality. The philosophic beliefs of those times can be interpreted as systems of thought designed to deal with the threat of anxiety. Stoics believed that anxiety was the result of too great an investment in personal accomplishments. The Greeks were the first to define *hysteria*, a result of anxiety, as a manifestation of physical symptoms with no medically sound physical cause. Christianity suggested that guilt was the source of anxiety, specifically guilt about failing to live up to one's high moral ideals. The existential philosophers of the mid-nineteenth century associated guilt with personal freedom of choice. Anxiety existed because individuals had not only the freedom to choose, but also the responsibility to do so.[8]

Scientific thinkers of the nineteenth century interpreted anxiety as an adaptive response to a threat that was present in all species. Freud differentiated anxiety as objective, a reaction to the external environment, or neurotic, the intrapsychic struggle that exists within each individual.[8] His extensive work laid the cornerstone for much of our contemporary thinking about anxiety and defined it as a clinical, diagnostic entity. Later psychiatric theorists believed that anxiety had its basis in dependency needs, security needs, or the need for power.[8] Spielberger et al. delineated the influence of both intrapsychic and environmental processes by defining trait and state dimensions of anxiety.[9]

Contemporary conceptualizations of anxiety incorporate a stimulus–response model. Response-oriented theorists define anxiety as the neurophysiologic response to a stimulus. This response, not the stimulus itself, is the focus of their work.[8] Hoehn-Saric and McLeod comprehensively discussed the physiology of anxiety.[10] In contrast, stimulus-oriented theories, such as the cognitive approaches of Lazarus[11] and Beck,[16] approach anxiety as a behavioral response to a pattern of thoughts, feelings, and situations that is unique to the individual. Their focus is on the stimuli and serves as the basis for most clinical work with anxiety. Though similar to fear, anxiety is an entity that persists even though the threat and resulting chaos has long since finished. The World Wide Web has afforded researchers unprecedented opportunities to examine anxiety and its effects. This unique prospect allows immediate access to source information that otherwise might be lost. Stanford researchers Spiegel and Butler collected data by means of a Web-based survey on acute stress reactions post 9/11.[4,11] Researchers measured anxiety factors that could be predictive for the development of later PTSD.[11]

We would be remiss not to include the Eastern view in the measurement of anxiety, particularly since increasing numbers of health care providers have been trained in this art. Anxiety is determined by assessing meridian disruption. The Eastern view recognizes anxiety as a stress reaction that creates a disturbance in the energy flow that may involve the liver, spleen, heart, lung, and kidney. Anxiety can be measured by using an instrument such as acupuncture, which works on unblocking the body's meridians using fine needle insertion. Use of Western medications for the initial phase of shock and stabilization is judiciously recommended.[12,13]

In summary, anxiety has been described as an experience with psychologic, somatic, and behavioral components. This experience can be characterized as an enduring personality characteristic, a situational response to life events, or a psychiatric diagnosis. The complexity and diversity of these interpretations of anxiety has implications for its measurement.

Issues in Measuring Anxiety

Several important issues must be addressed when selecting an instrument to measure anxiety. The first is to choose an instrument that is congruent with one's research question and conceptual framework. Questions to consider include how anxiety is defined in the framework of choice. Is it seen as a personality characteristic corresponding to anxious tendencies, as a change in response to an event or experience, or as a diagnostic indicator of psychopathology?[1,14] The answer is important because specific measures exist for each definition.

Another important conceptual question to consider is the specificity of measurement required by the research question and the research design. Historically, instruments developed from specific measures of anxiety to more global indices of psychologic health or distress that include anxiety as one dimension. Early instruments, such as the Taylor Manifest Anxiety Scale[15] and the Hamilton Anxiety Scale,[16] were specific measures of anxiety and only anxiety. Instruments such as the Brief Symptom Inventory[17] and the Profile of Mood States[18] are more global assessments of psychologic status and include anxiety as one component. Some clinicians believe it is difficult to differentiate between the affective symptoms of anxiety and those of depression. This concern has resulted in the development of anxiety/depression models[19] and instruments such as the Hospital Anxiety and Depression Scale.[20]

A third consideration is the target population to be studied. Characteristics such as age, psychologic and physical health status, language, education, and reading level must be considered. In terms of age, all the instruments in this chapter assess anxiety in adults. The reader is referred elsewhere for a comprehensive discussion of the measurement of anxiety in children and adolescents.[21,22] Several measures of anxiety assess or differentiate diagnostic anxiety disorders in psychiatric patient populations. Depending on the existence of psychometric data to support their use with other groups, they may or may not be appropriate for nonpsychiatric use.

The preexistence of a physical illness, acute or chronic, presents an interesting dilemma. Many disease processes and their treatment may result in symptoms that are similar to those considered physiologic indicators of anxiety: changes in pulse rate, respiratory rate, and blood pressure; alterations in eating and sleeping patterns; nausea, vomiting, and diarrhea; and fatigue and restlessness.[23] This is particularly true of individuals who have cardiac disease, respiratory disease, cancer, endocrine disorders, or hematologic disorders such as anemia.[8] Certain metabolic states, specific medications, and poorly controlled pain can all result in physical symptoms that mimic anxiety.[24] The choice of an instrument that minimizes or eliminates such indicators of anxiety is an important consideration with medically ill populations. The issues of primary language and educational or reading level also must be addressed. Several of the instruments to be presented were developed in countries other than the United States, therefore close review is necessary to be sure that the language used and cultural context are congruent with the researcher's target population.

A final issue is the method of measurement. Three main approaches are represented by the instruments: structured diagnostic interviews, observational rating scales, and self-report paper-and-pencil instruments. Content analysis of verbal data also is reviewed. In conclusion, the choice of conceptual framework, research design, and target population, as well as the knowledge and expertise of the researcher, all influence the choice of measurement approach. It is of value to recognize the World Wide Web as an instrument of measurement application, particularly as it relates to survey use in data collection. Information may be gathered quickly relative to the time of the occurrence. Qualitative data, rich in content, may be accessed using a comment section or chat room format. Nowhere is this more evident than in the follow-up investigations of 9/11. Recognizing that media, particularly television, can place people spread all over the world at the actual scene of an anxiety-producing event has far-reaching implications for outcomes research.[3,11,14] Use of the World Wide Web as a tool for obtaining data has yet to be adequately acknowledged by some health care providers.

Instruments

The discussion of instruments developed to measure anxiety is organized in terms of their specificity. Anxiety-specific measures are presented first, followed by those that measure anxiety and depression. Global indices of psychologic health or distress are then presented.

Taylor Manifest Anxiety Scale

The Taylor Manifest Anxiety Scale (TMAS), developed in 1950, is a screening test for the identification of research subjects. Taylor[15] describes its development as an alternative to the use of experimental manipulation, such as electric shock or stress-producing situations, to select subjects with varied levels of anxiety. This self-report scale consists of 50 item statements, indicative of anxiety, from the Minnesota Multiphasic Personality Inventory (MMPI). The response format is true/false. Additional items have been added to control for social desirability, lying, and rigidity of responses. Test–retest reliability has been reported as 0.81 to 0.88. Content judges established face validity, and the TMAS was found to have a correlation of 0.85 with the administration of the MMPI. This instrument was originally tested on college students and psychiatric patients. Its use has been expanded to include adults in general.

Hamilton Anxiety Scale

Another older instrument, the Hamilton Anxiety Scale, was developed in 1959 as a clinical interview rating scale of the psychic and somatic aspects of anxiety. The scale consists of 14 items or clinical symptoms with a 5-point rating response ranging from 0 (not present) to 4 (very severe). The original form did not include descriptive statements of these rating responses. However, Bech et al.[16] have developed a list of item definitions for each response choice. For example, item 5, Intellectual Retardation, is defined by:

0   The patient exhibits normal intellectual activity.
1   The patient has to make an effort to concentrate on his work.
2   Even with major effort it is difficult for the patient to concentrate on his work. Less initiative than usual. The patient at an early state experiences brain fatigue.
3   Marked difficulties with concentration, initiative, and decision making. The patient needs many breaks even when performing simple, routine jobs.

4   It is difficult for the patient to follow normal conversation, and he cannot read a
      newspaper or watch television.

In addition, they have developed a scoring system to differentiate generalized anxiety
from panic anxiety. The Hamilton Anxiety Scale has been used extensively since its development. An interrater reliability Spearman test correlation of 0.78 has been reported
for the revised form, with strong item-to-total score correlations. Validity data is reported with global assessment measures of anxiety used as the criterion.[15] Originally designed to be used with psychiatric patients diagnosed with anxiety disorders, its use has
expanded to adult patients and nonpatients, including a study of preoperative and postoperative anxiety experienced by cardiac surgery patients.[15]

State-Trait Anxiety Inventory (STAI)

Probably the most extensively used measure of anxiety, the STAI, comprises separate
self-report scales for measuring two distinct anxiety concepts: state and trait. *State anxiety*
is defined as "a transitory emotional state or condition," whereas *trait anxiety* is defined
as "relatively stable individual differences in anxiety proneness."[9] Each scale consists of
20 statements that subjects rate to describe how they generally feel (trait) or how they feel
at a particular moment in time (state). Subjects respond on a 4-point scale, from 1 (not at
all) to 4 (very much so). In studies conducted by Spielberger et al.,[9] test–retest reliability
coefficients of 0.73 to 0.86 and 0.86 to 0.92 have been reported for the trait subscale and
coefficients of 0.16 to 0.54 and 0.83 to 0.92 for the state subscale.[9] Alpha coefficient values obtained to measure internal consistency ranged from 0.83 to 0.92 for state and 0.86
to 0.92 for trait.[25] Concurrent validity was supported by correlating the STAI with the
Taylor and Institute for Personality and Ability Testing (IPAT) Anxiety Scales (0.79 to
0.83 and 0.75 to 0.76, respectively). Construct validity was determined by comparing like
subjects under stressful and nonstressful situations.[8] The STAI has been successfully used
with high school and college students,[9] psychiatric patients,[9] medical and surgical patients,[25–30] obstetric patients,[31,32] the chronically ill,[33,34] and the elderly.[35] The STAI is written at a fifth-grade reading level, but a children's version is available.

Anxiety Status Inventory (ASI/SAS)

Developed by Zung,[36] the Anxiety Status Inventory is actually two measures, the ASI and
the Self-rating Anxiety Scale (SAS). The ASI is a 20-item observer rating scale, and the
SAS, as implied in its name, is a 20-item self-report scale. The ASI uses a 4-point rating
scale to evaluate the severity of anxiety symptoms observed during a clinical interview,
from 1 (none) to 4 (severe). The SAS consists of positively and negatively worded statements that the respondent rates as having experienced within the last week from 1 (none
or a little of the time) to 4 (most or all of the time). Both scales measure clinical anxiety
in psychiatric patients. However, the author also reports studies that have included individuals without psychiatric illnesses.

The reliability coefficient comparing the ASI with the SAS is 0.66. Split-half coefficients for these scales were 0.83 and 0.71, respectively. Concurrent validity correlations
with the TMAS were 0.33 for the ASI and 0.30 for the SAS. Discriminant validity was supported in comparison studies of patients with anxiety disorder and controls.[36]

Brief Scale for Anxiety

Developed by Tyrer et al.,[37] the Brief Scale for Anxiety is another clinical interview rating
scale designed to assess the psychologic and somatic symptoms of anxiety. The interviewer rates the subject on each of 10 symptoms on a 7-point scale from 0 (no occurrence
of the symptom) to 7 (incapacitation by/lack of control of the symptom). The instrument

was originally created to identify anxiety in psychiatric patients who did not have a primary anxiety disorder, but the author indicates that this measure could also be used with medical and neurologic patients.[37] It also can be used to monitor changes in symptoms. Limited reliability and validity data are available.

Anxiety Scale (Gottschalk-Gleser Content Analysis Scales)

For a qualitative approach to the examination of anxiety, Gottschalk and Bechtel have developed a computer-based scale to analyze verbal samples.[38] The scale consists of six types of anxiety: death, mutilation, separation, guilt, shame, and diffuse/nonspecific, with three or four weighted choices under each type: self, animate others, inanimate objects, and denial. For example:

> *Shame anxiety.* References to ridicule, inadequacy, shame, embarrassment, humiliation, overexposure of deficiencies or private details, or threat of such experienced by:
>
> a. Self
> b. Animate others
> c. Denial

Reliability coefficients for the computerized version and hand coding were 0.85 for the total scale and 0.58 to 0.92 for the individual items. Validity data were not reported.

Hospital Anxiety and Depression Scale (HADS)

Developed by Zigmond and Swaith, this 14-item measure of anxiety and depression is unique in that it was specifically designed to assess these disorders in medically ill patients by excluding items related to somatic symptoms.[20] Using a 4-point rating format, the respondent assesses how he or she has felt during the past week. The HADS has been used in studies involving general medical outpatients, individuals experiencing chronic illnesses such as cancer[39] and cardiac conditions, and nonpatient community volunteers.[1] The authors report that HADS can be used to monitor change over time. Item-to-subscale reliability correlations are reported as being 0.41 to 0.76 for the anxiety items and 0.30 to 0.60 for the depression items. Spearman correlations between the scales and psychiatric ratings were 0.70 and 0.74 for anxiety and depression, respectively. The HADS has been translated into several languages, including Arabic, Dutch, French, German, Hebrew, Swedish, Italian, and Spanish.

Prototypical Anxiety and Depression Scales

Koeter and VanDenBrink developed the prototypical anxiety and depression scales to determine the existence of anxiety disorders among nonpsychotic psychiatric patients.[19] Twenty-one items were drawn from the more comprehensive 148-item Present State Examination-E, including 8 anxiety items and 13 depression items. The resulting scales are rated based on a clinical interview. The authors report high interrater reliability and internal consistency alpha coefficients of 0.59 to 0.60 for anxiety and 0.77 to 0.81 for depression. The validity of the scales was evaluated using the Hamilton Anxiety Scale and the Hamilton Depression Scale. Correlations for anxiety were 0.56 to 0.79 and 0.47 to 0.78 for depression.[19] The use of this measurement with other than psychiatric patients has not been reported.

Courtauld Emotional Control Scale (CECS)

Unlike any other scale presented here, the CECS was developed to measure emotional control of anxiety, anger, and depressed mood. This 21-item self-report scale assesses the extent to which respondents control their emotional responses to stress. The anxiety, anger, and depressed mood subscales consist of item statements that require rating on a 4-point scale. Watson and Greer report the use of the CECS with adult female cancer patients, male nonpatients, and personality type A cardiac patients.[40] Test–retest reliability correlations have been reported as 0.84 to 0.95 for the total scale and 0.84 for anxiety, with internal consistency alpha coefficients of 0.86 to 0.88 for the total scale and 0.88 for anxiety. Concurrent validity has been determined using the STAI for the anxiety subscale. It was found that individuals who scored high on the CECS tended to score low on direct measures of anxiety.[40]

Symptom Checklist-90-Revised (SCL-90-R)

As developed by Derogatis et al., the Symptom Checklist 90 was designed primarily to reflect the psychologic symptom patterns of psychiatric and medical patients.[41] In 1976, based on clinical experiences and psychometric analyses, the original instrument was modified and is now the SCL-90-R.[42] This self-report 90-item scale measures nine primary dimensions of psychologic status: (1) somatization, (2) obsessive-compulsive, (3) interpersonal sensitivity, (4) depression, (5) anxiety, (6) hostility, (7) phobic anxiety, (8) paranoid ideation, and (9) psychoticism. It also measures three global indices of overall distress. The respondent is asked to report how much he or she was distressed by the symptoms identified in the item statements. The 5-point responses range from 0 (not at all) to 4 (extremely). "Nervousness or shakiness inside" is one item on the SCL-90-R.

A companion observation rating scale, the SCL-90 Analogue, also is available. This scale consists of nine dimension-specific, 100-mm visual analogue scales with the anchor "not at all" at one end and "extremely" at the other. Brief defining paragraphs facilitate rating. Interrater reliability correlations are reported as 0.81 to 0.94 for all dimensions and 0.86 for anxiety. The authors report that the SCL-90-R is sensitive to the evaluation of intervention and drug studies. Test–retest reliability coefficients have been reported as 0.55 to 0.94 for the total scale and 0.80 to 0.84 for the anxiety dimension. The internal consistency alpha coefficient for the anxiety dimension was reported as 0.85.[42] The author reports face validity and concurrent validity with the MMPI. The SCL-90-R has been widely used to assess global distress and its specific dimensions.[43] Target populations have included psychiatric patients,[42,44] patients without a psychiatric illness,[42] and cancer patients.[45,46] Clinical profiles for the major psychiatric diagnoses exist.[42] Rief and Fichter suggested that modification of the dimension subscales has shown greater discriminant validity in identifying psychiatric disorders.[44] The SCL-90-R is available in Spanish.

Brief Symptom Inventory (BSI)

The BSI is a 53-item self-report version of the SCL-90-R.[47] It has the same dimension and global indices structure as its parent measure, and it is administered and scored similarly.[17] The authors report that the BSI can be used in a narrative form if the respondent is unable to read. The reliability test–retest correlations for the dimensions of the BSI are reported as 0.68 to 0.91, with internal consistency alpha coefficients of 0.71 to 0.83. Convergent validity of the BSI was determined using the clinical scales of the MMPI, with correlations ranging from 0.30 to 0.72. Correlations ranged from 0.32 to 0.49 over the nine dimensions.[47] Like its parent instrument, the BSI has been used extensively.[17,48] Target populations have included psychiatric patients and individuals without a diagnosed psychiatric illness,[17,47] medical patients, including individuals with asthma,[33] cancer,[49,50] hypertension,[17] HIV/AIDS;[17] and caregivers of individuals with dementia.[51]

General Health Questionnaire (GHQ-28)

The General Health Questionnaire was originally developed as a 60-item self-report instrument designed to detect the presence of general psychiatric disorders in the primary care setting. This measure contains four subscales: (1) somatic symptoms, (2) anxiety and insomnia, (3) social dysfunction, and (4) severe depression. Goldberg and Hillier developed a 28-item version of the original scale.[52] The respondents rate their experience of symptoms over the past few weeks. The phrases used for the 4-point rating scales vary with each item statement. The authors recognize the differences in language between Great Britain and the United States and provide the American user with suggested word substitutions for four of the items.[52] The following are examples of the anxiety items: "Been feeling run down and out of sorts?" and "Been getting a feeling of tightness or pressure in your head?" Concurrent validity for the revised GHQ-28 was determined through comparison with clinical interviews. Correlations were 0.51 to 0.75 for the subscales with a total scale correlation of 0.76. Predictive validity also was evaluated. Reliability data were not reported.[52] The GHQ-28 has been used with target populations of patients in primary care and general practice, particularly those experiencing acute psychiatric disorders.[53]

Affects Balance Scale (ABS)

Developed by Derogatis, the ABS is a 40-item self-report checklist that describes affect status in terms of four positive and four negative dimensions.[54] The positive dimensions are joy, contentment, vigor, and affection, and the negative dimensions are anxiety, depression, guilt, and hostility. For each descriptive adjective the respondent indicates on a 5-point scale the extent to which the adjective describes him or her, from 0 (never) to 4 (always). Examples of the adjectives included on the ABS are *nervous*, *timid*, *energetic*, *tense*, and *anxious*. The author has reported internal consistency reliability coefficients of 0.78 to 0.92. The construct validity of the ABS has been evaluated using group comparisons.[55] Sangal et al.[55] reported significantly less negative affects in improved anxiety disorder patients than in unimproved patients. Long-term survivors of breast cancer had significantly higher negative affect scores than short-term survivors.[56] Target populations for this instrument have included anxiety disorder patients[55,56] and cancer patients.[46] A global, balanced measure of affect, the Affect Balance Index, also can be calculated.

General Well-Being Schedule (GWB)

The GWB is an 18-item self-report measure of subjective feelings of psychologic well-being and distress.[53] The scale reflects both positive and negative feelings. Six dimensions cover anxiety, depression, general health, positive well-being, self-control, and vitality. The first four items use 6-point response scales representing intensity and frequency, and respondents rate their experience over the last month. A sample item is "Have you been bothered by nervousness or your nerves?" The remaining four items use 0-to-10 rating scales defined by adjectives at each end, such as "How *relaxed* or *tense* have you been?"

Test–retest reliability coefficients have been reported as 0.68 to 0.85, with an internal consistency reliability of the total scale of 0.91 to 0.95. The average concurrent validity correlation with three independent anxiety scales was 0.64.[53] The GWB has been successfully used with psychiatric day patients and adults who do not have a diagnosed psychiatric illness.

Profile of Mood States (POMS)

McNair et al. developed the Profile of Mood States to measure six identifiable mood or affective states: (1) tension-anxiety, (2) depression-dejection, (3) anger-hostility, (4) vigor-activity, (5) fatigue-inertia, and (6) confusion-bewilderment.[18] The POMS is a 65-item, self-report adjective rating scale, with a 5-point response from 0 (not at all) to 4 (extremely). The respondents describe their feelings over the past week. A total Mood Disturbance Score also can be calculated. Examples of the adjectives include *shaky, on edge, panicky,* and *uneasy.*

A test–retest reliability coefficient of 0.70 has been reported for the Tension-Anxiety subscale. Internal consistency reliability coefficients for this subscale are reported as 0.90 to 0.92 and 0.93 for the total scale. Concurrent validity of the POMS has been reported with a correlation of 0.80 between this instrument and the Hopkins Symptom Distress Scales (SCL-90, BSI).[21] Target populations for the use of the POMS have been outpatient psychiatric patients, healthy adults, and cardiac surgery patients.[28]

Brief Profile of Mood States (Brief POMS)

Cella et al.[57] developed an 11-item short form of the POMS as a reliable measure of general mood disturbance or distress. The result is the Brief POMS. Through extensive psychometric evaluation, the authors identified the best indicators of overall distress, resulting in a Total Mood Disturbance score. There are no somatic item statements in this measure.[58] The 5-point response format has been retained. The internal consistency reliability of the Brief POMS is reported as 0.92. Correlation with the POMS is 0.93. Significant group differences were found between pancreatic cancer and gastric cancer patients, supporting the discriminant validity of the Brief POMS. Although this measure was developed for use with cancer patients during all stages of treatment, the authors suggest that it could be used with individuals experiencing other chronic diseases.

Summary of Research Findings

A comprehensive summary of the current research findings on anxiety is beyond the scope of this chapter. An overview of the trends in recently published anxiety research, with discussion of selected studies, will give the reader some sense of this area of inquiry. Trends include the general assessment of anxiety, or anxiety as part of global distress, in specific populations; anxiety as a causal factor; anxiety as the direct focus of an intervention; and anxiety as a component of the outcome of an intervention.

General Assessment of Anxiety or Distress in Specific Populations

The assessment of anxiety specifically, or as a component of the global assessment of distress, is a common theme in the current research literature. In a much-cited study, Derogatis and his associates conducted a multisite assessment of the presence of psychiatric disorders among 215 newly admitted cancer patients.[45] Using a psychiatric interview and standardized psychologic tests, including the SCL-90-R, they found that 44% of their subjects manifested a clinical psychiatric diagnosis. Of this group, approximately 85% experienced a disorder with depression or anxiety as the central symptom. In a similar study, Stefanek et al. assessed the psychologic status of 126 oncology outpatients.[49] Using the BSI, they reported that approximately one third of the patients expressed moderate to high levels of depression and anxiety.

Gift[33] sought to describe the psychologic and physiologic aspects of acute dyspnea in asthmatics. Anxiety, as one component of psychologic status, was measured with the State scale of the STAI. See the end of the chapter for a summary of her study and its findings. Levels of anxiety and self-confidence experienced by pregnant women were the focus of a study by Pond and Kemp.[32] They compared 35 adolescent with 58 adult prenatal patients, measuring anxiety with the STAI. Although no significant differences were found between these groups, they found significant negative correlations for both state and trait anxiety during pregnancy and for self-confidence in all the women.

The effects of different coping patterns on the physical health, depression, and anxiety experienced by spouse caregivers of persons with dementia were studied by Neundorfer.[51] The BSI anxiety and depression subscales were used in the assessment of 60 spouse caregivers. The patient's memory and behavior problems, the caregiver's appraisal of the stressfulness of these problems, and the caregiver's appraisal of their options explained 43% of the variance in both depression and anxiety.

Myocardial infarction patients were assessed in a study of heart rate variability and psychologic outcomes by Buchanan et al.[29] The psychologic outcomes included anxiety, anger, denial, and depression, with anxiety being measured by the STAI. Anxiety was higher within 4 days of hospital admission but had significantly decreased 6 months later.

Wong and Bramwell[30] examined the relationship between uncertainty and anxiety after mastectomy for breast cancer among 25 women. Subjects completed measures of anxiety and uncertainty at 1 to 2 days before and 1 to 2 weeks after hospital discharge. Using the STAI, the researchers found a significant positive correlation between anxiety and uncertainty at the postdischarge testing. In a 6-month study of cancer patients with advanced disease, Payne[39] sought to identify the influence of site (home or hospital) and method of palliative chemotherapy on quality of life. The operationalization of quality of life included a measure of anxiety and depression, the HADS. Anxiety and depression accounted for 92% of the variance in quality of life.

Silver and her research team[6] examined the degree to which demographic factors, mental and physical health history, lifetime exposure to stressful events, September 11–related experiences, and coping strategies used after 9/11 predict psychological outcomes over time. A World Wide Web–based survey of 2729 participants completed the survey within 3 weeks of receiving. Surveys were again distributed at 2- and 6-month intervals. It was determined that the impact of a national trauma is not limited to those directly involved. The implementation of coping strategies shortly after the event with long-term utilization was identified as the key difference in positive versus negative psychologic and somatic outcomes.

Anxiety as a Causal Factor

Two studies in the recent literature are representative of the examination of anxiety as a causal factor. Annie and Groer studied the influence of state and trait anxiety on immunoglobulin A (IgA) concentrations in 30 women during pregnancy and at childbirth.[31] State anxiety appeared to account for some of the variance in IgA concentration at both points in time. The State subscale of the STAI was used to measure anxiety. Also using the State subscale of the STAI, Eaton and his associates explored the relationship of psychosocial variables, including anxiety, depression, family process, and health locus of control, to management and control of insulin-dependent diabetes in 127 subjects.[34] Their results showed that both anxiety and depression had weak positive correlations with blood sugar levels. Life stage had the most significant effect on management and control of diabetes.

Anxiety as the Direct Focus of an Intervention

The recent literature also includes intervention studies in which anxiety is the focus of intervention. Zimmerman and her colleagues evaluated the effects of music with suggestion on the anxiety levels of patients in coronary care units.[26] Seventy-five patients were randomly assigned to one of three groups: listening to music, listening to "white noise," or having a period of uninterrupted rest. The State subscale of the STAI was administered, and blood pressure, heart rate, and digital skin temperature were measured. The authors attribute the lack of significant findings to the fact that all three groups actually experienced an intervention.

Weintraub and Hagopian examined the effect of nursing consultation sessions on anxiety, side effects experienced, and helpfulness of self-care strategies used by patients receiving radiation therapy.[25] Fifty-six subjects were randomly assigned to either the health education control or nursing consultation group. Again, the STAI was used to measure anxiety. The researchers reported that the mean state anxiety scores were consistently lower, but not statistically significant, in the nursing consultation group.

In another intervention study with cancer patients, Holland et al. conducted a multisite, randomized clinical trial of alprazolam versus progressive muscle relaxation in the treatment of anxiety and depressive symptoms.[46] Four measures of anxiety and depression, including the ABS and the SCL-90-R, were used. See Exemplar Studies at the end of the chapter for a summary of this study and its findings.

Peterson conducted an anxiety intervention study with 72 patients about to undergo cardiac catheterization.[27] Subjects were randomly assigned to one of three groups: educational intervention, social intervention, or control. Anxiety was measured, using the STAI, before and after intervention. Both the educational and social intervention groups experienced a significant decrease in anxiety compared with the control group.

Anxiety as a Component of the Outcome of an Intervention

An interesting trend in the research literature is the inclusion of anxiety with a number of other related factors as the focus of an intervention. Fraser and Kerr examined the effects of back massage on the anxiety levels of elderly residents in a long-term care institution.[35] Twenty-one subjects were randomly assigned to three groups: back massage with normal conversation, conversation only, or no intervention. The STAI State subscale was the measure of anxiety, along with electromyographic recordings, systolic and diastolic blood pressure, and heart rate. There was a statistically significant difference in anxiety between the back massage group and the no-intervention group. The statistical significance of other relationships among study variables may have been affected by the sample size.

Cupples conducted study of the effect of timing and reinforcement of preoperative education on knowledge and recovery in patients having coronary bypass graft surgery.[28] Forty subjects were randomized to either the preadmission and postadmission preoperative education group or the postadmission-only education group. Postoperative anxiety was measured with the STAI. The Profile of Mood States measured postoperative mood. Preoperative knowledge of surgery and physiologic recovery also were monitored. Subjects in the experimental group were found to have more positive mood states than those in the control group.

Summary

The concept of anxiety has many diverse interpretations that subsequently influence the selection of a measurement instrument. Whether conceptualized as an enduring personality characteristic, a response to life events, or a psychiatric diagnosis, anxiety can be measured by one of the instruments presented in this chapter. The clear delineation of one's research question, conceptual framework, and research design will facilitate an appropriate choice. Selection of a measure that is appropriate to the target population also is important, particularly when the somatic symptoms of a preexisting physical problem can influence the validity of the measurement process. Anxiety is an important and universal experience that may influence, or be influenced by, many aspects of health and function. Trends in the recent literature demonstrate significant interest in examining this phenomenon in a variety of settings and with a variety of approaches. Readers are encouraged to recognize the advantages associated with World Wide Web–based research endeavors. Associated survey distribution can be immediate, as in the case of 9/11, is expedient, and can facilitate rich qualitative data collection. Expense advantages may also be a favorable association.

Exemplar Studies

Gift, A. Psychologic and physiologic aspects of acute dyspnea in asthmatics. *Nurs Res,* 1991, *40*(4):196–199.

This study compared psychologic and physiologic variables during intense dyspnea to those at times of no or low dyspnea in people with asthma. Thirty-six adults, 19 to 76 years old, were assessed on admission to the emergency room in acute dyspnea and again when they had no or low dyspnea just before discharge. Psychologic and physiologic variables measured included anxiety, overall psychologic distress, specific asthma-related distress, oxygen saturation, and airway obstruction. Clinical symptoms found to be elevated during high dyspnea were respiratory rate, pulse, wheezing, and accessory muscle use. The psychologic variables of anxiety, depression, somatization, and hostility were higher during high dyspnea, and peak expiratory flow rates and oxygen saturation were significantly lower. Subscales of the Asthma Symptom Checklist—pain/fear, fatigue, dyspnea, hyperventilation/hypocapnia, congestion, and rapid breath—also were higher during high dyspnea.

This study represents a comprehensive approach to the description of both psychologic and physiologic responses in an acute event, dyspnea, with a specific population, asthmatics. Two measures of anxiety, the STAI and the anxiety dimension of the BSI, were used to measure anxiety and were found to correlate significantly, thereby supporting their construct validity. The study clearly operationalizes the variables of interest.

Holland, J., Morrow, G., Fetting, J., et al. A randomized clinical trial of alprazolam versus progressive muscle relaxation in cancer patients with anxiety and depressive symptoms. *J Clin Oncol,* 1991, *9*(6):1004–1011.

This multisite, randomized study compared over a 10-day period the efficacy of the anxiolytic drug alprazolam (Xanax) with the use of progressive muscle relaxation for the treatment of anxiety and depressive symptoms among 147 cancer patients. Seventy patients took alprazolam (0.5 mg three times a day), while 77 listened to an audiotape of a training session three times a day. Four measures of anxiety and depression, including the ABS and the SCL-90-R, were administered at enrollment in the study and 10 days later. Both interventions resulted in a significant decrease in observer- and patient-reported anxiety and depressed mood symptoms. Patients receiving alprazolam demonstrated a slightly more rapid decrease in anxiety and a greater reduction of depressive symptoms. As both interventions are safe, inexpensive, and effective, a decision could be made in terms of the patient's preferences for a behavioral approach or medication.

This study compared a purely physiologic intervention, medication, with a behavioral approach, progressive muscle relaxation. A multimethod approach was used in measuring anxiety and depression, including interview-observation and self-report instruments. The findings that both interventions were successful in reducing anxiety and depression have important implications for patient care. Because either intervention is effective, patients can make a choice based on their own personal likes and dislikes.

VandeCreek, L., Rogers, E., & Lester, J. Use of alternative therapies among breast cancer outpatients compared with the general population, *Alternative Therapies in Health and Medicine,* 1999, 5(1):71-76.

This study of 112 randomly selected female breast cancer outpatients from a Midwestern university hospital concerned the creation of a profile that describes interest in and use of a wide variety of alternative therapies available to breast cancer outpatients. Related issues such as cost and reimbursement patterns were examined. Findings were compared with a published profile of the general public. An interview ascertained the use of alternative therapies and incorporated two questionnaires in the data collection: (1) mental adjustment to the cancer experience and (2) personal growth in response to the encounter with cancer.

Findings identified the three most commonly used alternative therapies as prayer (76%), exercise (38%), and spiritual healing (29%). Statistical exploration of the psychosocial responses to breast cancer revealed that younger breast cancer outpatients experience more anxiety. Compared with the general population, there is a unique profile of alternative therapy use in breast cancer outpatients.

Study results indicate that breast cancer outpatients create a unique profile of alternative therapy use. Generalization of the research findings is limited to the population studied. Further research is suggested that would explore related issues, such as perceived curative potential, trust in conventional therapies, and influence of choice.

References

1. Talbot, M. Hysteria, hysteria: The post-9/11 mystery rash. *New York Times Magazine,* June 2, 2002:42.
2. Belkin, L. The odds of that: Coincidence in an age of conspiracy. *New York Times Magazine,* August 11, 2002:32.
3. Silver, R.C., Holman, E., McIntosh, D., et al. Nationwide longitudinal study of psychological responses to September 11. *JAMA,* 2002, 288(10):1235-1244.
4. Spiegel, D., & Butler, L.D. Acute stress in response to the September 11 terrorist attacks. *Can Psychiatr Assoc Bull,* 34(4):29-32.
5. Walker, L.G. The measurement of anxiety. *Postgrad Med J,* 1990, 66(Suppl 2):511-517.
6. Goodwin, D.W. *Anxiety.* New York: Oxford University Press, 1986.
7. Kellerman, H., & Burry, A. *Handbook of psychodiagnostic testing.* 2nd ed. Boston: Allyn & Bacon, 1991.
8. Derogatis, L., & Wise, T. *Anxiety and depressive disorders in the medical patient.* Washington, DC: American Psychiatric Press, 1989.
9. Spielberger, C., Gorsuch, F., & Lushene, R. *STAI manual for the S-T-A-I ("Self-evaluation Questionnaire").* Palo Alto, CA: Consulting Psychologist Press, 1971.
10. Hoehn-Saric, R., & McLeod, D. *Biology of anxiety disorders.* Washington, DC: American Psychiatric Press, 1993.
11. Lazarus, R., & Folkman, S. *Stress, appraisal and coping.* New York: Springer, 1984.
12. Abbate, S. Gentle treatment for general anxiety disorder, post-traumatic stress, and episodic anxiety. *Acupunct Today,* 2002, 3(3).
13. Flaws, B., & Lake, J. *Chinese medical psychiatry.* Boulder, CO: Blue Poppy Press, 2001.
14. Schlenger, W., Caddell, J., Ebert, L., et al. Psychological reactions to terrorist attacks: Findings from the national study of Americans' reactions to September 11. *JAMA,* 2002, 288(5):581-636.
15. Taylor, J. A personality scale of manifest anxiety. *J Abnorm Soc Psychol,* 1953, 48(2):285-290.
16. Bech, P., Grosby, H., Husum, B., & Rafaelsen, S. Generalized anxiety or depression measured by the Hamilton Anxiety Scale and the Melancholia Scale in patients before and after cardiac surgery. *Psychopathology,* 1984, 17:253-263.
17. Derogatis, L. *BSI Administration, scoring and procedures Manual II.* Towson, MD: Clinical Psychometric Research, 1992.
18. McNair, D., Lorr, M., & Droppleman, L. *EDITS manual for the Profile of Mood States.* San Diego: Educational and Industrial Testing Service, 1981.
19. Koeter, M., & VanDenBrink, W. The relationship between depression and anxiety: Construction of a pro-

totypical anxiety and depression scale. *Psychol Med*, 1992, 22:597-606.

20. Zigmond, A.S., & Swaith, R.P. The Hospital Anxiety and Depression Scale. *Acta Psychiatr Scand*, 1983, 67:361-370.

21. Roberts, N., Vargo, B., & Ferguson, H.B. Measuring anxiety and depression in children and adolescents. *Psychiatr Clin North Am*, 1989, 12(2):837-860.

22. Hoehn-Saric, E., Maisami, M., & Wiegand, D. Measurement of anxiety in children and adolescents using semistructured interviews. *J Am Acad Child Adolesc Psychiatr*, 1987, 26:541-545.

23. Massie, M.J. Anxiety, panic and phobias. In J. Holland & J. Rowland (Eds.), *Handbook of psycho-oncology: Psychological issues in cancer*. New York: Oxford University Press, 1989.

24. Holland, J.C. Anxiety and cancer: The patient and the family. *J Clin Psychiatr*, 1989, 50(Suppl 11):20-25.

25. Weintraub, F., & Hagopian, G. The effect of nursing consultation on anxiety, side effects and self-care of patients receiving radiation therapy. *Oncol Nurs Forum*, 1990, 17(Suppl 3):31-38.

26. Zimmerman, L., Pierson, M., & Marker, J. Effects of music on patient anxiety on coronary care units. *Heart Lung*, 1988, 17(5):560-566.

27. Peterson, M. Patient anxiety before cardiac catheterization: An intervention study. *Heart Lung*, 1991, 20(6):643-647.

28. Cupples, S. Effects of timing and reinforcement of preoperative education on knowledge and recovery of patients having coronary artery bypass graft surgery. *Heart Lung*, 1991, 20(6):654-660.

29. Buchanan, L., Cowan, M., Burr, R., et al. Measurement of recovery from myocardial infarction using heart rate variability and psychological outcome. *Nurs Res*, 1993, 42(2):74-78.

30. Wong, C., & Bramwell, L. Uncertainty and anxiety after mastectomy for breast cancer. *Cancer Nurs*, 1992, 15(5):363-371.

31. Annie, C., & Groer, M. Childbirth stress: An immunologic study. *J Obstet Gynecol Neonatal Nurs*, 1991, 20(5):391-397.

32. Pond E., & Kemp, V. A comparison between adolescent and adult women on prenatal anxiety and self-confidence. *Maternal-Child Nurs J*, 1992, 20(1):11-20.

33. Gift, A. Psychologic and physiologic aspects of acute dyspnea in asthmatics. *Nurs Res*, 1991, 40(4):196-199.

34. Eaton, W., Mengel, M., Larson, D., et al. Psychosocial and psychopathologic influences on management and control of insulin-dependent diabetes. *Int J Psychiatr Med*, 1992, 22(2):105-117.

35. Fraser J., & Kerr, J. Psychophysiological effects of back massage on elderly institutionalized patients. *J Adv Nurs*, 1993, 18:238-245.

36. Zung, W. A rating instrument for anxiety disorders. *Psychosomatics*, 1971, 12(6):371-379.

37. Tyrer, P., Owen, R.T., & Cicchetti, D.V. The brief scale for anxiety: A subdivision of the comprehensive psycho-pathological rating scale. *J Neurosurg Psychiatr*, 1984, 47:970-975.

38. Gottschalk, L.A., & Bechtel, R.J. The measurement of anxiety through the computer analysis of verbal samples. *Comp Psychiatr*, 1982, 23(4):364-369.

39. Payne, S.A. A study of quality of life in cancer patients receiving palliative chemotherapy. *Soc Sci Med*, 1992, 35(12):1505-1509.

40. Watson, M., & Greer, S. Development of a questionnaire of emotional control. *J Psychosom*, 1983, 27(4):299-305.

41. Derogatis, L.R., Lipman, R., & Covi, L. SCL-90: An outpatient psychiatric rating scale—Preliminary report. *Psychopharmacol Bull*, 1973, 9:13-23.

42. Derogatis, L.R. *SCL-90-R Administration, scoring and procedures manual II*. Towson, MD: Clinical Psychometric Research, 1992.

43. Derogatis, L.R. SCL-90-R. In J.V. Mitchell (Ed.), *The ninth mental measurements yearbook*, (vol. II). Lincoln: University of Nebraska Press, 1985.

44. Rief, W., & Fichter, M. The Symptom Check List SCL-90-R and its ability to discriminate between dysthymia, anxiety disorders and anorexia nervosa. *Psychopathology*, 1992, 25:128-138.

45. Derogatis, L.R., Morrow, G., Fetting, J., et al. The prevalence of psychiatric disorders among cancer patients. *JAMA*, 1983, 249(6):751-757.

46. Holland, J., Morrow, G., Schmale, A., et al. A randomized clinical trial of alprazolam versus progressive muscle relaxation in cancer patients with anxiety and depressive symptoms. *J Clin Oncol*, 1991, 9(6):1004-1011.

47. Derogatis, L.R., & Melisaratos, N. The Brief Symptom Inventory: An introductory report. *Psychol Med*, 1983, 13:595-605.

48. Derogatis, L.R. The Brief Symptom Inventory. In J. Conoley & J. Kramer (Eds.), *The tenth mental measurements yearbook*. Lincoln: University of Nebraska Press, 1989, pp. 111-113.

49. Stefanek, M., Derogatis, L.R., & Shaw, A. Psychological distress among oncology patients. *Psychosomatics*, 1987, 28(10):537-539.

50. Zabora, J., Smith-Wilson, R., Fetting, J., & Enterline, J. An efficient method for psychosocial screening of cancer patients. *Psychosomatics*, 1990, 31(2):192-196.

51. Neundorfer, M. Coping and health outcomes in spouse caregivers of persons with dementia. *Nurs Res*, 1991, 40(5):260-265.

52. Goldberg, D.P., & Hillier, V.F. A scaled version of the general health questionnaire. *Psychol Med*, 1979, 9:139-145.

53. McDowell, I., & Newell, C. *Measuring health: A guide to rating scales and questionnaires*. New York: Oxford University Press, 1987.

54. Derogatis, L.R. *The Affects Balance Scale*. Baltimore, MD: Clinical Psychometric Research, 1975.

55. Sangal, R., Coyle, G., & Hoehn-Saric, R. Chronic anxiety and social adjustment. *Comp Psychiatr*, 1983, 24(1):75-78.

56. Derogatis, L.R., Abeloff, M., & Melisaratos, N. Psychological coping mechanisms and survival time in metastatic breast cancer. *JAMA*, 1979, 242(4):1504-1508.

57. Cella, D., Jacobsen, P., Orav, E., et al. A brief POMS measure of distress for cancer patients. *J Chron Dis*, 1987, 40(10):939-942.

58. Hoehn-Saric, R. Comparison of generalized anxiety disorder with panic disorder patients. *Psychopharmacol Bull*, 1982, 18(4):104-108.

59. VandeCreek, L., Rogers, E., & Lester, J., Use of alternative therapies among breast cancer outpatients compared with the general population. *Altern Ther Health Med*, (5)1:71-76.

24

Measuring Depression

Jeannie V. Pasacreta

Over the last 10 years, dramatic scientific advances have profoundly extended the trajectory for chronic medical and psychiatric illnesses. People are being diagnosed earlier and living longer with vastly increasing opportunities to experience simultaneous, interrelated, psychiatric and medical morbidity. One of the most common psychiatric sequelae that occur secondary to chronic medical illness is depression, which interferes significantly with recovery, quality of life, and survival. Similarly, chronic medical problems that often go unaddressed are far more prevalent among individuals with primary depression than among those without the diagnosis. Complex interacting forces—including but not limited to rising medical costs, managed care arrangements, and the stigma associated with mental illness—have placed a low priority on the recognition and treatment of depression in our health care system. As a result, our most vulnerable citizens have no access to comprehensive, integrated medical and psychiatric services; this creates long-term problems that drive health care costs up and diminish quality.

Misconceptions about depression are common across diverse patient populations. They stem from the fact that *depression* has a variety of meanings and is commonly used to describe a broad spectrum of human emotions and behaviors. This spectrum can range from expected, transient, and nonclinical sadness after upsetting life events to the clinically relevant extremes of suicidality and major depressive illness. Because depression is described as a common malady among individuals with chronic illness, researchers are in an optimal position to clarify the characteristics and consequences associated with this often elusive concept. The literature on primary depressive phenomena is large and reveals advances in the understanding of etiologic factors, classification, prevalence, course, and treatment. These strides are somewhat obscured when examining the literature on depression in medically ill patients, particularly because depression is often conceptualized differently from study to study. The ultimate goal of this chapter is to describe various models and measurement systems for delineating depression and provide some guidelines for choosing appropriate measurement strategies. The need to broaden the definition of depression beyond the discrete psychiatric varieties and clarify outcomes associated with depression secondary to medical illness is stressed as an important means of expanding knowledge in this area.

In the largest and most comprehensive study to date, nonpsychiatric physicians recognized major depressive disorder (MDD) in less than half of the depressed individuals they saw.[1] Only 19% of the patients in this study who were diagnosed with a depressive disorder received an antidepressant pharmacologic agent. No more than 6% of depressed patients in the community had consulted a psychiatrist. On average, depressed patients received 10 minutes or less of advice and education from nonpsychiatric physicians, whereas psychiatrists and psychologists offered some forms of psychotherapy in longer sessions.[1] According to psychiatric providers, a combination of psychotherapy and antidepressant medication was the most effective form of management, as assessed by symptom reduction and improved functioning. In this study, psychiatrists achieved better outcomes than medical practitioners.[1] Although these data apply to individuals in the general population, when they are placed within the context of trends among individuals living with a chronic illness, the need for the application of effective assessment and treatment strategies is compelling.

Terms that will be used throughout this chapter include *depressive syndromes*, which refers to a specific constellation of symptoms that make up a discrete psychiatric disorder. Types of depressive syndromes include major depression, dysthymia, subsyndromal depressive symptoms, depression resulting from a specific medical condition, and adjustment disorder with depressed features. The clinical significance of subsyndromal depressive symptoms in most settings remains elusive and is an important area for future study.

Theoretical Underpinnings of Depression: Measurement and Treatment Strategies

The term *depression* was adopted in 1905 by Adolf Meyer to describe pathologic disturbances of mood in an attempt to eliminate confusion created by the indiscriminate use of the word *melancholia*.[2] *Melancholia* was originally reserved to describe extreme states of mental dejection accompanied by self-deprecation and neurovegetative symptoms. The literal meaning of melancholia, black bile, suggested a state of gloom and darkness with explicit biologic connotations.[3] Adoption of the term *depression* failed to eliminate conceptual confusion. Varied definitions continue to be used interchangeably, and clinicians and researchers have not reached agreement on the basic concepts of depression, the best methods of classification and measurement, and whether depressive phenomena, etiology, and outcomes vary across diagnostic groups (i.e., primary major depression versus depression secondary to cancer, versus depression secondary to diabetes).

Despite extensive research, the mechanisms that underlie depressive phenomena, particularly when secondary to medical illness, are poorly understood.[4] There is growing consensus, however, that depression is often the consequence of multiple biologic, psychologic, cognitive, and sociologic interacting mechanisms.

The most widely accepted and tested theoretical models of depression are the cognitive and neurobiologic views. Cognitive theories of depression are based on the general premise that the process of acquiring knowledge and formulating beliefs is a primary determinant of mood and behavior. Cognitive approaches emphasize the mediating role that distorted thinking plays in determining affective state.[5] The cognitive schema proposed by Beck[6] draws on concepts from cognitive and social psychology, information processing and psychoanalytic theory. The theoretical underpinnings of cognitive behavioral therapy (CBT) view cognitive and emotional concomitance of affective syndromes as exaggerated and persistent forms of perceived defeat or deprivation causing distorted, negative thinking. CBT aims to prevent depressive episodes through a correction of basic assumptions, the depressionogenic schemata. CBT has been reported to be effective in the treatment of patients with mild to severe depression, especially when combined with pharmacotherapy.[6-8] These combined modalities have received the most empirical support.

Some investigators have questioned cognitive approaches by challenging the belief that cognitive and motivational problems induce depression. An alternative view is that cognitive and motivational problems are merely the consequence of depression and as such should be regarded as symptoms. Proponents of the cognitive view of depression readily acknowledge the multiplicity of factors underlying depressive disorders.[3,9]

The importance of genetic vulnerability has been conclusively demonstrated in bipolar illness and recurrent unipolar depressions.[3,10,11] Several genetically determined biochemical alterations have been implicated, particularly in the etiology of primary and severe depressive disorders. These biologic hypotheses have been based largely on psychopharmacologic inference.[3,11] Most biochemical explanations of depression hypothesized a decrease in brain serotonin or norepinephrine levels but failed to favor one class over the other.[11] The permissive amine hypothesis of affective disorders, which was heralded as an important development in the synthesis of biologic hypotheses of depression, suggests that a central serotonergic deficiency may represent the vulnerability to affective illness. Lowered catecholamines correspond to depression and increased catecholamines, to mania. Within this view, depression and mania are viewed along a continuum, rather than being polar opposites, with mania representing a more severe deviation from normal mood.[12] Neurobiologic theories of depression assume a primary neurochemical defect. The occurrence of severe depression in medically ill patients without a prior history suggests that an alteration in brain chemistry might occur secondary to continuous aversive stimulation, thereby emphasizing the need for an integrated approach to assessment and treatment.

In several studies that examine the occurrence of depression in medically ill patients, depression is equated with a crisis response. According to Caplan,[13] receiving catastrophic news about a medical diagnosis results in immediate problem-solving efforts; however, demands on the individual exceed the ability to respond, producing both physiologic and psychologic arousal. Problem-solving ability is consequently reduced by physiologic arousal, resulting in poor attention, poor concentration, poor judgment, a sense of disorganization, and erosion of self-concept. The inability to use adaptive skills results in dysphoria, manifested by depression and anxiety.

As a result of numerous theoretical orientations, many diagnostic and measurement systems that identify overlapping populations have been used to document depression in research studies. With the exception of the Beck Depression Inventory (BDI), most measurement systems are only loosely tied to a theoretical framework. Criteria-based systems are grounded in the medical model and thus loosely tied to biologic theories of depression. The link between theory and the measurement of depression becomes particularly vague when mild to moderate levels of depression or those secondary to a medical condition are described. The following sections describe the primary measurement systems used to ascertain the prevalence of depression among the general population, primary psychiatric, and nonpsychiatric patient groups. The notion is stressed that varied instruments produce varied results and issues relevant to special populations. Attention to the interplay among somatic and psychologic symptoms in medically ill subjects is offered, with suggestions for handling these issues in research.

Primary Measurement Systems for Delineating Depression

Three major systems are used to delineate depression, including criteria-based systems, rating scales specific to depression, and self-report scales that measure general psychologic profiles and include depression as a dimension.

Criteria-Based Systems

In 1951, the Washington University Department of Psychiatry began a strong tradition of research, paying careful attention to the criteria used to make specific psychiatric diagnoses. Research was based on the premise that in order to obtain reliable diagnoses that could be compared across studies, rules of case definition had to be decided and associated with standardized procedures of examination.[14] In 1972, the Feigner Criteria were published, along with a structured interview to elicit information needed to apply specific diagnostic criteria.[15] The Feigner Criteria were later modified by Spitzer, Endicott, and Robins,[16] who published specific criteria for making 25 psychiatric diagnoses, called the Research Diagnostic Criteria (RDC). The RDC consists of descriptions of the clinical features of select disorders with specific inclusion and exclusion criteria. It is supplemented by a structured interview, the Schedule for Affective Disorders and Schizophrenia (SADS).[16]

The literature that classifies depressive phenomena according to criteria-based systems originated in the discipline of psychiatry. Throughout much of the last century, the focus has been to classify depressions into discrete categories based on family history, symptoms, treatment, and course. Classification schemes are based on the medical model and *nosology*, or the grouping of symptoms into single disease states with prediction of course and response to treatment as the goal.[17] The current focus in psychiatry is to separate depressions into distinct heterogeneous categories, often with the intent of distinguishing the types that will respond to pharmacotherapy.

The second edition of the *Diagnostic and Statistical Manual of Mental Disorders* (DSM-II),[18] which was used until 1980, classified depression into two broad categories: (1) those presumed to be reactive to life events, which were characterized by antecedent psychosocial conditions and presumed to be psychogenic in nature (neurotic depression and psychotic depressive reaction), and (2) those not related to a precipitating life experience and presumed to be biologic or endogenous in nature.

The third edition of the *Diagnostic and Statistical Manual of Mental Disorders* (DSM-III and DSM III-Revised),[19,20] heralded a major change in approach using a criteria-based method for classifying depression based on the RDC approach. DSM III/DSM-III-R (revised) were descriptive, and they disregarded etiologic considerations. Clinically significant depression was defined in terms of a constellation of symptoms (syndrome). Depressive syndromes were classified according to course (single episode or recurrent), and recurrent episodes were defined as disorders. DSM-III further distinguished depressive phenomena into bipolar and depressive types. The essential feature of the bipolar type is the presence of manic or hypomanic episodes in an individual or close relative. Depressed mood may or may not be present. "Major depressive episode/disorder" described a syndrome characterized by depressed mood, a change from previous functional level, and loss of interest or pleasure with accompanying neurovegetative symptoms (i.e., insomnia, psychomotor retardation, diminished appetite), suicidality, guilt, and worthlessness. A "melancholic type" of major depression was described in DSM-III as the most severe type of depression, believed to be particularly responsive to somatic therapy. Dysthymia, or "depressive neurosis," is a diagnosis reserved for chronic depression that interferes with function but does not fulfill the severity criteria for major depression. Depressive symptoms must be present almost continuously for a period of two years or longer.

The diagnostic manual currently in use is the DSM-IV-TR (text revised)[21] and continues to use the criteria-based system developed in DSM-III. Criteria for a major depressive episode are that five or more of the following symptoms have been present during the same 2-week period and represent a change from previous functioning: (1) depressed mood most of the day, nearly every day, as indicated by either subjective report or observation made by others; (2) markedly diminished interest or pleasure in all, or almost all, activities most of the day, nearly every day; (3) significant weight loss when not dieting, or weight gain or decrease or increase in appetite nearly every day; (4) insomnia or hypersomnia nearly every day; (5) psychomotor agitation or retardation nearly every day; (6) fatigue or loss of energy nearly every day; (7) feelings of worthlessness or excessive guilt nearly every day; (8) diminished ability to think or concentrate, or indecisiveness, nearly every day; and (9) recurrent thoughts of death, recurrent suicidal ideation without a specific plan, or a suicide attempt or specific plan for committing suicide.

At least one of the symptoms must be either (1) depressed mood or (2) loss of interest or pleasure. The symptoms must cause clinically significant distress or impairment in social, occupational, or other areas of functioning. Symptoms that are clearly due to a general medical condition are excluded. The symptoms cannot be due to the direct physiologic effects of a drug of abuse, other medication, or a general medical condition. Symptoms cannot be due to bereavement.

The diagnostic criteria for mood disorder due to a medical condition[21] includes prominent and persistent disturbance in mood predominating in the clinical picture and is characterized by either (or both) of the following: (1) depressed mood or markedly diminished interest or pleasure in all, or almost all, activities and (2) elevated, expansive, or irritable mood. There must be evidence from the history, physical examination, or laboratory findings that the disturbance is the direct physiologic consequence of a general medical condition and that the disturbance cannot be better accounted for by another mental disorder (e.g., adjustment disorder with depressed mood in response to the stress of having a general medical condition). Finally, the disturbance does not occur exclusively during the course of a delirium, and the symptoms cause clinically significant distress or impairment in social, occupational, or other important areas of functioning.

A DSM-IV-TR category of depressive phenomena particularly germane to a description of depression in medically ill patients, as they frequently receive this diagnosis,[21] is adjustment disorder with depressed features. In general, adjustment disorder is associated with an explicit precipitant and is transient and milder in nature than a major depressive episode. It is not considered a primary mood disturbance, thus the diagnosis is not considered in epidemiologic studies, and knowledge development in the area of subsyndromal depressive symptoms has been hindered.

DSM-IV-TR,[21] by excluding depressive symptoms related to a physical condition, has made it more difficult to classify and thus diagnose and treat patients who experience depression secondary to a medical diagnosis. Although the purpose of this change was to make standardized criteria for psychiatric diagnosis more rigorous to enhance reliability, the change excluded a group of the medically ill from further study and thus eventual effective treatment. None of the interview schedules designed to obtain criteria-based diagnoses have been standardized on medically ill populations.[22]

Most investigations of depression in the medically ill point to a small number of patients with major depressive syndromes or dysthymia and a much larger number with symptoms of lesser intensity. The immediate and long-term significance of depressive symptoms, because they are not of the type or intensity to be included in rigorous syndromic diagnoses, remains unclear.

Rating Scales

Rating scales have been used primarily as screening instruments or as a means of quantifying the severity of depression, particularly in intervention studies as an indicator of treatment response. Screening is a process whereby a disorder is presumptively identified in a particular population. Screening studies have based the definition of a case of depression on the attainment of a certain score on one of many depression rating scales. For a rating scale to be used for research purposes, Nunnally recommends a coefficient alpha of at least 0.6. If a rating scale is used as a screening instrument in the clinical setting, coefficient alpha should be at least 0.8.[23] For some rating scales, norms exist that have been established using homogeneous samples (e.g., normal controls, psychiatric inpatients, medically ill patients). Fundamentally, norms provide an interpretive point of reference and allow for assessment of an individual in terms of an existing standard. Several issues are inherent in the use of rating scales to measure depression. Primarily, differing scale construction leads to serious difficulty when comparing studies that used different instruments.[2] It is virtually impossible to assume the measurement of like concepts when using different measures. In addition, self-report measures may produce high false-positive or false-negative diagnoses (when using criteria-based diagnoses as the standard), depending on the cutoff points used, which may differ in separate investigations even when the same scale was used.[24] Some individuals may not be willing or able to report affective symptoms during a severe depressive state.[25]

Some investigators have used depression symptom scales as sole diagnostic instruments in patients with possible depression associated with medical illness.[26,27] Rating scales can be self-report scales or observer rated. The singular use of self-report instruments to measure depression has been questioned,[28] suggesting that the positive predictive power of various self-report instruments is limited (i.e., the probability that a patient with a scale score greater than a certain value will have a criteria-based depression). In a study regarding the predictive value of the BDI,[28] researchers screened 768 consecutive cancer outpatients for depression. Five hundred eighty-nine subjects completed the BDI, 117 of whom had scores of 10 or greater. Only 12 of those 117 patients met the criteria for major depression according to DSM-III. The prevalence rate of depression in this sample was only 2%. The authors concluded that the predictive power of the BDI among cancer patients was poor and that other screening instruments be used with caution because they inflate the prevalence of depression in patients with cancer.

As stated, most depression rating scales have corresponding cutoff points that distinguish patients with clinical depression (scoring above cutoff point) from those without it (scoring below cutoff point). When used in this regard, rating scales are considered screening instruments. Assessment of the relationship between symptom scale scores and clinical depression, as it is understood in primary psychiatric patients, suggests that such scales are poorly correlated.[28] The underlying assumption regarding the practice of correlating scale scores with criteria-based diagnoses to determine their validity is that criteria-based diagnoses of depression are inherently better than other methods in the medically ill. Data regarding untoward outcomes associated with depressive syndromes, as well as less severe depressive symptoms, are slowly emerging and challenge the singular use of the medical paradigm in determining the types of depression that are clinically significant among medically ill patients. Only when the full range of depressive symptoms experienced by these populations is studied and understood will effective treatments, both pharmacologic and psychotherapeutic, be tested and developed.

Rating scales are devised as (1) self-report scales in which the subject fills out responses on a structured scale without assistance from an interviewer; (2) observer-assisted scales in which the subject responds to the scale with assistance from an interviewer, who may read questions from the scale; and (3) clinical observer scales in which ratings are based on clinical observation and interview by a trained individual. Each variety of rating scale has its advantages and disadvantages. Self-report measures, for example, may yield inaccurate information from severely depressed individuals. Subjects who are severely depressed may be unable to respond on their own due to problems with apathy, psychomotor retardation, and poor concentration, to name just a few. On the other hand, observer-rated scales may be subject to observer bias and reliability problems; thus, stringent interviewer training is imperative. The issues mentioned stress the need to plan carefully regarding the type of instrument that will be used to measure depression in research and to anticipate potential problems and solutions before they occur.

The Use of General Psychologic Profiles to Measure Depression

In several studies that examine the occurrence of depression, self-report instruments are used that reveal general psychologic profiles and include depression as a specific dimension.[29,30] Examples of multidimensional inventories that have been used in this regard include the Hospital Anxiety and Depression Scale (HAD),[31] the Hopkins Symptom Checklist-90 (SCL-90),[32] and the Brief Symptom Inventory (BSI).[33] Several factors account for the use of multidimensional rather than depression-specific scales. Multidimensional scales provide information regarding other emotional states that may accompany depression in select populations. This may be useful in descriptive studies as well as to note the differential effects of research interventions. In addition, numerous studies equate the occurrence of depression in medically ill patients with a crisis response[34] and associate its existence with other psychologic states. An ongoing debate regarding the ability to clearly separate symptoms of anxiety and depression has contributed to the use of scales that measure general as opposed to specific distress in some patients. Some investigators view less severe, reactive, or situational depressions as indistinguishable from anxiety disorders. Historically, this viewpoint is based on the work of Lewis[35] and the observation of high overlap in the symptomatic presentation of the two classes of disorders and their similar responses to therapeutics. Several investigators, however, have reviewed evidence for both unitary and distinct positions, reporting strong support for the distinction of anxiety and depression as separate entities.[36–39]

The Conceptualization of Depression

In current clinical practice and research, there are two major paradigms for conceptualizing depression: the general phenomena of depressive symptoms and specific psychiatric, depressive disorders. While the general medical sector tends to conceptualize depression according to the former definition, much of the mental health specialty sector conceptualizes depression according to the latter.[40]

The psychiatric specialty, with its focus on categorizing depressions into discrete psychiatric syndromes, has hindered inquiry into less severe depressive symptoms. This point is certainly not meant to minimize the importance of having standardized criteria by which to make valid and reproducible diagnoses (so that risk factors, treatments, and course of illness can be better understood, predicted, and monitored). However, as criteria for depressive syndromes have become more stringent (as per the changes from DSM-II to DSM-III to DSM-III-R to DSM-IV), more individuals, particularly those with depression subsequent to a medical disorder, are being excluded from diagnostic groups. Although this may be appropriate because of the intrinsic differences between primary and secondary depression, examining the course and consequences associated with less severe depressive symptoms is needed so that treatment for the broad spectrum of depression can be tested and expanded. The relevance of this view is supported by several studies that associate untoward outcomes with persistent depressive symptoms in the medically ill.

In a study by Mossey and colleagues,[41] the effects of persistent depressive symptoms on hip fracture recovery were examined. Depressive symptoms were measured using the Center for Epidemiologic Studies-Depression scale (CES-D). After controlling for age, prefracture physical function, and cognitive status, which were found to be predictors of recovery, subjects consistently reporting few depressive symptoms were three times more likely than those with persistently elevated CES-D scores to achieve independence in walking, nine times more likely to return to prefracture levels in at least five of seven physical function measures, and nine times more likely to be in the highest quartile of overall physical function. These findings emphasize the significance of persistently elevated depressive symptoms in the recovery process and the importance of routine screening, evaluation, and treatment of depressed mood states.

The preceding study used CES-D scores over 16 to define elevated depressive symptoms, and although the authors did not evaluate subjects for the presence of criteria-based depressive syndromes, it can be assumed that a large percentage of them would not have met specified criteria. This assumption is based on a study by Schulberg and colleagues,[42] which analyzed the efficiency of the CES-D against a criterion measure—the Diagnostic Interview Schedule (DIS), which permits clinicians to formulate psychiatric diagnoses according to DSM-III criteria. Sixty-two percent of high-scoring medical patients (from a total sample of 294) were assigned no psychiatric diagnosis by the DIS. The authors suggested that considerably higher than usual cutoff scores be used to improve the efficiency of the CES-D. Although this may improve the ability of the instrument to predict psychiatric syndromes, it minimizes the clinical significance of less severe symptom profiles as well as the importance of exploring their associated risk factors, course, outcomes, and treatment response.

Routine psychiatric evaluations of 100 adult patients undergoing allogeneic bone marrow transplantation for acute leukemia were reviewed to examine the possible relationship of psychiatric and psychosocial factors to duration of survival following the procedure.[43] Three variables were found to independently affect outcome: illness status (first remission versus other status), presence of depressed mood, and the extent of perceived social support. Patients with depressed mood ($n = 13$) as a prominent symptom at the pretransplant evaluation had significantly shorter survival after transplantation. Only one patient in the depressed group had a diagnosis of major depression. The authors admit that their sample was small and that the mechanism by which depressed mood affects outcome remains highly speculative. The important point was that depressive symptoms of lesser magnitude than those associated with stringent psychiatric diagnoses were being coupled with unfavorable outcomes in medically ill patients. Study that expands the conceptual and operational nature of depression in special populations is warranted.

Landmark research commonly known as the Medical Outcomes Study examined and compared outcomes associated with depressive disorders, depressive symptoms, chronic medical conditions, and no chronic conditions.[40] Data were collected from 11,242 outpatients at three health care sites. The study associated significant morbidity with depressive symptoms and pointed to the need to expand the study of depression among the medically ill to include depressive symptoms that do not qualify for disorder status. According to the authors:

> Patients with either current depressive disorder or depressive symptoms in the absence of disorder tended to have worse physical, social and role functioning, worse perceived current health status and greater bodily pain than patients with no chronic conditions. The poor functioning uniquely associated with depressive symptoms with or without depressive disorder was comparable to or worse than that uniquely associated with eight major chronic medical conditions. For example, the unique association of days in bed with depressive symptoms was significantly greater than the comparable association with hypertension, diabetes and arthritis. Depression and chronic medical conditions had unique and additive effects on patient functioning.[40,p914]

In addition to the clear relationship between depression and medical outcomes, the impact of comorbid depression and quality of life is well established. Depression may result from the increased strain of having a chronic medical condition rather than directly from the disease itself.[41] A number of studies suggest that depressed mood is related to difficulties in adaptation to medical complications[42–46] and diminished quality of life.[40] Most studies use the Medical Outcomes Survey short form—36 (MOS-SF36), which was developed as part of the Medical Outcomes Study to measure quality of life in medically ill samples.[40] The Medical Outcomes Study provides a framework for measuring the additive, synergistic impact of depression and quality of life.

Depression, Somatic Symptoms, and Functioning

The effects of medical treatments inflict transient or permanent physical changes, somatic symptoms, and functional impairments in patients. Excessive psychologic distress can exacerbate side effects of treatment agents.[41] Conversely, treatment side effects can dramatically impact recipient mood and affect.[42] Because of the expected nature of somatic and affective changes secondary to many medical problems and their treatments, symptoms of depression that reach clinical significance often go unnoticed and untreated. Somatic symptoms imposed by various illnesses and treatments often coexist with somatic symptoms that are characteristic of depressive syndromes (Figure 24-1). The coexisting and competing nature of somatic and affective symptoms (treatment of physical problems often assumes priority in the medical treatment setting) has led to an underrecognition of clinically significant depression as well as to the assumption that depression is an appropriate response to a physically and emotionally disruptive chronic illness.

Although it is true that transient symptoms of depression occur with some regularity throughout the chronic illness trajectory, severe depressive symptoms or a constellation of depressive symptoms (syndrome) is not expected or typical. The frequent inability to recognize symptoms of depression that go beyond the expected may arise from difficulties separating somatic changes resulting from illness from those associated with severe depression. The need to measure somatic symptoms and depression separately to ascertain an accurate prevalence of depression is crucial. Early attempts to measure the impact of physical symptoms experienced by medically ill patients focused on one dimension of the individual's life—physical performance. Karnofsky and Burchenal[43a] developed a scale that rates physical activity from 1 to 100% in increments of 10%. The

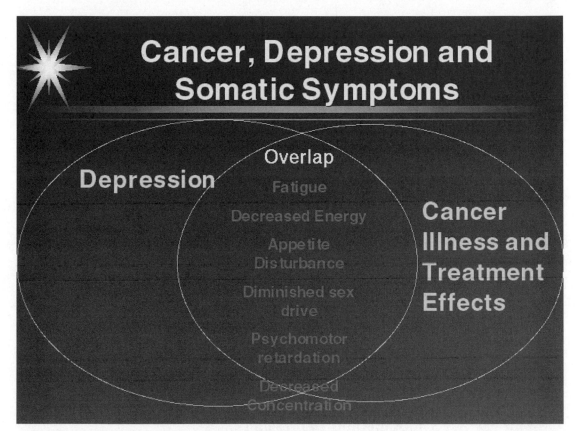

Figure 24.1   Cancer, Depression and Somatic Symptoms

Karnofsky Performance Scale, extensively used by cooperative cancer research groups, has been shown to correlate with tumor response and survival. The scale was originally developed in response to an urgent need for a brief measure that could demonstrate response to cancer treatment protocols. The value of instruments such as the Karnofsky in adequately describing the multiple dimensions of human functioning and their relationship to concepts such as affect and quality of life has been questioned.[44] Many prevalence studies of depression secondary to medical illness utilized Karnofsky measures alone. Their findings in regard to the highly interrelated nature of somatic symptoms and affect represent a limited view and underscore the extreme difficulty in assigning symptoms to a medical or psychologic etiology. Use of a more comprehensive measure of somatic symptoms and functional status outcomes as well as expanding data collection times to reflect varied patient experiences are some suggestions that may expand our understanding of the dynamic balance between somatization, affect, and functional outcomes and help to clarify factors associated with and consequential to degrees of depressive phenomena.

Because of difficulties diagnosing depression in the medically ill (associated with the overlap of somatic and affective symptoms), some investigators have suggested that somatic items be excluded from criteria-based systems in this population. Such modification threatens the validity of the modified system and increases the severity of criteria for a depressive syndrome in patients with cancer.[45] To counter these problems, Endicott proposed that alternative symptoms be used to replace those most likely to be affected by the medical condition and its treatment. Depending on the type of cancer and type of treatment, an investigator can decide that one symptom, such as appetite loss, is not to be used and substitute some other common depressive symptom in its place (e.g., tearfulness or depressed appearance). If several of the associated clinical features are apt to be affected by the cancer or its treatment, or both, the investigator must decide which list of alternative symptoms will be used. Endicott[45] stressed that training procedures for clinical evaluators must ensure that modified criteria be used similarly and consistently for all subjects. It is important that replacement symptoms be of equal validity and reliability to those that are being replaced.[28]

Some studies of depression among the medically ill conclude that depression is best evaluated by the severity of dysphoric mood; the degree of feelings of hopelessness, guilt, and worthlessness; and the presence of suicidal thoughts.[45,47] Theoretically, excluding somatic items sounds reasonable. However, some investigators question the necessity of removing somatic items,[28] stating that doing so may threaten established instrument validity. When criteria developed by Endicott[45] were used to diagnose depression in patients with cancer (because the physical conditions and resultant symptoms were considered an interfering variable), the number identified as depressed was about the same as the number diagnosed by the older DSM-III criteria. Only two patients were not concordant. According to Kathol and colleagues,[28] these findings suggest that "although somatic symptoms are less satisfactory as predictors of the syndrome of major depression, in fact when coupled with the psychological complaints, most of the same patients will meet the criteria for depression whether somatic symptoms are replaced by psychological symptoms or not." According to this view, somatic symptoms may not confound depression among cancer patients provided that a sufficient number of psychologic symptoms are present.

Organic Mental Symptoms and Depression

Organic mental impairment can have a direct causal relationship to depression in some patients. Certain drugs, including chemotherapy, steroids and commonly prescribed medications, such as those for anxiety and pain, can produce depression in some individuals.[46] Pancreatic and neurologic cancers, cerebral metastasis, uncontrolled pain, and certain metabolic, nutritional, and endocrine derangements are also associated with a depressionogenic effect.[46] These problems present special challenges to the study of depression among the medically ill and highlight the need to screen for organic impairment with a well-established, valid, and reliable instrument.

Prevalence of Depression in the General Population

Historically, prevalence rates for depressive disorders have varied greatly because of imprecise nosology, unrepresentative sampling, and unreliable measurement. The National Institute of Mental Health (NIMH) Epidemiological Catchment Area Program (ECA)[48] addressed many of these problems in a landmark study of mental disorders in the United States. The ECA program involved approximately 20,000 community residents in five areas of the United States. The NIMH Diagnostic Interview Schedule (DIS) developed by Robins and colleagues[49] was the primary assessment device used in this study. This instrument leads to valid and reliable diagnoses, and most notably, nonpsychiatric personnel can be trained to conduct the interviews.

According to the ECA study, lifetime prevalence rates (proportion of the general population with a disorder at any time in their lives) of major depression varied from 3.7 to 6.7 per 100.[48] The prevalence of dysthymia ranged from 2.1 to 3.8 per 100.[48] Lifetime rates of a major depressive episode were significantly higher for women than men, as were rates of dysthymic disorder. In other studies, point prevalence estimates (measurement limited to one point in time) for major depression in females ranged from a low of 2.0 per 100[49,50] to a high of 22.6 per 100.[51] The point prevalence of depressive symptoms (individuals scoring above set cutoff points on a variety of depression rating scales) is reported to range from 9 to 20%.[4]

The prevalence rates just listed are important for several reasons. First, the consistently higher rates of depressive disorders among women highlights the importance of exploring the occurrence of depressive phenomena among female groups. Secondly, the wide range of point prevalence rates points to the special care that must be taken when comparing point prevalence rates among specialty populations to those found in the general public. Third, some studies of depression in medically ill patients have compared high point prevalence among their samples to lifetime rates in the general population; these comparisons pose obvious interpretive difficulties. Finally, because most epidemiologic studies of depression have examined the prevalence of the major affective disorders or because those disorders have served as the criteria against which more subtle symptoms are evaluated, inquiry has been slow to develop into the occurrence and consequences associated with more subtle depressive symptoms in the general public and particularly in the medically ill.

Case Finding of Depressed People in Clinical Settings

Depression is one of the most common psychiatric diagnoses in nonpsychiatric populations. Given that 50% to 60% of people seeking help for depression are treated exclusively in the primary care setting, accurate detection in this setting is important.[52] One strategy that may improve detection is the use of psychiatric screening or case-finding instruments as part of the routine health evaluation. Several case-finding instruments are relatively short and can be easily self-administered by patients with at least grade-school to middle-school reading ability. For patients without such reading skills, instruments can be administered by trained office staff. Several of the instruments are available in different languages, including Spanish. All are easily scored, except for the Medical Outcomes Study Depression Screen, which requires a calculator.

Characteristics of case-finding instruments often enable clinicians to decrease the number of intensive diagnostic interviews without missing those who might potentially benefit from a full diagnostic interview. Research has demonstrated that among 100 patients in a clinic with an average prevalence of 5% for major depression, the clinician would have to do a diagnostic interview in only 31 patients to identify the 4 with major depression, and only 1 person with major depression would be missed. It is unlikely that many busy clinicians could or would want to do diagnostic interviews in all 100 patients so that they would not miss 1 case of depression. Further, when using a case-finding instrument, the clinician can expect to miss about 20% of patients with depression; current practice often misses 50% of such patients.[53,54]

Recent data suggest that primary care clinicians miss as many as 35% to 65% of patients with major depression.[53–55] Clinician recognition may be unaffected by a patient's sex or level of education, may be slightly lower among younger patients, and may be higher among patients with the most severe and disabling disease.[53,55,57] Fewer than 20% of people with major depression in the primary care setting have severe disease, and data suggests that 25% of these people are still being missed.[56] Although case-finding instruments detect a higher proportion of those with major depression (80%) than primary care clinicians do (35% to 65%), it is unclear whether they miss the same spectrum of disease most commonly missed by clinicians. Because sensitivity tends to increase with increasing severity of disease, it is likely that case-finding instruments will most often miss those with mild disease and that they will not miss as many as 25% of persons with severe disease.[58]

Targeting high-risk patients with a higher underlying prevalence of depression for case finding is an intuitively appealing strategy because it offers greater efficiency by improving the positive predictive value of the case-finding instrument. However, gains in efficiency are related to the magnitude of the risk factor and the prevalence of that risk factor in the patient population.[59,60] For example, the strongest demographic risk factor for depression is female sex (relative risk, 2).[61,62] In primary care practices, women patients outnumber men by a ratio of 60:40.[63] If only women were screened with a case-finding instrument that was 80% sensitive and 72% specific, the positive predictive value would increase only marginally, from 13% to 16%. This minimal gain would be associated with a 20% decrease in sensitivity for the case-finding strategy and a potential for missing 40% of depressed patients. A more potent (relative risk, 3) and less common (10%) risk factor is known previous depressive illness.[64] If the "highly attuned" clinician limited case-finding to patients with this risk factor, he or she would increase the positive predictive value of the case-finding strategy to 29%, but overall sensitivity would be greatly reduced. Seventy-five percent of patients with major depression and no past known depressive illness would not be screened.

Incorporating case-finding instruments for depression into practice has some pitfalls. Routine screening for depressive disorders may lead clinicians to focus only on depression and ignore other common psychiatric disorders. Patients with anxiety disorders and alcohol abuse may have positive scores on depression instruments. Unless these disorders are ruled out, patients may be mistakenly labeled as depressed or may not be recognized as having depression comorbid with another psychiatric condition. Case-finding instruments designed to detect multidimensional psychiatric phenomena may be less likely to bias the clinician toward focusing only on depression. One recently developed instrument, the Primary Care Evaluation of Mental Disorders, is a multidimensional questionnaire that assess several specific psychiatric disorders.[65] It includes questions related to depression, anxiety, somatization disorder, and alcohol abuse. Positive responses to any of the four sections trigger specific structured interview questions that are used to make definitive diagnoses. Such multidimensional instruments may minimize undue emphasis on depression and identify comorbid psychiatric disorders.

Special Methodologic Considerations

Timing of Depression Measurement

Given that a multisymptom crisis response occurs close to the time of a chronic medical diagnosis, it seems reasonable that investigators allow adequate time for patients to adjust to their situation before examining the nature of ongoing or residual depressive phenomena. Studies that do not consider this issue leave the difference between a transient crisis reaction and ongoing depression unclear. Because depression is characterized by change, a longitudinal design may best shed light on the course of depression over time.

Current understanding of the interplay of psychologic and physical symptoms among patients receiving aggressive treatments or with aggressive and/or highly symptomatic conditions is quite limited. Studies usually do not measure psychologic and physical symptoms prospectively or frequently enough to address the cyclical, interrelated, and highly variable nature of affective and physical symptoms. Some studies, especially among the elderly, have documented considerable variability of mood and its correlates across consecutive days and even within the same day.[66-71] Although their foci vary widely, these and similar studies have documented the association of short-term fluctuations in psychologic status with longer-term outcomes, such as physical health and psychologic well-being. Moldofsky and Chester[70] found that within-day variability in pain and mood in arthritis patients predicted differential health outcomes and service utilization two years later. Thus, multiple repeated assessment (experience sampling method) (ESM) of physical and psychologic symptoms can be a powerful tool in examining associations between physical and psychologic status and selected health-related outcomes. There is a critical need for prospective longitudinal research capable of identifying not only individuals at risk for depression but also critical time periods when depression is most likely to manifest itself. Using a methodology that assesses psychologic and physical symptoms frequently enough to allow for the variability inherent in certain conditions is essential. Such information could provide a foundation for the development and timing of interventions in vulnerable populations.

ESM, a procedure developed in 1975 by Csikszentmihalyi and his colleagues,[66] was designed to study the subjective experience of people interacting in natural environments and to provide repeated measurements of a person's activities, feelings, and thoughts in real time. Methods for obtaining repeated-measures data vary widely, but all are a variant on ESM. ESM uses multiple daily or within-day assessments to sample symptoms, affective states, activities, and events. A major limitation of cross-sectional measures is that they are unable to obtain unbiased, quantitative information on daily life contexts and activities, which may be fundamental for an understanding of patients' subjective experience.[72] In contrast, the most heuristic value of the ESM lies in its ability to describe the patterns or stream of an individual's daily experiences.[73] The ESM uses repeated self-assessments to study patients' thoughts, mood, motivation, physical symptoms, and activities in their natural settings. By providing a longitudinal series of data for each individual, the ESM offers a rich data source with potential to analyze individual variability and change over time. In addition, considering longitudinal study designs, the ESM provides additional strength over time-series methods. Time-series analysis generally assumes an equal interval between measurement points. However, the random schedule of the ESM increases the reliability of subjects' responses resulting from the random nature of measurement timing.[74]

Measurement Issues in the Seriously Ill

Attention to conceptual and methodologic issues regarding depression among medically ill patients is vital if research is to inform clinicians of the true nature of these phenomena. In clinical and research settings, detection and case identification are particularly difficult. This is due to several factors, including the high prevalence of clinically significant "subsyndromal" depressive symptoms in medically ill samples (depressive symptoms not severe enough or of sufficient duration to be classified as a psychiatric disorder), the overlapping nature of physical and neurovegetative symptoms of depression, and the biases produced by different sample sites, each of which offers unique benefits and limitations. Because of these issues, recognition of depression is seriously impeded in clinical settings. Similarly, the nature and outcomes of depression in the medically ill remain unclear despite an abundance of research in this area.[75] Although it has been suggested that depression is different from classic forms of major depression in the medically ill, methodologic inadequacies inhibit elaboration and thorough understanding of those differences. The use of innovative and multidimensional study methodologies, guided by testing specific theories of putative causal pathways, are needed to successfully extend our current knowledge base and conceptual models.[76]

From a practical perspective, medical inpatients and the seriously ill are a relatively captive audience who often enjoy contact with researchers, although some may be unwilling or unable to participate because of the severity of their conditions. Examination of patients in acute settings offers some advantages to studying the relationships between medical illnesses and depression. There is a wide range in severity of symptoms, from minor to life threatening. Similarly, there is a wide range in severity of depressive symptoms. These shifts provide optimal variance and opportunity to observe the dynamic interchange between physical and psychologic phenomena over a small time span. This is also reflected in high rates of service use and large changes in outcomes over short periods of time.[77]

There may be limitations to the study of depression among the seriously ill. The difficulties in case identification discussed above may be highlighted by the severity of medical illnesses (with their associated and potentially confounding symptoms) and the low prevalence of prior mood disorder. The presence of acute physical illness places people under severe physiologic, psychologic, and social stress. In addition, patients may be hospitalized and as such removed from their home environments, and usual social support systems. They are exposed to psychosocial stressors unique to the hospital setting (e.g., dependency on hospital staff; unfamiliar and sometimes painful diagnostic and therapeutic procedures; altered eating, bathing, and sleep routines; and uncertain prognosis). The generalizability of findings from depressed subjects in such special circumstances may be limited. In addition, data-collection personnel, especially because they are seeing subjects, often may be perceived as supportive and as such can significantly affect the phenomena they are measuring.

Given these issues, research on depression in the seriously ill offers and requires special considerations. Determination of the validity of different approaches to case identification may benefit from the severity and variety of depressive and medical disorders.[40] Similarly, study of health service utilization (in its relation to depression and medical burden) may profit from high rates of illness and service use. Finally, the severity of subjects' illness may highlight biologic, psychologic, or psychosocial pathogenic relationships between depression and medical conditions, although specific findings may not prove relevant to patients in other settings.

Researchers should given consideration to the following issues:

1. Case identification is a crucial first step. The approach to depressive symptoms potentially confounded by medical illnesses must be defined explicitly. Choice of an inclusive approach avoids premature exclusion of relevant phenomena; exploratory analyses can examine the effects of other approaches to the relationships of interest.

2. The use of similar research instruments across sample sites greatly facilitates comparison of results. Each subject group offers its own leverage for answering particular questions. Psychiatric inpatients highlight the contributions of severe psychopathology (useful, for example, in identifying biologic markers). Medical inpatients are well suited to studies examining the validity of different approaches to case identification, investigating health service utilization, or highlighting the contribution of acute, severe, life-threatening medical disorders to affective illness. Medical outpatients have many advantages regarding generalizability and public health significance. Community samples are needed to determine the biases of all the above groups, which are each defined by service utilization.

3. The study of relationships between depression and medical illness may promote understanding of pathogenic mechanisms in depression associated with physical illness. Research questions can be guided a biopsychosocial conceptual framework. This context demands

multidimensional study methodology to identify the routes by which medical illness influences depression in particular patient groups. Multivariate models should examine direct and indirect effects to medical illness on depression in particular patient groups while considering intervening variables, such as functional impairment and social support. Guided multiple regressions or structural equation modeling will allow for the determination of the strengths of associations.

4. Of particular importance, especially if complex multivariate analyses are used, is that specific theoretical models should guide and direct research. The development and testing of such models is a major challenge that should be addressed by current research.

Individuals are living longer with a variety of chronic illnesses and often within the context of aggressive and physically and psychologically debilitating treatments. These trends promise to continue, and therefore further study is needed to ensure improved detection and treatment approaches.

Overview of Selected Instruments to Measure Depression

Ten instruments representing each of the measurement systems described earlier will be described in this section. Instruments were chosen that have been widely used, have abundant data regarding their psychometric properties, and can be used with a variety of populations.

Structured Clinical Interview for DSM-IV (SCID)

The SCID is a semistructured interview for making major psychiatric diagnoses according to DSM-IV-TR.[78] It is meant to be administered by a trained psychiatric clinician and includes an introductory overview followed by a list of symptoms and criteria representing the major psychiatric diagnostic classes contained in DSM-IV-TR. Because of its modular construction, the SCID can be used in studies for which only certain diagnoses are of interest, such as major depression. Using a decision tree approach, the SCID guides the clinician in testing diagnostic hypotheses as the interview is conducted. The output of the SCID is a record of the presence or absence of each of the disorders being considered for a current (past month) or lifetime diagnosis. SCID questions are grouped by diagnosis and by criteria needed to meet a particular diagnosis. A fundamental principle of the SCID is that although one or more structured questions are asked about each diagnostic criterion, ratings are of the criteria and not necessarily the specific answers to the questions.[78] If the interviewer suspects that a symptom is present, he or she does not allow denial of the symptom to go unchallenged. For example, if a subject appears quite depressed during an interview, depressed mood may be coded as present even if the subject denies it. Specific ratings for diagnostic criteria are coded as 1, 2, or 3: 1 means the symptom described in the criterion is absent; 2 indicates a subthreshold condition (e.g., 10 days of depression rather than the required 2 weeks); 3 means that the symptom described in the criteria is present. A rating of 0 indicates that there is inadequate information to provide a rating. There are two standard editions of the SCID. SCID-P is designed to be used with adult subjects who are identified psychiatric patients. The SCID-NP is for use in studies in which the subjects are not identified as psychiatric patients (e.g., community surveys, family studies, research in primary care). Optimally, an interviewer using the SCID should have enough clinical experience with psychopathology and diagnosis to conduct a psychiatric interview without an interview guide. Training of experienced clinicians can be accomplished with the SCID user's guide, which explains all versions of the SCID and gives instructions for using diagnostic modules.

A test–retest reliability study of the SCID was conducted on 592 subjects in four patient and two nonpatient sites in the United States, as well as one patient site in Germany.[79] Agreement between interviewers was expressed in terms of k, a statistic that corrects for chance agreement. For the patient sample, k was 0.64 for current and lifetime diagnoses of major depression. For the nonpatient samples, agreement was much lower regarding diagnosis of major depression, with a k of 0.42. These reliability estimates raise questions about the sources of diagnostic disagreement, such as interviewer training and information variance (i.e., raters getting varied supplemental information in addition to the clinical interview).

Diagnostic Interview Schedule (DIS)

The DIS is a criteria-based system designed to make DSM-IV-TR diagnoses.[80] The depressive disorders section of the DIS can be used to evaluate the presence of depressive disorders, including major depression and dysthymia. This highly structured, comprehensive interview permits the formulation of psychiatric diagnoses according to DSM-IV-TR criteria. Questions H1 to H44 pertain to the diagnosis of major depression and dysthymia and can be used separate from other diagnostic sections of the interview schedule. The DIS questions start with a historic frame of reference, such as, "Have you ever had a period in your life when you had a particular symptom?" After this initial question, it is then determined whether the symptom causes sufficient change in a person's life or behavior to be clinically significant, and whether the symptom is caused by drugs, alcohol, or physical disorders. All clinically significant symptoms not entirely explained by physical causes are coded on a structured form, and the respondent is asked to date the last occurrence of the most recent episode. Several studies of the DIS method of obtaining diagnoses have addressed the reliability of lifetime diagnoses and demonstrate adequate reliability for depressive disorders. The DIS has been validated for use in medically ill patients. Nonpsychiatric personnel can be trained to conduct the interviews; face-to-face and telephone-administered versions of the depression section of the DIS have been found to be equivalent.

The Beck Depression Inventory (BDI)

The BDI is a depression rating scale, widely used to screen for clinical depression. It has become one of the most widely used scales for assessing depression and is based on the cognitive model that describes depression as the "activation of primitive negative schemas that lead to a selective negative bias in interpreting experiences."[5] The scale first appeared in 1961 and was based on clinical descriptions of symptoms frequently occurring in depressed psychiatric patients.[80] The current instrument is a unidimensional self-report scale designed to measure the behavioral manifestations and depth of depression.[81] The BDI requires that scale statements be read to subjects, who select the most appropriate choice for themselves from the statements. Because of this feature, the BDI is open to observer bias and is an interviewer-assisted scale rather than a self-report scale in the true sense of the term. The scale is intended for use with psychiatric populations as a measure of the symptom severity of depressed mood and as a screening instrument for use with nonpsychiatric populations.

The BDI was developed in part to deal with discrepancies in clinical judgment and ambiguities associated with psychiatric nosology. The tool consists of 21 "symptom-attitude categories" that were clinically derived by Beck and his associates.[82] Each category represents a characteristic manifestation of depression. The respondent rates himself or herself using a 4-point discrete scale. Examples of individual items on the BDI include (0) I do not feel sad; (1) I feel sad; (3) I am sad all the time and I can't snap out of it; (3) I am so sad or unhappy that I can't stand it; (0) I don't get more tired than usual; (1) I get tired more easily than I used to; (2) I get tired from doing almost anything; (3) I am too tired to do anything. Items are summed to produce a total depression score ranging from 0 to 63. Scores are interpreted as follows: 0–9: normal range; 10–15, mild depression; 16–19, mild-moderate depression; 20–29: moderate-severe depression; 30–63, severe depression. Beck's design of the BDI was apparently based on the observation that intensity of distress, severity of depression, and numbers of symptoms are correlated and that the frequency of depressive symptoms is distributed across the continuum from nondepressed to severely depressed. The scale is intended for use within psychiatric populations as a measure of the symptom severity of depressed mood and as a screening instrument for nonpsychiatric populations. The guidelines for BDI cutoff scores are 0–10, none to mild depression; 11–18, mild to moderate depression; 19–29, moderate to severe depression; 30–36, severe depression.[82]

Cavanaugh and colleagues[27] assessed medical inpatients, depressed psychiatric patients, and normal individuals using the BDI. They analyzed their data using a latent trait model. The results indicated that the BDI measures one underlying general syndrome of depression. Six cognitive items on the BDI were able to discriminate the severity of depression in each group. The two items that discriminated best, dissatisfaction and social interest, were related to the subject's pleasure capacity. One item, crying, discriminated well for depression in medical patients only.

The BDI has been factor analyzed by several different groups. The results of these studies have been summarized by Beck and colleagues.[82] Investigators conclude that the BDI can be broken down into three highly intercorrelated factors: negative attitude toward self, performance impairment, and somatic disturbance. The items composing these factors may shift according to the diagnostic group studied.

Reliability estimates of the BDI were reported by Beck and associates.[82] Internal consistency is reported as 0.86, and test–retest reliability ranged between 0.48 and 0.86. Concurrent validity has been established with other widely used measures of depression, including the Hamilton (0.73); the Zung (0.76); and the MMPI depression subscale (0.76).

Center for Epidemiological Studies of Depression Scale (CES-D)

The CES-D[83] was developed by the Center for Epidemiologic Studies at NIMH specifically to meet the need for a brief, inexpensive measure of depression suitable for use in community surveys.[83–85] The instrument is not explicitly tied to a theoretical framework but can screen for clinical depression in large epidemiologic studies. The CES-D consists of 20 items that were selected from other depression scales, including the BDI, the Schedule for Affective Disorders, and the MMPI. Six major symptoms areas were identified, and several items from the other scales were selected to identify each category. The areas include depressed mood, guilt/worthlessness, helplessness/hopelessness, psychomotor retardation, loss of appetite, and sleep disturbance. The scale range of answers is from 0 to 3; in all cases, except for four questions, higher scores indicate more impairment. For those four questions, the scores are reversed. As stated, the total score has a range from 0 to 60, and this single total score is used as an estimate of the degree of depressive symptomatology. Sizeable proportions of varied populations scoring higher than 15 on the CES-D have been found to experience major depressive or dysthymic disorders.[42] Examples of individual items on the CES-D include "Were you bothered by things that usually don't bother you?" "Have you had trouble keeping your mind on what you were doing?" and "Have you felt depressed?" "Have you had crying spells?" All questions refer to the two weeks before the interview.

The reliability of the CES-D has been tested on clinic populations[83] and on probability samples of households in three communities, including Kansas City, MO, Washington County, MD, and Alameda County, CA.[83,85,86] Results of these investigations indicated that the scale has high internal consistency reliability, acceptable test–retest stability, and good construct validity in both clinical and community samples. Some evidence of criterion validity has been demonstrated in clinic samples.[83]

The Symptom Checklist-90 (SCL-90)

The SCL-90 is a 90-item self-report symptom inventory designed to assess the psychologic status of individuals, including medical patients.[32] The scale measures multidimensional psychologic distress, including nine primary symptom dimensions, such as depression. The instrument is able to communicate information relative to the nature and intensity of depression on a continuous (low to severe) basis rather than on a discrete basis. The scale asks, "How much were you distressed by . . ." and then lists 90 items, including poor appetite, feeling hopeless about the future, feeling no interest in things, and feeling blue. Each item is rated on a 5-point scale ranging from 0 (not at all) to 4 (extremely).

The SCL-90 is scored to obtain nine dimensions and three global indices. The nine dimensions are somatization, obsessive-compulsive, interpersonal sensitivity, depression, anxiety, hostility, phobic anxiety, paranoid ideation, and psychoticism. The depression dimension reflects a broad range of signs and symptoms of clinical depressive syndromes. Symptoms of dysphoric affect and mood, withdrawal of interest in usual life activities, and loss of vital energy are reflected in this dimension, as are feelings of hopelessness and futility. The global indices include the General Severity Index (GSI), the Positive Symptom Distress Index (PSDI), and the Positive Symptom Total (PST). The function of the global measures is to communicate in a single score the level or depth of symptomatic distress experienced by an individual. Internal consistency (Cronbach's alpha) for the SCL-90 ranges from a low of 0.79 to a high of 0.90.[32] Test–retest reliability (stability) coefficients range from 0.68 to 0.83. Factor analyses provide empirical support for 7 to 9 dimensions.[32]

The Brief Symptom Inventory (BSI)

The BSI[33] is a 53-item self-report symptom inventory designed to assess the psychologic status of individuals, including medical patients.[88] It is a short version of the SCL-90, and psychometric evaluation reveals it to be an acceptable short alternative to that test.[87] The scale measures multidimensional psychologic distress along nine primary symptom dimensions, including depression. The instrument is able to communicate information relative to the nature and intensity of depression on a continuous (low to severe) scale rather than on a discrete basis. The scale asks, "How much were you distressed by . . ." and then lists 53 items, such as poor appetite, feeling hopeless about the future, and feeling no interest in things. Each item is rated on a 5-point scale ranging from 0 (not at all) to 4 (extremely).

The BSI is scored to obtain nine dimensions and three global indices. The nine dimensions are the same as those for the SCL-90. The depression dimension reflects a broad range of signs and symptoms of clinical depressive syndromes, including symptoms of dysphoric affect and mood, and withdrawal of interest in usual life activities.[87] The global indices are the same as those for the SCL-90. The function of the global measures is to communicate in a single score the level or depth of symptomatic distress experienced by an individual. The GSI is the single best indicator of current distress levels and should be utilized in most instances where a single summary measure is required.[33] The GSI combines information on the numbers of symptoms and the intensity of perceived distress.[87]

Internal consistency (Cronbach's alpha) for the BSI ranges from a low of 0.71 to a high of 0.85. Test–retest reliability (stability) coefficients range from 0.68 to 0.91. The stability for the global indices are 0.80 (PST), 0.87 (PSDI), and 0.90 (GSI).[87] Validity was examined by comparing the BSI dimensions with the MMPI, resulting in positive correlations greater than 0.30.[33] Factor analysis provides empirical support for 7 to 9 dimensions.[33]

Geriatric Depression Scale (GDS)

The GDS is a 30-item self-report questionnaire that assesses symptoms of depression in the elderly. The GDS is used with elderly individuals and is sensitive to depression among elderly people with from mild to moderate dementia and physical illness.[88] The GDS-L is a self-report questionnaire consisting of yes/no categories that takes about 5 minutes to complete. The range of scores is 0 to 30, with higher scores indicating greater depression. Examples of scale questions include "Are you hopeful about the future?" and "Do you frequently feel like crying?" Reliability estimates of the scale demonstrate good internal consistency (Cronbach's alpha = 0.94) and test–retest reliability of 0.86.[88] Several beneficial features of the GDS: (1) Binary response options usually make the scale easily comprehended by older adults; (2) the GDS does not include potentially confounding somatic items; (3) it can be completed in approximately 5 minutes; (4) it contains more criteria characteristic of late-life depression than do other depression rating scales; and (5) it is one of the few depression rating scales validated in an older hospitalized population.[89]

As a screening instrument for major depression, a cutoff score of 11 yields sensitivity of 92% (the ability of the instrument to distinguish subjects with and without depressive disorder); specificity of 89% (the instrument's accuracy in selecting individuals with depressive disorders, as opposed to other disorders); positive predictive power of 56% (ability to predict those with depressive disorder); and a negative predictive value of 99% (ability to predict those without depressive disorder).[89]

Hamilton Depression Rating Scale (HDRS)

The HDRS was developed during the late 1950s as a standardized scale for the measurement of the severity of depressive symptoms.[90] Since its initial publication, the HDRS has been cited as the most widely used scale for patient selection and follow-up in research studies of treatments for depression.[91] The HDRS is commonly used to measure change over time, therefore, individual items are often examined to study the differential effects of various treatments. The scale was initially designed to yield a total score based on 17 of its 21 items, although many investigators have used all 21 items. The HDRS was designed to quantify the severity of depression based on face-to-face clinical interview. The HDRS treats depression as a unitary concept, and attempts to identify factors have yielded conflicting results. The HDRS has been shown to have a high degree of overall scale reliability, and considerable evidence exists for its concurrent, discriminant, and construct validity.[92–96] Despite its many advantages, however, the HDRS has several limitations as a research tool. First, interrater reliability of individual items on the scale have been criticized[93,96] and in one study ranged from a low of –0.02 to a high of 0.76.[96] Clinicians are instructed to consider the frequency and intensity of a symptom when assigning it a value on an anchored rating scale, yet operationally defined response categories are absent, which leads to a range of interpretations. Also fostering interpretive differences is the fact that questions are directed at a time frame of a few days to a week, in which time symptoms may fluctuate. The HDRS relies heavily on the expertise of an interviewer with extensive psychiatric background, which limits its use in large-scale or epidemiologic studies.[91,96] Additionally, three items on the scale (insight, psychomotor agitation, and psychomotor retardation) have demonstrated such poor test–retest correlation that some recommend their exclusion from the instrument.[96] To remedy some of the aforementioned problems, a structured-interview version of the HDRS has been developed, with an alpha reliability of 0.82 for the 17-item HDRS, a 14-item version exists (with insight, psychomotor agitation, and psychomotor retardation removed having a test–retest reliability of 0.67).[91,96] Interviewers without psychiatric backgrounds can be trained to use the schedule, and telephone and face-to-face interviews have yielded similar results.[97] The scale is heavily weighted with somatic items, however, thereby limiting its utility with medically ill subjects.

Hospital Anxiety and Depression Scale (HAD)

The HAD is a brief, self-administered rating scale designed to detect anxiety and depression among individuals with medical illnesses.[31] It is intended to screen for clinically significant depression among medically ill patients and to measure and monitor the severity of depression through repeat administration. The HAD focuses on the psychologic rather than the somatic manifestations of depression, excluding items that are characteristic of both depression and medical illness, such as appetite and sleep disturbance. The HAD contains 14 items, seven pertaining to depression, seven to anxiety. Examples of scale items pertaining to depression are "I still enjoy the things I used to enjoy"; "I have lost interest in my appearance"; "I can enjoy a good book or radio or TV program." Assessment of the overall severity of depression is rated on a four-point (0 to 3) scale. The range of scores for the depression subscale of the HAD is 0 to 21. A score between 8 and 10 indicates the probable presence of clinically significant depression.[31]

The depression subscale emphasizes anhedonia, which some consider the symptom of depression that is most characteristic of the biochemical subtype and thus predictive of response to antidepressants.[98] Evidence for the concurrent validity of the HAD has been reported in psychiatric patients,[99] in a heterogeneous group of patients with physical illness,[100] and in patients attending a genitourinary clinic.[101] The validation studies demonstrate that the HAD functions as two scales measuring two distinct psychologic states. In one study of the HAD, an exploratory factor analysis was carried out in 568 cancer patients.[102] Two distinct but correlated factors emerged that corresponded to the anxiety and depression subscales. The internal consistency of the two subscales using coefficient alpha was also high (anxiety, 0.93; depression, 0.90), which justifies the HAD for use as a screening instrument.

One criticism of the HAD is that its brevity has excluded important aspects of the states of anxiety and depression. This does not just apply to somatic symptoms, which have been deliberately excluded; elements of depression such as hopelessness, guilt, and low self-esteem are not assessed because the scale measures only features of anhedonia.

The Zung Self-Rating Depression Scale (SRS)

The SRS is a widely used 20-item self-report scale that subjects are supposed to complete without assistance.[103] The SRS has been used as a screening instrument for major depressive disorder according to psychiatric diagnostic criteria and as an instrument to measure the severity of depressive symptoms.[103] The scale was devised so that of the 20 items, 10 were worded symptomatically positive and ten symptomatically negative. Subjects are instructed to indicate the frequency with which they experience a symptom or feeling described (a little, some, a good part or most of the time). The scale includes affective, behavioral and somatic features. Sample items are "I feel downhearted and blue;" "I still enjoy sex;" "I find it easy to do the things I used to do;" and I have crying spells or feel like it." The maximum contribution of behavioral and somatic features to the full score is 50%.

Comparisons of Zung scores to criteria for major depression based on DSM-III-R demonstrated a sensitivity (the ability of the instrument to distinguish subjects with and without depressive disorder) of 97%, specificity (the instrument's accuracy in selecting individuals with depressive disorders as opposed to other disorders) of 63%, positive predictive value (ability to predict those with depressive disorder) of 77%, and a negative predictive value (ability to predict those without depressive disorder) of 95%.[103]

Although the SRS is a self-report scale designed to be completed without supervision, some authors have questioned this premise. In one study, patients were easily confused by the reversed direction of scale items. Since psychomotor retardation, poor concentration, and indecisiveness are common among depressed individuals, the time required to complete the scale alone was often inordinate. Based on these issues, an interviewer assisted approach may be beneficial.

Summary and Conclusions

Despair, hopelessness, lack of compliance with medical and psychiatric treatment, social isolation, and even premature death are but a few of the consequences frequently associated with depression. Despite significant strides in the understanding and treatment of certain types of depression, our understanding—particularly of less severe, secondary depression—has been obscured by methodologic problems and inconsistencies. Although it has been difficult to bridge the gap between depressive disorders and less severe depressive symptoms with our current state of knowledge, recommendations made in this chapter are important steps in clarifying the nature of depressive phenomena.

All too often, psychologic services for depressed patients are considered dispensable. They are viewed as expensive and without tangible need or benefit. Documentation of the nature of depression, its response to systematically tested interventions, and its cost in terms of exaggerating the impact of chronic illness and increasing days in bed and time off work, deserves ongoing, careful investigation. Only when the theoretical, methodologic, and measurement issues addressed in this chapter receive meticulous attention will the nature and consequences associated with depressive phenomena be realized and the development of effective treatments be viewed as a research and clinical priority.

Exemplar Study

Pasacreta, J.V. Depressive phenomena, physical symptom distress and functional status among women with breast cancer. *Nurs Res*, 1997. *46*(4): 214–221.

The nature and scope of depression and its relationship to physical symptom distress and functional status were examined in 79 women 3 to 7 months after breast cancer diagnosis. Psychiatric diagnostic criteria for depressive disorders and a depression rating scale (the CES-D) were used to measure depression. Nine percent of the sample had depressive disorder, and 24% had elevated depressive symptoms. Women with elevated depressive symptoms had more physical symptom distress ($p < 0.0001$) and more impaired functioning ($p < 0.0001$) than subjects with depressive disorders and without depression. Multiple regression was used to examine the contribution of key variables to functional status. Two variables accounted for 35% of the variance in functional status: symptom distress (28%) and depressive symptoms (7%). Correlations between major study variables suggest some conceptual overlap, but the absence of multicollinearity did not affect the results of the multiple regression procedure and indicated the distinct nature of the variables. In fact, patients who received chemotherapy had similar levels of depressive symptoms but significantly higher levels of symptom distress compared with those who did not receive chemotherapy. This highlights the separate nature of depressive symptoms and physical symptom distress in this sample. Findings are consistent with others reporting that depressive symptoms, even in the absence of disorder, have poor functioning. Future study demands attention to these issues.

References

1. Wells, K.B. Sturm, R., & Sherbourne, C.D. *Caring for depression: A RAND study*. Cambridge, MA: Harvard University Press, 1996, p. 243.
2. Snaith, R.P. The concepts of mild depression. *Br J Psychiatry*, 1987, 150:387-393.
3. Akiskal, H.S., & McKinney, W.T. Overview of recent research in depression: Integration of ten conceptual models into a comprehensive clinical frame. *Arch Gen Psychiatry*, 1975, 32:285-305.
4. Simon, G.E., VonKorff, M. Recognition, management, and outcomes of depression in primary care. *Arch Fam Med*, 1995, 4:99-105.
5. Gerber, P.D., Barrett, J. et al. Recognition of depression by internists in primary care: A comparison of internist and gold standard psychiatric assessments. *J Gen Intern Med*, 1989, 4:7-13.
6. Beck, A.T., Rush, A.J., Shaw, B.F., et al. *Cognitive therapy of depression. A treatment Manual*. New York, NY: Guilford Press, 1979.
7. Beck, A.T. Cognitive therapy: A 30-year retrospective *Am Psychol*, 1991, 46:368-375.
8. American Psychiatric Association. Practice guidelines for major depressive disorder in adults. *Am J Psychiatry*, 1993, 150:1-21
9. Wright, A.T., & Beck, J.H. Cognitive therapy of depression: Theory and practice. *Hosp Comm Psychiatry*, 1983, 34:1119-1126.
10. Gershon, E., Dunner, D., Goodwin, F. Toward a biology of affective disorders. *Arch Gen Psychiatry*, 1971, 25:1-15.
11. Sachar, E.J., & Baron, M. The biology of affective disorders. *Ann Rev Neurosci*, 1979, 2:505-518.
12. Prange, A., Wilson, I., & Lynn, C.W. L-tryptophan in mania: Contribution to a permissive hypothesis of affective disorders. *Arch Gen Psychiatry*, 1974, 3:56-62.
13. Caplan, G. Mastery of stress: Psychosocial aspects. *Am J Psychiatry*, 1981, 138:413-420.
14. Robins, L.N. The development and characteristic of the NIMH Diagnostic Interview Schedule. In M.M. Weissman, J.K. Meyers, & C.E. Ross (Eds.), *Community surveys*, vol. 4. New York: Neale Watson Academic Publications, 1981.
15. Feighner, J.P., Robins, E., & Guze, S.B. Diagnostic criteria for use in psychiatric research. *Arch Gen Psychiatry*, 1972, 26:57-63.
16. Spitzer, R.L., Endicott, J., & Robins, L.N. *Schedule for affective disorders and schizophrenia*. New York: New York Psychiatric Institute, 1978. Biometrics Research Division, Evaluation Section.
17. Feinstein, A.R. A critical overview of diagnosis in psychiatry. In V.M. Rakoff, H.C. Stancer, & H.B. Kedward (Eds.), *Psychiatric diagnosis*. New York: Brunner-Mazel, 1977, pp. 189-206.
18. American Psychiatric Association. *Diagnostic and statistical manual of mental disorders (DSM-II)*. 2nd ed. Washington, DC: American Psychiatric Association, 1968.
19. American Psychiatric Association. *Diagnostic and Statistical Manual of Mental Disorders (DSM-III)*. 3rd ed. Washington, DC: American Psychiatric Association, 1980.
20. American Psychiatric Association. *Diagnostic and Statistical Manual of Mental Disorders (DSM-III-R)*. 3rd ed., revised. Washington, DC: American Psychiatric Association, 1987.
21. American Psychiatric Association. *Diagnostic and Statistical Manual of Mental Disorders (DSM-IV-TR)*. 4th ed., text revised. Washington, DC: American Psychiatric Association, 2000.
22. Rodin, G., & Voshart, K. Depression in the medically ill: An overview. *Am J Psychiatry*, 1986, 14:696-705.
23. Nunnally, J.C. *Psychometric theory*. New York: McGraw Hill, 1978.
24. Meyers, J.K., & Weissman, M. Use of a self-report symptom scale to detect depression in a community sample. *Am J Psychiatry*, 1980, 137:1081.
25. Prusoff, B.A., & Klerman, G.L. Differentiating depressed from anxious neurotic outpatients. *Arch Gen Psychiatry*, 1974, 30:302-308.
26. Nielsen, A.C., & Williams, T.A. Depression in ambulatory medical patients: Prevalence by self-report questionnaire and recognition by nonpsychiatric physicians. *Arch Gen Psychiatry*, 1980, 37:999-1004.
27. Cavanaugh, S., Clark, D., & Gibbons, R.D. Diagnosing depression in the hospitalized medically ill. *Psychosomatics*, 1983, 24:809-815.
28. Kathol, R.G., Noyes, R., Williams, J., et al. Diagnosing depression in patients with medical illness. *Psychosomatics*, 1990, 31:436-449.
29. Koenig, R., Levin, S.M. & Brennan, M.J. The emotional status of cancer patient as measured by a psychological test. *J Chron Dis*, 1967, 20:923-930.
30. Craig, T.J., & Abeloff, M.D. Psychiatric symptomatology among hospitalized cancer patients. *Am J Psychiatry*, 1974, 26:133-136.
31. Zigmond, A.S., & Snaith, R.P. The Hospital Anxiety and Depression Scale. *Acta Psychiatr Scand*, 1978, 67:361-370.
32. Derogatis, L.R. SCL-90 administration, scoring and procedures manual. 2nd ed. Baltimore, MD: Procedures Psychometric Research, 1983.
33. Derogatis, L.R., & Spencer, P.M. *The Brief Symptom Inventory (BSI): Administration, scoring and procedures manual—I*. Baltimore, MD: Johns Hopkins University School of Medicine, 1982.
34. Holland, J.C. Clinical course of cancer. In J.C. Hol-

land & J.H. Rowland (Eds.), *Handbook of psychooncology: Psychological care of the patient with cancer*. New York: Oxford University Press, 1989, pp. 75–100.

35. Lewis, A.J. Psychological medicine In R.B. Scott (Ed.), *Price's textbook of the practice of medicine*. London: Oxford University Press, 1966.

36. Derogatis, L.R., Klerman, G.L., & Lipman, R.S. Anxiety states and depressive neurosis—Issues in nosological discrimination. *J Nerv Mental Dis*, 1972, 155:392-403.

37. Prusoff, B.A., Klerman, G.L., & Paykel, E.S. Concordance between clinical assessments and patients' self report in depression. *Arch Gen Psychiatry*, 1972, 26:546.

38. McNair, D.M., & Fisher, S. Separating anxiety from depression. In M.A. Lipton, A. DiMascio, & K.F. Killiam (Eds.), *Psychopharmacology: A generation in progress*. Norwalk, CT: Appleton-Lange, 1978.

39. Lesser, I.M., & Rubin, R.T. Diagnostic considerations in panic disorders. *J Cl Psychiatry*, 1986, 217(Suppl): 4-10.

40. Wells, K.B., Stewart, A., Hays, R.D., et al. The functioning and well being of depressed patients: Results from the Medical Outcomes Study. *JAMA*, 1989, 262:914-919.

41. Mossey, J.M., Knott, K., & Craik, L. The effects of persistent depressive symptoms on hip fracture recovery. *J Gerontol*, 1990, 45:163-168.

41a. Andrykowski, M.A., Redd, W.H., & Hatfield, A.K. The development of anticipatory nausea: A prospective analysis. *J Consult Clin Psychol*, 1985, 4:447-454.

42. Schulberg, H.C., Saul, M., McClelland, M.A., et al. Assessing depression in primary medical and psychiatric practices. *Arch Gen Psychiatry*, 1985, 42:1164-1170.

42a. Burish, T.G., & Lyles, J.N. Effectiveness of relaxation training in reducing adverse reactions to cancer chemotherapy. *J Behav Med*, 1981, 4:65-78.

43. Colon, E., Callies, A.L., Popkin, M., & McGlave, P.B. Depressed mood and other variables related to bone marrow transplantation survival in acute leukemia. *Psychosomatics*, 1991, 32:420-425.

43a. Karnofsky, D.A., & Burchenal, J.H. The clinical evaluation of chemotherapeutic agents in cancer. In C.M. Macleod (Ed.), *Evaluation of chemotherapeutic agents*. New York: Columbia University Press, 1949.

44. Frank-Stromborg, M. Single instruments for measuring quality of life. In M. Frank-Stromborg (Ed.), *Instruments for clinical nursing research*. Norwalk, CT: Appleton & Lange, 1988.

45. Endicott, J. Measurement of depression in patients with cancer: Proceedings of the working conference on methodology in behavioral and psychosocial cancer research. *Cancer*, 1984, 53(Suppl):2243.

46. Breitbart, W., & Holland, J.C. Psychiatric complications of cancer. *Curr Ther Hematol-Oncol*, 1988, 3:268-274.

47. Bukberg, J., Penman, D., & Holland, J.C. Depression in hospitalized cancer patients. *Psychosom Med*, 1984, 46:199-212.

48. Robins, L.N., Helzer, J.E., & Weissman, M.M. Lifetime prevalence of specific psychiatric disorders at three sites. *Arch Gen Psychiatry*, 1984, 41:949-958.

49. Robins, L.N., Helzer, J.E., Croughnan, J., et al. *NIMH Diagnostic Interview Schedule: Version III*. Rockville, MD: National Institutes of Mental Health, 1981.

50. Essen-Moller, E., & Hagness, O. The frequency and risk of depression within a rural population in Scandia. *Acta Psychiatr Scand*, 1961, 162(Suppl):28-32.

51. Orley, J., & Wing, J.K. Psychiatric disorders in two villages. *Arch Gen Psychiatry*, 1979, 36:513-520.

52. Schurman, R.A., Krooner, P.D., Mitchell, J.B. The hidden mental health network. Treatment of mental illness by nonpsychiatric physicians. *Arch Gen Psychiatry*, 1985, 42:89-94.

53. Coulehan, J.L., Schulberg, H.C., & Block, M.R. The efficiency of depression questionnaires for case finding in primary medical care. *J Gen Intern Med*, 1989, 4:541-547.

54. Attkisson, C.C., & Zich, J.M., (Eds.). *Depression in primary care: Screening and detection*. New York: Routledge, 1990.

55. Pérez-Stable, E.J., Miranda, J., Muñoz, R.F., & Ying, Y.W. Depression in medical outpatients. Underrecognition and misdiagnosis. *Arch Intern Med*, 1990, 150:1083.

56. Coyne, J.C., Schwenk, T.L., & Fechner-Bates, S. Nondetection of depression by primary care physicians reconsidered. *Gen Hosp Psychiatry*, 1995, 17:3-12.

57. Ormel, J., Koeter, M.W., van den Brink, W., & van de Willige, G. Recognition, management, and course of anxiety and depression in general practice. *Arch Gen Psychiatry*, 1991, 48:700.

58. Gerety, M.B., Williams, J.W., Jr., Mulrow, C.D., et al. Performance of case-finding tools for depression in the nursing home: Influence of clinical and functional characteristics and selection of optimal threshold scores. *J Am Geriatr Soc*, 1994, 42:1103.

59. Baron, J.A. The clinical utility of risk factor data. *J Clin Epidemiol*, 1989, 42:1013.

60. Boyko, E.J., & Alderman, B.W. The use of risk factors in medical diagnosis: Opportunities and cautions. *J Clin Epidemiol*, 1990, 43:851.

61. Kessler, R.C., McGonagle, K.A., Zhao, S., et al. Lifetime and 12-month prevalence of DSM-III-R psychiatric disorders in the United States. *Am J Psychiatry*, 1994, 51:8-19.

62. Regier, D.A., Boyd, J.H., Burke, J.D., Jr., et al. One-month prevalence of mental disorders in the United States. *Arch Gen Psychiatry*, 1988, 45:977.

63. Barker, L.R., Burton, J.R., Zieve, P.D., (Eds.). *Principles of ambulatory medicine*. Baltimore, MD: Williams & Wilkins, 1986.

64. Crum, R.M., Cooper-Patrick, L., & Ford, D.E. Depressive symptoms among general medical patients: Prevalence and one-year outcome. *Psychsom Med*, 1994, 56:109.

65. Spitzer, R.L., Williams, J.B., Kroenke, K., et al. Utility of a new procedure for diagnosing mental disorders in primary care. The PRIME-MD 1000 study. *JAMA*, 1994, 272:1749.

66. Csikszentmihalyi, M., & Graef, R. The experience of freedom in daily life. *Am J Comm Psychol*, 1980, 8:401-414.

67. Lawton, M.P., Devoe, M.R., & Parmalee, P. The relationship of events and affect in the daily life of an elderly population. *Psychol and Aging*, 1995, 10:469-477.

68. Larson, R.J., Zuzanek, J., & Mannell, R. Being alone

versus being with people: Disengagement in the daily experience of older adults. *J Gerontol*, 1985, 40:375-381.

69. Lawton, M.P., Devoe, M.R., & Parmalee, P. The relationship of events and affect in the daily life of an elderly population. *Psychol Aging*, 1985, 10:469-477.

70. Moldosfky, H., & Chester, W.J. Pain and mood patterns in patients with rheumatoid arthritis. *Psychosom Med*, 1970, 32:309-318.

71. Zautra, A.J., Finch, J.F., Reich, J.W., & Guarnaccia, C.A. Predicting the everyday life events of older adults. *J Pers*, 1991, 59:507-538.

72. Barge-Schaapveld, D.Q.C.M., Nicloson, N., van der Hoop, R. G., & DeVries, M.W. Changes in daily life experience associated with clinical improvement in depression. *J Affect Disord*, 1995, 34:139-154.

73. Larson, R., & Csikszentmihalyi, M. The experience sampling method. *New Directions Method Soc Behav Sci*, 1983, 3:41-56.

74. Hormuth, S.E. The sampling of experiences in situ. *J Pers*, 1986, 54:262-293.

75. Lyness, J.M., King, D.A., Cox C., et al. The importance of subsyndromal depression in older primary care patients: Prevalence and associated functional disability. *J Am Geriatr Soc*, 1999, 47(6):647.

76. Lyness, J.M., Caine, E.D., Conwell, Y. et al. Depressive symptoms, medical illness, and functional status in depressed psychiatric inpatients. *Am J Psychiatry*, 1993, 150(6):910.

77. Barge-Schaapveld, D.Q.C.M., Nicloson, N., Berkhof, J., & DeVries, M.W. Quality of life in depression: Daily life determinants and variabilty. *Psychiatry Res*, 1999, 88:173-189.

78. Spitzer, R.L., Williams, J.B.W., Gibbon, M., First, M.B. The structured clinical interview for DSM-IV-TR (SCID) I: History, rationale and description. *Arch Gen Psychiatry*, 2000, 49:624-629.

79. Williams, J.B.W., Gibbon, M., First, M.B., et al. The structured clinical interview for DSM-III-R (SCID) II: Multi site test-retest reliability, *Arch Gen Psychiatry*, 1992, 49:630-636.

80. Beck, A.T., Ward, C., & Mendelson. An inventory for measuring depression. *Arch Gen Psychiatry*, 1961, 4:53-63.

81. Beck, A.T., & Beamsderfer, A. Assessment of depression: The depression inventory. In: *Modern Problems in Pharmacopsychiatry*, 7, New York: Basel & Karger, 1974.

82. Beck, A.T., Steer, R.A., & Gurbin, M.G. Psychometric properties of the Beck Depression Inventory: Twenty-five years of evaluation. *Clin Psychol Rev*, 1988, 8, 77-100.

83. Radloff, L.S. The CES-D Scale: A self-report depression scale for researching the general population. *Appl Psychol Measures*, 1986, 1:385-401. Rodin, G. & Voshart, K. Depression in the medically ill: An overview. *Am J Psychiatry*, 1986, 14:696-705.

84. Comstock, G.W. & Helsing, K.J. Symptoms of depression in two communities. *Psychol Med*, 1976, 6:551.

85. Weissman, M.M., Sholomskas, D., Pottenger, M., et al. Assessing depressive symptoms in five psychiatric populations: A validation study. *Am J Epidemiol*, 1977, 106:203-214.

86. Roberts, R.E. Reliability of the CES-D scale in different ethnic contexts. *Psychiatr Res*, 1980, 2:125-134.

87. Derogatis, L., & Melisaratos, N. The Brief Symptom Inventory: An introductory report. *Psychol Med*, 1983, 13:595-605.

88. Derogatis, L. The SCL-90-R, BSI and matching clinical rating scales. In M. Maruish (Ed.), *Psychological testing, planning and outcome assesssment*. New York: Lawrence Erlbaum Assoc., 1993.

89. Yesavage, J.A., Brink, T.L. & Rose, T.L. Development and validation of a geriatric depression screening scale: A preliminary report. *J Psychiatr Res*, 1978, 17:699-706.

90. Hamilton, M.A. A rating scale for depression. *J Neurol Neurosurg Psychiatry*, 1960, 23:56-62.

91. Williams, J.B.W. A structured interview guide for the Hamilton Depression Rating Scale. *Arch Gen Psychiatry*, 1988, 45:742-747.

92. Carroll, B.J., Fielding, J.M., & Blashki, T.G. Depression rating scales: A critical review. *Arch Gen Psychiatry*, 1973, 28:361-366.

93. Cicchetti, D.V., & Prusoff, B.A. Reliability of depression and associated clinical symptoms. *Arch Gen Psychiatry*, 1983, 40:987-990.

94. Korner, A., Nielson, B.M., Eschen, F., et al. Quantifying depressive symptomatology: Inter-rater reliability and inter-item correlations. *J Affect Disord*, 1990, 20:143-149.

95. Maier, W., Heuser, I., Philipp, M. et al. Improving depression severity assessment. II. Content, concurrent and external validity of three observer depression scales. *J Psychiatr Res*, 1988, 22:13-19.

96. Potts, M.K., Daniels, M., Burnam, A., & Wells, K.B. A structured version of the Hamilton Depression Rating Scale: Evidence of reliability and ease of administration. *Psychiatr Res*, 1990, 24:335-350.

97. Simon, G.E., Revicki, D., & VonKorff, M. Telephone assessment of depression severity. *J Psychiatr Res*, 1993, 27:247-252.

98. Klein, D.G. Endogenomorphic depression. *Arch Gen Psychiatry*, 1974, 31:447-454.

99. Bramley, P.N., Easton, A.M.E., & Morley, S. The differentiation of anxiety and depression by rating scales. *Acta Psychiatr Scand*, 1988, 77:136-139.

100. Aylard, P.R., Gooding, G.H., & McKenna, P.J. A validation study of three anxiety and depression self assessment scales. *J Psychosom Res*, 1987, 31:261-268.

101. Moorey, S., Greer, S., Watson, M., et al. The factor structure and factor stability of the hospital anxiety and depression scale in patients with cancer. *Br J Psychiatry*, 1991, 158:255-259.

102. Zung, W.W.K. A self-rating depression scale. *Arch Gen Psychiatry*, 1965, 12:63-70.

103. Zung, W.W.K., Broadhead, W.E., & Roth, M.E. Prevalence of depressive symptoms in primary care. *J Fam Prac*, 1993, 37:337-344.

104. Pasacreta, J.V. Depressive phenomena, physical symptom distress and functional status among women with breast cancer. *Nurs Res*, 1997, 46(4):214.

25

Measuring Healthy Lifestyle

Ann Malone Berger and Susan Noble Walker

Since the mid-1970s, increasing interest in the relationship between lifestyle behavior and health has been evident in nursing and other disciplines. Researchers have examined the patterns of healthy lifestyle and the stages and processes of lifestyle behavior change to further our understanding of health-related behaviors. Since the publication of the Canadian LaLonde[1] report in 1974, national and international public health initiatives have emphasized disease prevention and health promotion and focused on lifestyle behaviors and individuals' responsibility to influence their own health. In most industrialized nations today, the leading causes of illness and death have shifted from communicable diseases to those chronic diseases that are strongly linked with personal lifestyle.

In the 1979 *Surgeon General's Report on Health Promotion and Disease Prevention*,[2] it was estimated that at least 50% of all deaths in the United States each year were the result of unhealthy lifestyles. After the release of that report, an agenda was developed of national health objectives to be achieved by 1990. It emphasized lifestyle modification as one major strategy to enhance health and prevent illness.[3] Although the objectives clearly focused more heavily on disease prevention than on health enhancement, the idea of health as a positive concept was introduced. Throughout the 1980s, data systems were established and expanded to track progress toward meeting the objectives, and nearly half of the objectives were wholly or partially accomplished by 1990.[4] Much of the major decline in death rates from heart disease, stroke, and unintentional injuries was attributed to reduction in risk factors associated with lifestyle behaviors, such as cigarette smoking, alcohol consumption, dietary fat intake, and sedentary lifestyle.

In 1991, *Healthy People 2000*[5] challenged the nation to move beyond measuring the health of the population by death rates to defining good health by reduction of unnecessary suffering, illness, and disability and by improvement in quality of life. That report suggested that personal responsibility is the key to good health and set forth objectives for the year 2000 in three broad categories: health promotion, health protection, and preventive services. The health-promotion objectives concerned "individual lifestyle-personal choices made in a social context-that can have a powerful influence over one's health prospects."[5] The current U.S. public health initiative, *Healthy People 2010*,[6] sets forth a comprehensive health-promotion and disease-prevention agenda for the nation, with 467 objectives organized in 28 focus areas. Focus areas with objectives concerning healthy lifestyle choices include nutrition and overweight, physical activity and fitness, mental health, and tobacco use. Each objective has a target outcome to be achieved by the year 2010. The National Center for Health Statistics (NCHS) coordinates the monitoring of progress on these objectives, using data from more than 150 different sources, including federal government departments and nongovernmental organizations. These data are available to researchers through DATA2010, an interactive database system accessible through the NCHS Web site.[7] If the vision for healthy people in healthy communities set forth in *Healthy People 2010* is to be achieved, it is essential to have a clear understanding of the nature of a healthy lifestyle and of why and how individuals acquire and maintain healthy lifestyle behavior patterns.

The Concept of Healthy Lifestyle

Although the term *healthy lifestyle* is used frequently in everyday conversation and in the public media, its use in scientific discourse has been far from consistent. It has been described in the literature in various ways; sometimes narrowly, as simply avoiding of bad health habits, and sometimes broadly, including all behaviors that have an impact on health status. Healthy lifestyle is central to the *American Journal of Health Promotion's* definition of health promotion, as "the science and art of helping people to change their lifestyle to move toward a state of optimal health."[8] Issues surrounding the conceptualization of healthy lifestyle and the related concepts of health and health promotion have been addressed thoughtfully and quite comprehensively by several nursing authors,[8–12] who have recognized the considerable ambiguity that currently exists. Healthy lifestyle has been conceptualized within the broader contexts of lifestyle and of health behavior. Both contexts provide important information contributing to the definition of the concept of healthy lifestyle.

Healthy Lifestyle as a Component of Lifestyle

The themes of personal responsibility and individual choice of behavior patterns are evident in definitions of both global and healthy lifestyle. For their study of the influence of selected lifestyle or personal practices on physical health, Wiley and Camacho defined lifestyle as "discretionary activities which are a regular part of an individual's daily pattern of living."[13] Ardell[14] advocated a wellness lifestyle to enable individuals to realize their highest potential for well-being. He described lifestyle as "the aggregation of all individual decisions affecting health status," incorporating "all those behaviors over which we have control, including those actions which affect our health risks."[14]

Many definitions also recognize that lifestyle choices take place in an environmental context. Bruhn[15] described lifestyle as (1) a person's way of life, with some aspects chosen and others determined by socioenvironmental factors, (2) long-term patterns encompassing behaviors and attitudes as well as a philosophy or outlook on life, and (3) components that are acquired and modified throughout life. He viewed health behaviors as an integral part of lifestyle and outlined characteristics of illness and wellness lifestyles. Abel addressed the need for a definition that could be operationalized in empirical research, and suggested that "health lifestyles comprise patterns of health-related behavior, values, and attitudes adapted [sic] by groups of individuals in response to their social, cultural and economic environment."[16] Milio characterized lifestyles as "patterns of choices [concerning personal behavior] made from the alternatives that are available to people according to their socioeconomic circumstances and to the ease with which they are able to choose certain ones over others."[17] Pender suggested that health as a positive life process may be experienced and expressed through lifestyle patterns, "person/environment interactional patterns that become increasingly complex throughout the lifespan."[18] She proposed five dimensions of lifestyle patterns through which health may be expressed-affect, attitudes, activity, aspirations, and accomplishments-and noted that some can be directly observed, whereas others must be self-reported.

Healthy Lifestyle as a Component of Health Behavior

The term *health behavior* first appeared in the literature when Kasl and Cobb differentiated sick role behavior and illness behavior from health behavior.[19] They defined health behavior as "any activity undertaken by a person believing himself to be healthy, for the purpose of preventing disease or detecting it in an asymptomatic stage."[19] Since that time, the term has been used in various ways and applied in a variety of populations. Although some authors, like Kasl and Cobb, restrict the definition of health behavior to action or activity, others expand the definition to encompass various cognitive elements of behavior. Gochman provides a broadly constructed definition of health behavior as "personal attributes such as beliefs, expectations, motives, values, perceptions, and other cognitive elements; personality characteristics, including affective and emotional states and traits; and overt behavior patterns, actions, and habits that relate to health maintenance, to health restoration, and to health improvement.[20] He notes that such a definition includes mental events and feeling states that must be measured indirectly, as well as overt actions that can be observed directly. Although health behavior was initially conceptualized as applicable only to those who were healthy,[19] its relevance for those with chronic illnesses conditions has since been recognized. Various authors advocate the value of health-promoting behaviors for those with diabetes,[21] cancer,[22] multiple sclerosis,[23] and Parkinson's disease.[24]

Laffrey, Loveland-Cherry, and Winkler[25] summarized the definitions of health behavior found in the nursing and public health literature as including the use of health care services, compliance with medically prescribed regimens, routine activities of one's life, actions taken to prevent illness, and actions taken to achieve a higher level of well-being. They associated these diverse definitions of health behavior with two major paradigms that reflect different views of health: the pathogenic or disease paradigm, in which health behavior is conceptualized as preventing or detecting disease, and the health paradigm, in which health behavior is conceptualized as promoting higher levels of health or wellness. In the disease paradigm, health behavior is variously labeled as illness-preventing, risk-reducing, or health-protecting. The original definition by Kasl and Cobb[19] reflects this preventive orientation. An extensive body of evidence linking certain lifestyle behaviors (such as cigarette smoking, physical inactivity, and alcohol consumption) to disease and death has accumulated since the 1960s.[26,27] Preventive health behaviors may be isolated acts, such as obtaining an influenza vaccination, or lifestyle, components such as performing monthly breast self-examination or regularly wearing seat belts.

Within the health paradigm, health behavior is labeled health-promoting or wellness-enhancing. Although a preventive orientation dominates much of the literature on health behavior, a promotive orientation is increasingly prominent. It is strongly evident in the salutogenic framework for health proposed by Antonovsky,[28] in the high-level wellness literature,[29,30] and in the work in nursing of Laffrey[31] and Pender.[32] As an expression of the actualizing tendency, health-promoting behaviors are pursued because they are satisfying and enjoyable rather than to avoid disease or premature death.[14,32] Health-promoting behaviors are continuous activities considered to be an integral part of one's lifestyle. Walker et al. defined health-promoting lifestyle behavior as "a multidimensional pattern of self-initiated actions and perceptions that serve to maintain or enhance the level of wellness, self-actualization, and fulfillment of the individual.[33] The Alameda County Study of Health and Ways of Living, begun in 1965 at the Human Population Laboratory, provided perhaps the first definitive link between lifestyle behaviors and positive health consequences (defined as physical, mental, and social well-being). That work was important because it suggested that "certain behaviors have generalized health, rather than just specific disease, consequences."[34] Support for the association of health behaviors with high-level wellness, a holistic outcome, is more theoretical than empirical at this time. As health disciplines embrace wellness and quality of life as outcomes valued as highly as declines in morbidity and mortality rates, more research undoubtedly will address such connections.

Dimensions of Healthy Lifestyle

Interest in the concepts of health promotion and healthy lifestyle has expanded in the scientific arena, including that of nursing science. A literature review identified only one nursing research report concerned with preventive health behavior or health-promotion behavior published between 1958 and 1980, and thirty between 1980 and 1992.[35] In contrast, a search of CINAHL identified 130 research articles published between 1993 and early 2003 concerned with preventive health behavior or health-promoting lifestyle behavior and 62 concerned with health risk appraisal. There has been much discussion among nurse researchers as to whether (1) health-promoting behavior should be differentiated from illness-preventing behavior; (2) preventive behavior might be subsumed as a category of promotive behavior; (3) illness-preventing, health-maintaining, and health-promoting behaviors might be placed on a continuum of promotiveness; or (4) health-protecting and health-promoting behaviors might be viewed as two complementary components of a healthy lifestyle.[9,11,25,31,32,35] It is recognized that particular lifestyle behaviors, such as exercise, may be undertaken by some individuals to prevent cardiovascular disease, by others to promote a feeling of well-being, and by still others for reasons that are unrelated to health, such as socializing. For some research purposes the nature of motivation for healthy lifestyle behaviors is important, whereas for others it is not. Consensus has not been achieved concerning the dimensionality of healthy lifestyles. Categories of preventive and promotive behaviors mentioned in the literature as components of healthy lifestyles can be summarized as:

Self-responsibility for health	Stress management, rest, and sleep
Physical activity and exercise	Accident or injury prevention
Nutrition	Smoking avoidance or cessation
Interpersonal relationships/support	Spiritual growth, fulfillment of potential
Safe use of medications and alcohol	Sexual behaviors

Continued identification of the dimensions of healthy lifestyle is important to further the development of instruments as well as knowledge in this area.

Summary

Some defining characteristics of a healthy lifestyle emerge repeatedly, although not unanimously, from the literature. Healthy lifestyle includes complex multidimensional patterns of behavior that have cognitive, affective, or emotional, as well as action or activity elements. Healthy lifestyle behavior is self-initiated, voluntary, and individually chosen from available options and influenced by socioenvironmental and other contextual factors. It is a continuing and consistent long-term, but modifiable, pattern of behavior integrated into daily living as a way of life. Healthy lifestyle serves to prevent illness and maintain or enhance wellness, whether engaged in for health consequences or not, and regardless of the individual's current state of health.

Issues in Instrument Selection

Relatively few instruments measure healthy lifestyle behaviors. Early tools were developed as health risk appraisals (HRAs) and focused on risk reduction through adoption of preventive behaviors specific to particular diseases, such as smoking and lung cancer. More recent instruments measure both risk potential and health-promoting lifestyle behaviors, or health-promoting lifestyle alone.

When selecting an instrument, it is important to consider the lifestyle dimensions assessed, relevance for the population being studied, length, method of administration and reporting results, and cost for use. The researcher should look for evidence of reliability and validity, including the populations in which they were evaluated and the instrument's ability to discriminate among distinct groups,[16] cultural sensitivity,[36] and, for intervention research, sensitivity to change over time.[37] Caution must be exercised to ensure that a tool developed for one population is not automatically transferred to a second with different characteristics, such as race, culture, or age. With HRAs, it is important to consider whether the tool identifies individual characteristics that affect life expectancy based on current scientific knowledge.[38]

It is recognized that, although some healthy lifestyle behaviors may be observed directly, self-report is necessary for comprehensive measurement of the concept. Kirscht[39] points out that self-report is needed because many behaviors cannot be observed at all or cannot be observed on enough occasions to provide reliable data. The accuracy of self-report is generally good but may be threatened by inaccurate recall or by intentional false responses resulting from sensitive issues or perceived social desirability. Information on health issues obtained by telephone interviews has been shown to be as reliable and valid as information obtained by face-to-face or mail interview.[40] A few self-reported behaviors, such as smoking and drug use, can be validated with biologic measures. Reliability and validity can be enhanced by the specificity of measurement tools and by multiple modes of assessment of the same behavior when feasible.[39,41]

A major issue in selecting instrumentation is that if lifestyle represents patterns of coherent behaviors, then measurement must go beyond single health behaviors to clusters of behaviors that show linkages. Clusters of behaviors have been demonstrated in several studies, with correlations among preventive health behaviors that vary across studies but are generally of low to moderate magnitude.[39,42] Higher correlations have been shown among promotive health behaviors.[33] There clearly is not yet sufficient internal consistency of items or statistical association among a comprehensive set of preventive and promotive healthy lifestyle behaviors to permit measurement by any single scale.

Instruments designed to measure healthy lifestyle operationalize the concept in a variety of ways, some narrower and some broader. Instruments described in this chapter provide more comprehensive measurement of either or both of the health-protecting and health-promoting behavioral components of a healthy lifestyle, rather than measurement of single behaviors or behavioral sets (such as nutrition or smoking). They are arranged in sequence from those that emphasize preventive behaviors to those that emphasize promotive behaviors.

Health Risk Appraisal

Most HRAs are derived from the original Centers for Disease Control and Prevention (CDC) version developed by the U.S. government in the late 1970s or from the Carter Center revision in 1988. HRAs were developed primarily to assist health professionals in practice settings to educate and counsel patients to modify hazardous behaviors. HRAs also have been used as a screening tool, a research tool, and a baseline or outcome measure to evaluate health-promotion programs.

An HRA is a personalized estimation of one's risk for dying or major illness in the next 10 years from each of the most frequent causes of death. Risks are calculated by a computer program that compares the individual's characteristics to national mortality statistics using equations developed by epidemiologists and updated on a routine basis. These risks are communicated to the client through a personalized or group report, as illustrated in Figure 25.1. The report accounts for both controllable and uncontrollable risk factors but emphasizes that the individual should focus on modifiable risk factors. Although the HRA estimates the probability of specified outcomes among groups of persons with similar characteristics, it cannot predict the precise outcome for each individual.

In HRAs, risk is expressed in terms of both risk age and health score. The ideal score is a risk age lower than real age or a health score of 100 points. Risk age is calculated first on the basis of current risk factors and a second time as if the risk factors were reduced as much as possible by adopting healthier lifestyle behaviors. The second "target" risk

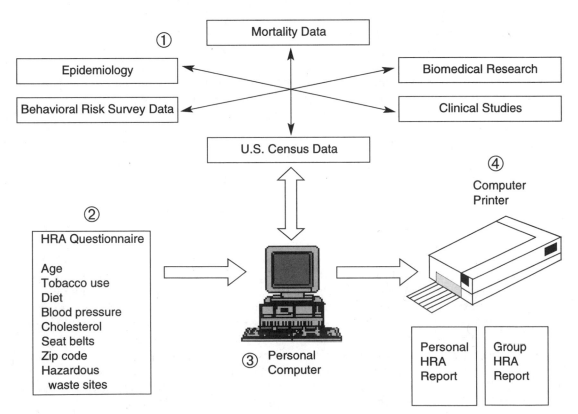

Figure 25.1   Components of a health risk appraisal. Adapted with permission of the Healthier People Network, Inc., Atlanta, GA.

age shows the potential health benefit to the individual of improving lifestyle through the elimination of risky behaviors. Estimates of risks are imperfect because of individual variance in susceptibility to disease. Risk age provides useful feedback to stimulate individual behavior change, but the health score appears most suitable in research, particularly when it involves inferential statistical analysis. Health scores range from 0 to 100 (maximum incorporation of risk-reducing behaviors into one's lifestyle).[43] Gustafson[44] states that the effectiveness of the HRA should be measured by how it influences individuals to make recommended behavior changes to improve their health score.

The HRA has a high degree of face validity, and its use as an awareness and educational tool in health-promotion programs is strongly supported in the literature. Establishing the reliability, validity, and effectiveness of HRAs is critical to future use and development of this technology for research purposes. When it is used to predict risk or evaluate a program, questions remain unanswered. In the most rigorous scientific sense, reliability and validity are minimally acceptable because many health risk factors have yet to be determined.[45] Test-retest reliability coefficients have ranged from 0.99 on many items to considerably lower levels (0.23-0.65) for self-reported blood pressure, cholesterol levels, and dietary patterns.[45] Item reliability is enhanced when clinical screening includes the actual measurement of blood pressure, cholesterol, and body weight and height at the time of HRA administration.[46]

To be scientifically credible, the HRA must identify high-risk individuals. The validity of risk estimates depends on the ratio of known to unknown plus chance etiologic factors related to the leading causes of death. Validity is based on the accuracy of the algorithms derived from death certificate data, epidemiologic and clinical data, and respondents' self-reports of risk factors. Results are limited by the availability and accuracy of statistics used to estimate risks and by the method used to handle missing data.[47,48] When comparing the CDC version with the Carter Center version, Gazmararian et al.[48] found that, although the CDC version was a more accurate predictor of 10-year mortality, the predictive validity of each version was sufficient to warrant their continued use.

In the early 1990s, there was steady growth and widespread distribution of HRAs. Many areas in HRAs still can be further developed. No risk indicators are available yet for many common and serious health problems, and only healthy people receive reliable risk estimates from the HRAs, as they are not designed to be used with people already diagnosed with chronic diseases. In summary, HRA technology has demonstrated adequate reliability, validity, and effectiveness to encourage continued development for use in research.

The Healthier People Network (HRA)

The CDC-HRA was first developed by the CDC and made available in 1980. *Healthier People* version 4.0, a revised version of the CDC-HRA, was a microcomputer-based HRA. It was updated and published in 1991 as a result of a joint venture between the CDC and the private sector (Carter Center of Emory University). After the Carter Center discontinued its involvement in 1991, the Healthier People Network (HPN) was founded to continue the scientific development and distribution of the HRA. This nonprofit organization is supported by federal contracts, foundation grants, and user fees.[49] The goals of the HPN are to update the HRAs in a timely manner as scientific knowledge changes and to disseminate them to health-promotion professionals so they can inform the public of their health risks. The HPN HRA software program uses an individual's health-related behaviors and personal characteristics, U.S. mortality statistics, and epidemiologic data to compute that individual's probability of dying in the next 10 years from 42 causes of death. Version 6.0 of the HRA Midlife Questionnaire became available in 1997 using probability data from the 1990 census. A set of 43 questions cover topics such as demographics, blood pressure, cholesterol, driving, smoking, alcohol use, and gender-specific health issues. A sample item is "On the average, how close to the speed limit do you usually drive?" Most questions have a forced-choice answer format, and some require a fill-in-the-blank response. After completion of computer analysis based on the latest mortality data, the two-page report to the participant highlights health risks affecting life expectancy and pinpoints risks that the individual can control. The report also provides information and general recommendations about preventive services. The HPN report should always be interpreted to the client by a qualified health professional. A group report also is available to assess the health status of an employee group as a basis for establishing priorities for an organization's health-promotion program efforts.

In addition to the software program, a camera-ready copy of the four-page questionnaire and a manual are provided. The manual outlines the computer program's structure and risk calculations and includes step-by-step operating instructions. The HPN HRA Midlife Questionnaire will be revised and released as soon as 2000 census data is analyzed to recalculate health risks and odds of death. A Spanish-language version is available.

A Health Risk Appraisal for Older Adults (HRA-OA)

The HPN also has developed an HRA for older adults.[49] Participants complete a printed questionnaire that is processed by a HPN computer program to generate a printed report. The HRA-OA, printed in 14-point type, consists of the 43 questions of the Midlife Adult HRA, plus additional questions for people ages 55–90. Whereas the calculations for the Midlife questions are based on mortality statistics, the added questions for the HRA-OA focus on functional status and morbidity. These questions are divided into eight modules: existing conditions—29 questions; home safety—13 questions; functional status—22 questions; nutrition—26 questions; social support—12 questions; mental health—20 questions; vision, hearing, and dental—22 questions; and demographics—8 questions.

The individualized report consists of a standard report for the Midlife HRA questions plus a report for the following outcomes: risk for institutionalization, hearing impairment, home environment hazards, functional status, nutrition, burns and fire-related injury, physical disability, adverse drug reactions, tetanus, falls, influenza/pneumonia, existing conditions, vision impairment, mental health, and social support.

The outcomes, precursors, and questions appropriate for the older adult population were selected after an extensive literature review. A draft of the questionnaire was field-tested in five states with various populations with 1400 subjects. The HRA-OA was well received by the participants, most of whom completed the questionnaire in less 1/2 hour. The results of the field-test reports were compiled and analyzed to arrive at norms, which are used to develop the morbidity and functional status estimates and report modules.

Other Instruments

Youth Risk Behavior Survey (YRBS)

The YRBS is a survey instrument developed by the CDC for use within the Youth Risk Behavior Surveillance System (YRBSS).[50] The YRBS is a school-based epidemiologic surveillance system designed to monitor progress toward 16 national health objectives and 3 of the 10 leading health indicators for 2010[6] and to provide comparable national, state, and local data across six categories of behavior.[51,52] The Division of Adolescent and School Health (DASH) in the CDC conducts a biennial survey to measure the prevalence of the identified priority health risk behaviors among a national probability sample of students in grades 9-12. The CDC also provides fiscal and technical assistance to state and local education departments who wish to use the YRBS to assess the prevalence of these health risk behaviors among youth in their locales.

The YRBS focuses on those behaviors established during youth that contribute to the leading causes of mortality, morbidity, and social problems during both youth and adulthood. Those six priority areas of health risk behavior include (1) behaviors that may result in violence and unintentional injuries (motor vehicle crashes); (2) alcohol and other drug use; (3) tobacco use; (4) sexual behaviors that may result in HIV infection, other sexually transmitted diseases, and unintended pregnancies; (5) unhealthy dietary behaviors; and (6) inadequate physical activity. The 2003 YRBS High School Questionnaire is a self-administered, 87-item, multiple-choice questionnaire with a standard scannable "bubble sheet" that can be used to record responses. It has a seventh-grade reading level and was designed for use with adolescents during a typical 45-minute school class period. It includes 7 demographic items and 80 behavioral items; varied response options include yes/no, age when a behavior was started, and frequency of behaviors within the past 30 days or the past 12 months. An example of an item is "How old were you when you had your first drink of alcohol other than a few sips?" (never, 8 years old or younger, 9 or 10, 11 or 12, 13 or 14, 15 or 16, 17 or older).

Results are reported for aggregates rather than individuals. The process of development of the YRBS produced content validity through the use of panels of experts who delineated priority behaviors consistent with national health objectives and devised questions to measure those behaviors. No empirical evidence of validity or reliability is available. However, development included four waves of field-testing with national, state, and local samples of high school students that strengthened the tool through various revisions of wording, response categories, and recall periods before its release in 1990. The CDC, in collaboration with representatives from universities, relevant national organizations, and federal agencies, modified the questionnaire for college populations. The resulting National College Health Risk Behavior Survey (NCHRBS) was conducted through the mail in 1995 with a scientific sample of students enrolled in public and private, 2- and 4-year colleges and universities.[53] The CDC plans to repeat the NCHRBS in 2003.

Index of Health Practices

The Index of Health Practices was developed as one component of a more extensive questionnaire used within the Human Population Laboratory Studies in Alameda County, California, in the 1960s.[26] It is the first measure of health behaviors to be used as a public health screening instrument. The index contains seven items pertaining to habits of sleep, eating, exercise, alcohol consumption, and smoking. The items were developed from a literature review; however, little empirical evidence to support the selected items was available at the time. The index was designed to measure health habits in a study examining the relationship between "good" health habits and physical health status. Based on data from that survey of 6928 adults, the researchers reported that responses to the items were highly reliable. Although the small number of items gives rise to concerns about the instrument's sampling validity as a comprehensive measure of healthy lifestyle, the criterion-oriented validity for this tool appears to be excellent. Health practices measured by this index have been correlated with physical health status and with mortality. The tool's restricted number of items and lack of detail concerning the assessed health habits limit its usefulness.

Lifestyle Assessment Questionnaire (LAQ)

The LAQ, developed in 1976 by the National Wellness Institute, has been a popular and useful lifestyle assessment instrument for research. *Wellness* is described by the developer of this instrument as a continuous, active process rather than as a single goal or achievement. The process involves becoming aware of various areas in one's life, identifying the areas that need improvement, and then making choices that will help to attain a higher level of health and well-being. The LAQ contained four sections: (1) a TestWell® Wellness Inventory (assessment of lifestyle behaviors), (2) an HRA, (3) personal data, and (4) personal growth (an opportunity to obtain a bibliography of publications on 43 topics). The complete LAQ was available in both paper-and-pencil and computer versions, but these are no longer available for purchase.

The TestWell® Wellness Inventory component of the LAQ is now available online, with adult (50 and 100 items), teen (50 and 100 items), college (50 and 100 items) and older adult (50 items) versions.[54] It is based on a six-dimensional model of wellness, with physical, emotional, occupational, intellectual, spiritual, and social areas. Each version's question set consists of 10 sections: physical activity, nutrition, self-care, safety, social and environmental wellness, emotional wellness and sexuality, emotional management, intellectual wellness, occupational wellness, and spirituality and values. A example of an item is "I am satisfied with the balance between my work time and leisure time." Each item is scored on a scale ranging from 1 (almost never) to 5 (almost always). Item scores are summed to obtain a subscale score for each section, and subscale scores then are summed to obtain a total score. Content validity was established by a panel of health-promotion experts for the original LAQ items, and components of reliability and validity of the TestWell Wellness Inventory have been reported with high school and graduate students.[55]

Wellness Index and Wellness Inventory

Wellness Associates is a nonprofit educational organization that is the successor to the Wellness Resource Center founded by Dr. John W. Travis in 1975. In the *Wellness Workbook*, Travis and Ryan[30] describe a model of wellness that views the individual and environment as interacting in a Wellness Energy System, with system output consisting of 12 dimensions of wellness: self-responsibility and love, breathing, sensing, eating, moving, feeling, thinking, playing and working, communicating, sex, finding meaning, and transcending. These dimensions are depicted on 12 sections of a Wellness Wheel that reflects how well an individual's energy is balanced. Dimension scores to be recorded on the Wellness Wheel can be obtained from a full-length Wellness Index or an abbreviated Wellness Inventory.

The Wellness Index is a 380-item self-scoring questionnaire for adults that is included in the Wellness Workbook[30] and available as a separate booklet.[56] The number of items in each of the 12 sections varies from 19 in the wellness and thinking section to 71 in the wellness, self-responsibility, and love section. Responses are recorded on a 5-point scale ranging from 0 (no, never, or hardly ever) to 4 (yes, always, or usually). The Wellness Inventory (3rd edition) is a 120-item abridged form of the questionnaire that contains 10 items in each of the 12 sections and is available both in a 12-page pamphlet[57] and an interactive computer version.[58] The response format also is abridged to a 3-point scale ranging from 0 (no, rarely) to 2 (yes, usually). Items on the Wellness Index and Wellness Inventory are described as wellness attributes that reflect both awareness and action based on awareness. A sample item is "I meditate or relax myself for at least 15 (to 20) minutes each day." Both questionnaires can be self-scored, and scores for each of the 12 wellness dimensions are transferred onto the Wellness Wheel to assess balance. The interactive computer version of the Wellness Inventory displays both the individual's score and level of satisfaction, with answers in each section. The experience of completing either of these tools is designed to educate more than to test the individual. These questions are recommended for initial wellness assessment sessions to increase clients' awareness of healthy lifestyle and assist in developing priorities and plans for lifestyle change. They have not been subjected to psychometric evaluation for use in research. The authors do not present their methodology for item or scale development and state that "much wellness information is subjective and 'unprovable' by current scientific methods."[28,pxxvii] No information about reliability or validity is available.

Personal Lifestyle Questionnaire (PLQ)

The PLQ was developed by Muhlenkamp and Brown[59–61] to measure the extent of individuals' participation in health-related or health-promotion activities; these terms are not conceptually defined. The 24-item instrument includes three to five items in each of six categories of health practices: exercise, substance use, nutrition, relaxation, safety, and general health promotion. Items are scored on a 4-point Likert scale ranging from 1 (never) to 4 (almost always). An example of an item is "See a health-care provider for a check-up at least yearly." A subscale score may be obtained for each of the six categories; a total score, called Lifestyle, is computed by adding the scores obtained on the six subscales. The authors indicated that they have more confidence in the use of the total score than in the subscale scores,[59] and validity and reliability data support that conclusion.[59–60]

Development of the item pool for the PLQ is not described. Construct validity was assessed by means of a factor analysis of the responses of 380 subjects to determine the validity of the six theorized categories. Seven factors emerged, five of which were almost identical to the original subscales. Intercorrelations between subscale scores ranged from 0.003 to 0.42.[59] Only 0.002% of the variance on the PLQ total score was attributed to social desirability in a sample of 175 nursing clinic clients.[60] Convergent validity of the scale was assessed by administering it with the National Wellness Institute's Lifestyle Assessment Questionnaire; correlation coefficients of 0.83 and 0.72 were obtained in two separate samples. Concurrent validity was assessed in a sample of 127 individuals by correlating the PLQ score with an HRA-modifiable risk score (risk that can be lowered by changing health behaviors), with an r of –0.25.[59] Internal consistency of the total scale was acceptable, with alpha coefficients of 0.74 and 0.76 in samples of 133 and 383 subjects. Subscale coefficients ranged from 0.24 to 0.75, so that some would not be acceptable for use in inferential research. The PLQ's test-retest reliability coefficient was 0.78 over a 4-week period and 0.88 over a 3-week period with small samples.[59,60] The PLQ may be a useful short instrument to measure a combination of preventive and promotive health practices among adults when restricted to use of the total score. The PLQ is available from the Graduate Program and Research Office, College of Nursing, Arizona State University, Tempe.

The PLQ was evaluated by Mahon, Yarcheski, and Yarcheski for use with adolescents.[62] In a sample of 222 adolescents aged 15 to 21, factor analysis yielded two factors based on a priori criteria. Factor I (labeled, general health practices) included 13 of 17 items from the exercise, nutrition, relaxation, safety, and general health-promotion subscales, and Factor II included all 4 of the substance abuse items. Internal consistency of the general health practices subscale was acceptable with an alpha coefficient of 0.72, but that of the substance abuse subscale was unacceptably low at 0.58. The authors recognize the limitations of such a short scale, but suggest that the general health practices scale derived from the PLQ may be useful for assessing positive health practices among adolescents.

Health-Promoting Lifestyle Profile II (HPLPII)

The Health-Promoting Lifestyle Profile (HPLP), developed by Walker et al.[33] for use in testing the Health Promotion Model, has been widely used. It measures health-promoting lifestyle, conceptualized as a "multidimensional pattern of self-initiated actions and perceptions that serve to maintain or enhance the level of wellness, self-actualization, and fulfillment of the individual."[33] The item pool for the original HPLP was developed from a 100-item yes/no checklist designed as a clinical nursing tool. Items concerned with prevention or detection of specific diseases were deleted because they lacked concept validity. Empirical validation resulted in the elimination of all items concerned with undesirable health behaviors (e.g., smoking and excessive alcohol consumption). Factor analysis isolated six dimensions used as subscales, and second-order factor analysis yielded a single factor, interpreted as health-promoting lifestyle, the multidimensional construct measured by the instrument. A Spanish-language version of the tool became available in 1990. It was found to be culturally relevant, reliable (total alpha 0.93, subscale alphas 0.70-0.87), and valid as evidenced by factor analysis that explained 45.9% of the variance in the measure.[63]

A revised and updated version, the HPLPII, replaced the HPLP in 1995.[64] This 52-item summated behavior-rating scale uses a 4-point ordinal response format to measure the frequency of self-reported health-promoting behaviors. Responses range from 1 (never) to 4 (routinely). The HPLPII consists of a total scale and six subscales (8 to 9 items each) that measure the dimensions of health-promoting lifestyle: health responsibility, physical activity, nutrition, interpersonal relations, spiritual growth, and stress management. A sample item is "Eat 3-5 servings of vegetables each day." A score for overall health-promoting lifestyle is obtained by calculating a mean of the individual's response to all 52 items; six subscale scores are the means of responses to subscale items. The use of mean scores retains the 1-to-4 measurement of item responses and allows meaningful comparisons of scores across subscales.

Psychometric evaluation of the HPLPII was undertaken in a community sample of 712 adults.[64] Construct validity was examined with traditional factor analysis employing principal axis extraction followed by oblique rotation. A six-factor solution resulted in the Spiritual Growth and Interpersonal Relations subscale items loading together, the other four subscale items loading cleanly on separate factors at levels of 0.43 or greater, and a nuisance factor with no significant loadings. Spiritual Growth and Interpersonal Relations were recognized as closely aligned concepts, both involving a sense of connectedness and belonging. A seven-factor solution included six factors that were interpretable as hypothesized and the nuisance factor. Confirmatory factor analysis using LISREL was employed to evaluate the hypothesized six-dimensional structure of health-promoting lifestyle, with the subscales permitted to correlate with each other. Fit indices indicated that the model fit the data well (GFI 0.980; AGFI 0.940; RMSR 0.034). Convergent validity was assessed by comparing it to the PLQ; the correlation of the HPLPII and the PLQ total scores among a subset of 80 adults was 0.678. Social desirability explained only 1.4% of the variance in responses on the HPLPII among a subset of 80 adults. Concurrent criterion-related validity was evidenced by the relationship of health-promoting lifestyle to the outcomes of perceived health status and quality of life. The correlation of the HPLPII with the Medical Outcomes Study Short-Form General Health Survey general health perception scale was 0.269 in a subset of 158 adults, and correlation with the Quality of Life Index was 0.464 in a subset of 49 adults. The total scale was found to have high internal consistency, with an alpha coefficient of 0.943, and the subscales had acceptable internal consistency with alpha coefficients ranging from 0.793 to 0.872 among a sample of 712. Test-retest stability among 26 undergraduate nursing students at a 3-week interval was $r = 0.892$. The HPLP and HPLPII have been used with numerous healthy populations: the full range of adult age groups and clinical disorders such as, heart disease, hypertension, cancer, schizophrenia, diabetes, AIDS, and multiple sclerosis. A Spanish-language version of the HPLPII became available in 2002. The HPLPII is copyrighted and can be obtained from Dr. Susan Noble Walker, College of Nursing, University of Nebraska Medical Center, Omaha. Pender reports that psychometric testing of an adolescent version of the HPLPII is in progress.[32]

Summary

In the 1970s HRAs were developed by epidemiologists to assess lifestyle behaviors associated with an increased risk of preventable death. During the 1980s, an emerging emphasis on health promotion was accompanied by the development of a few instruments to measure lifestyle behaviors believed to be associated with health and wellness. Most instruments presented in this chapter have established reliability and validity. Most are designed for use with adults and late adolescents. The development of additional instruments to measure the healthy lifestyle behaviors of children and adolescents is needed to further understanding of behavior patterns during these critical developmental periods.

Healthy lifestyle behavior is an area of interdisciplinary interest. Research has initially focused largely on descriptive studies and the testing of conceptual frameworks. Findings from a few studies point to the existence of discrete clusters of behavior in various samples.[9,42,60,65] Many investigations examine only a few preventive and/or promotive behaviors, and little is currently known about how the full range of healthy lifestyle behaviors relate to one another. More work is needed to further understanding of how change in one dimension of healthy lifestyle may facilitate or impede simultaneous or subsequent change in others. The development of childhood health beliefs and behaviors and of family patterns of behavior also are important areas for investigation. Research in the past decade has included intervention and outcome studies. However, these have tended to target only one or occasionally two behaviors rather than the full constellation of healthy lifestyles behaviors and have focused more on the adoption of behavior(s) rather than long-term maintenance and lifestyle change.

Linkages between individual lifestyle behaviors and health outcomes have become more apparent, but knowledge alone has not been sufficient to produce lasting behavior change. Researchers have proposed a variety of paradigms to explain why people engage in healthy lifestyle behavior, including the Health Belief Model,[66] the Health Promotion Model,[32] the Theory of Reasoned Action,[67] the Transtheoretical Model,[68] the Resource Model of Preventive Health Behavior,[10] and others that focus on the determinants of individual behavior. Research is just beginning to build has built a knowledge base concerning the linkages between demographic, cognitive/perceptual and socio-environmental factors, and patterns of healthy lifestyle in individuals and populations. Several literature reviews have summarized the findings published to date.[32,35,39,69,70–71] Although theoretical models that describe the determinants and process of health behavior change are readily available, their utility in guiding the design of behavior change interventions is only beginning to be investigated. There is heightened interest in and funding available to support research focusing on healthy lifestyle behavior change to reduce morbidity, mortality, and functional decline associated with chronic conditions; to control health care expenditures; and to improve the well-being of individuals throughout the lifespan.

Exemplar Study

Frank-Stromborg, M., Pender, N., Walker, S., & Sechrist, K. Determinants of health-promoting lifestyle in ambulatory cancer patients. *Soc Sci Med*, 1990, *31*(10):1159-1168.

This study sought to determine the degree to which cognitive-perceptual and modifying variables identified in the Health Promotion Model[32] explained the occurrence of health-promoting behaviors in a sample of 385 adults undergoing cancer treatment. A secondary purpose was to determine the potential for illness-specific, cognitive-perceptual, and modifying variables to explain further the occurrence of health-promoting behaviors in adults with cancer. Multiple regression analyses revealed that 23.5% of the variance in health-promoting lifestyle was explained by three cognitive-perceptual variables from the model (definition of health, perceived health status, and perceived control of health) and four modifying variables (education, income, age, and employment). When illness-specific variables were added to the analysis, initial reaction to the diagnosis of cancer was found to be a significant contributor to the regression. The study results support the importance of both general health-related and cancer-specific cognitive-perceptual factors in explaining the occurrence of health-enhancing behaviors among ambulatory cancer patients. Researchers concluded that these factors may therefore be suitable targets for interventions to encourage the adoption of healthy lifestyles. This study is exemplary in that it uses a conceptual model to frame the study, increases understanding of health-promoting lifestyles in adults with cancer, and establishes a rationale for future theory testing and research in clinical populations.

References

1. LaLonde, M. *A new perspective on the health of Canadians*. Ottawa: Government of Canada, 1974.
2. U.S. Department of Health Education and Welfare. *Healthy people: The Surgeon General's Report on Health Promotion and Disease Prevention*. Washington, DC: U.S. Government Printing Office, 1979.
3. U.S. Department of Health and Human Services (DHHS). Public Health Service. *Promoting health: Preventing disease: Objectives for the nation*. Rockville, MD: U.S. Department of Health and Human Services, 1980.
4. National Center for Health Statistics. *Health, United States, 1989 and prevention profile*. Hyattsville, MD: U.S. DHHS, 1990.
5. U.S. DHHS. *Healthy People 2000: National health promotion and disease prevention objectives*. Washington, DC: U. S. Government Printing Office, 1991.
6. U.S. DHHS. *Healthy People 2010, With understanding and improving health and objectives for improving health*. 2nd ed. 2 vols. Washington, DC: U.S. Government Printing Office, November 2000. Access date 7 Mar 2003. http://www.healthypeople.gov.
7. CDC, National Center for Health Statistics. Healthy people: Tracking the nation's health. Updated 15 Jan 2003. Access date 7 Mar 2003. www.cdc.gov/nchs/hphome.htm.
8. O'Donnell, M.P. Definition of health promotion. *Am J Health Prom*, 1986, 1:4-5.
9. Brubaker, B.H. Health promotion: A linguistic analysis. *Adv Nurs Sci*, 1983, *5*(3):1-14.
10. Kulbok, P.A. Social resources, health resources, and preventive health behavior: Patterns and predictors. *Public Health Nurs*, 1985, *2*(2):67-81.
11. Pender, N. Health and health promotion: Conceptual dilemmas. In M. Duffy & N. Pender (Eds.), *Conceptual issues in health promotion*. Indianapolis, IN: Sigma Theta Tau, 1987, pp. 7-23.
12. Pender, N.J., Barkauskas, V.H., Hayman, L., et al. Health promotion and disease prevention: Toward excellence in nursing practice and education. *Nurs Outlook*, 1992, *40*(3):106-112.
13. Wiley, J., & Camacho, T. Life-style and future health: Evidence from the Alameda County study. *Prev Med*, 1980, 9:1-21.
14. Ardell, D.B. The nature and implications of high level wellness, or why "normal health" is a rather sorry state of existence. *Health Values Achiev High Lev Wellness*, 1979, *3*(1):16-24.
15. Bruhn, J.G. Life-style and health behavior. In D.S. Gochman (Ed.), *Health behavior: Emerging research perspectives*. New York: Plenum, 1988.
16. Abel, T. Measuring health lifestyles in a comparative analysis: Theoretical issues and empirical findings. *Soc Sci Med*, 1991, *32*(8):899-908.
17. Milio, N. *Promoting health through public policy*. Philadelphia: Davis, 1981.

18. Pender, N.J. Expressing health through lifestyle patterns. *Nurs Sci Q*, 1990, *3*(3):115-122.
19. Kasl, S., & Cobb, S. Health behavior, illness behavior. *Arch Environ Health*, 1966, *12*:246.
20. Gochman, D.S. Health behavior: Plural perspectives. In D.S. Gochman (Ed.), *Health behavior, emerging research perspectives*. New York: Plenum, 1988.
21. Miller, J.F. Categories of self-care needs of ambulatory patients with diabetes. *J Adv Nurs*, 1982, *7*(1):25.
22. Frank-Stromborg, M. Health promotion behaviors in ambulatory cancer patients: Fact or fiction? *Oncol Nurs Forum*, 1986, *13*(4):37-43.
23. Stuifbergen, A.K. Barriers and health behaviors of rural and urban persons with MS. *Am J Health Behav*, 1999, *23*(6):415-425.
24. Fowler, S.B. Hope and a health-promoting lifestyle in persons with Parkinson's disease. *J Neurosci Nurs*, 1997, *29*(2):111-116.
25. Laffrey, S.C., Loveland-Cherry, C.J., & Winkler, S.J. Health behavior: Evolution of two paradigms. *Public Health Nurs*, 1986, *3*(2):92-100.
26. Belloc, N.B., & Breslow, L. Relationship of physical health status and health practices. *Prev Med*, 1972, *1*(3):409-421.
27. U.S. Preventive Services Task Force. *Guide to clinical preventive services*. Baltimore, MD: Williams & Wilkins, 1989.
28. Antonovsky, A. *Unraveling the mystery of health*. San Francisco: Jossey-Bass, 1987.
29. Ardell, D.B. *High level wellness*. Berkeley, CA: Ten Speed Press, 1986.
30. Travis, J.W., & Ryan, R.S. *Wellness workbook for health professionals*. 2nd ed., rev. Berkeley, CA: Ten Speed Press, 1988.
31. Laffrey, S.C. An exploration of adult health behaviors. *West J Nurs Res*, 1990, *12*(4):434-447.
32. Pender, N. *Health promotion in nursing practice*. 4th ed. Upper Saddle River, NJ: Prentice Hall, 2002.
33. Walker, S.N., Sechrist, K.R., & Pender, N.J. Health-promoting lifestyle profile: Development and psychometric characteristics. *Nurs Res*, 1987, *36*(2):76-81.
34. Berkman, L., & Breslow, L. *Health and ways of living*. New York: Oxford University Press, 1983.
35. Kulbok, P.A., & Baldwin, J.H. From preventive health behavior to health promotion: Advancing a positive construct of health. *Adv Nurs Sci*, 1992, *14*(4):50-64.
36. Lange, J.W. Methodological concerns for non-Hispanic investigators conducting research with Hispanic Americans. *Res Nurs Health*, 2002, *25*:411-419.
37. Lipsey, M.W. *Design sensitivity*. Newbury Park, CA: Sage, 1990.
38. Acquista, V.W., Wachtel, T.J., Gomes, C.I., et al. Home-based health risk appraisal and screening program. *J Comm Health*, 1988, *13*(1):43-52.
39. Kirscht, J.P. Preventive health behavior: A review of research and issues. *Health Psychol*, 1983, *2*(3):277-301.
40. Frey, J.H. *Survey research by telephone*. Beverly Hills, CA: Sage, 1983.
41. Kirscht, J. Process and measurement issues in health risk appraisal. *Am J Public Health*, 1989, *79*(12):1598-1599.
42. Rakowski, W., Julius, M., Hickey, T., & Halter, J. Correlates of preventive health behavior in late life. *Res Aging*, 1987, *9*(3):331-355.

43. Killeen, M.L. What is the health risk appraisal telling us? *West J Nurs Res*, 1989, *11*(5):614-620.
44. Gustafson, D.H. Health risk appraisal: Its role in health services research. *Health Serv Res*, 1987, *22*(4):453-465.
45. Edington, D.W., & Yen, L. Reliability, validity, and effectiveness of health risk appraisals. *Directory Health Risk Appraisals*, 1992, *1*(1):27-38.
46. Berlin, J., Thorington, B., McKinlay, J., & McKinlay, S. The accuracy of substitution rules for health risk appraisals. *Am J Health Prom*, 1990, *4*(3):214-219.
47. DeFriese, G.H., & Fielding, J.E. Health risk appraisal in the 1990s: Opportunities, challenges, and expectations. *Ann Rev Public Health*, 1990, *11*:401-418.
48. Gazmararian, J., Foxman, B., Yen, L., et al. Comparing the predictive accuracy of health risk appraisal: The Centers for Disease Control versus Carter Center program. *Am J Health Prom*, 1991, *81*(10):1296-1301.
49. The Healthier People Network. HRA. Access date 7 Mar 2003. www.mindspring.com/~hpnhra/hra.html.
50. Measuring the health behavior of adolescents: The Youth Risk Behavior Surveillance System and recent reports on high-risk adolescents. *Public Health Rep*, 1993, *108*(suppl 1):1-96.
51. Grunbaum, J.A., Kann, L., Kinchen, S.A., et al. Youth Risk Behavior Surveillance—United States, 2001. *J Sch Health*, 2002, *72*(8):313-28.
52. CDC, National Center for Chronic Disease Prevention and Health Promotion: Adolescent & School Health. *YRBSS: Youth Risk Behavior Surveillance System*. Updated 11 Feb 2003. Access date 7 Mar 2003. www.cdc.gov/nccdphp/dash/yrbs/.
53. Youth Risk Behavior Surveillance: National College Health Risk Behavior Survey—United States, 1995. *MMWR*, 1997, *46*(SS-6):1-54.
54. National Wellness Institute. *Your on-line wellness inventory: Testwell.org*. Updated 28 Aug 2001. Access date 7 Mar 2003. www.testwell.org.
55. Owen, R.T. The reliability and validity of a wellness inventory. *Am J Health Prom*, 1999, *13*(3):180-182.
56. Travis, J.W. *Wellness Index* (2nd ed.). Berkeley, CA: Ten Speed Press, 1988.
57. Travis, J.W. *Wellness Inventory*. 3rd ed. Asheville, NC: Wellness Associates Publication, 1988.
58. Wellness Associates. *Wellness Inventory*. Access date 7 Mar 2003. www.wellnessinventory.net.
59. Muhlenkamp, A.F., & Brown, N.J. The development of an instrument to measure health practices. Paper presented at the American Nurses' Association Council of Nurse Researchers Conference, Minneapolis, MN, 1983.
60. Muhlenkamp, A.F., Brown, N.J., & Sands, D. Determinants of health promotion activities in nursing clinic clients. *Nurs Res*, 1985, *34*(6):327-332.
61. Brown, N.J., Muhlenkamp, A., Fox, L., & Osborn, M. The relationship among health beliefs, health values, and health promotion activity. *West J Nurs Res*, 1983, *5*(2):155-163.
62. Mahon, N.E., Yarcheski, A., & Yarcheski, T.J. Psychometric evaluation of the Personal Lifestyle Questionnaire for Adolescents. *Res Nurs Health*, 2002, *25*:68-75.
63. Walker, S.N., Kerr, M.J., Pender, N.J., & Sechrist, K.R. A Spanish language version of the Health-

Promoting Lifestyle Profile. *Nurs Res*, 1990, *39*(5):268-273.

64. Walker, S.N., & Hill-Polerecky, D.M. (1995). Psychometric evaluation of the revised Health-Promoting Lifestyle Profile. Paper presented at the 123rd Annual Meeting of the American Public Health Association, San Diego, CA, October 29-November 2, 1995.

65. Langlie, J.K. Interrelationships among preventive health behaviors: A test of competing hypotheses. *Public Health Rep*, 1979, *94*(3):216-225.

66. Rosenstock, I. Historical origins of the health belief model. *Health Educ Monographs*, 1974, *2*(4):328-335.

67. Fishbein, M., & Ajzen, I. *Beliefs, attitudes, intention, and behavior: An introduction to theory and research.* Reading, MA: Addison-Wesley, 1975.

68. Prochaska, J.O., & DiClemente, C.C. *The transtheoretical approach: Crossing traditional boundaries of change.* Homewood, IL: Dow Jones-Irwin, 1984.

69. Gillis, A.J. Determinants of a health-promoting lifestyle: An integrative review. *J Adv Nurs*, 1993, *18*:345-353.

70. Palank, C.J. Determinants of health-promotive behavior: A review of current research. *Nurs Clin North Am*, 1991, *26*(4):815-831.

71. Gochman, D.S. (Ed). *Handbook of health behavior research I: Personal and social determinants.* New York: Plenum Press, 1997.

III

Instruments for Assessing Health-Promotion Activities

26

Measuring Self-Care Activities

Marylin J. Dodd

Many individuals and families have performed self-care in the past. Today many more health care consumers are taking increased interest in their health and assume greater responsibility for their own care. Three main reasons for this resurgence of interest can be identified. The first concerns dissatisfaction with current cost-control systems and measures, maldistribution of physicians and medical facilities, and iatrogenic outcomes. The second reason is the shift from acute to chronic health problems. The third is the gradual change in value and belief systems in which clients desire more control over themselves, their environment, and their social systems, including health care systems.[1,3]

Since the 1960s, health care professionals have incorporated self-care philosophy into their practice. However, in this era of dwindling community health resources and cost containment, the concept of self-care has taken on a central and critical importance in the attainment of quality health-promotion and illness-related care. Healthy individuals, patients, and families simply must manage more by themselves. The mandate is clear for health care professionals to provide health information and teach skills to everyone.

The concept of self-care has a wide range of meaning, given the various perspectives from which self-care is viewed in the health care system and by professional practitioners. These views range from a conservative ideology,[4,5] with emphasis on minimal dependence on the current health care system, to a less conservative view,[6] in which the health care professional, such as the nurse, plays a significant role not only in assisting the patient in acquiring self-care skills but also in managing the patient's self-care.

The meaning of self-care varies according to its proponents. There are notable similarities in ideology as well as differences. Similarities include the performance of activities for oneself in relation to matters that affect health. There is recognition that this performance requires both knowledge and skills, ranging from simple to complex, on the part of the one providing self-care. Access to medical technology is considered a part of self-care. Another common belief is the need for client input in setting client goals and program planning and evaluation. A major difference is the extent to which the client performs self-care activities independently of the health care system and its professionals. Inherent in this difference are issues of control and the extent to which the patient should have unsupervised access to medical technology. The researcher desiring to measure self-care must consider these varying definitions and select an instrument congruent with the purposes of determining self-care.

What emerges from a review of the literature on self-care is the individual's readiness to learn about a health- or disease-related situation,[7] knowledge of what to do,[8] beliefs in ability,[9,10] and possession of the functional ability to perform self-care activities.[11,12] Suggestions on how to assess the individual's readiness to learn, instruments to determine knowledge about the situation, and the psychophysiologic capabilities to initiate self-care are not within the scope of this chapter. These concepts are found elsewhere in this text. The focus of the chapter is a review of tools to measure actual self-care activities.

In Orem's self-care deficit theory of nursing, the concept of self-care is central and is defined as "the practice of activities that maturing and mature persons initiate and perform, within time frames, on their own behalf in the interests of maintaining life, healthful functioning, continuing personal development, and well-being.[6,p461] She clearly emphasizes the crucial role of the nurse in assisting patients to meet their self-care demands when actual or potential deficits exist.

Orem's conceptualization of self-care as consisting of three categories is useful in organizing this review.[6] According to Orem, self-care is undertaken to meet three types of self-care requisites: (1) universal, (2) developmental, and (3) health-deviation. Universal self-care requisites focus on life processes and the maintenance of human structure and function, such as sufficient air, water, and food. Developmental self-care requisites focus on human developmental processes and events during various stages of the life cycle and on events that may adversely affect development. Health-deviation self-care requisites arise from disabilities, deviations, or defects in human structure and function and from medical diagnosis and treatment of disease conditions. The greatest preponderance of self-care research and many of the methodologic issues that the researcher must consider have involved health-deviation self-care.

Health-Deviation Self-Care Requisite

Progress has been made in this area of self-care during the past several years. First, well-conceptualized studies, including explicit definitions of self-care, are more numerous. Second, the measure of self-care activities is not limited to only a few interview or questionnaire items[9,13] embedded in an instrument that also assesses patients' attitudes, values, knowledge, disease and treatment parameters, and functional (psychomotor) abilities. Third, self-care instruments[14] are described more clearly, and their psychometric properties (reliability and validity data) are more frequently reported.

While the majority of experimental studies have focused on disease outcomes, that is, normal glucose, blood pressure, or cholesterol levels, increasing numbers of studies explicitly measure the self-care activities patients perform to obtain the desired disease and treatment outcomes. Specific self-care instruments include use of behaviors to manage side effects of treatment in people diagnosed with cancer,[15] diet modification, weight reduction, exercise, and smoking cessation in people diagnosed with heart conditions.[16,17] Two important instruments are comprehensively discussed. (B. Riegel, personal communication, March 31, 2003),[15,17] and others are summarized in Appendix 26A.[18–28]

Self-Care Diary (SCD)

The SCD was developed by Nail and her colleagues[15] to measure the incidence and severity of selected side effects of cancer treatment and the use and efficacy of self-care activities used to manage those side effects. The patient is instructed as to when (date) to complete the diary and what time frame to consider (i.e., "since your treatment" or "in the past three days"). For each of the 16 side effects, the patient indicates whether or not she or he experienced the side effect in the time frame given. If the patient responds negatively, she or he is directed to the next side effect item. If the patient responds affirmatively, she or he is asked to rate the severity of the side effect (not at all, a little, moderately, quite a lot, or extremely), to indicate which of the listed self-care activities she or he used to manage the side effect, and to indicate how effective the activities were on a 6-point scale with descriptors. The number of self-care activities listed for specific side effects varies from 3 to 17, and there is space to write in self-care activities not included in the list. A place also is provided to list a side effect not included in the instrument and list the self-care activities used to manage it. Patients complete the diary at home and return it to the investigators in a stamped, self-addressed envelope.

The scoring of the SCD is descriptive, and the incidence and severity of side effects are obtained by summing and averaging. Similarly, the number of self-care activities and their efficacy can be summed and averaged. Individual side effects and self-care activities also can be derived, depending on the purpose of investigators.

Reliability and validity data are available for the SCD. The overall side effect severity scores at day 2 and day 5 were correlated at $r = 0.80$, demonstrating an acceptable level of test–retest reliability.[15] The list of side effects and self-care activities was derived from literature on patients' experiences with chemotherapy. Further content validity was provided by two patients who were undergoing treatment and three experienced oncology clinical nurse specialists. Nail and her colleagues describe two scoring issues related to the SCD.[15] First, many patients in their study used multiple combinations of self-care activities, but the methodology employed in this study did not lend itself to measuring the efficacy of combinations of self-care activities. Second, the evaluation of the efficacy of a single self-care activity is limited to the fact that combinations are used and no data were collected on the sequence of initiation of self-care activities. Because combinations of activities were used, no data were collected on the sequence of initiation of self-care activities, and the order in which the self-care activities are performed is unknown, a patient who moves from using an effective self-care activity to using an ineffective activity will receive the same score as a patient taking the opposite path.

The SCD was designed to be used with cancer patients receiving chemotherapy. The investigators describe their sample as predominantly Caucasian, married, middle-aged women with a diagnosis of breast cancer.

Self-Care of Heart Failure Index (SCHF)

The SCHF was developed by Riegel and associates (B. Riegel, personal communication, March 31, 2003).[17] Self-care was defined as a two-phase process of *maintaining health* through positive health practices and *managing heart failure* through a process of recognizing heart failure symptoms, evaluating heart failure symptoms, and evaluating the treatments chosen. Items were developed to reflect both self-care maintenance and self-care management. A total of 22 items evaluated on a 4-point scale (never, sometimes, frequently, always) were tested.

Self-Care Maintenance

Items addressing self-care maintenance focus on 7 health behaviors that are important for persons with heart failure (e.g., daily weights, and exercising at least 3 times each week).

Self-Care Management

Self-care management was assessed using the single most common symptom of heart failure, shortness of breath. Ninety-seven percent of a hospitalized sample of 97 patients reported shortness of breath in the prior 3 months. Four theoretically derived scores were generated, reflecting the process of self-care management: (1) heart symptom recognition (1 item), (2) symptom evaluation (7 items), (3) treatment implementation (3 items), and (4) treatment evaluation (1 item). A self-care self-confidence scale measures confidence in the ability to self-manage heart failure (4 items).

Work is ongoing to finalize a scoring algorithm that produces a summary score useful for research purposes. The proposed scoring algorithm (1) recognizes the ability to stay asymptomatic through self-care maintenance behaviors and (2) weights all five self-care management scores equally. Specifically, all patients are given up to 4 points for self-care maintenance. Patients who are symptomatic get up to 20 points for self-care management. Thus, the symptomatic patients get 12 points for effectively managing the diagnosis and avoiding shortness of breath for the prior 3 months. An additional 8 points are available for components of self-care management (symptom importance [up to 4 points], and self-confidence [up to 4 points]). Thus, asymptomatic patients also accumulate up to 24 points reflecting heart failure self-care ability. This scoring algorithm permits a summary score on all patients, regardless of their symptom status.

During pilot testing with a sample of 97 patients with heart failure, the self-care maintenance scale demonstrated an alpha coefficient of 0.60. Factor analysis revealed two factors explaining 50.2% of the variance in Self-Care Maintenance: healthy behaviors (29.7% of the variance in scores) and medication compliance (20.5% of the variance in scores). The alpha coefficient of the healthy behavior items was 0.65. Medication compliance behaviors were routine in most patients, but the healthy behaviors, including daily weighing, were uncommon. One item, talking to the doctor whenever you need guidance, loaded on both factors. The investigators state that "further testing is needed to determine if items in the Maintenance scale need to be revised or eliminated."

In pilot testing with the same sample of 97 patients, the self-care management scale, heart failure symptom recognition, symptom evaluation, and treatment implementation loaded together and was named *Decision-making* (alpha coefficient of 0.80). Treatment evaluation loaded with self-efficacy and was subsequently named *Appraisal* (alpha coefficient of 0.79). The investigators note that although the scores for symptom recognition, symptom evaluation, treatment implementation, and treatment evaluation are theoretically derived and provide interesting clinical information, these scores do not form individual subscales and alpha coefficients should *not* be calculated separately on them (B. Riegel, personal communication, March 31, 2003).[17]

Scoring of the SCHF provides three cumulative subscale scores (self-care maintenance, decision-making, and appraisal).

Discriminant analysis was used to determine how people with heart failure who recognized shortness of breath differed from those who did not. Patients who readily recognized shortness of breath ($n = 31$) were significantly more likely to implement a treatment ($p = 0.004$), and were higher in self-efficacy ($p = 0.008$) than individuals who failed to recognized this symptom ($n = 48$). Discriminant analysis was also used to determine how the decision-making abilities of people with heart failure predicted self-care. Decision-making ability was measured with selected items from the Executive Functions Scale[29] and grouped into three categories based on the difficulty experienced in decision making. The totals of the items reflecting self-care management ranged from 4.43 to 19 out of a possible score of 20, and differed significantly among the three groups ($F = 4.80$, df = 2, $p = 0.01$). Degrees of freedom (df) is related to the parameters of the Analysis of Variance

(ANOVA); F is the ANOVA symbol for a data analysis technique. Those individuals who found decision making easiest ($n = 16$) had the highest scores (mean 13.18 +/− 1.83), and those in the intermediate category, that is, unable to make a decision, ($n = 31$) had the worst scores (mean 10.21 +/− 3.25). Those who found decision making most difficult ($n = 45$) had an average score of 11.07 +/− 3.35.[17]

The investigators have identified the methodologic issues of their ongoing work to establish the SCHF for research use. The SCHF has shown sufficient promise to date. In earlier work, the investigators developed a longer instrument (65 items) as a clinical tool, the Self-Management of Heart Failure Scale.[30] Although this scale has more items than the SCHF, the SCHF is a more comprehensive measure of self-care.

Universal Self-Care Requisite

The definition of the universal self-care requisite includes the life processes and the maintenance of human structure and function, such as sufficient air, water, and food. In this chapter both prevention and screening activities are incorporated in this definition. These preventive and screening activities include breast self-examination, smoking behaviors, and frequency of annual checkup. Many of the methodologic issues of earlier research with health-deviation self-care are evident in studies of universal self-care. For example, a conceptual framework for the study and the definition of self-care often are not given; measurement of universal self-care activities includes only a few interview or questionnaire items in an instrument; and the interview items or self-reports are inadequately described.

Universal Self-Care Instruments

Examples of instruments to assess self-care in terms of activities to meet universal self-care demands include Denyes' Self-Care Practice instrument[18,23] and the Universal Self-Care Inventory.[31,32] In Chapter 25, "Measuring Healthy Lifestyle," by Berger and Walker, a number of instruments for health-promotion self-care are described. Given the emphasis of Chapter 25, only one instrument of particular interest is described here, and other instruments are summarized in Appendix 26A.

Children's Self-Care Performance Questionnaire

The Children's Self-Care Performance Questionnaire was developed by Moore to measure self-care practices of children and adolescents. The first version of this questionnaire measures both universal and developmental self-care requisites.[33] Orem's[6] self-care deficit theory of nursing provided the framework for the study of 471 students (9 to 18 years of age) who participated in the development and testing of the questionnaire. The Children's Self-Care Performance Questionnaire is a 35-item instrument, designed in a 5-point Likert-scale format with word descriptors (1, never; 2, rarely; 3, sometimes; 4, often; 5, always). Scoring is additive and the possible range of scores is 35 to 175, with higher scores associated with more self-care practices.

Reliability and validity data have been documented for the Self-Care Performance Questionnaire. Internal consistency reliability estimates are adequate, and the coefficient alpha equals 0.83. Content validity was established with a panel of seven experts on Orem's theory. The items in the Self-Care Performance Questionnaire were found to be based on categories specified by Orem, with item categories being assigned by two content experts. Concurrent validity was demonstrated in the moderate correlations of the questionnaire with another self-care behavior instrument (0.54, $p < 0.001$)[18] and a self-care agency questionnaire (0.58, $p < 0.001$).[34] And finally, construct validity was obtained with a LISREL factor analysis that yielded 10 factors corresponding to Orem's self-care requisites.

Subsequent work by Moore and her colleagues has included the mother of the child and the provision of her dependent care to that child.[28] The Dependent Care Agent Questionnaire is summarized in Appendix 26A.

The most recent version of the Children's Self-Care Performance Questionnaire includes a section on health deviation self-care requisites of the pediatric oncology population.[28] This 51-item version has two sections. The first section includes the universal and developmental self-care requisites (35 items) and the second includes the health deviation self-care requisites (16 items) of children with cancer. The word descriptors on the 5-point Likert scale remain unchanged from the first version of the questionnaire. Scoring of the questionnaire should be performed by adding the Likert responses for each item, after first reversing the scoring for 12 of the items.[28]

Content validity for the entire instrument was established by basing items on information from healthy children and children with cancer, both groups of these children were asked what they do to promote health, such as make themselves more healthy, and organizing the items to reflect Orem's theory.[6] In addition, pediatric nurses evaluated the questionnaire. Construct validity was established by using LISREL, and identified factors that corresponded with Orem's theory.[33] LISREL is a statistical technique that yields clusters of related factors.

Developmental Self-Care Requisite

The definition of developmental self-care requisite includes human developmental processes and events during various stages of the life cycle and events that may adversely affect development. This area of self-care has received the least amount of attention by researchers. In a dissertation, Denyes[35] developed a self-care agency instrument in a sample of healthy adolescents. Later, she extended this work to include the measurement of self-care practices that included both universal and developmental self-care requisites.[18] This instrument and others are summarized in Appendix 26A.[18–28]

Summary

Enhancing self-care abilities is an important goal in the current practice environment. Self-care as a concept for clinical practice is flourishing. However, the empiric development and testing of self-care theory lag behind, in part because of the atheoretical use of self-care tools to measure this important concept. Greater effort is needed in this area, especially in developmental, family, and community self-care instruments.

Exemplar Study

Nail, L.M., Jones, L.S., Green, D., et al. Use and perceived efficacy of self-care activities in patients receiving chemotherapy. *Oncol Nurs Forum*, 1991, *18*(5):883–887.

This study exemplifies the evolution in the measurement of self-care. Nail and her colleagues have improved on earlier instruments that measured self-care by listing the 16 possible side effects of chemotherapy and their related self-care activities. Their modification has made it easier for participants to answer by checking a response, rather than the earlier "fill-in-the-response" format. The design is descriptive, with repeated measures of side effects and self-care activities. The methods are carefully detailed. The Self-Care Diary retained the incidence and severity of side effects and the efficacy of self-care activities included in earlier instruments that measured self-care.

The investigators have demonstrated good psychometric characteristics for the Self-Care Diary, with test–retest reliability and two forms of content validity. More frequent self-care activities were performed by participants for the side effects of fatigue, sleep difficulty, nausea, decreased appetite, and changes in food taste and smell. The efficacy of the self-care activities was rated by participants as moderate to moderately high in relief of the side effects. The issue of evaluation of the efficacy of single self-care activities when participants use combinations of self-care activities to manage a side effect remains unresolved.

References

1. Green, L.W., Weelin, S.H., Schauffler, H.H., et al. Research and demonstration issues in self-care: Measuring the decline of medicocentrism. *Health Educ Monogr*, 1977, 5(2):161-189.
2. Norris, C. Self-care. *Am J Nurs*, 1979, 79(3):486.
3. McCorkle, R. Nurses as advocates for self-care. *Cancer Nurs*, 1983, 6(1):17-19.
4. Levin, L. Patient education and self-care: How do they differ? *Nurs Outlook*, 1978, 26:170-175.
5. Fry, J. Self Care: Its place in the total health care system, a report by an independent working party. London: Royal College of General Practitioners Archives, Personal Papers, 1973.
6. Orem, D.T., with one chapter by S.G. Taylor & K.M. Renpenning. *Nursing: Concepts of practice*. St. Louis, MO: Mosby, (1995).
7. Steiger, N.J., & Lipson, J.G. *Self-care nursing*. Bowie, MD: Brady, 1985.
8. Lorig, K., Laurin, J., & Gines, G.E.S. Arthritis self-management. *Nurs Clin North Am*, 1984, 19(4):637-645.
9. Hurley, A.C. Measuring self-care ability in patients with diabetes: The Insulin Management Diabetes Self-Efficacy Scale. In O. Strickland & C.F. Waltz (Eds.), *Measurement of nursing outcomes, Vol. 4. Measuring client self-care and coping skills*. New York: Springer, 1990, pp. 28-44.
10. Gortner, S., & Jenkins, L. Self-efficacy and activity level following cardiac surgery. *J Adv Nurs*, 1990, 15:1132-1138.
11. Rameizl, P. CADET, a self-care assessment tool. *Geriatric Nurs*, 1984, 7(1):43-47.
12. Karl, C.A. The effect of an exercise program on self-care activities for the institutionalized elderly. *J Gerontol Nurs*, 1982, 8(5):282-285.
13. Kubricht, D.W. Therapeutic self-care demands expressed by outpatients receiving external radiation therapy. *Cancer Nurs*, 1984, 7(1):43-52.
14. Dropkin, M.J. Compliance in postoperative head and neck patients. *Cancer Nurs*, 1979, 2(5):379-384.
15. Nail, L.M., Jones, L.S., Greene, D., et al. Use and perceived efficacy of self-care activities in patients receiving chemotherapy. *Oncol Nurs Forum*, 1991, 18(5):883-887.
16. Jaarsma, T., Halfens, R., Tan, F., et al. Self-care and quality of life in patients with advanced heart failure: The effect of a supportive educational intervention. *Heart Lung*, 2000, 29:319-330.
17. Riegel, B., Carlson, B., Moser, D., & Sheposh, J. Preliminary testing of the research version of the self-management of heart failure scale. Paper presented at Heart Failure Society of America, Washington, DC, 2000.
18. Denyes, M.J. Orem's model used for health promotion: Directions for research. *Adv Nurs Sci*, 1988, 11:13-21.
19. Frey, M.A. & Denyes, M.J. Health and illness self-care in adolescents with IDDM: A test of Orem's theory. *Adv Nurs Sci*, 1989, 12:67-74.
20. McCaleb, A., & Edgel, A. Self-concept and self-care practices of healthy adolescents. *J Pediatr Nurs*, 1994, 9:233-238.
21. Cull, V. Exposure to violence and self-care practice of adolescents. *Fam Comm Health*, 1996, 19:31-41.
22. McCaleb, A., & Cull, V.V. Sociocultural influences and self-care practices of middle adolescents. *J Pediatr Nurs*, 2000, 15(1):30-35.
23. Etter, J.F., Bergman, M.M., & Perneger, T.V. On quitting smoking: Development of two scales measuring the use of self-change strategies in current and former smokers. *Addict Behav*, 2000, 25(4):523-538.
24. Saunders, J. *Nursing self-care and HIV disease*. (KO8 NR00033, funded by National Institute for Nursing Research, Bethesda, MD, 1990-1995.) Duarte, CA: City of Hope, 1990-1995.
25. Valente, S.M., Saunders, J., & Uman, G. Self-care, psychological distress, and HIV disease. *J Assoc of Nurses in Aids Care*, 1993, 4(4):15-25.
26. Moore J.B., & Mosher, R.B. Adjustment responses of children and their mothers to cancer: Self-care and anxiety. *Oncol Nurs Forum*, 1997, 24(3):519.
27. Moore, J.B., & Gaffney K.F. Development of an instrument to measure mothers' performance of self-care activities for children. *ANS Adv Nurs Sci*, 1989, 12(1):76-83.
28. Gaffney, K.F., Moore, J.B. Testing Orem's theory of self-care deficit: Dependent care agent performance for children. *Nurs Sci Q*, 1996, 9(4):160.
29. Coolidge, F., & Griego, J. Executive functions of the frontal lobes: Psychometric properties of a self-rated scale. *Psychol Rep*, 1995, 77:24-26.
30. Riegel, B., Carlson, B., & Glaser, D. Development and testing of a clinical tool measuring self-management of heart failure. *Heart Lung*, 2000, 29(1):4-15.
31. Gazda, K. Coronary revascularization: The early impact on quality of life. Unpublished master's thesis. Wayne State University, Detroit, MI, 1986.
32. Horsburgh, M.E., Beanlands, H. Locking-Cusolito, H., et al. Personality traits and self-care in adults awaiting renal transplant. *West J Nurs Res*, 2000, 22(4):407.
33. Moore, J.B. Measuring the self-care practice of children and adolescents: Instrument development. *J Matern Child Nurs*, 1995, 23(3):101-108.
34. Kearney, B.Y., & Fleischer, B.J. Development of an instrument to measure exercise of self-care agency. *Res Nurs Health*, 1979, 2(1):25-34.
35. Denyes, M.J. Development of an instrument to measure self-care agency in adolescents. University of Michigan, *Dissertation Abstracts International*, 1981, 41(5):1716B.

Appendix 26A. Additional Measures of Self-Care

Instrument	Description	Psychometric Indices
Denyes Self-Care Practice Instrument Developed by Denyes[18]	Measure of general self-care actions and universal self-care requisites of adolescents using Orem's self-care as the framework[18] 17-item self-report instrument, scale of frequency of actions yields a total self-care practice score	Used primarily with adolescents and has test–retest reliability of 0.84 to 0.92 in this population[18-21] Cronbach's alpha reliability coefficient for a sample of 426 adolescents was 0.87[22]
Self-Change Strategies (SCS) Developed by Etter, Bergman, & Perneyer[23]	Measures strategies for smoking cessation used by current and former smokers (SCS-CS) 19-item questionnaire version for current smokers (SCS-CS) 17-item questionnaire version for former smokers (SCS-FS) Eight items and 2 strategies were common to both versions of the questionnaire Subject asked to rate the frequency of self-change strategies on a 5-point Likert scale (1 = never, 5 = all the time). Total scores obtained by summing the items on both versions	Content validity demonstrated in the questionnaire items based on qualitative data of 120 current and former smokers; further validity was obtained in a sample of 638 smokers and ex-smokers. Construct validity established with factor analysis, 5 factors explaining 66% of the variance in both CS and FS groups; test re–test reliability (4-week interval) from 0.59 to 0.86; consistency reliability coefficients exceeded the criterion of alpha = 0.7
Self-Care Activity Report Scale (SCARS) Developed by Saunders et al.[24,25]	Measures changes in self-care in relation to a specific situation or important event (e.g., becoming HIV-positive, motor vehicle accident, change in beliefs) 4 parts: (I) description of important event (II) 31 items, changes in usual activities (III) 23 symptoms listed; subject checks appropriate symptoms experienced, what was done to manage them, and effectiveness of intervention (IV) list of support groups; subject to check one(s) attended and rate helpfulness	Scores include total changes in self-care Consistency reliability: Cronbach's alpha (tested in HIV group): total change score: 0.88; positive change score: 0.82; negative change score: 0.67 Factor analysis for 2 factors: (I) promoting health (alpha 0.85); (II) overcoming health barriers and risks (alpha 0.76) Test-retest reliability (Pearson's correlation): 0.90 Must modify for other study populations

Dependent Care Agent Performance Questionnaire (long version including child with cancer section) Developed by Moore & Mosher[26]	55-item instrument based on a previously established 39-item instrument[27] to which 16 items were added specifically for mothers of children with cancer. A 5-point Likert-scale format with possible scores ranging from 55 to 275 (higher scores indicate high levels of dependent care agent performance or practice)	Internal consistency coefficient Cronbach's alpha of 0.93 in a sample of 74 mothers Same methods used for establishing content and construct validity as with the earlier 39-item instrument, and were satisfactory.[26]
Dependent Care Agent Questionnaire Developed by Gaffney & Moore[28]	Measures health promotion and self-care activities provided by an adult on behalf of a child; 39 items, 5-point Likert scale with word descriptors Scores are derived by summing, with a range of possible scores 39 to 195 Higher scores reflecting a greater level of dependent care agent performance	Internal consistency coefficient in sample of 380 subjects, alpha of 0.88, with item-total correlations ranged from 0.27 to 0.63. Content validity—content areas identified by mothers and Orem's theory Construct validity using factor analysis Factors congruent with Orem's theory Hypothesis testing with basic conditioning factors was supported

Superscript numbers correspond to studies cited in the References.

27

Measuring Breast and Colorectal Cancer Screening Beliefs and Behaviors

Susan M. Rawl and Victoria L. Champion

Two cancers that can be cured, if detected early, are breast and colorectal cancer (CRC). Together, breast cancer and CRC account for 43% of the new cancer cases diagnosed each year. A focus on prevention and early detection is imperative to decrease the significant burden of cancer on society. Early detection of breast cancer and CRC through routine screening has the potential to save thousands of lives annually. Regular mammography and a variety of CRC screening tests facilitate early-stage diagnosis, which, in turn, contribute to mortality reductions.[1] Over 90% of people diagnosed with localized-stage breast or colorectal cancer realize at least a 5-year survival, whereas those diagnosed with distant disease have only a 20% chance of living 5 years.[2] Removal of adenomatous polyps, the precursors to colorectal cancer, has been shown to decrease CRC incidence by 75% to 90%.[3]

Unfortunately, participation rates for both breast cancer and CRC screening fall short of desired levels. Although the percentage of U.S. women who have had at least one mammogram is rising, there is still a cadre of women who have never been screened, and the rate of routine repeat mammography screening needed to produce further mortality reductions is poor.[4] The CRC screening participation rates among the general population are quite low. Nationally, only 44% of people report ever having had a sigmoidoscopy and only 34% had a sigmoidoscopy or colonoscopy within the past 5 years.[5] Because of the high incidence rates for both breast cancer and CRC and the efficacy of early screening, increasing adherence to screening for both cancers is of utmost importance.

The focus of this chapter is to describe instruments to measure breast cancer and CRC screening-related beliefs and behaviors. First, evidence is presented on the efficacy of breast cancer screening (breast self-examination [BSE], clinical breast examination [CBE], and mammography), CRC screening (fecal occult blood tests [FOBT], sigmoidoscopy, and colonoscopy), and adherence to screening guidelines. Selected theories that have guided development of breast cancer and CRC screening measures are reviewed. Finally, instruments to measure breast cancer and CRC screening beliefs and behaviors are described in the order listed in the appendices.

Breast Cancer Screening

Breast cancer is the most common cancer in U.S. women, and its incidence is steadily increasing. Estimates are that 212,600 breast cancer cases will be discovered in 2003, with an expected 40,200 deaths.[3] The most effective method to combat mortality is through early diagnosis by appropriate and regular use of mammography, CBE, and BSE.

Regular use of mammography offers excellent protection against mortality through early detection of breast cancer, with mortality reductions demonstrated in numerous studies conducted over the last 30 years. Eight major randomized controlled trials have been conducted for screening with mammography, collectively including more than 500,000 women.[6-17] Together, these trials provide strong support for mortality decreases of up to 30% in women 50 and over who are appropriately screened with mammography. Despite high levels of awareness of breast cancer screening, adherence to recommended mammography screening guidelines remains inadequate. The most recent data from the National Health Interview Survey show that 35% to 38% of women aged 40 or older have not had a mammogram in the last year.[18] Only 54% to 57% of women in this age group reported having had both a mammogram and a CBE in the last 12 months. Both the American Cancer Society and National Cancer Institute recommend annual screening with mammography for women 50 or older.[19,20]

Although mammography currently is the method of choice for early breast cancer detection, several factors indicate that BSE will continue to play a role in this effort. Both the American Cancer Society and the National Cancer Institute recommend that mammography be supplemented by yearly CBE and monthly BSE. Approximately 17% of lumps in the Breast Cancer Detection Project (BCDP) were detected by women between annual exams. A new analysis suggests mortality benefit for BSE even when mammography and CBE are completed.[21] Based on mathematical models, it was proposed that the high survival rate for women with interval tumors in the BCDP data set may result from the fact that 85% of the women practiced regular BSE. One study found that even when women were screened every year with high-quality mammography and CBE, 13% of cancers surfaced between screenings.[22]

Colorectal Cancer Screening

The American Cancer Society estimates that more than 147,500 people will be diagnosed with CRC in 2003, with more than 57,100 resulting deaths.[3] Although the 5-year survival rate for localized disease exceeds 90%, only about 37% of CRC is diagnosed at this stage.[23] Of the cancers that may be controlled through early detection, CRC presents a unique opportunity for both primary and secondary prevention. Epidemiologic and genetic studies suggest that CRC results from complex interactions among inherited susceptibility and environmental and lifestyle factors. Adenomatous polyps, precursors to CRC, may take between 7 and 12 years to progress from normal mucosa to adenoma to cancer.[24,25] Evidence also suggests that the removal of such polyps can reduce CRC incidence. The National Polyp study reported a 76% to 90% reduction in the incidence of CRC for the next 6 years after polyps were removed.[25] Considering that CRC is the second leading cause of cancer death in the United States, the impact of early detection could indeed be substantial.

Scientists estimate that deaths from CRC could be reduced by 50% if current screening guidelines were properly implemented.[26] Randomized trials have demonstrated the efficacy of screening with FOBT in reducing mortality by over 30%.[27] This mortality reduction was achieved primarily because FOBT led to endoscopic screening with flexible sigmoidoscopy or colonoscopy. Endoscopic screening allows for removal of precancerous (adenomatous) polyps, which has been found to decrease CRC incidence by 75% to 90%.[28]

Guidelines for CRC screening have been published by the American Cancer Society,[29] the Agency for Healthcare Research and Quality,[28] and the American College of Gastroenterology.[30] Recommendations for specific screening tests depend on risk factors related to family history, comorbid conditions, and genetic abnormalities. Individuals who have no known risk factors other than age are deemed to be at average risk for developing CRC. For average-risk people, screening recommendations start at age 50 and include five options: (1) annual FOBT, (2) flexible sigmoidoscopy every 5 years, (3) annual FOBT plus flexible sigmoidoscopy every five years, (4) colonoscopy every 10 years, or (5) double-contrast barium enema every 5 to 10 years.

Data from the Behavioral Risk Factor Surveillance System indicate that only 44% of screening-eligible people received an FOBT and/or endoscopic screening in the recommended time frame.[31] For individual tests, 20.6% of respondents had had an FOBT in the preceding year and only 33.6% reported having had a sigmoidoscopy or colonoscopy within the preceding 5 years.[31] Adherence to CRC screening guidelines is lower than those for mammography. From 1987 to 1998, FOBT participation among women rose from 21% to 26% while endoscopic screening rose from 6% to 10%.[5,32,33]

Theoretical Construct for Measuring Screening Beliefs and Behavior

Theories provide a framework for explaining behavior. It follows, then, that studies to increase cancer screening behaviors are most useful when they are developed from a solid theoretical framework. The use of theory allows investigators to select mediating, moderating, and outcome measures that are most relevant to the health behavior of interest. Three theories often have informed the selection and development of measures used in screening behavior research. These include the health belief model (HBM), the transtheoretical model (TTM), and social cognitive theory (SCT).

The HBM was one of the first theories to gain widespread use in studies of breast cancer and CRC screening.[34,35] Four concepts are most commonly associated with the HBM: (1) perceived susceptibility, (2) perceived seriousness, (3) perceived benefits, and (4) perceived barriers. *Perceived susceptibility* was defined as a person's perceived risk of developing a disease, while *severity* was defined as perceived consequences of the disease on the person's well-being. Cancer is universally regarded as a serious disease with potentially severe consequences and, as a result, there is little variability in measures of perceived severity. Perceived benefits and barriers were defined as positive and negative effects related to a specific health action. Rosenstock and colleagues added self-efficacy to the HBM.[35] *Self-efficacy* can be defined as a person's confidence in his or her ability to take action.

The TTM was developed and tested by Prochaska and colleagues to understand how individuals progress toward adapting behaviors that result in optimal health.[36] Core constructs include stages of change, processes of change and decisional balance. Stages of change refer to behavior and include precontemplation, contemplation, preparation, action, maintenance, and termination. *Precontemplation* is defined as a stage in which a person does not intend to take action in the immediate future, usually defined as 6 months. *Contemplation* is defined as stage in which a person decides to take action within the next six months. *Preparation* is the stage in which an individual prepares to take action in the immediate future. This may involve making an appointment or other preparation for action, such as obtaining an FOBT kit. *Action* is defined as the point at which an individual has taken specific action to create behavioral change. *Maintenance* follows action and is defined as the period of time in which a person works to maintain behavior and the point at which behavior is so ingrained that there is no chance of relapse. The TTM has been used with mammography screening behavior and is being applied to colorectal screening. Studies using this model have used stage of change as both a predictor of behavioral change and outcome.

Social cognitive theory includes the concepts of outcome expectations and efficacy expectations that act in concert to predict behavior.[37] *Outcome expectations* are defined as beliefs that a given action will result in a desired outcome, whereas *efficacy expectation*, or *self-efficacy*, is the belief that one has the ability to complete an action necessary to produce the outcome. The concept of self-efficacy has been integrated into later versions of the HBM. Although these theories are frequently used in screening research, the current trend is to combine theoretical frameworks to obtain maximum predictive potential. Several of the screening studies described in this chapter have measured concepts from multiple theories.

Instruments for Breast Cancer Screening

Instruments used to study screening behaviors of BSE and mammography fall into two primary categories: beliefs and actual behavior. Beliefs are the constructs guided by theory that have been used to predict screening behavior. The major beliefs reviewed in the following section are perceived benefits and barriers to screening and perceived self-efficacy. Fear is discussed as an emerging construct being used to predict breast cancer screening. We also review instruments to measure both BSE and mammography behaviors. Perceived susceptibility and cancer fatalism are discussed in a later section as they relate generally to other types of screening, in addition to breast cancer screening.

Measuring Beliefs about BSE and Mammography

Benefits, Barriers, and Self-Efficacy for BSE

Several theories include the concepts of perceived benefits and barriers to breast cancer screening, as well as perceived self-efficacy, to predict breast cancer screening. Because these beliefs are specific to the screening behavior, scales differ depending on whether the outcome behavior is BSE or mammography. We will first review the scales that deal with BSE, and then move to the scales that address mammography.

Champion developed some of the earliest measures of benefits and barriers to BSE.[38] In this initial report, conceptual definitions for each of the variables were developed based on extensive literature reviews. Content validity was tested by submitting items to judges who were familiar with the HBM. Items were scaled on a 5-point Likert scale with responses varying from "strongly agree" (5) to "strongly disagree" (1). The scales for benefits and barriers each contained 8 items. Construct validity was assessed by exploratory factor analysis and multiple regression. Scale revision was completed in 1993 with the addition of a new scale to measure perceived ability to complete BSE.[39] The confidence scale was the first attempt at development of a measure of self-efficacy.

After initial revision, all scales were reviewed by a panel of three experts, one of whom was involved with the original development of the HBM. Instruments were tested for validity and reliability using a random sample of 581 women. The internal consistency correlation coefficients represented improvement over the previously reported scales. Test–retest reliabilities ranged from 0.45 to 0.70, again evidencing only moderate test–retest reliability. Construct validity was assessed using exploratory factor analysis, with resulting deletion of four items. All remaining items loaded at 0.45 or above on the respective factors. Predictive validity was established by examining relationships between the respective HBM scales and BSE behavior. Predictive validity was demonstrated by the significant correlation of all scales with the BSE behavior. Champion and Menon used both benefit and barrier scales and reported on a self-efficacy to BSE scale that demonstrated an alpha of 0.90.[40] Construct validity for self-efficacy to BSE was demonstrated by the significant relationship with BSE behavior.

Cultural adaptation and translation of the HBM scales into other languages has been successful, with good psychometrics reported with Jordanian and Korean women.[41,42] When translated into the Arabic language, Cronbach alphas of 0.79 and 0.77 were reported for benefits and barriers, respectively, along with an alpha of 0.89 for BSE self-efficacy.[41] For the Korean women, alphas were 0.79 for benefits, 0.74 for barriers, and 0.91 for BSE self-efficacy.[42] All three scales demonstrated predicative validity by significant correlations with either BSE frequency or proficiency.

Lauver and Angerame developed a BSE belief and attitude scale using the literature and previously constructed items.[43] A 5-point response set ranged from "strongly agree" to "strongly disagree." Several constructs were measured: general efficacy of BSE, specific efficacy of BSE, confidence in doing BSE, and attitudinal items addressing remembering, interference, comfort, fear, and pain. A total of 64 women were recruited for teaching sessions from employees in an industrial occupational setting. Cronbach alpha for the subscales ranged from 0.65 to 0.89. BSE frequency scores were compared using Spearman ranked-correlation coefficients. Competence, remembering, and comfort scales had moderately strong positive relationships with frequency (0.35 to 0.58), and the interference scale had a negative correlation of –0.44. Correlations between efficacy and frequency were not significant. Fear and pain subscales had weak, nonsignificant relations.

Benefits, Barriers, and Self-Efficacy for Mammography

In 1999, Champion published her first benefits and barriers scales that were used to predict mammography screening.[44] Concepts from the original BSE scales were used with additions that reflected issues specific to mammography. The benefits scale included 5 items that focused on perceived health benefits of completing mammography. Sample benefit items included "having a mammogram will help me worry less about breast cancer" and "decrease my chances of dying from breast cancer." Item responses were a 5-point Likert scale from "strongly agree" (5) to "strongly disagree" (1). The internal consistency alpha coefficient was 0.75. Barriers to mammography included 11 items, such as fear of finding something wrong and being too old to need a mammogram. An alpha of 0.88 was obtained. For both scales, predictive validity was established through testing of theoretical relationships, and construct validity was supported through factor analysis.

Several researchers have used the benefits and barriers scales in other studies. Han and colleagues used an adaptation of the Champion scale with a 5-item benefit scale and 9-item barrier scale.[45] Alphas were 0.89 and 0.78, respectively. Both scales differentiated women who had never reported a mammogram from those who reported having at least one mammogram. Subsequent work conducted by Champion and colleagues have used these validated scales.[40,46-49]

In 2003, Champion developed a scale to measure self-efficacy for obtaining a mammogram.[50] Self-efficacy was defined as perceived confidence in one's ability to obtain a mammogram. Based on Bandura's definition of self efficacy,[37] 20 items were developed and submitted to five content experts. After deleting items as suggested by content experts, 10 items were used with 1390 women enrolled in a longitudinal intervention study to increase mammography use. The 10-item scale was measured on a 5-point Likert format and demonstrated a Cronbach alpha of 0.88. Confirmatory analysis indicated that all items correlated with the latent variable. Logistic regression results supported the theoretical relationships indicating that women with higher self-efficacy were more likely to be screened with mammography.[51]

Lagerlund and colleagues reported on a benefits to mammography scale and emotional barriers to mammography scale.[52] The benefits scale contained 7 items reflecting perception of health benefits to mammography and had an alpha of 0.62. Emotional barriers contained 9 items with an alpha of 0.58. Both scales differentiated attenders from nonattenders at a breast cancer screening clinic. Other researchers have used various combinations of questions to measure perceived benefits and barriers to mammography. For instance, Crane et al. identified items from Janz and Becker to include in a scale measuring susceptibility, severity, benefits, barriers, and control.[53,54] The benefit items had an alpha reliability of 0.67. Barriers were individually assessed for their relation to mammography. Perceived benefits were not significantly related to mammography. The one barrier related to mammography was transportation. Other researchers have measured constructs without constructing scales. Friedman and coworkers used only a few items to measure self-efficacy, benefits, and barriers.[55] No alphas were reported.

Mammography Pros and Cons

A different approach to measuring benefits and barriers involved using the TTM. Rakowski et al. reported on a decisional balance summary index that was composed of two variables, pros and cons to mammography behavior.[56,57] The pros related to perceived benefits for obtaining mammography, and the cons related to barriers to obtaining a mammogram. A set of 12 items were developed and assessed using a 5-point Likert scale ranging from "strongly agree" (5) to "strongly disagree" (1). Factor analysis with varimax rotation yielded the two components. The pros scale had a coefficient alpha of 0.72, and the cons scale had a coefficient alpha of 0.71. A summary decision balance score was created by converting both pros and cons to t-scores and subtracting the cons t-scores from the pros t-scores. In order to test the theoretical relationships, women were categorized by stage. Stages included (1) precontemplation (no prior mammogram and no intent to have one in coming year), (2) contemplation (no mammogram in prior year but intending to have one), (3) action (on schedule for a mammogram according to NCI/ACS guidelines), (4) maintenance (current and two prior mammograms on NCI/ACS schedule), and (5) relapse (one or more mammograms in the past but not planning to have one in the future). The decisional balance scale differentiated women as to stage of mammography adoption. Further testing of the pros and cons scale by Rakowski confirmed results.[58]

Other researchers have used the concepts of pros and cons. Rimer, using the decisional balance construct, identified 8 items, with 7 pro items and 1 con item.[59] The decisional balance was strongly associated with mammography. Clemow et al. used 19 items to form a pros and cons scale building on Rakowski's and Rimer's 1996 work.[60–62] The pros measure had a Cronbach alpha of 0.79; the cons scale had an alpha of 0.75. Pros and cons were significantly related to mammograms obtained.

Fear

Two additional concepts have appeared in the literature when addressing compliance with breast cancer screening. The first is the emotional construct of fear. Originally, fear of breast cancer was operationalized as a barrier to obtaining mammography. Witte clearly separated fear from barriers by defining the construct as a negatively toned emotion accompanied by a high level of physiologic arousal stimulated by a threat that is perceived to be significant and personally relevant.[63] Champion and colleagues constructed a scale to measure this state of heightened anxiety in response to breast cancer.[64] Initially, 10 items were developed and evaluated by content analysis from an expert panel. The scale was analytically tested with a sample of 1390 women who were enrolled in a prospective intervention trial to increase mammography adherence. Principal component analysis revealed that 8 items fit well on one factor and 55% of the variance was related to the factor. All further analysis used the 8-item scale. The alpha coefficient was 0.91 and test–retest was 0.70. Construct validity was supported by fear predicting adherence to mammography, as theoretically specified.

Measuring Behavior: Breast Self-Examination and Mammography

Several researchers have developed frequency and proficiency scales to measure actual BSE behavior. Instruments that address frequency and proficiency are described next.

Breast Self-Examination Frequency

Frequency of BSE is usually measured by a self-report questionnaire in which women are asked to indicate the number of times they completed BSE in the last 12 months. Champion and others reported in several research articles their measurement strategies for frequency of BSE.[39,40,65] Frequency was measured by asking a woman to indicate the number of times she completed BSE within a 12-month period.

Breast Self-Examination Proficiency

Champion also developed a scale to measure self-reported proficiency as assessed with a 9-item scale.[39,66] Women responded to questions assessing length of time taken for examination, pattern of examination, position of hands, areas covered, and use of a mirror. An observational checklist was used by trained observers to assess proficiency. A total of 10 procedural components were included.

To evaluate an intervention protocol, attempts to determine the validity of BSE evaluation tools were undertaken by a group of researchers at the Fred Hutchinson Cancer Research Center.[67] Observer assessment of BSE practice included five items: (1) covered 8 or more areas of the breast, (2) used finger pads, (3) used firm pressure, (4) used massage and search pattern, and (5) used mirror plus supine position. When the five unweighted points were scored, 44.6% of women scored five points or more and were rated as having excellent BSE technique. Calculation of the observation score allowed differentiation of regular practitioners from those who were not regular practitioners (chi square = 15.2, $p \leq 0.004$). In addition, women were asked to palpate three models that had a total of 15 lumps of varying sizes embedded within them. BSE technique was associated with ability to detect lumps ($p \leq 0.006$). For each two-step increase in the technique scale, one additional lump was detected. Difference in lumps detected before and after instruction was significant ($p \leq 0.002$). Irregular BSE practitioners did not increase post-training scores. Testing supported using at least five observation steps in determining BSE proficiency.

Coleman developed a scoring system to measure eight components of BSE proficiency as specified by a BSE training technology called Mamma Care.[68] These eight components related to (1) area, (2) pressure type, (3) motion, (4) part (fingers or hands), (5) pattern, (6) number of fingers, (7) number of motions, and (8) duration. Using these components, a scoring system was developed and validated. A paired-comparisons procedure was used to provide each component a BSE weight. The weights were then combined to produce a value on an interval scale. A paired-comparisons survey instrument presenting each of the eight components in all possible combinations was constructed.[69] Experts in teaching the Mamma Care method of BSE completed the tool by checking which pairs were critical for correct BSE technique.

All the health professionals involved in this assessment had been trained in the Mamma Care method of teaching BSE, and three expert judges were instrumental in developing the Mamma Care method. Weights for each item were calculated by dividing the total number of responses (28 choices times 20 experts) each component received by the overall total response. Raw scores for each of the steps were calculated. For instance, the area score was the total percentage of breast area actually palpated divided by the number of square inches of breast surface present. Duration was the actual time of examination in minutes converted to a maximum of 1. Each subject's pressure was divided by 6 and a value of 1 given if light, medium, and deep pressures were used and less than 1 given for the other choices according to rank. The other five components (motion, number of motions, pattern, part of fingers, and number of fingers) were given a score of 0 or 1, with 1 being the preferred choice. Raw scores were then multiplied by the weighted scores, and all scores summed for a performance score to produce a set of weights with the following values: area, 0.216; duration, 0.06; motion, 0.14; part, 0.13;

pattern, 0.1225; number of fingers, 0.075; number of motions, 0.0725; and pressure type, 0.185.

To validate the scoring system, both pre- and post-tests were completed by women who were taught BSE individually using self-modeling and by women taught BSE in a group using a breast model. Instructors were trained in teaching the Mamma Care method of BSE.[68] Observer scores were trained to 95% agreement on the number of palpations and 95% agreement on the number of squares examined by the standard observer. Pre- and post-test values demonstrated discrimination. Proficiency included using all components on a checklist to evaluate persons in a clinical area. Necessary components for the checklist were (1) correct position, (2) examination of all areas, (3) adequate pressure, (4) use of a circular motion with the application of each type of pressure, (5) use of the pads of the three middle fingers, (6) use of a vertical strip pattern, (7) squeezing the nipple to check for discharge, and (8) examining the breast for symmetric dimpling or retraction. Using a weighted scale might be appropriate in research settings when an accurate picture of proficiency is needed.

A study by Atkins and colleagues assessed the relative effectiveness of different search patterns on area of breast covered and number of lumps detected.[70] To assess area covered, a videotape of each subject's BSE was recorded after a training session. A slide and matching schematic score sheet with a breast board divided into numbered 3-cm squares was provided to compare with the BSE tape. Each square that was palpated with distal finger pads of the first three fingers was counted. Percentage of coverage was calculated by dividing the number of squares palpated by the total number of squares represented in the area. The mean interrater reliability was 0.82. In addition, a measure of lump detection representing the total number of actual lumps detected in two silicon breast models was used, with the score ranging from 0 to 10. A false-positive score also was calculated, representing the total number of false-positive lumps identified in two silicon breast models. Duration scores were obtained by recording duration of the exam on both the breast board and the model.

These methods of measuring area covered and number of lumps detected were used to assess differences in search patterns by comparing concentric circle, radial spoke, and vertical strip patterns. Results indicated that these methods of scoring distinguished the vertical strip pattern in terms of most breast area covered.

Mammography Utilization

Mammography behavior has been measured in many ways. The NCI Breast Cancer Screening Consortium used a series of items, including whether the woman had ever heard of a mammogram, ever had a mammogram, the number of mammograms in the last five years, and the timing of the most recent mammograms.[71,72]

Mammography Stage of Adoption

Stage of mammography behavior as defined by the TTM has been used by several researchers, starting with Rakowski, Fulton, and Feldman.[57] This group borrowed questions from the NCI Breast Cancer Screening Consortium. Five stages were defined as (1) precontemplation—no prior mammogram and no intent to have one in coming year; (2) contemplation—no mammogram in prior year but intending to have one; (3) action—on schedule for a mammogram according to NCI/ACS guidelines; (4) maintenance—current and two prior mammograms on NCI/ACS schedule; and (5) relapse—one or more mammograms in the past but planning to have another on the NCI/ACS schedule. Champion and Skinner used variations of the staging questions to measure mammography adoption and stage of mammography adoption.[50,73–76]

Mammography Adherence

Mammography adherence can be measured by simply asking a woman if she has received a mammogram within the specified guidelines issued by ACS or NCI. Many researchers use a dichotomous question and specify the timeframe.[49,77–79] Additionally, mammography adherence can be defined as the action stage when staging algorithms are used.

Instruments for Colorectal Cancer Screening

In this chapter, instruments used to study beliefs and behaviors of CRC screening with FOBT, sigmoidoscopy, and colonoscopy have been organized the same way as breast screening measures. Health beliefs reviewed here are perceived benefits and barriers to CRC screening. If sufficient information was available on individual items and psychometrics of measures for other health beliefs, these are also presented. We also review instruments to measure FOBT, sigmoidoscopy, and colonoscopy behaviors. Perceived susceptibility and fatalism will be discussed later in the chapter because they are relevant to cancer screening in general.

Measuring Beliefs about FOBT, Sigmoidoscopy, and Colonoscopy

Benefits and Barriers for FOBT, Sigmoidoscopy, and Colonoscopy

The development of measures of benefits and barriers for CRC screening have been guided by the same theoretical frameworks as those for breast screening. Research on CRC screening, although still in its infancy, is being solidly built on the foundation provided by 20 years of scientific progress in the area of breast cancer screening. Based on the extensive work of Champion, Rawl and colleagues modified and tested six HBM scales to measure benefits of and barriers to three different types of CRC screening tests: FOBT, sigmoidoscopy, and colonoscopy.[80] The six scales were developed after extensive review of existing literature and analysis of data provided by focus groups conducted with screening-naïve and experienced individuals. Focus groups were conducted with people who had been screened and subsequently diagnosed with adenomatous polyps and first-degree relatives of patients with CRC.[81] Benefit and barrier scales were tested with larger samples of these two groups.

Internal consistency was assessed for each of the six scales and alphas were 0.65 or above. Construct validity was supported through exploratory factor analyses, with benefit and barrier scale items being unidimensional and factor loadings all being 0.35 or above. Known groups validity was supported through analyses of variance tests comparing beliefs of screening-naïve and experienced individuals. People who had previous experience with FOBT, sigmoidoscopy, or colonoscopy perceived fewer barriers than those who had never had these screening tests. Benefits were related to previous participation in sigmoidoscopy and colonoscopy, but not to FOBT.[80]

Wardle and colleagues developed and tested scales to measure benefits and barriers to sigmoidoscopy.[82] Benefits of sigmoidoscopy were measured using a 7-item scale with 5-point Likert response options ranging from "strongly agree" to "strongly disagree." Barriers were measured using a 6-item scale with the same response options. Cronbach alphas of 0.83 were reported for both scales. These investigators also developed and tested a 4-item scale to measure fatalism; an alpha of 0.77 was obtained for this scale. Principal component analyses were used to establish validity for all scales.[82]

Pros and Cons of Colorectal Cancer Screening

As described earlier, pros and cons are similar to the HBM construct of benefits and barriers. These constructs have been derived from the TTM of behavior change and were first developed for mammography by Rakowski.[56] Manne and colleagues adapted Rakowski's pros and cons measures for CRC screening. Internal consistency reliability was assessed and Cronbach alphas of 0.76 and 0.80 were reported for the 9-item pros and the 19-item cons of CRC screening scale, respectively.[83]

Factors Related to CRC Screening Adherence

Vernon and colleagues were among the first to develop and validate an instrument to measure health beliefs related to CRC screening. Theoretical constructs from the HBM, the theory of reasoned action, and social cognitive theory were operationalized by these researchers. Multitrait scaling analyses were conducted and good psychometrics were reported for scales to measure salience and coherence, self-efficacy, worry, and intention. Reliability coefficients (alphas) for all scales were above 0.70, and validity was supported through exploratory and confirmatory factor analyses as well as discriminant analyses.[84]

Measuring Behavior: FOBT, Sigmoidoscopy and Colonoscopy

CRC Screening Utilization

CRC screening behaviors have been measured in many ways. National surveys such as the Behavioral Risk Factor Surveillance Survey (BRFSS) revised measures of utilization of FOBT, sigmoidoscopy, and colonoscopy to better capture participation in these screening tests in the general population.[3,5,23] The BRFSS includes a brief description of each screening test and uses a series of items, including whether people have ever had an FOBT, and if so, when their last stool blood test was done. The same two questions are asked regarding endoscopic screening with sigmoidoscopy/colonoscopy combined. People are asked if they have ever had a sigmoidoscopy or colonoscopy and, if so, when they had their last exam.

CRC Screening Adherence

FOBT, sigmoidoscopy and colonoscopy adherence can be measured by simply asking a person if she or he has had the test within the specified timeframe recommended by ACS. Many researchers use a dichotomous question and specify the timeframe.[77,80,83] Additionally, FOBT, sigmoidoscopy, or colonoscopy adherence can be defined as the action stage when staging algorithms are used.

CRC Screening Stage of Adoption

Stage of adoption of CRC screening behaviors, as defined by the TTM, have been modified from those originally developed for mammography by Rakowski and colleagues.[50,57,73–76] Rawl, Champion, and colleagues have adapted these for CRC screening and defined four stages for each test separately. After descriptions of each test are provided, four items assess whether people (1) have ever done or had the test, (2) have thought about doing or having the test, (3) are planning to do or have the test in the next 6 months, and (4) have a test kit at home now or have an appointment to have a sigmoidoscopy/colonoscopy. Another item assesses time since last test.[85,86]

The *FOBT stages of adoption* are defined as (1) *precontemplation*—has never done an FOBT OR had one more than 15 months ago AND does not intend to do one in the next 6 months; (2) *contemplation*—has never done an FOBT OR had one more than 15 months ago AND intends to do one in the next 6 months; (3) *preparation*—has never done an FOBT OR had one more than 15 months ago AND has an FOBT kit at home now; and (4) *action*—has done FOBT within the last 15 months.[85,86]

Sigmoidoscopy stages of adoption are defined as (1) *precontemplation*—has never had a sigmoidoscopy OR had one more than 5 years ago AND does not intend to have one in the next 6 months; (2) *contemplation*—has never had a sigmoidoscopy OR had one more than 5 years ago AND intends to have one in the next 6 months; (3) *preparation*—has never had a sigmoidoscopy OR had one more than 5 years ago AND has an appointment to have one; and (4) *action*—has had a sigmoidoscopy within the last 5 years.[85,86] Other researchers have defined similar stages for sigmoidoscopy, excluding the preparation stage.[87]

Colonoscopy stages of adoption are defined as (1) *precontemplation*—has never had a colonoscopy OR had one more than 10 years ago AND does not intend to have one in the next 6 months; (2) *contemplation*—has never had a colonoscopy OR had one more than 10 years ago AND intends to have one in the next 6 months; (3) *preparation*—has never had a colonoscopy OR had one more than 10 years ago AND has an appointment to have one; and (4) *action*—has had a colonoscopy within the last 10 years.[85,86]

Manne and colleagues have developed another approach to measuring CRC stages of adoption.[83] Their measures are used to categorize individuals into one of five stages for CRC screening and combines stages for all three screening tests. The interaction between CRC screening tests can be addressed using this more complex staging algorithm. Validation of their staging algorithm was evidenced by results of logistic regression analyses. Cons were correlated with stage of adoption in the expected directions.[83]

Beliefs Relevant to Both Breast and Colorectal Cancer Screening

Two theoretical constructs that may be relevant to many cancer screening behaviors are perceived susceptibility and cancer fatalism. Measurement of these constructs are discussed here through specific examples of application to both breast and CRC screening.

Perceived Susceptibility

Perceived susceptibility, or perceived risk, is defined by the HBM as a subjective estimate of contracting a disease.[54] One of the earliest attempts to measure perceived susceptibility to breast cancer as defined by the HBM was reported in 1984.[38] *Susceptibility* was defined as perceived personal risk of developing breast cancer. Both internal consistency reliability and test–retest reliability were reported, and validity was established through factor analysis and regression of BSE on perceived susceptibility. Internal consistency for the initial scale was 0.77, and test–retest was 0.86. The same scale was refined for an African American sample in 1997.[66] Perceived susceptibility demonstrated an alpha of 0.83 and test–retest reliability of 0.65. The latest revision occurred in 1999, when the scale was decreased to 3 items with a standardized alpha of 0.87 and test–retest of 0.62.[44] Validity was demonstrated through confirmatory factor analysis and testing of theoretical relations. This work demonstrated that the 3-item scale performed as well as the initial 5-item scale. Champion's scales have been used with different cultures. Mikhail and colleagues translated the scales into Arabic.[41] Good internal consistency reliability (0.85) and predictive validity were demonstrated. Perceived susceptibility was also tested with a Mexican American group of women, with whom a Cronbach alpha of 0.73 was obtained.[88] Lee and colleagues translated and tested Champion's scales with Korean women and reported an alpha of 0.92 for the perceived susceptibility scale.[42]

Other researchers have developed measures for perceived risk in relation to breast cancer. Lerman and colleagues measured perceived risk with three items placed on a 5-point Likert scale.[89] Psychometrics were not reported. Lagerlund et al. reported on perceived susceptibility in a Swedish population.[52] *Perceived susceptibility* was defined as perceived risk of contracting a health disorder. Three items were developed using a 6-point Likert response scale. This scale differentiated attenders from nonattenders at a breast cancer screening clinic. Internal consistency was reported at 0.69. Finally, other authors have measured perceived risk by defining both relative risk (compared to other women your age) and absolute risk (risk on a scale of 0–100).[79,90–92] Both relative and absolute risks were usually measured using single items and were not consistent across studies.

Perceived susceptibility or risk of developing CRC has been operationalized in the same variety of ways as breast cancer. Rawl modified Champion's 3-item perceived susceptibility to breast cancer for CRC and used it in preliminary studies, in which alphas of 0.75 to 0.77 were obtained.[80] Vernon and colleagues used a similar 3-item scale to assess perceived susceptibility and reported internal consistency reliability of 0.79.[84] Others have used single-item measures of absolute and relative risk by asking people to estimate their chance of getting CRC sometime during their lifetime or to compare themselves with others who share some characteristic such as age, gender, or family history.[83,93,94]

Fatalism

Fatalism is another concept that is often identified as a barrier to cancer screening and has been related to cultural and socioeconomic factors, especially for African Americans.[95] Powe examined cancer fatalism among African Americans as a perception of helplessness when considering cancer. She developed a 15-item questionnaire that assessed four attributes of fatalism: fear, predetermination, pessimism, and inevitable death.[96,97] The instrument was tested with elderly Caucasians and African Americans in relation to CRC screening. A Cronbach alpha of 0.84 was reported, and all items loaded on one factor at 0.20 or above.[95]

Validity of Self-Reported Screening

The validity of measuring screening behaviors via participant self-report has been questioned, but because of the difficulty in obtaining objective measures, researchers often rely on self-report. Self-report measures include the inherent biases of acquiescence and social desirability. Further, BSE is a complex behavior that cannot be measured by a single question. BSE scales to measure both frequency and proficiency are reported with varying degrees of validity. The issue of validity of measurement for BSE extends to both frequency and proficiency, with no real standard by which to compare measures.

Mammography self-report, although costly and time intensive, can be verified by medical records. There are two main sources of error in self-report of mammography. The first is nondeliberate recall or simple errors in remembering. Secondly, women may intentionally misreport mammography if they perceive having mammograms to be socially desirable behavior. Various studies have attempted to determine accuracy of mammography self-report. King and colleagues found that HMO populations had about a 94% accuracy in self-report as verified by medical records.[98] A more recent study found that the question of ever having a mammogram was verified 100% of the time, 24% of women recalled the exact date of their last mammogram, and another 40% correctly reported within one month.[99] Others have found much lower verification rates, especially with non-Caucasian samples.[78,100,101] Researchers must be aware that self-report, regardless of validity and reliability of measures, may suffer from reporting biases.

Validating self-report of CRC screening has shown similarly mixed results. Gordon and colleagues reported high levels of concordance between self-report and HMO medical records for both FOBT (over 90%) and sigmoidoscopy (80%), while others have found low rates of concordance in low-socioeconomic status and African American respondents in community settings.[102–104]

Challenges

One of the most critical challenges in measurement of beliefs and behaviors for breast cancer or CRC screening is consistency in measurement. More than half the time, researchers develop their own measures without consideration of prior work. This creates a proliferation of both conceptual and operational definitions that make comparisons across studies impossible. Additionally, validity and reliability of even well-designed scales must constantly be reexamined in new populations. Breast self-examination measurement must include not only frequency but proficiency. The frequency of BSE *without* measurement of proficiency is practically worthless. For self-report of mammography or CRC screening tests, it is essential that participants clearly understand the procedure or behavior being assessed. Women may confuse mammography with chest x-ray if a definition is not clear. The problem becomes even more acute when evaluating participation in CRC screening. Even with detailed descriptions, people have difficulty understanding the difference between sigmoidoscopy and colonoscopy.

Precise and consistent, standardized measurement of constructs related to screening can provide a strong foundation for scientific progress in the prevention and early detection of cancer.

References

1. American Cancer Society. *Cancer facts & figures 2002.* Atlanta, GA: American Cancer Society, 2002.
2. Jemal, A., Thomas, A., Murray, T., et al. Cancer statistics 2002. *CA Cancer J Clin,* 2002, *52*(4):23-47.
3. American Cancer Society. *Cancer facts & figures 2002.* Atlanta, GA: American Cancer Society, 2003.
4. Champion, V., Skinner, C.S., Saywell, R.M., Jr., et al. *A comparison of tailored mammography interventions* (funded research R01NR04081). Bethesda, MD: National Institute of Nursing Research, 1999.
5. Centers for Disease Control. Trends in screening for colorectal cancer—United States, 1997 and 1999. *MMWR Morb Mort Wkly Rep,* 2001, *50*(9):162-170.
6. Shapiro, S. Periodic screening for breast cancer: The HIP randomized controlled trial. *J Natl Cancer Inst Monographs,* 1997, *22*:27-30.
7. Shapiro, S., Venet, W., Strax, P., et al. Ten- to fourteen-year effect of screening on breast cancer mortality. *J Natl Cancer Inst,* 1982, *69*(2):349-355.
8. Tabar, L., Gad, A., Holmberg, L.H., et al. Reduction in mortality from breast cancer after mass screening with mammography. *Lancet,* 1985, 829-832.
9. Tabar, L., Fagerberg, G., Duffy, S.W., et al. Update of the Swedish two-county program of mammographic screening for breast cancer. *Radiol Clin North Am,* 1992, *30*(1):187-210.
10. Tabar, L., Faberberg, G., Day, N.E., & Holmberg, L. What is the optimum interval between mammographic screening examinations? An analysis based on the latest results of the Swedish two-county breast cancer screening trial. *Br J Cancer,* 1987, *55*(5):547-51.
11. Nystrom, L., Rutqvist, L.E., Wall, S., et al. Breast cancer screening with mammography: Overview of Swedish randomised trials. *Lancet,* 1993, *341*:973-978.
12. Andersson, I., Aspegren, K., Janzon, L., et al. Mammographic screening and mortality from breast cancer: The Malmo Mammographic Screening Trial. *BMJ,* 1988, *297*:943-948.
13. Frisell, J., Eklund, G., Hellstrom, L., et al. Randomized study of mammography screening—Preliminary report on mortality in the Stockholm trial. *Breast Cancer Res Treat,* 1991, *18*:49-56.
14. Roberts, M.M., Alexander, F.E., Anderson, T.J., et al. Edinburgh trial of screening for breast cancer: Mortality at seven years. *Lancet,* 1990, *335*:241-246.
15. Miller, A.B., Howe, G.R., & Wall, C. The national study of breast cancer screening protocol for a Canadian randomized controlled trial of screening for breast cancer in women. *Clin Invest Med—Medecine Clinique et Experimentale,* 1981, *4*(3-4):227-258.
16. Miller, A.B., Baines, C.J., To, T., & Wall, C. Canadian National Breast Screening Study: 1. Breast cancer detection and death rates among women aged 40 to 49 years. *Can Med Assoc J,* 1992, *147*(10):1459-1476.
17. Miller, A.B., Baines, C.J., To, T., & Wall, C. Canadian National Breast Screening Study: 2. Breast cancer detection and death rates among women aged 50 to 59 years. *Can Med Assoc J,* 1992, *147*(10):1477-1488.
18. Smith, R.A., Cokkinides, V., & Eyre, H.J. American Cancer Society guidelines for the early detection of cancer. *CA: Cancer J Clin,* 2003, *53*(1):27-43.
19. American Cancer Society. *Cancer facts & figures 2001.* Atlanta, GA: American Cancer Society, 2001.
20. Eastman, P. NCI adopts new mammography screening guidelines for women. *J Natl Cancer Inst,* 1997, *89*(8):538-539.
21. Schwartz, M. Validation of a model of breast cancer screening: An outlier suggests the value of breast self-examination. *Med Decision Making,* 1992, *12*(3):222-228.
22. Seidman, H., Gelb, S.K., Silverberg, E., & Lubera, J. Survival experience in the breast cancer detection demonstration project. *CA: Cancer J Clin,* 1987, *37*(5):258-290.
23. Ries, L.A.G., Eisner, M.P., Kosary, C.L., et al. *SEER Cancer Statistics Review, 1973-1997.* Bethesda, MD: National Cancer Institute, 2002.
24. Winawer, S.J., Zauber, A.G., O'Brien, M., et al. The National Polyp Study. *Cancer,* 1992, *70*(5):1236-1245.
25. Winawer, S.J., Zauber, A.G., Ho, M.N., et al. Prevention of colorectal cancer by colonoscopic polypectomy. The National Polyp Study Workgroup. *N Engl J Med,* 1993, *329*(27):1977-1981.
26. National Cancer Institute. *Conquering colorectal cancer: A blueprint for the future.* Colorectal Cancer Progress Review Group, 2000.
27. Mandel, J.S., Bond, J.H., Church, T.R., et al. Reducing mortality from colorectal cancer by screening for fecal occult blood. Minnesota Colon Cancer Control Study. *New Engl J Med,* 1993, *328*(19):1365-71.
28. Winawer, S.J., Fletcher, R.H., Miller, L., et al. Colorectal cancer screening: clinical guidelines and rationale. *Gastroenterology,* 1997, *112*(2):594-642.
29. Smith, R.A., von Eschenbach, A.C., Wender, R., et al. American Cancer Society guidelines for the early detection of cancer: update of early detection guidelines for prostate, colorectal, and endometrial cancers. *CA: Cancer J Clin,* 2001, *51*(1):38-75.
30. Rex, D., Johnson, D., Lieberman, D., et al. Colorectal cancer prevention 2000: Screening recommendations of the American College of Gastroenterology. *Am J Gastroenterol,* 2000, *95*(4):868-877.
31. Centers for Disease Control. Screening for colorectal cancer—United States, 1997. *MMWR Morb Mort Wkly Rep,* 1999, *48*(6):116-121.
32. Ries, L.A.G., Eisner, M.P., Kosary, C.L., et al. *SEER Cancer Statistics Review, 1973-1997.* Bethesda, MD: National Cancer Institute, 2002.
33. Breen, N., Wagener, D.K., Brown, M.L., et al. Progress in cancer screening over a decade: Results of cancer screening from the 1987, 1992, and 1998 National Health Interview Surveys. *J Natl Cancer Inst,* 2001, *93*(22):1704-1713.
34. Hochbaum, G.M. *Public participation in medical screening programs: A socio-psychological study.* Washington, DC: U.S. Dept. of Health, Education, and Welfare, 1958.
35. Rosenstock, I.M., Strecher, V.J., & Becker, M.H. Social learning theory and the Health Belief Model. *Health Ed Qtly,* 1988, *15*(2):175-183.
36. Prochaska, J.O., Velicer, W.F., Rossi, J.S., et al. Stages of change and decisional balance for 12 problem behaviors. *Health Psychol,* 1994, *13*(1):39-46.
37. Bandura, A. Self-efficacy. In *Social foundations of thought and action: A social cognitive theory.* Englewood Cliffs, NJ: Prentice-Hall, 1986, pp. 390-449.

38. Champion, V. Instrument development for health belief model constructs. *Adv Nurs Sci*, 1984, 6(3):73-85.

39. Champion, V.L. Instrument refinement for breast cancer screening behaviors. *Nurs Res*, 1993, 42(3):139-143.

40. Champion, V.L., & Menon, U. Predicting mammography and breast self-examination in African American women. *Cancer Nurs*, 1997, 20(5):315-322.

41. Mikhail, B.I., & Petro-Nustas, W.I. Transcultural Adaptation of Champion's Health Belief Model Scales. *J Nurs Schol*, 2001, 33(2):159-165.

42. Lee, E.H., Kim, J.S., & Song, M.S. Translation and Validation of Champion's Health Belief Model Scale With Korean Women. *Cancer Nurs*, 2002, 25(5):391-395.

43. Lauver, D., & Angerame, M. Development of a questionnaire to measure beliefs and attitudes about breast self-examination. *Cancer Nurs*, 1988, 11(1):51-57.

44. Champion, V.L. Revised susceptibility, benefits, and barriers scale for mammography screening. *Res Nurs Health*, 1999, 22(4):341-348.

45. Han, Y., Williams, R., & Harrison, R. Breast cancer screening knowledge, attitudes, and practices among Korean American Women. *Oncol Nurs Forum*, 2000, 27(10):1585-1591.

46. Champion, V.L., & Huster, G. Effect of interventions on stage of mammography adoption. *J Behav Med*, 1995, 18(2):169-187.

47. Champion, V.L. The relationship of selected variables to breast cancer detection behaviors in women 35 and older. *Oncol Nurs Forum*, 1991, 18(4):733-739.

48. Miller, A.M., & Champion, V.L. Attitudes about breast cancer and mammography: Racial, income, and educational differences. *Women Health*, 1997, 26(1):41-63.

49. Rawl, S., Champion, V., Menon, U., et al. The impact of age and race on mammography practices. *Health Care Women Int*, 2000, 21:583-597.

50. Champion, V.L., Menon, U., Maraj, M., et al. Comparison of tailored interventions to increase mammography screening in nonadherent older women. *Prev Med*, 2003, 12(1):61-71.

51. Champion, V.L., Skinner, C.S., & Menon, U. Development of a self-efficacy scale for mammography. (Submitted.)

52. Lagerlund, M., Hedin, A., Sparen, P., et al. Attitudes, beliefs, and knowledge as predictors of nonattendance in a Swedish population-based mammography screening program. *Prev Med*, 2000, 31:417-428.

53. Crane, L.A., Kaplan, C.P., Bastani, R., & Scrimshaw, S.C.M. Determinants of adherence among health department patients referred for a mammogram. *Women Health*, 1996, 24(2):43-64.

54. Janz, N.K., & Becker, M.H., The Health Belief Model: A decade later. *Health Ed Qtly*, 1984, 11(1):1-47.

55. Friedman, L.C., Weinberg, A.D., Woodruff, A., et al. Breast cancer screening behaviors and intentions among asymptomatic women 50 years of age and older. *Am J Prev Med*, 1995, 11(4):218-223.

56. Rakowski, W., Dube, C.E., Marcus, B.H., et al. Assessing elements of women's decisions about mammography. *Health Psychol*, 1992, 11(2):111-118.

57. Rakowski, W., Fulton, J.P., & Feldman, J.P. Women's decision making about mammography: A replication of the relationship between stages of adoption and decisional balance. *Health Psychol*, 1993, 12:209-214.

58. Rakowski, W., Ehrich, B., Goldstein, M.G., et al. Increasing mammography among women aged 40-74 by use of a stage-matched, tailored intervention. *Prev Med*, 1998, 27(5 Pt 1):748-756.

59. Rimer, B.K., Schildkraut, J.M., Lerman, C., et al. Participation in women's breast cancer risk counseling trial. Who participates? Who declines? *Cancer*, 1996, 77(11):2348-2355.

60. Clemow, L., Costanza, M.E., Haddad, W.P., et al. Underutilizers of mammography screening today: Characteristics of women planning, undecided about, and not planning a mammogram. *Ann Behav Med*, 2000, 22(1):80-88.

61. Rakowski, W. Transtheoretical model of behavioral change: Application to clinical practice. *Mind/Body Med*, 1996, 1(4):207-220.

62. Rimer, B.K., Conaway, M.R., Lyna, P.R., et al. Cancer screening practices among women in a community health center population. *Am J Prev Med*, 1996, 12(5):351-357.

63. Witte, K. Putting the fear back into fear appeals: The extended parallel process model. *Comm Monographs*, 1992, 59(4):329-349.

64. Champion, V.L., Menon, U., et al. A breast cancer fear scale: Psychometric development. (Under review.)

65. Champion, V., & Scott, C. Effects of a procedural/belief intervention on breast self-examination performance. *Res Nurs Health*, 1993, 16(3):163-170.

66. Champion, V.L., & Scott, C.R. Reliability and validity of breast cancer screening belief scales in African American women. *Nurs Res*, 1997, 46(6):331-337.

67. Mahloch, J., Paskett, E., Henderson, M., et al. An evaluation of BSE frequency and quality and their relationship to breast lump detection. *Adv Cancer Control: Screen Prev Res*, 1990, :269-280.

68. Coleman, E.A. Practice and effectiveness of breast self-examination: A selective review of the literature (1977-1989). *J Cancer Ed*, 1991, 6(2):83-92.

69. Shepperd, S.L., Solomon, L.J., Atkins, E., et al. Determinants of breast self-examination among women of lower income and lower education. *J Behav Med*, 1990, 13(4):359-371.

70. Atkins, E., Solomon, L.J., Worden, J.K., & Foster, R.S. Relative effectiveness of methods of breast self-examination. *J Behav Med*, 1991, 14(4):357-367.

71. Zapka, J.G., Stoddard, A., Maul, L., & Costanza, M.E. Interval adherence to mammography screening guidelines. *Med Care*, 1991, 29:697-707.

72. National Cancer Institute Breast Cancer Screening Consortium. Screening mammography: A missed clinical opportunity? *JAMA*, 1990, 264(1):54-58.

73. Champion, V., & Springston, J. Mammography adherence and beliefs in a sample of low-income African American women. *Int J Behav Med*, 1999, 6(3):228-240.

74. Champion, V.L., Skinner, C.S., & Foster, J.L. The effects of standard care counseling or telephone/in-person counseling on beliefs, knowledge, and behavior related to mammography screening. *Oncol Nurs Forum*, 2000, 27(10):1565-1571.

75. Champion, V.L., Skinner, C.S., Menon, U., et al. Comparisons of tailored mammography interventions at

two months postintervention. *Ann Behav Med*, 2002, *24*(3):211-218.

76. Skinner, C.S., Champion, V.L., Menon, U., & Seshadri, R. Race and education differences in mammography related perceptions among 1,336 nonadherent women. *J Psychosoc Oncol*, In Press.

77. Black, W.C., Haggstrom, D.A., & Welch, H.G. All-cause mortality in randomized trials of cancer screening. *J Natl Cancer Inst*, 2002, *94*(3):167-173.

78. Champion, V.L., Menon, U., McQuillen, D.H., & Scott, C. Validity of self-reported mammography in low-income African-American women. *Am J Prev Med*, 1998, *14*(2):111-117.

79. Lerman, C., Daly, M., Sands, C., et al. Mammography adherence and psychological distress among women at risk for breast cancer. *J Natl Cancer Inst*, 1993, *85*(13):1074-1080.

80. Rawl, S., Champion, V.L., Menon, U., et al. Validation of scales to measure benefits and barriers to colorectal cancer screening. *J Psychosoc Oncol*, 2001, *19*(3/4):47-63.

81. Rawl, S.M., Menon, U., Champion, V.L., et al. Colorectal cancer screening beliefs: Focus groups with first-degree relatives. *Cancer Pract*, 2000, *8*(1):32-37.

82. Wardle, J., Williamson, S., McCaffery, K., et al. Increasing Attendance at Colorectal Cancer Screening: Testing the Efficacy of Mailed, Psychoeducational Intervention in a Community Sample of Older Adults. *Health Psychol*, 2003, *22*(1):99-105.

83. Manne, S., Meropol, N., Rakowski, W., et al. Correlates of colorectal cancer screening compliance and stage of adoption among siblings of individuals with early onset colorectal cancer. *Health Psychol*, 2002, *21*(1):3-15.

84. Vernon, S.W., Myers, R.E., & Tilley, B.C. Development and validation of an instrument to measure factors related to colorectal cancer screening adherence. *Cancer Epidemiol Biomark Prev*, 1997, *6*(10):825-832.

85. Rawl, S., & Champion, V. *Increasing screening in families with colorectal cancer* (funded research 1R21CA093454). Bethesda, MD: National Cancer Institute, 2002.

86. Rawl, S., Champion, V., & Rex, D. *Telehealth intervention to increase colorectal cancer screening* (funded research 1R15NR007999). Bethesda, MD: National Institute of Nursing Research, 2003.

87. Brenes, G.A., & Paskett, E.D. Predictors of stage of adoption for colorectal cancer screening. *Prev Med*, 2000, *31*:410-416.

88. Borrayo, E.A., & Guarnaccia, C.A. Differences in Mexican-born and U.S.-born women of Mexican descent regarding factors related to breast cancer screening behaviors. *Health Care Women Int*, 2000, *21*:599-613.

89. Lerman, C., Audrain, J., & Croyle, R.T. DNA-testing for heritable breast cancer risks: lessons from the traditional genetic counseling. *Ann Behav Med*, 1994, *16*(4):327-333.

90. Burnett, C.B., Steakley, C.S., Slack, R., et al. Patterns of breast cancer screening among lesbians at increased risk for breast cancer. *Women Health*, 1999, *29*(4):35-55.

91. Daly, M.B., Lerman, C.L., Ross, E., et al. Gail model breast cancer risk components are poor predictors of risk perception and screening behavior. *Breast Cancer Res Treat*, 1996, *41*:59-70.

92. Lerman, C., Daly, M., Masny, A., & Balshem, A. Attitudes about genetic testing for breast-ovarian cancer susceptibility. *J Clin Oncol*, 1994, *12*(4):843-850.

93. Lipkus, I.M., Lyna, P.R., & Rimer, B.K. Colorectal cancer risk perceptions and screening intentions in a minority population. *J Natl Med Assoc*, 2000, *92*(10):492-500.

94. Blalock, S.J., DeVellis, B.M., Afifi, R.A., & Sandler, R. Risk perceptions and participation in colorectal cancer screening. *Health Psychol*, 1990, *9*(6):792-806.

95. Powe, B.D. Cancer fatalism among African-Americans: A review of the literature. *Nurs Outlook*, 1996, *44*:18-21.

96. Powe, B.D. Cancer fatalism among elderly Caucasians and African Americans. *Oncol Nurs Forum*, 1995, *22*:1355-1359.

97. Powe, B.D. Fatalism among elderly African Americans: Effects on colorectal cancer screening. *Cancer Nurs*, 1995, *18*(5):385-392.

98. King, E.S., Rimer, B.K., Trock, B., et al. How valid are mammography self-reports? *Am J Pub Health*, 1990, *80*(11):1386-1388.

99. Barratt, A., Cockburn, J., Smith, D., & Redman, S. Reliability and validity of women's recall of mammographic screening. *Austr N Z J Pub Health*, 2000, *24*(1):79-81.

100. Hiatt, R.A., Perez-Stable, E.J., Quesenberry, C., et al. Agreement between self-reported early cancer detection practices and medical audits among Hispanic and non-Hispanic white health plan members in northern California. *Prev Med*, 1995, *24*(3):278-285.

101. Fulton-Kehoe, D., Burg, M.A., & Lane, D.S. Are self-reported dates of mammograms accurate? *Pub Health Rev*, 1992, *93*(20):233-240.

102. Gordon, N., Hiatt, R., & Lampert, D. Concordance of self-report data and medical record audit for six cancer screening procedures. *J Natl Cancer Inst*, 1993, *85*(7):566-570.

103. Lipkus, I.M., Rimer, B.K., Lyna, P.R., et al. Colorectal screening patterns and perceptions of risk among African-American users of a community health center. *J Comm Health*, 1996, *21*(6):409-427.

104. Price, J. Perceptions of colorectal cancer in a socioeconomically disadvantaged population. *J Comm Health*, 1993, *18*:347-362.

105. Rakowski, W., Clark, M.A., Pearlman, D.N., et al. Integrating pros and cons for mammography and pap testing: Extending the const. *Prev Med*, 1997, *26*:664-673.

106. Velicer, W.F., DiClemente, C.C., Prochaska, J.O., et al. Decisional balance measure for assessing and predicting smoking status. *J Pers Soc Psychol*, 1985, *48*(5):1279-1289.

107. National Cancer Institute Cancer Screening Consortium for Underserved Women. Breast and cervical cancer screening among underserved women: Baseline survey results from six states. *Arch Fam Med*, 1995, *4*(7):617-624.

108. Skinner, C.S., Champion, V.L., Gonin, R., & Hanna, M. Do perceived barriers and benefits vary by mammography stage? *Psychol Health Med*, 1997, *2*(1):65-75.

109. Black, M.E.A., Stein, K.F., & Loveland-Cherry, C.J. Older women and mammography screening behav-

ior: Do possible selves contribute? *Health Educ Behav,* 2001, *28*(2):200-216.

110. Myers, R.E., Vernon, S.W., Tilley, B.C., et al. Intention to screen for colorectal cancer among white male employees. *Prev Med,* 1998, 27(2):279-87.

111. Rawl, S., Menon, U., Champion, V., et al. Do benefits and barriers differ by stage of adoption for colorectal cancer screening? (submitted).

112. Lerman, C., Kash, K., & Stefanek, M. Younger women at increased risk for breast cancer: perceived risk, psychological well-being, and surveillance behavior. *J Natl Cancer Inst Monogr,* 1994, *16*:171-176.

113. Powe, B.D., & Weinrich, S. An intervention to decrease cancer fatalism among rural elders. *Oncol Nurs Forum,* 1999, *26*(3):583-588.

Appendix 27A. Measures of Breast Cancer Screening Beliefs

Instrument	Description/Constructs Measured	Psychometrics
Champion Health Belief Model Scales[38,40–43,45,49,66,78,88]	**Breast Self-Examination (BSE) Beliefs:** *Perceived Benefits of BSE:* 4-item Likert scale to assess perceived positive outcomes of performing monthly BSE *Perceived Barriers to BSE:* 11-item Likert scale to assess perceived negative aspects of BSE. Sample items included BSE is embarrassing, takes too much time, not necessary if provider does breast exam, breasts are too large, etc. *Perceived Self-Efficacy for BSE:* 10-item Likert scale to assess confidence in performing BSE. Sample item: "I am able to find a breast lump which is the size of a pea." **Mammography Beliefs:** *Perceived benefits of mammography:* 5-item Likert scale to assess perceived positive outcomes of mammography. Sample item: "Having a mammogram will help me find breast lumps early." *Perceived barriers to mammography:* 11-item Likert scale to assess perceived emotions, physical, or structural concerns related to mammography. Sample items included mammography is embarrassing, takes too much time, is costly, painful, etc. *Perceived Self-Efficacy for Mammography:* 10-item Likert scale to assess confidence in obtaining a mammogram. Sample item: "I can remember to schedule a mammogram."	Internal consistency: $\alpha = 0.69$ Test–retest: $r = 0.48$ Confirmatory factor analyses[66] Internal consistency: $\alpha = 0.83$ Test–retest: $r = 0.52$ Confirmatory factor analyses[66] Internal consistency: $\alpha = 0.90$ Test–retest: $r = 0.65$ Confirmatory factor analyses[66] Internal consistency: $\alpha = 0.75$; Test–retest: $r = 0.61$ Construct validity: exploratory and confirmatory factor analyses Predictive validity[4] Internal consistency: $\alpha = 0.88$; Test–retest: $r = 0.71$ Construct validity: exploratory and confirmatory factor analyses Predictive validity[4] Internal consistency: $\alpha = 0.88$ Construct validity: Confirmatory factor analysis, logistic regression for theoretical relationships

Mammography Pro and Con Scales[56,57,60,62,105]	**Mammography Pro and Con Scales:** *Pros of Mammography:* 5- to 6-item Likert scales derived from transtheoretical model to assess positive perceptions of mammography. Similar to HBM construct of benefits. Sample item from pro scale: "Having a regular mammogram will give you a feeling of control over your health." *Cons of Mammography:* 5- to 7-item Likert scales derived from transtheoretical model to assess negative perceptions toward and avoidance of mammography (cons). Similar to HBM construct of barriers. Sample item from con scale: "You would probably not have a mammogram unless you had a problem with your breasts."	Validity of pro and con constructs supported via principal component analyses. Reliability indices for pro scales: Internal consistency (5 items): $\alpha = 0.72$ 6 items: $\alpha = 0.77$ Reliability indices for con scales: Internal consistency (5 items): $\alpha = 0.77$ 7 items: $\alpha = 0.78$
Decisional Balance Index[57,60,106]	Summary index derived from two variables, pros and cons, which denote positive and negative features of the target behavior. Positive decisional balance = pros outweigh cons, negative decisional balance = cons outweigh pros. Pro and con indexes converted to standardized scores, then to t scores. Decisional balance measure computed by subtracting con t scores from pro t scores	Construct validation of pro and con scales supported via principal component analyses. Validation of decisional balance constructs supported by examination of relationships to stage of adoption; decisional balance became more favorable as woman moved through stages of adoption
Champion Breast Cancer Fear Scale[64]	*Breast Cancer Fear:* 8-item Likert scale designed to assess fear of breast cancer, specifically, the subjective response and physiologic arousal to the threat	Internal consistency: $\alpha = 0.91$ Test–retest: $r = 0.70$. Construct validity established via principal component analyses and regression analyses to test relationships to relevant HBM variables

27B. Measures of Breast Cancer Screening Behaviors

Instrument	Description/Constructs Measured	Psychometrics
BSE Frequency[39,40,65]	**Breast Self-Examination (BSE) Frequency** *Frequency:* Self-reported frequency of BSE; number of times BSE completed in last 12 months	Single item measure
BSE Proficiency[39,40,65,67,68,70]	**Breast Self-Examination Proficiency** *Self-Reported Proficiency:* Assessed with 9-item scale, including self-report of length of time taken to examine breasts, pattern, positioning, use of hands, areas of breast covered, and whether mirror was used *Observed Proficiency:* Observational checklist used by trained observer to assess proficiency. Included 10 procedural components deemed critical to correct BSE technique. Perfect score = 24 points *Frequency & Proficiency:* Self-report log/diary in the form of a 12-month calendar kept by women. Allowed for checking off completion of BSE steps and techniques each month. Range of 0–96 points possible over 12 months Observer assessment covered 5 items, such as areas of breast covered, use of finger pads, pressure, search pattern, and mirror Developed scoring system to measure eight components of BSE proficiency as specified by Mamma Care: area covered, pressure type, motion, part of fingers, pattern, number of fingers, number of motions and duration	Pre- and post training indicated significant difference ($p = 0.002$) Weights given to each component and pre- and post test validity indicated significant differences
Mammography Utilization[71,72,79,107]	Self-reported utilization questions developed by NCI Breast Cancer Consortium regarding whether woman had ever heard of a mammogram, ever had a mammogram, number of mammograms had in last 5 years, timing of most recent mammogram	Single item measures

| Mammography Stage of Adoption[44,57,78,108] | **Mammography Stage of Adoption:** Assessed by combining responses to mammography utilization questions regarding whether woman ever heard of a mammogram, ever had a mammogram, number of mammograms had in last 5 years, timing of most recent mammogram, and intent to have a mammogram in the next 6 months

Precontemplation: Never had a mammogram and not thinking about having one in the next 6 months
Contemplation: Never had a mammogram but thinking about having one in next 6 months
Action: Had a mammogram in last 15 months
Relapse precontemplation: Last mammogram > 15 months ago and not thinking about having one
Relapse contemplation: Last mammogram > 15 months ago and thinking about having one in next 6 months | Staging algorithms based on combinations of utilization items
Construct validity: Women in various stages differed from each other in directions predicted by theory: precontemplators and contemplators were less likely to agree with benefits of mammography and more likely to agree with barrier items than those in action[108] |
| Mammography Adherence[49,78,79,109] | **Mammography Adherence:** Dichotomous variable indicating whether woman had had a mammogram in specified timeframe. Timeframe can vary from last 12 months, last 15 months, last 24 months, or time since intervention receipt/delivery. Adherence often determined based on whether mammogram was obtained within appropriate timeframe in accordance with American Cancer Society recommendations (depending on woman's age) | Only 48% of self-reported mammograms were verified by medical record data[78] |

27C. Measures of Colorectal Cancer Screening Beliefs

Instrument	Description/Constructs Measured	Psychometrics
CRC Screening Benefits & Barriers Scales[80]	**Colorectal Cancer Screening Beliefs**	
	Benefits of FOBT. 5-item Likert scale assessing perceived benefits to doing a stool blood test at home. Sample item: "A stool blood test will help find CRC early."	Internal consistency: $\alpha = 0.65$ Construct validity supported via exploratory factor analyses, known groups validity
	Barriers to FOBT. 8-item scale assessing perceived barriers to doing a stool blood test at home. Sample items assess fear of positive results, embarrassment, lack of time, no need for FOBT because I have no problems/symptoms, unpleasant nature of collecting stool sample, and so on	Internal consistency: $\alpha = 0.72$ Construct validity supported via exploratory factor analyses, known groups validity
	Benefits of sigmoidoscopy. 5-item Likert scale assessing perceived benefits of having a sigmoidoscopy. Sample item: Having a sigmoidoscopy will decrease my chance of dying from CRC	Internal consistency: $\alpha = 0.67$ Construct validity supported via exploratory factor analyses, known groups validity
	Barriers to sigmoidoscopy. 8-item Likert scale assessing perceived barriers to having a sigmoidoscopy. Sample items include those listed above under barriers to FOBT *plus* pain, lack of understanding about what will be done during the test, dietary restrictions, laxative, and enema (bowel prep)	Internal consistency: $\alpha = 0.65$ Construct validity supported via exploratory factor analyses, known groups validity
	Benefits of colonoscopy. 5-item Likert scale assessing perceived benefits of having a colonoscopy. Sample item: "Having a colonoscopy will help you not worry as much about CRC."	Internal consistency: $\alpha = 0.70$ Construct validity supported via exploratory factor analyses, known groups validity
	Barriers to colonoscopy. 10-item Likert scale assessing perceived barriers to having a colonoscopy. Sample items include those listed above under barriers to FOBT & sigmoidoscopy *plus* fear of complications and lack of transportation	Internal consistency: $\alpha = 0.77$ Construct validity supported via exploratory factor analyses, known groups validity
Attitudes Toward Sigmoidoscopy[82]	**Attitudes Toward Sigmoidoscopy**	
	Benefits of sigmoidoscopy. 7-item Likert scale assessing positive attitudes toward sigmoidoscopy. Sample item: "The test would be reassuring," "If I don't go, I might later wish I'd been tested."	Internal consistency: $\alpha = 0.83$ Validity supported via principal components analyses
	Barriers to sigmoidoscopy. 6-item scale assessing negative attitudes toward sigmoidoscopy. Sample items: "The test would be uncomfortable," "embarrassment would put me off."	Internal consistency: $\alpha = 0.83$ Validity supported via principal components analyses
	Fatalism. 4-item Likert scale assessing fear of cancer/fatalism. Sample items: "I would rather not know," "What will be, will be."	Internal consistency: $\alpha = 0.77$ Validity supported via principal components analyses
	Sigmoidoscopy Priority. 3-item scale assessing whether screening is a priority. Sample items: "I'm too busy to have the test," "There is no need for healthy people to have the test."	Internal consistency: $\alpha = 0.72$ Validity supported via principal components analyses

Pros and Cons of Colorectal Screening[83]	**Pros and Cons**	
	Pros of CRC screening: 9 items rated on a 5-point Likert scale (5 = strongly agree, 1 = strongly disagree) derived from the transtheoretical model to assess positive perceptions of CRC screening. Similar to HBM construct of benefits. Sample item from pros scale: "Regular colon cancer tests will help me live a long life."	Internal consistency: α = 0.76 Face validity supported
	Cons of CRC Screening: 19-items rated on a 5-point Likert scale (5 = strongly agree, 1 = strongly disagree) derived from the transtheoretical model to assess negative perceptions toward and avoidance of CRC screening. Similar to HBM construct of barriers. Sample item from cons scale: "Too many things can go wrong with tests for colon cancer."	Internal consistency: α = 0.80 Face validity supported
Factors Related to CRC Screening Adherence[84,110]	**Factors Related to CRC Screening Adherence**	
	Salience and coherence: 4-item scale measuring perceptions about the technical effectiveness & personal benefit (benefits). Sample items: "Doing CRC screening makes sense to me," "Going through screening is an important thing for me to do."	Internal consistency: α = 0.88 Validity supported via exploratory and confirmatory factor analyses, discriminant analyses
	Self-efficacy: 4-item scale measuring perceptions of confidence in ability to get CRC screening. Sample item: "Going through CRC screening would be difficult for me to do."	Internal consistency: α = 0.82 Validity supported via exploratory and confirmatory factor analyses, discriminant analyses
	Worries/concerns: 2-item scale measuring perceived negative consequences of CRC screening (barriers). Sample item: "I am worried that screening will show I have CRC or polyps."	Internal consistency: α = 0.72 Validity supported via exploratory and confirmatory factor analyses, discriminant analyses
	Intention: 2-item scale measuring intent to undertake CRC screening. Sample item: "I intend to undergo CRC screening."	Internal consistency: α = 0.79 Face validity supported

27D. Measures of Colorectal Cancer Screening Behaviors

Instrument	Description/Constructs Measured	Psychometrics
CRC Screening Utilization[1,3,23,31]	Self-reported utilization questions developed for the Behavioral Risk Factor Surveillance Survey regarding whether people have ever done a stool blood test using a home kit, and if so, when their last stool blood test was done. Two similar items assess whether respondents ever had sigmoidoscopy or colonoscopy (combined) and timing of last endoscopy procedure	Single item measures
CRC Screening Adherence	Dichotomous variable indicating whether person had a screening test in specified timeframe. Timeframe for FOBT can vary from last 12 months, last 15 months, last 24 months, or time since intervention receipt/delivery. Adherence may be determined based on whether test was obtained within appropriate timeframe in accordance with American Cancer Society recommendations. Adherence to endoscopic screening dependent on risk stratification	Single item measures
CRC Screening Stage of Adoption[85-87,111]	**Stage of Adoption for CRC Screening** After descriptions of each test are provided, four items (for EACH test) assess whether people: (1) have ever done/had the test, (2) have thought about doing or having the test, (3) are planning to do/have the test in the next 6 months, and (4) have a stool blood test kit at home now or have an appointment to have a sigmoidoscopy/colonoscopy. Another item assesses time since last test **FOBT Stage of Adoption** is defined as: (1) *Precontemplation*—never done an FOBT OR had one more than 15 months ago AND does not intend to do one in the next 6 months; (2) *Contemplation*—never done an FOBT OR had one more than 15 months ago AND intends to do one in the next 6 months; (3) *Preparation*—never done an FOBT OR had one more than 15 months ago AND has an FOBT kit at home now; (4) *Action*—done FOBT within the last 15 months. **Sigmoidoscopy Stage of Adoption** is defined as: (1) *Precontemplation*—never had a sigmoidoscopy OR had one more than 5 years ago AND does not intend to have one in the next 6 months; (2) *Contemplation*—never had a sigmoidoscopy OR had one more than 5 years ago AND intends to have one in the next 6 months; (3) *Preparation*—never had a sigmoidoscopy OR had one more than 5 years ago AND has an appointment to have one; (4) *Action*—had a sigmoidoscopy within the last 5 years	Staging algorithms based on combinations of utilization items Construct validity: People in various stages differed from each other in directions predicted by theory. Precontemplators and contemplators were less likely to agree with benefits of FOBT, sigmoidoscopy and colonoscopy and more likely to agree with barrier items than those in action[111] May be difficult to stage for endoscopy since provider recommendation for follow-up is dependent on findings

	Colonoscopy Stage of Adoption is defined as: (1) *Precontemplation*—never had a colonoscopy OR had one more than 10 years ago AND does not intend to have one in the next 6 months; (2) *Contemplation*—never had a colonoscopy OR had one more than 10 years ago AND intends to have one in the next 6 months; (3) *Preparation*—never had a colonoscopy OR had one more than 10 years ago AND has an appointment to have one; (4) *Action*—had a colonoscopy within the last 10 years. **Sigmoidoscopy Stage of Adoption:** *Precontemplation*: No sigmoidoscopy in last 5 years and not planning to have one in next 12 months *Contemplation*: No sigmoidoscopy in last 5 years and planning to have one in next 12 months *Action*: Had sigmoidoscopy in last 5 years	Construct validity supported Theoretical predictions consistent with findings. Women in precontemplation and contemplation perceived more barriers and had lower perceived susceptibility/risk than those in action
Colorectal Screening Stage of Adoption[83]	**Colorectal Screening Stage of Adoption** *Precontemplation*: Has not had any screening and has no plan for any in the next year *Relapse/risk for relapse*: Has had one or more screening test in the past but is now off schedule AND does not plan to have a screening test in the next year, OR is presently on schedule but does not plan to have the test that would place the person on schedule in the next year *Contemplation*: Has not had a prior screening test but intends to have one in the next year OR is off schedule after having prior screening but intends to have one in the next year *Action*: Has had a colonoscopy on schedule and plans on having another in a timeframe that would keep them on schedule OR has had an FOBT and a sigmoidoscopy on schedule and plans to have both tests in the same time period that would keep them on schedule *Maintenance*: Has had two or more colonoscopies on a regular schedule and plans to have another on schedule OR has had two or more FOBTs and two or more sigmoidoscopies on a regular schedule and plans to have both tests in the time period that would keep them on schedule	Construct validity supported Theoretical predictions consistent with findings; people in precontemplation and contemplation reported more cons compared to those in action; addresses interdependence of screening tests

27E. Measures of Cancer Beliefs Relevant to Breast and Colorectal Cancer Screening

Instrument	Description/Constructs Measured	Psychometrics
Perceived Susceptibility or Risk: Breast Cancer Champion, 1984[38,44,79,90,91,112]	**Breast Cancer** *Perceived susceptibility/risk:* 3-item Likert scale assesses perceived beliefs of personal threat or harm related to breast cancer. Sample item: "My chances of getting breast cancer in the next few years are great." *Perceived relative risk:* "Compared to other women your age, would you say your chances of getting breast cancer are: much lower, lower, about the same, higher, or much higher?" *Perceived absolute risk:* "On a scale of 0–100, where 0 = no chance of getting breast cancer and 100 = definitely will develop breast cancer, rate your chances of getting breast cancer sometime during your lifetime."	Internal consistency: α = 0.87 Test-retest: r = 0.62 Construct validity: exploratory and confirmatory factor analyses Predictive validity (Champion, 1999)[44] Single item measure. Inconsistently related to screening behavior across studies Single item measure. Inconsistently related to screening behavior across studies
Perceived Susceptibility/ Risk: CRC[83–86,93,94]	**Colorectal Cancer (CRC)** *Perceived susceptibility/risk:* 3-item Likert scale modified from Champion's to assess perceived beliefs of personal threat or harm related to CRC. Sample item: "My chances of getting CRC in the next few years are great." *Perceived susceptibility:* 3-item scale measuring subjective personal risk of developing CRC or polyps. Sample item: "I think it is very likely that I will develop CRC or polyps." *Perceived relative risk:* "Compared to other people your age, race and sex/with similar family history, what do you think is your chance of getting colorectal cancer in your lifetime?" Response options: below average, average, or above average;[83] 5-point Likert scale with 1 = much lower and 5 = much higher.[93,94] *Perceived absolute risk:* "What is your chance of getting CRC sometime during your lifetime?" Response options: below average, average, above average;[83] 5-point Likert scale with 1 = very unlikely to 5 = very likely;[93] 0–100 rating scale.[94]	Internal consistency: α = 0.75 to 0.77 in preliminary studies Internal consistency: α = 0.79 Validity supported via exploratory and confirmatory factor analyses, discriminant analyses Single item measures. Inconsistently related to screening intention or behavior Single item measures. Inconsistently related to screening intention or behavior
Cancer Fatalism[95–97,113]	*Cancer Fatalism:* 15-item dichotomous scale that measured fear, predetermination, pessimism, and inevitable death	Internal consistency: 0.84 Construct validity: Exploratory factor analysis

28

Measuring Information-Seeking Behaviors and Decision-Making Preferences

Caroline Bagley-Burnett

Information is a key to understanding the problems, challenges, and frustrations with which an individual is faced throughout his or her lifespan. Individuals often have to seek out new information to promote health, prevent illness, or make treatment decisions. Information is essential in decision making and is considered by many to be a means of coping with and reducing stress and maintaining control.[1–10] For these reasons, it is important for health care providers (1) to understand the concept of information seeking, (2) to possess a knowledge of the behaviors exhibited by patients seeking information, (3) to develop the skills necessary to assess the amount and type of information patients want, (4) to recognize the contextual and situational variables that influence a patient's desire for information, and (5) to recognize situations in which a patient wants or does not want to participate in decision making.

The purposes of this chapter are to present relevant background on the concept of information-seeking and decision-making preferences as found in both consumer and health care literature, to describe the development of instruments used to measure aspects of information seeking and decision making, to evaluate the utility of these instruments for their ability to fulfill their designed purpose, to summarize pertinent research findings that have used selected instruments, and to discuss the contribution of the work toward enhancing health care professionals' understanding of patients' information-seeking behaviors and decision-making preferences.

Consumer Information-Seeking Behavior

A review of the consumer and health-care literature from 1975 to the present reveals that the concept of information seeking is both complex and not easily understood. Research in this area can be found in the consumer literature as early as the 1920s. Early studies that focused on consumer prepurchase information-seeking activities were one component of marketing theory. The literature was sparse until the 1960s, when studies that address the prepurchase activities of consumers surfaced.[11,12]

Since then, interest in consumer prepurchase behavior has increased significantly. There are several reasons for this increase. Manufacturers, retailers, and advertisers benefit from data on consumer prepurchase behavior. These data enable them to target the interests of consumers and result in increased product sales. The consumers' and women's movements have highlighted individuals' rights to information, resulting in an increased demand to be informed. Researcher interest in what motivates people to seek information and make health care decisions has increased. Legislators, health care professionals, and policymakers have shown increased interest in information-seeking behavior. At the national and state levels, laws have been enacted that mandate informed consent, adequate disclosure concerning treatment alternatives for diseases such as breast cancer, and the inclusion of patient package inserts for such drugs as oral contraceptives and estrogens. A few health insurance companies reimburse for health education and may prorate insurance rates accordingly. Organizations such as the American Cancer Society, the National Cancer Institute, and many drug companies, have developed their own information sources for use by consumers. Changes in the economic climate, including income and employment levels, periods of high inflation, skyrocketing medical costs, reduced provider payments, and cutbacks in federal funding, have contributed to an increased preference for more information.

The changes outlined have given consumers improved access to more complete and often complex information. Physicians and nurses are more likely to offer explanations about diagnoses, treatments, side effects, and expected outcomes. This access to and improved availability of information may enable consumers to participate in independent health care decisions, to ask more questions, and to seek information from several sources. Sources of information may include physicians, nurses, pharmacists, television, radio, newspaper, magazines, and to a lesser degree family and friends.[13,14]

Discrepancies[13,14] still exist between what consumers say they want to know and how much information physicians believe their patients want to know. Faden et al.[15] reported that physicians consistently underestimate the amount of information people want about treatments and their side effects. Studies performed with patients receiving patient package inserts show similar results.[13] Research has focused on distinguishing between the amount of information patients say they want and whether, once they have received that information, they choose to use it in health care decision making.

Studies suggest that, although individuals have a desire for information, they frequently report different preferences for participation in actual treatment decisions.[16–21] Caution must be exercised in generalizing these findings or in assuming that more information is better, all people desire complete information, patients want to participate in health care decisions, and more information reduces stress and enhances the ability to cope with this stress. Recent research has focused on how much information individuals want, variables that influence the amount of research desired, and whether a person wants to make the decisions and in what situations. These studies have provided insight into the relationship of such variables as age, sex, and race and psychosocial, cultural, economic, and educational backgrounds to the desire for information and participation in decision making.[22–29] Other factors that influence information-seeking and decision-making preferences, such as previous illness, severity of illness, and personal and significant others' experiences with the health care system, need to be explored.

The problem today, then, is not so much the availability of information as the identification of the type of information a person wants, a recognition of how much and under what circumstances information is needed, a determination of the circumstances in which the individual wishes to use the information, the extent of participation desired, and a clarification of the relationship between sociodemographic variables and the information seeking process. In addition, more research is needed (1) to determine the effects of shared decision making on patient satisfaction and health care outcomes, (2) to determine effective approaches for assessing patient preferences, and (3) to evaluate how best to engage patients in decisions about their health care decisions.[30,31]

As a result of the research conducted on consumer prepurchase information-seeking behavior, a body of knowledge has accumulated that has conceptual relevance to research conducted in the health-care field. For example, Payne[32] and Englander and Tyszka[33] have used an information display board method. This method consists of an information display matrix that has rows listing alternatives and columns describing the attributes of each alternative.[33] They found that people proceeded in either an intradimensional or interdimensional manner; that is, when faced with several alternatives and the choice of characteristics within each alternative, the person might choose to exhaust all characteristics with one alternative (intradimensional) or might choose to explore all the alternatives (interdimensional) before investigating characteristics within each alternative. Unfortunately, the authors did not identify individual characteristics of people or contextual variables that might predict the type of approach chosen. They did find that, when faced with many alternatives, people tend to limit the intradimensional search component, thus sacrificing some depth of knowledge about an alternative, to seek more limited information on the large number of alternatives. Conversely, when faced with only two alternatives, people tended to extend the depth of search. When faced with many alternatives, people attempted to eliminate or collapse the categories to decrease the total number of options to be evaluated. The apparent purpose is to decrease both the complexity of the task and the strain or tension experienced in the evaluation process.

Fast and colleagues[34] investigated the effects of consumer education on search. They described a theoretical model that posited a relationship between consumer education and type of information source used during search. The dependent variable was time allotted to search from four information sources: advertising, sellers, friends and acquaintances, and independent product test reports (such as those found in *Canadian Consumer, Consumer Reports, Consumers' Research,* and *Protect Yourself* magazines). The independent variables in the model include consumer education (e.g., high school, community, or general continuing education programs), wage rate, age, educational level, prior experience, perceived risk, and urgency of purchase. The following findings have particular application to information seeking and decision making in health care.

Friends or relatives were the only search source used in situations that were perceived as high urgency or where there was previous product ownership. In some situations the authors found that prior experience was negatively associated with search. High school continuing education, community workshops, and general public continuing education were not significantly related to information sources chosen for search. There was a significant relationship between reading consumer literature and using product test reports during search. Written product information was preferred over formal classroom presentations.

Although the findings of this study relate to search behavior associated with purchase of major household appliances, the authors define these goods as "high-involvement" items. That is, the items are high cost, involve complex technology, and are potentially uncertain and risky purchases. Framed in this manner, findings from this study have direct relevance to information search and decision making in health care. Health care decisions may involve high-cost, complex technology and uncertainty and risk. Testing of the findings from this study in health care information search and decision-making situations is warranted.

Instruments

Reference to information-seeking activities and decision-making preferences in the health care literature did not appear until the 1960s. These accounts were predominantly clinical anecdotes.[1] Gradually, however, more studies addressed various facets of information-seeking activities and decision-making preferences for consumers of health care.[1,3,17,18,21,22,25,26,35,36]

Little has been written on theories of information-seeking behaviors. Lazarus's theory of stress and coping often is used as a conceptual framework when studying the concept of information-seeking activities. He maintains that knowledge reduces stress and thereby enhances coping.[7] It seems logical, therefore, that people who actively seek information enhance their ability to cope with a particular situation.

Mills and Krantz conceptualized information as a form of cognitive control because it often results in the interpretation of an aversive event so that the threat is lessened.[37] Lenz conceptualized search as an interpersonal process with the primary sources of information being others to whom one has direct access or can be referred.[1] According to Lenz, this process contains six steps: (1) a stimulus, (2) goal setting, (3) a decision regarding whether to seek information actively, (4) search behavior, (5) information acquisition and codification, (6) decision regarding the adequacy of the information acquired, and (7) outcomes.[1]

Hopkins[3] conceptualized information search as a process that occurs throughout a series of related stressful episodes and is characterized by the polar extremes of avoidance and hypervigilance. It is defined as a coping strategy with varying levels of intensity measured quantitatively on the Information Preference Questionnaire.

Research in the area of information-seeking activities and decision-making preferences has increased in the last 5 years. Instruments have been developed that measure search behavior, identify factors influencing information-seeking behavior, and describe situations in which individuals wish to participate in decision making.[38] Many studies have recently addressed the issues of patient information search and desire to participate in decision making, but valid and reliable standardized instruments that are clinically useful are few. Studies are now needed that strengthen instrument validity and reliability. This can be accomplished through collaborative research efforts, use of multiple instruments in the same study, and research conducted with diverse populations.

The following sections review existing scales; their testing, scoring, validity, and reliability; the populations in which they have been tested; and strengths and limitations. Studies using the scales are evaluated.

Miller Behavioral Style Scale (MBSS)

Individuals cope with life experiences in a variety of ways. Use of a defense mechanism, (e.g., denial) may protect and provide the person with time to adjust to stressful events with which he or she is faced. Coping with new situations is influenced by an individual's past experiences, choice of defense mechanisms, and successful outcomes from previous exposure to stressful events. Information has been suggested by some as a means of coping with these stressful events. Personality psychologists have long debated the question of whether individuals exhibit consistent and stable differences in their abilities and inclinations either to seek information or to distract themselves under stress.[39] Recognition of the complexity of information-search behavior has forced researchers to address not only information-seeking activities but also the psychologic and behavioral profile of consumers to meet their needs better. The following discussion summarizes almost two decades of work conducted by Miller and colleagues that focuses on the development, testing, and revisions of the MBSS and more recently the Monitoring Process Model (MPM). The MPM was developed to distinguish how "high and low monitor" and individuals cope with stresses that are of a long-term nature; high monitors tend to scan for threats and is associated with more distress.[40]

Miller and Grant described the development of a scale designed to classify people in terms of their preference for information in a stressful situation.[41] They conceptualize informational preferences under threat as a coping style or dimension. This style categorizes people into monitors (information seekers) or blunters (distractors) on the basis of their choice when faced with a threatening situation. Monitoring involves being alert for and sensitized to the negative aspects of an event. Blunting involves distraction from and cognitive avoidance of objective sources of danger.[4] Miller et al. have conducted considerable research designed to determine when an individual employs a certain coping style and when and if it reduces stress. They have demonstrated that the effectiveness with which people cope with stressful situations is determined by their coping style and by the fit of their preferred strategy to the specific properties of the situation.[4]

Miller developed a self-report scale, the Miller Behavioral Style Scale (MBSS), an instrument designed to measure informational preferences. This scale was not initially developed for use in health care situations. The scale describes four vignettes that represent potentially stress-producing events. Each vignette has eight statements that describe different ways in which an individual might respond. Four of the statements are monitoring responses and four are blunting responses. The following is one vignette.[4]

> Vividly imagine that you are on an airplane. Thirty minutes from your destination the plane unexpectedly goes into a nose dive and then suddenly levels off. The pilot announces that everything is okay, although the rest of the ride may be rough. You are not, however, convinced that all is well.[4]

An example of a monitoring response is, "I would listen carefully to the engines for unusual noises and would watch the crew to see if their behavior was out of the ordinary." An example of a blunting response would be, "I would watch the end of the movie even if I had seen it before."

Subjects are instructed to check statements that best describe behaviors they are likely to use in a stressful situation. Two methods of scoring the MBSS have been described. The first method involves summing the number of positive responses to the "monitor" items and subtracting the sum of positive responses to the "blunting" items.[42] This method yields a single score ranging from −20 to 20. A negative score suggests a tendency to avoid information. The second method of scoring uses separate monitor and blunter scores. Higher scores on each scale indicates more of the behavior being measured.[42] Test-retest reliability across a 4-month period has been reported for the monitor and blunter scales ($r = 0.72$ and $r = 0.75$, respectively).

The MBSS has been shown to predict preference for information versus distraction in response to threatening situations.[4] Chorney et al.[43] have used the instrument in an experimental setting to determine how monitors and blunters perform on a cold pressor task. (The cold pressor task subjectively measures an individual's tolerance level and pain threshold of the extremities to temperature.) A sample of 92 male undergraduate psychology students volunteered for this study. Monitors performed better when the experimental strategy encouraged monitoring, and blunters did better when the situation was compatible with blunting. Their results confirm those of other studies that report the importance of matching an individual's cognitive strategies with his or her coping styles. They conclude that the MBSS "appears to provide a useful, straightforward measure of an important coping style, one which here and elsewhere has been shown to predict performance differences in stress situations."[43]

Miller has used the MBSS with people faced with a short-term aversive stimulus, such as a gynecologic examination, and those faced with a chronic disease, such as cancer or hypertension. She found that blunters who received a lot of information actually reported an increase in anxiety prior to colposcopy. Monitors did not report an increase in anxiety in the same situation. The investigators concluded that this increase in anxiety exhibited by the blunters was a result of receipt of information counter to their preferences.

Barsevick and Johnson[44] examined the information-seeking behaviors of 36 women undergoing colposcopy, a stressful medical procedure. The specific aims of their study were to examine the relationship between (1) preference for information and information-seeking behavior during colposcopy, (2) preference for behavioral involvement and information-seeking behavior during colposcopy, and (3) information-seeking behavior and positive and negative emotional responses during colposcopy.[44]

The MBSS and Krantz Health Opinion Survey (KHOS) were the primary instruments used by the investigators. They observed that women who ask questions or request written information do not always have characteristic preferences for information or involvement in health care.[44] The authors found no significant relationship between scores on the MBSS and the number of questions asked by women undergoing colposcopy or their request for an information sheet. They reported a low correlation between the MBSS and KHOS ($r(36) = 0.33, p < 0.05$). The authors suggested that according to the findings, the MBSS is not a sensitive indicator of preference for information and involvement in health care situations.[44] However, other more recent studies have found the MBSS to be a valid and reliable measure of coping styles and preferences for information. The MBSS/MPM has been used in a variety of settings (e.g., genetic testing and counseling for breast cancer, BRCA 1 and BRCA 2, women at risk for ovarian cancer, and in settings with severe long-term medical threats).[40,45-52]

The MBSS is a widely used measure designed to identify the relationship between information use and coping styles, that is, monitors (information seekers) and blunters (avoiders). This body of work has contributed significantly to our understanding of individuals' processing of information in stressful situations and provides clinicians with a useful measure to determine individual coping styles and preferences for information, thus facilitating tailored interactions.

Information Styles Questionnaire (ISQ)

Cassileth et al. developed the ISQ.[6] This instrument is a self-report tool designed to ascertain the preferences of cancer patients for information about their disease and their desire to participate actively in their treatment. The questionnaire has six sections; five contain individual questions designed to obtain general data about desire for information and preference for involvement in self-care. For example, in one of the questions respondents choose from five possible response options that describe their preference for information. These options range from 1 (no more details than needed) to 5 (as many details as possible). Another question asks the person whether he or she desires other information; if the answer is yes, the person is asked to explain. The patient is asked to choose from the following statements the one that best describes his or her point of view: "I prefer to leave decisions about my medical care and treatment up to my doctor" and "I prefer to participate in decisions about my medical care and treatment." An additional question asks the person to select one of the following statements: "I only want the information needed to care for myself," "I want additional information only if it is good news," and "I want as much information as possible, good or bad." The sixth section contains a list of 12 items designed to elicit specific types of information needed on a scale from "absolutely need," "would like to have," to "do you want" the information. A sample of the statements used to elicit specific information follows: what all the possible side effects are, what treatment will accomplish, whether or not it is cancer, and what the likelihood of cure is.

The instrument was pilot-tested with 50 people, and the items "were shown to use wording that patients found meaningful and comprehensible and were able to discriminate among patients' viewpoints."[6,p832] The issues of instrument validity and reliability were not addressed. In addition, no specific information described the development of the instrument or the rationale for item choice.

Subsequently, the ISQ has been used with 256 cancer patients from a major urban medical center[6] and 109 cancer patients from a small community hospital. Fitzpatrick compared the frequencies of information styles and participation preferences between his sample[53] and that of Cassileth et al.[6] In general, the results appear similar in both groups; however, no statistical tests were performed to determine whether significant differences existed between the responses of the two groups.[53] As the issues of validity and reliability of the instrument were not addressed, it would have been useful to compare the two groups.

Fitzpatrick[53] stated that the results of his research essentially replicate those of Cassileth et al.[6] This statement is significant, as Cassileth et al. observed that a potential source of bias was the setting from which the patients came. Unfortunately, no detailed demographic comparison was made between the two groups. Such a comparison might have provided some clues concerning the magnitude of potential bias. Fitzpatrick indicated that demographic variables may, in fact, account for some of the observed differences. Issues of the validity and reliability of the ISQ should be addressed. The instrument should be compared with other scales to determine its discriminant validity. Further, testing of the ISQ with other samples to compare specific demographic, psychologic, and sociologic variables will contribute to establishing the instrument's reliability.

The ISQ appears to be a comprehensive instrument designed to elicit many aspects of information preferences. Its clinical utility lies in its structure. The ISQ can be used relatively easily and yields useful information.

Krantz Health Opinion Survey (KHOS)

Krantz et al. developed the KHOS to measure preference for health care information, self-treatment, and active involvement in health care. The instrument has two subscales, one measuring information preference and the second measuring the degree of behavioral involvement.[54] The original instrument consisted of 40 items that addressed the issues of how informed a person wants to be and how active a role he or she desires to play in his or her health care.

Krantz et al.[54] reported that extensive testing was undertaken to determine the instrument's validity and reliability. The initial 40-item instrument was pilot-tested on 200 undergraduate students. Fourteen items were eliminated because they had a correlation of less than 0.20 with the total score or because they had a narrow distribution of response alternatives. The 26 items were retested with a sample of 159 undergraduates. Factor analysis was used to identify components of the instrument and yielded two subscales. The 10 items not correlating with these two subscales were eliminated. The two subscales are the Information Subscale (I-Scale) and the Behavior Involvement Subscale (B-Scale). The I-Scale contains seven items measuring desire to ask questions and wanting to be informed about medical decisions. The following is an example of a statement found on the I-Scale:[54] "I usually don't ask the doctor or nurse many questions about what they're doing during a medical examination."

The B-Scale contains nine items that measure attitudes toward self-treatment and active behavioral involvement of patients with their care. The following is an example of the statements found on the B-Scale:[54] "Clinics and hospitals are good places to go for help, since it's best for medical experts to take responsibility for health care." The scale then yields a total score, which is a composite of the two subscales, and individual I-Scale and B-Scale scores. The binary, agree-disagree format was designed so that high scores represent positive attitudes toward self-directed or informed treatment.[54]

Discriminant validity was established by administering the KHOS in conjunction with the Crowne-Marlowe Social Desirability Scale and the Health LOC Scale to a Sample of 100 male and 100 female undergraduates. A second sample consisted of 38 undergraduates who received the KHOS and the Minnesota Multiphasic Personality Inventory (MMPI) Hypochondriac Scale. A third sample ($n = 87$) received the KHOS and the Ullman Repression-Sensitization (R-S) Scale. A fourth sample ($n = 87$) received the KHOS and the Ullman Repression-Sensitization (R-S) Scale. A fifth sample ($n = 80$) received the KHOS two times during a 7-week interval to determine test-retest reliability.[54]

Application of the KR 20 test strongly confirmed the reliability of the KHOS and its component subscales (KR = 0.77). The authors remark that females in general tended to score higher than males on all parts of the KHOS. The authors do not discuss the possible significance of this finding.

The B-Scale and I-Scale were not correlated significantly with one another. The KHOS and the Wallston Health Locus of Control Scale had a correlation of 0.31, and the correlations were 0.26 and 0.23 for the B-Scale and I-Scale, respectively. The authors suggest that these low correlations indicate that the two subscales are probably measuring relatively independent processes. The KHOS does not show significant correlations with the R-S, the MMPI, and the Crowne-Marlowe Social Desirability Scale.

Additional studies were conducted to establish predictive, construct, and discriminant validity of the KHOS. For these studies, Krantz et al. administered the KHOS to a sample of 149 students, including 56 randomly selected residents of a college residence hall, 81 students reporting to a college infirmary for routine treatment of minor illnesses, and 12 students enrolled in a medical self-help course at the same school.[54] It was predicted that the criterion group, the students attending a medical self-help course, would score higher on the behavioral involvement, information, and total scores of the KHOS because their involvement in such a course was believed to demonstrate greater interest in obtaining information about health.

The scores of the self-help and clinic samples were compared to those of the residence hall students using one-way analyses of variance and Dunnett's t-test. One-tailed tests were used, as directional predictions were specified. The total KHOS scores and the B-Scale scores were higher for the self-help group than for the residence hall group and significant at the $p < 0.005$ level. The clinic users did not differ on the total KHOS score or the I-Scale but were significantly lower on the B-Scale ($p < 0.05$). Krantz et al. established discriminant validity of the instrument in its ability to predict correctly the differences between the criterion group of high-self-care students and the general population and in the fact that the low B-Scale scores were correlated with high use of clinic facilities.

The authors reported on three studies designed to established reliability and validity of the KHOS. They noted that the scale is predictive of behaviors that relate to seeking routine medical care for minor illnesses that require short-term interventions. It has not been established whether the instrument is valid or reliable in predicting illness-seeking behavior in long-term chronic or traumatic illness. Results of these studies suggest that people who prefer to be more active in their own health care are more likely to care for themselves when faced with a minor illness than to seek care from a physician.

Since its initial design, the KHOS has been used in a variety of other settings. Auerbach et al. used the scale with 40 patients scheduled for dental surgery.[55] The study attempted to provide construct validation data for the I-Scale of the KHOS. The study subjects were asked to complete several measures in conjunction with the KHOS (e.g., Rotter Internal Locus of Control Scale and Corah Dental Anxiety Scale). The results demonstrated that the KHOS subscales are positively correlated with the total KHOS (I-Scale = 0.73, p = 0.0001; B-Scale = 0.63, p = 0.0001), but the subscales are not related to each other or to other scales. These results are consistent with those described by Krantz et al.[54]

Studies reporting use of the information subscale of the KHOS appear more frequently in the literature than those reporting use of the behavioral involvement measure.[28,53–55] Turk-Charles et al.[28] reported use of the information measure in a study of individuals' information-seeking behaviors in medical establishments. They report Cronbach's alpha coefficient of 0.70, consistent with that initially reported by Krantz. Nease and Brooks[56] conducted a study to compare the KHOS and the Autonomy Preference Index (API) measures for patients' desire for information and participation in decision-making. Findings from their work suggest that the KHOS and API are correlated, with the decision-making subscales being more so than the information subscales. They suggest that although both are measures assess an individual's desire for information, the KHOS information subscale primarily focuses on behaviors engaged in by an individual to obtain information, whereas the API focuses on the information desired. Since both measures have been used fairly extensively, researchers and clinicians should carefully examine each in the context of proposed use.

The appeal of the KHOS instrument is its brevity, ease of scoring, and bidimensional approach in identifying a person's desire for information and relevant behavioral components. This instrument has clinical utility and has been used in a variety of settings and with different populations as part of an initial assessment.

Preference to Participate in Treatment Decisions: The Control Preferences Scale (CPS)

Development of the CPS has evolved from more than two decades of research. This section summarizes some of the seminal work in the development of the CPS and describes the development of the CPS.

Initially, a field study was conducted to elicit how decisions were made by patients with life-threatening illnesses. Four patterns of control over decision-making emerged. These patterns include:

1. *Provider-controlled decision making*. Health personnel have final control over the design of treatment, and the patient and family are involved to varying degrees in the actual implementation of treatment.

2. *Patient-controlled decision making.* The patient exercises final control over the type of treatment received.
3. *Family-controlled decision making.* The family has final control over what treatment the patient receives.
4. *Jointly controlled decision making.* Control over the design of therapy is shared by one or more of the participants in decision making.[8]

The preliminary work led Degner and Russell[8] to hypothesize that people with cancer have preferences about keeping, sharing, or giving away control over treatment decisions that can be measured along a continuum. They also were interested in finding out to whom cancer patients would delegate decision-making authority, a physician or family member. Therefore, they designed a study to answer the following research question: "Do patients facing life-threatening illness such as cancer have preexisting preferences about the roles they might play in treatment decision-making?"[8,p368]

Eight vignettes were developed that described varying degrees of control over treatment decisions. The vignettes were reviewed for clarity by four oncology nurses and four oncology physicians. They were then tested on 10 patients and revised.

Sixty adult cancer patients were selected from two oncology clinics. Clinic staff were asked to identify patients that could be classified as keepers, sharers, and givers of decision-making authority. Twenty subjects were identified for each category. Subjects were equally divided by age (39 years of age or younger and 40 years of age and older).

Two alternatives for decision control were chosen from the four patterns identified from the field study. Physician and family were chosen as alternatives for decision-making authority. Four vignettes per each alternative were used. Patient preferences were elicited by having subjects examine each of the sample vignettes in pairs. For example, vignettes A and B were examined against each other, and one was selected as preferred and placed on top of the other. A third card was selected and examined against the vignette that had previously been placed on top. Priority of preference was again determined. This process was continued until a preference sequence was achieved for each of the four vignettes within the two alternatives.

Degner and Russell[8] reported that most patients preferred a pattern of shared control. Patients also reported a preference for giving control to a physician rather than a family member. The authors cite the following study limitations: patients sampled were at varying points along the disease trajectory; females with breast cancer were overrepresented, and lung and bowel cancers were underrepresented in the sample compared to the population of adults with cancer. Therefore, generalization of the findings is limited to the study sample.[8]

Degner and Sloan[16] conducted companion studies designed to determine "the prevalence of differing preferences about roles in treatment decision making in the context of cancer, whether these preferences differed when people anticipate having cancer versus are actually diagnosed with cancer, and which demographic and disease treatment factors were the most important predictors of these preferences."[16,p942] The authors also were interested in determining whether illness distress affected preference in treatment decisions. The symptom distress scale was the instrument used to assess the subject's degree of perceived distress.

Degner and Sloan surveyed 436 newly diagnosed cancer patients and 482 members of the general public (householders) in the Canadian province of Manitoba between January and June 1988.[16] A card-sorting method, revised as a result of findings from the previous study, was used to determine preferences in decision-making participation. There were two alternative sets, a patient-physician and a family-physician dimension. Each set consisted of five cards. Each card depicted a different role in decision making and an illustrative cartoon. The method used with the study subjects to determine preference was the same as that used in the study conducted in 1988 by the researchers, as described.

Differences in preferences were observed between patients with a diagnosis of cancer and householders. Fifty-nine percent of newly diagnosed cancer patients preferred that physicians assume responsibility for treatment decisions. The most common choice selected by cancer patients was that a physician should consider the patient's opinion. Sixty-four percent of householders reported that they would want to play an active role in treatment decisions. Both groups reported a desire for physician and family to share decision making if the patient became too ill. This finding suggests that distress from a diagnosis of cancer may influence the desire to participate in treatment decisions. Older subjects in both groups reported wanting less control in treatment decision making. Differences between groups on education and gender variables were observed. In the cancer patient groups being more highly educated and female was associated with a preference for more control in treatment decision making. This finding was not observed among the householders.

From this seminal work, Degner and colleagues formulated the control preferences construct.[57] "The control preferences construct, which emerged from grounded theory, was defined as the 'degree of control an individual wants to assume when decisions are being made about medical treatment.' "[57,p24] The CPS is composed of five cards, each of which depict a different role individuals may desire in health care decision making. These five roles range along a continuum from assuming a very active role ("I prefer to make the decision about the treatment I will receive") a collaborative role ("I prefer that my doctor and I share responsibility for deciding which treatment is best for me"), and a passive role ("I prefer to leave all decisions regarding treatment to my doctor").[57]

Degner and colleagues have conducted extensive research in the validation of this scale. Reference 57 contains a complete discussion of the process undertaken in the development and validation of the CPS. The scale has been used extensively in studies in which patient decision-making preferences and patient values were studied. Several studies have compared individuals' preferred and actual role in decision making and others have used the scale solely to identify an individual's preferred role.[58-62]

The CPS had extensive clinical and research utility. Clinicians will find it is easy to administer, useful with persons of differing levels of education, and fast, providing the clinician with information about the degree of health care decision-making participation an individual prefers. The CPS provides researchers with a simple but valid and reliable measure. The responses can be scored in a similar manner to a Likert scale, thus enabling use with regression models for ordinal data. Differences between preferred and actual preferences (i.e., those preferences an individual states s/he wants compared to those actually chosen) can be assessed using the CPS.[57]

Autonomy Preference Index (API)

Ende and colleagues[18] developed the API to measure "patients' preferences for two identified dimensions of patient autonomy: decision-making and the acquisition of information."[18,p23] Ende et al. observed that increased attention has been given to the provision of information to patients to facilitate independent health care decisions. However, they note that little research has focused on whether patients actually want to make the decisions once they have accumulated information. These observations are consistent with those made by Beisecker.[17,64] Therefore, determining why patients want information and what they actually do with it once they obtain it seem to be fertile areas for research.

The API, a 23-item questionnaire was developed using a modified Delphi technique that involved the use of 13 experts interested in patient autonomy. The experts represented medicine, sociology, and ethics. Two dimensions emerged from this process. The dimensions were patients' preferences for making decisions and patients' desire for information. The Decision-Making Preference Scale consists of 15 items, 6 of which are general and 9 of which are related to 1 of 3 clinical vignettes. Each vignette describes a clinical condition representing increasing illness severity (mild upper respiratory tract illness, moderate hypertension, and severe myocardial infarction). The Information Seeking Scale consists of eight items.

Content validity was established by field-testing and reviewing the items with patients. "Each item was then discarded, modified and retested, or retained based on feedback from patients, the item's ability to discriminate among patients, and its reliability."[18,p23] Concurrent and convergent criterion validity of the decision-making scale were established. Concurrent validity of the decision-making scale was tested by asking respondents to choose one of five statements that best described their attitude toward medical care. The statements ranged from "patient should have complete control" to "doctor should have complete control." Patients' responses to this item correlated with the decision-making scores ($r = 0.54$, $p < 0.0001$).

Criterion validity was assessed by administering part of the instrument to a "highly" motivated group of diabetics who were adept at self-care. The authors assumed that diabetic patients possessing these characteristics would be a good comparison group with the study sample. The diabetic population scored higher on the decision-making scale than the study population ($p < 0.1$). It is suggested that the assertion that criterion validity was established should be interpreted cautiously because no attempt was made to validate the "highly" motivated characteristics of the diabetics. No validity testing was conducted on the information-seeking scale.

Instrument reliability was established through test-retest on a sample of 50 patients. Test-retest reliability scores were computed for the decision-making scale and for the information-seeking scale. Pearson's product-moment correlation was 0.84 and 0.83 for each scale. Cronbach's alpha coefficient was 0.82 for each scale.

Administration of the questionnaire takes approximately 10 minutes. Each scale is scored separately. The range of scores is from 0 (very low) to 100 (very high) preference for either decision making or information seeking. The vignettes are scored on a scale of 0 to 10, where 0 represented no desire to participate in decision making, 5 represented a desire to participate that was equal to the physician's, and 10 equaled patient desire for complete control. This approach to determining the amount of decision making desired by patients is similar to that reported by Beisecker. The scores from each of the scales can be correlated with demographic variables.

Ende et al. report the findings from their research that was designed to answer the following questions:[18,p23] (1) To what extent do patients prefer to take an active role in their own care? (2) What patient characteristics influence these preferences? and (3) How are these preferences affected by varying disease severity?

The authors approached 803 randomly selected general medical clinic patients for inclusion in the study. Thirty-nine percent (312 patients) agreed to participate. Comparisons were made among refusers and nonrefusers on selected demographic variables to determine whether significant differences existed between these groups. No significant differences were observed. In addition, a random selection of refusers was mailed a copy of the API with a response rate of 45%. No significant differences were observed on mean decision-making and information-seeking scores between the study participants and the refusers who returned the questionnaire. Therefore, the authors believe that they had a representative sample.

No correlation was observed between patients' desire for information and their preferences for decision making. Findings from their study suggest that, in general, patients do not want to participate in medical decision making. An inverse relationship between desire to participate and severity of illness was observed. Seventy-five percent of patients reported a preference for making decisions during a minor illness (upper respiratory infection), whereas the remaining 25% reported a preference for making decisions during a major illness (high blood pressure or myocardial infarction). A positive relationship was observed between being younger and higher educational level and preference for decision making ($p = 0.001$ and $p = 0.05$, respectively). A negative relationship was observed between marital status (e.g., separated or divorced) and skilled or semiskilled occupation and medical decision making ($p = 0.10$ [level of significance set at 0.15]).

Only younger age and higher education were positively correlated with information seeking. Of particular interest is that in regression models for both scales, less than 20% of the variance was accounted for. This finding alone has significant importance for future research in this area, as well as for the clinical application of the findings. Clearly, a lot is still unknown concerning patients' desire for information and participation in decision making. The authors correctly point out that, although approaches to ascertaining individual preferences can be standardized to a point, there remains a large degree of individual variance that can be addressed only by assessing these preferences at the time of the physician-patient encounter.

Ende and colleagues[65] sought to explore additional reasons why patients may desire information but choose not to take an active role in health-care decisions. They hypothesized that, although sociodemographic variables and role disparity between physicians and patients may influence these preferences, the role of being a patient may override these reasons in influencing behavior. Therefore, the authors designed a study that sought to answer the following research questions:[65] (1) When physicians are patients, how involved in decision making do they prefer to be? (2) To what extent are their preferences affected by the severity of illness? (3) How do their preferences for autonomy compare with those of regular patients?

The sample consisted of 151 physicians. Ninety percent were general internists. A sample of 315 patients was selected from individuals returning to a general medicine outpatient practice. Each subject was asked to complete the 23-item API. The only difference in the scales given to the physicians and patients was that physicians were instructed to answer the questions as if they were patients.

Both physician patients and nonphysician patients indicated a high preference for information. Interestingly, patients reported a significantly higher preference for information than physicians. Physician patients reported a significantly higher preference to participate in decision making than patients. This difference was observed in response to general desire to participate in decision making and to the three specific vignettes. Of particular interest, however, is that both groups scored less than 50 on the general decision-making scale and less than 5 on each item from the vignettes. These findings indicate that both groups prefer decisions to be made by the provider. The desire to participate in decision making decreased with the severity of illness for both the physician patients and the patients. These findings are consistent with the authors' results in earlier work[18] and with those of others.

Gibson and colleagues[66] adapted the API for use in patients with a diagnosis of asthma. The items in the Asthma Autonomy Questionnaire were consistent with those in the API, changing the scenarios to be asthma-specific. The authors do not report reliability data from their study, but they do report that their results are similar to those reported earlier by Ende. Adams and colleagues[67] also published findings from use of the Gibson API adapted for asthma patients. The report a total Cronbach alpha coefficient of 0.87, again with similar findings as previously reported. The API continues to be used in a variety of clinical settings (e.g., in primary care settings, patients with AIDS, and with caregivers) and has been demonstrated to have stable reliability and validity. The API has been shown to correlate with the KHOS (see previous section).[56]

Ende and colleagues[65] contributed significantly to the body of knowledge concerning individuals' preferences for information and desire for participation in decisions. In addition, their findings suggest that "patient role" and severity of illness are significant variables influencing desire to participate in medical care decisions. Overall, findings from these studies continue to support the earlier work of Ende et al. Patients, on average, report a desire for information even if they report low preferences for actual participation in decision making. The more severe the illness, the less preference for participation in decision making. Age and educational level are related to desire for more participation.

Decisional conflict is a state of uncertainty about the course of action to take, characterized by verbalizing uncertainty, vacillation between choices, delay in making decisions, and questioning personal values and beliefs when faced with making a decision.[68] O'Connor developed the Decisional Conflict Scale (DCS), which is composed of three subscales. The three subscales are (1) decisional uncertainty (three items); (2) factors contributing to uncertainty (9 items); and (3) perceived effective decision making (4 items). The DCS has been used in a number of health care situations in which indivduals must make difficult decisions. The author has evaluated the measure with individuals deciding to undergo influenza immunizations and breast cancer screening and my Meropol and colleagues[63] in decision making in cancer patients considering phase 1 clinical trials. Total scale Cronbach's alpha ranges from 0.78 to 0.92. This measure has clinical utility, especially in situations in which patients are faced with difficult and complicated decisions.[69]

Summary

This chapter has presented a review of the literature on consumer and health care information-seeking behaviors and decision-making preferences. Instruments developed to measure these concepts have been discussed. This review has revealed a number of patterns. Age, gender, education level, and severity of illness have emerged as significant variables relative to the desire for information and participation in decision making.[17,19,43,64] Discrepancies between desire for information and desire for participation in decision making also have been observed in several studies.[8,17,18,20] Significant advances have been made in understanding the complex nature of information-seeking behaviors and decision-making preferences. However, both Degner and Russell[8] and Ende et al.[18] observed that only about 20% of the variance had been accounted for by sociodemographic variables inserted in models designed to elicit relationships, such as variables and preferences for information seeking and decision making. Both suggest that much remains unknown in this area and that individual assessment at the time of the patient-physician encounter continues to be an important aspect of determining the amount of information desired and preference for participation in decision making.

Several directions emerge for future research in the area of information seeking and decision making. First, refinement of instruments is essential. Adaptation of the instruments to enhance their clinical utility is a high priority. Research using several instruments together will promote the establishment of discriminant validity. Reliability will be enhanced by the use of instruments in different populations. Of particular importance is to use these instruments in samples of minority, low-income, and other special populations. More research is needed to determine the impact that situational variables, such as severity of illness or setting, have on search and decision-making behaviors. Finally, attempts should be made to determine the predictive ability of these instruments in specific individuals and groups who have similar patterns of search and decision-making preferences. Collaborative research efforts provide one approach to achieve these outcomes.[70]

References

1. Lenz, E.R. Information seeking: A component of client decisions and health behavior. *Adv Nurs Sci*, 1984, *6*(3):59-72.
2. Janis, I.L., & Mann, L. *Decision-making: A psychological analysis of conflict, choice and commitment.* New York: The Free Press, 1977.
3. Hopkins, M.B. Information seeking and adaptational outcomes in women receiving chemotherapy for breast cancer. *Cancer Nurs*, 1986, *9*(5):256-262.
4. Miller, S.M., Leinbach, A.L., & Brody, D.S. Coping styles in hypertensives: Nature and consequences. *J Consult Clin Psychol*, 1989, *57*:333-337.
5. Wallston, K.A., Kaplan, G.D., & Maides, S.A. Development and validation of the health locus of control (HLC) scale. *J Consult Clin Psychol*, 1976, *44*(4):580-583.
6. Cassileth, B.R., Zupkis, R.V., Sutton-Smith, K., & March, V. Information and participation preferences among cancer patients. *Ann Intern Med*, 1980, *92*(6):832-836.
7. Lazarus, R.S. *Psychological stress and the coping process.* New York: McGraw-Hill, 1966.
8. Degner, L.F., & Russell, C.A. Preferences for treatment control among adults with cancer. *Res Nurs Health*, 1988, *11*:367-374.
9. Degner, L.F. Ethics and decision-making: Lessons from the "Cancer Wars." *Can J Nurs Res*, 2002, *34*(3):9-13.
10. Miller, S.M. Monitoring versus blunting styles of coping with cancer influence the information patients want and need about their disease: Implications for cancer screening and management. *Cancer*, 1995, *76*(2):167-177.
11. Newman, J.W., & Lockman, B.D. Measuring prepurchase information seeking. *J Consumer Res*, 1975, *2*(3):216-220.
12. Kiel, G.C., & Layton, R.A. Dimensions of consumer information seeking behavior. *J Market Res*, 1981, *18*:233-236.
13. Fleckenstein, L., Joubert, P., Lawrence, R., et al. Oral contraceptive patient information: A questionnaire study of attitudes, knowledge and preferred information sources. *JAMA*, 1976, *235*(13):1331-1336.
14. Silliman, R.A., Dukes, K.A., Sullivan, L.M., & Kaplan, S.H. Breast cancer care in older women: Sources of information, social support and emotional health outcomes. *Cancer*, 1998, *83*(4):706-711.
15. Faden, R.R., Lewis, C., Becke, C., et al. Disclosure standards and informed consent. *J Health Polit Policy Law*, 1981, *6*(2):255-257.
16. Degner, L.F., & Sloan, J.A. Decision-making during serious illness: What role do patients really want to play? *J Clin Epidemiol*, 1992, *45*(9):941-950.
17. Beisecker, A.E., & Beisecker, T.D. Patient information seeking behaviors when communicating with doctors. *Med Care*, 1990, *28*(1):19-28.
18. Ende, J., Kazis, L., Ash, A., & Moskowitz, M.A. Measuring patients' desire for autonomy: Decision-making and information seeking preferences among medical patients. *J Gen Int Med*, 1989, *4*(1):23-30.
19. Blanchard, C.G., Labrecque, M.S., Ruckdeschel, J.C., & Blanchard, E.B. Information and decision-making preferences of hospitalized adult cancer patients. *Soc Sci Med*, 1988, *27*(11):1139-1145.
20. Strull, W.M., Lo, B., & Charles, G. Do patients want to participate in medical decision-making? *JAMA*, 1984, *252*(21):2990-2994.
21. Deber, R.B., Kraetschmer, N., Irvine, J. What role do patients wish to play in treatment decision making? *Arch Intern Med*, 1996, *156*(13):1414-1420.
22. Degner, L.F., Kristjanson, L.J., Bowman, D., et al. Information needs and decisional preferences in women with breast cancer. *JAMA*, 1997, *277*(18):1485-1492.
23. Davison, B.J., Gleave, M.E., Goldenberg, et al. Assessing information and decision preferences of men with prostate cancer and their partners. *Cancer Nurs*, 2002, *25*(1):42-49.
24. Silliman, R.A., Troyan, S.L., Guadagnoli, E., et al. The impact of age, marital status, and surgeon-patient interactions on the care of older women with breast carcinoma. *Cancer*, 1997, *80*:1326-1334.
25. Rees, C.E., & Bath, P.A. Information-seeking behaviors of women with breast cancer. *Oncol Nurs Forum*, 2001, *28*(5):899-907.
26. Kravitz, R.L., & Melnikow, J. Engaging patients in medical decision making: The end is worthwhile, but the means need to be more practical. *BMJ*, 2001, *323*:584-585.
27. Catalan, J., & Brener, N. Whose health is it? Views about decision-making and information-seeking from people with HIV infection and their professional carers. *AIDS Care*, 1994, *6*(3).
28. Turk-Charles, S., Meyerowitz, B.E., & Gatz, M. Age

differences in information-seeking among cancer patients. *Int J Aging Hum Dev*, 1997, 45(2):85-98.

29. Johnson, J.D., Roberts, C.S., Cox, C.E., et al. Breast cancer patients' personality style, age, and treatment decision making. *J Surg Onc*, 1996, 63:183-186.

30. Guadagnoli, E., & Ward, P. Patient participation in decision-making. *Soc Sci Med*, 1998, 47(3):329-339.

31. Frosch, D.L., & Kaplan, R.M. Shared decision making in clinical medicine: Past research and future directions. *Am J Prev Med*, 1999, 17(4):285-294.

32. Payne, J.W. Task complexity and contingent processing in decision-making: An information search and protocol analysis. *Organiz Behav Hum Perform*, 1976, 16:366-369.

33. Englander, T., & Tyszka, T. Information seeking in open decision situations. *Acta Psychol*, 1980, 45:169-170.

34. Fast, J., Vosburgh, R.E., & Frisbee, W.R. The effects of consumer education on consumer search. *J Consum Affairs*, 1989, 23(1):65-90.

35. Messerli, M.L., Garamendi, C., & Romano, J. Breast cancer: Information as a technique of crisis intervention. *Am J Orthopsychiatr*, 1980, 50(4):728-731.

36. Dodd, M.J., & Mood, D.W. Chemotherapy: Helping patients to know the drugs they are receiving and their possible side effects. *Cancer Nurs*, 1981, 4(4):311-315.

37. Mills, R.T., & Krantz, D.S. Information, choice, and reactions to stress: A field experiment in a blood bank with laboratory analogue. *J Perspect Soc Psychol*, 1979, 37(4):608-620.

38. Wallston, K.A., Smith, R.A.P., King, J.E., et al. Desire for control and choice of antiemetic treatment for cancer chemotherapy. *West J Nurs Res*, 1991, 13(1):12-23.

39. Miller, S.M. Monitoring and blunting: Validation of a questionnaire to assess styles of information seeking under threat. *J Person Soc Psychol*, 1987, 52(2):345-353.

40. Schwartz, M.D., Lerman, C., Miller, S.M., et al. Coping disposition, perceived risk, and psychological distress among women at increased risk for ovarian cancer. *Health Psychol*, 1995, 14(3):232-235.

41. Miller, S.M., & Grant, R.P. The blunting hypothesis: A view of predictability and human stress. In P. Soden, S. Bates, & W. Dockens (Eds.), *Trends in behavior therapy.* New York: Academic, 1979.

42. Miller, S.M., & Mangan, C.E. The interacting effects of information and coping style in adapting to gynecologic stress: Should the doctor tell all? *J Pers Soc Psychol*, 1983, 45:223-236.

43. Chorney, R.L., Efran, J.S., Ascher, L.M., & Lukens, M.D. *The performance of monitors and blunters on a cold pressor task.* Paper presented before the Eastern Psychological Association, 1982.

44. Barsevick, A.M., & Johnson, J.E. Preference for information and involvement, information seeking and emotional responses of women undergoing colposcopy. *Res Nurs Health*, 1990, 13:1-7.

45. Lerman, C., Schwartz, M.D., Miller, S.M., et al. A randomized trial of breast cancer risk counseling: Interacting effects of counseling, educational level and coping style. *Health Psychol*, 1996, 15(2):75-83

46. Tercyak, K.P., Lerman, C., Peshkin, B.N., et al. Effects of coping style and BRCA1 and BRCA2 test results on anxiety among women participating in genetic coun-

seling and testing for breast and ovarian cancer risk. *Health Psychol*, 2001, 20(3):217-222

47. Miller, S.M., Fang, C.Y., Manne, S.L., et al. Decision making about prophylactic oophorectomy among at-risk women: Psychological influences and implications. *Gyn Oncol*, 1999, 75(3):406-412.

48. Rees, C.E., & Bath, P.A. Information-seeking behaviors of women with breast cancer. *Onc Nurs Forum*, 2001, 28(5)899-907..

49. Rees, C.E., & Bath, P.A. The psychometric properties of the Miller Behavioral Style Scale with adult daughters of women with early breast cancer: A literature review and empirical study. *J Adv Nurs*, 2000b, 32:366-374.

50. Garvin, B.J., & Kim, C.J. Measurement of preference for information in U.S. and Korean cardiac catheterization patients. *Res Nurs Health*, 2000, 23(4):310-318.

51. Johnson, J.D., Roberts, C.S., Cox, C.E., et al. Breast cancer patients' personality style, age, and treatment decision-making. *J Surg Oncol*, 1996, 63:183-186.

52. Miller, S.M., Rodoletz, M., Schroeder, C.M., et al. Applications of the monitoring process model to coping with severe long-term medical threats. *Health Psychol*, 1996, 15(3):216-225.

53. Fitzpatrick, R.J. *Emotional distress, locus of control, and information preferences among cancer patients.* Unpublished doctoral dissertation, University of Tennessee, Knoxville, 1983.

54. Krantz, D.S., Baum, A., & Wideman, M.V. Assessment of preferences for self-treatment and information in health care. *J Person Soc Psychol*, 1980, 39(5):977-990.

55. Auerbach, S.M., Martelli, M.F., & Mercuri, L.G. Anxiety, information, interpersonal impacts and adjustment to a stressful health care situation. *J Person Soc Psychol*, 1983, 44(6):1284-1296.

56. Nease, R.F., & Brooks, W.B. Patient desire for information and decision making in health care decisions: The Autonomy Preference Index and the Health Opinion Survey. *J Gen Intern Med*, 1995, 10(11):593-600.

57. Degner, L.F., Sloan, J.A., & Venkatesh, P. The control preferences scale. *Can J Nurs Res*, 1997, 29(3):21-43.

58. Harrison, D.E., Galloway, S., Graydon, J.E., et al. Information needs and preference for information of women with breast cancer over a first course of radiation therapy. *Patient Ed Couns*, 1999, 38(3):217-225.

59 Christensen, A.J., Ehlers, S.L., Raichle, K.L., et al. Predicting change in depression following renal transplantation: Effect of patient coping preferences. *Health Psychol*, 2000, 19(4):348-353.

60. Bilodeau, B.A., & Degner, L.F. Information needs, sources of information, and decisional roles in women with breast cancer. *Oncol Nurs Forum*, 1996, 23(4):691-696.

61. Beaver, K., Luker, K.A., Owens, R.G., et al. Treatment decision making in women newly diagnosed with breast cancer. *Cancer Nurs*, 1996, 19(1):8-19.

62. Davison, B.J., Degner, L.F., & Morgan, T.R. Information and decision-making preferences of men with prostate cancer. *Oncol Nurs Forum*, 1995, 22(9):1401-1408.

63. Beisecker, A.E Aging and the desire for information and input in medical decisions: Patient consumerism

in medical encounters. *Gerontologist*, 1988, *28*(3):330-335.

64. Meropol, N.J., Weinfurt, K.P., Burnett, C.B., et al. Perceptions of patients and providers regarding phase 1 cancer clinical trials: Implications for physician-patient communication. *J Clin Oncol*, 2003, *21*(13):2589-2596.

65. Ende, J., Kazis, L., Ash, A., & Moskowitz M.A. Preferences for autonomy when patients are physicians. *J Gen Int Med*, 1990, *5*(6):506-509.

66. Gibson, P.G., Talbot, P.I., Toneguzzi, R.C., and the Population Medicine Group 91C. Self-management, autonomy, and quality of life in asthma. *Chest*, 1995, *107*(4):1003-1008.

67. Adams, R.J., Smith, B.J., & Ruffin, R.E. Patient preferences for autonomy in decision making in asthma management. *Thorax*, 2001, *56*(2):126-132.

68. O'Connor, A.M. Validation of a decisional conflict scale. *Medical Decis Making*, 1995, *15*(1):25-30.

69. O'Connor, A.M., Pennie, R.A., & Dales, R.E. Framing effects on expectations, decisions, and side effects experienced: The case for influenza immunization. *J Clin Epidemiol*, 1996, *49*(11):1271-1276.

70. O'Connor, A.M. Consumer/patient decision support in the new millennium: Where should our research take us? *Can J Nurs Res*, 1999, *30*(4):257-261.

29

Measuring Alterations in Taste and Smell

Roberta Anne Strohl

It has been estimated that more than 2 million Americans have some impairment in taste or smell. The study and measurement of these disorders have not reflected the frequency of their occurrence. Disturbances in these senses are difficult to measure. Easy-to-use, reliable, and valid tools do not exist. These factors, coupled with the non-life-threatening nature of taste and smell impairment, have led them to be called "the neglected senses." Although not as debilitating as alterations in sight or hearing, taste and smell abnormalities can contribute to nutritional compromise. People who are unable or unwilling to eat because of the unpleasant tastes of food may not tolerate the treatment they require. Nutritional compromise may contribute to increased side effects and decreased response to therapy. Particularly in individuals treated with combined modality therapy, the inability to eat may have dire consequences. To discuss the alterations of taste and smell and their measurement, it is necessary to describe the normal taste and smell responses.

Normal Taste Sensation

Ziporyn,[1] Guyton,[2] and Schiffman[3] have extensively reviewed what is known of taste sensation. Adults have approximately 10,000 taste buds located on the tongue, palate, pharynx, tonsils, epiglottis, and in some people in the mucosa of the cheek and lips. Taste buds respond to four primary sensations: sweet, sour, salty, and bitter. Sweet receptors are found on the anterior surface and tip of the tongue, sour and salty on the two lateral sides, and bitter on the circumvallate papillae of the posterior surface. Sour and bitter tastes are perceived most acutely on the palate, whereas salty and sweet tastes are most sensitive on the tongue. Each taste bud is not exclusively sensitive to a single sensation, and all respond in varying proportions to sweet, sour, salty, and bitter. It is believed that a center in the brain detects all the variations of taste and the sum of these stimuli produce a distinguishable taste.[1-3] Stevens[4] demonstrated this ability to taste mixtures by mixing compounds in concentrations proportional to their individual detection thresholds and measuring the detection threshold of the mixture compared to water. He found that there was no limit to the number of compounds that could be at least partially integrated. He proposed that there are multiple parallel channels for processing the intensity and quality of taste.

Sweet taste originates from a mostly organic group of chemicals, including sugars, alcohols, glycol, ketones, amides, sulfonic acids, and inorganic salts of beryllium and lead. Sour taste results from acids, and salty taste results from ionized salts. Bitter taste is caused by organic substances, such as alkaloids and long-chain acids. Intense bitter taste is objectionable, often a protective mechanism, as many poisons have a bitter taste. From birth there appears to be a preference for sweet taste. Berridge[5] looked at photos of newborns in reaction to taste. From hours after birth different taste sensations elicited different responses. Sweet taste causes a positive or hedonic response characterized by lip smacking and relaxation of muscles, while bitter sensations resulted in aversive gapes and complex grimaces.

Taste buds consist of both gustatory receptor cells and supporting cells. Each taste bud consists of approximately 48 cells. The life span of a taste cell is about 10 days. Cell renewal is made possible by mitotic division in the surrounding epithelium. At the center of each taste bud is a taste pore. Microvilli or taste hairs protrude from the surface of the taste cells and are believed to form the receptor surface for taste. The container-like structure of the taste bud provides a minute cup for solutions to be tasted, allowing substances to mix with saliva for tasting. Taste nerve fibers, stimulated by the taste buds, are located in the taste cells.[1-3]

When a substance in solution comes in contact with a taste bud, the taste response is initiated. Functioning as a chemical sieve, the taste bud allows the substance to stimulate the taste nerve. Various physiologic mechanisms change the diameter of a taste pore and alter its permeability, transmitting the stimulus along nerve fibers.[1-3]

Taste impulses from the anterior two thirds of the tongue pass first into the fifth nerve, then through the chorda tympani to the facial nerve and into the tractus solitarius in the brain stem. Sensations from the circumvillate papillae on the back of the tongue and posterior mouth transmit impulses through the glossopharyngeal nerve to a lower level of the tractus solitarius. The vagus nerve transmits taste signals from the base of the tongue and pharynx.[2]

All fibers synapse in the nuclei of the tractus solitarius and send second-order neurons to the thalamus. Third-order neurons transmit the signal to the lower tip of the postcentral gyrus in the parietal cortex; taste is perceived here. Neurons that travel from the pons to the lateral hypothalamus and free endings of the trigeminal nerve in the oral cavity and tongue also participate in the taste response.[2-3]

Normal Smell Sensation

The sense of smell is less well understood. The olfactory membrane is located in the superior part of each nostril and has a surface area of approximately 2.4 cm^2. Olfactory cells are derived from the central nervous system and are specialized bipolar neurons. The olfactory receptor cells renew themselves about every 30 days. Each person has about 100 million olfactory cells. The cells form an olfactory bulb, which terminates in olfactory hairs or cilia and line the mucous coating of the nasal cavity.[1-3]

The primary sensations of smell have not yet been identified, although sensations are believed to be analogous to the sweet, sour, bitter, and salty stimuli of taste. The chemical process of olfactory stimulation is unknown, and no general agreement about the basic qualities and classifications of smell exist. Attempts to classify smell have been numerous, starting with Plato, who cited only pleasant and unpleasant smells. Linnaeus, in 1752, reported seven smell classifications: aromatic, fragrant, ambrosial, alliaceous (garlicky), hircine (goaty), repulsive, and nauseous. Currently, it is postulated that separate olfactory cells respond to seven primary smells: camphoraceous, musky, floral, pepperminty, etheral, pungent, and putrid. It is unlikely that this list accurately reflects all the primary smell sensations. There may be as many as 50 primary smell sensations.[1,2]

The means of olfactory cell stimulation is unclear. A substance must be volatile to reach the cells. It also must be somewhat water- and lipid-soluble to pass through the nasal mucus, the olfactory cilia, and the tips of the olfactory cells. Smell occurs in cycles, and inspiration is critical for this response. It is believed that olfactory cells respond with a change in membrane potential (much as taste cells do), which then stimulates the olfactory nerve. Wave theories propose that smell is triggered by direct stimulation radiating from an odorous source. Steric theories suggest that chemical reactivity occurs when particles of an odorant react with receptor cells.[1,2]

When stimulated, the nerve fibers send the smell response to larger bundles that leave the epithelium through perforations in the cribriform plate. Axons are sent to the olfactory bulb. These terminate in dendrites in the glomerulus, which is located near the bulb's surface. Some of the axons form the olfactory tract; others lead back to tufted cells that return axons to the glomerulus. This circular pathway amplifies the message.[1]

Olfactory nerve fibers terminate in two areas of the brain, the medial and lateral olfactory areas. The medial area, located in the midportion of the brain, is superior and anterior to the hypothalamus. The lateral olfactory area, in the cerebral cortex, consists of the uncus, prepyriform area, the lateral portion of the anterior perforated surface, and part of the amygdaloid nuclei. The lateral area is believed to be responsible for the association of smell with other sensations. Although taste and smell are separate sensations, they are closely related.[2] Loss of the ability to smell during a cold has taught us that the sense of taste also is diminished.

Disorders of Taste and Smell

Given the complexity of taste and smell sensations, it should not be surprising that there are numerous situations in which taste and smell can be altered. Although it is beyond the scope of this chapter to discuss them all, the terminology used to describe taste and smell abnormalities includes:[3]

Ageusia: absence of taste
Anosmia: absence of smell
Dysgeusia: distortion of normal taste
Dysosmia: distortion of normal smell
Hypergeusia: increased sensitivity of taste
Hyperosmia: increased sensitivity of smell
Hypogeusia: lessened sensitivity of taste
Hyposmia: lessened sensitivity of smell

Schiffman[3] classifies taste and smell disorders into four causal categories: (1) disorders resulting from local atrophy of receptor sites; (2) physical damage to neural projections; (3) surgical or traumatic disturbances of cell renewal by disease, drugs, or radiation; and (4) changes in the receptor cell environment resulting from alterations in saliva or olfactory mucosa (damage due to drugs or environmental pollutants, such as benzene, carbon disulfide, or ethyl acetate). Sensory changes as a result of disease have been studied most extensively, therefore the chapter will focus on that area.

Changes in Taste and Smell Resulting from Disease States

A number of diseases, including renal disease, diabetes, anorexia, cancer, and trauma, are associated with alterations in taste and smell. More work has been done in the area of taste abnormalities than smell abnormalities, partly because of the difficulty in measuring and lack of understanding of the sense of smell. Patients with cancer have been found to report alterations in taste and smell as a result of both the disease and its treatment. As the author's clinical practice is in oncology, this area is emphasized. A review of the literature reveals that more research in this area is needed and that there is not a singular explanation for the changes in taste and smell reported by persons with cancer. Changes related to cancer, treatment-related factors, and coexisting diseases, are presented in Table 29.1.[6-43] Changes related to aging also are common, including taste bud epithelial thinning; zinc deficiency as a result of normal dietary changes and the aging process; and decreased vascular supply to taste cells. With aging the number of taste buds decreases. Taste sensations in edentulous patients may improve if dentures are removed.[44-53]

Table 29.1 Changes in Taste and Smell Related to Various Conditions

Nature of Change	Alteration/Explanation	Reference
Cancer		
Lowered bitter threshold	Tumor may secrete substance that stimulates bitter taste buds; results in meat aversion	6–13
Increase in sucrose threshold	Depression of cell renewal by tumor; decrease in taste cell numbers; decrease in stimulus received by taste receptors	12–13, 15–19
Weight loss	Correlates with extent of tumor; taste abnormalities improve as tumor regresses; without tumor response, abnormalities increase	8,9
Increase in salt threshold	Unknown	17,18
Studies in which no abnormalities found	—	11
Alteration in smell	Unknown; patients reported unusual smell in chemotherapy and/or radiation clinic	19,20
Loss of smell and taste in graft vs. host disease	An unusual manifestation of graft vs. host disease involving the oral cavity	21,22
Cancer surgery		
Removal of tongue	Loss of sweet and salty receptors	23
Removal of palate	Loss of sour and bitter receptors	23
Laryngectomy	Loss of olfactory component of taste	23
Cancer chemotherapy		
Loss of taste	Stomatitis complicated by infection and coating of tongue alters receptor sites; taste cells with high mitotic index altered by drugs that halt cell growth; 2–4 years after stem cell transplant half of survivors had taste loss	21
Metallic taste	Associated with cytoxan, vincristine, methotrexate	21
Food aversions	Conditioned response related to the association of nausea and vomiting with chemotherapy	21,22
Loss of taste in the anterior two thirds of the tongue in herpes zoster	Involvement of mandibular division of trigeminal nerve	23,25–27

(continues)

Table 29.1 *continued*

Nature of Change	Alteration/Explanation	Reference
Head and neck irradiation		
Damage to microvilli of taste cell	Taste may be partially restored 20–60 days post-treatment and return to normal 60–120 days after treatment	28–33
Loss of saliva and related salivary gland damage:		
Profound taste loss	Occurs at dose > 3000 rad (sweet taste may persist longer as there are more sweet taste buds)	
Loss of smell	Related to irradiation of nasal passage and damage to olfactory receptor site	
Some hypogeusia may be permanent		
Diabetes	Taste loss evidenced by higher thresholds for all sensations except sour, which is related to the degree of peripheral neuropathy, particularly autonomic neuropathy involving taste nerve	3,34,35
Renal disease	Hypogeusia due to low zinc levels; persistent generalized unpleasant taste; alteration in cranial nerves related to renal failure; decrease in salivary flow; change in calcium and phosphorus saliva content	36–39
Anorexia	Taste loss related to altered zinc and copper levels	40
Head trauma	Smell alteration related to fracture of cribriform plate, laceration of olfactory nerves, and hemorrhage in frontal lobe; hemorrhage into taste center of brain	41,42
Allergic rhinitis	Higher olfactory thresholds needed. Higher thresholds in patients with nasal polyps and sinusitis related to damage of receptors and decrease in air flow	44
Liver disease	Lower tolerance to bitter taste and decreased appetite; etiology unclear	45
Alcoholism	Decreased smell threshold correlated with MRI indication of decreased cortical sulcus volume	43,46
	Preference for high concentration of sweet	47
Depression	19 of 47 patients reported symptoms of unpleasant taste unrelated to drug use	42
Schizophrenia	A change in the functional integrity of the odor identification pathway via the limbic system to orbitofrontal cortex may be the cause	48

Although research in both the measurement and etiology of taste and smell disturbances is needed, the complexity of these senses and the numerous ways in which responses can be altered make these difficult to investigate. Some of the currently available testing methods are quite complex, necessitating collaborative research to identify and document clinical changes.

Measurement of Taste

Instrument selection depends on study intent. The instruments described here either document taste changes and aversions for particular foods or food groups or they actually record taste and smell thresholds. Many of these instruments are complicated and may require collaborative researcher and clinician efforts.

Documenting Taste Changes

The initial assessment of taste problems should include a brief intake questionnaire. One suggestion based on my clinical experience follows:

Have you noticed changes in the way food tastes?
When did you notice this change?
Have you changed the way you season food? If so, how?
Have the tastes of any particular foods changed?
Do any foods taste better than others?
What foods have you stopped eating, and why?
Are the taste changes constant?

Dobell et al.[53] used a questionnaire to examine and compare the food preferences of 50 renal patients undergoing chronic hemodialysis and continuous ambulatory peritoneal dialysis with age- and sex-matched controls ($n = 30$). Two questionnaires were administered, one assessing food preferences for 88 items and one assessing factors influencing dietary habits. The 88 foods were grouped into 14 classes. Thirty-three patients received hemodialysis, and 17 received peritoneal dialysis. Analysis of variance compared groups in terms of food preference and chi-square analysis compared dietary habits. The study determined that sweet foods ($p = 0.002$), vegetables ($p = 0.003$), red meats ($p = 0.010$), and fish and poultry ($p = 0.015$) were more objectionable to patients on dialysis than for controls. Red meats ($p = 0.010$), fish and poultry ($p = 0.032$), and eggs ($p = 0.005$) were less pleasant for patients receiving hemodialysis than for those on peritoneal dialysis. Red meat was the most unpopular food for all dialysis patients. The most common factor affecting dietary intake was a loss of interest in food and/or cooking, perhaps related to fatigue.[53]

Markley et al.[54] placed foods in six categories: breads, fruits, vegetables, meats, milk and dairy, and miscellaneous, including coffee, condiments, and carbonated beverages. Dysgeusia was classified into four alterations in taste: Type I, one food or beverage in any single group; Type II, more than one food or beverage but not all items in a group; Type III, all common items in one group; and Type IV, all foods and beverages.

These classifications may be useful to compare weight loss related to taste alterations caused by the progression of taste cell loss that occurs with head and neck irradiation. In patients with anorexia nervosa, taste changes can be classified using this approach, and recovery can be documented as the patient progresses through therapy.

The Radiation Side Effects Profile (RSEP)

In a study of the self-care strategies of patients receiving radiation therapy, Hagopian[55] developed a tool to measure not only the side effects experienced but also the self-care strategies used by patients to reduce the severity of the radiation side effects. One item on the RSEP documents taste changes and related symptoms contributing to loss of appetite or sore throat or mouth. Patients first rate the severity of each symptom on a 4-point scale from 0 (none) to 3 (very bad) and then rate the effectiveness of the self-care strategies used to alleviate the symptom using the scale, from 0 (not at all helpful) to 3 (very helpful). This rating of effectiveness constituted the Helpfulness Index.

A Severity Index indicating the severity of side effects and the helpfulness of self-care measures is determined by summing the scores. Self-care measures were classified into categories, including diet modification in which people with taste changes indicated self-care measures, such as trying different foods and seasonings and avoiding sweets.[56,57]

The summary score for the Severity Index may be of limited usefulness as it includes symptoms other than those related to taste. Test–retest reliability was determined for both the Severity Index and Helpfulness Index with Pearson's product–moment correlation values obtained at 1-week intervals during the first and second week of treatment . and again during the fourth and fifth week of therapy. With 56 subjects, the correlation coefficient between week 1 and week 2 on the Severity Index was 0.59 ($p > 0.001$). In the fourth and fifth week, in 28 subjects, the correlation coefficient was 0.83 ($p > 0.001$). For the Helpfulness Index in week 1 and week 2 the correlation coefficient was 0.46 ($p > 0.0007$). For weeks 4 and 5 it was 0.56 ($p > 0.001$). Content validity was obtained with a physician and clinical nurse expert to determine the representativeness of the side effects. The judges were asked to rate the clinical relevance of side effects on a scale of 1 (irrelevant) to 4 (extremely relevant). The index of the content validity or proportion of items receiving a 3 or 4 was 0.84. Construct validity was obtained for the Helpfulness Index as well. This tool has been used in other studies to document side effects in those receiving radiation therapy.[55]

Wall and Gabriel Checklist

Wall and Gabriel[18] compared taste alterations in children with leukemia to a group of healthy children. Children with leukemia were oriented to the four taste qualities using posters showing sweet, sour, salty, and bitter food. A checklist of 62 foods commonly eaten by children was used to determine taste preferences. This checklist was pretested with children and their parents in the community. Parents identified what foods the child preferred before the illness and how their choices had changed since diagnosis. Parents of healthy children were given the same checklist of foods. Reliability was determined for the list of preferred foods. Children were asked to respond to three questions: (1) Do you like to eat? (2) What are your favorite foods? and (3) What foods do you not like? Parents rated each food as 0 (dislike), 1 (tolerate), and 2 (like). For evaluation purposes, the 62 foods were divided into the four basic food groups. Scores were summed for each food group by adding the scores and dividing by the number of foods in the group. Significant differences existed only in the meat group ($p < 0.0125$).

This study is the best controlled investigation of taste changes found in this review. The methods used could be adapted to an adult population to help to determine patterns of food likes and dislikes. Repeating this study during the course of the treatment process should further elucidate patterns of taste changes and their relationships to treatment. Interviewing patients to determine the nature of any taste changes is a logical first step. Although this is subjective, it will identify changes that may significantly influence the child's eating behaviors. Listing foods from all groups may help to cue patients to a pattern in taste alterations.

Documenting Taste Response and Thresholds

Schecter et al.[58] used a single-blind study to investigate the effects of zinc sulfate on taste and smell dysfunction. In this trial, subjects were initially given a placebo. If no change in taste or smell occurred, the subject was given oral doses of zinc sulfate, and each subject served as his or her own control. Subjects who improved on placebo were not given zinc. In this study, patients who did not improve with placebo improved with zinc. Reliability and validity information was not presented.

Before any taste testing is done, an oral cavity examination should be performed to identify other factors that can influence or impede testing, such as candidiasis, stomatitis, xerostomia, herpes zoster, and oral cavity tumors. Although these factors do not preclude testing, they must be noted. The most commonly used technique for documenting taste is the measurement of detection and recognition thresholds. Subjects are presented with two bottles, one of which is water and the other, the substance being tested.[59,60]

Three drops of varying concentrations of the test substance are placed on the subject's tongue (usually approximately 10 concentrations). The subject rinses between tests. The point at which the substance is detected as being different from water is the *detection threshold*. The point at which the substance is recognized as sweet, sour, salty, or bitter is the *recognition threshold*. The recognition threshold usually is at a slightly higher concentration than the detection threshold. Normal subjects generally are used as the comparison group. Subjects are matched by age and should be matched for other factors, such as smoking history. Loss of the recognition threshold is believed to occur as a natural process of aging in both taste and smell, when enough receptors exist to detect a stimulus but not enough to make subtle distinctions.[58]

Taste Scale

Henkin et al.[59] developed a scale to document taste activity using the forced-choice, three-drop concentration technique. Taste detection and recognition thresholds were assessed. The measurements were transformed to a bottle-unit scale with each concentration designated as a bottle-unit and the change from one concentration to the next a bottle-unit change. Ranges at which normal subjects were able to recognize and detect substances have been determined. Patients who are expected to experience taste loss during therapy, such as those undergoing radiation, may be given the test weekly during therapy to document loss. Recovery after treatment also can be determined in this manner, recalling that it may take 3 to 6 months for taste to recover or that there may be permanent taste loss.

Using the Henkin method, Wall and Gabriel[18] found significant differences in detection thresholds for sweet ($p < 0.05$) and salty ($p < 0.05$) and in recognition thresholds for all modalities: sweet ($p < 0.05$), salty ($p < 0.05$), sour ($p < 0.05$), and bitter ($p < 0.05$).

Taste testing by the Henkin method has been criticized as revealing only certain forms of sensory loss and does not control for the area tested or the number of taste buds stimulated. It is possible to test specific areas by applying taste solutions with cotton-tip swabs to identify taste loss, but not thresholds. The application of solutions to specific areas is known as spatial testing and may be valuable in elucidating specific areas of taste loss after head and neck surgery or trauma.[59]

Rodin et al.[60] studied taste abnormalities in bulimic subjects. Subjects use a computerized visual analogue scale to rate the relative strength and pleasure of salty, sweet, sour, and bitter tastes in a variety of concentrations. Scores for the various concentrations were compared to deionized water. Researchers found no difference between bulimics and controls. When a spatial taste test was performed to stimulate discrete areas of the mouth and tongue, differences were found. In this study bulimics had a lower sensation of all tastes on the palate. Taste receptors on the palate may have been damaged by repeated contact with stomach acids during purging. The use of specific area testing and the ability of subjects to record their own responses using a computer-generated visual analogue scale are interesting attributes that could be translated into other research areas, such as testing with children.

Taste Magnitude Estimation

Citric acid in concentrations of 0.1, 0.01, and 0.001 M is used to evaluate sensitivity to the changing magnitude of a stimulus.[61] Three cups contain a small amount of citric acid in differing concentrations. Subjects take a small sip without swallowing, hold a small amount of solution in their mouth, and rate the concentrations in the proper order.[60] Patients with taste loss may require higher concentrations of solution to be able to taste them and may not be able to detect changes in the magnitude of stimuli. Small[6] found that patients with temporal lobe removal for epilepsy required higher concentrations for sensation than did normal controls.

Taste Magnitude Matching

Subjects are asked to judge stimuli from two sensory continua on a common intensity scale. Audible tones varying in loudness are interspersed with taste stimuli that vary in concentration. Patients are asked to assign numbers that reflect the intensities of the tastes and the tones.[61] The purpose of this is to test patients' ability to rank the strength of stimuli. Patients with taste loss may not perceive changes in intensity and will match taste concentrations with abnormally weak tones. Comparing the taste magnitude to audible sensations does not rely on patients' memory of previous sensations.

Sucrose Threshold

Sucrose solutions of 0.32, 0.1, 0.032, and 0.01 M and distilled water are used to determine the patient's sucrose threshold. A tastant and distilled water are given to the patient in separate cups. The patient is instructed to take small sips from each cup and identify which contains the tastant. The patient does not swallow any of the samples and rinses his or her mouth between trials with distilled water. Threshold is reached when the patient can identify three consecutive samples of the same concentration. The normal human threshold is 0.032 M. Reports of increased threshold for sucrose tolerance have been reported in persons with cancer.

Electrogustometry

A 5-mm stainless steel probe is used to test electric taste thresholds in the four quadrants of the tongue as well as on both sides of the soft palate. This is an excellent way to quantify the area of involvement in taste dysfunction.[59] Threshold values in these six areas are compared with standardized measurements made on normal subjects at Nihon University School of Medicine in Japan. This mean threshold value for the Japanese is 8 U. Thresholds for electric taste do not exactly mimic those for the four chemical tastes, but they are reproducible. Additional information on taste-testing techniques for determining thresholds, and other taste and smell testing tools, such as the Henkin, Spatial Testing and Magnitude Estimation, and Magnitude Matching may be obtained from the National Institute of Health's National Institute on Deafness and other designated centers that study chemosensory disorders. These centers focus on the regeneration of sensory and nerve cells, prevention of the effects of aging, and development of new diagnostic tests, treatment and rehabilitation. The centers are:

Richard L. Doty, Ph.D.
University of Pennsylvania Smell and Taste Research Center
Hospital of the University of Pennsylvania
3400 Spruce Street
Philadelphia, PA 19104-4283
215-662-6580

Marion E. Frank, Ph.D.
Taste and Smell Center
Connecticut Chemosensory Clinical Research Center
University of Connecticut Health Center
Farmington, CT 06032
203-679-2459

Gary Beauchamp, Ph.D.
Monell Chemical Senses Center
3500 Market Street
Philadelphia, PA 19104
215-898-6666

Thomas E. Finger, Ph.D.
Rocky Mountain Taste and Smell Center, Box 111
University of Colorado Health Sciences Center
4200 East 9th Avenue
Denver, CO 80262
303-270-6464

Maxwell M. Mozell, Ph.D
SUNY Health Sciences Center of Syracuse
Clinical Olfactory Research Center
766 Irving Avenue
Syracuse, NY 13210
315-464-4538

Measurement of Smell

Interviews may help to clarify the origin and nature of smell disorders. In the author's clinical practice, the following questions have been helpful in assessing alterations in smell:

Have you noticed a change in smell?
Can you describe the change?
When did it occur?
Have certain odors become unpleasant?
Does the area where you are being treated have an odor?
Are there smells that have become more pleasant?
Have you noticed any loss of smell?

Smell Threshold Testing

Thresholds for smell are determined in the same manner as those for taste. A simple test frequently used to test the first cranial nerve can be used to assess the status of smell. Substances such as coffee, peanut butter, or chocolate are placed in the bottom of a small gauze-covered jar. The blindfolded patient is given both an empty jar and one containing the stimulus to smell. The subject is given a list of possibilities from which to identify the odor. Each nostril is tested separately. Some investigators place the subject's head into a box containing a volatilized agent to exclude personal body odors.[2,3]

Forced-Choice Three-Sniff Technique

The Forced-Choice Three-Sniff Technique has been used by Henkin[59] and other investigators.[62] Stimuli are pyridine (onion- or garlic-like), nitrobenzene (bitter almond), and thiophene (burnt rubber). Measurements are transformed to the same bottle-unit logarithmic scale as the one used for taste testing. Hyposmia is defined as one bottle-unit threshold above normal. Cowart et al.[44] used a two-alternative, forced-choice technique to document hyposmia in allergic rhinitis. Olfactory thresholds were significantly higher in allergic patients than in controls ($p < 0.001$) as 23.1% of subjects demonstrated a significant loss of smell.

University of Pennsylvania Smell Identification
Test (UPSIT)

The most widely used test to assess smell is the UPSIT. This test has allowed convenient and accurate measurement of smell without complex equipment. It is a 40-item "scratch-and-sniff" microencapsulated odorant test. The test is commonly used in 1500 clinics in North America and has been used to validate other instruments. It is sensitive to a wide range of smell deficits caused by sinusitis, chemical exposure, Alzheimer's disease, cystic fibrosis, alcoholism, and lesions of the cerebral cortex.

The test is self-administered and may be sent to the patient by mail. It consists of four envelope-sized booklets each containing 10 "scratch-and-sniff" odorants. The stimuli are released by scratching the strip with a pencil. Above each odorant is a multiple-choice question with four alternatives for each item. For example: "This odor smells most like (a) chocolate (b) banana, (c) onion, or (d) fruit punch." Age- and gender-related norms have been established. The internal consistency reliability of the UPSIT is 0.922. Fractionated versions of the test consist of 10-, 20-, and 30-item fractionations that have been tested for internal consistency and resulted in 0.752, 0.855, and 0.898, respectively.[62]

Testing Smell in Children

Sheene and Wright[63] grouped 40 microencapsulated odorants into groups of five each and asked children to identify each odorant by selecting responses from one of five photographs. The results were used to select 5 odorants: baby powder, bubble gum, candy cane, fish, and orange. Children 3 1/2 years to 5 years 5 months identified odorants correctly 92% of the time. Most normal children age 5 and older were able to identify these odors. This study indicated that children age 5 to 12 could be tested for smell.

Summary

Tests such as the UPSIT have made it easier to study and measure smell, but the literature, and particularly the nursing literature, lacks studies measuring alterations in taste and smell. Although they are not life-threatening, these disruptions can result in significant nutritional compromise. More research is needed to document the nature and prevalence of alterations in taste and smell.

Exemplar Study

Wall, D., & Gabriel, L. Alterations of taste in children with leukemia. *Cancer Nurs*, 1983, 6(6):447–449.

This study compares the alterations of taste in children receiving chemotherapy to a group of healthy children. The study investigated taste acuity changes, the effects of chemotherapy, the effects of relapse or remission, and changes in food preference and appetite. The Henkin method, used successfully in children and adults with a variety of disease states, was used to measure taste. The questionnaire of changes of food likes and dislikes was compiled and received content validity from pediatric dieticians. Pretesting of the questionnaire was performed with parents of healthy children with 87.8% agreement on the list of preferred food. This study is exemplary because of the validity established for the instrument and the use of children as subjects.

References

1. Ziporyn, T. Taste and smell: The neglected senses. *JAMA*, 1982, 247(3):277-282.
2. Guyton, A. *Textbook of medical physiology*. Philadelphia: Saunders, 1986.
3. Schiffman, S. Taste and smell in disease. Part I. *N Engl J Med*, 1983, 308(21):1275-1280.
4. Stevens, J.C. Detection of very complex mixtures. *Ann NY Acad Sci*, 1998, 855:831-833.
5. Berridge, K.C. Measuring hedonic impact in animals and infants: Microstructure of affective taste reaction patterns. *Neurosci Biobehav Rev*, 2000, 24 (2):173-198.
6. Small, D.M., Zatorre, R.J., & Jones-Gotman, M. Changes in taste intensity perception following an-

terior temporal lobe removal in humans. *Chem Senses*, 2001, 26:425-432.
7. Murray, R.G. Ultrastructure of taste receptors. In L.M. Beidler (Ed.), *Handbook of sensory physiology*. New York: Springer-Verlag, 1971, p. 31.
8. DeWys, W.D. Abnormalities of taste as a remote effect of a neoplasm. *Ann NY Acad Sci*, 1974, 230:427-432.
9. DeWys, W.D., & Walters, K. Abnormalities of taste sensation in cancer patients. *Cancer*, 1975, 36(5):1888-1896.
10. DeWys, W.D. Changes in taste sensation in cancer patients: Correlation with caloric intake. In *The chem-*

ical senses and nutrition. New York: Academic, 1977, p. 381.

11. DeWys, W.D. Nutritional care of the cancer patient. *JAMA*, 1980, *244*(4):374-376,

12. Vickers, Z., Nielsen, D., & Theologides, A. Food preferences of patients with cancer. *J Am Diet Assoc*, 1981, *79*(4):441-446.

13. Trant, A.S., Serin, J., & Douglass, H. Is taste related to anorexia in cancer patients? *Am J Clin Nutr*, 1982, *36*(1):45-58.

14. Brewin, T. Can a tumor cause the same appetite perversion or taste change as a pregnancy? *Lancet*, 1980, *2*:907-908.

15. Hall, J.C., Staniland, J.R., & Giles, G.R. Altered taste thresholds in gastrointestinal cancer. *Clin Oncol*, 1980, *6*(2):137-142.

16. Bruera, E., Carraro, S., Roca, E., et al. Association between malnutrition and caloric intake, emesis, psychological depression, glucose taste and tumor mass. *Cancer Treat Rep*, 1984, *68*(6):873-876.

17. Barale, K., Aker, S.N., & Martinsen, C.S. Primary taste thresholds in children with leukemia undergoing marrow transplantation. *J Parenter Enter Nutr*, 1982, *6*(4):287-290.

18. Wall, D.W., & Gabriel, L. Alterations of taste in children with leukemia, *Cancer Nurs*, 1983, *6*(6):447-449.

19. DeWys, W., Costa, A.G., & Henkin, R. Clinical parameters related to anorexia. *Cancer Treat Rep*, 1981, *65*:49-53.

20. Hall, B., Hardesty, I., & Hogan, R. Nutrition alteration in less than body requirements related to nausea and vomiting. In J. McNally, E. Somerville, C. Miaskowski, & M. Rostad (Eds.), *Guidelines for oncology nursing practice*. Philadelphia: Saunders, 1991, pp. 173-179.

21. LeVeque, F.G. An unusual presentation of chronic graft versus host disease in an unrelated bone marrow transplantation. *Oral Surg Oral Med Oral Pathol*, 1990, *69*(5):581-584.

22. Erdman, L., Larsen, J., Hagglund, H., & Garduf, A. Health-related quality of life, symptom distress and sense of coherence in adult survivors of allogeneic stem cell transplantation. *Eur J Cancer Care*, 2001, Jun10(2):124-130.

23. Kashima, H., & Kalinowski, B. Taste impairment following laryngectomy. *Ear Nose Throat J*, 1979, *58*(2):88-92.

24. Donovan, M.L., & Pierce, S.G. *Cancer care nursing*. New York: Appleton-Century-Crofts, 1976.

25. Bernstein, I.L., & Bernstein, I.D. Learned food aversions and cancer anorexia. *Cancer Treat Rep*, 1981, *65*(5):43-47.

26 Aker, F. The role of taste and taste dysfunction in oral diagnosis. *Quintessence Int*, 1980, *11*(11):81-83.

27. Garg, R.K., Agrawal, A., Nag, D., & Jha, S. Herpes zoster associated with facial, auditory and trigeminal involvement. *J Assoc Phys India*, 1992, *40*(1):45-46.

28. Donaldson, S.F. Nutritional consequences of radiotherapy. *Cancer Res*, 1977, *37*(7):2407-2410.

29. Shatzman, A.R., & Mossman, K.L. Radiation effects on bovine taste bud membranes. *Radiat Res*, 1982, *92*(2):353-358.

30. Mossman, K.L., & Henkin, R.I. Radiation-induced changes in taste acuity. *Int J Radiat Oncol Biol Phys*, 1978, *4*(7/8):663-670.

31. Johnson, C.A., Keane, T.S., & Prudo, S.M. Weight loss in patients receiving radical radiation therapy for head and neck cancer: A prospective study. *J Parenter Enter Nutr*, 1982, *6*(5):399-406.

32. Bolze, M.S., Fosmire, G.J., Stryker, J.A., et al. Taste acuity, plasma zinc levels and weight loss during radiotherapy: A study of relationships. *Radiology*, 1982, *144*(1):163-168.

33. Mossman, K. Long-term effects of radiotherapy on taste and salivary function in man. *Int J Radiat Oncol Biol Phys*, 1982, *8*(2):991-998.

34. Hardy, S.L., Brennand, C.P., & Wyse, B.W. Taste thresholds of individuals with diabetes mellitus and of control subjects. *J Am Diet Assoc*, 1981, *79*(3):286-288.

35. Abbasi, A. Diabetes: Diagnostic and therapeutic significance of taste impairment. *Geriatrics*, 1981, *36*(12):73-79.

36. Russell, R.M., Cox, M.E., & Solomons, W. Zinc and the special senses. *Ann Intern Med*, 1983, *99*(2):227-239.

37. Mahajan, S.K., Prasad, A.S., Lambuian, J., et al. Improvement of uremic hypogeusia by zinc: A double-blind study. *Am J Clin Nutr*, 1980, *33*(7):1517-1521.

38. Zetin, M., & Stone, R.A. Effects of zinc in chronic hemodialysis. *Clin Nephrol*, 1980, *13*(1):20-26.

39. Ciechanover, M., Peresecenschi, G., Aviram, A., et al. Malrecognition of taste in uremia. *Nephron*, 1980, *26*(1):20-23.

40. Casper, R.C., Kirschner, B., Sandstead, H.H., et al. An evaluation of taste function in anorexia nervosa. *Am J Clin Nutr*, 1980, *33*(8):1801-1807.

41. Nakajima, Y., Utsumi, H., & Takahaski, H. Ipsilateral disturbance of taste due to pontine hemorrhage. *J Neurol*, 1983, *229*(2):133-139.

42. Goto, W., Yakamoto, T., & Kaneko, M. Primary pontine hemorrhage and gustatory disturbance: Clinicoanatomic study. *Stroke*, 1983, *14*(4):507-513.

43. Kampov-Polevoy, Agarbutt, J.C., & Janowsky, D. Evidence of preference for a high-concentration sucrose solution and excessive alcohol consumption. *Am J Psychol*, 1997, *154*(2):269-270.

44. Cowart, B., Flynn-Rodden, K., McGeady, M., & Lowry, L. Hyposmia in allergic rhinitis. *J Allerg Clin Immunol*, 1993, *91*(3):747-751.

45. Deems, R., Friedman, M., Friedman, L, et al. Chemosensory function, food preference, and appetite in human liver disease. *Appetite*, 1993, *20*(3): 209-216.

46. Ditraglia, G., Press, D., Butters, N., et al. Assessment of olfactory deficits in detoxified alcoholics. *Alcohol*, 1991, *8*(2):109-115.

47. Miller, S., & Naylor, G. Unpleasant taste, a neglected symptom in depression. *J Affect Dis*, 1989, *17*(3):291-293.

48. Kopala, L., Clark, C., & Hyrwitz, T. Olfactory deficits in neuroleptic-naive patients with schizophrenia. *Schizophr Res*, 1993, *8*(3):245-250.

49. Koopman, C.F., & Coulthard, S.W. The oral cavity and aging. *Otolaryngol Clin North Am*, 1982, *15*(2):293-300.

50. NIH. Variation in taste thresholds with human aging. *JAMA*, 1982, *247*(6):775-779.

51. Schiffman, D. Taste and smell in disease. Part II. *N Engl J Med*, 1983, *308*(22):1337-1339.

52. Prasad, A., Fitzgerald, J., Hess, J., et al. Zinc deficiency in elderly patients. *Nutrition*, 1993, *9*(3):218-224.

53. Dobell, E., Chan, M., Williams, P., et al. Food preferences and food habits of patients with chronic renal failure undergoing dialysis. *J Am Diet Assoc*, 1993, *93*(10):1129-1135.

54. Markley, E.J., Matts-Kulig, D.A., & Henkin, R. A classification of dysgeusia. *J Am Diet Assoc*, 1983, *83*(5):578-583.

55. Hagopian, G.A. Development of a radiation side effects profile. In O.L. Strickland & C.F. Waltz (Eds.), *Measurement of nursing outcomes. vol. 4: Measuring client self-care and coping skills*. New York: Springer, 1990, pp. 45-57.

56. Norcoss-Weintraub, F., & Hagopian, G. The effect of nursing consultation sessions on patient's well-being in a radiation oncology department. *Oncol Nurs Forum*, 1990, *17*(3):31-36.

57. Hagopian, G. The effect of a radiation therapy newsletter on patient's knowledge, self-care behaviors, and side effects. *Oncol Nurs Forum*, 1991, *18*(7):1199-1207.

58. Schecter, P.J., Friedewald, W.T., Bancert, D.A., et al. Idiopathic hypogeusia: A description of the syndrome and a single-blind study with zinc sulfate. *Int Rev Neurobiol*, 1972, (suppl 1):125-129.

59. Henkin, R., Schecter, P., & Friedewald, W. A double-blind study of the effects of zinc sulfate on taste and smell dysfunction. *Am J Med Sci*, 1976, *272*(3):285-289.

60. Rodin, J., Bartoshuk, L., Peterson, C., et al. Bulimia and taste: Possible interactions. *J Abnorm Psychol*, 1990, *99*(1):32-39.

61. Bartoshuk, L. Clinical evaluation of taste. *Ear Nose Throat J*, 1989, *68*(5):331-337.

62. Doty, R., Frye, R., & Agrawal, R. Internal consistency and reliability of the fractionated and whole University of Pennsylvania Smell Identification test. *Percept Psychophys*, 1989, *45*(5):381-384.

63. Sheene, P.R., & Wright, H. Olfactory performance during childhood: Development of an odorant identification test for children. *J Pediatr*, 1992, *121*(6):908-911.

IV

Instruments for Assessing Clinical Problems

30

Measuring Bowel Elimination

Kathryn K. Chambers and Susan C. McMillan

A variety of instruments and methods have been developed to provide quantitative data about human bowel function. Early attempts to objectively evaluate elimination involved simple questioning. However, wide differences in health status among populations, absence of dietary considerations, and reliance on patient recall of defecation performance resulted in questionable data.[1]

By the mid-1960s, research into the effects of diet on bowel performance precipitated the development of measurement tools and techniques for quantifying the frequency of defecation, stool consistency, stool wet weight, and intestinal transit time.[2-9] Further studies of gastrointestinal motility produced methods for quantifying intraluminal pressures within the alimentary tract.[10-14] Focusing on these parameters, numerous studies were conducted on normal subjects and those with elimination problems.

Other investigators have developed questionnaires and surveys that have provided subjective data describing attitudes and behaviors related to elimination and evaluating bowel patterns among various populations.[15-18] Depending on study objectives and the population under investigation, however, both subjective and objective dimensions of bowel elimination may need to be measured.

Because bowel function can be affected by neurophysiologic, psychologic, and cultural conditions, a comprehensive approach to the measurement of the concept of elimination must include all such parameters. Bowel function varies not only among subjects with different underlying conditions, it also can vary in the same subject at different times. Instrument selection, therefore, is critical, and it is generally believed that a thorough study will require the use of more than one instrument.

Instruments that result in quantitative data provide objective measures of bowel function, but interpretations are limited by the normal variability of colonic function[19] and the influence of multiple variables.[20] In contrast, instruments that result in qualitative data (descriptive data) provide subjective measures that attempt to identify various bowel patterns or describe the concept of elimination per se. Instrument choice ultimately is determined by research goals, populations under study (normal versus abnormal bowel function), number of subjects, and resources available.

Objective Scales Yielding Quantitative Data

Objective measures can be categorized according to the parameters considered relevant to the investigation of bowel function. The following instruments and methods have been used to investigate both normal subjects and those with problems of elimination, such as bowel syndromes, megacolon, diverticulitis, Crohn's disease, constipation related to medication, and diarrhea associated with enteral feedings.

Bowel Transit Time

Methods that have been used to measure gut transit time may be classified as radiologic, colorimetric, particulate, chemical, and isotopic.

Radiologic Measures

Hinton et al. developed a simple technique using radiopaque pellets of barium-impregnated polyethylene.[2] A known number of pellets are swallowed, usually 20, and the disappearance of the pellets from the gut or the appearance of the pellets in the stool are observed by serial radiographs. Results are expressed as the time taken for the passage of the first and of 80% of the markers. Recovery rate using 30 subjects was 99.3%. Replicate studies were performed with only descriptive data and variability in transit time up to 2 days in the same subject. Comparison studies with other markers, again using descriptive data only, were difficult to assess because of the inherent differences in the various methods. For instance, radiopaque pellets were compared to glass beads and were shown to have a shorter mean transit time (MTT), probably because the beads have a higher specific gravity than the pellets. Comparisons with chemical markers were less than optimal because some of the chemical was found in the urine as well as the stool.

Payler et al. used Hinton's method for measuring intestinal transit time while studying the effect of bran on intestinal transit and found reproducibility poor, with variability in transit times even in the same subject.[4] To provide more accurate and reproducible data, Cummings et al. compared MTT using radiopaque pellets in two different ways and compared this to Hinton's method of 80% excretion as an expression of transit time (80% TT).[3] MTT was measured using a constant amount of marker fed to subjects over a period of weeks (MTT-C) and again measured by giving single doses of similar markers to the subjects (MTT-S). The MTT-S method was found to be preferable to the 80% TT if a single-dose technique was used. The MTT-S correlated more closely with the MTT-C ($r = 0.87$) than did the 80% TT ($r = 0.78$) and gave a value for transit that is more physiologic. Although the MTT-C method provided more information about transit in individuals (data that reflect the way residue passes through the gut, i.e., colon), it can be tedious and is not suitable for studies on an epidemiologic scale.

Although it has limitations, an alternative method for measuring transit time through the gut was developed and tested by Cummings and Wiggins.[5] It requires the collection of only one stool after 4 days of ingestion of markers. It is suitable for use in epidemiologic studies on an outpatient basis. This method compared favorably with MTT-C ($r = 0.78$, $p < 0.001$) and MTT-S ($r = 0.94$, $p < 0.001$) and proved a satisfactory alternative method for validating transit techniques. Once transit times begin to exceed 4 days, its accuracy falls off, and it would not be suitable for studying the constipated patient.

A 1992 study also correlated two radiologic methods, one using daily studies and one using a single radiologic study on day 7.[21] Significant positive correlations further support the value of the single measures of both segmental and total transit time while exposing the patient to lower doses of radiation.[21] Other studies have also confirmed that transit time correlates highly with subjective patient data regarding constipation and infrequent bowel movements.[22-25]

Defecography, also known as *proctography*, involves the insertion of a thick barium paste into the rectum and making a videorecording of the expulsion. The time for rectal evacuation is calculated from the moment of first passage of barium through the anal canal until evacuation is complete. A group of 58 patients with idiopathic constipation was compared with 20 controls.[22] The significant differences in evacuation time and in the amount of barium remaining in the rectum between the patients and controls supports the validity of this method.

The usefulness of defecography was examined in constipated patients by using a commercially prepared barium paste inserted into the rectum.[25] The patient was seated on a specially prepared stool for defecation and the defecogram was recorded on videotape and continuous fluoroscopy. Recording started when the patient began straining to defecate. Anorectal angle changes were measured and subjects were evaluated for leakage of contrast at rest; presence of rectocele, rectal intussuception, or prolapse; and the completeness of rectal evacuation. Correlation of this method with anorectal manometry produced weak to moderate correlations. An important result of this study was that it found 27% of the patients to have a significant rectocele, which correlated with a decreased number of stools and decreased rectal emptying. The investigators concluded that defecography could be useful in classification of patients with impaired evacuation.[25]

Colorimetric Measures

Various dyes have been used to mark stool and then calculate passage through the intestinal tract. Simplicity makes this method especially attractive, and it has been used in a variety of research settings.[26-29] Two widely used dyes are brilliant blue (100 mg/capsule) and carmine (500 mg/capsule). Dosing usually requires three capsules per each experimental day. Transit time is computed as the time from ingestion of the marker until most of the color has appeared in the feces. This requires daily stool collection and careful examination of the stool, which may lend itself to misinterpretation.

Rogers et al. compared the use of radiopaque pellets and dye in measuring bowel transit time and, after rigorous analysis of variance, concluded that the two methods gave identical information.[29] This comparison supports the validity of both methods. Colorimetric measures provide mouth-to-anus transit time but cannot provide data about passage through the different parts of the gastrointestinal tract. These measures would, therefore, be limited in usefulness when studying the diseased colon or other bowel disorders to ascertain segmental function. They lend themselves well to the study of diarrhea, as the specific gravity of radiologic markers may affect the transit time in the diarrheal stool.

Particulate Measures

Particulate measures are tedious and require complex and careful analysis of stool specimens. Furthermore, complete recovery can be seriously altered by stool adsorption of the reagent secondary to dietary fiber composition. Polyethylene glycol (PEG) can be ingested by subjects (1-g doses) after dilution in water and then analyzed in stools with a spectrophotometer. The use of PEG as a transit time measure was compared to other standard measures, including dyes, pellets, and isotopes.[29] Mean recovery for 242 doses was 85.3% (± 12.6%). Low recovery was attributed to binding of PEG by stool components. A separate analysis of MTT values from all markers revealed no significant differences in transit time estimates among marker types.

Chemical Measures

One of the major limitations of the use of radiopaque pellets is that total excretion may not represent pool sizes and turnover rates of unexcreted intestinal content. Thus, pellet excretion may not have any significant relationship to the usual clinical descriptions of bowel habits. Patients may report daily bowel movements, but pool sizes could be very large and turnover small, that is, a large proportion of the colonic contents may not be excreted for long periods.[7] Because chemical markers are incorporated into the food intake, their excretion can indicate the completeness of stool collections and permit corrections for variations in fecal flow. Chromic oxide (Cr-203) has been used widely in humans since 1947 for these purposes because it is nontoxic, readily measurable in the feces, and appears to be completely unabsorbable. Subjects are given 60-mg tablets of chromic oxide with meals (not to exceed 300 mg/day). Fecal collections are pooled and stored at 4°C until the collection period is completed. Although measurements demonstrated reliability (replicate demonstrations showed a coefficient of variation of 2.8% ± 1.5%), analysis is time-consuming.[8]

Dick reported on the use of cuprous thiocyanate as a continuous marker for feces that is insoluble under physiologic conditions but could be decomposed by relatively mild chemical treatments.[6] The marker is administered with each meal, with a total daily dose of 1 g; stools are collected and stored and then analyzed for copper content. Analysis requires the addition of nitric acid followed by atomic absorption spectroscopy. Copper recovery over 79 four-day periods on 14 subjects was 99.7%. Although not statistically analyzed, a histogram comparing the recoveries of cuprous thiocyanate to barium sulfate and chromium oxide demonstrated a higher percentage of recovery with cuprous thiocyanate.

In an investigation into the effects of fiber on bowel function, Wrick et al. compared various markers for transit time, one of which was Chromium (Cr[III]) mordanted onto isolated bran fiber, and found no significant differences in transit time estimates between Cr(III) and PEG or radiopaque pellets.[29] Chromium-mordanted bran is prepared and placed into capsules, each dose providing 35 to 45 mg Cr, and ingested daily. Fecal Cr recovery is assessed by atomic absorption spectrophotometry. Complete stool collection is required, and a lengthy preparation procedure for spectroscopy is necessary.[29] Mean fecal Cr recovery from 244 doses of Cr(III)-mordanted bran was 84% ± 16.9%. Incomplete conversion to chromic oxide (during preparation for spectroscopy) and marker overlap between testing periods were two explanations offered by these investigators for results lower than 100%. Apparently, the cellulose in the mordanted bran altered the colonic microflora so that there was a microbial interaction with the mordant, which somehow influenced the recovery of Cr. This limitation needs to be considered with subjects who may have slow turnover of intestinal pool.

Isotopic Measures

Isotopic measures have the advantage of quantifying transit rates separately through the small and large intestines, whereas other transit time measures are suitable for total mouth-to-anus assessments only. Hansky and Connell first used Cr-51 to investigate transit times by labeling sodium chromate (Na_2CrO_4).[9] A gelatin capsule filled with 0.5 g of chromic oxide with an activity of 1 to 2 microcuries is swallowed by the subject, and a scintillation counter permits quantification according to the amount of Cr-51 present in stools. A mean percentage recovery of radioactivity of 83.5% was demonstrated, but more important, this technique permits the quantitative measurement of the rate of passage of the maximum bulk of the markers.

Waller used Cr-51 as a marker while investigating small- and large-bowel transit times in subjects with constipation and diarrhea.[30] Other markers were used concurrently, but comparative statistical analysis was not performed. Transit times for all markers were similar. However, Cr-51 provided differential measurements for colonic function in diarrheal and constipated states that would not have been ascertained using standard measures and would be useful when investigating segmental gastrointestinal transit.

Between 1990 and 1993 three studies with four different isotopic markers were conducted.[31-33] Iodine-131-cellulose, ^{99m}Tc-radiolabeled resin, ^{111}In-labeled particles, and ^{99m}Tc-labeled aluminum magnesium sulfate were used in the studies to assess gastric and bowel transit time. All three studies found significant differences between constipated patients and controls, thereby supporting the validity of the use of isotopic markers by correlating it with another method of evaluating bowel motility. Although they did find a positive association (60%) between scintigraphy and anorectal manometry in the constipated group, there was an overall poor level of agreement when nonconstipated persons were included. These researchers concluded that although scintigraphy has the advantage of low radiation exposure, its inability to distinguish between patients with slow-transit constipation and defecatory complaints makes its clinical value uncertain.

Stool Consistency
Penetrometer Cone
A quantitative technique for assessing stool consistency, devised by Exton-Smith et al., uses a penetrometer cone, which is lowered until it is touching the stool, released, and then allowed to penetrate the stool for 5 seconds.[34] Distance of penetration is measured in units of 0.1 mm. Several readings are taken along the column of the stool and are averaged. The total range of penetrometer readings is 0 to 240, with a mean of 80.6 for hard stools and 128.9 for soft stools. Further work is being carried out to refine the method and to establish a normal range of values.

Stool Ash Analysis
In a clinical study assessing lactose intolerance with tube-fed patients, Walike and Walike found that stool ash analysis validated subjective ratings of stool consistency made by nurse clinicians.[15] Stool content was analyzed for sodium, potassium, percentage of fat, nitrogen, phosphate, percentage of ash, and wet and dry weight. Stool weight, percentage of water, and sodium were significantly higher with the lactose-containing diet and correlated well with stool consistency ratings.

Frequency of Defecation
Because self-reporting has been considered unreliable by most investigators, Hinton et al. devised a collection technique that provided accurate measurements of frequency as well as a convenient way to transport specimens to the laboratory for further analysis.[2] This method continues to be used today with a few minor alterations. It entails the use of a polyethylene bag that is suspended over the toilet to collect the stool specimen while allowing the urine to pass freely. The plastic bag is then sealed with a rubber band and inserted into a specimen cup and labeled with the appropriate information. Assuming subject compliance, this method should provide objective, quantifiable data about stool frequency.

Stool Wet/Dry Weight and Volume
Numerous investigations have shown that dietary constituents, medications, and colonic function affect fecal characteristics.[5,10,11,19,27] Statistical analysis of fecal measurements often

includes the calculation of coefficients of variation for each subject for each measurement. Statistical comparisons of these measures to other variables (transit time, dietary fiber, medications) are then determined to explore any relationships further.[19] Although no special instruments for measuring these parameters are described in the literature, techniques for such assessments are clearly delineated.[19]

Gastrointestinal Motility Measures

Manometer

Various invasive measures have been used to assess quantitatively the motility of the alimentary tract. Early studies using miniature balloons connected through polyethylene tubing to a metal capsule optical manometer of high sensitivity provided intraluminal pressure readings in both normal patients and those with dysfunctional conditions.[10,11] The same technique has been used to compare the effects of codeine and senna on the motor activity of the left colon.[12] Any type of cardiovascular, respiratory, or somatic movement will affect the tracings and can interfere with accurate interpretations. An assessment of colonic activity is given by the product of the total duration of activity and the mean amplitude of the slow waves. Analysis for observer error initially produced a mean standard deviation of $\pm 3.2\%$. This was considered too great an error, and therefore the standard deviations of duplicate analyses were calculated, and the mean of these standard deviations was $\pm 1.8\%$ ($p = 0.01$).

Pezim et al.[35] used anorectal manometry to compare patients with constipation to patients with normal bowel function. A multilumen polyvinyl catheter with sideholes was placed in the rectum, with the patient in the left lateral decubitus position. Measurements were taken at rest and with contraction. There was no difference in the resting pressure between the groups of patients, and maximum pressure of the anal canal contraction was greater in the group of patients who had normal bowel function (177 ± 7 mmHg vs. 144 ± 8 mmHg, $p < 0.01$). Anal manometry did not detect a significant difference between groups of patients, despite the difference in contraction pressures. The researchers conclusion was that although the test alone could not distinguish between constipated and nonconstipated patients, it could be useful in conjunction with other tests to detect certain disease states.[35]

Balloon Expulsion

Balloon expulsion is a simple test used in evaluation of dysfunctional elimination. Preston and Lennard-Jones compared a group of patients with a diagnosis of slow-transit constipation to a control group that had no constipation.[36] Transit time was measured with radiopaque markers; one passed 10 of the 20 markers, and the rest had not passed 20 markers after 5 days. For the expulsion test, a lubricated balloon connected to a catheter was inserted into the rectum and inflated with 50 cc of water. A pressure probe was inserted into the balloon to ensure that straining was occurring during attempts to expel the balloon. None of the patients in the group with slow-transit constipation were able to expel the balloon, in contrast to the control group, who were all able to expel the balloon spontaneously. The conclusion was that the constipated patients had a failure of relaxation of the muscles of the pelvic floor. Although similar studies have continued to show that patients with normal bowel function can expel a filled balloon, they have not demonstrated that all patients who are constipated cannot. Researchers have concluded that this simple test may add valuable data about various patients' types of constipation.[25,35]

Thermistor Probe

Kagawa-Busby et al. studied the effects of diet temperature on the tolerance of enteral feedings and evaluated gastric motility and intragastric temperature by inserting a nasogastric feeding tube with a thermistor probe for recording temperature and a polyethylene cannula for pressure recordings.[14] No reference was made to evaluations of the validity or reliability of the instruments used. Observation periods were predetermined and identical for all subjects; thus, analysis of observer error was not relevant. However, this does not exclude the possibility of misinterpretation of readings by omission.

Subjective Scales Yielding Quantitative Data

Elimination studies frequently attempt to measure the effects of certain variables (diet, medications, bowel diseases) on stool consistency and require the quantification of subjective data. Walike and Walike assessed stool consistency among tube-fed patients on lactose-containing versus lactose-free diets. Descriptive ratings were performed by nurse clinicians and validated by concurrent stool ash analysis.[15] Descriptive parameters were plotted against time and categorized between both diets (Figure 30.1). Patients on the lactose-containing tube feedings had at least one and a half times as many stools as the lactose-free group. The lactose-containing group also had predominantly loose to liquid stools compared to the soft to hard stools of the lactose-free group.

To evaluate the effectiveness of dioctyl sodium sulfosuccinate as a prophylactic measure in preventing constipation among hospitalized patients, Goodman et al. used a scale for grading stool consistency.[16] Six descriptive categories were used, including A (watery); B (soft-formed, normal stool); and C (watery, hard-formed stool).

The scales used by Walike and Walike and by Goodman et al. offer ways to categorize stool consistency. However, there was no mention of interrater reliability or validity testing by either group of investigators. It is apparent that selection criteria will vary for a given population; that is, stool characteristics for subjects with tube-fed diets will differ from those of subjects who may be at risk for constipation. This makes the establishment of a standardized scale for measuring stool consistency difficult and it emphasizes the importance of selecting appropriate criteria for the population under study.

Although some subjectively reported measures may be reports of clinicians, others require reports of patients. One such self-report measure was used in concert with anorectal manometry.[37] An unnamed 3-item scale of severity of abdominal pain, distension, and bowel habit disturbance was used. These symptoms were scored on a 0-to-10 scale and summated for a severity score of 0 to 30. Evidence of validity was provided by demonstrating a decrease in subjective symptoms (from 23.5 to 9.6) after hypnotherapy. Test–retest reliability with a 9- to 12-day delay was assessed on a group of controls. No differences were found in the two measures, thereby supporting the reliability of the self-report measure.

	DIET									
	LACTOSE-FREE					LACTOSE-CONTAINING				
Watery						XX	XXX	XX		
Liquid						XX		X		
Very loose, semiliquid	X			X			XX		XXX	
Loose, very soft		X	X							
Day	2	4	6	8	10	2	4	6	8	10

Figure 30.1 Comparison of stool frequencies and consistencies on two diets for one subject. Each X represents one stool.

A more sophisticated measure, the Bowel Disease Questionnaire (BDQ), was designed to differentiate among nonulcer dyspepsia, irritable bowel syndrome, organic gastrointestinal disease, and health.[38] The 46 gastrointestinal symptoms-related items were developed based on a careful review of the literature, including other previously published instruments; this provided beginning evidence of construct validity. An additional 25 questions addressing past illnesses and use of the health care system also were included. The BDQ was administered to 361 subjects: 115 with functional bowel disease (either nonulcer dyspepsia or irritable bowel syndrome), 101 with organic gastrointestinal disease, and 145 healthy adults. The mean completion time for the BDQ was 17 minutes. Variables that identified nonulcer dyspepsia were found to be (1) upper abdominal pain more than six times in a year, (2) no increase in bowel movements when pain begins, (3) stools that were not loose or watery, and (4) no doctor visits for colonic symptoms. Variables that identified functional bowel disease included (1) more bowel movements when pain begins, (2) more than three bowel movements daily, (3) presence of mucus, (4) frequent feeling of incomplete evacuation, (5) vomiting, and (6) heartburn. The ability of the instrument to differentiate among the groups of patients supports its validity as a diagnostic tool. Test–retest with delay using 42 subjects supports its reliability (median kappa for all questions was 0.78 with a range of 0.52 to 1.0).

Constipation Assessment Scale (CAS)

The CAS is an eight-item self-report tool designed to measure the presence and severity of constipation. The CAS was developed on a careful review of the literature, which offers beginning evidence of construct validity.[39] It is a 3-point summated rating scale resulting in a total score that ranges from 0 (no constipation) to 16 (severe constipation).

Validity of the CAS was studied using contrasted groups, including a control group ($n = 32$) of adult cancer patients at risk for constipation because of morphine or vinca alkaloids. A significant difference between the two groups ($p < 0.0001$) provided evidence of construct validity. Further evidence of validity was provided by the ability of the scale to differentiate between the levels of intensity reported by the patients receiving morphine and those receiving vinca alkaloids ($p < 0.01$).[39] A later study using 30 controls and 30 cancer patients receiving morphine reconfirmed the ability of the scale to differentiate ($p < 0.0001$) between groups.[40]

The reliability of the CAS has been studied with both test–retest and internal consistency methods. Test–retest ($n = 16$) with a 1-hour delay resulted in a strong correlation ($r = 0.98$, $p = 0.000$). Internal consistency using Cronbach's alpha was evaluated twice using two groups of cancer patients with very acceptable results (alpha = 0.70 and 0.78) for such a short scale.[39,40]

Diarrhea Assessment Scale (DAS)

DAS is a newly developed scale designed for use with patients receiving radiation therapy to the pelvic area.[41] However, it appears to be a generic measure of the presence and severity of diarrhea. To provide beginning evidence of construct validity, the DAS was developed on a careful review of the literature to include four characteristics of diarrhea: (1) frequency, (2) consistency, (3) urgency, and (4) abdominal discomfort. The patient rates each of these on a 0-to-3 scale; scores are summed, providing a range of 0 (no diarrhea) to 12 (severe diarrhea).

Construct validity of the DAS was studied using the known-groups technique. The scores of a group of apparently healthy adults ($n = 20$) were compared with those of a group of men receiving radiation therapy for cancer of the prostate ($n = 20$). A significant difference ($p < 0.0001$) between groups supports the validity of the scale. The mean score for the patient group was 7.85 (SD = 1.35). Reliability was estimated with the combined sample (*n* = 40). The resulting reliability coefficient (Cronbach's alpha 0.87) was acceptably high for such a short scale.[41] Further research on this tool is warranted, but it appears promising.

Subjective Scales Yielding Qualitative Data

Andersson et al. Scale

Andersson et al. developed a scale to evaluate bowel habits while investigating the effects of dietary restriction of fat and the use of antidiarrheal agents after bowel resection in patients with Crohn's disease.[17] The bowel habits were evaluated according to the following scale:

> *Satisfactory or good.* Three or less bowel movements/24 hours, usually after breakfast and causing no social inconvenience
> *Fair.* Four to six movements/24 hours, mostly in relation to meals and with *minor* inconvenience
> *Poor.* Seven or more bowel movements/24 hours, considerable social inconvenience, and/or incapacity for work

Drossman et al. Questionnaire

Using a broader approach, Drossman et al. developed a brief, self-administered questionnaire to identify bowel patterns among the general population.[18] The questionnaire contained several areas of inquiry for comparative analysis and provided demographic data as well as information about subject attitudes and behavior related to bowel function. Based on their responses to questions about stool frequency, abdominal pain, or awareness of changes in bowel patterns, subjects could be classified into several categories. Examples are:

> *Category A: alternating bowel function.* Subject responded affirmatively to questions about loose, frequent stools alternating with hard, infrequent stools and to similar questions
> *Category B: abdominal pain.* Included in this category were subjects with more than six episodes of lower abdominal pain in the last year under various circumstances, such as abdominal pain relieved by bowel movement, loose stools associated with pain

Selection criteria for the categories were based on reports from other investigations into dysfunctional bowel syndromes and were both objective and subjective. Subject attitudes regarding bowel dysfunction were assessed by such questions as "Does stress affect your bowel pattern?" with response options of "never," "sometimes," and "always."

Drossman's instrument allows the researcher to identify by questionnaire a range of bowel patterns in the general population and to categorize subjects into groups with specific types of bowel dysfunction. It was administered to 789 subjects, and the results were in agreement with data reported from other investigations into comparable bowel patterns.

Summary

A variety of types of instruments and methods are available to assess bowel function. These include both objective and subjective measures. The use of several measures may be necessary to obtain data that accurately reflects the concept of elimination and human bowel patterns. Further, considering the normal variability of colonic function, interpretations of these data will need to reflect the dynamic status of this basic human process.

Exemplar Study

McMillan, S.C., & Williams, F. Validity and reliability of the Constipation Assessment Scale. *Cancer Nurs*, 1989, *12*(3):183–189.

This study exemplifies the measurement of constipation, a pervasive problem in many nursing settings. The purpose of the study was to develop and study the Constipation Assessment Scale (CAS). The authors developed the scale based on characteristics of constipation identified by a careful review of the literature. This evidence of content validity is supplemented with evidence of construct validity accomplished through comparison of known groups. These comparisons support the validity of the CAS in assessing both the presence and severity of constipation. In addition, estimates of both internal consistency and test–retest reliability are provided. Patients are able to complete the CAS in about 2 minutes, making the scale clinically useful. The readability level of the scale is at the sixth-grade level, which further supports the clinical usefulness of the CAS.

References

1. Godding, E.W. Physiological yardsticks of bowel function and the rehabilitation of the constipated bowel. *Pharmacology*, 1980, *20*(Suppl 1):88-103

2. Hinton, J.M., Lennard-Jones, J.E., & Young, A.C. A new method for studying gut transit times using radiopaque markers. *Gut*, 1969, *10*(10):842-850.

3. Cummings, J.H., Jenkins, D.J.A., & Wiggins, H.S. Measurement of the mean transit time of dietary residue through the human gut. *Gut*, 1976, *17*17(3):210-218.

4. Payler, D.K., Pomare, E.W., Heaton, K.W., & Harvey, R.F. The effect of wheat bran on intestinal transit. *Gut*, 1975, *16*(3):209-213.

5. Cummings, J.H., & Wiggins, H.S. Transit through the gut measured by analysis of a single stool. *Gut*, 1976, *17*(3):219-223.

6. Dick, M. Use of cuprous thiocyanate as a short-term continuous marker for feces. *Gut*, 1969, *10*(5):408-415.

7. Davignon, J., Simmonds, W.J., & Aherns, E.H., Jr. Usefulness of chromic oxide as an internal standard for balance studies in formula-fed patients for assessment of colonic function. *J Clin Invest*, 1968, *47*(1):127-129.

8. Bolin, D.W., King, R.P., & Klosterman, E.W. A simplified method for the determination of chromic oxide when used as an index substance. *Science*, 1952, *116*(5):634-638.

9. Hansky, J., & Connell, A.M. Measurement of gastrointestinal transit using radioactive chromium. *Gut*, 1962, *3*(4):187-193.

10. Connell, A.M. The motility of the pelvic colon. Part I. *Gut*, 1961, *2*(2):175-179.

11. Connell, A.M. The motility of the pelvic colon. Part II. *Gut*, 1962, *3*(4):342-349.

12. Waller, S.L. Comparative effects of codeine and senna on the motor activity of the left colon. *Gut*, 1975, *16*(5):407-410.

13. Meunier, P., Rochas, A., & Lambert, R. Motor activity of the sigmoid colon in chronic constipation: Comparative study with normal subjects. *Gut*, 1979, *20*(12):1095-1101.

14. Kagawa-Busby, K.S., Heitkemper, M.M., Hansen, B.C., et al. Effects of diet temperature on tolerance of enteral feedings. *Nurs Res*, 1980, *29*(5):276-280.

15. Walike, B.C., & Walike, J.W. Relative lactose intolerance. *JAMA*, 1977, *238*(9):948-951.

16. Goodman, J., Pang, J., & Bessman, A.N. Dioctyl sodium sulfosuccinate—An ineffective prophylactic laxative. *J Chronic Dis*, 1976, *29*(1):59-63.

17. Andersson, H., Bosaeus, I., Hellberg, R., & Hulten, L. Effect of a low-fat diet and antidiarrheal agents on bowel habits after excisional surgery for classical Crohn's disease. *Acta Chir Scand*, 1982, *148*(3):285-290.

18. Drossman, D.A., Sandler, R.S., McKee, D.C., & Lovitz, A.J. Bowel patterns among subjects not seeking health care: Use of a questionnaire to identify a population with bowel dysfunction. *Gastroenterology*, 1982, *83*(3):529-534.

19. Wyman, J.B., Heaton, K.W., Manning, A.P., & Wicks, A.C.B. Variability of colonic function in healthy subjects. *Gut*, 1978, *10*(2):147-150.

20. Slavin, J.L., Sempos, C.T., Brauer, P.M., & Marlett, J.A. Limits of predicting gastrointestinal transit time from other measures of bowel function. *Am J Clin Nutr*, 1981, *34*(10):2111-2116.

21. Bouchoucha, M., Devroede, G., Arhan, P., et al. What is the meaning of colorectal transit time measurement? *Dis Colon Rectum*, 1992, *35*:773-782.

22. Sloots, C.E., Poen, A.C., Kerstens, R., et al. Effects of prucalopride on colonic transit, anorectal function and bowel habits in patients with chronic constipation. *Aliment Pharmacol Ther*, 2002, *16*:759-767.

23. Guimaraes, E.V., Goulaart, E.M., & Penna, F.J. Dietary fiber intake, stool frequency and colonic transit time in chronic functional constipation in children. *Braz J Medi Biol Res*, 2001, *34*:1147-1153.

24. Lu, C. L., Chen, E.Y., Chang, F.Y., et al. Effect of a calcium channel blocker and antispasmodic in diarrhoea-predominant irritable bowel syndrome. *J Gastroent Hepatol*, 2000, *15*:925-930.

25. Glia, A., Lindberg, G., Nilsson, L.H., et al. Clinical value of symptom assessment in patients with constipation. *Dis Colon Rectum*, 1999, *42*(11):1401-1410.

26. Glia, A., Lindberg, G., Nilsson, L.H., Mihocsa, L,. Akerlund, J.E. Constipation assessed on the basis of colorectal physiology. *Scand J Gastroenterol*, 1998, *33*:1273-1279.

27. Wrick, K.L., Robertson, J.B., Van Soest, P.J., et al. The influence of dietary fiber source on human intestinal transit and stool output. *J Nutr*, 1983, *113*(8):1464-1479.
28. Kelsay, J.L., Behall, K.M., & Prather, E.S. Effect of fiber from fruits and vegetables on metabolic responses of human subjects: Bowel transit time, number of defecations, fecal weight, urinary excretions of energy and nitrogen and apparent digestibilities of energy, nitrogen and fat. *Am J Clin Nutr*, 1978, *31*(7):1149-1152.
29. Rogers, H.J., House, F.R., Morrison, P.J., & Bradbrook, I.D. Comparison of the effect of drugs upon some commonly used measures of bowel transit time. *Br J Clin Pharmacol*, 1978, *6*(6):493-497.
30. Waller, S.L. Differential measurement of small and large bowel transit times in constipation and diarrhea: A new approach. *Gut*, 1975, *16*(5):371-378.
31. McLean, R.G., Smart, R.C., Gaston-Parry, D., et al. Colon transit scintigraphy in health and constipation using oral iodine-131-cellulose. *J Nuc Med*, 1990, *31*:985-989
32. Stivland, R., Camilleri, M., Vassallo, M., et al. Scintigraphic measurement of regional gut transit in idiopathic constipation. *Gastroenterology*, 1991, *101*: 107-115.
33. Wald, A., Farrukh, J., Rehder, J., & Holeva, K. Scintigraphic studies of rectal emptying in patients with constipation and defecatory difficulty. *Digest Dis Sci*, 1993, *38*:343-358.
34. Exton-Smith, A.N., Bendall, M.J., & Dent, F. A new technique for measuring the consistency of feces. A report in the elderly. *Age Ageing*, 1975, *4*(1):58-62.
35. Pezim, M.E., Pemberton, J.H., Levin, K.E., et al. Parameters of anorectal and colonic motility in health and severe constipation. *Dis Colon Rectum*, 1993, *36*(5):484-491.
36. Preston, D.M., & Lennard-Jones, J.E. Anismus in chronic constipation. *Dig Dis Sci*, 1985, *30*(5):413-418.
37. Prior, A., Colgan, S.M., & Whorwell, P.J. Changes in rectal sensitivity after hypnotherapy in-patients with irritable bowel syndrome. *Gut*, 1990, *31*:896-898.
38. Talley, N.J., Phillips, S.F., Melton, L.J., et al. A patient questionnaire to identify bowel disease. *Ann Int Med*, 1989, *111*(8):671-674.
39. McMillan, S.C., & Williams, F. Validity and reliability of the Constipation Assessment Scale. *Cancer Nurs*, 1989, *12*(3):183-188.
40. McMillan, S.C., & Levy, M. Reassessment of the validity and reliability of the Constipation Assessment Scale. An unpublished study, 1990. Contact address: University of South Florida College of Nursing, MDC Box 22, Tampa, FL 33617.
41. Casey, L., & Zachariah, B. A pilot study to develop a diarrhea assessment scale. Unpublished study, 1993. Contact address: James A. Haley Veterans Hospital, 119, Tampa, FL 33613.

31

Measuring Cardiac Parameters

Susan J. Quaal

Since the beginning of anesthesia in 1846, clinicians have relied on their senses of sight, hearing, smell, taste, and touch to monitor the patient, aided in later years by simple technical devices such as the stethoscope. For example, diagnosis of fluid overload is marked by clinical signs of weight gain, distended neck veins, peripheral edema, and chest x-ray findings. However, these markers do not provide the precision needed to accurately diagnose and treat these patients. The true hemodynamic profile is difficult to measure accurately solely from the physical assessment. Modern medical technology measures cardiac parameters via transducers and signal processors that convert one form of energy to another.[1,2] Most of these techniques have enhanced our understanding of the mechanism of the patient's decompensation and helped to guide appropriate therapeutic interventions. As critical care medicine has rapidly evolved, patient monitoring capabilities have also become increasingly complex. The basic principle underlying measurement of cardiac parameters stems from the ability of catheters, placed into arteries and veins, to acquire diagnostic information about the cardiovascular system during the two phases of the cardiac cycle—systole and diastole. Contraction and relaxation of the heart produces characteristic rises and falls in pressure waveforms.[3] These fluctuations result from (1) changes in blood volume (blood entering a chamber or vessel causes the pressure to rise, whereas blood exiting a chamber or vessel causes the pressure to fall) or (2) changes in myocardial fiber tension (contraction causes the pressure to rise, relaxation causes the pressure to fall).

The cardiovascular system has three types of pressures:[4] hemodynamic, kinetic energy, and hydrostatic. Hemodynamic pressure is the energy imparted to the blood by contraction of the left ventricle. This type of pressure is preserved by the elastic properties of the arterial system. Kinetic energy is the energy associated with motion and affects the pressure measured during direct arterial blood pressure monitoring. Hydrostatic pressure is the pressure a column of fluid exerts on the container wall. In the vascular system, hydrostatic pressure is proportional to the height of the column of blood between the heart and the peripheral vasculature. In a standing person, the pressure in the leg is higher than the pressure in the arm because of the difference in hydrostatic pressure.[5]

Patient pulse pressures are transduced into amplified electrical signals, from which parameters such as blood pressure, stroke volume, cardiac output, intracardiac and pulmonary artery pressures, estimates of vascular resistance, and mixed venous oxygen saturation can be computed. Physiologic measurement is the assignment of numbers or units of measure to hemodynamic data. Numeric data are important but must not be used in isolation. Just as a clinical diagnosis cannot be made on one laboratory value, optimal clinical decisions cannot be made on numeric hemodynamic data alone. Correlation of hemodynamic data must be undertaken in conjunction with all the patient's clinical indicators.[6]

Issues of physiologic measurement are not any different from issues related to psychosocial and behavioral measurement. There is equal concern with validity, reliability, and generalizability of findings. Collection and accurate measurement of cardiac parameters is the responsibility of the clinician, who must be knowledgeable of the characteristics and correct measurement of hemodynamic waveforms. It is critically important that these physiologic measurements be carried out with rigor and consistency. Measurement characteristics should include (1) validity or accuracy, which is the degree to which the measured value represents the actual value also called (fidelity), (2) reliability or measurement accuracy over time, (3) sensitivity or precision (the ability of the instrument to measure repeatedly the smallest degree of change), and (4) stability, or the ability of the instrument to return to zero point after an input stimulus and lack of drift (ability of the instrument to remain stable at a given setting).[7] Techniques for measuring cardiac parameters must be described in great detail when designing and publishing a physiologic research study. This ensures exact replication of the study. Ideally, a biomedical instrument that measures cardiac parameters should (1) be noninvasive, (2) directly measure the variable, (3) not change or alter the variable being measured, (4) be applicable in a variety of settings, (5) provide a quantitative value, (6) provide continuous measures that are accurate and reliable, (7) have a rapid response time (frequency response) or a wide range of values, (8) be sensitive to small changes in physiologic variables, (9) maintain calibration without drift or noise, and (10) be cost-effective and easy to operate.[8]

Before using any of the measurements and associated instrumentation, the researcher must be familiar with manufacturer-recommended operation and safety instructions. It is also the responsibility of the researcher to obtain any required certification of the instrument or measurement procedure before collecting data.

The Concept of Blood Pressure

As the left ventricle contracts, blood is ejected into the aorta. The highest pressure generated at the peak of the pulse wave is *systolic pressure*. Arterial pressure falls to a trough level at the end of diastole, which is termed *diastolic pressure*. As pressure rises in the aorta, a pulse wave is generated and propagated throughout the arterial tree. Physical characteristics of the arterial system cause this pulse wave to change in contour as it propagates from the aorta to the arteries and capillaries (Figure 31.1) The upstroke becomes steeper and the pulse wave becomes more triangular. The incisura or dicrotic notch, marking the closure of the aortic valve, is prominent in recordings from the aortic arch but becomes slurred in the distal arteries.[4] These changes occur as the high-frequency vibrations produced during aortic valve closure are quickly damped by the viscous and inertial properties of the blood and vascular wall.[9] Energy imparted to the blood by ventricular contraction is reflected back toward the heart from various sites in the circulation. These

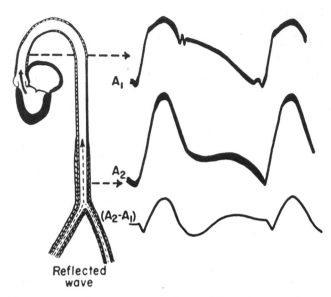

Figure 31.1 Changes in arterial pressure waveforms. The primary pulse contour (A_1) is recorded from the aortic arch. A_2 is the pulse recorded from the distal aorta. The difference between these pulses ($A_2 - A_1$) is the reflected pulse wave that travels toward the heart from the arterioles. (Reprinted from *Physiology of the Heart and Circulation*. Little, p. 243, 1985, with permission of Elsevier.)

backward pressure waves merge with the forward-moving waveform to produce the characterized arterial pressure waveform contour.

Systolic pressure in the lower extremities may be 20 to 30 mm Hg higher than in the upper extremities. The difference between systolic and diastolic pressure is termed *pulse pressure*, which is approximately 50 mm Hg. *Mean pressure* is the average pressure during the cardiac cycle and can be approximated for central arterial pressure by using the following formula: mean pressure = diastolic pressure × ⅓ pulse pressure.[10]

Arterial pressure is regulated by two predominant mechanisms: (1) a system of rapidly acting vascular reflexes and resistances and (2) a group of slower mechanisms that adjust the body's fluid volume and indirectly affect arterial pressure. As a result, substantial changes in body position and level of muscular activity, as well as alterations in circulating blood volume, are tolerated without causing a significant deviation in blood pressure.[9,10] Blood pressure measurement can be performed either *indirectly* with a cuff, stethoscope, and sphygmomanometer or *directly* by placing an intraarterial catheter.[11]

Indirect Blood Pressure Measurement

The term *indirect* is appropriate because pressure in the blood pressure cuff is measured, rather than that in the blood vessel itself. A nondistensible cuff containing an inflatable bladder is placed on the subject's arm, with the middle of the bladder placed directly over the brachial artery.[12]

The bladder (connected to a needle-valved rubber bulb by a piece of rubber tubing) is inflated by pumping the rubber bulb. The pressure in the cuff bladder is reflected on a mercury or aneroid manometer. Inflation of the bladder compresses the artery so that blood flow diminishes to the point of obliteration distal to the cuff. When the needle valve of the inflation bulb is released, the bladder within the cuff deflates and the cuff pressure falls. When the cuff pressure decreases to the peak pressure generated by left ventricular contraction, blood resumes flowing through the brachial artery on an intermittent basis. Sharp tapping or knocking sounds termed *Korotkoff* sounds are generated with each systole.[13]

Korotkoff sounds are named for the Russian physician who first described the auscultatory method in 1905.[9] Early investigators proposed that Korotkoff sounds were the result of a water hammer or breaker effect. Using a simulated artery of translucent latex, Sacks[14] studied the production of Korotkoff sounds in a vessel filled with colored fluid and found that the vessel was never fully occluded; some colored fluid was always present. During the production of the Korotkoff sounds, the collapsed cross-section of the vessel traveled longitudinally beneath the cuff, coincident with the pulse wave. Moreover, the sounds appeared to be generated when the collapsed section of the vessel arrived at the distal end of the cuff. Such finds have led some investigators to conclude that Korotkoff sounds are the result not of turbulence within the vessel, but rather of dynamic instability of the vessel wall, which occurs when fluid oscillations imposed on it become amplified. This instability is the result of the elastic property of the artery wall. When this elastic property is diminished, as in fixed vessel disease, a greater change of auscultatory error is believed to exist. In summary, consensus does not exist in the literature regarding the exact cause of Korotkoff sounds.[15] Therefore the American Heart Association (AHA)[16] recommends that phase 1, 4, and 5 pressure readings be documented when the sounds of phase 5 extend to zero. The clinical significance of such findings in uncertain. The five phases are:[13]

Phase 1: Pressure level at which the first faint, clear tapping sounds are heard (systolic blood pressure).
Phase 2: Time during cuff deflation when a murmur or swishing sounds are heard.
Phase 3: Period during which sounds are crisper and increase in intensity.
Phase 4: Time when a distinct, abrupt muffling of sound occurs. The phase reflects the diastolic pressure in children and in adults with hyperkinetic states that allow for audible sounds throughout the deflation period.
Phase 5: Pressure level when the last sound is heard and after which all sound disappears. This phase reflects the diastolic pressure in the adult.

Procedure for Recording an Indirect Blood Pressure

Recommendations for human blood pressure determination by sphygmomanometers are as follows:[17]

1. Situate the individual in a quiet environment with the arm resting at heart level. Put him or her at ease, and allow a 50-minute rest period.
2. Place the manometer at eye level, sufficiently close to read the calibrations marking the gauge or column.
3. Select the appropriately sized cuff. Bladder width should be at least 40% of arm circumference, bladder length should be at least 80% of arm circumference.
4. Locate the brachial artery along the inner upper arm by palpation.
5. Wrap the cuff smoothly and snugly around the arm, centering the bladder over the brachial artery. The lower margin should be 2.5 cm above the antecubital space. (Do not rely on cuff marking; find the center by folding the bladder in half.)

6. Determine the level of maximal inflation by observing the pressure at which the radial pulse is no longer palpable as the cuff is rapidly inflated (palpate systolic) and by adding 30 mm Hg. (Note the presence of an irregular pulse.)
7. Rapidly and steadily deflate the cuff. Then wait 15 to 30 seconds before reinflating.
8. Position the stethoscope over the palpated brachial artery below the cuff at the antecubital fossa. Ear pieces should point forward. The bell head of the stethoscope should be applied with light pressure, ensuring skin contact at all points. Heavy pressure may distort sounds.
9. Rapidly and steadily inflate the cuff to the maximal inflation level, as determined in step 6.
10. Release the air in the cuff so that the pressure falls at a rate of 2 to 3 mm Hg per second.
11. Note the systolic pressure at the onset of at least two consecutive beats (phase 1) for both adults and children. Blood pressure levels should always be recorded in even numbers and read to the nearest 2 mm Hg mark on the manometer.
12. Note the diastolic pressure at muffling (phase 4) for children and cessation of sounds (Phase 5) for adults. Phase 5, at which the last sounds are heard, is the diastolic pressure in adults. Listen for 10 to 20 mm Hg below the last sound heard to confirm disappearance, and then deflate the cuff rapidly and completely.
13. Record systolic/diastolic pressure. When phase 4 pressure is recorded, the pressure at phase 5 also should be recorded. Example: 108/64/52 or 110/66/0 mm Hg.
14. Record the patient's position, the cuff size, and the arm used for the measurement.
15. Wait for 1 to 2 minutes before repeating the pressure measurement in the same arm to permit the release of blood trapped in the arm veins.

Reliability, Validity, and Measurement Error

To be detected by a stethoscope, Korotkoff sounds must be at a frequency within an audible range. In low-flow states, resulting from a primary reduction in cardiac output or increased peripheral vascular resistance, transmission of sounds is impaired. Sound transmission also can be decreased in obese patients or in those with severe peripheral edema.[18] Common sources of variation in blood pressure measurement are listed in Table 31.1. Indirect blood pressure measurements may be unreliable and invalid due to factors related to patient, blood pressure bladder and cuff and the examiner.

The Patient

The examiner must attempt to measure an indirect blood pressure reading that is representative of the patient's ordinary and reproducible circumstances. Ideally, blood pressure should be recorded in a quiet room at a comfortable temperature after the patient has rested for 5 minutes. Frohlich et al.[17] stated that "the patient's arm should be bared, unrestricted by clothing, with the palm of the hand exposed upward and the elbow flexed at the heart level. Ideally, the person should not have eaten or smoked for 30 minutes prior to the blood pressure measurement." (p10)

Frohlich et al.[17] comment on the effect of arm position and measurement accuracy:

The pressure of the arm increases as the arm is lowered from the level of the heart (phlebostatic axis); conversely, raising the arm above this position lowers the pressure measurement. The effect is largely explained by hydrostatic pressure or by the effect of gravity on the column of blood. Therefore, when measuring indirect blood pressure, the patient's arm should be positioned so that the location of the stethoscope head (preferably, the bell) is at the level of the heart. This location of the heart is arbitrarily taken to be at the junction of the fourth intercostal space and the lower left sternal border. Attention to the position of the brachial artery in relation to the heart is particularly important when the patient is standing upright. No corrections for position need to be made if the patient is lying supine on a flat surface with the head slightly raised, since the arm by the side of the body is sufficiently close to the level of the heart. When the patient is seated, placing the arm on a nearby tabletop a little above waist level will result in a satisfactory position. If

Table 31.1   Common Sources of Variation in Blood Pressure Measurement

Source	Cause	Effect	Remedy
Manometer	Loss of mercury	Reading impaired	Have medical equipment dealer add more mercury to zero mark
	Clogged air vent at top of manometer tube	Mercury column will respond sluggishly to pressure	Clean or replace air vent
	Loose air vent nut	Mercury column will bounce	Tighten knurled nut at top
Bladder	Too narrow	High reading	Determine bladder and cuff size
	Too wide	Low reading	Use proper technique
	Not centered over artery	High reading	Use proper technique
Cuff	Loose application	High reading	Use proper technique
	Applied over clothing	Reading impaired	Use proper technique
	Too wide	Low reading	Use pediatric cuff
Tubing	Too wide	Low reading	Check for leaks and replace
Stethoscope	Eartips not forward	Auditory impairment, low systolic, high diastolic	Use proper technique

Modified from American Heart Association of Metropolitan Chicago. *Manual for instructors in the measurement of blood pressure.* 1976. Chicago: American Heart Association, 1984, 33:879-881.

the position of the arm cannot be appropriately adjusted, a correction of the hydrostatic pressure must be made: For each 1 cm of vertical height above or below the heart level, 0.8 mm Hg must be added or subtracted, respectively, to the observed pressure.

Korotkoff sounds may not always disappear but may continue to be heard until cuff pressure drops to zero in children and in patients with aortic valvular insufficiency or high cardiac output (anemia, thyrotoxicosis, or pregnancy) and marked vasoconstriction. Phase 4, during which the pitch of Korotkoff sounds changes, should then be used as the marker for diastolic pressure.[19]

Cuff and Bladder

Length and width of bladder and ratio of one to the other are known factors influencing indirect blood pressure measurement. False low blood pressure readings result if the blood pressure cuff is too small, and false high readings occur if the cuff is too large. The AHA[16] recommends a bladder width of 40% of the arm circumference, and the cuff should be long enough to encircle at least 80% of the arm in adults. The correct ratio of bladder width to arm circumference is 0 : 4. The bladder width multiplied by 2.5 defines the ideal arm circumference of that particular cuff. Therefore the ideal arm circumference for a bladder width of 12 cm is 12.0×2.5, or 30 cm. Thigh cuffs should be used for obese individuals whose arm circumferences are greater than 41 cm.[13]

Banner and Gravenstine[20] determined the effect of snugness of cuff wrap on the accuracy of blood pressure measurement. The study was performed in six healthy volunteers. In both studies, control values were obtained from the right upper arm with cuffs of appropriate size and snug fit. The first study had two phases. In the first phase, cuffs of appropriate size were wrapped snugly around the upper left arm of seated subjects. The effects of two other degrees of cuff snugness were evaluated by placing a 250-ml intravenous fluid bag between the cuff and arm over the triceps, measuring blood pressure, then draining the bag of half of its contents and then all of its contents without rewrapping the cuff (loose and very loose fits). The second phase was identical except that the cuffs used on the left arm were one size too small. These researchers found that appropriately sized cuffs, whether wrapped tightly or loosely, gave correct blood pressure readings. Cuffs snugly wrapped, but too small for the subject, gave high readings averaging 10 mm Hg over actual. Loose wrapping of small cuffs gave variable results in individual subjects that exaggerated systolic blood pressure from 2 to 80 mm Hg.

Direct (Invasive) Blood Pressure Measurement

Direct arterial pressure is measured via a transducer connected to a small plastic catheter, which is inserted into a peripheral artery. Transduced pressures provide systolic, diastolic, and mean values, as well as displayed arterial waveform. Gorny[21,p68] described invasive blood pressure monitoring as follows:

> Direct blood pressure measurement is used when continuous hemodynamic monitoring for the evaluation of changing patient status, evaluation of related therapy and continuous blood sampling, such as for arterial blood gas measurement, are required. The intraarterial method is preferred to the indirect auscultation technique in patients with low cardiac output states when pulses may be poorly palpable and Korotkoff sounds may be difficult to hear.
>
> Invasive monitoring provides a moment-to-moment pictures and a visual display of BP trends. During direct BP monitoring, intravascular pressure changes caused by cardiac contraction associated with the transmission of electrical impulses within the cardiac cycle are measured. An artery is cannulated with a catheter, which is connected to a fluid-filled tubing and transducer system. The transducer converts the pressure signals caused by the back and forth movement of the arterial wall sensed as the artery-catheter interface into electrical energy that is displayed as waveforms on an oscilloscope.

Arterial catheters can be placed by direct threading, the Seldinger technique, or the transfixing method. Direct technique involves inserting the catheter until arterial pressure is transmitted to the catheter, and the needle is removed while the catheter is advanced. The Seldinger technique makes use of a wire over which the catheter is threaded. The transfixation technique requires a puncture by the catheter through the posterior blood vessel wall, which is subsequently drawn into the blood vessel.[22]

Cannulation sites include the radial, brachial, axillary, femoral, dorsalis pedis, and posterior tibial arteries. The radial artery is the most commonly used peripheral site because of its easy accessibility. The indwelling arterial polyurethane catheter is then connected to a disposable transducer that converts the patient's arterial pressure to an electrical signal that is transmitted via an electrical cable to the bedside monitor that displays the blood pressure waveform and quantifies systolic and diastolic values.[23]

Reliability and Validity

Gardner and Hujcs[22,p12] point out that the "accuracy of blood pressure readings depends on establishing an accurate reference point from which all subsequent measurements are made." Zeroing a hemodynamic monitoring system is accomplished by positioning a fluid-filled stopcock at the phlebostatic axis, turning it off to the patient or open to air, and activating the bedside monitor zero function. All pressure contributions from the atmosphere are negated and only pressure values that exist within the heart chamber of vessel are measured.[24] It is the stopcock that is opened to air, not the transducer, which is leveled to the patient's phlebostatic axis.[23–25]

The phlebostatic axis is a point of junction between a frontal and transverse chest plane located by drawing an imaginary line from the fourth sternal intercostal space and extending it around to the right side of the chest. A second imaginary line is drawn vertically from the midaxillary line down to bisect the first transverse line. Zeroing should be performed at least once a shift, after raising or lowering the head of the bed, and before implementing any treatment changes based on the invasive arterial pressure.[26,27,28]

To measure direct invasive blood pressure accurately, the fluid-filled catheter system must be able to transmit the patient's pressure with fidelity or accuracy of reproduction. Physiologic waveforms are dynamic, not static. Thus, a hemodynamic monitoring system must have excellent fidelity, termed *dynamic response*, which refers to an oscillatory response produced by the system after it is excited. This is similar to vibrations produced by striking a bell. Another example of dynamic response is the bouncing action of a tennis ball when it is thrust against a hard surface. A lesser height is reached with each successive bounce. The number of oscillations per second is referred to as its *natural frequency*.

Frequency response of a catheter-plumbing hemodynamic monitoring system can be obtained by stimulating the system with high pressure and observing the system's oscillatory response. The system's in-line fast-flush device can be used to excite the system by opening and quickly closing the device. This action temporarily interrupts pressure waveform transmission and applies a step change of square-wave pressure, followed by oscillations that revert back to the arterial pressure waveform.[22,24,25,26]

Natural frequency is determined by measuring (in millimeters) the distance between two consecutive oscillatory peaks, termed a *period*, and dividing this distance by the strip recorder paper speed (25 mm/sec; Figure 31.2). Optimal natural frequency is about 25 Hz, which would be no more than one little box (1 mm) between each two successful vertical oscillations. Figure 31.3 illustrates an optimal dynamic response of 25 Hz. Figure 31.4 illustrates a damped system. False low systolic and high diastolic readings occur with an overdamped system.[22,23]

Decisions regarding pharmacologic and other interventions often are contingent on the patient's blood pressure, so it is imperative that direct measurement occur only after acceptable natural frequency has been validated. Measures to maximize natural frequency are (1) remove all air bubbles from the monitoring system, (2) minimize the potential for clot formation at the catheter tip by using a continuous-flush system, (3) keep catheter and connecting tubing length under 5 feet, and (4) eliminate loose-fitting connections.[22,23,29–31]

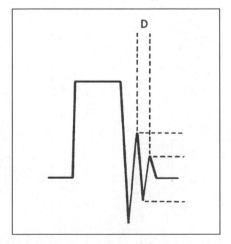

Figure 31.2 Illustration of the fast-flush dynamic response (square-wave) assessment. Natural frequency is estimated by measuring the distance (D) between two consecutive peaks (the "period") and dividing by the paper speed (25 mm/sec).

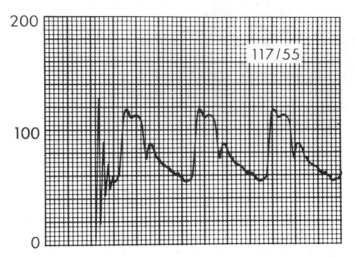

Figure 31.3   An optimal natural frequency of 25 Hz. There is one small box between any two successive oscillations divided by the paper speed (25 mm/sec).

Discrepancies between Direct and Indirect Blood Pressure Measurements

Discrepancies occur between indirect and direct methods of blood pressure measurement as the result of methodology, instrumentation, and natural physiologic causes. Research has suggested that indirect blood pressure measured generally underestimates the systolic value and overestimates the diastolic value.[32] However, the most important contributing factor of discrepancy between these two methods can be attributed to methodology. Arm position, cuff size, obesity, and edema all can contribute to indirect measurement error. It is recommended that a palpatory reading be recorded as the systolic pressure if it is found to be higher than the auscultatory reading.[13] When using the

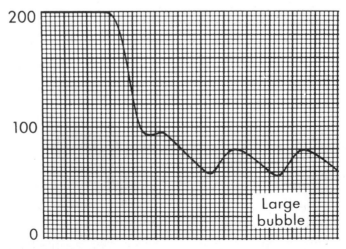

Figure 31.4   A damped response caused by a large air bubble in the software-connecting tubing.

direct technique, the system must be zeroed and natural frequency assessed with correction to 25 Hz to achieve reliable measurement.[23,29,32,33,34]

Thermal Dilution Cardiac Output Measurement

Cardiac output is the amount of blood ejected by the heart per unit of time and is normally 4 to 8 liters/minute. Tissue viability depends on an adequate delivery of oxygen and nutrients from the circulating blood. Therefore, cardiac output is an important parameter in assessing the patient with myocardial failure and as an indicator of response to therapy.

Thermal dilution technique for measurement of cardiac output was described by Fegler in 1954.[35] A specific quantity (5–10 ml) of normal saline dextrose solution at a known temperature is injected into the blood stream via a special pulmonary catheter with a thermistor positioned at its distal tip. The change in temperature as this bolus of fluid is warmed by the blood is recorded by the distal tip thermistor and is recorded by cardiac output computer as a temperature-time curve that is inversely proportional to the blood flow. Thermol dilution cardiac output (TDCO) determinations measure flow over only a few seconds. Therefore, three to five repeated measurements are made, and the mean of these values is used to reflect the average cardiac output.[36,37,38]

Reliability and Validity

Temperature of both blood and injectate solution must be accurate and stable. A newer closed injectate system with an inline thermistor that measures injectate temperature as it leaves the syringe has reduced but not eliminated this source of measurement error. Daily and Schroeder[37] caution that heat from the injectate, whether iced or room temperature, is lost through handling the injectate syringe and throughout the catheter itself as it travels to the right atrium. A warm environment or the use of heat lamps can appreciably alter the injectate temperature. Ways to minimize injectate heat transfer or loss are listed in Table 31.2. The injectate must be administered rapidly (10 ml in < 4 seconds) and evenly. Table 31.2 highlights strategies to maximize the accuracy of thermodilution-calculated cardiac output.[37]

Iced versus Room-Temperature Injectate

Multiple studies, representing diverse patient populations, have compared 10 ml of room-temperature and iced injectate in TDCO, and report high correlations.[32–38] Gillman[39] cautioned that a change in injectate temperature once it is measured introduces a 3% to 6% error. The associated error for inaccurate injectate volumes was found to be 1% per 0.1 ml using 10 ml injectate, and 2% per 0.1 cc using 5 cc. All crystalloid solutions were found to be acceptable.

Pulmonary Artery Wedge Pressure Measurement

Development of a flow-directed catheter has allowed indirect assessment of left ventricular function via the pulmonary artery wedge pressure (PAWP) measurement. At the tip of this catheter is a balloon that, when inflated, causes the catheter tip to become buoyant and advanced in the direction of blood flow. When positioned in a capillary, the catheter obstructs forward blood flow and a pressure-sensing device at the distal tip reflects left atrial pressure, which is important in assessing left ventricular function when clinical signs of heart failure are present. Normal values are 6 to 12 mm Hg.[40–42]

Table 31.2 Strategies to Maximize Accuracy of Thermodilution-Calculated Cardiac Output (CO)

Strategy	Discussion
Rapid, even injection technique	Slow or uneven technique produces inaccurate data Cardiac output curve reveals slow or uneven upstroke
Examine each CO curve for technical adequacy	Each curve should be printed out, rather than depending solely on digital value
Delay CO computerized analysis until after injection is completed	In patients with very low stroke volumes, blood moves very slowly from the right atrium to the pulmonary artery; thus the CO computer can complete analysis before maximum temperature difference has been sensed if the analysis is begun prior to the end of the injection
Minimize injectate heat transfer or loss	
Use closed-injectate system with an inline temperature probe	Reduces exposure to environment; minimizes hand contact with injectate. Inline temperature probe measures injectate temperature after it leaves syringe
Inject an initial volume of injectate to "cool the catheter"	Reduces heat loss of subsequent injections; do not use initial injection for CO measurement
Use room-temperature, not iced, injectate	Similar results found between iced and room-temperature CO determinations; room-temperature injectate less likely to cause slowing of heart rate. May need to use iced injectate in hypothermic patients to ensure minimum temperature difference of 12 degrees
Keep injectate solution, tubing, and catheter away from direct sunlight or heat lamps	May cause artificial reading

Reliability and Validity

Accuracy of PAWP measurement is crucial and can be obtained only through a program of excellence in quality assurance, which minimally must consist of zeroing, referencing, and dynamic response.[30] Additional factors that ensure accuracy include confirmation of catheter location by capillary blood gases and a chest x-ray to validate placement in lung zone III.

Zeroing and Referencing

Zeroing and referencing are two independent activities performed simultaneously as the most basic quality assurance components. Zeroing and referencing have been described as the "single most important steps in setting up a pressure measurement system" and "cause of the largest pressure measurement error in the clinical situation."[23]

Zeroing is performed by opening the system to air and therefore establishing atmospheric pressure as zero. *Referencing* is accomplished by placing the air-fluid interface stopcock opened to air at the right heart level to negate the weight effect of fluid (hydrostatic pressure) in the catheter tubing.[38] The phrase *zeroing the transducer* is a misnomer. It is the stopcock that is opened to air, not the transducer, which is leveled to the patient's phlebostatic axis. Pressure-monitoring systems should be zeroed and referenced at least once per shift, after the head of the bed is raised or lowered and before extrapolating pressure date that is used in clinical patient management decision making.[28]

Dynamic Response Testing and Natural Frequency Assessment

Pulmonary artery wedge pressures are static, not dynamic. The catheter and connecting software's ability to transmit pressure accuracy to the transducer depends on its dynamic response, which was discussed under arterial pressure measurement.[41,42]

Capillary Blood Gases

Proper placement of the inflated balloon tip pulmonary artery catheter in the capillary bed can be validated by capillary (c) blood gases, as compared to arterial (a) blood gases. A properly "wedged" catheter seals off any forward blood flow. Thus a "capillary blood gas" will be higher in oxygen and lower in carbon dioxide than an arterial blood gas sample. Catheter placement in the PAWP position is validated if the following criteria are met when comparing a capillary to arterial blood gas sample.[40]

$$PcO_2 - PaO_2 \geq 19 \text{ mm Hg}$$
$$PaCo_2 - PcCo_2 \geq 11 \text{ mm Hg}$$
$$Phc - pHa > 0.08$$

New Technologies in the Assessment of Hemodynamic Parameters

The goal of hemodynamic monitoring is to maintain adequate tissue perfusion. Since organ blood flow cannot be directly measured in clinical practice, arterial blood pressure, pulmonary artery pressure, and cardiac output are the estimators of tissue perfusion. New technologies, which provide improved and less invasive methods for hemodynamic monitoring, continue to be developed. Examples include novel measurements of preload, oxygen delivery and consumption, intermittent bolus thermodilution, right ventricular ejection fraction, Doppler cardiac output, and exhaled carbon dioxide cardiac output monitoring.[42-59]

Exemplar Studies

Ahrens, T., Pennick, J.C., & Tucker, M.K. Frequency and requirements for zeroing transducers in hemodynamic monitoring. *Am J Crit Care*, 1995, 4:466-471.

This article reports the results of two studies, a bench study and a clinical study. The drift from zero in a hemodynamic monitoring system was examined from the time of setup and daily for a period of 1–10 days. In the bench study, no transducer had a drift more than ± 2 mm Hg, and 19 of 50 transducers remained exactly at zero. When drift occurred, it usually happened in the first 24 hours and never after 72 hours. In the clinical study, 98.7% of transducers showed no drift.

McGhee, B.H., & Woods, S.I. Critical care nursing knowledge of arterial pressure monitoring. *Am J Crit Care*, 2002, 40:43-51.

A total of 391 critical care nurses having at least 4 years of nursing experience (94.1%) completed an 18-item criterion-referenced questionnaire in arterial blood pressure physiology, technical aspects of arterial blood pressure monitoring, and waveform interpretation in selected pathophysiologic conditions. Results of this study conducted at two university-affiliated hospitals suggested a knowledge deficit in arterial pressure monitoring, one of the most basic aspects of hemodynamic monitoring.

Bridges, E. Monitoring pulmonary artery pressures: Just the facts. *Crit Care Nurse,* 2000, 20:59-78.

This paper reviewed six studies that evaluate critical care nurses' knowledge of pulmonary artery (PA) pressure monitoring. Mean test scores ranged from 31% to 65%. An important finding from these studies is that the areas associated with the lowest scores— knowledge and the ability to apply information related to the collection and interpretation of data obtained with a PA catheter—have been consistent during the past 10 years. Areas consistently associated with the lowest scores include interpretation of normal and abnormal waveforms and technical factors that affect the accuracy and reliability of PA pressure measurement.

References

1. Boldt, J. Clinical review: Hemodynamic monitoring in intensive care. *Crit Care,* 2002, 6:52-59.
2. Ginosar, Y., & Sprung, C. The Swan-Ganz catheter: Twenty-five years of monitoring. *Crit Care Clin,* 1996, 12:771-776.
3. Campbell, B. Arterial waveforms; monitoring changes in configuration. *Heart Lung,* 1997, 26:204-214.
4. McGhee, B.H., & Bridges, E.J. Monitoring arterial blood pressure: What you may not know. *Crit Care Nurse,* 2002, 22:60-79.
5. Rhodes, R., & Tanner, G. *Medical physiology.* Boston: Little, Brown, 1995.
6. Adams, K.F. Guiding heart failure care by invasive hemodynamic measurements. *J Card Failure,* 2002, 8:63-70.
7. Waltz, C.F., Strickland, O.L., & Lenz, E.R. *Measurement in nursing research* (2nd ed.). Philadelphia: Davis, 1991.
8. Carr, J.J., & Brown, J.M. *Introduction to biomedical equipment technology* (2nd ed.). New York: Prentice Hall, 1993.
9. Little, R.C. *Physiology and biophysics of the circulation.* Chicago: Yearbook Publishers, 1972.
10. Asmar, R., Darne, B., el Assaad, M., & Topoachin, J. Assessment of outcomes other than systolic and diastolic blood pressure: Pulse pressure, arterial stiffness and heat rate. *Blood Press Monit,* 2001, 6:329-333.
11. Bridges, E.J., & Middleton, R. Direct arterial vs oscillometric monitoring of blood pressure: Stop comparing and pick one (a decision-making algorithm). *Crit Care Nurs,* 1997, 17:58-66, 68-72.
12. Hoover, L. Comparison of blood pressure readings between cuff pressures and radial arterial catheters with changes in transducer level and patient position. *Am J Crit Care,* 2000, 9:220-221.
13. Anderson, F.D., Cunningham, S.G., & Maloney, J.P. Indirect blood pressure measurement: A need to reassess. *Am J Crit Care,* 1993, 2:272-279.
14. Sacks, A.H. Indirect blood pressure measurements. A matter of interpretation. *Angiology,* 1979, 30:683-695.
15. McCutcheon, E.P., & Rusherm, R.F. Korotkoff sounds: An experimental critique. *Circ Res,* 1967, 20:249-262.
16. Perloff, D., Grim, C., Flack, A.L., et al. Human blood pressure determination by sphygmomanometry. *AHA medical/scientific statement.* Dallas: American Heart Association, 1993.

17. Frohlich, E.D., Grim, C., Labarthe, D.R., et al. *Recommendations for human blood pressure determination by sphygmomanometers* (vol. V). AHA publication no 70-1005 (SA). Dallas: American Heart Association, 1987, pp. i-34.
18. Henneman, E.A., & Henneman, P.L. Intricacies of blood pressure measurement: Reexamining the ritual. *Heart Lung,* 1989, 18:263-271.
19. Druding, M.C. Integrating hemodynamic monitoring and physical assessment. *Dimensions Crit Care Nurs,* 2000, 19:25-30.
20. Banner, T.E., & Gravenstine, J.S. Comparative tightness of fit on accuracy of blood pressure measurements. *J Clin Monit,* 1991, 7:281-284.
21. Gorny, D.A. Arterial blood pressure measurement technique. *AACN Clin Issues Crit Care Nurs,* 1993, 4:66-80.
22. Gardner, R.M., & Hujcs, M. *Fundamentals of physiologic monitoring.* AACN Clinical Issues in Critical Care Nursing. Philadelphia: Lippincott, 1993, 4:11-24.
23. Gardner, P.E., & Bridges, E.J. Hemodynamic monitoring. In S.L. Woods, E.S. Sivarajan-Froelicher, C. Halpenny, & S. Motzer (Eds.). *Cardiac nursing* (3rd ed.). Philadelphia: Lippincott. 1995, pp. 424-458.
24. Quaal, S.J. Quality assurance in hemodynamic monitoring. *AACN Clin Issues Crit Care Nurs,* 1993, 4:197-206.
25. Lumina Imperial-Perez, F., & McRae, M. *Arterial pressure monitoring.* Aliso Viejo, CA: AACN, 1998.
26. Bridges, E.J., Bond, E.F., Ahrens, T., et al. Ask the expert. *Crit Care Nurse,* 1997, 17:100-101.
27. Courtois, M., Fatal, P.G., Kovacs, S.J., et al. Anatomically and physiologically based reference level for measurement of intracardiac pressures. *Circulation,* 1995, 92:1994-2000.
28. Ahrens, T., Pennick, J., & Tucker, M. Frequency requirements for zeroing transducers in hemodynamic monitoring. *Am J Crit Care,* 1995, 4:466-471.
29. Kechelisen, M. Hemodynamic monitoring series: Pulmonary artery pressure monitoring. AACN Protocols for Practice. Stanford, CT: Appleton & Lange, 1997.
30. Quaal, S.J. Improving the accuracy of pulmonary artery catheter measurements. *J Cardiovasc Nurs,* 2001, 15:71-82.
31. Daily, E. Hemodynamic waveform analysis. *J Cardiovasc Nurs,* 2001, 15:6-22.
32. Rebenson-Piano, M.A., Holm, K., & Powers, M. An examination of the differences that occur between

direct and indirect blood pressure measurement. *Heart Lung*, 1987, *16*:385-389.

33. Dietz, B., & Smith, T.T. Enhancing the accuracy of hemodynamic monitoring. *J Nurs Care Qtly*, 2002, *17*:27-34.

34. Quaal, S.J. *Hemodynamic monitoring series: Intraaortic balloon pumping*. AACN Protocols for Practice. Aliso Viejo, CA: AACN, 2003.

35. Fegler, G. Measurement of cardiac output in anesthetized animals by thermodilution method. *J Exp Physiol*, 1954, *39*:153-164.

36. Gawlinski, A. Measuring cardiac output: Intermittent bolus thermodilution method. *Crit Car Nurse*, 2000, *20*:118-124.

37. Daily, E.K., & Schroeder, J.S. *Techniques in bedside hemodynamic monitoring* (4th ed.). St. Louis: Mosby-Yearbook, 1989, pp. 34-48.

38. Gawlinski, A. Facts and fallacies of cardiac output measurements. AACN's 1993 National Teaching Institute Proceedings, 1993, pp. 50-51.

39. Gillman, P. Bolus thermodilution cardiac output: Reliable parameter or best guess? AACN's 1993 National Teaching Institute Proceedings, 1993, pp. 52-53.

40. Morris, A.H., & Chapman, R.H. Wedge pressure confirmation by aspiration of pulmonary capillary blood. *Crit Care Med*, 1985, *13*:736-740.

41. Kleinman, B., Powell, S., & Gardner, R.M. Equivalence of fast flush and square wave testing of blood pressure monitoring systems. *J Clin Monit*, 1996, *12*:149-154.

42. Bridges, D.J. Monitoring pulmonary artery pressures: Just the facts. *Crit Care Nurse*, 2000, *20*:59-78.

43. Frazier, S.K., & Moser, D.K. Cardiac power output during transition from mechanical to spontaneous ventilation in canines. *J Cardiovasc Nurs*, 2001, *15*:23-32.

44. Quaal, S.J. *Hemodynamic monitoring series: Intraaortic balloon pumping*. AACN Protocols for Practice. Aliso Viejo, CA: AACN, 2003.

45. Tibby, S.M., & Murdoch, I.A. Monitoring cardiac function in intensive care. *Arch Dis Child*, 2003, *88*:46-52.

46. Bigatello, L.M., & George, E. Hemodynamic monitoring. *Minerva Anestesiol*, 2002, *68*:219-225.

47. Pickering, T.G. Principles and techniques of blood pressure measurement. *Cardiol Clin*, 2002, *20*:207-223.

48. Ott, K., Johnson, K., & Ahrens, T. New technologies in the assessment of hemodynamic parameters. *J Cardiovasc Nurs*, 2001, *15*:41-56.

49. Hamilton, T.T., Humber, L.M., & Jessen, M.E. Pulse CO: A less-invasive method to monitor cardiac output from arterial pressure after cardiac surgery. *Ann Thorac Surg*, 2002, *74*:1408-1412.

50. Cheney, J.C., & Dereak, S. Minimally invasive hemodynamic monitoring for the intensivist: current and emerging technology. *Crit Care Med*, 2002, *30*:2338-2345.

51. Campbell, D.I. Cardiac output determination using compliance. *Anesthesia*, 2002, *57*:1137-1140.

52. Linton, N.W.F., & Linton, R.A. Is comparison of changes in cardiac output, assessed by different methods, better than only comparing cardiac output to the reference method? *Br J Anaesth*, 2002, *88*:336-339.

53. Murias, G.E., Villagra, A., Vatua, S., et al. Evaluation of a noninvasive method for cardiac output measurement in critical care patients. *Intensive Care Med*, 2002, *28*:1470-1474.

54. Friedman, Z., Berkenstadt, H., Margalit, N., et al. Cardiac output assessed by arterial thermodilution during exsanguination and fluid resuscitation: Experimental validation against a reference technique. *Eur J Anaesthesiol*, 2002, *19*:337-340.

55. Kaplan, A. The potential to replace more invasive monitoring techniques. *Crit Care Med*, 2002, *30*:1933-1934.

56. Sega, E., Katzenelson, R., Berkenstadt, H., & Perel, A. Transpulmonary thermodilution cardiac output measurement using the axillary artery in critically ill patients. *J Clin Anesth*, 2002, *14*:210-213.

57. Kauffman, K.E. Newer trends in monitoring: The esophageal Doppler monitor. *AANA J*, 2000, *68*:421-428.

58. Boulnois, J.L., & Pechoux, T. Non-invasive cardiac output monitoring by aortic blood flow mastermind with the Dynamo 3000. *J Clin Monit Comput*, 2000, *15*:127-140.

59. Cariana, P., Relli, M.M., Braschi, A., et al. Noninvasive cardiac output assessment during heart surgery. *J Clin Monit*, 2002, *17*:147-149.

32

Measuring Physiologic Parameters in Obstetric Nursing

Jana Lauderdale

Physiologic measures are used throughout obstetric nursing to guide the management of care provided to childbearing women. As the author's professional expertise lies in the area of women's health, this chapter examines various assessment tools used in obstetric nursing, emphasizing the strengths, limitations, reliability, and validity of each tool. The chapter assists nurses interested in maternal-child research, as well as other health care providers. Selected instruments used for antepartum, labor and delivery, newborn nursery, and postpartum care are discussed in light of their use to both client management and nursing research.

Antepartal Tools

Diabetes, preeclampsia, systemic lupus erythematosus, chronic hypertension, sickle cell disease, and Rh isoimmunization are all conditions that can contribute to the development of uteroplacental insufficiency (UPI). Freeman[1] reports that at least two thirds of antepartum fetal deaths are due to UPI. Therefore, any woman who is at risk of developing UPI, previously had a stillborn child, or has noted a decrease in the amount or absence of fetal movement is considered a candidate for antepartum fetal assessment.

Since the 1980s a myriad of changes have taken place in obstetric care. The use of ultrasound and increased knowledge of maternal-fetal physiology have given physicians and nurses unprecedented access to the fetus for purposes of assessment. Fetal assessment is one component in the process of prenatal care and involves early identification of current or potential problems. Two tools commonly used in antepartum fetal assessment, the nonstress test and the biophysical profile, are discussed.

The Nonstress Test (NST)

The NST is one of the most widely applied tools for antepartum fetal assessment. The purpose of the test is to observe fetal heart rate (FHR) acceleration in response to fetal movement. Accelerations of the FHR imply an intact central and autonomic nervous system that is not being affected by a decrease of oxygen to the fetus (i.e., intrauterine hypoxia). The NST can be administered as early as 27 weeks of gestation and is especially useful in the presence of pregnancy-induced hypertension, diabetes, intrauterine growth retardation, multiple gestation, and spontaneous rupture of membranes. Its advantages are:

Noninvasive
Quick
Relatively inexpensive
Easy to perform
Easy to interpret
Can be performed in an outpatient setting
No known contraindications

Disadvantages of the NST

False-positive rate for nonreactive findings resulting from fetal sleep cycles, medications, and fetal immaturity
Precise tracings inconsistently obtained
Woman must lie relatively still for at least 20 minutes

The woman is placed in a semi-Fowler's position, with a pillow placed under the right hip to displace the uterus to the left and to avoid supine hypotension. An electronic fetal monitor is used to obtain a tracing of the FHR and fetal movement. The examiner applies belts to the woman's abdomen. One belt holds a device that detects uterine or fetal movement. The other belt holds a device that detects the FHR. Recordings are obtained for approximately 30 to 40 minutes. Each fetal movement is documented so that simultaneous FHR changes may be assessed.

The results of the NST are interpreted as follows:

Reactive test. Normal NST. A reactive NST shows at least two accelerations of FHR with fetal movements of 15 beats per minute, lasting 15 seconds or more, over 20 minutes.
Nonreactive test. Abnormal NST. The NST is considered nonreactive when fewer than two accelerations occur over 20 to 40 minutes. If accelerations do occur, the test is considered nonreactive if their amplitude is less than 15 beats per minute, or if they do not last 15 seconds.
Unsatisfactory test. Test yields uninterpretable data or inadequate fetal activity.

The reactive NST appears to indicate fetal well-being. A nonreactive NST indicates the need for further testing.[2] In many cases the NST results are compared with the results of a biophysical profile or a contraction stress test to evaluate all possible parameters.[3]

Chez and Chez's[4] study was one of the first comprehensive investigations to assess the reliability of obstetric nurses' interpretations of NSTs.[4] Out of the 1000 National Association of American College of Obstetrics and Gynecology (NAACOG) member nurses surveyed, 412 interpreted five NST strips. Participants were self-identified as nurses with a primary clinical focus of labor and delivery or antepartum. The study's three purposes were (1) to determine whether nurses could correctly interpret NST strips, (2) to determine whether demographic variables correlated with the accuracy of interpretation, and (3) to compare the responses of obstetric nurses to those of an obstetrician (the same strips had been interpreted by obstetricians in a previous study).

Eighty-four to 98% of the nurses agreed on the interpretation for each of the five strips. Nurses' responses differed significantly from physicians' interpretations of strips as reactive or nonreactive on only one strip, on which 92% of the nurses concurred compared to 98% of the obstetricians. Nurses' interpretations were not related to experience, education, formal courses in electronic fetal monitoring, or other demographic variables. The findings emphasize nurses' ability and expertise in interpreting NST strips as being equivalent to that of obstetricians.[4]

Internal validity of the Chez and Chez[4] study might be affected by the history and maturation of the participants, as the study involving physicians was already several years old at the time of the comparison study. The researchers found intraobserver (within-participant) reliability in the majority of study participants.

Limitations of the NST instrument that may affect the reliability of the test include the high percentage of false-positive results (from 50% to 80%), that is, a fetus with a nonreactive NST has a normal outcome.[5] What represents normal fetal activity is under discussion and may contribute to the high false-positive rate. One approach to counteracting this limitation would be to limit testing prior to 30 weeks' gestation. This effectively reduces fetal activity variation. Studies indicate that fetal nonreactivity may be more closely associated to gestational age rather than fetal compromise.[6,7] Another means to standardize test interpretation would be to hold regular periodic joint reviews of tracings by physicians and nurses.

The Biophysical Profile (BPP)

The BPP utilizes ultrasound to evaluate fetal status based on multiple criteria of fetal behavior. Manning and Harman[8] indicate that the most commonly used tool evaluates five variables according to established criteria. Table 32.1 describes each variable and the

Table 32.1 Biophysical Profile: Technique and Interpretation

Variable	Normal	Abnormal
Fetal breathing movements	≥ 1 episode of ≥ 30 sec. in 30 min.	Absent or no episode of ≥ 30 sec. in 30 min.
Gross body movements	≥ 3 discrete body or limb movements in 30 min. (episodes of active continuous movement considered as single movement)	≤ 2 episodes of body or limb movements in 30 min.
Fetal tone	≥ 1 episode of active extension with return to flexion of fetal limb(s) or trunk. Opening and closing of hand considered normal tone	Either slow extension with return to partial flexion or movement of limb in full extension or absent fetal movement
Reactive fetal heart rate (FHR)	≥ 2 episodes of FHR acceleration or of beats per min (bpm) lasting ≤ 15 sec., associated with fetal movement in 20 min.	≤ 2 episodes of acceleration of FHR or acceleration of ≥ 15 bpm in 20 min.
Qualitative amniotic fluid volume	≥ 1 pocket of fluid measuring ≥ 1 cm in two perpendicular planes	Either no pockets or a pocket ≤ 1 cm in two perpendicular planes

Manning, F.A. Fetal assessment based on fetal biophysical profile scoring: Experiences in 12,620 referred high-risk pregnancies. *Am J Obstet Gynecol*, 1985, *151*(3):343-350. Used with permission.

criteria used for evaluation. Clinical management decisions are based on a composite of all five scores rather than a single variable. The score assists physicians and nurses in determining whether a fetus is at risk at the time of testing. A score of 0 is considered abnormal, and a score of 2 is normal. A total score of 10/10 indicates a normal BPP and a functional, nonhypoxemic fetal central nervous system. A score of 8/10 indicates a fetus not at risk of death or damage within 1 week. As the BPP score decreases to 6/10, there is an increased risk of developing perinatal complications. A score of 4/10 or less signifies fetal asphyxia and indicates the need for an immediate delivery.[3]

Manning and Harman[8] believe that an evaluation of the total score for BPP requires not only interpretive knowledge of the score but also integration of this information with the clinical situation. The evaluation of less than all the pertinent data could lead to needless intervention or preventable harm.

To use this instrument in clinical antepartum assessment or in perinatal nursing research, one must be cognizant of influences that may affect outcome. Gebauer and Lowe[9] described these influences as endogenous or exogenous variables. Endogenous variables include fetal age, fetal behavioral states, maternal or fetal infection, hypoglycemia and hyperglycemia, and postmaturity.

Gestational age and the behavior of the fetus were reported as being interdependent.[9] Fetal behavioral states include body and eye movements and heart rate patterns in relation to four states that can change from quiescence to vigorous activity. Specific parameters have been identified for fetuses beyond 35 weeks. However, for fetuses under 35 weeks, state behaviors have been found to be unstable over time. Nijhuis[10] reported that preterm fetuses were not capable of true state transitions. This suggests that to interpret a BPP score on a fetus less than 35 weeks, one must take into account the behavioral state according to fetal age.

How the fetus reacts in the presence of an infection continues to be questioned. BPP abnormalities that have thus far been associated with infection include absence of fetal heart rate reactivity and fetal breathing.[9]

Maternal hypoglycemia or hyperglycemia have been reported to affect primarily fetal breathing movements, which in turn affect the BPP score results.[11] Hypoglycemia tends to decrease fetal breathing movements, whereas hyperglycemia has been shown to increase fetal breathing movements, which suggests the importance of testing during periods of maternal normoglycemia.[12]

Additional issues to consider include the maternal presence of either therapeutic or nontherapeutic drugs. Therapeutic drugs that depress the central nervous system also decrease both fetal breathing movements and fetal heart rate variability, thus lowering the BPP score.[13]

Ingestion of nontherapeutic drugs, such as cocaine and nicotine, also have been shown to have a suppressive effect on the BPP score. Effects vary from fetal hypoxemia to reduced fetal breathing activity.[2,8–14] The final issue to be raised by Gebauer and Lowe[9] concerns postdated pregnancy and its possible effect on the BPP score. Manning and Harman[8] support the use of the BPP to identify the compromised postdate fetus (a fetus beyond 40 weeks' gestation). However, as Gilson et al.[15] point out, although the BPP is sensitive in diagnosing a postdate fetus, the test is not sensitive enough to confirm which fetus will present with adverse perinatal effects.

All antepartum tests have some level of error in prediction. Most tests are accurate in predicting a healthy fetus, but less accurate at predicting the compromised fetus, indicating that several tests may be required to increase the validity of prediction.[16]

However, according to Vintzileos et al.,[12] the BPP has been shown to be the most accurate test for identifying a compromised fetus.

Labor and Delivery Tools

Perinatal nurses must keep constant pace with the ever-changing philosophies and new technologies of childbirth. Research in the area of labor and delivery have varied in focus. However, one proven area of research focuses on the pain of childbirth. What causes it? How can it be controlled? These are questions that have been and are still being investigated.

According to the gate-control theory, pain occurs as a result of a mechanism in the dorsal horn of the spinal column that serves as a gate. This gate increases or reduces the flow of nerve impulses from the periphery to the central nervous system. Gates may be opened or closed by central nervous system activities, such as anxiety and excitement, or through selective localized activity.[17] The gate-control theory has implications for childbirth. Tactile stimulation can control pain. Activities to accomplish this include sacral pressure, backrub, conditioning, and distraction.

In childbirth, there is a physiologic basis for the discomfort. In the first stage of labor, pain arises from dilation or stretching of the cervix. During the second stage of labor, pain results from hypoxia of the contracting uterine muscle cells and distention of the vagina and perineum. Pain during the third stage results from uterine contraction and cervical dilation as the placenta is expelled.[17]

Several factors can affect a woman's perception of childbirth pain. These include cultural background, presence of a support person, fatigue and sleep deprivation, previous experience with pain, anxiety, whether she has had childbirth education, maternal position during labor, and the environment of the childbirth setting.

Women's accounts of childbirth pain are difficult to assess. The methods reported often result in conflicting information. Study results must be reviewed in light of the source of the data, that is, were the data based on the woman's perception or based on physiologic indicators of pain? One tool that has been applied to the area of assessing maternal comfort during childbirth is the Maternal Comfort Assessment Tool.

Maternal Comfort Assessment Tool

The Maternal Comfort Assessment Tool estimates the level of maternal comfort during maximum slope of labor (cervical dilation from 4 to 9 cm) while assuming one of two positions, upright or recumbent.[18] The tool measures the laboring woman's focus of attention, including eye contact, breathing pattern and vocal behavior, muscle tension and activity, and verbalizations during contractions. Vital signs, cervical changes, duration, frequency, and intensity of contractions, medications, and use of monitoring equipment also are recorded. Scores for each observable behavior are totaled, with the highest possible comfort score for each contraction being 14, the lowest 0. Comfort scores for a series of three contractions are recorded hourly.

Prestudy interrater reliability for the Maternal Comfort Assessment Tool was found to have an agreement percentage of 89%. In addition, interrater reliability was calculated by taking a series of three contractions from each of five randomly selected clients. The agreement percentage was found to be 91%.[18]

Other factors that may affect the reliability and validity of this tool include how psychologic factors such as maternal feelings of independence and control influence the tool scores. Another issue of concern is that this tool has been tested only on low-risk clients. High-risk clients may bring a different perspective to the tool's application.[18]

Electronic Fetal Monitoring (EFM)

EFM is an auditory and visual assessment tool that provides continuous data for uterine activity and fetal heart response evaluation. Data include baseline heart rate, beat-to-beat variability, and fetal heart rate changes over time. EFM not only gathers clinical management data, but because of its self-documenting properties, it also can be used to obtain research data in combination with direct hands-on assessment, verbal client information, and the client's vital sign assessment. All clients in labor need some form of fetal monitoring to detect potential problems. The choice of form this takes is based on multiple factors. The need for EFM has been a source of debate for years. When first introduced in the 1960s, EFM's intended use was to detect the compromised fetus during labor and delivery. As Ellison et al.[19] report, EFM is fairly reliable in recognizing the dying fetus, but less reliable in identifying fetuses with hypoxia-ischemia involving the central nervous system. In a study comparing the effectiveness of EFM with periodic auscultation, it was reported that more accurate predictions about 5-minute Apgar scores (newborn assessment at birth) were made with EFM than with auscultation. This suggested that better data regarding neonatal well-being could be provided by EFM.[20] Larson goes on to suggest that one of the primary contributions of EFM may be its "ability to enable clinicians to make better predictions and judgments" regarding neonatal well-being.[20] Other researchers concur with this belief, finding that EFM has significantly improved the outcome of labor and delivery by calling increased attention to the importance of FHR and to the labor process.[19]

EFM uses a tocodynamometer to record uterine contractions and a Doppler ultrasound device to monitor the FHR. Although uterine pressure measurements accurately reflect the frequency of contractions, one disadvantage to its use is that EFM does not correlate with baseline or maximum intrauterine pressure during contractions. A second disadvantage is that FHR variability obtained with external monitoring does not correlate well with the true variability obtained by the internal scalp electrode.

In internal FHR monitoring, the fetal electrocardiogram (ECG) is recorded on the electronic fetal monitor. This is accomplished through the use of a fetal scalp electrode. This method provides an accurate representation of the baseline FHR variability. A fluid-filled catheter or a pressure transducer can be used in conjunction with the EFM. This catheter, or transducer, provides a quantitative measure of intrauterine pressure during a contraction.

Specific conditions that can alter or effect the reliability and validity of information obtained with electronic fetal monitoring equipment comes from a variety of sources. The labor room environment itself can affect monitor operation. Environmental specifications for proper operation include an operating temperature of 0°C to +55°C; a storage temperature of –40°C to +75°C, and a relative humidity of 5% to 95%.[21] Table 32.2 describes areas that must be considered when data from the EFM do not agree with coexisting physiologic measures.

Newborn Assessment Tools

Immediately following birth, numerous physiologic adaptations take place in the newborn. Care focuses on assessing and stabilizing the newborn. Assessment involves the collection of data from several parameters. Assessment as an ongoing process enables caregivers to compare initial findings with data obtained at a later time. Two assessment tools, the Apgar scoring tool and the Dubowitz tool, are discussed in the following sections.

Table 32.2   Troubleshooting Inconsistent Electronic Fetal Monitoring Data

Dilemma	Possible Cause	Resolution
Poor pen tracing	Active fetus, maternal movement, loose belt, insufficient gel, maternal obesity	Readjust belt, reposition transducer, relax client, apply gel
FHR higher than normal range	Recording maternal heart rate, fetal arrhythmia, or fetal death	Compare maternal pulse to signal, listen to FHR with fetoscope
Tracing burned into paper	Stylet heat too high, jammed paper	Turn stylet knob counterclockwise to lower heat, check paper feed
Tocotransducer		
No contraction	Machine recording, negative pressures	Adjust uterine waveform, activity baseline
Waveform hard to differentiate	Check placement of toco	Place toco over fundus, or where uterine movement is strongest
Inverted waveform	Maternal activity may alter toco position during contractions	Reposition toco
ECG-spiral electrode		
Occasional vertical lines on tracing	Faulty cable, or spiral electrode, or no ECG signal	Check leg plate and wires, apply new electrode
Equipment malfunction	Connection of leads to leg plates incorrect, connect interference, i.e., excess fetal hair can sometimes cause poor tracing	Reconnect leads or apply new electrode
Intrauterine catheter		
Straight line on tracing	Check cable plug, pressure transducer defective	Plug in cable, replace transducer
No contraction waveform or pressure changes during contraction	Plugged catheter, uterine perforation	Flush catheter, test monitor, check uterine activity during valsalva
Tracing indicates peak of waveform	Monitor not calibrated	Calibrate monitor to zero only transducer
Waveform artifacts	Tip of catheter in uterine wall or dry area	Pull catheter out 2 to 3 cm, flush clear with normal saline

Adapted from Hewlett-Packard Medical Products Booklet. Palo Alto, CA: Hewlett-Packard, 1990.

Apgar Scoring Tool

Virginia Apgar, an anesthesiologist, introduced the Apgar scoring tool in 1953.[22] The purpose of the Apgar score is to evaluate the physical condition of the newborn at birth and any potential resuscitation requirement. The score is based on five indicators of neonatal adjustment to extrauterine life: heart rate, respiratory effort, reflex irritability, muscle tone, and color. The newborn is rated 1 minute after birth and again at 5 minutes, and receives a total score ranging from 0 to 10 assessed in the following manner:

1. Heart rate is auscultated or palpated.
2. Respiratory rate is assessed by counting the number of respirations for 1 full minute.
3. Muscle tone is determined by evaluating the degree of flexion and resistance to straightening of the extremities and the rapidity with which they return to a state of flexion.
4. Reflex irritability is evaluated by rubbing the back or flicking the soles of the feet.
5. Color of the neonate's skin is evaluated for cyanosis and pallor.

Even though it has been widely accepted since the 1950s, its value has been repeatedly questioned.[23] Apgar[24] herself reminded us that the tool should in no way substitute for a careful examination or repeated observations over the first few hours of life.

Livingston[25] examined the interrater reliability of the Apgar score in both term and preterm infants. Fifty-two infants were included in the study; 11 were premature, and 41 were term. Apgar scores were assigned to each infant and then compared to scores recorded in the mother's chart.

Percentage agreement at 1 and 5 minutes for each of the five indicators was calculated. In the preterm infant group, the agreement of 1-minute scores ranged from a high of 82% for tone and respiratory rate to a low of 55% for heart rate. At 5 minutes, the agreement was highest for heart rate (100%) and lowest for reflex irritability (36%). The mean percent agreement of the five indicators was 69% at both 1 minute and 5 minutes. The poor interrater reliability estimates could result from recall errors in recording. The Apgar scores were recorded after resuscitative efforts and were based on the recorder's memory of the infant's condition at 1 and 5 minutes.

Percentage agreement for the term infants was lowest for reflex irritability (81%) and highest for heart rate (98%). At 5 minutes, percentage agreement for heart rate, tone, and reflex irritability was 98%; for color and respiratory rate, percentage agreement was 95%. The mean percentage agreement was 89% at 1 minute and 97% at 5 minutes.

Even though the findings of this study suggest that use of the Apgar in premature infants is questionable, the score still provides valuable data on the neonate during the first few minutes of life. Reliability may be improved by periodic review and interrater checks, the use of a timing device, and education in how to use the Apgar.[25,26]

Finally, observer bias on the part of the person delivering the infant can be an issue. As Apgar scores have become equated with the quality of health care, it is recommended that the one delivering the infant not be the one to assign the Apgar score.[27]

The Dubowitz Assessment Tool

The Dubowitz assessment tool was developed by Lilly Dubowitz and coworkers in the 1960s and continues to be a reliable tool for determining the appropriate gestational age of the neonate regardless of birth weight. The tool is used to assess intrauterine growth alterations and preterm neonates by measuring physical characteristics and neuromuscular tone indices on admission to the newborn nursery.

The tool contains 21 criteria (10 neurologic and 11 external physical criteria). Each category is scored, and the scores summed to a total score. Total scores range between 0 to 69, indicating gestational ages between 26 and 46 weeks.

The original study by Dubowitz and associates[28] was carried out on 167 infants in a large metropolitan hospital. Only if an infant had an absent Moro reflex or was too ill was she or he excluded. All infant assessments were made by one investigator and within 5 days of delivery. The majority of assessments were made in the first 24 hours. The external score correlated with gestation 91% of the time. Neurologic scores correlated with gestation 89% of the time. A combined total correlation of 95% produced a stronger result than either alone.

The reliability of this tool can be increased by using it with neonates between the gestational ages of 28 and 42 weeks. Before assessing, Olds et al.[29] suggests the need to document preexisting maternal conditions that can affect the neonate assessment results. Conditions such as diabetes, which appears to accelerate fetal physical growth, may retard maturation. Pregnancy-induced hypertension, which retards fetal physical growth, also may speed maturation. Other characteristics that may affect the neuromuscular outcome scores include the active muscle tone and edema seen in neonates of women with pregnancy-induced hypertension, respiratory depression resulting from certain maternal analgesia and anesthesia, and the flaccid and edematous neonate that often results from respiratory distress syndrome.[29]

Postpartum Assessment Tool

The postpartum period (puerperium) is the 6 weeks between the birth of the newborn and the return of the reproductive organs to the nonpregnant state. Unfortunately, today the time spent with clients following delivery is brief, ranging from a few hours for a normal birth to 4 days for a cesarean birth. Even though the time may be short, the information shared between nurse and client can be substantial in terms of client education and research possibilities.

REEDA Tool

One tool used for postpartum assessment of episiotomy healing was developed by Davidson.[30] This tool appraises the perineum or incision for signs of *r*edness, *e*dema, *e*cchymosis, *d*ischarge, and *a*pproximation—thus, the tool came to be known as the REEDA scale. Each category is assessed and a number assigned, for a total score range from 0 to 15. The higher the score, presumably, the more tissue trauma.

Hill's[31] investigation of the psychometric properties of the REEDA evaluated interrater reliability and construct validity of the tool. A total of 94 women participated. Eighty-six women received an episiotomy, and the remaining eight delivered with an intact perineum. Perineal assessments were conducted on 56% of the women during the first 24 hours after delivery, with the remaining assessments completed during the second 24 hours. During the rater training period it was discovered that the trainers had difficulty assessing redness and ecchymosis. This continued during data collection. After 39 participants were assessed, it was decided to add a sixth category, called discoloration, so that a differentiation between redness and ecchymosis was not needed.

To determine interrater reliability between raters and for the addition of the category of discoloration, the kappa statistic was used. Correlations for the total REEDA score between raters were only moderate. Correlations using discoloration were higher than those for redness and ecchymosis, indicating higher rater agreement by using the descriptor discoloration. To evaluate construct validity of the REEDA, the known-groups technique was used. Results indicated support for the construct validity for this tool.

Hill[31] believes that with moderate interrater reliability and the problem of "redness and ecchymosis assessment," the REEDA tool may be less than reliable for research purposes. Other issues affecting reliability and validity include measurement discrepancies (i.e., the scale measures edema in terms of width, not considering length or depth), inconsistent correlations between the descriptors *edema* and *pain,* and the fact that only three properties of wound healing were reported to be useful in this study. Construct validity questions have been raised regarding use of the REEDA in the immediate postpartum period. The use of the descriptor *approximation* as an index of better healing and decreased pain is questioned.[31] Further investigation is needed to determine the strengths and limitations of the use of the REEDA scale in clinical practice or research.

Summary

The chapter has examined and discussed the application of various tools used throughout the perinatal nursing area, emphasizing the strengths and limitations of each. It is hoped that the review has familiarized the reader with some of the tools available not only for clinical use but also for research. It also was our intent to stimulate critical thinking regarding the reliability and validity issues that need consideration and further investigation before a tool is appropriate for research purposes.

Exemplar Study

Andrews, C., & Chrzanowski, M. Maternal position, labor and comfort. *Appl Nurs Res,* 1990, 3(1):1–7.

Based on the knowledge we have regarding the potentially negative effects to both mother and fetus of laboring in the recumbent position, Andrews and Chrzanowski developed a study to ascertain whether women laboring in an upright position reported less discomfort and had a shorter-phase maximum slope as indicated by their labor pattern. These women were compared to women laboring in the recumbent position. The study utilized the Maternal Comfort Assessment Scale.

The study findings were that women who labor in the upright position had a significantly shorter labor ($t(38) = 3.2, p = 0.003$). The length of the phase of maximum slope correlated positively with age and race. Young black women indicated having shorter phases. Comfort scores were found to vary only slightly between the two groups ($t(38) = 1.42, p = 0.163$).

References

1. Freeman, R.K. The contraction stress test. In R. Eden & F. Boehm (Eds.), *Assessment and care of the fetus.* Norwalk, CT: Appleton & Lange, 1990.
2. Manning, F.A. Fetal assessment based on fetal biophysical profile scoring: Experiences in 12,620 referred high-risk pregnancies. *Am J Obstet Gynecol,* 1985, 151(31):343-350.
3. Gegor, C., & Paine, L. Antepartum fetal assessment techniques: An update for today's perinatal nurse. *J Perinat Neonat Nurs,* 1992, 5(4):1-15.
4. Chez, B.F., & Chez, R. Interpretations of nonstress tests by obstetric nurses. *J Gynecol Neonat Nurs,* 1990, 19(3):227-232.
5. Kisilevsky, B.S. Human fetal responses to sound as a function of stimulus intensity. *Obstet Gynecol,* 1989, 73:971-976.
6. Bishop, E. Fetal acceleration test. *Am J Obstet Gynecol,* 1981, 141:905-909.
7. Keegan, K. The nonstress test. *Clin Obstet Gynecol,* 1987, 30:921-935.
8. Manning, F.A., & Harman, C.R. The fetal biophysical profile. In R.D. Eden & F.H. Boehm (Eds.), *Assessment and care of the fetus.* Norwalk, CT: Appleton & Lange, 1990.
9. Gebauer, C., & Lowe, N. The biophysical profile: Antepartal assessment of fetal well-being. *J Gynecol Neonat Nurs,* 1993, 22(2):115-125.
10. Nijhuis, J.G. Behavioral states: Concomitants, clinical implications and the assessment of the condition of the newborn's system. *Eur J Obstet Gynecol Reproduct Biol,* 1986, 21:301-308.
11. Gabbe, S.G. Antepartum fetal evaluation. In S. Gabbe, J. Niebyl, & J. Simpson (Eds.), *Obstetrics: Normal and problem pregnancies.* New York: Churchill Livingstone, 1991, pp. 377-424.
12. Vintzileos, A.M., Campbell, W.A., Nochimson, D.J., & Weinbaum, P.J. The use and misuse of the fetal biophysical profile. *Am J Obstet Gynecol,* 1987, 157:527-533.
13. Carlan, S., & O'Brien, W.F. The effect of magnesium sulfate on the biophysical profile of normal term fetuses. *Obstet Gynecol,* 1991, 7:681-684.
14. McLeod, W., Brien, J., Loomis, C., et al. Effects of maternal ethanol ingestion on fetal breathing movements, gross body movements and heart rate at 37 to 40 weeks gestational age. *Am J Obstet Gynecol,* 1983, 145:251-257.
15. Gilson, G.J., O'Brien, M.E., Vera, R.W., et al. Prolonged pregnancy and the biophysical profile: A birthing center perspective. *J Nurs Midwifery,* 1988, 33:171-177.
16. Schifrin, B.S., & Clement, D. Why fetal monitoring remains a good idea. *Contemp Obstet Gynecol,* 1990, 35(2):70-86.
17. Bobak, I., & Jensen, M. *Maternity and gynecologic care. The nurse and the family* (5th ed.). St. Louis, MO: Mosby Year Book, 1993.
18. Andrews, C.M., & Chrzanowski, M. Maternal position, labor and comfort. *Appl Nurs Res,* 1990, 3(1):1-7.
19. Ellison, P., Foster, M., Sheridan-Pereira, M., & MacDonald, D. Electronic fetal heart monitoring, auscultation, and neonatal outcome. *J Obstet Gynecol,* 1991, 164(5):1281-1289.
20. Larson, E.B. Fetal monitoring and predictions by clinicians: Observations during a randomized clinical trial in very low birth weight infants. *Obstet Gynecol,* 1989, 74:584-589.
21. Hewlett-Packard Medical Products Booklet. Palo Alto, CA: Hewlett-Packard, 1990.
22. Apgar, V. A proposal for a new method of evaluation of the newborn infant. *Curr Res Anesthes Analges,* 1953, 32:260-267.
23. Sykes, G.S., Molloy, P.M., Johnson, P., et al. Do Apgar scores indicate asphyxia? *Lancet,* 1982, 1:494-496.
24. Apgar, V., & James, L. Further observations of the newborn scoring system. *Am J Dis Child,* 1962, 104:419-428.
25. Livingston, J. Interrater reliability of the Apgar scores in term and preterm infants. *Appl Nurs Res,* 1990, 3(4):164-165.
26. Auld, P., Rudolph, A., Avery, M., et al. Responsiveness and resuscitation of the newborn. The use of the Apgar score. *Am J Dis Child,* 1961, 101:69-80.

27. Apgar, V. The newborn (Apgar) scoring system. Reflections and advice. *Pediatr Clin North Am*, 1966, *13*:645-650.
28. Dubowitz, L., Dubowitz, B., & Goldberg, C. Clinical assessment of gestational age in the newborn infant. *J Pediatr*, 1970, *77*(1):1-10.
29. Olds, S., London, M., & Ladewig, P. *Maternal newborn nursing. A family centered approach* (4th ed.). Reading, MA: Addison-Wesley, 1992.
30. Davidson, N. Evaluating postpartum healing. *J Nurs Midwifery*, 1974, *19*:7-10.
31. Hill, P. Psychometric properties of the REEDA. *J Gynecol Neonat Nurs*, 1990, *35*(3):162-165.

33

Measuring Dyspnea

Mary L. Scott

Dyspnea, or shortness of breath, is a common symptom or sensation of pathologic cardiopulmonary conditions requiring clinical assessment and intervention. It may be present during exercise or at rest in acute and chronic diseases. Recently, the American Thoracic Society developed a consensus statement that assists in a more accurate definition of dyspnea.[1] This definition refers to improvements made in the understanding of dyspnea and the interactions noted between physiologic and behavioral components that can produce respiratory discomfort. The definition also includes the unique descriptions given by patients that describe their own understanding of the sensations related to breathlessness. The statement further suggests that "breathing discomfort" is subjective in nature, the intensity of the sensations are variable, and physiologic, psychologic, social, and environmental factors may begin a cascade of "secondary physiologic and behavioral responses."[1, p322]

Dyspnea occurs most frequently in people with primary pulmonary disease (asthma and chronic obstructive pulmonary disease [COPD]), coronary artery disease, and neuromuscular disorders affecting the respiratory muscles. This complex symptom can occur in conditions resulting in increased ventilation, alteration in the physical properties of the lung, or increased respiratory work. It may be present with pregnancy, obesity, or psychologic conditions characterized by anxiety.[2] It also has been described in persons with cancer, post-bypass surgery, congestive heart failure, cocaine addiction, rheumatoid arthritis, hyperthyroidism, and other medical-surgical conditions.[3] Carrieri-Kohlman et al.[4] enhance this description by describing dyspnea as a "multifaceted process influenced by personal, situational, health status and environmental factors."[4,p226] Furthermore, the perception of the symptom also is influenced by age, gender, personality, perceived self-efficacy, concurrent illness disease severity, and length of time the symptom has been experienced.[4] Emotions, moods, and social support can also influence dyspnea perception and the coping mechanisms of the individual who is dealing with the symptom.

Dyspnea is a complex symptom indicating an awareness of an excessive effort to breathe based on the level of physical exertion experienced. Pathophysiologic bases may differ with the nature of the cardiopulmonary disease state. Behavior and emotion can influence expression of the sensation. It is currently thought that the major mechanisms creating the dyspneic experience involve "corollary discharges of respiratory motor activity and feedback from chemoreceptors and mechanoreceptors in the lung and chest wall.[1, p325] In addition, the neural pathways are not clearly understood, and no single mechanism can account for all clinical situations in which dyspnea occurs.

Conceptual Considerations

Dyspnea has been defined as difficult, labored, and uncomfortable breathing.[5,6] The sensation is subjective and involves personal perception and reaction to the sensation. In sum, dyspnea is complex, sensory, perceived, and interpreted by the individual experiencing it,[7] indicating that it should be rated by the person experiencing it. One's degree of physical compensation may or may not reflect subjective interpretation, and any objective measurement may or may not correlate with subjective feelings. At one end of the continuum are individuals who describe severe dyspnea and demonstrate minor pathophysiologic alterations. At the other are individuals describing minimal dyspnea but demonstrating marked change in pulmonary function. This finding has been supported by investigators who have observed and attempted to quantify dyspnea in a variety of disease states.[5-9] These investigators agree that pulmonary function disturbances differ by disease and that no one measurement of lung function can define respiratory capacity. Therefore, the observation of increased respiratory rate (tachypnea) or increased depth of respiration (hyperpnea) should not be confused with dyspnea.[3] Patients with primary pulmonary disease experience abnormal breathing mechanics.[10] Diseases such as pulmonary fibrosis, asthma, and emphysema illustrate the relationship between inspiratory effort and dyspnea. In pulmonary fibrosis, the lungs and thorax are stiffer than normal, and inspiratory muscles must increase their tension to produce the same tidal volume. When the thoracic volume is abnormally large, as in emphysema and chronic asthma, it is necessary for the patient to breathe near-maximum inspiratory levels and use accessory inspiratory muscles to overcome a high resistance to airflow at normal lung volumes. In acute asthma, dyspnea is correlated with sternocleidomastoid muscle retraction. In emphysema, a large lung volume is created by the loss of elastic tissue recoil at rest. Dyspnea in these patients is related to a decreased capacity to respond to the ventilatory stimulus.

Improvement in treatment now includes pharmacologic and nonpharmacologic approaches to both acute and chronic dyspnea. These new approaches assist in treating dyspnea in various disease states by reducing ventilatory demand, decreasing central drive, reducing ventilatory impedance, reducing resistive load and altering central perception.[1] Pharmacologic interventions may involve the use of bronchodilators, methylxanthines, anxiolytic drugs, glucocorticosteriods, and opioids.[11] Some nonpharmacologic approaches involve the controversial use of supplemental oxygen and complementary and alternative measures (acupuncture, acupressure, and other behavioral approaches).[12] Nutritional changes, specific exercise training, and patient education can assist in the overall approach and management of dyspnea.[1,12,13]

In cancer patients, dyspnea may be the result of disease or treatment.[11] It may be present before a malignancy is diagnosed, or it may develop at any point during the illness. Patients with primary lung or mediastinal tumors and those with neck or central nervous system tumors involving the respiratory centers are at high risk for developing altered ventilatory patterns. Individuals with cancer who have received radiation to the chest or neck or who have received antineoplastic agents that can cause pulmonary toxicity may develop dyspnea. Complications, such as pleural effusion, ascites, pneumonia, or pulmonary emboli, also may produce dyspnea. Patients with concurrent histories of pulmonary disease, cigarette smoke exposures, congestive heart failure, environmental/ occupational exposures, or anemia may exhibit dyspnea, as well as those who have had surgery of the head, neck, chest, or lung. In a recent prospective study of ambulatory terminally ill cancer patients, Bruera and colleagues assessed the frequency of moderate to severe dyspnea and its correlates.[15] Vital capacity, peak flow, maximal inspiratory pressure, and oxygen saturation were measured in 135 patients. Patients also used visual analogue scales to rate dyspnea, anxiety, and fatigue/tiredness. The extent of lung involvement by either primary or metastatic tumor was determined from the medical record, and associated with the intensity and presence of dyspnea. The results of this study indicated that the intensity of dyspnea and anxiety were higher in patients who experience moderate dyspnea. Additional findings from this study indicate that respiratory muscle weakness is an independent correlate of dyspnea intensity. It can be suggested that trials using medications that increase inspiratory muscle strength may be beneficial to this patient population. The authors also found that a univariate correlation between fatigue/tiredness and anxiety may suggest that the interaction between fatigue/ tiredness and dyspnea can be explained by the interaction between anxiety and fatigue/ tiredness.

A study of perceived dyspnea in 30 lung cancer patients highlights the need for careful and thoughtful assessment of this sensation.[14] This study described patterns of dyspnea, identified coping and adaptive strategies used by lung cancer patients, and determined the relationship between activity and dyspnea. A convenience sample was interviewed twice over a 2-month interval. At time 1, the American Thoracic Society Questionnaire (including the Grade of Breathlessness Scale [GBS]), the Dyspnea Interview Schedule, the Dyspnea Visual Analog Scale (DVAS), and the Karnofsky Performance Scale (KPS) were completed.[17] At time 2, the GBS, KPS, and DVAS were administered. Interviews using the American Thoracic Society Questionnaire and Dyspnea Interview Schedule provided themes, patterns, and precipitants. Patients reported significant dyspnea and fatigue and experienced losses in concentration, memory, and appetite during periods of shortness of breath.

This study demonstrated that dyspnea is a significant problem for patients with lung cancer. It also pointed to the need to evaluate dyspnea carefully with multiple instruments. The DVAS, GBS, and KPS are easy to administer, reliably measure the subjective symptoms of dyspnea, and facilitate appropriate planning for intervention.

Roberts et al.[18] report that only pain and eating problems are identified more frequently than dyspnea in late-stage cancer patients. Using self-report surveys, chart audits, and interviews with patients and the nurses caring for them, Roberts and colleagues studied the meaning of dyspnea in late-stage cancer. They concluded that, although patients appeared to be coping, they were isolated, inconsistently managed, and inadequately supported. Furthermore, they concluded that dyspnea was overlooked among late-stage cancer patients, that patients did not report their symptoms of dyspnea, and that nurses caring for these patients did not have a clear understanding of the symptom or its management. The researchers reported that medical intervention was inconsistent and that narcotic use, described as beneficial in terminal dyspnea, was not utilized. Reducing physical activity was reported as the primary dyspnea control strategy.

In a descriptive study, Heinzer, Bish, and Detwiler promote the idea that a holistic approach is needed for patients with COPD, and that the management of dyspnea should include both physiologic and psychologic interventions. Using four open-ended research questions and the Modified Borg Scale (MBS), the authors described the perceptions of dyspnea in hospitalized COPD patients who had experienced acute dyspneic episodes during their inpatient admissions. Fear, anxiety, panic, and helplessness were identified as common feelings, with the presence of the nurse being very calming during these episodes. The nurse's recognition of the legitimacy of the episode was also noted to be helpful. It was the opinion of the authors that the use of the MBS was valuable as a clinical assessment instrument in the acute care environment.[19]

Physical and Psychosocial Variables Correlated with Dyspnea Perception

The patient's description of the dyspnea sensation varies with diagnosis and extent of disease. Persons with obstructive disease (e.g., emphysema, chronic bronchitis) recognize that they have great difficulty moving air in and out of their lungs. Individuals with restrictive disease (e.g., pulmonary fibrosis or infiltrative disease) complain of "hard breathing"[20] with little exertion and appear to experience sensations that would be normal for a higher level of exercise. However, some of the above individuals and others with pulmonary vascular disease, heart disease, or respiratory muscle weakness may describe a feeling or sense of suffocation, which is different from the shortness of breath sensation previously described.

Efforts have been made to correlate physiologic parameters with breathing difficulty. Blood gas levels and static lung volumes do not appear to correlate with the development of dyspnea.[21–23] Blood gases, however, are affected by the level of ventilation. Although respiratory work and the oxygen cost of breathing are elevated in pulmonary disease, investigators have discovered that they do not correlate with reported dyspnea or cause perceived dyspnea.[24–26]

Pulmonary function studies have been used to try to correlate pulmonary dysfunction and severity of dyspnea with specific lung diseases. Restrictive disease decreases vital capacity and limits perfusion. Forced vital capacity and diffusing capacity have been shown to correlate moderately with the severity of dyspnea experience in restrictive diseases. In obstructive diseases, the maximal voluntary ventilation (MVV)—the largest liter volume that can be breathed per minute voluntarily—has the highest reported correlation with dyspnea.

The Dyspnea Index is a percentage of the MVV and expresses the minute ventilation at a specific level of exercise.[24] For a normal person walking 2 miles per hour on level ground, this measurement is ±12%.[24] Studies have shown that if the dyspnea index is less than 30%, shortness of breath usually does not occur. Subjects with an index greater than 50% are likely to be short of breath at abnormally low exercise levels. However, Fishman and Leslie[25] and Gottfried et al.[26] found that patients with obstructive lung disease may not complain of dyspnea even with a dyspnea index of 50% or greater.[23]

Because testing for MVV is difficult to reproduce, the 1-second forced expiratory volume (FEV_1) is the most convenient and useful measure of evaluating prolonged expiration and degree of airway obstruction. The FEV_1 is correlated slightly lower with dyspnea than the MVV and depends on individual effort and cooperation.

Researchers are now beginning to study how physical activity correlates with patients diagnosed with COPD who experience the dyspnea symptom complex.[13,27] Building on Leidy's earlier efforts to define functional performance in patients with COPD,[28] Belza et al. were able to demonstrate functional status and walking abilities in 63 COPD patients.[27] Multiple physiologic and psychosocial testing instruments were used to measure functional performance, functional capacity, the symptom experiences of dyspnea and fatigue, health-related quality of life, and health status.

To determine the threshold at which dyspnea is perceived, measurements of resistive and elastic loads have been added to breathing tests to aid clinicians in understanding how some patients can experience airflow obstruction without breathlessness. Studies have shown that for patients with chronically high airway resistance, increased changes in resistance are needed to experience dyspnea. Asthmatics probably experience high thresholds for and decreased perception of dyspnea because of more frequent episodes of bronchospasm and greater responsiveness to histamine.[8]

Emotional states can profoundly affect levels of dyspnea in those with airway constriction secondary to pulmonary disease.[20,29-32] Fatigue, depression, anxiety, helplessness, loss of vitality, preoccupation, nervousness, and fear have been reported to accompany dyspnea.[14,29-32] The presence of panic, worry, and anger can confound measurement of dyspnea as a solitary symptom. Gift and Cahill[29] examined the psychologic and physiologic factors associated with acute dyspnea in patients with COPD. They concluded in an in-depth pilot study that clinical symptoms and physiologic responses change during dyspnea. Clinical symptoms included the number of respirations per minute, the depth of respirations, the presence or absence of sighing and paradoxical breathing, and the use of accessory muscles. The Vertical Visual Analogue Scale (VVAS) was used to measure dyspnea. The Spielberger State Anxiety Inventory (SAI) and Brief Symptom Inventory (BSI) also were administered. Physiologic measures included arterial blood gas and serum cortisol levels. Medication use also was recorded. This study demonstrated the coexistence of a psychophysiologic component with dyspnea. Gift and Cahill emphasized that the patient's emotional status needs to be given special attention, particularly anxiety and depression. Correlations between breathlessness and various psychosocial phenomena have been studied in adult asthmatics. Gift and Cahill[29] have demonstrated that the dyspnea experienced by patients with asthma is generally acute and that asthma-related dyspneic events are not generalizable to patients whose dyspnea is chronic and present during rest or minimal exercise.

Carrieri et al.[30] studied dyspnea in 39 children with documented asthma and episodes of wheezing. Most of the children used inhalers with bronchodilator medications, and six received periodic oral steroids. These researchers developed an interview guide for specific use in this study. It contained open-ended questions, forced-choice response formats, and three measures of dyspnea intensity. The guide explored participants' physical sensations, emotional sensations, breathing on both good and usual days, intensity of dyspnea, and coping strategies. Measures of dyspnea intensity included a word descriptor scale, a visual analogue scale, and a color shade scale. These scales had been previously used to evaluate pain in children. The visual analogue was adapted by using happy and sad circular faces and easy-to-understand anchors at each end of the 100-mm line. The shaded color scale was presented to the children following a question about what color the child's breathing was when it was bad. A 4-point color shade ranged from light to dark. Carrieri et al.[30] demonstrated that children with asthma were able to rate the intensity of their dyspnea and describe the asthma sensation qualitatively.

Experiments to Produce the Sensation of Dyspnea

Efforts to study the sensation of dyspnea and to understand ventilatory regulation have focused on producing unpleasant respiratory sensations resembling breathlessness. Early investigations employed breathholding and examined perceptions of additional respiratory loads.[21] Transcutaneous vagal nerve and chest wall blocks also have been performed to try to produce the sensation of dyspnea and evaluate its effect.[25] Studies with asthmatics to determine the relationship between the psychology and physiology of dyspnea have added to a basic understanding of the neural, chemical, and muscular functions of dyspnea, but their relationship to dyspnea continues to be vague.[8]

Treadmill and standardized walking tests (2, 6, and 12 minutes) have been used to produce and evaluate dyspnea as it relates to exercise.[21,32–34] Butland et al.[35] demonstrated high correlation coefficients between 2-, 6-, and 12-minute walking tests, indicating that they are similar measures of exercise tolerance (6 minutes versus 12 minutes, $r = 0.9555$; 2 minutes versus 12 minutes, $r = 0.864$; 2 minutes versus 6 minutes, $r = 0.892$). Patients are encouraged to cover as much ground as possible in the prescribed time period. After the walk, patients must indicate their level of dyspnea using a 10-cm visual analogue scale that ranges from "Extremely short of breath" to "No shortness of breath."[35] Standardized walking tests are clinically easy to perform and have been tested for validity. They may be used by clinicians to correlate pulmonary function and physical disability in patients over long periods.

Another method of assessing treatment effects on daily functions of patients with chronic airflow limitations is to measure activity and medication. Guyatt et al.[36] studied patients with chronic airflow limitation (CAL) and asked them (1) to perform a 6-minute walk test, (2) to rate their dyspnea after the walk test, and (3) to complete three questionnaires that measured dyspnea associated with daily activities. Patients received four 2-week treatments with salbutamol and oral theophylline. At the end of each treatment period, outcomes were measured by FEV_1 and forced vital capacity. Three instruments were completed: the Rand Instrument, the Oxygen Cost Diagram, and the Chronic Respiratory Disease Questionnaire. A global rating of changes in dyspnea also was assessed. This study was rigorously performed under exacting conditions. The results of the study demonstrated that the dimension of dyspnea measured by the Chronic Disease Respiratory Questionnaire was a more responsive and valid measure of shortness of breath in daily activities than the other two functional status measures. The study also indicated that dyspnea following the walk test is best measured in conjunction with the 6-minute walk. The investigators also concluded that they successfully demonstrated the feasibility and usefulness of the comparison of functional status measures in the randomized control trial setting.

In an interesting study measuring the affective response of exercise in COPD, Carrieri-Kohlman et al. studied two groups of patients with COPD.[13] One group was nurse monitored and the other group was nurse coached. Using a 200-mm vertical analogue scale, dyspnea intensity and dyspnea-related anxiety were measured. The Spielberger State Anxiety Inventory was used to measure trait and state anxiety and to assess the patient's stable predisposition to anxiety. Pulmonary Function Tests and Arterial Blood Gases were also done. Patients did treadmill walking and walking at home to maintain four walks weekly. Results indicated that both groups had decreased dyspnea with activities of daily living. Dyspnea-related anxiety was also decreased after only a few sessions, and an increase in expended calories was noted in the nurse-coached group.[13]

Instruments

The results of the dyspnea studies over the past several years have succeeded in broadening the approach to the study of the phenomenon. A dyspnea component has been included in many quality of life studies. A comprehensive assessment of dyspnea can include cognitive awareness patterns, ideas, and beliefs and an evaluation of behaviors that ascertain a patient's understanding of the underlying disease process.

This has led to the idea that staging systems for COPD patients would be helpful. These staging systems would have different cutoff points for severity of disease based on FEV_1 predicted values as an objective index and the level of dyspnea, as defined by the patient, as a subjective index. Examples of this effort can be seen in the studies done by Hajiro et al., Alaini et al., and Parshall.[37-39] Standardization of methods and ease of use of instrumentation will assist in the continuation of this process and hopefully lead to an improvement in predicting and providing care for patients experiencing the symptom.

The subjective nature of dyspnea and the lack of consistent, observable signs and symptoms have made measurements difficult.[40] Verbal reports of breathlessness and psychophysiologic magnitude estimation techniques have been used to measure dyspnea.[32,41-43] Studies have measured dyspnea from a time perspective, that is, the amount of dyspnea perceived daily and the amount of dyspnea produced at a specific time in the experimental setting.[8,18]

Retrospective determinations of daily activity and associated breathing difficulty are one method of evaluating dyspnea. Scales equating dyspnea with activity have proved to be reliable and correlate well with measures of pulmonary function. Several instruments have been developed to measure dyspnea in specific timeframes and to evaluate the relationship between dyspnea and specific activities.

Baseline Dyspnea Index (BDI) and Transition Dyspnea Index (TDI)

Two indices have been used to correlate lung function and exercise capacity: the Baseline Dyspnea Index (BDI) and the Transition Dyspnea Index (TDI).[44-46] Tested for reliability on patients with COPD, the BDI grades the severity of dyspnea at a single point in time. The TDI documents changes in dyspnea from a baseline assessment. The BDI and the TDI both contain three classification axes: functional impairment (activities of daily living), magnitude of task in exertional capacity (intensity of activity), and magnitude of subject effort (effort or difficulty breathing). Each main axis contains five categories, rated 0 to 4. Scores are summed for a baseline score that ranges from 0 to 12. Each main axis in the TDI contains seven scores, ranging from –3 (major deterioration) to +3 (major impairment). These scores are summed to form a transition score (–9 to +9). The BDI and the TDI, along with spirometry and a 12-minute walking distance, were used to measure dyspnea, lung function, and exercise capacity in patients with obstructive pulmonary disease. Mahler et al.[47] concluded that the BDI and the TDI can be used to quantify dyspnea severity and identify changes over time. Using Jaspen's multiserial correlation coefficient (m), the study demonstrated statistically significant relationships between the mean Baseline Dyspnea Score and the 12-minute walking test ($m = 0.54$) and forced vital capacity ($m = 0.63$).

In another study, the BDI and the TDI were used to assess the effects of theophylline on dyspnea, lung function, and exercise performance on 12 male ambulatory patients with nonreversible airway obstruction.[48] Arterial gas tensions, steady-state, maximal exercise performance, and the 12-minute walking distance were measured. Results demonstrated that theophylline reduced dyspnea but did not improve lung function, gas exchange, or exercise performance.

The BDI and TDI have been used in patients with pulmonary disease and cardiac disorders. Content validity, concurrent validity, construct validity, and sensitivity for both instruments were accomplished in several studies. The BDI is easy to administer and useful for measuring baseline dyspnea levels. The TDI may be best used to measure the effects of disease progression and the outcomes of treatment.

Borg Scale of Perceived Exertion/Modified Borg Scale

The Borg Scale of Perceived Exertion is a 15-point rating scale, with content validity established from Borg's work related to exertion, fatigue, psychophysiologic relationships, perceived intensity of work, and work curves.[49] Several studies established concurrent validity, test–retest reliability, and sensitivity.[8,50–53] This instrument is particularly helpful to understand perceived exertion and effort during exercise. It also assists investigators in correlating physiologic parameters of lung disease during exercise testing.

The Modified Borg Scale is a 10-item scale, revised from the original 15-point scale. It is a quantifiable rating scale that assesses dyspnea perception at one specific time point by a particular stimulus.[51] In a study of breathlessness perception in asthmatics, Burdon et al.[8] used the Modified Borg Scale to study perceived breathlessness. The patient is asked to rate words describing increasing degrees of breathlessness by numbers between 0 and 10. The 10-item scale examines perceived breathlessness as it relates to changes in specific pulmonary function studies. Exercise testing and physiologic parameters of lung disease can be assessed, but routine activities of daily living cannot be determined.

Burdon et al.[8] documented that breathlessness increased as the FEV_1 decreased. This suggested a strong close linear relationship between the two indices (mean $r = 0.88 \pm 0.15$ SD). The researchers did, however, note considerable variation in the severity of breathlessness for any degree of airflow obstruction (mean intercept 0.50 ± 0.89 SD). A significant relationship ($p < 0.01$) between bronchial responsiveness and magnitude of respiratory distress was found.

In a study using a modified Borg Scale (MBS) to assess the degree of dyspnea in patients with COPD and asthma in an emergency department, Kendrick et al.[54] were able to demonstrate that this scale was efficient for nurses and patients to use in evaluating dyspnea. Peak flow rates were correlated to the MBS, and both measures were used in the triage process. The authors did indicate, however, that it is important to provide careful and specific instructions to patients when using the scale, especially when patients are in a compromised state. Kendrick et al.[54] added the term *breathlessness* for clarification and have since made the scale part of the nursing assessment documentation.

Both the Borg Scale and the Modified Borg Scale can be used for dyspnea measurement in patients with COPD and asthma. These scales are not helpful to investigators interested in understanding responses to routine activities. Additional measures are described in Appendix 33A.

Visual Analog Scales (VAS)

As with other sensations, Visual Analog Scales (VAS) have been used to measure dyspnea.[47] The VAS is a 100-mm measured line with descriptive phrases at each end. Respondents mark a point corresponding with his or her discomfort and symptom severity. McGavin et al.[61] correlated these scales to standardized exercise tests and pulmonary function studies to aid in determining relationships between exercise and breathlessness. Harries et al.[33] studied the relationships between standardized walking tests, lung function, and the VAS. Subjects were divided into groups according to pulmonary diagnosis: 70 had been diagnosed with bronchitis, and 33 were emphysematous. A significant correlation existed between the walking test and VAS ($r = 0.7, p < 0.00001$) for patients with emphysema.

In a study of 16 asthmatic patients in acute respiratory distress and 30 COPD patients, Gift[62] compared a vertical visual analog scale (VVAS) as a measure of dyspnea to the standard horizontal visual analog scale. Both scales were 100 mm in length with anchor terms being "no shortness of breath" at the left or lower end of the line and "shortness of breath as bad as can be" at the right or upper end. The VVAS was found to be easier to use. Concurrent and construct validity were confirmed by two groups of patients (asthmatics and COPD patients) and comparison to peak expiratory flow rates. The VVAS appears to be easy to understand and use by patients experiencing dyspnea. It can assist the clinical evaluation and monitoring of dyspnea and assess the effectiveness of specific interventions to decrease dyspnea.[63]

The VVAS and a scale of subjective symptoms and objectively observed signs of accessory muscle use have been combined by Gift into the Dyspnea Assessment Guide (DAG).[63] To use the DAG, the patient indicates the degree of dyspnea experienced on the vertical visual analog scale and completes the subjective symptom section by circling answers from the list provided. Accessory muscle use is assessed in the semi-Fowler's position. Sternocleidomastoid muscle contraction in combination with clavicle lifting during inspiration is assessed. Gift suggests that the DAG can be useful to evaluate clinical interventions, such as position changes, anxiety-reducing techniques, and energy-conservation measures.

Carrieri-Kohlman et al.[13] used a 200-mm vertical VAS in the study evaluating the nursing intervention-related exercise training and dyspnea. This was chosen to assist the subjects' rating while they were walking on the treadmill, and was anchored with "Not at all" on the bottom and "Worst possible" on the top.

Conceptual Model for Dyspnea

The use of some of the previously described instruments and those presented in Appendix 32A to measure dyspnea have assisted authors in developing conceptual models for dyspnea. Both models describe dyspnea as a complex phenomenon. Gift's model[2] identifies five components of dyspnea: sensation, perception, distress, response, and reporting. *Sensation* is described as the detection of dyspnea by receptor and neural pathways. *Perception* is the individual's interpretation of dyspnea based on past experiences and current expectations. *Distress* refers to the psychologic aspects of dyspnea. *Response* is the individual's coping style and strategies. *Reporting* includes the descriptors of dyspnea and the decision to report or not report shortness of breath.

A second model, by McCord and Cronin-Stubbs,[40] focuses on a plan for operationalizing dyspnea. The authors believe that interventions to manage dyspnea can be directed toward four constructs: antecedents, mediators, reactions, and consequences or outcomes pertinent to dyspnea are identified, assessed, and evaluated.

McCarley[55] has proposed yet another model that has a focus for chronic dyspnea. The development of the model is based on the contention that existing models did not differentiate between acute and chronic dyspnea. The model is based on three components: "physiologic antecedents, dyspnea, and consequences."[53,p234] The basic construct is that dyspnea is always present, but from time to time it may vary in intensity. Further, it is proposed that the baseline gradually increases over time and that acute bouts may occur intermittently. The model also indicates that there are long-term consequences of chronic dyspnea (different from acute dyspnea) that influence physical, psychologic, and sociocultural factors.

Carrieri-Kohlman et al. have proposed a model for the management of dyspnea that considers the fear involved.[13] This model indicates that anxiety associated with the symptom stimulus would decrease with repeated "exposure to the symptom and concomitant 'coaching' about coping strategies that can be used to decrease dyspnea."[13,p137] This theory is the basis for the study using exercise training sessions previously described.

All these models include the realization that psychologic and physiologic components are usually present in dyspnea and should be evaluated. The models assist in considering the themes of dyspnea discussed by Wickham,[12] namely:

- Dyspnea is equivalent to pain in its complexity and subjective experience. Resulting anxiety and the cyclic nature of untreated dyspnea can cause great difficulties for patients and families.
- In some patients, dyspnea can be an invisible problem. This is especially true in patients with cancer at the end of life.
- Dyspnea can be a profound and lonely experience. All aspects of physical functioning can be affected and negative emotions can occur.
- The terms used to describe dyspnea and breathlessness can be difficult for patients to understand. Descriptors that distinguish one cause of dyspnea from another can assist in the overall understanding of the symptom and lead to standardizing assessment and treatment.

Summary

Acute and chronic dyspnea have been studied in a wide variety of adult and pediatric patient populations. Instruments are available to measure and quantify various aspects of this symptom. Self-reports and self-report checklists, interview guides, visual analogue scales, scales measuring perceived exertion and activity, and physiologic pulmonary studies now comprise the armament for dyspnea measurement. These instruments can provide investigators with data to further define and test interventions to assist patients to cope with this problem.

References

1. American Thoracic Society. Dyspnea mechanisms, assessment, and management: A consensus statement. *Am J Resp Crit Care Med*, 1999, *159*:312-340.
2. Carrieri, V., Janson-Bjerklie, S., & Jacobs, S. The sensation of dyspnea: A review. *Heart Lung*, 1984, *13*(4):436-447.
3. Gift, A. Dyspnea. *Nurs Clin North Am*, 1990, *24*(4):955-965.
4. Carrieri-Kohlman, V., Douglas, M., Gormley, J., & Stulbarg, M. Desensitization and guided mastery: Treatment approaches for the management of dyspnea. *Heart Lung*, 1993, *22*(3):226-234.
5. Comroe, J. Some theories in the mechanism of dyspnea. In J. Howell and E. Campbell (Eds.), *Breathlessness*. Oxford: Blackwell Scientific Publications, 1966, p. 1.
6. Comroe, J. *Physiology of respiration* (2nd ed.). Chicago: Yearbook Publishers, 1974.
7. Widimsky, J. Dyspnea. *Coret Vasa*, 1979, *21*(2):128-141.
8. Burdon, J., Juniper, E., Killian, K., et al. The perception of breathlessness in asthma. *Am Rev Respir Dis*, 1982, *126*(5):825-828.
9. Janson-Bjerklie, S., Ruma, E., Stulbarg, M., & Carrieri V. Predictors of dyspnea intensity in asthma. *Nurs Res*, 1987, *36*:179-183.
10. Ball, W., & Summer, W. Clinical manifestations and diagnosis of pulmonary disease. In A. Harvey, R. Johns, V. McKusick, et al. (Eds.), *The principles and practice of medicine*. New York: Appleton-Century-Crofts, 1980, p. 353.
11. Janssens, J., Benoit, M., & Titelion. Management of dyspnea in severe chronic obstructive pulmonary disease. *J Pain Symp Manage*, 2000, *19*(5):378-387.
12. Wickham, R. Dyspnea: Recognizing and managing an invisible problem. *Oncol Nurs Forum*, 2002, *29*(6):925-933.
13. Carrieri-Kohlman, V., Gormley, J., Eiser, S., et al. Dyspnea and the affective response during exercise training in obstructive pulmonary disease. *Nurs Res*, 2001, *50*(3):136-146.
14. Krzhsko, A., Erdel, S., Griener, M., & Lawrance, A. Guidelines for nursing care of patients with altered ventilation. *Oncol Nurs Forum*, 1983, *10*(2):113-119.
15. Bruera, E., Schmitz, B., Pither, J., et al. The frequency and correlates of dyspnea in patients with advanced cancer. *J Pain Symp Manage*, 1999, *19*(5):357-362.
16. Brown, M., Carrieri, V., Janson-Bjerklie, S., & Dodd, M. Lung cancer and dyspnea: The patient's perception. *Oncol Nurs Forum*, 1986, *13*(5):19-24.
17. American Thoracic Society. Recommended respiratory disease questionnaire for use with adults in epidemiological research. *Am Rev Respir Dis*, 1978, *118*(Appendix):7.
18. Roberts, D., Thorne, S., & Pearson, C. The experience of dyspnea in late-stage cancer: Patients' and nurses' perspectives. *Cancer Nurs*, 1993, *16*(4):310-320.

19. Heinzer, M.V., Bish, C., & Detwilder, R. Acute dyspnea as perceived by patients with chronic obstructive pulmonary disease. *Clin Nurs Res*, 2003, *12*(1):85-101.

20. Carrieri, V., & Janson-Bjerklie, S. Strategies patients use to manage the sensation of dyspnea. *West J Nurs Res*, 1986, *8*(3):284-305.

21. Epler, G., Saber, F., & Gaensler, E. Determination of severe impairment disability in interstitial lung disease. *Am Rev Respir Dis*, 1980, *121*(4):647-659.

22. McDadden, E., Kiser, R., & Degroot, W. Acute bronchial asthma. *N Engl J Med*, 1973, *288*(5):221-226.

23. Morgan, W. Pulmonary disability and impairment. *Am Thorac Soc News Basis RD*, 1982, *10*(1):1-18.

24. Carrieri, V., & Janson-Bjerklie, S. Dyspnea. In V. Carrieri, A. Lindsey, & C. West (Eds.), *Pathophysiological phenomena in nursing*. Philadelphia: Saunders, 1986, p. 191.

25. Fishman, A.P., & Leslie, J.F. Dyspnea. *Bull Eur Physiol Respir*, 1979, *15*(5):789-804.

26. Gottfried, S., Altose, M., Kelson, S., & Cherniak, N. Perception of changes in airflow resistance in obstructive pulmonary disorders. *Am Rev Respir Dis*, 1981, *124*(5):566-570.

27. Belza, B., Steele, B., Hunziker, J., et al. Correlates of physical activity in chronic obstructive pulmonary disease. *Nurs Res*, 2001, *50*(4):195-202.

28. Leidy, N.K. Functional performance in people in chronic obstructive disease. *Image: J Nurs Schol*, 1995, *27*(1):23-34.

29. Gift, A., & Cahill, C. Psychophysiologic aspects of dyspnea in chronic obstructive disease: A pilot study. *Heart Lung*, 1990, *19*(3):252-257.

30. Carrieri, V., Kieckhefer, G., Janson-Bjerklie, S., & Souza, J. The sensation of pulmonary dyspnea in school age children. *Nurs Res*, 1991, *40*(2):81-86.

31. Gift, A., Plaut, S., & Jacox, A. Psychologic and physiologic factors related to dyspnea in subjects with chronic obstructive pulmonary disease. *Heart Lung*, 1989, *15*(6):595-601.

32. Gift, A., & Pugh, L. Dyspnea and fatigue. *Nurs Clin North Am*, 1993, *28*(2):373-384.

33. Harries, D., Booker, H., Rehaln, M., & Collins, J. Measurement and perception of disability in chronic airways obstruction. *Am Rev Respir Dis*, 1983, *127*(4)(Suppl):119-120.

34. Bilman, M., Rambhatla, K., Blair, G., & Sieck, G. Breathlessness index, a simple and repeatable exercise test for patients with chronic obstructive pulmonary disease. *Am Rev Respir Dis*, 1983, *127*(4)(Suppl):109.

35. Butland, R., Pang, J., Gross, E., et al. Two-, six-, and 12-minute walking tests in respiratory disease, *Br Med J*, 1982, *284*(6320):1607-1608.

36. Guyatt, G., Townsend, M., Berman, L., & Pugsley, S. Quality of life in patients with chronic airflow limitation. *Br J Dis Chest*, 1987, *81*(1):45-54.

37. Hajiro, T., Nishimura, K., Tsukino, M., et al. A comparison of the level of dyspnea vs. disease severity in indicating the health-related quality of life of patients with COPD. *Chest*, 1999, *116*(6):1632-1637.

38. Ailani, R., Ravakhah, K., Digiovine, B., et al. Dyspnea differentiation index: A new method for rapid separation of cardiac vs. pulmonary dyspnea. *Chest*, 1999, *116*(4):1100-1105.

39. Parshall, M. Adult emergency visits for chronic cardiorespiratory disease: Does dyspnea matter? *Nurs Res*, 1999, *48*(2):62-70.

40. McCord, M., & Cronin-Stubbs, D. Operationalizing dyspnea: Focus on measurement. *Heart Lung*, 21(2):167-179.

41. Nield, M., Kim, M., & Patel, M. Use of magnitude estimation for estimating the parameters of dyspnea. *Nurs Res*, 1989, *38*(2):77-80.

42. Nield, M., & Kim, M. The reliability of magnitude estimation for dyspnea measurement. Nurs Res, 1991, 40(1):17-19.

43. Burki, N., Davenport, P., Safdar, R., & Zechman, F. The effects of airway anesthesia on magnitude estimation of added inspiratory resistive and elastic loads. *Am Rev Respir Dis*, 1983, *127*(1):2-4.

44. Mahler, D., Weinberg, D., Wells, C., & Feinstein, A. Measurement of dyspnea: Description of two new indexes, interobserver agreement, and physiologic correlations. *Am Rev Respir Dis*, 1982, *125*(Suppl):138.

45. Mahler, D., & Wells, C., Evaluation of clinical methods for rating dyspnea. *Chest*, 1988, *93*(1):580-586.

46. Mahler, D., Rosiello, R., Harver, A., et al. Comparison of clinical dyspnea ratings and psychophysical measurements of respiratory sensation in obstructive pulmonary disease. *Am Rev Respir Dis*, 1987, *135*(6):1229-1233.

47. Mahler, D., Harver, A., Rosiello, R., & Daubenspeck, J. Measurement of respiratory sensation in interstitial lung disease. *Chest*, 1989, *96*(4):767-771.

48. Mahler, D., Mattay, R., Berger, H., et al. Sustained-release theophylline reduces dyspnea in non-reversible obstructive airway disease. *Am Rev Respir Dis*, 1983, *127*(Suppl):87.

49. Borg, G. Perceived exertion as an indicator of somatic stress. *Scand J Rehab Med*, 1970, *2*(2-3):92-98.

50. Gottfried, S., Altose, M., Kelson, G., & Cherniak, N. Perception of changes in airflow resistance in obstructive pulmonary disorders. *Am Rev Respir Dis*, 1981, *124*(5):566-570.

51. Wilson, R., & Jones, R. A comparison of the visual analog scale and modified Borg scale for the measurement of dyspnea during exercise. *Clin Sci*, 1989, *76*(3):277-279.

52. Moody, L. Measurement of psychophysiologic response variables in chronic bronchitis and emphysema. *Appl Nurs Res*, 1990, *3*(1):36-38.

53. Moody, L., McCormick, K., & Williams, A. Disease and symptom severity, functional status and quality of life in chronic bronchitis and emphysema. *J Br Med*, 1990, *13*(3):297-306.

54. Kendrick, K., Baxi, S., Smikth, R. Usefulness of the modified Borg scale in assessing the degree of dyspnea in patients with COPD and asthma. *J Emerg Nurs*, 2000, *26*(3):216-222.

55. McCarley, C. A model of chronic dyspnea. *Image: J Nurs Schol*, 1999, *31*(3):231-236.

56. Janson-Bjerklie, S., Carrieri, V., & Hudes, D. The sensation of pulmonary dyspnea. *Nurs Res*, 1986, *35*(3):154-159.

57. Joyce, C., Zutshi, D., Hrubes, V., & Mason, R. Comparison of fixed interval and visual analogue scales for rating chronic pain. *Eur J Clin Pharmacol*, 1975, *8*(6):415-420.

58. Killian, K., Mahutte, C., Howell, J., & Campbell, E. Effect of timing, flow, lung volume and threshold pressure on resistive load detection. *J Appl Physiol*, 1980, *49*(6):958-963.

59. Killian, K., Burens, D., & Campbell, E. Effect of breathing patterns on the perceived magnitude of added loads to breathing. *J Appl Physiol*, 1982, *52*(3):578-584.

60. Killian, K., Campbell, E., & Howell, J. The effect of increased ventilation on resistive load discrimination. *Am Rev Respir Dis*, 1979, *120*(6):1233-1238.

61. McGavin, C., Artivinli, M., Nave, H., & McHardy, G. Dyspnoea, disability, and distance walked: Comparison of estimates of exercise performance in respiratory disease. *Br Med J*, 1978, *2*(3):241-243.

62. Gift, A., Plaut, S., & Jacox, A. Psychologic and physiologic factors related to dyspnea in subjects with chronic obstructive pulmonary disease. *Heart Lung*, 1986, *15*(6):595-601.

63. Gift, A. Dyspnea assessment guide. *Crit Care Nurs*, 1991, *9*(8):79.

64. Stoller, J., Ferranti, R., & Feinstein, A. Further specification and evaluation of a new index for dyspnea. *Am Rev Respir Disease*, 1986, *143*(2):129.

65. Comstock, G. Progress report on comparison of respiratory questionnaires in Washington County, MD. *Am Rev Respir Dis*, 1978, *118*(appendix 1):1.

66. Comstock, G., Tockman, M., Helsing, K., & Hennesy, K. Standardized respiratory questionnaires: Comparison of the old with the new. *Am Rev Respir Dis*, 1979, *119*(1):45-49.

67. Kinsman, R., Fernandez, E., Schochet, M., et al. Multidimensional analysis of the symptoms of chronic bronchitis and emphysema. *J Behav Med*, 1983, *6*(4):339.

68. Guyatt, G., Berman, L., Townsend, M., et al. A measure of quality of life for clinical trials in chronic lung disease. *Thorax*, 1987, *42*(5):773.

Appendix 33A. Additional Measures of Dyspnea

Instrument	Description	Psychometric Indices
University of California, San Diego Questionnaire (1)	24-item questionnaire Measures dyspnea over past week 6-point rating scale for each of 21 tasks	Reliable and valid Limitations: intensity of dyspnea associated with ambulatory activity depends on work performance and patient's weight
Standardized Respiratory Disease Questionnaire (ATS-DLD-78) Developed by the American Thoracic Society (20,56,65,66)	Used to evaluate the behavioral manifestations of dyspnea; obtain data on pulmonary symptomatology; and elicit demographic data Self-report or interview guide questionnaire can be used to obtain history of pulmonary disease, environmental and occupational exposures, medication use, smoking	Concurrent validity established Reliability and concurrent validity documented (sample of 946 white males) Limitations: collects comprehensive data but not over time; rigor of psychometric testing questioned
Dyspnea Interview Schedule (20) Developed by Janson-Bjerklie	48-item semistructured interview guide Asks questions about perceived dyspnea, aggravating and alleviating factors, prodromal indicators, physiologic/psychologic/behavioral correlates Elicits data about adaptive mechanisms, social support, effects of dyspnea on activities of daily living Shorter, 9-item version (Clinic Interview) developed: items from original tool, dyspnea description, precipitants, prodromal indicators, correlates, adaptive mechanisms Provides useful insight into the sensation of dyspnea	Both instruments require replication in diverse settings
Five-Level Scale of Breathlessness (18,53) Developed by the American Thoracic Society	Included in the Standardized Respiratory Interview Guide or Self-Report Questionnaire 5-point rating scale that correlates dyspnea with activity Scale is retrospective, can be used with persons experiencing chronic SOB and aids clinicians in determining baseline dyspnea levels	Content validity established Concurrent validity confirmed (sample = 45 patients with COPD) Limitation: reliability remains to be documented; uses ambulation as a major indicator of dyspnea; does not evaluate consequences of other activities
Chronic Disease Assessment Tool (CDAT) (52,53)	2-part questionnaire: Part I: 5 sections containing 106 items (general health and medical history, environmental risk, health impact measurement survey, quality of life index, demographics); Part II: open-ended questions addressing physical assessment and pulmonary function Allows measurement of psychophysiologic responses, functional status, and quality of life for many chronic diseases	Content validity established Internal consistency, reliability, and concurrent validity established (sample = 45 patients with chronic bronchitis or emphysema) (44) CDAT does address the symptom triad of dyspnea, fatigue, depression to determine applicability to clinical practice and research

Appendix 33A. Additional Measures of Dyspnea (*cont.*)

Instrument	Description	Psychometric Indices
The Bronchitis-Emphysema Checklist (35,52,64)	Delineates symptom categories in an 89-item self-report checklist Symptoms include fatigue, helplessness-hopelessness, decathexis, poor memory, peripheral sensory complaints, sleep difficulty, irritability, anxiety, alienation, dyspnea	Content validity established (sample = 29 patients with chronic bronchitis and emphysema) (67) Internal consistency, reliability, construct validity established (sample = 146 patients with chronic bronchitis or emphysema) (56) Internal consistency and reliability supported (sample = 68 patients with pulmonary disease) (52)
Pulmonary Functional Status and Dyspnea Questionnaire (27)	Two scales used to obtain information regarding the impact of respiratory distress on functional performance as related to daily activities Self-administered Dyspnea is evaluated with 3 general appraisal questions that indicate global dyspnea scores	Reliability and validity established May require replication in diverse settings
Magnitude Estimation (40, 41, 44–48,56–60)	Psychophysiologic technique estimating relationship between subjective and physical magnitude of the sensation Increase in dyspnea is estimated from subject's own reference points as loads are added	Reliable and valid with some concerns Construct validity established
St. George Respiratory Questionnaire (SGRO) (37)	Self-administered 76 items Measures symptoms, activity, and impact of disease on daily life Dyspnea included in overall symptom category	Reliable and valid Translated into several languages
Modified Baseline Dyspnea Index (MDI) Developed by Stoller et al. (64)	Developed to improve the Baseline Dyspnea Index (BDI) and to determine differences between functional impairment at work and at home Interview guide with a 5-point rating scale 3 subscales Scoring for a functional impairment subscale yields total score for functional impairment at work and at home	Content and concurrent validity established (sample = 32 patients with stable COPD) Requires documentation of reliability testing and testing with larger sample sizes to compare sensitivity of MDI with BDI Advantages: may assist clinicians in developing interventions specific to patients' problems

Oxygen Cost Diagram (46–48)	Variation of Visual Analog Scale (VAS) Determines point at which a specific activity level corresponds with the subject's perception of dyspnea 100-mm vertical line used, with everyday activities placed in proportion to their oxygen cost Point where SOB limits exercise is marked by subjects	Correlates with BDI and 12-minute walk test Content validity, interrater reliability, concurrent validity, and sensitivity established (sample of patients with pulmonary or cardiac disorders, pulmonary infiltrates, COPD, asthma, cystic fibrosis, interstitial lung disease, chronic airflow obstruction) (38,39) Limitation: emphasis on ambulation
Chronic Respiratory Disease Questionnaire (36,65)	20-item, 7-point Likert rating scale 4 subscales examine changes in quality of life over 2-week period: dyspnea (subjects asked to specify 5 important, frequent activities that cause shortness of breath (SOB)); fatigue; emotional function; mastery or control	Content validity established (sample = 100 patients with COPD) (65), resulting in a reduction from 123 original items to 20 items Test–retest reliability and concurrent validity established (sample = 25 patients with COPD) (36)

Numbers in parentheses correspond to studies cited in the References.

34

Measuring Fatigue

Barbara F. Piper

Fatigue Definitions

One of the challenges to measuring fatigue may be to agree on a universal definition.[1,2] Despite the numerous interdisciplinary definitions and descriptions that exist, no single definition or set of diagnostic criteria have been adopted.[3] Several factors are responsible for this lack of definitional clarity. One major factor is the fact that fatigue's underlying mechanisms, although posited, remain largely unknown. Some have proposed that an animal model must be developed to study fatigue for this to occur.[4] Another factor is that fatigue, like pain, is a complex, multicausal, and multidimensional sensation.[5] As a consequence, some have argued that investigators and measures have had difficulty in differentiating between fatigue's signs, symptoms, or indicators (e.g., reduction in force; tired eyes, legs, or whole body); its outcomes, responses, or effects (e.g., decreased activity, functional status, capacity, stamina, or endurance)[6] and signs or symptoms that may or may not be related to fatigue, such as depression, weakness,[7] asthenia, malaise, and exertion.[8] When fatigue is viewed as a subjective sensation, it is defined simply as whatever the person says it is[1,2] and best measured by self-report. Fatigue has been defined[5] by its underlying biologic nature, such as diaphragmatic,[9,10] motor,[11] or neuromuscular fatigue;[12] by its underlying cause (i.e., central, peripheral, attentional,[13] pathologic, physiologic, or psychologic); by its unknown etiology; and by the exclusion of all other possible diseases (i.e., chronic fatigue syndrome or idiopathic chronic fatigue[14,15]).

Because of this complexity, some propose, at least for cancer-related fatigue, that fatigue no longer be referred to or defined as simply a symptom, but rather it should be designated a syndrome, one that includes the diversity of signs and symptoms associated with an abnormal condition[5,16,17] and/or disease state.[18] Thus, it is probably premature to adopt a universal definition or set of diagnostic criteria[19,20] until more testing of these definitions and criteria can be undertaken and a better understanding of underlying mechanisms is appreciated.[5]

There is emerging consensus among health care professionals and study evidence that fatigue experienced by clinical populations differs significantly from the transient, more easily relieved sense of tiredness experienced by healthy individuals.[1,2,8,21–26] As a result, several evidence-based practice guidelines now combine both the perception of fatigue with a decline in functioning in their definitions[26–28] to distinguish it from the tiredness more commonly seen in healthy populations.[29,30]

Dimensions of Fatigue

Not only is there is emerging consensus that fatigue is multidimensional.[5,26,31,32] but there is also emerging consensus as to what these dimensions may be.[1,5,6] Commonly cited dimensions include severity,[33] behavioral,[33] affective,[33] cognitive,[2,4] symptom or sensory,[1,34–38] temporal,[12,15,33,37,39,40] and physiologic.[8] Less commonly cited dimensions include situational,[38] biochemical,[8] psychologic,[38,41] psychosocial,[42] and personality.[41] Studies are needed to determine how these dimensions may vary across different clinical populations and treatments, and how they may be related to underlying fatigue mechanisms.

Despite the fact that most fatigue scales measure fatigue's intensity,[43–47] clinically it's been difficult to incorporate even a simple 0–10 numeric rating scale (NMR) that measures fatigue's intensity.[48] Fatigue continues to be underreported, underassessed, underdiagnosed, and undertreated.[3,27,46] Numerous patient-, provider-, and setting-related barriers have been identified.[49] Measuring fatigue in clinical settings may require mandate similar to the one issued by the Joint Commission on Hospital Accreditation for pain documentation, for fatigue documentation to occur.[49]

Although symptom intensity drives practice, measuring intensity alone may be insufficient.[50,51] Other methods must be used to capture its multidimensional properties.[2,43,46,51,52]

The multidimensional measurement of fatigue is important because it is believed to more comprehensively assess fatigue and may enhance differentiation among underlying causative mechanisms,[14] thereby guiding more appropriate fatigue management strategies.[5] These measurement assumptions, however, need more study.

It is important to measure the temporal dimension and patterns of fatigue as these can better prepare patients for when they might experience fatigue and guide treatment planning. In patients followed daily over the first three weeks after a myocardial infarction, five different patterns of fatigue over time were documented,[40] suggesting that patients should not be treated uniformly. Similarly, in cancer patients, different fatigue patterns have been documented depending on the form of treatment prescribed (i.e., radiation therapy or chemotherapy).[5] Among chemotherapy patients, different fatigue patterns have been shown to vary according to how the chemotherapy is administered (i.e., short daily or weekly intravenous bolus infusions versus continuous or monthly infusions).[53]

Unfortunately, many have arbitrarily assumed that scales that measure fatigue multidimensionally are too burdensome for clinical use because of their length. As a consequence, such measurement has largely been relegated to research studies.

Not all patients, however, may need an in-depth, multidimensional assessment or measurement of fatigue. It is critical to begin to identify those at high risk for chronic fatigue (i.e., one or more months)[5] to tailor resources and therapies accordingly.[52] Two studies have validated none (0), mild (1–3), moderate (4–6), and severe (7–10) intensity levels for fatigue in cancer patients receiving therapy,[30,54] suggesting that a score of 4 or higher on a 0–10 NMR scale may be a useful indicator for identifying high-risk patients who require more in-depth workup and multidimensional fatigue assessment.[27,30,52]

Although these intensity levels constitute the best currently available data for evidence-based practice, they need to be tested in other clinical populations for their validity. In the interim, published studies of fatigue reports must describe the ranges in fatigue scores, because reporting only mean or median values may underestimate fatigue severity[55] and fail to identify high-risk patients who might benefit from further workup and intervention. The most commonly identified dimensions and the instruments that measure these dimensions are listed in Table 34.1.[5,21,42,45–47,54,56–91,184–187]

Underlying Fatigue Theories and Models

A number of theories have been proposed to explain the underlying mechanisms of fatigue.[5,6,8,34,41,92–96] They include central and peripheral[94,97] and neurophysiologic mechanisms;[94,95] physiologic,[8,99] psychologic,[8,99] situational,[5,34,41] personality,[41] and environmental factors;[8,41,99] symptom and activity patterns,[8,96,99] developmental, social, and innate host factors;[41,98,99] and energy variable interactions.[8,96,99] Models schematically depicting these theories include the Central/Peripheral Nervous System Model,[94] the Circadian Rhythmicity Model,[100] the Energy Analysis Model,[96] an Integrated Fatigue Model (IFM),[8,99] Levine's Energy Conservation Model,[101] the Distressing Symptoms Model,[102] a Stress/Coping Model,[34] the UCSF Symptom Management Model,[103] Psychobiologic-Entropy Model,[6,104] statistically developed structural equation models,[105] and muscle ATP metabolism, vagal afferent, and serotonergic dysregulation and hypopituitary axis (HPA) models.[4,27,106]

Each of these models and theories are in various stages of development and hypothesis testing.[5] Although the central/peripheral nervous system and IFM models are arguably the most widely recognized models developed to investigate fatigue, model selection to guide research designs depends on the research questions posed and the investigator's discipline or perspective. No one theory or model can be universally recommended at this time.

Despite the fact that many of these theories have not been as well developed or tested as have theories of pain, a number of similarities exist that may shed light on the underlying mechanisms of fatigue. One similarity is that both fatigue and pain are complex, multidimensional sensations[5,107] that may be explained in part by their underlying central and peripheral nervous system mechanisms.[5,108] It is well known that the nervous system plays a significant role in the transduction, transmission, perception, and modulation of pain and the response to pain. As a better understanding has emerged of the underlying neurophysiologic mechanisms for pain, so too have improved conceptualizations and measurements of pain's multidimensions evolved.[107,108] The nervous system is postulated to play a significant role in the perception and modulation of fatigue.[5,94] As a consequence, it may be useful to examine what is known about the underlying mechanisms of pain, particularly when pain and fatigue occur together as a symptom complex (i.e., two symptoms) or a symptom cluster (i.e., three or more).[49,109]

Central nervous system mechanisms proposed for fatigue[5] include lack of motivation, impaired recruitment of motor neurons,[26,28] intermittent conduction blocks in partially demyelinated central motor pathways,[26,28] and inhibition of voluntary effort.[93,110,111] The action of sensory pathways on the reticular formation is thought to be critical to the understanding of these central fatigue mechanisms.[112]

Chemoreceptors in fatigued muscles are thought to send feedback impulses to the reticular formation in the central nervous system.[5] These impulses result in motor pathway inhibition anywhere from the voluntary centers in the brain to the spinal motor neurons.[112] This inhibition of voluntary effort can be overridden by feedback stimuli from nonfatigued muscles that stimulate the facilitory portion of the reticular formation, resulting in decreased inhibition and decreased fatigue.[112]

Table 34.1 Proposed Dimensions of Fatigue

Proposed Dimension(s)	Proposed Indicator(s)	Instruments Measuring This Dimension
Affective, Emotional, or Psychologic Dimension: Includes emotional manifestations/responses to fatigue (5)	Degree of emotional distress or response to fatigue (i.e., increased irritability, frustration, resentment, and depression) Emotional meaning attributed to fatigue (i.e., unpleasant) Reduced motivation	Cancer Fatigue Scale (56) Cancer-Related Fatigue Distress Scale (57,58) Fatigue Assessment Questionnaire (59) Fatigue Impact Scale (42) Global Fatigue Index (60) Multidimensional Assessment of Fatigue (61–63) Mental Fatigue Inventory (64) Multidimensional Fatigue Symptom Inventory (65) Piper Fatigue Scale-Revised (46) Schwartz Cancer Fatigue Scale (47,66)
Behavioral Dimension: Includes signs and symptoms that reflect changes in physical performance, impact of fatigue symptoms on activities of daily living (ADLs) or the amount of effort or exertion that needs to be expended (5)	Impact of fatigue on ADLs, physical performance, or functional status Reflected by an increased degree of effort that needs to be expended Reflected by perceptions that it takes longer to complete tasks and declines in performance (e.g., card sorting, posture, communication style) Reflected in decreased ability to socialize or perform roles and/or consequences of fatigue	Brief Fatigue Inventory (45,54,67) Dutch Fatigue Exertion Scale (68) Fatigue Impact Scale (42) Fatigue Symptom Inventory (69,70) HIV-Related Distress Scale (71) Multidimensional Assessment of Fatigue (61–63) Multidimensional Fatigue Inventory (184–187) Multidimensional Fatigue Symptom Inventory (65) Piper Fatigue Scale-Revised (46)
Cognitive or Mental Dimension: Includes signs and symptoms that reflect the impact of fatigue on thought or concentration processes (5)	Ability to concentrate, remember, think clearly, or direct attention Ability to perform certain tasks In chemotherapy patients, may be referred to as "chemo-brain" (82) and neurocognitive dysfunction (83,84)	Chalder Fatigue Scale (72) Fatigue Assessment Questionnaire (59) Fatigue Impact Scale (42) Fatigue Symptom Checklist (FSCL) (73–75) and Modified FSCL (76,77) Lee's Visual Analogue Scale for Fatigue (78) Mental Fatigue Inventory (64) Multidimensional Fatigue Symptom Inventory (65) Neurocognitive tests, e.g., Forward-Backward Digit Span Tests (79–81) Piper Fatigue Scale-Revised (46) Schwartz Cancer Fatigue Scale, 28 items (47)

Table 34.1 *Continued*

Proposed Dimension(s)	Proposed Indicator(s)	Instruments Measuring This Dimension
Physiologic Dimension: Includes the underlying mechanisms of fatigue (5)	Reflects the anatomic, biochemical, genetic, metabolic, neurophysiologic, and neuroendocrinologic mechanisms of fatigue	Studies have measured loss of force/work-generating capacity, shifts in power spectrum of electromyelogram, and muscle slowing (conduction velocity and contractile speed) Others have measured changes in serum melatonin (85), heart rate, and oxygen consumption (86); hematocrit levels (87) and hemoglobin levels (88,89), temperature (21), accumulation or depletion of metabolites (90), fluid and electrolyte shifts, and noninvasive measurement of phosphate-containing compounds (90)
Sensory or Physical Dimension: Includes fatigue signs and symptoms and their intensities (5)	Signs and symptoms may be localized to a specific body part, muscle group, or fiber (e.g., tired eyes, chest, or shoulders) or may be more generalized over the whole body (e.g., feeling tired, drained, having no energy, feeling weak or exhausted, or feeling "bone tired" (91) Includes motor or muscle fatigue indices Other terms used for this dimension include general, physical, or somatic fatigue	Included in almost all fatigue self-report scales
Temporal Dimension: Includes signs and symptoms that relate to the timing, onset, pattern, duration of fatigue (5)	Timing/circadian pattern (when occurs) Onset /duration (days, weeks, months, years) Pattern (abrupt, brief, momentary, insidious, transient—short term/acute, i.e., < than 1 month; intermittent, seldom, frequent, constant, continuous, or chronic i.e., > than 1 month Changes in pattern over time	Fatigue Symptom Inventory (69,70) Multidimensional Assessment of Fatigue (61–63) Piper Fatigue Scale-Revised (46) Schwartz Cancer Fatigue Scale, 28-item version (47)

Numbers in parenthesis correspond to studies cited in the References.

Similar inhibition–facilitation mechanisms operate in attention fatigue states,[5,6] because the ability to concentrate, focus, and direct attention involves the active inhibition of competing stimuli.[113] Because mental effort is required to maintain this directed attention, prolonged mental effort can lead to fatigue in the underlying neural mechanisms that block competing or distracting stimuli.[113] Inability to perform cognitively,[23] think clearly, direct attention, or concentrate are manifestations of this mental or cognitive fatigue process.[79]

In multiple sclerosis (MS) patients, metabolic disregulation processes are hypothesized to affect cognitive fatigue as fluctuations in brain glucose metabolism are reported,[114] and have been implicated in MS patients experiencing motor and muscle fatigue.[115] In one study, patients' subjective fatigue scores significantly correlated with overall central lesion burden as measured by brain magnetic resonance imaging (MRI), suggesting a central nervous system origin in these patients.[7]

Peripheral nervous system mechanisms proposed for fatigue[5] include impaired peripheral nerve function, neuromuscular junction transmission, abnormal coactivation of agonists and antagonists associated with spasticity,[26,28] and impaired fiber activation.[94] Impaired neuromuscular junction transmission has been implicated in causing fatigue in myasthenia gravis patients,[116] whereas disturbances in the neurotransmitter acetylcholine have been associated with causing fatigue in botulism patients.[117]

Both central and peripheral nervous system mechanisms may be involved in the overwhelming fatigue that patients experience who have chronic fatigue syndrome, cancer, autoimmune disorders, and MS.[5] It has been postulated that the central and peripheral release of endogenous cytokines by leukocytes, lymphocytes, and activated macrophages may be responsible for fatigue in these patients because of the effects these cytokines may have on the central and peripheral nervous systems, metabolism, and other body functions.[7,118–120] Cytokines are thought to interact with these systems to produce many of the common manifestations seen in fatigue. Receptors for hormones and neurotransmitters have been found to be present on immune and nervous system cells,[121–123] suggesting that these systems may be able to communicate and interact with one another to perhaps explain the possible origins of some fatigue manifestations that are seen clinically.

Cytokines also have been implicated in causing fatigue in cancer patients[5,27] receiving radiation[124,125] and biotherapies[120] and in patients exhibiting signs and symptoms of cognition disorders[120] and anemia.[126] The exogenous administration of cytokines, such as interferon, has been postulated to produce fatigue, anorexia, and cognition disorders through direct effects on the frontal lobe, brain structural neurons, or neurotransmitters.[127] Peripheral neuropathies are reported with high-dose interferon therapies.[128] Similarly, the release of endogenous gamma interferon and tumor necrosis factor (TNF) in response to interleukin-2 administration has been implicated in causing alterations in neuroendocrine secretion,[129] brain electrical activity,[130] and blood-brain barrier permeability.[131] In addition to their effects on the nervous system, TNF and interleukin-1 have been implicated in causing the progressive muscle wasting associated with cancer cachexia,[132] sleep induction, and fatigue.[133,134] Thus, these particular cytokines may cause fatigue secondary to their effects on the body's metabolic functions.[132]

Possible metabolic causes of fatigue include malnutrition;[135] depletion of energy sources, such as phosphocreatine and glycogen; and changes in amino acids;[118,136,137] decreased oxygen carrying capacity or supply;[138] and steroid use.[135] Although altered or depleted energy stores are thought to enhance the occurrence of fatigue,[8,10] the relationships between fatigue and abnormalities in metabolism, cachexia,[132] type and extent of nutritional intake (i.e., anorexia and body mass indices), and L-carnitine deficiencies[139] have not been well-studied.

Neurotransmitters may mediate fatigue.[8,118,140] Decreased arousal, cognitive fatigue, and tiredness can result from disruption of serotonergic pathways.[141] Fatigue is an important symptom of disturbed circadian rhythm,[100,142,143] and studies are in progress in cancer patients to explore the relationships that may exist between circadian rhythms, fatigue, and melatonin secretion.[24]

Selecting a Fatigue Instrument

For a subjective fatigue scale or a biologic measure to be used in busy practice settings and in research studies, it must be valid, reliable, and sensitive to change over time; easy to administer and score; and not unduly burdensome or fatiguing to administer. Clinically, eliciting the perceived and observed effects of fatigue on the performance of daily activities or physical performance is critical.[29] Busy health care professionals can ask patients three simple questions to assess the severity of fatigue: (1) Are you experiencing fatigue? (2) If yes, how severe is the fatigue on a 0–10 scale? and (3) How is the fatigue interfering with your activities of daily living?[5]

Assessment, measurement and treatment of fatigue are now considered standard care for many patients.[15,16,27,28] As a consequence, practice settings must work toward incorporating a scale for measuring fatigue into documentation forms. It is important to screen all patients at baseline as they undergo their initial diagnostic workup, since even before treatment has begun, patients may experience fatigue.[13] Screening should be repeated at all subsequent visits, including follow-up visits when patients no longer receive active treatment.[5,27]

For research studies, the research questions and the theoretical model that drive the study dictate the measurement strategies to be used. The method(s) selected should depend on the dimension(s) an investigator is most interested in studying[144] and how frequently fatigue will be measured (i.e., several times during the day versus weekly or monthly).

Measurement reliability and validity are critical if the study outcomes are to be credible and generalizable. Single-item, single-dimension intensity rating scales, such as the 0–10 NMR scale, have been reported to be less reliable than multiple-item fatigue measures.[78] However, they can be clinically useful in two settings: (1) to screen and rescreen patients periodically to identify individuals who need more in-depth fatigue workups as well as multidimensional measurement and (2) when fatigue must be measured frequently (e.g., during a 24-hour period).

Using multiple fatigue measures together, a process called triangulation,[145] can enhance the reliability and validity of study findings, but it must be used judiciously to avoid respondent fatigue. Methods that are too lengthy, redundant, or cumbersome can confound fatigue findings and lead to subject refusal to participate in studies and to subject attrition over time in longitudinal studies.

The timing of measurement must be addressed in the study design and published reports. For example, will the time of day for measurement be held constant across all subjects to control for circadian patterns? How do the usual diurnal fluctuations of self-report and physiologic indicators covary and affect measurement strategy? Will self-report and physiologic measures be administered within a short time of one another to enhance validity? Will subjects be less compliant if asked to complete measures when they are most fatigued? Unfortunately, the administration timing of fatigue measures often is not made explicit in published studies. When timing is mentioned, more commonly it is addressed in studies that have used repeated measures throughout the day to capture circadian patterns[117,146] or in studies that control for the effects of treatment (i.e., two hours after radiation therapy).[147] Ideally, laboratory studies or physiologic measures should be performed concurrently or within a few hours of self-report measures.

To investigate differences between healthy or control subjects and clinical populations, it is important to use an instrument that effectively discriminates fatigue between these groups (discriminant validity) and has established normative data in healthy subjects. In addition, what constitutes mild, moderate, and severe levels of fatigue; cut scores (i.e., the point at which treatment or additional workup and referral are needed), and effect sizes must be reported. In addition, an instrument needs to be sensitive (i.e., responsive) to changes in fatigue over time when longitudinal designs and repeated measures are used. Last, sample characteristics must be considered because age, educational level, language, culture, and visual, hearing, and motor coordination can affect measurement strategy, subject compliance, and findings.

There are now several valid and reliable instruments that measure the subjective perception of fatigue. There are single-item, single-dimensional scales that measure intensity of fatigue either on a single-item 0–10 NMR scale (Table 34.2)[30,153–156] or a multi-item, single-dimension intensity rating scale (Table 34.3).[22,33,43–45,54,57,58,60–64,66–68,70,148,149,155,162–172] Whether using a single item or a multi-item scale makes a difference in measuring fatigue, the single-dimensional intensity scale has not been well studied.

With the current focus on measuring quality of life (QOL) and symptoms in addition to fatigue, subjective fatigue has been measured by single or multiple items within specific subscales on instruments originally designed to measure other phenomena of interest, such as mood states,[148,149] symptom distress,[150] QOL,[43,91,151,152] and anemia.[43,151] A few of these scales are described in Table 34.3. Multidimensional scales are described in Table 34.4.[21,30,33,37,41–44,46,47,56,59,65,66,69–73,76–78,98,147,153,155–161,166,171–187]

Historic Overview of Fatigue Measurement and Research

To better appreciate the current status of fatigue measurement and research findings, it is helpful to review past major fatigue developments. These are summarized in Table 34.5.[6,8,21,24,27,33,35–37,41,49,73–75,89,92,93,95,97,100,109,147,150,152,158,172,179,188–208]

Summary of Research Findings

In designing studies to measure fatigue, it is important to consider variables that others have found are associated with or predictive of fatigue. This section describes some of these variables.

Age

Age may be a risk factor for certain types of fatigue[5] depending on the disease or treatment. For example, the mean age range for chronic fatigue syndrome (CFS) is 27–42 years.[14] Among women newly diagnosed with breast cancer, older women may be more vulnerable to attentional fatigue following surgery than are younger women.[209] In contrast, older men and women treated with chemotherapy have less fatigue.[210] Other studies have found no association between age and fatigue.[211,212]

Anemia

In HIV/AIDS patients, anemia is a common consequence of disease, its complications, and its treatments.[3] Anemia ranges from 20% to 70%, depending on the form of treatment

Table 34.2 Single-Item, Single-Dimension Scales for Fatigue

Instrument/Scales	Description	Psychometric Indices
Likert-type scales Numeric rating scales (e.g., 0–10 NMR) Visual Analog Scales	Measure intensity of subjective fatigue Efficient to use clinically Appropriate for repeated measurements during a 24-hour period Not suitable for in-depth studies of fatigue as measures only fatigue intensity (153)	Correlate well with other single dimension, multi-item intensity scales (e.g., Profile of Mood States Fatigue-Inertia Subscale, Pearson-Byars Fatigue Feeling Tone Checklist) and the multidimensional Piper Fatigue Scale-Revised (30)
Rhoten Fatigue Scale (154,155)	Single-item, 11-point graphic rating scale (not tired, full of energy to totally exhausted) Developed to measure fatigue in 5 surgical patients Simple to administer and score	Minimal psychometric testing (156) Further testing warranted

Numbers in parenthesis correspond to studies cited in the References.

Table 34.3 Multiple-Item, Single-Dimension Fatigue Scales

Instrument/Scales	Description	Psychometric Indices
Brief Fatigue Inventory (BFI) (45,67,54)	9-item, 0–10 fatigue intensity scale; includes items such as usual and worst levels of fatigue (e.g., weariness, tiredness) in the past 24 hours, and interference in general activity Averaging 9 items gives a global fatigue severity score Scoring established for 1–3 (mild), 4–6 (moderate), and 7–10 (severe) fatigue levels	Internal consistency (0.96) in cancer patients Concurrent, construct and discriminant validity in cancer patients (45) Further testing warranted
Cancer-related Fatigue Distress Scale (57,58)	20-item scale Each item measured on a 0–10 scale Third-grade reading level Developed to measure fatigue distress in cancer patients	Internal consistency (0.98) Construct validity Further testing warranted
Dutch Exertion Fatigue Scale (68)	9-item self-report scale that measures fatigue that occurs with exertion during daily household, personal hygiene, and social activities Each item scored on a 0–4 scale, then recoded as a dichotomous variable Total scores range between 0 and 9 Cut scores have been established	Internal consistency (0.91) Construct and criterion-related validity Further testing warranted
Dutch Fatigue Scale (68)	9-item self-report scale Each item measured on a 0–4 scale then converted to a dichotomous score Total scores range between 0 and 9 Cut scores established Tested initially in congestive heart failure patients	Internal consistency adequate Construct and criterion-related validity adequate Further testing warranted
EORTC-QLQ-C30 Fatigue Subscale (162)	3-item fatigue scale incorporated into the European Organization for Research and Treatment of Cancer 30-item Quality of Life Scale Measures intensity of fatigue (e.g., during the past week, did you need to rest, have you felt weak, were you tired?) Each item scored on a 4-point Verbal Rating Scale (not at all, a little, quite a bit, and very much) Not suitable for in-depth studies of fatigue as a limited number of responses are possible and only fatigue intensity measured (153)	Internal consistency of fatigue scale (0.80) Evidence of discriminant validity Translated and tested in several cancer patient samples, particularly in Europe Further testing warranted

Table 34.3 Multiple-Item, Single-Dimension Fatigue Scales

Instrument/Scales	Description	Psychometric Indices
Fatigue Severity Scale (FSS) (22,155,163–165)	9-item self-report scale, originally developed to measure fatigue in patients with multiple sclerosis or systemic lupus erythematosus (70) Responses indicate degree of agreement on a 7-point Likert scale with each statement (1 = strongly disagree, to 7 = strongly agree) The 9 items combined into a total fatigue score	Internal consistency established. Correlates well with visual analogue scales Discriminates between patients and controls Detects clinically predicted changes in fatigue over time Tested and translated into several languages (165); considered a good measure of fatigue in patients with chronic fatigue syndrome (166) Further testing warranted
Functional Assessment of Cancer Therapy Fatigue Subscale (FACT-F) (43,153,167)	The FACT-F consists of both the 28-item FACT-General that measures health-related quality of life and the 13-item Fatigue Severity Scale The Fatigue Severity Scale includes items such as "feel weak all over" and "have energy" Each item is rated on a 5-point Likert scale ranging from 0 = "not at all" to 4 = "very much so"	The FACT-F has good internal consistency and test–retest reliability (0.90 and 0.95) Tested in cancer patients; may have some items that are difficult for patients to understand or to translate into other languages (45) Good concurrent and discriminant validity Construct validity not reported Further testing warranted
Global Fatigue Index (GFI) (66)	The GFI uses 15 of the 16 items of the MAF (61–63), a scale derived from the original Piper Fatigue Scale (33) to measure fatigue in rheumatoid arthritis patients	Construct validity Single dimension confirmed by factor analysis (60) Internal consistency (0.96) and divergent validity good. Further testing warranted
Mental Fatigue Inventory (64)	9-item measure of mental fatigue symptoms (e.g., poor concentration) 5-point Likert scale (0 "not at all," 4 "very much")	Reported to have good internal consistency and beginning discriminant validity in British patients with chronic fatigue syndrome, depression, and healthy controls Further testing warranted
Medical Outcomes Study—Short Form-36 Vitality Subscale (168–170)	A generic measure of health-related quality of life Has a 4-item vitality subscale that includes the following questions measured over the past 4 weeks: Did you feel full of pep? Did you have a lot of energy? Did you feel worn out? Did you feel tired? Measures fatigue intensity	Has good construct and discriminant validity and internal consistency reliability estimates (168) Colloquialisms may be a problem in translation Further testing warranted
Multidimensional Assessment of Fatigue Scale (60–63, 155)	Revised version of original Piper Fatigue Scale (33) 16 items supposedly measure 4 dimensions of fatigue (severity-2 items, distress-1, degree of interference in ADLs-11, timing-2) Easy to administer and relatively easy to score Severity, distress and interference items scaled from 0 to 10; frequency item is categoric (0–4) (44,171)	Internal consistency: Cronbach's alpha: 0.93 (rheumatoid patients), 0.88 (cancer patients) Not recommended for use in cancer patients (44) Factor structure not stable across studies Two to four factors may result (155) and some consider the scale unidimensional (44,60) Further testing warranted

548

Pearson-Byars Fatigue Feeling Tone Checklist (172)	10-item Adjective Rating Scale Subjects rate whether they feel "same as," "worse than," or "better than" Adjectives are rated on a 1 = "very peppy," to 10 = "ready to drop" scale Numbers summed to give a total fatigue score (8–20)	Good internal consistency (0.82–0.97) and test–retest reliability (45) Limitations: Colloquialism, and patients may have difficulty knowing how to respond to certain items 3-point rating scale may not provide enough variability to assess different levels of fatigue (45) Further testing warranted
Profile of Mood States Fatigue (POMS-F) and Vigor Subscales (POMS-V) (148,149)	The POMS-F is a 7-item fatigue severity scale that includes such items as "bushed" and "worn out" The POMS-V is an 8-item vigor scale that includes such items as "alert," "full of pep" Both subscales rated using a 5-point Likert scale	Both scales are brief but have colloquialisms that may hinder translation (45) A shorter 30-item POMS and respective vigor and 5-item fatigue scale is available (149) The 5-item F-POMS-Short Form performed well with internal consistency, stability, construct and concurrent validity, and responsiveness in one cancer study (44) Further testing warranted

Numbers in parenthesis correspond to studies cited in the References.

Table 34.4 Multidimensional Fatigue Scales

Instrument/Scales	Description	Psychometric Indices
Cancer Fatigue Scale (56)	15-item scale with 3 subscales: physical, affective, cognitive Each item rated on a 1 (not at all) to 5 (very much) scale Score range 0–28 (physical), 0–16 (affective), and 0–16 (cognitive) Maximum score: 60 Designed for cancer patients	Good internal consistency (0.76–0.87), construct and concurrent validity Further testing warranted
Chalder Fatigue Scale (72)	11-item, self-report scale that measures intensity of mental (4 items) and physical (7 items) fatigue symptoms Items rated on a 4-point, 0–3 Likert scale ("better than usual," to "much worse than usual") Scores on each item are summed to give a total fatigue score (173)	Construct validity via factor analyses (173) Cronbach's alpha (0.89) Face validity and reasonable discriminant validity in adult (174), pediatric (175), and general practice patients (176) Has not demonstrated an ability to discriminate between different subtypes of individuals with fatigue (166) Further testing warranted
Fatigue Assessment Questionnaire (59)	20-item scale with 3 subscales: physical, affective, cognitive Each item measured on a 4-point scale Measures intensity and distress during the past week and previous month Developed to measure fatigue in cancer patients	Good construct validity and reliability Further testing warranted
Fatigue Attribution Scale (177)	20-item scale with 3 subscales: normalizing, psychologic, somatic Each item scored on a 4-point Likert scale for symptom frequency (0 = not at all to 3 = all the time) Developed to measure fatigue in French primary care patients	Low reliability of subscales (somatic [0.64], psychologic [0.53], and normalcy [0.37]) Factor analysis showed 3 factors, with somatic subscale having the strongest psychometric properties Instrument needs further development and testing before it can be recommended
Fatigue Impact Scale (42)	40-item scale to measure fatigue's impact on function: cognition (10 items), physical (10 items), and psychosocial (20 items) in MS patients Items rated according to degree a fatigue-related problem exists (0 "no problem" to 4 "extreme problem") Maximum score = 160	Grade 8 reading level High internal consistency reliabilities (Cronbach's alpha > 0.87) Confirmatory factor analysis and additional testing warranted
Fatigue/Stamina Scale (178)	25-item Likert scale: fatigue (11 items) and physical stamina (14 items)	Cronbach's alphas: 0.89 (fatigue), 0.87 (stamina) Significant Pearson's correlations: fatigue scale and Profile of Mood States fatigue/inertia scale = 0.79; stamina scale and POMS vigor/activity scale = 0.62 Stamina significantly and inversely related to fatigue Further testing warranted

Measure	Description	Reliability/Validity
Fatigue Symptom Checklist (FSCL) (41–43, 77, 147, 179, 180)	30-item scale with three fatigue symptom factors: (1) decline in motivation or concentration (mental fatigue), (2) general feelings of fatigue, (3) specific feelings of fatigue incongruity (e.g., stiff shoulders) Fatigue feelings (e.g., want to lie down) more frequent than mental fatigue or specific feelings of incongruity The more numerous the fatigue symptoms, the higher the fatigue intensity (73,181) Dichotomous (yes/no) & modified scaling has been developed (rating the presence, absence, and intensity of each symptom on 1–4 or 1–5 Likert scale) (98,180) Items tailored to specific subjects (21,37) Two forms developed and tested based on the original FSCL in a series of childbearing studies: a Fatigue Identification Form and a Fatigue Continuum Form (77)	Reliability and validity estimates not always reported in studies Principal component analysis (construct validity) on modified FSCL in studies of pregnant and postpartum women: 6 factors extracted (subjective weariness, decreased concentration, psychologic, physical, head and neck, and physical/generalized) (76) Further testing warranted
Fatigue Symptom Inventory (69,70)	13-item scale with 3 subscales: intensity (4 items) duration (2 items) and interference (7 items) Each item measured on an 11-point numeric rating scale (0–10) Developed specifically for cancer patients	Good concurrent and discriminant validity (70) Low test–retest reliability (182), good internal consistency (0.94) (70) Further testing warranted
HIV-Related Fatigue Scale (71)	58-item scale thought to measure three dimensions of HIV-related fatigue: intensity, circumstances surrounding fatigue, and fatigue consequences Developed by incorporating items from 5 previously developed fatigue scales Most items evaluated using a 1–10 rating scale with word anchors 1 ("not at all") to 10 ("a great deal") for the past week	Good internal consistency (0.94) for total scale and for 3 subscales (0.73–0.95) Further testing warranted
Lee's Visual Analog Scale for Fatigue (VAS-F)(44,78,155,158)	18-item scale with 2 subscales: energy (5 items) and fatigue (13 items) All items use visual analogue scales (VAS) although others have changed the VASs to numeric rating scales (1–10) with word anchors added (44,171)	Internal consistency (Cronbach's alpha): 0.91–0.96 (fatigue); 0.94–0.96 (energy) Concurrent validity established by Pearson's correlations (VAS-F compared to Stanford Sleepiness Scale and the POMS fatigue-inertia and vigor-activity subscales) Reliabilities (patients with myocardial infarction) 0.86 (fatigue), 0.83 (energy) (183) In the revised scale, construct validity and good internal consistency obtained Stability was achieved for the energy subscale in one study (44) In another study, three factors were found: "no fatigue," "fatigue," and "energetic" (155) Further testing warranted

Table 34.4 *Continued*

Instrument/Scales	Description	Psychometric Indices
Multidimensional Fatigue Inventory (184–187)	20 items using 5-point Likert scaling 5 subscales/dimensions: general, physical, mental fatigue, reduction in motivation, and reduction in activity Each subscale has 4 items No summated grand total of the 20 items Takes approximately 10 minutes to complete	Internal consistency reliabilities for the 5 subscales adequate (44,185,186) Construct and concurrent validity estimates established and at times vary by different patient populations (44,182) Suggested by some that with the exception of the mental fatigue scale, the remaining subscales behave similarly, thus blurring the distinction or relevancy between these dimensions (153) Further testing warranted
Multidimensional Fatigue Symptom Inventory (65)	Two versions: An 83-item scale with 5 subscales: global fatigue, somatic, affective, behavioral, and cognitive; takes 5–10 minutes to complete A 30-item scale with 5 subscales: general fatigue, physical, emotional, mental, and vigor Each item is measured on a 5-point scale (0 = "not at all" to 4 = "extremely") over the previous 7 days	Good internal consistency and test–retest reliabilities for both scales Good evidence for concurrent, convergent, divergent, and construct validity Tested only in women with breast cancer Further testing warranted
Piper Fatigue Scale-Revised (PFS-R) (46,157,158)	22-item scale with 4 subscales revised from originally developed PFS (33): behavioral/severity, affective meaning, sensory, and cognitive/mood. Plus 3 open-ended items that measure perceived causes of fatigue, relief measures, and associated symptoms Each item measured on an 11-item (0–10) numeric rating scale Total fatigue and subscale scores are calculated and range between 0 and 10 Easy to score and administer Scores for mild (1–3), moderate (4–6), and severe (7–10) established in breast and prostate cancer patients (30) Takes 2–5 minutes to complete	Consistently good reliability and validity estimates across different patient and cultural samples (159,160) (B.F. Piper, personal communication, June 12, 2003) Most widely used and translated scale Further testing warranted (46,156)

Profile of Fatigue-Related Symptoms (161)	54-item measure of chronic fatigue syndrome (CFS) symptoms 4 scales: emotional distress, cognitive difficulty, somatic symptoms, fatigue Each item assessed "during the past week" on a 7-point rating scale (0 not at all, 6 extremely)	4 factors confirmed by factor analysis Estimates good for convergent validity, test–retest reliability, internal consistency (British subjects with CFS/postviral fatigue syndrome) Further testing warranted
Schwartz Cancer Fatigue Scale (47,66)	Two versions: A 28-item scale with four subscales: physical, emotional, cognitive, and temporal Each item measured on a 5-point scale A shorter version of 6 items, each measured by a 5-point scale (1 = not at all to 5 = extremely) Shorter version measures two dimensions of cancer-related fatigue: physical and perceptual	Good reliability and construct and discriminant validity estimates for both versions Further testing warranted

Numbers in parenthesis correspond to studies cited in the References.

Table 34.5   Historic Overview of Fatigue Measurement and Study

1920–1929	Muscio (35) states that fatigue is composed of multiple unrelated phenomena and suggests that fatigue cannot be defined; Poffenberger develops the first single-item measure of tiredness (188)
1930–1939	No major developments occurred or reported.
1940–1949	Cameron (92) and Bartley (189) state that fatigue's complexity makes definition difficult; first fatigue textbook written (36)
1950–1959	First physiologic theory proposed that fatigue is caused by central and peripheral nervous system mechanisms (97); first multi-item intensity scale, the Fatigue Feeling Tone Checklist, tested in airmen (172); first report linking the occurrence of fatigue with pain (190); first anecdotal interventions reported (191)
1960–1969	First international fatigue conference held (192) with noted fatigue theorists (73,95)
1970–1979	First multidimensional fatigue scale, the Fatigue Symptom Checklist tested in healthy Japanese workers (73–75,179); nurses conduct the first patient fatigue studies (21,147,193); first study to document that an increased feeling of fatigue occurs at a specific intensity level (74); the first symptom distress scale developed (150); first study to document that MS patients have more severe fatigue than normal controls and that this is related to the patient's mobility status (193); first fatigue study in radiation therapy patients published (147) that sought to identify a biologic marker for fatigue; first study to examine the relationship between an environmental stimulus (e.g., noise) and fatigue (37); first review article on postoperative fatigue (194); first study describing fatigue in chemotherapy patients published (195); second classic fatigue textbook published (196)
1980–1989	Key fatigue publications (8,41,93) and emergence of quality of life (QOL) and its importance (152); first nonpharmacologic cancer studies to treat fatigue reported (27); first biotherapy and fatigue studies conducted (197,198); emergence of chronic fatigue syndrome; initial testing of the Piper Fatigue Scale (33); fatigue accepted as a nursing diagnosis (199); first national scientific nursing meeting held for fatigue, pain, and nausea (200)
1990–1999	Managed care emergence with emphasis on outcomes and evidence-based practice guidelines; first state of the science paper on cancer-related fatigue (6); first studies linking anemia, epoetin alfa, fatigue, and QOL (89); national cancer fatigue initiatives begun in United States (201), Canada, and Europe cosponsored by cancer nursing organizations (i.e., Oncology Nursing Society, Canadian Oncology Nursing Organization, and European Oncology Nursing Society and pharmaceutical firms (i.e., OrthoBiotech and Janssen-Cilag); Cancer Fatigue Coalition formed (OrthoBiotech) (202); First national multidisciplinary scientific cancer fatigue meeting held in Houston, TX at M.D. Anderson Cancer Center; additional nonpharmacologic trials reported (27) and pharmacologic studies to treat fatigue initiated (203)
2000–present	Additional non-anemia-related drug intervention studies to treat fatigue in cancer (204,205) and HIV/AIDS initiated (158); first neurotransmitter–circadian rhythm cancer fatigue studies reported (24,100); first report on cancer fatigue and symptom clusters (109); first cancer fatigue and sleep (206) and energy conservation intervention studies reported (207); first cancer survivor and cytokine study published (208); first evidence-based cancer fatigue guidelines published that continues to be revised annually (27); first NIH consensus conference on cancer pain, fatigue, and depression (49)

and the extent of disease[3] and has been found to be significantly associated with fatigue in one large study.[213] Anemia is a common side effect of chemotherapy treatments[214] and end-stage renal disease (ESRD).[215] Almost all ESRD patients[215] and 50% to 60% of cancer patients will experience anemia.[216, 217] Anemia has been associated with increased fatigue,[45] decreased QOL, and decreased ability to perform activities of daily living.[88] Anemia may affect cognitive function and mental fatigue in cancer and chronic renal disease patients[214,215] and may adversely affect cancer survival.[88] When patients respond to epoetin alfa treatment,[89, 218] less fatigue and fewer declines in functional status and improvements in QOL are reported, suggesting that effective treatment of anemia can be associated with the amelioration of fatigue in some circumstances.

Comorbidities

In cancer[2,173] and MS patients,[28] the presence of comorbidities has been linked to higher fatigue levels. Thyroid disorders such as hypothyroidism have been postulated to be associated with fatigue, but this has not been well-studied. Thyroid disorders often go undiagnosed[219, 220] and untreated. In one study that examined this variable as a possible late effect of treatment, 70% of cancer survivors had subclinical or clinical hypothyroidism, as measured by serum thyroid-stimulating hormone levels, compared to a 31% to 78% prevalence rate reported in other studies.[212] Surprisingly, patients who were receiving hormone replacement therapy for their hypothyroidism were more fatigued than those diagnosed with hypothyroidism who were not being treated. Further study examining these relationships is needed.[219]

Disease Variables

There are conflicting data as to whether disease stage and severity, extent, or duration of illness are related to fatigue. Some studies have found positive relationships,[2,3,28,220–225] while others have not.[26,211,212,226,227] In one systemic lupus erythematosus (SLE) study, fatigue scores were 33% higher in women with active versus inactive disease; yet women with quiescent disease report significant fatigue, suggesting that the relationship between SLE disease activity and fatigue may be nonlinear.[220]

Deconditioning, Muscle Wasting, and Weakness

Patients who are fatigued often are counseled to get more rest which may not be in their best interest. Such reliance on rest can lead to an ever increasing downward spiral of inactivity, deconditioning, and increased fatigue.[6,12,26] Loss of muscle strength and mass are thought to increase the risk for fatigue[10,26] but have not been well studied in relationship to fatigue. Weakness may precede the feeling of fatigue, depending on the reasons for weakness (e.g., muscle deconditioning, therapeutic regimen, or disease state).[11]

Sarcopenia, or a loss in muscle mass, is associated with androgen ablation therapy in men with metastatic prostate cancer[228] due to decreased testosterone levels that result from therapy. Similar relationships between muscle wasting and fatigue have been proposed in testosterone-deficient men treated for HIV/AIDS.[3]

Depression and Anxiety

Although mood disturbances such as anxiety and depression are frequently reported to be associated with fatigue,[12,139,220,229–231] there are conflicting findings. Some studies have found positive correlations,[22,33,62,87,180,181,232,233] but others have not.[22,181,234]

Many somatic symptoms of depression can overlap with the somatic symptoms of fatigue caused by disease states or treatments.[52] Fatigue is often a presenting symptom of depression. Sleep disturbances, such as insomnia, multiple awakenings during sleep, and early waking, are common in depression and may contribute to fatigue. In contrast, fatigue can occur in the absence of depression or may cause depression itself because of its negative impact on perceived quality of life. Although depression may occur with fatigue, it is important to differentiate between the two as care and therapies will differ depending on the condition or circumstance.[5] Fatigue also can predict negative mood,[235] and is significantly associated with greater psychologic distress,[213] illustrating the strong interplay that may exist between these states.[235]

Methodologically, many depression inventories have been designed specifically for use in psychiatric populations and are not easily tailored to measure reactive depression in the general population. Since most depression inventories contain both somatic and cognitive/affective items to diagnose depression, false-positives can result when these inventories are used to diagnose depression in the medically ill.[52,236,237]

When depression was assessed in one study using only the nonsomatic items of the Center for Epidemiologic Survey of Depression Inventory (CES-D), Smets and Visser[238] documented different trajectory patterns of fatigue and depression over time in cancer patients receiving radiotherapy. Other studies continued to find significant correlations between depression and fatigue even after controlling for the more somatic items on depression scales,[7] which suggests that there may be common underlying mechanisms for the two states.

Considering the frequency with which anxiety and depression go undiagnosed and untreated clinically,[220] more attention should to be given to diagnosing and treating these problems, particularly when considering treatment options for fatigue. Holland and colleagues[239] have suggested that health care professionals begin to use the term *psychologic distress* when assessing and treating these disorders to reduce the societal stigma associated with them.

Environment

Environmental factors, such as altitude or the use of assistive equipment to conserve energy, have not been well studied.[5] Since dyspnea can precede and be correlated with fatigue in COPD patients,[240,241] environmental conditions that exacerbate dyspnea, such as "tobacco smoke, strong odours and the weather"[242] may need to be assessed when measuring and managing fatigue in these patients. Heat sensitivity affects 60% to 80% of patients with MS and has been associated with worsening fatigue and neurologic function with as little as a 0.5-degree Fahrenheit change in core body temperature.[26,28] This suggests that maintaining a controlled temperature environment may be important when measuring changes in fatigue over time in these patients.

Medications

Most medications are associated with fatigue. These include antihistamines, anticholinergic agents, beta-blockers,[41] centrally acting alpha-blockers, and central nervous system depressants such as narcotics and hypnotics.[12,27] In one SLE study, higher fatigue levels were significantly associated with the administration of hydroxychloroquine, but not with prednisolone or azathioprine.[220] In MS patients, medications used to treat MS symptoms and other comorbidities are associated with fatigue.[28] In the elderly, as the number of medications increases, so too does the level of fatigue.[243]

Morbidity and Mortality

Fatigue in some circumstances may affect morbidity[244] and mortality.[245-248] In one cardiac study,[249] fatigue was the strongest predictor of a subsequent myocardial infarction. Clearly, more attention should be given to including these outcome variables in fatigue studies. Treatment of anemia with epoetin alfa in cancer patients has been linked to improvements in fatigue and quality of life, and may also be linked to improved survival rates in patients who respond to epoetin alfa treatment.[88,250]

Race, Ethnicity, and Culture

Few studies have examined racial, ethnic, or cultural factors and how these may be related not only to the incidence of fatigue, but also to its patterns and expression.[68,159,160,251] In one study, higher levels of fatigue were reported in non-Caucasian versus Caucasian pregnant women,[252] and in another study, more gastrointestinal symptoms were attributed to fatigue by Korean women than by their American counterparts.[253] Although several fatigue studies have been conducted in different cultures, most have addressed English-speaking, Caucasian samples,[53,228,240,254] with few published exceptions.[2,159,160,251,255,256]

Sex

Female gender may be a risk factor;[5] for others it is not,[212] or the findings are conflicting.[5,138] Females are more likely to receive a fatigue diagnosis in cancer,[210,257,258] CFS,[14] and HIV/AIDS[213] than males. In one study, men were significantly more tired than women.[259]

Socioeconomic Level

Few studies have examined the relationship between socioeconomic factors and fatigue. Although a higher socioeconomic level is considered a risk factor for CFS, the data are conflicting.[14,212]

Symptom Burden and Distress

Fatigue can occur as a primary symptom by itself, but more often it occurs in conjunction with other symptoms, such as pain,[228,260] insomnia,[6,56,261] or dyspnea.[56,228,240] As a consequence, increased attention is now being given to identifying symptoms that most frequently occur together as a symptom complex or cluster with fatigue and under what circumstances.[108]

Many studies have documented that as the number of symptoms and distress from these symptoms other than fatigue increase, fatigue intensity levels increase.[13,96,146,262,263] In one study, path analysis revealed that symptom distress, defined as problems with nausea, vomiting, and sleep, offered the best direct explanation for fatigue in women receiving chemotherapy for early-stage breast cancer.[262] In another study, unrelieved symptom distress two weeks post surgery for early-stage breast cancer predicted attentional fatigue in older women three months post surgery.[13] Patients with lung cancer, COPD, asthma, and pulmonary hypertension have difficulty distinguishing dyspnea from fatigue when they occur together,[264] which reinforces the need to measure and treat symptom complexes. In patients with AIDS, fatigue was significantly correlated with the number of AIDS-related physical symptoms, including pain.[265] Similarly, significant correlations between fatigue and the number and severity of other symptoms are reported in ESRD patients.[138]

In general, sleep disorders have not been well studied in clinical populations,[12] nor has insomnia and its specific relationship to fatigue and other variables.[266] In the general population, insomnia is associated with an increased risk of anxiety and depression,[267] decreased daytime performance,[268] and decreased functional status.[269] Consistent across studies is the finding that disturbances in sleep are related to increases in fatigue severity.[98,163] In one study, fatigued HIV/AIDS patients were significantly more likely to "sleep and nap more and have decreased mid-morning alertness (i.e., cognitive fatigue) than HIV-seronegative individuals."[3]

Two studies using wrist actigraphy in cancer patients have documented positive relationships between the number of nighttime awakenings and higher daytime fatigue levels.[261,270] Similarly, 50% of ESRD patients report restless sleep patterns.[271] Problems with sleep in ESRD are significantly correlated not only with fatigue[139] but also with higher fatigue levels.[259]

Poor sleep quality affects nearly two thirds of SLE patients, and moderate correlations with fatigue have been documented.[220] Sleep disruptions and anxiety about sleep were the most significant proximal variables linked to fatigue in SLE patients,[272] suggesting that further studies are warranted in this area.

Treatment

Interest is growing in studying fatigue not only as an acute effect of medical treatment, such as surgery,[273] but also as a more long-term or late effect of treatment,[160,212,274] deliveries,[275] and disease and/or treatment.[169] Most studies currently are cross-sectional.[228] Limited longitudinal data exist that examine the relationships over time between fatigue and late treatment effects. One Norwegian study of Hodgkin's disease patients in remission for more than 5 years brought patients in for follow-up fatigue studies and documented higher fatigue levels in patients who had treatment-induced pulmonary dysfunction.[212]

Quality of Life, Functioning, and Employment Status

Many patients report that fatigue negatively affects their QOL,[202,241] physical well-being, ability to walk long distances, and ability to socialize and work.[241,276] Studies are needed that examine the extent to which fatigue affects patients' abilities not only to return to work but how long it takes them to return to work, as well as its effects on maintaining or resuming full-time work status.[5] Fatigue can decrease work capacity in cancer patients, as measured by symptom-limited cycle ergometry.[212,269]

Increased levels of fatigue are associated with decreases in activities of daily living and performance status. Two studies have documented marked declines in physical functioning in cancer patients when fatigue intensity scores are at level 7 on a 0 to 10 NMR scale.[45,46] When compared to seronegative individuals, 50% of HIV/AIDS patients state that fatigue interferes with their activities of daily living, and these patients were significantly more likely to be unemployed.[213] Several studies in HIV infection and cancer have documented the negative effects that fatigue has on all domains of QOL.[3,91,151,213]

Objective and Biologic Markers

Unfortunately, few studies have included biologic or physiologic measures in their designs. Thus, the ability to correlate perceptions of fatigue to physiologic measures is limited. Identifying correlations between subjective and objective indicators of fatigue remains difficult[139] and has not been consistently fruitful, possibly because of problems in the measurement's timing and the potential for measurement error.[11] As more valid and reliable measures of fatigue are incorporated into studies and the coordination between the timing of subjective and objective testing is improved, progress will be made[23] to determine whether this lack of correlation reflects imprecise measurement or a true lack of association.[11]

Changes in oral and forehead temperatures in MS patients[21] and weight declines in cancer patients[96,147] have been found to correlate with self-reports of fatigue. Other empiric studies have documented negative correlations between self-reports of fatigue and pH, oxygen saturation, and cardiac ejection fractions in congestive heart failure patients[277] and decreases in physical activity and grip strength behaviorally in arthritis patients,[61] but the preponderance of fatigue self-report studies show no relationship to physiologic measures.[146] Similar findings are reported in studies that have examined relationships between other symptoms and their possible physiologic indicators.[278]

In one study, no significant correlations were found between fatigue and hemoglobin, hematocrit, albumin, and total protein values in HIV/AIDS patients,[279] whereas in another study, higher fatigue levels and more hours slept at night were associated with lower CD4+ counts and higher serum lactate dehydrogenase levels.[221] Conflicting data exist that link levels of anemia with fatigue. In one dialysis study, fatigue improved with epoetin alfa treatment in a randomized clinical trial,[280] whereas no relationship was found between epoetin alfa and fatigue in descriptive studies,[146,250] which suggests that design or methodologic issues may be involved. Similarly, no correlations have been documented between surrogate markers for liver disease and fatigue in hepatitis C infection.[227,281] In MS patients, subjective reports of mental and physical fatigue have not correlated with objective measures of cognitive functioning[282,283] or changes in motor activity,[203] whereas decreased central nervous system glucose metabolism has correlated.[284]

Selected cytokines have been found to correlate with fatigue in radiation therapy patients[124,125] and breast cancer survivors,[169] but there are conflicting results when cytokine studies have been conducted in MS patients.[7,26]

Studying these relationships is complicated not only by the diurnal fluctuations that may affect the timing and measurement of these indicators, but also by the complex nature of their relationships. For example, "physiological variables can be profoundly abnormal without the patient having any symptoms."[278] In contrast, a wide variety of symptoms may be present, as in the case of chronic fatigue syndrome and other disorders, but no physiologic abnormality or etiology can be documented.

Because of the inconsistent relationship between symptoms and physiologic indicators, Wilson and Cleary conclude that it is unlikely that treatments directed only at biologic factors, even if they can be identified, will be completely effective in the relief of symptoms.[278] These authors suggest that other things, such as social and psychologic factors, patient expectations, and relationships to health care providers, may need to be explored as well.[278] Whether this holds true for the study of fatigue remains to be seen.

Summary

Many advances have been made in the measurement and study of fatigue, but studies continue to be needed in a number of areas. In addition to those previously mentioned, priority should be given to basic fatigue research, to identify the possible underlying mechanisms for fatigue in clinical populations.[5]

Studies are needed to identify fatigue patterns over time and to see how these may be related to demographic, disease, and treatment variables. Fatigue intensity scores should be reported not only as means, percents, and median values, but also in terms of no, mild, moderate, and severe levels with relevant correlation and regression analyses. This will enable professionals to predict better who is at risk for fatigue and when in the course of disease or treatment the trajectory of fatigue can be expected to occur.[5] More studies are needed that establish what constitutes clinically and statistically significant changes in fatigue scores over time,[158,285] as well as how to control for or measure symptom response shift[286,287] or reframing over time,[288] when patients change their internal standard or meaning of fatigue based on experience. Studies also are needed to evaluate whether measuring fatigue multidimensionally furnishes any additional or essential information over and above simply asking the patient about intensity alone, and when and for whom this would be true.

Future studies must include patients who are receiving palliative or terminal care[289-291] and individuals who are receiving preventive care because they are at high risk for disease or its recurrence. Evidence-based practice guidelines and diagnostic criteria should be tested in practice.[19,20,27] Since fatigue may complex or cluster with other symptoms, studies are needed that document these relationships and changes in these relationships over time. In summary, much work remains to be done to incorporate the measurement of fatigue into practice settings, to identify underlying fatigue mechanisms, and to prescribe effective therapies.

The exemplar study described below was selected because it represents a well-designed fatigue intervention study, employs a number of reliable and valid multidimensional measures, identifies what constitutes a clinically and statistically significant improvement in fatigue over time, employs appropriate and sophisticated statistical procedures, and uses physiologic measures to determine objective correlates of subjective fatigue.

Exemplar Study

Breitbart, W., Rosenfeld, B., Kaim, M., & Funesti-Euch, J. A randomized, double-blind, placebo-controlled trial of psychostimulants for the treatment of fatigue in ambulatory patients with human immunodeficiency virus disease. *Arch Intern Med,* 2001, *161*:411-420.

Purposes: The primary purpose of this RCT was to compare the efficacy of two psychostimulant medications, methylphenidate hydrochloride (Ritalin) and pemoline (Cylert) to placebo in treating fatigue in HIV/AIDS patients. Secondary purposes included evaluating medication adherence, safety, and tolerability, and treatment efficacy on quality of life and psychologic distress outcomes.

Conceptual Framework: Implied, none made explicit.

Design Methods: Phase I dose-escalating, double-blind, placebo-controlled 6-week RCT.

Sample Methods: In addition to other exclusion and inclusion criteria, all patients at baseline had to have persistent fatigue (present for at least 2 weeks or more) rated 5 on a 0–10 NMR scale. A total of 213 subjects underwent screening; 144 were randomized to one of three study arms and 109 completed the 6-week study. Subjects were included in the final analyses if they had completed 3 of the 7 assessment visits.

Setting: One large New York City (NYC) Medical Center.

Instruments: Fatigue measures included the Revised Piper Fatigue Scale (PFS-R)[46] (primary dependent variable) and the Lee Visual Analogue Scale for Fatigue Severity (VAS-F).[78] Other variables measured included physical functioning (Karnofsky Performance Status), muscular endurance (timed isometric unilateral straight leg-raising task), health-related quality of life (MOS-SF-36), symptoms (Brief Symptom Inventory), depression (Beck Depression Inventory), side effects and adverse events (Systematic Assessment for Treatment Emergent Events and Extra-pyramidal Symptoms Rating Scale), complete blood counts, and blood chemistry panels. Baseline and end-of-study neuropsychological testing was conducted, but these results were not reported in this article.

Procedures: Subjects were recruited from a variety of NYC agencies and were seen in person weekly for 6 weeks in addition to being contacted between visits several times per week by the research nurse. Subjects were paid $25 for each visit. All fatigue and assessment measures, including weights and pill counts, were completed weekly.

Data Analyses: Pearson product-moment correlations, fatigue change scores over time (baseline to end of 6 weeks), ANOVA, MANOVA, ANCOVA, and hierarchic linear modeling were used to compare regression slopes of fatigue and rate of fatigue change scores over time, by treatment arm, and by disease status.

Findings: Randomization produced equivalent groups on all demographic, clinical, and medical variables. Blinding was effective, and 91% were medication adherent. The three groups differed significantly in terms of fatigue improvement scores (PFS-R total and affective and sensory scores) (range in effect sizes: 0.24–0.28) and VAS-F energy scores (effect size: 0.23). No significant group differences were noted for PFS-R cognitive or severity scores or for VAS-F total or fatigue subscale scores. Patients were classified as having clinically significant improvements in their fatigue scores over time if their PFS-R total scores decreased by 5 or more points or their VAS-F total fatigue scores decreased by 50 mm or more. Using these criteria, 41% of patients taking methylphenidate and 38% taking pemoline had improved fatigue scores over time compared to 15% in the placebo group. There were statistically significant and more rapid decreases in PFS-R total scores for both psychostimulant groups than for the placebo group. Changes between the two psychostimulant groups' fatigue scores did not significantly differ. Thus, there were no significant interaction effects, indicating that the improvements in fatigue scores in the two treatment groups were not related to "disease severity, extent of depressive symptoms, concomitant antidepressant medications, sex, race, or risk transmission factor" (p. 416). Changes in Beck Depression Inventory scores, Brief Symptom Inventory Global Distress Scores, and MOS-SF-36 subscales were significantly correlated with improved PFS-R total and VAS-F total fatigue scores. Thus, both psychostimulants appear to be equally effective in reducing HIV/AIDS-related fatigue. "The strongest, most consistent, and statistically significant group differences were evident on . . . the PFS" (p. 418). There was no treatment effect demonstrated on the timed endurance test.

Limitations: Short duration of study, limited method to monitor medication adherence, small sample size and attrition rates, and absence of reported lab values.

Practice and Research Implications: Weekly multidimensional measurement of fatigue was not found to be unduly burdensome to the patients in this study. The reported effect sizes and the clinically significant change score indicators need to be examined and replicated in other samples and studies. The study's inclusion and exclusion methods provide useful guidance to future designs. The positive effects that the psychostimulants had on fatigue need replication and extension. The fact that 38% to 41% of the subjects responded with decreased fatigue scores in the treatment groups is excellent, but it also suggests that other mechanisms may be operating to cause fatigue in this group of patients, suggesting that multimodal or combination therapies might be pursued in future studies.

Selected Internet Resources

www.cancersymptoms.org
www.consensus.nih.gov/ta/022/022_statement.htm
www.nccn.org
www.nationalmssociety.org/sourcebook-fatigue.asp
www.thebody.com/treat/fatigue.html

References

1. Glaus, A. Assessment of fatigue in cancer and no-cancer patients. *J Supportive Care Cancer*, 1993, 1:305-315.
2. Glaus, A., Crow, R., & Hammond, S. A qualitative study to explore the concept of fatigue/tiredness in cancer patients and healthy individuals. *J Supportive Care Cancer*, 1996, 4:82-86.
3. Groopman, J.E. Fatigue and cancer and HIV/AIDS. *Oncology*, 1998, 12(3):335-344.
4. Gutstein, H.B. The biologic basis of fatigue. *Cancer* (September 15 Suppl), 2001, 92(6):1678-1683.
5. Piper, B.F. (2003). Fatigue. In V. Carrieri-Kohlman, A.M. Lindsey, & C.M. West (Eds.), *Pathophysiological*

phenomena in nursing (3rd ed.). Philadelphia: Saunders, 2003, pp. 209-234.

6. Winningham, M.L., Nail, L.M., Burke, M.B., et al. Fatigue and the cancer experience: The state of the knowledge. *Oncol Nurs Forum*, 1994, 21(1):23-36.

7. Columbo, B., Martinelli Boneschi, F., Rossi, P., et al. MRI and motor evoked potential findings in nondisabled multiple sclerosis patients with and without symptoms of fatigue. *J Neurol*, 2000, 247:506-509.

8. Piper, B.F., Lindsey, A.M., & Dodd, M.J. Fatigue mechanisms in cancer patients: Developing nursing theory. *Oncol Nurs Forum*, 1987, 14(6):17-23.

9. Aubier, M., Farkas, G., De Troyer, A., et al. Detection of diaphragm fatigue in man by phrenic stimulation. *J Appl Physiol*, 1981, 50(3):538-544.

10. Burns, S.M. Preventing diaphragm fatigue in the ventilated patient. *Dimensions Crit Care Nurs*, 1991, 10(1):13-20.

11. Schwid, S.R., Thornton, C.A., Pandya, S., et al. Quantitative assessment of motor strength and fatigue in MS. *Neurology*, 1999, 53(1):743-750.

12. Epstein, K.R. The chronically fatigued patient. *Med Clin North Am*, 1995, 79(2):315-327.

13. Cimprich, B., & Ronis, D.L. Attention and symptom distress in women with and without breast cancer. *Nurs Res*, 2001, 50(2):86-94.

14. Ang, D.C., & Calabrese, L.H. A common-sense approach to chronic fatigue in primary care. *Cleve Clin J Med*, 1999, 66(6):343-351.

15. Fukuda, K., Straus, S.E., Hickie, I., et al. The chronic fatigue syndrome: A comprehensive approach to its definition and study. International Chronic Fatigue Syndrome Study Group. *Ann Intern Med*, 1994, 121:953-958.

16. Cella, D., Peterman, A., Passik, S., et al. Progress toward guidelines for the management of fatigue. *Oncology*, 1998, 12(Suppl 11A):369-377.

17. Winningham, M.L. The puzzle of fatigue: How do you nail pudding to the wall? In M.L. Winningham & M. Barton-Burke (Eds.), *Fatigue in cancer*. Sudbury, MA: Jones & Bartlett, 2000.

18. Miaskowski, C. The Lesage/Portnoy article reviewed. *Oncology*, 2002, 16(3):385-386.

19. Cella, D., Davis, K., Breitbart, W., & Curt, G. Cancer-related fatigue: Prevalence of proposed diagnostic criteria in a United States sample of cancer survivors. *J Clin Oncol*, 2001, 19(14):3385-3391.

20. Sadler, I.J., Jacobsen, P.B., Booth-Jones, M., et al. Preliminary evaluation of a clinical syndrome approach to assessing cancer-related fatigue. *J Pain Symptom Manage*, 2002, 23(5):406-416.

21. Freel, M.I., & Hart, L.K. *Study of fatigue phenomena of multiple sclerosis patients*. (Grant No. 5R02-NU-00524-2), Division of Nursing, USDHEW, 1977.

22. Krupp, L.B., LaRocca, N.G., Muir-Nash, J., & Steinberg, A.D. The Fatigue Severity Scale: Application to patients with multiple sclerosis and systemic lupus erythematosus. *Arch Neurol*, 1989, 46:1121-1123.

23. Krupp, L.B., & Elkins, L.E. Fatigue and declines in cognitive functioning in multiple sclerosis. *Neurology*, 2000, 55:934-939.

24. Payne, J.K., Rabinowitz, I., & Piper, B.F. Physiological biomarkers of cancer treatment-related fatigue

(Poster Abstract 191). *Oncol Nurs Forum*, 2002, 29(2):376.

25. Poulson, M.J. The art of oncology: When the tumor is not the target: Not just tired. *J Clin Oncol*, 2001, 19(21):4180-4181.

26. Silwa, J.A. Neuromuscular rehabilitation and electrodiagnosis: 1. Central neurologic disorders. *Arch Phys Med Rehab*, 2000, 81:S3-S112.

27. Mock, V., Atkinson, A., Barsevick, A., et al. *Cancer-related fatigue: NCCN practice guidelines in oncology* (v.1.2003). Retrieved online from www.nccn.org.

28. Multiple Sclerosis Council for Clinical Practice Guidelines. *Fatigue and multiple sclerosis: Evidence-based management strategies for fatigue in multiple sclerosis*. Retrieved online from www.pva.org/NEWPVASITE/publications/pdf/fatigue/.pdf, 1998.

29. Curt, G.A. Impact of fatigue on quality of life in oncology patients. *Semin Hematol*, 2000, 37(4 Suppl. 6):14-17.

30. Piper, B.F., Dodd, M.J., Ream, E., et al. Improving the clinical measurement of cancer treatment-related fatigue. *Better health through nursing research: International State of the Science* [Abstract. p. 99], Washington, DC: ANA, 1999.

31. Potempa, K.M. Chronic fatigue. *Ann Rev Nurs Res*, 1993, 11:57-76.

32. Ream, E., & Richardson, A. Fatigue: A concept analysis. *Int J Nurs Stud*, 1996, 33(5):519-529.

33. Piper, B.F., Lindsey, A.M., & Dodd, M.J. The development of an instrument to measure the subjective dimension of fatigue. In S.G. Funk, E.M. Tornquist, M.T. Champagne, et al. (Eds.), *Key aspects of comfort: Management of pain, fatigue, and nausea*. New York: Springer, 1989, pp. 199-208.

34. Fletchner, H., & Bottomley, A. Fatigue assessment in cancer clinical trials. *Expert Rev Pharmacoeconomics Outcomes Res*, 2002, 2(1):67-76.

35. Muscio, B. Is a fatigue test possible? *Br J Psychol*, 1921, 12:31-46.

36. Bartley, S.H., & Chute, E. *Fatigue and impairment in man*. New York: McGraw-Hill, 1947.

37. Putt, A.M. Effects of noise on fatigue in healthy middle-aged adults. *Commun Nurs Res*, 1977, 8:24-34.

38. Milligan, R.A., & Pugh, L.C. Fatigue during the childbearing period. In J.J. Fitzpatrick & J.S. Stevenson (Eds.), *Annual review of nursing research* (vol. 12). New York: Springer, 1994, pp. 33-49.

39. Berger, A. Patterns of fatigue and activity and rest during adjuvant breast cancer chemotherapy. *Oncol Nurs Forum*, 1998, 25(1):1-62.

40. Lee, H., Kohlman, G.C.V., Lee, K., & Schiller, N.B. Fatigue, mood, and hemodynamic patterns after myocardial infarction. *Appl Nurs Res*, 2000, 13(2):60-69.

41. Potempa, K., Lopez, M., Reid, C., & Lawson, L. Chronic fatigue. *Image*, 1986, 18:165-169.

42. Fisk, J.D., Ritvo, P.G., Ross, L., et al. Measuring the functional impact of fatigue: Initial validation of the Fatigue Impact Scale. *Clin Infect Dis*, 1994, 18(Suppl 1):S79-S83.

43. Cella, D. The Functional Assessment of Cancer Therapy-Anemia (FACT-AN) Scale: A new tool for the assessment of outcomes on cancer anemia and fatigue. *Sem Hematol*, 1997, 34(Suppl 2):13-19.

44. Meek, P.M., Nail, L.M., Barsevick, A., et al. Psycho-

metric testing of fatigue instruments for use with cancer patients. *Nurs Res*, 2000, *49*(4):181-190.

45. Mendoza, T.R., Wang, X.S., Cleeland, C.S., et al. The rapid assessment of fatigue severity in cancer patients: Use of the Brief Fatigue Inventory. *Cancer*, 1999, *85*(5):1186-1196.

46. Piper, B.F., Dibble, S.L., Dodd, M.J., et al. The Revised Piper Fatigue Scale: Psychometric evaluation in women with breast cancer. *Oncol Nurs Forum*, 1998, *25*(4):677-684.

47. Schwartz, A.L. The Schwartz Fatigue scale: Testing reliability and validity. *Oncol Nurs Forum*, 1998, *25*(4):711-717.

48. Dean, G.E., & Stahl, C. Increasing the visibility of patient fatigue. *Semin Oncol Nurs*, 2002, *18*(1):20-27.

49. National Institutes of Health. *Final state-of-the-science statement: Symptom management in cancer: pain, depression and fatigue*, 2002. Retrieved online from www.consensus.nih.gov/ta/022/022_statement.htm.

50. Wang, X.S., Mendoza, T.R., Gao, S.Z., & Cleeland, C.S. The Chinese version of the Brief Pain Inventory (BPI-C): Its development and use in a study of cancer pain. *Pain*, 2000, *67*(203):407-416.

51. Gift, A.G., & Shepard, C.E. Fatigue and other symptoms in patients with chronic obstructive pulmonary disease: Do women and men differ? *J Obstet Gynecol Neonatal Nurs*, 1999, *28*(2):201-208.

52. Piper, B.F. The Groopman article reviewed. *Oncology*, 1998, *12*(3):345-346.

53. Richardson, A., Ream, E., & Wilson-Barnett, J. Fatigue in patients receiving chemotherapy: Patterns of change. *Cancer Nurs*, 1998, *21*(1):17-30.

54. Cleeland, C.S., & Wang, X.S. Measuring and understanding fatigue: NCCN proceedings. *Oncology*, 1999, *13*(11a):1-7.

55. Small, S.P., & Lamb, M. Measurement of fatigue in chronic obstructive pulmonary disease and in asthma. *Int J Nurs Stud*, 2000, *37*:127-133.

56. Okuyama, T., Akechi, T., Kugaya, A., et al. Factors correlated with fatigue in disease-free breast cancer patients: Application of the Cancer Fatigue Scale. *Support Care Cancer*, 2000, *8*(3):215-222.

57. Holley, S. Cancer-related fatigue: Suffering a different fatigue. *Cancer Pract*, 2000, *8*(2):87-94.

58. Holley, S.K. Evaluating patient distress from cancer-related fatigue: An instrument development study. *Oncol Nurs Forum*, 2000, *27*(9):1425-1431.

59. Glaus, A., Crowe, R., & Bohme, C. Development of a Fatigue Assessment Questionnaire (FAQ) for cancer patients. *Ann Oncol*, 1996, *7*(Suppl 5):134.

60. Bormann, J., Shively, M., Smith, T.L., & Gifford, A.C. Measurement of fatigue in HIV-positive adults. Reliability and validity of the Global Fatigue Index. *J Assoc Nurs AIDS Care*, 2001, *12*(3):75-83.

61. Tack (Belza), B. *Dimensions and correlates of fatigue in older adults with rheumatoid arthritis*. Unpublished doctoral dissertation, University of California, San Francisco, 1990.

62. Belza, B.L., Henke, C.J., Yelin, E.H., et al. Correlates of fatigue in older adults with rheumatoid arthritis. *Nurs Res*, 1993, *42*(2):93-99.

63. Belza, B.L. Comparison of self-reported fatigue in rheumatoid arthritis and controls. *J Rheum*, 1995, *22*(4):639-643.

64. Bentall, R.P., Wood, G.C., Marrinan, T., et al. A brief mental fatigue questionnaire. *Br J Clin Psychol*, 1993, *32*(Pt 3):375-379.

65. Stein, K.D., Martin, S.C., Hann, D.H., & Jacobsen, P.B. A multidimensional measure of fatigue for use in cancer patients. *Cancer Pract*, 1998, *6*(3):143-152.

66. Schwartz, A., & Meek, P. Additional construct validity of the Schwartz Cancer Fatigue Scale. *J Nurs Meas*, 1999, *7*(1):35-45.

67. Wang, X.S., Giralt, S.A., Mendoza, T.R., et al. Clinical factors associated with cancer-related fatigue in patients being treated for leukemia and non-Hodgkin's lymphoma. *J Clin Oncol*, 2002, *20*(5):1319-1328.

68. Tiesinga, L.J. *Fatigue and exertion fatigue: From description through validation to application of the Dutch Fatigue Scale (DUFS) and the Dutch Exertion Fatigue Scale (DEFS)*. Dissertation Thesis, University of Gronigen, The Netherlands, 1999.

69. Hann, D.M., Deniston, M.M., & Baker, F. Measurement of fatigue in cancer patients: Further validation of the Fatigue Symptom Inventory. *Qual Life Res*, 2000, *9*(7):847-854.

70. Hann, D.M., Jacobsen, P.B., Azzarello, L.M., et al. Measurement of fatigue in cancer patients: Development and validation of the Fatigue Symptom Inventory. *Qual Life Res*, 1998, *7*:301-310.

71. Barroso, J., & Lynn, M.R. Psychometric properties of the HIV-related fatigue scale. *J Assoc Nurs AIDS Care*, 2002, *13*(1):66-75.

72. Chalder, T., Berelowitz, G., Pawlikowska, T., et al. Development of a fatigue scale. *J Psychosom Res*, 1993, *37*(2):147-153.

73. Yoshitake, H. Rating the feelings of fatigue. *J Sci Labour*, 1969, *45*(7):422-432.

74. Yoshitake, H. Relations between the symptoms and the feeling of fatigue. *Ergonomics*, 1971, *14*:175-186.

75. Yoshitake, H. Three characteristic patterns of subjective fatigue symptoms. *Ergonomics*, 1978, *21*(3):231-233.

76. Pugh, L.C. Childbirth and the measurement of fatigue. *J Nurs Meas*, 1993, *1*(1):57-66.

77. Pugh, L.C., Milligan, R., Parks, P.L., et al. Clinical approaches in the assessment of childbearing fatigue. *J Obstet Gynecol Neonatal Nurs*, 1999, *28*(1):74-80.

78. Lee, K.A., Hicks, G., & Nino-Murcia, G. Validity and reliability of a scale to assess fatigue. *Psychiatr Res*, 1991, *36*:291-298.

79. Cimprich, B. Attentional fatigue following breast cancer surgery. *Res Nurs Health*, 1992, *15*:199-207.

80. DeLuca, J., Johnson, S.K., & Natelson, B.J. Information processing efficiency in chronic fatigue syndrome and multiple sclerosis. *Arch Neurol*, 1993, *50*(3):301-304.

81. McDonald, E., Cope, H., & David, A. Cognitive impairment in patients with chronic fatigue: A preliminary study. *J Neurol Neurosurg Psychiatr*, 1993, *56*:812-815.

82. Chemobrain: Chemotherapy side effect? *Patient Perspect*, 1996, April 1-2.

83. Meyers, C.A. Neurocognitive dysfunction in cancer patients. *Oncology*, 2000, *14*(1):75-79; discussion 79, 81-82, 85.

84. Olin, J.J. Cognitive function after systemic therapy for breast cancer. *Oncology*, 2001, *15*(5). Retrieved

online from www.cancernetwork.com/journals/oncology/o0105c.htm.

85. Arendt, D., Borbely, A.A., Franey, C., & Wright, J. The effects of chronic, small doses of melatonin given in the late afternoon on fatigue in man: A preliminary study. *Neurosci Lett*, 1984, *45*:317-321.

86. Burton, R.R. Human responses to repeated high G simulated aerial combat maneuvers. *Aviat Space Environ Med*, 1980, *51*:1185-1192.

87. Jamar, S.C. Fatigue in women receiving chemotherapy for ovarian cancer. In S.G. Funk, E.M. Tournquist, M.T. Champagne, et al. (Eds.), *Key aspects of comfort: Management of pain, fatigue, and nausea*. New York: Springer, 1989, pp. 224-233.

88. Littlewood, T.J., Bajetta, E., Nortier, J.W.R., et al. Effects of epoetin alfa on hematologic parameters and quality of life in cancer patients receiving nonplatinum chemotherapy: Results of a randomized, double-blind, placebo-controlled trial. *J Clin Oncol*, 2001, *19*(11):2865-2874.

89. Glaspy, J., Bukowski, R., Steinberg, D., et al. Impact of therapy with epoetin alfa on clinical outcomes in patients with nonmyeloid malignancies during cancer chemotherapy in community oncology practice. *J Clin Oncol*, 1997, *15*:1218-1234.

90. Miller, R.G., Giannini, D., Milner-Brown, H.S., et al. Effects of fatiguing exercise on high-energy phosphates, force and EMG: Evidence for three phases of recovery. *Muscle Nerve*, 1987, *10*:810-821.

91. Ferrell, B.R., Grant, G.E., Dean, G.E., et al. "Bone tired": The experience of fatigue and its impact on quality of life. *Oncol Nurs Forum*, 1996, *23*(10):1539-1537.

92. Cameron, C. A theory of fatigue. *Ergonomics*, 1973, *16*:633-646.

93. Ciba Foundation Symposium 82. *Human muscle fatigue: Physiological mechanisms*. London: Pittman Medical, 1981.

94. Gibson, H., & Edwards, R.H.T. Muscular exercise and fatigue. *Sports Medicine*, 1985, *2*:120-132.

95. Grandjean, E.P. Fatigue: Its physiological and psychological significance. *Ergonomics*, 1968, *11*:427-436.

96. Irvine, D., Vincent, L., Graydon, J.E., et al. The prevalence and correlates of fatigue in patients receiving treatment with chemotherapy and radiotherapy. *Cancer Nurs*, 1994, *17*(5):367-378.

97. Merton, P.A. Voluntary strength and fatigue. *J Physiol*, 1954, *123*:553-564.

98. Pugh, L.C. *Psychophysiological correlates of fatigue during childbirth*. Unpublished doctoral dissertation, University of Maryland, Baltimore, 1989.

99. Piper, B.F. Fatigue. In M.E. Ropka & A. Williams (Eds.), *Handbook of HIV nursing & symptom management*. Boston: Jones & Bartlett, 1998.

100. Dean, G.E. *Circadian rhythms and the experience of fatigue in women before and after surgery for breast cancer*. Unpublished Dissertation, University of California, Los Angeles School of Nursing, 2002.

101. Levine, M. *Introduction to clinical nursing* (2nd ed.). Philadelphia: F.A. Davis, 1973.

102. Lenz, E.R., Pugh, L.C., Milligan, R.A., et al. The middle-range theory of unpleasant symptoms: An update. *Adv Nurs Sci*, 1997, *19*(3):14-27.

103. Dodd, M.J., Jansen, S. Facione, N., et al. Advancing the science of symptom management. *J Adv Nurs*, 2001, *33*(5):668-676.

104. Winningham, M.L. The foundations of energetics: Fatigue, fuel, and functioning. In M.L. Winningham & M. Barton-Burke (Eds.), *Fatigue in cancer: A multidimensional approach*. Sudbury, MA: Jones & Bartlett, 2000.

105. Vercoulen, J.H.M.M., Swanink, C.M.A., Galama, J.M.D., et al. The persistence of fatigue in chronic fatigue syndrome and multiple sclerosis: Development of a model. *J Psychosom Res*, 1998, *45*(6):507-517.

106. Andrews, P.L.R., & Morrow, G.R. Approaches to understanding the mechanisms involved in fatigue associated with cancer and its treatments: A speculative review. *Eur Sch Oncol Sci Updates: Fatigue Cancer*, 2001, *5*:79-93.

107. McGuire, D.B. Comprehensive and multidimensional assessment and measurement of pain. *J Pain Symptom Manage*, 1992, *7*(5):312-319.

108. National Institute of Nursing Research. *Symptom management: Acute pain. A report of the NINR priority expert panel on symptom management acute pain*. Bethesda, MD: U.S. Department of Health & Human Services, 1994.

109. Dodd, M.J., Miaskowski, C., & Paul, S.M. Symptom clusters and their effect on the functional status of patients with cancer. *Oncol Nurs Forum*, 2001, *28*(3):465-470.

110. Maclaren, D.P.M., Gibson, H., Parry-Billings, M., & Edwards, R.H.T. A review of metabolic and physiological factors in fatigue. *Exerc Sport Sci Rev*, 1989, *17*:29-66.

111. Poteliakoff, A. Adrenocortical activity and some clinical findings in acute and chronic fatigue. *J Psychosom Res*, 1981, *25*:91-95.

112. Asmussen, E. Muscle fatigue. *Med Sci Sports Exerc*, 1979, *11*:313-321.

113. Kaplan, S., & Kaplan, R. *Environment and cognition*. New York: Praeger, 1982.

114. Benton, D., Parker, P., & Donohoe, R. The supply of glucose to the brain and cognitive functioning. *J Biosoc Sci*, 1996, *28*(4):463-479.

115. Kent-Braun, J.A., Sharma, K.R., Weiner, M.W., & Miller R.G. Effects of exercise on muscle activation and metabolism in multiple sclerosis. *Muscle Nerve*, 1994, *17*:1162-1169.

116. Vollestad, N.K., & Sejersted, O.M. Biochemical correlates of fatigue. *Eur J Appl Physiol*, 1988, *57*:336-347.

117. Cohen, F.L., & Hardin, S.B. Fatigue in patients with catastrophic illness. In S.G. Funk, E.M. Tournquist, M.T. Champagne, et al. (Eds.), *Key aspects of comfort: Management of pain, fatigue, and nausea*. New York: Springer, 1989, pp. 208-216.

118. Elkins, L.E., Krupp, L.B., & Sherl, W. The measurement of fatigue and contributing neuropsychiatric factors. *Sem Clin Neuropsychiatry*, 2000, *5*(1):58-61.

119. Jones, T.H., Wadler, S., & Hupart, K.H. Endocrine-mediated mechanisms of fatigue during treatment with interferon-alpha. *Semin Oncol*, 1998, *25*:54-63.

120. Piper, B.F., Rieger, P.T., Brophy, L., et al. Recent advances in the management of biotherapy-related side effects: Fatigue. *Oncol Nurs Forum*, 1989, *16*:27-34.

121. Ader, R., Felten, D.L., & Cohen, N. *Psychoneuroimmunology* (2nd ed.). San Diego: Academic Press, 1991.
122. Blalock, J.E., & Smith, E.M. A complete loop between the immune and neuroendocrine systems. *Fed Proceed*, 1985, *44*:108-112.
123. Kavelaars, A., Kuis, W., Knook, L., et al. Disturbed Neuroendocrine-immune interactions in chronic fatigue syndrome. *J Clin Endocrinol Metab*, 2000, *85*(2):692-696.
124. Geinitz, H., Zimmermann, F.B., Stoll, P., et al. Fatigue, serum cytokine levels, and blood cell counts during radiotherapy of patients with breast cancer. *Int J Radiat Oncol Biol Phys*, 2001, *51*(3):691-698.
125. Greenberg, D.B., Gray, J.L., Mannix, C.M., et al. Treatment-related fatigue and serum interleukin-1 levels in patients during external beam irradiation for prostate cancer. *J Symptom Manage*, 1993, *8*(4):196-200.
126. Barlogie, B., & Beck, T. Recombinant human erythropoetin and the anemia of multiple myeloma. *Stem Cells*, 1993, *11*:88-94.
127. Adams, F., Quesada, J.R., & Gutterman, J.U. Neuropsychiatric manifestations of human leukocyte interferon therapy in patients with cancer. *JAMA*, 1984, *252*(1):938-941.
128. Bernsen, P.L.J.A., Wong-Chung, R.D., & Janssen, J.T. Neurologic amyotrophy and polyradiculopathy during interferon therapy. *Lancet*, 1985, *1*(8419):50.
129. Besedovsky, H.O., del Rey, A.E., & Sorkin, E. Immune-neuroendocrine interactions. *J Immunol*, 1985, *135*(Suppl 2):750S-754S.
130. Krueger, J.M., Walter, J., Dinnarello, C.A., et al. Sleep-promoting effects of endogenous pyrogen (interleukin-1). *Am J Physiol*, 1984, *246*(6, pt 2):R994-R999.
131. Denicoff, K.D., Rubinow, D.R., Papa, M.Z., et al. The neuropsychiatric effects of treatment with interleukin and lymphokine-activated killer cells. *Ann Intern Med*, 1987, *107*(3):293-300.
132. St. Pierre, B.A., Kasper, C.E., & Lindsey, A.M. Fatigue mechanisms in patients with cancer: Effects of tumor necrosis factor and exercise on skeletal muscle. *Oncol Nurs Forum*, 1992, *19*(3):419-425.
133. Chao, C.C., DeLa Hunt, M., Hu, S., et al. Immunologically mediated fatigue: A murine model. *Clin Immunopath*, 1992, *64*:161-165.
134. Moldofsky, H., Lue, F.A., Eisen, J., et al. The relationship between interleukin-1 and immune functions to sleep in humans. *Psychosom Med*, 1986, *48*:309-318.
135. Decramer, M., Laquet, L.M., Fagard, R., & Rogiers, P. Corticosteroids contribute to muscle weakness in chronic airflow obstruction. *Am J Respir Crit Care Med*, 1994, *150*:11-16.
136. Newsholme, E.A., & Blomstrand, E. The plasma level of some amino acids and physical and mental fatigue. *Experimentia*, 1996, *52*:413-415.
137. Parry-Billings, M., Blomstrand, E., & McAndrew, N. A communicational link between skeletal muscle, brain, and cells of the immune system. *Int J Sports Med*, 1990, *11*:S122-S128.
138. Nardini, S. Respiratory muscle function and COPD. *Monaldi Arch Chest Dis*, 1995, *50*:325-336.
139. McCann, K., & Boore, J.R.P. Fatigue in persons with renal failure who require maintenance haemodialysis. *J Adv Nurs*, 2000, *32*(5):1132-1142.
140. Korszun, A., Sackett-Lundeen, L., Papadopoulos, E., et al. Melatonin levels in women with fibromyalgia and chronic fatigue syndrome. *J Rheum*, 1999, *26*:2675-2680.
141. Heliman, K.M., & Watson, R.T. Fatigue. *Neurol Net Comm*, 1997, *1*:283-287.
142. Roscoe, J.A., Morrow, G.R., Hickok, J.T., et al. Temporal relationships among fatigue, circadian rhythm and depression in breast cancer patients undergoing chemotherapy treatment. *Support Care Cancer*, 2002, *10*:329-336.
143. van de Luit, L., van der Meulen, J., Cleophas, T.J.M., & Zwinderman, A.H. Amplified amplitudes of circadian rhythms and nighttime hypotension in patients with chronic fatigue syndrome: Improvement by inopamil but not by melatonin. *Angiology: J Vasc Dis*, 1998, *49*(11):903-908.
144. Kent-Braun, J.A. Noninvasive measures of central and peripheral activation in human muscle fatigue. *Muscle Nerve*, 1997, *5*:S98-S101.
145. Polit, D.F., & Hungler, B.P. *Nursing research: Principles and methods*. Philadelphia: Lippincott, 1987.
146. Cardenas, D.D., & Kutner, N.G. The problem of fatigue in dialysis patients. *Nephron*, 1982, *30*:336-340.
147. Haylock, P.J., & Hart, L.K. Fatigue in patients receiving localized radiation. *Cancer Nurs*, 1979, *2*(6):461-467.
148. McNair, D.M., Lorr, M., & Droppleman, L.F. *POMS: Manuel for the Profile of Mood States*. San Diego: CA: Educational and Industrial Testing Service, 1971.
149. McNair, D.M., Lorr, M., & Droppleman, L.F. *EdITS manual for the Profile of Mood States*. San Diego: CA: EdITS/Educational and Industrial Testing Service, 1992.
150. McCorkle, R., & Young, K. Development of a symptom distress scale. *Cancer Nurs*, 1978, *1*:373-378.
151. Cella, D. Factors influencing quality of life in cancer patients: Anemia and fatigue. *Semin Oncol*, 1998, *25*(3)(Suppl 7):43-46.
152. Ferrell, B., Wisdom, C., & Wenzel, C. Quality of life as an outcome variable in the management of cancer pain. *Cancer*, 1989, *63*:2321-2327.
153. Stone, P., Richards, M., & Hardy, J. Fatigue in patients with cancer. *Eur J Cancer*, 1998, *34*(11):1670-1676.
154. Rhoten, D. Fatigue and the postsurgical patient. In C.M. Norris (Ed.), *Concept clarification in nursing*. Rockville, MD: Aspen, 1982, pp. 277-300.
155. Winstead-Fry, P. Psychometric assessment of four fatigue scales with a sample of rural cancer patients. *J Nurs Measurement*, 1998, *6*(2):111-122.
156. Wu, H.S., & McSweeney, M. Measurement of fatigue in people with cancer. *Oncol Nurs Forum*, 2001, *28*(9):1371-1384.
157. Schumann, L., & Rodriguez, T. The challenge of evaluating fatigue. *J Am Acad Nurse Practitioners*, 2000, *12*(8):329-338.
158. Breitbart, W., Rosenfeld, B., Kaion, M., & Furesti-Esch, J. A randomized double-blind placebo-controlled trial of psychostimulants for the treatment of fatigue in ambulatory patient with human immunodeficiency virus. *Arch Intern Med*, 2001, *161*(3):411-420.

159. Lee, E.H. Construct validity of the Revised Piper Fatigue Scale in Korean women with breast cancer. *J Korean Acad Nurs*, 1999, *29*:485-493.

160. Lee, E.H. Fatigue and hope: Relationships to psychosocial adjustment in Korean women with breast cancer. *Appl Nurs Res*, 2001, *14*(2):87-93.

161. Ray, C., Phillips, L., & Weir, W.R.C. Quality of attention in chronic fatigue syndrome: Subjective reports of everyday attention and cognitive difficulty, and performance on tasks of focused attention. *Br J Clin Psychol*, 1993, *32*:357-364.

162. Aaronson, N.K., Ahmedzai, S., Bergmen, B., et al. The European Organization for research and Treatment of cancer QLQ-30: A quality-of-life instrument for use in international clinical trials in oncology. *J Nat Cancer Inst*, 1993, *85*(5):365-376.

163. Krupp, L.B., Jandorf, L., Coyle, P.K., & Mendelson, W.B. Sleep disturbances in chronic fatigue syndrome. *J Psychosom Res*, 1993, *37*(4):325-331.

164. Schwartz, J.E., Jandorf, L., & Krupp, L.B. The measurement of fatigue: A new instrument. *J Psychosom Res*, 1993, *37*(7):753-762.

165. Kleinman, L., Bodet, M.W., Hakim, Z., et al. Psychometric evaluation of the fatigue severity scale for use in chronic hepatitis C. *Qual Life Res*, 2000, *9*(5):499-508.

166. Taylor, R.R., Jason, L.A., & Torres, A. Fatigue rating scales: An empirical comparison. *Psychol Med*, 2000, *30*(4):849-856.

167. Yellen, S.B., Cella, D.E., Webster, K., et al. Measuring fatigue and other anemia-related symptoms with the Functional Assessment of Cancer Therapy (FACT) measurement system. *J Pain Symptom Manage*, 1997, *13*(2):63-74.

168. Andrykowski, M.A., Curran, S.L., & Lightner, R. Off-treatment fatigue in breast cancer survivors: A controlled comparison. *J Behav Med*, 1998, *21*(1):1-18.

169. Bower, J.E., Ganz, P.A., Desmond, K.A., et al. Fatigue in breast cancer survivors: Occurrence, correlates, and impact on quality of life. *J Clin Oncol*, 2000, *18*(4):743-753.

170. Ware, Jr., J.E., Snow, K.K., Kosinski, M., & Gandek, B. SF-36 Health Survey: Manual and interpretation guide. Boston: Nimrod Press, 1993.

171. Aaronson, L.S., Teel, C.S., Cassmeyer, V., et al. Defining and measuring fatigue. *Image: J Nurs Schol*, 1999, *31*(1):45-50.

172. Pearson, R.G., & Byars, G.E. *The development and validation of a checklist for measuring subjective fatigue.* Report No. 56-115. Randolph Air Force Base, TX: School of Aviation Medicine, U.S. Air Force, 1956.

173. Loge, J.H., Ekeberg, O., & Kaasa, S. Fatigue in the general Norwegian population: Normative data and associations. *J Psychosom Res*, 1998, *45*:53-65.

174. Bonner, D., Ron, M., Chalder, T., & Wessely, S. Chronic fatigue syndrome: A follow up study. *J Neurol Neurosurg Psychiatr*, 1994, *57*:617-621.

175. Walford, G.A., Nelson, W., & McCluskey, D.R. Fatigue, depression, and social adjustment in chronic fatigue syndrome. *Arch Dis Child*, 1993, *68*(3):384-388.

176. Ridsdale, L., Evans, A., Jerrett, W., et al. Patients with fatigue in general practice: A prospective study. *BMJ*, 1993, *307*(6896):103-106.

177. Cathebras, P., Jacquin, L., le Gal, M., et al. Correlates of somatic causal attributions in primary care patients with fatigue. *Psychother Psychosom*, 1995, *63*:174-180.

178. Reeves, N., Potempa, K., & Gallo, A. Fatigue in early pregnancy: An exploratory study. *J Midwifery*, 1991, *36*(5):303-309.

179. Saito, Y., Kogi, K., & Kashiwagi, S. Factors underlying subjective feelings of fatigue. *J Sci Labour*, 1970, *46*(4):205-224.

180. Piper, B.F. *Subjective fatigue in women receiving six cycles of chemotherapy for breast cancer.* (Unpublished doctoral dissertation. University of California 1992, San Francisco.)

181. Srivastava, R.H. Fatigue in end-stage renal disease patients. In S.G. Funk, E.M. Tournquist, M.T. Champagne, et al. (Eds.), *Key aspects of comfort: Management of pain, fatigue and nausea.* New York: Springer, 1989, pp. 217-224.

182. Flechtner, H., & Bottomley, A. Fatigue and quality of life: Lessons learned from the real world. *Oncologist*, 2003, *8*(Suppl 1):5-9.

183. Lee, H.O. *Fatigue in myocardial infarction patients.* Unpublished doctoral dissertation. (University of California 1993, San Francisco.)

184. Schneider, R.A. Concurrent validity of the Beck Depression Inventory and the Multidimensional Fatigue Inventory-20 in assessing fatigue among cancer patients. *Psychol Rep*, 1998, *82*:883-886.

185. Schneider, R.A. Reliability and validity of the Multidimensional Fatigue Inventory (MFI-20) and the Rhoten Fatigue Scale among rural cancer out patients. *Cancer Nurs*, 1998, *21*(5):370-373.

186. Smets, E.M., Garssen, B., Bonke, B., & De Haes, J.C. The Multidimensional Dimensional Fatigue Inventory (MFI): psychometric qualities of an instrument to assess fatigue. *J Psychosom Res*, 1995, *39*(3):315-325.

187. Smets, E.M., Garssen, B., Cull, A., & de Haes, J.C. Application of the multidimensional fatigue inventory (MFI) in cancer patients receiving radiation. *Br J Cancer*, 1996, *73*(2):241-245,

188. Poffenberger, A.T. The effects of continuous work upon output and feelings. *J Appl Psychol*, 1928, *12*(5):450-467.

189. Bartley, S.H. What do we call fatigue? In E. Simonson & P.C. Weiser (Eds.), *Psychological aspects and physiological correlates of work and fatigue.* Springfield, IL: Charles C. Thomas, 1976, pp. 409-414.

190. Dorpat, T.L., & Holmes, T.H. Mechanisms of skeletal muscle pain and fatigue. *Arch Neurol Psychiatr*, 1955, *74*(1):638-640.

191. Snow, E.W., Machlan, L.O., Jr., Warnell, C.E., & Utt, T.P. The tired patient. *Med Times*, 1959, *87*:1500-1504.

192. Hashimoto, K., Kogi, K., & Grandjean, E. (Eds.), *Methodology in human fatigue assessment.* London: Taylor & Francis, 1971.

193. Hart, L.K. Fatigue in the patient with multiple sclerosis. *Res Nurs Health*, 1978, *1*(4):147-157.

194. Rose, E.A., & King, T.C. Understanding postoperative fatigue. *Surg Gynecol Obstet*, 1978, *147*:97-101.

195. Meyerwitz, B.E., Sparks, F.C., & Sparks, I.K. Adjuvant chemotherapy for breast cancer. *Cancer*, 1979, *43*:1613-1618.

196. Kinsman, R.A., & Weiser, P.C. Subjective symptomatology during work and fatigue. In E. Simonson & P.C. Weiser (Eds.), *Psychological aspects and physiological correlates of work and fatigue.* Springfield, IL: Charles C. Thomas, 1976, pp. 336-405.

197. Davis, C.A. *The impact of fatigue on functional status of patients receiving interferon therapy for malignant melanoma.* (Unpublished master's thesis, Yale University School of Nursing 1983, New Haven, CT.)

198. Rieger, P.A. (Trahan). *Interferon-induced fatigue.* Unpublished master's thesis. (University of Texas Health Science Center 1986, Houston.)

199. Voith, A.M., Frank, A.M., & Pegg, J.S. Nursing diagnosis: Fatigue. In R.M. Carroll-Johnson (Ed.), *Classification of nursing diagnoses: Proceedings of the eighth conference.* Philadelphia: Lippincott, 1989, pp. 453-458.

200. Funk, S.G., Tornquist, E.M., Champagne, M.T., et al. (Eds.), (1989). *Key aspects of comfort: Management of pain, fatigue, and nausea.* New York: Springer, 1989.

201. Mock, V., Nail, L.M., & Grant, M. Implementing the FIRE® planning grant. *Oncol Nurs Forum,* 1998, 25(8):1389-1390.

202. Curt, G.A. The impact of fatigue on patients with cancer: Overview of fatigue 1 and 2. *Oncologist,* 2000, 5(Suppl 2):9-12.

203. Sheean, G.L., Murray, N.M.F., Rothwell, J.C., et al. An open-labelled clinical and electrophysiological study of 3,4 diaminopyridine in the treatment of fatigue in multiple sclerosis. *Brain,* 1998, 121:967-975.

204. Morrow, G.R., Hickok, J.T., Raubertas, R.F., & Flynn, P.J. Effect of an SSRI antidepressant on fatigue and depression in 738 cancer patients treated with chemotherapy: A URCC CCOP study [Abstract 1531]. *Proceed Am Soc Clin Oncol,* 2001, 20:384a.

205. Schwartz, A.L., Thompson, J.A., & Nehal, M. Interferon-induced fatigue in patients with melanoma: A pilot study of exercise and methylphenidate. *Oncol Nurs Forum,* 2002, 29(7):1-13. Retrieved online from www.ons.org/xp6/ONS/Library.xml/ONS-Publications.xml/ONF.xml/ONF2002.xn.

206. Berger, A.M., VonEssen, S., Kuhn, B.R., et al. Feasibility of a sleep intervention during adjuvant breast cancer chemotherapy. *Oncol Nurs Forum,* 2002, 29(10):1431-1441.

207. Barsevick, A.M., Sweeney, C., Beck, S., et al. A randomized trial of energy conservation training versus attentional control during cancer treatment (Poster Abstract 195). *Oncol Nurs Forum,* 2002, 29(2):377.

208. Bower, J.E., Ganz, P.A., Aziz, N., & Fahey, J. Fatigue and proinflammatory cytokine activity in breast cancer survivors. *Psychosom Med,* 2002, 64:604-611.

209. Cimprich, B. Age and extent of surgery affect attention in women treated for breast cancer. *Res Nurs Health,* 1998, 21:229-238.

210. Redeker, N.S., Lev, E.L., & Ruggiero, J. Insomnia, fatigue, anxiety, depression, and quality of life of cancer patients undergoing chemotherapy. *Schol Inq Nurs Pract,* 2000, 14(4):275-298.

211. Bakshi, R., Miletich. R.S., Henschel, K., et al. Fatigue in multiple sclerosis: Cross-sectional correlation with brain MRI findings in 71 patients. *Neurology,* 1999, 53:1151-1153.

212. Knobel, H., Loge, J.H., Lund, M.B., et al. Late medical complications and fatigue in Hodgkin's Disease survivors. *J Clin Oncol,* 2001, 19(13):3226-3233.

213. Breitbart, W., McDonald, M.V., Rosenfeld, B., et al. Fatigue in ambulatory AIDS patients. *J Symptom Manage,* 1998, 15(3):159-167.

214. Gordon, M.S. *Impact of anemia on cognitive function in patients with cancer: The anemia disease state slide lecture kit.* Springfield, NJ: Scientific Therapeutics Information, Inc. Retrieved online from www.stimedinfo.com.

215. Tong, E.M., & Nissenson, A.R. Erythropoietin and anemia. *Semin Nephrol,* 2001, 21:190-203.

216. Bron, D., Meuleman, N., & Mascaux, C. Biological basis of anemia. *Semin Oncol,* 2001, 28(2Suppl 8):1-6.

217. Groopman, J.E., & Itri, L.M. Chemotherapy-induced anemia: Incidence and treatment. *J Nat Cancer Inst,* 1999, 91(19):1616-1634.

218. Gabrilove, J.L., Cleeland, C.S., Livingston, R.B., et al. Clinical evaluation of once-weekly dosing of epoetin alfa in chemotherapy patients: Improvements in hemoglobin and quality of life are similar to three-times-weekly dosing. *J Clin Oncol,* 2001, 19(11):2875-2882.

219. Canaris, G.J., Manowitz, N.R., Mayor, G., & Ridgway, E.C. The Colorado thyroid disease prevalence study. *Arch Intern Med,* 2000, 160:526-534.

220. Tench, C.M., McCurdie, I., White, P.D., & D'Cruz, D.P. The prevalence and associations of fatigue in systemic lupus erythematosus. *Rheumatology,* 2000, 39:1249-1254.

221. Darko, D.F., McCutchan, J.A., Kripke, D.F., et al. Fatigue, sleep disturbances, disability and indices of progression of HIV infection. *Am J Psychiatry,* 1992, 149:514-520.

222. Jacobs, L.D., Wende, K.E., Brownscheidle, C.M., et al. A profile of multiple sclerosis: The New York multiple sclerosis consortium. *Multiple Sclerosis,* 1999, 5:369-376.

223. Kroenke, D.C., Lynch, S.G., & Denney, D.R. Fatigue in multiple sclerosis: Relationship to depression, disability, and disease pattern. *Multiple Sclerosis,* 2000, 6:151-157.

224. Neidig, J.L., Nickel, J., & Smith, B. Self-reported symptoms in HIV infection. *Proceedings of the International Conference on AIDS* (Vancouver), (Abstract TuB176, p. 231).

225. Tayer, W.G., Nicassio, P.M., Weisman, M.H., et al. Disease status predicts fatigue in systemic lupus erythematosis. *J Rheumatol,* 2001, 28(9):1999-2007.

226. Goh, J., Coughlan, B., Quinn, J., et al. Fatigue does not correlate with the degree of hepatitis or the presence of autoimmune disorders in chronic hepatitis C infection. *Eur J Gastroent Hepatol,* 1999, 11(8):833-838.

227. Nelles, S., Abbey, S., Stewart, D.E., et al. Fatigue assessment in patients with hepatitis C [Abstract]. *Gastroenterology,* 1996, 110:A1276.

228. Stone, P., Richardson, A., Ream, E., et al. Cancer-related fatigue: Inevitable, unimportant and untreatable? Results of a multi-centre patient survey. *Ann Oncol,* 2000, 11:971-975.

229. Loge, J.H., Abrahamsen, A.F., Ekeberg, O., & Kaasa, S. Fatigue and psychiatric morbidity in Hodgkin's disease survivors. *J Pain Symptom Manage,* 2000, 19:91-99.

230. Moody, L., McCormick, K., & William, A.R. Psychophysiologic correlates of Quality of life in chronic bronchitis and emphysema. *West J Nurs Res,* 1991, 13(30):336-352.

231. Schwartz, C.E., Coulthard-Morris, L., & Zeng, Q. Psychosocial correlates of fatigue in multiple sclerosis. *Arch Phys Med Rehab,* 1996, 77:165-170.

232. Dean, G.E., Spears, L., Ferrell, B.R., et al. Fatigue in

patients with cancer receiving interferon alpha. *Cancer Pract*, 1995, 3(3):164-172.

233. Bruera, E., Brenneis, C., Michaud, M., et al. Association between asthenia and nutritional status, lean body mass, anemia, psychological status, and tumor mass in patients with advanced breast cancer. *J Pain Sympt Manage*, 1989, 4:59-63.

234. Pickard-Holley, S. Fatigue in cancer patients: A descriptive study. *Cancer Nurs*, 1991, 14:13-19.

235. Small, S.P., & Graydon, J.E. Perceived uncertainty, physical symptoms, and negative mood in hospitalized patients with chronic obstructive pulmonary disease. *Heart Lung*, 1992, 21(6):568-574.

236. Kalichman, S.C., Sikkema, K.J., & Somlai, A. Assessing persons with human immunodeficiency virus (HIV) infection using the Beck Depression Inventory: Disease processes and other confounds. *J Pers Assess*, 1995, 64:86-100.

237. Visser, M.R.M., & Smets, E.M.A. Fatigue, depression, and quality of life in cancer patients: How are they related? *J Supportive Care Cancer*, 1998, 6(2):101-108.

238. Smets, E.M., Visser, M.R., Willems-Groot, A.F., et al. Fatigue and radiation therapy: (B). Experience in patients 9 months following treatment. *Br J Cancer*, 1998, 78(7):907-912.

239. Holland, J.C., Anderson, B., Booth-Jones, M., et al. *Distress management: NCCN practice guideline in oncology* (v.1.2003), Retrieved online from www.nccn.org.

240. Lee, R., Graydon, J., & Ross, E. Effects of psychological well-being, physical status and social support on oxygen-dependent COPD patients' level of functioning. *Res Nurs Health*, 1991, 14:323-328.

241. Ream, E., & Richardson, A. Fatigue in patients with cancer and chronic obstructive airways disease: A phenomenological inquiry. *Int J Nurs Studies*, 1997, 34(1):44-53.

242. Small, S., & Lamb, M. Fatigue in chronic illness: The experience of individuals with chronic obstructive pulmonary disease and with asthma. *J Adv Nurs*, 1999, 30(2):469-478.

243. Liao, S., & Ferrell, B.A. Fatigue in an older population. *J Am Geriatr*, 2000, 48(4):426-430.

244. Dunbar, S.B., Kimble, L.P., Jenkins, L.S., et al. Association of mood disturbance and arrhythmic events in patients after cardioverter defibrillator implantation. *Depress Anxiety*, 1999, 9(4):163-168.

245. Irvine, D., Basinhi, A., Baker, B., et al. Depression and risk of sudden cardiac death after acute myocardial infarction: Testing for the confounding effects of fatigue. *Psychosom Med*, 1999, 61(6):729-737.

246. Kukell, W.A., McCorkle, R., & Driever, M. Symptom distress, psychosocial variables, and survival from lung cancer. *J Psychosoc Oncol*, 1986, 4:91-104.

247. Levy, S.M., Herberman, R.B., Maluish, A.M., et al. Prognostic risk assessment in primary breast cancer by behavioral and immunological parameters. *Health Psychol*, 1985, 4:99-113.

248. Temoshok, L. In consultation: Discussion of psychosocial factors related to outcome in cutaneous malignany melanoma: A matched samples design. *Oncol News Update*, 1987, 2:6-7.

249. Appels, A., Kop, W.J., & Schouten, E. The nature of depressive symptomatology preceding myocardial infarction. *Behav Med*, 2000, 26(2), 86-89.

250. Caro, J.J., Salas, M., Ward, A. & Goss, G. Anemia as an independent prognostic factor for survival in patients with cancer: A systematic, quantitative review. *Cancer*, 2001, 91:2214-2221.

251. Chan, C.W., & Molassiotis, A. The impact of fatigue on Chinese cancer patients in Hong Kong. *Supportive Care Cancer*, 2001, 9(1):18-24.

252. Pitzer, M.S. Patterns of fatigue and psychological factors during pregnancy: Their relationship to preterm labor/birth. *Nursing research: Global health perspectives: Proceedings of the 1991 International Nursing Research Conference*. Washington, DC: American Nurses' Association, 1991.

253. Piper, B., Lee, H.O., & Kim, O. Fatigue-transcultural implications for nursing interventions. In A.P. Pritchard (Ed.), *Cancer nursing: The balance. Proceedings of the Sixth International Conference on Cancer Nursing*. London: Scutari Press, 1991, pp. 140-144.

254. Stone, P., Hardy, J., Broadley, K., et al. Fatigue in advanced cancer. *Eur J Cancer*, 1999, 34:1670-1676.

255. Akechi, T., Kugaya, A., Okamura, H., et al. Fatigue and its associated factors in ambulatory cancer patients: A preliminary study. *J Pain Symptom Manage*, 1999, 17(1):42-48.

256. Roca, R.R., Ubeda, B.I., Fuentelsaz, G.C., et al. Impact of caregiving on the health of family caregivers. *Aten Primaria*, 2000, 26(4):217-223.

257. Heinonen, H., Volin, L., Uutela, A., et al. Gender-associated differences in the quality of life after allogeneic BMT. *Bone Marrow Transplant*, 2001, 28(5):503-509.

258. Knobel, H., Loge, J.H., Nordoy, T., et al. High level of fatigue in lymphoma patients treated with high dose therapy. *J Pain Symptom Manage*, 2000, 19(6), 446-456.

259. Brunier, G.M., & Graydon, J. The influence of physical activity on fatigue in patients with ESRD on hemodialysis. *ANNA Journal*, 1993, 20(4):457-531.

260. Gaston-Johansson, F., Fall-Dickson, J.M., Bakos, A.B., & Kennedy, M.J. Fatigue, pain, and depression in pre-autotransplant breast cancer patients. *Cancer Practice*, 1999, 7(5):240-247.

261. Berger, A.M., & Farr, L. The influence of daytime inactivity and nighttime restlessness on cancer-related fatigue. *Oncol Nurs Forum*, 1999, 26(10):1663-1671.

262. Berger, A.M., & Walker, S.N. An explanatory model of fatigue in women receiving adjuvant breast cancer chemotherapy. *Nurs Res*, 2001, 50(1):43-52.

263. Irvine, D.M., Vincent, L., Graydon, J.E., & Bubela, N. Fatigue in women with breast cancer receiving radiation therapy. *Cancer Nurs*, 1998, 21(2):127-135.

264. Jansen-Bjerklie, S., Carrieri, V.K., & Hudes, M. The sensations of pulmonary dyspnea. *Nurs Res*, 1986, 35:154-159.

265. Wilson, I.B., & Cleary, P.D. Clinical predictors of functioning in persons with acquired immunodeficiency syndrome. *Med Care*, 1996, 34:610-623.

266. Lee, K. Sleep and fatigue. *Ann Rev Nurs Res*, 2001, 19:249-273.

267. Ford, D.E., & Kamerow, D.B. Epidemiologic study of sleep disturbances and psychiatric disorders. *JAMA*, 1989, 262:1479-1484.

268. Morin, C.M. *Insomnia: Psychological assessment and management*. New York: Guilford Press, 1993.

269. MacVicar, S.B., & Winningham, M.L. Promoting the functional capacity of cancer patients. *Cancer Bull*, 1986, *38*:235-239.

270. Berger, A.M., & Higgenbotham, P. Correlates of fatigue during and following adjuvant chemotherapy: A pilot study. *Oncol Nurs Forum*, 2000, *27*(9):1443-148.

271. Devins, G.M., Edworthy, S.M., Paul, L.C., et al. Restless sleep, illness intrusiveness, and depression symptoms in three chronic illness conditions: Rheumatoid arthritis, end-stage renal disease, and multiple sclerosis. *J Psychosom Res*, 1993, *37*(2):163-170.

272. McKinley, P., Ouellette, S.C., & Winkel, G.H. The contributions of disease activity, sleep patterns, and depression to fatigue in systemic lupus erythematosus. *Arthr Rheum*, 1995, *38*(6):826-834.

273. Petersson, B., Wernerman, J., Waller, S.O., et al. Elective abdominal surgery depresses muscle protein synthesis and increases subjective fatigue: Effects lasting more than 30 days. *Br J Surg*, 1990, *77*(7):796-800.

274. Jacobsen, P.B., & Stein, K. Is fatigue a long-term side effect of breast cancer treatment? *J Moffitt Cancer Center*, 1999, *6*(3):256-263. Retrieved online from www.medscape.con/Moffitt/CancerControl/1999/v06.n02/cc0603.04.jaco/cc0603.04.jaco-01.html.

275. Parks, P.L., Lenz, E.R., Milligan, R.A., & Han, H.R. What happens when fatigue lingers for 18 months after delivery? *J Obstet Gynecol Neonatal Nurs*, 1999, *28*(1):87-93.

276. Vogelzang, N., Brietbart, W., Cella, D. et al. Patient, caregiver, and oncologist perceptions of cancer-related fatigue: Results of a tri-part assessment survey. *Semin Hematol*, 1997, *34*(Suppl 2):4-12.

277. Schaefer, K.M. A description of fatigue associated with congestive heart failure: Use of Levine's conservation model. In M. Parker (Ed.), *Nursing theories in practice*. Publication No. 15-2350. New York: National League for Nurses, 1990, pp. 217-237.

278. Wilson, I.B., & Cleary, P.D. Linking clinical variables with health-related quality of life: A conceptual model of patient outcomes. *JAMA*, 1995, *273*(1):59-65.

279. O'Dell, M.W., Meighen, M., & Riggs, R.N. Correlates of fatigue in HIV infection prior to AIDS: A pilot study. *Disabil Rehab*, 1996, *18*(5):249-254.

280. Laupacis, A., Muirhead, N., Keown, P., & Wong, C. A disease-specific questionnaire for assessing quality of life in patients on hemodialysis. *Nephron*, 1992, *60*(3):302-306.

281. Mahls, T.C., Daniels, K., Dahhan, W., & Donnelly, K. Fatigue in patients with chronic hepatitis C [Abstract]. *Gastroenterology*, 1996, *110*:A1254.

282. Krupp, L.B., Masur, D., Schwartz, J., et al. Cognitive functioning in late Lyme borreliosis. *Arch Neurol*, 1991, *48*:1125-1129.

283. Paul, R., Beatty, W., Schneider, R., et al. Cognitive and physical fatigue in multiple sclerosis: Relations between self-report and objective performance. *Appl Neuropsychol*, 1998, *5*:143-148.

284. Roelcke, U., Kappos, L., Lechner-Scott, J., et al. Reduced glucose metabolism in the frontal cortex and basal ganglia of multiple sclerosis patients with fatigue: A 18F-fluorodeoxyglucose positron emission tomography study. *Neurology*, 1997, *48*:1566-1571.

285. Schwartz, A.L., Meek, P.M., Nail, L.M., et al. Measurement of fatigue: Determining minimally important clinical differences. *J Clin Epidemiol*, 2002, *55*(3):239-244.

286. Sprangers, M.A.G., Van Dam, F.S.A.M., Broersen, J., et al. Revealing response shift in longitudinal research on fatigue: The use of the Thentest approach. *Acta Oncologica*, 1999, *38*(6):709-718.

287. Visser, M.R., Smets, E.M., Sprangers, M.A., & de Haes, H.J. How response shift may affect measurement change of fatigue. *J Pain Symptom Manage*, 2002, *20*:12-18.

288. Bernhard, J., Lowy, A., Maibach, R., & Hurny, C. Response shift in the perception of health for utility evaluation: An explorative investigation. *Eur J Cancer*, 2001, *37*:1729-1735.

289. Krishnasamy, M. Fatigue in advanced cancer-meaning before measurement? *Int J Nurs Studies*, 2000, *37*(5):401-414.

290. Porock, D., Kristjanson, L.J., Tinnell, K., et al. An exercise intervention for advanced cancer patients experiencing fatigue: A pilot study. *J Palliat Care*, 2000, *16*(3):30-36.

291. Vanio, A. & Auvinen, A. Prevalence of symptoms among patients with advanced cancer: An international collaborative study, symptom prevalence group. *J Pain Symptom Manage*, 1996, *2*(1):3-10.

35

Measuring Mobility and Potential for Falls

Ann Marie Spellbring and Judith W. Ryan

Falls are a major cause of morbidity, immobility, and mortality. Although falls occur across the lifespan, research on falls has focused on older adults because both the risk for falling and the potential for negative sequelae increase as an individual ages. Falls are the second leading cause of death from trauma in the United States and for those over 65 years of age, falls are responsible for one third of deaths caused by injury.[1] This chapter presents an approach in the conceptualization of falls, discusses methodologic issues related to measuring the incidence of falls in various settings, reviews specific measures used in falls and mobility research that identify risk factors for falls and characteristics of those who fall, and summarizes the future directions of falls and mobility research. Those who fall will be referred to in this chapter as fallers.

Falls

Conceptualization

Falls among older adults are usually multifactorial in nature. They generally are a result of the underlying physiologic changes associated with aging, physical illnesses, effects of medications, social factors, and/or environmental hazards. Falls may be precipitated by any of these individually or, more often, in interaction with each other.[2] A significant contribution to the conceptualization of falls has been presented by Hogue.[3] She views falls as occurring when the performance level of an individual is inadequate for the demands of environmental tasks. This conceptualization is supported by the adaptation and aging model proposed by Lawton and Nahemow,[4] in which personal competence (a person's capacities) and environmental press (the demands of the environment that activate behavior) interact to stimulate behavior. For example, when an individual is frail (less competent), it takes very little or perhaps no stimulation from the environment to initiate a fall. On the other hand, if the environment is particularly demanding, such as sleet and ice on steps, even highly competent individuals have difficulty and may be unable to prevent a fall.

Definition

The lack of agreement on a standard definition of falls in falls research has contributed to the inability to compare and contrast studies easily. The researcher must be particularly attentive to what is or is not included in the fall definition for each study. Unfortunately, even the 2001 "Guideline for the Prevention of Falls in Older Persons" developed by the American Geriatrics Society does not include a recommended definition of falls.[5] Most definitions of a fall include the elements of a change in body position and the lack of intention to do so,[6] as well as a loss of balance that cannot be corrected. In a consensus report of the Kellogg International Work Group on the Prevention of Falls by the Elderly[2] and supported in 1990 by the report of the Institute of Medicine's Committee on Health Promotion and Disability Prevention for the Second Fifty Years,[7,p7] the following standardized definition of a fall has been proposed: "A fall is an event which results in a person coming to rest inadvertently on the ground or other lower level and other than as a consequence of the following: sustaining a violent blow, loss of consciousness, sudden onset of paralysis, as in a stroke or an epileptic seizure." Although this definition has several exclusions, it is not uncommon for researchers to include some of what this definition excludes in their research on falls.

Falls Classification Systems

In addition to the difficulties posed by the lack of a standard definition of falls, it also is important for the researcher to explore specifically the various causes of the fall. Some authors refer to the intrinsic causes (pertaining to the individual),[8,9] but others have reported on the situational or extrinsic causes of falls (pertaining to the environment).[10] Appendix 35.1 describes major classification systems developed by Isaacs;[11] Wild, Nayak, and Isaacs;[12] Morse;[13] and Lach et al.[14]

The description of the fall event and its consequences is an additional area of measurement. Nevitt,[15] in a prospective year-long study of 325 elderly persons with a previous history of falling, suggests describing falls in terms of the following categories: (1) antecedents—the illness, medications, or symptoms preceding the fall as well as the behavioral and environmental circumstances; (2) mechanics—orientation of the fall (forward or backward), impact surfaces, what surface is landed on and what body part receives impact; and (3) consequences—ability to rise unaided, type and severity of injury, fear of falling, treatment, and activity and functional limitations.

Methodologic Issues

In addition to the lack of standard definition for falls and the multifactorial causes of falls, Cumming, Kelsey, and Nevitt[16] have addressed several methodologic challenges in the study of falls. One such issue regarding falls in community settings is the reliance on self-report information because most of these types of falls are unwitnessed and the information about a fall most often must come from the person who fell. Falls are a fairly common event and if no serious injury occurs, the person may forget the event and its details. Cummings, Nevitt, and Kidd[17] report that 13% to 32% of people who fell did not report their fall when they were interviewed 3 to 12 months later about falls that had occurred during that study period.

Falls research has been conducted in a variety of settings, which has made comparisons among studies somewhat difficult. The three major arenas for falls research are acute care hospitals, long-term care settings, and the community. Characteristics of the samples differ, as would be expected, but methodologies used often are setting specific. In determining risk factors and causes of falls, incident reports and chart review can be used readily in the institutional settings, but more dependence on recall or memory is required in the home environment. It has been proposed that falls among healthy adult populations in the community are caused by situational and environmental threats, whereas falls in the more frail institutionalized populations often are more attributable to individual characteristics.[7]

It is important to decide the unit of measure of the research. Some studies have identified the number of individuals who have fallen, whereas others have identified the rate of falls as the outcome measure. Much of the research on falls has been done to describe the characteristics of the faller by comparing risk factor prevalence in those who fell and those who did not fall. An alternative approach is to study the rate of falls in those with specific risk factors and those without.

Determining a fall rate also is of methodologic concern. No commonly established standard for reporting fall rates has been adopted. Researchers present fall rates differently, often not indicating how the rate was determined, which can lead to misleading conclusions or comparative problems for the reviewer. Sometimes fall rate is offered simply as a percentage of falls per number of subjects. Morse[13] recommended that the following formula be used as the standard for determining fall rate (number of falls per 1000 patient bed days):

$$\frac{\text{Number of patient falls}}{\text{Number of patient bed days}} \times 1000 = \text{Fall rate}$$

The number of patient bed days is determined by the daily total occupancy of the units for each day of the study. This formula yields a higher rate when the same subjects fall repeatedly because it uses the number of falls and not the number of fallers.

Instruments to Measure Falls

Fall research has focused on identifying the characteristics of fallers and attempting to predict risk for falls. These studies have been done retrospectively or prospectively with various methods of data collection, such as incident reports, patient interviews, medical records, and observations.

The clinical nursing literature has been especially prolific on establishing high-risk profiles for those at risk for falling.[18] These risk profiles have been especially helpful in developing appropriate interventions to modify risks. Falls account for the majority of all incident reports in hospitalized patients. The profiles of those at risk for falling have varied from study to study, but there is considerable overlap and similarity among studies. Instruments have been developed to address either the intrinsic or extrinsic factors that put a person at risk to fall.

Intrinsic Risks for Falls

Intrinsic risks pertain to characteristics that are unique to the individual that might put him or her at risk for falls, such as changes in cognition, gait and balance, or vision. A review[18] was conducted of 20 fall risk assessment scales from 1984 through 2001 for content and validation. It included 14 nursing assessment tools and 6 functional assessment tools. The findings support those reported in Appendix 35.2[19-48] with the addition of "incontinence or toileting issues" as a commonly measured behavior. In addition, the "Guideline for the Prevention of Falls in Older Persons"[5] includes the same risk factors in its univariate analysis of the most common factors identified in the 16 studies included in their analysis. Appendix 35.2 includes selected intrinsic risk factors for falls, as identified in various studies across clinical settings.[7]

Hendrich Risk Assessment Tool

Hendrich et al.[49] created a risk assessment tool based on a study of 338 hospitalized patients. It includes recent history of falls (not slip/trip), altered elimination, confusion/disorientation, depression, dizziness/vertigo, poor mobility/weakness, and primary cancer diagnosis. In addition, an "other" category is available to identify any unique vulnerability of the patient (e.g., excessive blood loss). The tool takes less than a minute to administer, with the seven items (differently weighted) having a maximum score of 25 points. The author identifies the patient at high risk for falling as one who scores three points or greater. The interrater reliability with this tool was 97.5%. Sensitivity was reported at 77% and specificity at 72%. A subsequent revision of the tool has also been reported.[50]

Schmid's Fall Risk Assessment Tool

Schmid[51] developed a fall risk assessment tool for hospitalized patients. It included assessment of mobility, mentation, elimination, fall history, and current medications. Content validity was verified by a task force of nurses who concurred on item selection and analysis. Criterion-related validity was established by examining risk scores on 334 patients who fell during a 5-week period. Construct validity was established by comparing patients assessed "at risk" for falls with patients assessed "not at risk." Test–retest reliability was established by a nurse assessing fall risk on admission and repeating the measure 4 hours later. Initially, weights were assigned to significant risk areas. A remanipulation of the data with different weightings of the fall risk tool increased test–retest reliability to 100%. Interrater reliability was established by comparing the percentage of agreement among the raters who independently administered the risk assessment to the same patient. The authors report an 88% agreement for the total score but suggest that the tool should be tested in other populations.

Spellbring's Assessment for High Risk to Fall Instrument

Spellbring[52] developed a 13-item Assessment for High Risk to Fall Instrument for use by nurses to identify elderly patients at risk of falling in the acute care setting. Categories addressed include mental and functional health status; history of previous falls; vision, hearing, and communication impairment; sleep patterns; mood fluctuation; hypotension; medications; and observation of gait and balance ability. Interrater reliability was determined by the percentage of agreement between registered nurses administering the instrument simultaneously. Thirty elderly medical-surgical patients were assessed within 24 hours of admission to the nursing unit. The mean time for completing the instrument was 17 minutes. Reliability ranged from 0.76 to 1.00 per item, with an overall reliability of 0.90 for total categories.

STRATIFY

Oliver et al.[53] developed a risk assessment tool called STRATIFY (St. Thomas Risk Assessment Tool in Falling Elderly Inpatients) with a prospective study used to identify risk factors in phase one and then test them in two additional phases at two hospitals' elderly care units (a large urban teaching hospital in London and a smaller, "district" general hospital). The tool includes five factors: fall as a presenting complaint, a combined Barthel index transfer and mobility score of 3 or 4, agitation, frequent toileting, and visual impairment. Each factor was scored 1 point, with a cutoff of 2 points for being at high risk for falls. The ability to correctly predict a fall within the next week after an assessment score of 2 or more had 93% sensitivity and 88% specificity at the large teaching hospital and 92% sensitivity and 68% specificity at the general hospital. No interrater reliability was reported.

Morse Fall Scale

Morse, Morse, and Tylko[54] developed a 6-item index, the Morse Fall Scale, to identify fall risk among 200 hospitalized patients. The scale consists of (1) history of falling, (2) secondary diagnosis, (3) ambulatory aids, (4) use of intravenous therapy, (5) gait, and (6) mental status. The six items are weighted, with a score range of 0 to 125. A score of 16 or above identifies the individual as a high-risk fall candidate. However, the authors caution that the final selection of a high-risk-to-fall score should be a matter of judgment, not a predetermined summed score.

Interrater reliability was established with 21 nurses rating six patients for an r of 0.96. The reliability estimates were only for five of the six items ($r = 0.82–1.0$). Mental status was omitted because of difficulty in obtaining consent from confused patients. A test for internal consistency revealed weak interitem correlations, with a coefficient alpha of 0.16 indicating that the items are independent, as might be expected in a short instrument for a multifaceted problem such as falls.

Validation of the scale was established by randomly splitting the cases, obtaining scale weights from 50% of the cases, and retesting the discriminatory power on the remaining 50%. The percent of patients correctly classified was 79%, which was not significantly different from the original. Validity also was tested prospectively on 2689 patients in three different clinical settings (acute care hospital, long-term care, and rehabilitation hospital), with increasingly higher scores obtained for patients from acute care to long-term care to rehabilitation settings.

Extrinsic Risks for Falls

The assessment of environmental hazards, or extrinsic factors, as part of a fall risk profile is well established both in the literature and clinical practice. Studies have indicated that 18% to 50% of falls are due to environmental conditions.[12,34,55–58] Common hazards cited include scatter rugs, loose carpets, slippery surfaces, and raised door thresholds;[56,58] low beds and toilet seats;[59] inadequate lighting;[12,56] cracked sidewalks and unsafe stairs;[57,60] raised bed rails;[61,62] and wheelchairs, walkers, and hemicanes.[63,64]

Tinetti and Speechley[65] identify three areas of general agreement when environmental factors are explored: (1) the more frail a person is, the more susceptible he or she is to even minor hazards; (2) an individual's specific disabilities are more likely to predict the amount of hazard a particular environmental condition presents; and (3) a person's experience with a specific environmental condition reduces the risk from it. Although these are commonly accepted areas of agreement among researchers on falls, controlled research studies that investigate the role of environmental hazards in falls are sparse. Most of the instruments used to measure environmental hazards are checklists constructed from the researcher's clinical experience and have not been standardized. In addition, the checklists are generally more qualitative than quantitative (e.g. "Are stairways adequately lighted?"). One such instrument, constructed by Tideiksaar,[66] is an environmental assessment useful in both home and institutional settings.

It is rare that the environment is directly assessed by researchers, and instead, subjects have described what they felt may have contributed to their falls. Conclusions about environment-related falls will remain uncertain until studies that also include the environment of nonfallers are conducted.

The Home Environment Survey

Rodriguez and colleagues[67] have developed a home environment hazards assessment instrument for their case-controlled study of falls in the elderly. They identified six environmental areas of importance: (1) floors: surface and tripping hazards; (2) furniture: use for sitting and walking support; (3) lighting: adequacy and ease of use; (4) bathroom: grab bars and slip-resistant surfaces; (5) storage areas: height; and (6) stairway conditions. The survey uses both direct observation of the home and interview of subjects to assess the environment. This instrument was assessed for face, predictive, and concurrent validity and internal consistency and repeatability. Although the study is not published, the authors state that the initial results from the validation study indicated that both the reliability and validity of the instrument are effective.

Near Falls

A relatively new area of investigation in fall research is the study of *near falls*, or events that are characterized by an unintentional loss of balance in which the person starts to go down but no fall occurs. The study of this phenomenon is challenged by subjects who do not have a clear definition of the term and the limited recall of persons who experience these events but, without a fall, have no real marker for remembering. Ryan, Dinkel, and Petrucci[68] created a 5-item measure to train elderly subjects in defining the term *near falls*. It includes common scenarios in which older persons may find themselves and requires them to distinguish between near falls, falls, and neither. Near falls may be an early predictor of high risk to fall or they may indicate a person who is more fit and hence able to regain balance and prevent the fall.[69]

Measures of Mobility

Mobility has been defined[70] as the "ability of a person to move purposefully within the environment." It depends on the integration of multiple physical, cognitive, and psychologic characteristics. For the most part, the literature has been conclusive about the extent to which impaired mobility related to gait and balance disturbances has contributed to falls. Morse[13] indicates that changes in gait and balance that occur with advancing age are more reliable indicators of liability to fall than is chronologic age. Physical performance measures of gait and balance are gaining increased attention in the literature. Specific performance tests for mobility have been able to identify fall risk not apparent in routine physical examinations.[71,72] The following measures are used to assess gait and balance capabilities and can serve as screening tools for those at risk for falls.

Berg Balance Scale

The Berg Balance Scale[73] was developed for screening the elderly at risk for falls. It evaluates performance on 14 items (1 sitting and 13 standing) related to balance functions frequently encountered in daily life, such as reaching, bending, and standing. Scoring is done on a 5-point scale (0 to 4). Total scores range from 0 to 56, with the lower scores indicating higher risk to fall. A cutoff score of 49 or less was identified for those at risk of falling. The scale takes about 15 minutes to administer and does require training of the testers. Interrater reliability was reported at 95% for the scale, which had a sensitivity of 77% and specificity of 86%.

Mobility Skills Scale

Hogue, Studenski, and Duncan[74] have developed a useful tool, the Mobility Skills Scale, to identify those at high risk for falls because of physical mobility impairments. The advantage of the tool is that it can be used in a variety of settings by health care professionals while they are routinely caring for patients. The Mobility Skills Scale contains seven items and takes 5 to 10 minutes to administer. The physical mobility tasks include (1) sitting balance, (2) sitting reach, (3) bending down to pick up pencil, (4) rising from a chair, (5) standing reach, (6) gait without an assistive device, and (7) descending stairs. Scale scores range from 0 to 7, reflecting the number of items that can be performed independently. The Mobility Skills Scale was tested for reliability and validity with 69 homecare patients with a mean age of 72 in the participant's own home. The interrater reliability for the individual items on this scale was acceptable (kappa = 0.79 to 0.92). The scale discriminated nonfallers from one-time fallers and repeated fallers (Krudskal Wallis Analysis of Variance, $H = X^2 (2) = 12.2$, $p = 0.005$). This instrument has a logical increase in difficulty for performing each subsequent task. This was confirmed with a coefficient of scaling reproducibility of 0.915, thereby demonstrating that subjects who could perform the most difficult items on the scale could also perform the easier tasks. The author suggests that the Mobility Skills Scale may be useful to screen for fall risk and detect mobility assistance needs.

Tinetti's Performance-Oriented Assessment of Balance and Gait

Tinetti and colleagues developed an assessment of balance and gait that reproduces the maneuvers required during daily activities.[36,72] A shorter version of this tool is also available.[75] Predictive items related to balance are unsteady sitting down, inability to stand on one foot, unsteady turning, and unsteady when nudged on sternum. Predictive gait measures include increased trunk sway, increased path deviation, and speed. These maneuvers are predictive when used in combination. The test takes 20 minutes to administer and requires training of the testers. Interrater and test–retest reliability for items that were timed are all over 0.95. The sensitivity was 80% and the specificity was 74%. The kappa statistic for individual maneuvers that were not timed are all over 0.50.

Dayhoff's Postural Control Scale

Dayhoff[76] has proposed a briefer and more clinically useful version of the Tinetti scales for hospitalized patients. Tinetti's 22-item assessment was reduced to 14 items related to three factors in postural control: automatic balance, voluntary control of balance, and gait. Subjects are scored on a 4-point scale according to their level of performance on each item. Examples of skills assessed include sitting balance, rising from chair, and step length. Criterion-related validity of self-report of a fall or no fall over 3 months before measurement reduced the 14 items to 6. Interrater reliability for each of the six items on the scale, using an ANOVA model for estimating generalizability coefficients, was acceptable with a range of 0.46 to 0.98 (mean 0.80). Internal reliability (coefficient alpha) was 0.88 for the sample.

Modified Gait Abnormality Rating Scale (GARS-M)

The Modified Gait Abnormality Rating Scale[77] is a 7-item modified assessment of gait designed to predict risk of falls among community-dwelling, frail older adults. Subjects were 52 male veterans with a mean age of 74.8 years. The subject's gait was scored by trained raters from a videotape of each walking 25 feet past the camera, turning around, and returning the 25 feet at a self-selected pace that was timed. The items were scored on a scale of 0 to 3 and consisted of the following categories: variability, guardedness, staggering, foot contact, hip range of motion, shoulder extension, and arm-heel-strike synchrony.

Intrarater reliability was a kappa of 0.493, 0.583, and 0.676, indicating moderate to substantial agreement for each of the three raters. The intraclass correlations coefficients for the raters were: 0.968, 0.950, and 0.984. Interrater reliability using kappa was 0.577 and 0.603 for the first and second trials. Construct validity was demonstrated when subjects with higher GARS-M scores had a history of falling while lower scorers did not have a fall history. Subjects with a history of falls had shorter stride length, walked slower, and had higher GARS-M scores than those who did not have a history of falls. The correlation between stride length and GARS-M score was $r = -0.754$ and between walking speed and GARS-M was $r = -0.679$, indicating concurrent validity.

The Timed Up & Go Test (TUG)

Shumway-Cook and colleagues[78] refined an earlier piloted[79] test of functional mobility. It requires that the person being assessed be timed while rising from a straight chair, walking 3 meters, turning around, returning to the chair, and sitting down. The cutoff time limit is 13.5 seconds or longer, with an overall correct prediction of falls rate of 90%. The test was then repeated with the person counting backward from a randomly selected number between 20 and 100. This "cognitive" variation had a 15-second or longer cutoff, with an overall correct prediction of falls rate of 87%. A third test was given while the person was carrying a full cup of water. This "manual" variation had a cutoff point of 14.5 seconds or longer, with a 90% correct prediction of falls rate. Interrater reliability was very high: 0.98 or above for each of the three variations. The TUG alone had 87% sensitivity and 87% specificity.

Roberts and Mueller Balance Scale

The Roberts and Mueller Balance scale[80] was designed to reflect the two factors related to balance—base of support and visual cues—and consists of eight stances: bipedal stance with eyes open and closed, monopedal stance with eyes open and closed, and the same four stances repeated on a beam. The time, in seconds, that subjects were able to maintain each of the stances up to a maximum of 30 seconds was summed for a total score, which ranged from 0 to 240. Higher scores indicate greater balance.

Validity and reliability were established with 61 persons aged 65 and over residing in the community. Construct validity was established by a factor analysis, and four factors were extracted: monopedal factor, bipedal factor without visual cues, visual factor, and beam factor. Standardized alpha coefficients for the four factor scores ranged from 0.60 to 0.76, with an overall coefficient of 0.82.[81] Interrater reliability was 0.99.[82]

Summary

Research and literature on falls in the elderly has demonstrated that falls are a multifactorial concept and should be considered from a physiologic, psychologic, and sociologic perspective.[4,7,65,83] The nursing literature has been very productive in establishing high-risk profiles of those who fall. Physical performance measures to assess gait and balance can serve as screening tools for those at risk for falls. It is important for future research to focus on the effectiveness of interventions targeted to specific risks. This holds an important and significant relevance to an aging population.

Websites

Websites that provide useful information on fall safety issues are listed here:

www.cpsc.gov/cpscpub/pubs/701.html from the U.S. Consumer Product Safety Commission—Home safety checklist.

www.patientsafety.gov/fallprev/fallrisk.html from the Veterans Health Administration.

www.aaos.org from the American Association of Orthopaedic Surgeons.

www.injuryresearch.bc.ca The British Columbia Injury Research and Prevention Unit provides descriptions for a wide variety of injury-related instruments under its icon "Tool Repository."

Exemplar Studies

Hendrich, A., Nyhuis, A., Kippenbrock, T., & Soja, M.E. Hospital falls: Development of a predictive model for clinical practice. *Appl Nurs Res,* 1995, *8*(3):129-139.

This study exemplifies the measurement of the most common variables related to risk for falling. These researchers began with an instrument of 22 risk factors and performed a retrospective chart review in a large (1000+ bed) acute care tertiary hospital. The tool differentiated characteristics that placed patients at high risk to fall and yielded the final risk model of seven significant risk factors. The seventh variable, primary cancer diagnosis, was subsequently replaced with "poor judgment in the absence of confusion." This study used a clear definition of a fall. Reliability and validity testing was rigorously addressed and the measure was sturdy in predicting fall risk. Additional strengths of this measure are that it includes the prominent risk factors for falls, has attributes that make it easily usable by clinicians, and serves as a basis for a fall prevention program.

Shumway-Cook, A., Brauer, S., & Woollacott, M. Predicting the probability for falls in community-dwelling older adults using the timed up & go test. *Phys Ther,* 2000, *80*(9):896-903.

This study exemplifies a simple quantitative measure of gait and mobility capacity that can be readily used in the clinical and research setting as a measure to predict fall risk. The basic test requires less than a minute to administer and the equipment required includes a chair, tape measure, and stopwatch. Two additional versions were also tested: one requiring mental distraction of the subject and one requiring a simultaneous manual task. There was little difference in the three versions as to time required. This study was based on prior studies and refined the measure even more usefully. Interrater reliability was excellent, and the ability to correctly predict falls or not to fall was 87%. This tool addresses just one dimension of vulnerability to fall (mobility), and it does require an ambulatory person to perform it.

References

1. Langlois, J.A., Smith, G.S., Baker, S.P., & Langley, J.D. International comparisons of injury mortality in the elderly: Issues and differences between New Zealand and the U.S. *Int J Epidemiol,* 1995, *24*:136-143.
2. Gibson, M.J., Andres, R.O., Isaacs, B., et al. The prevention of falls in later life. *Danish Med Bull,* 1987, *34*(4):1-10.
3. Hogue, C.C. Managing falls: The current bases for practice. In S.G. Funk, E.M. Tornquist, M.T. Champagne, & R.A. Weise (Eds.), *Key aspects of elder care: Managing falls, incontinence and cognitive impairment.* New York: Springer, 1992, p. 41.
4. Lawton, M.P., & Nahemow, L. Ecology and the aging process. In C. Eisdorfer & M.P. Lawton (Eds.), *The psychology of adult development and aging.* Washington, DC: American Psychological Association, 1973, p. 619.
5. Guideline for the prevention of falls in older persons. American Geriatrics Society, British Geriatrics Soci-

ety, and American Society of Orthopaedic Surgeons Panel on Falls Prevention. *J Am Geriatr Soc,* 2001, *49*(5):664-672.
6. Tinetti, M.E., Williams, T.F., & Mayewski, R. Fall risk index for elderly patients based on number of chronic disabilities. *Am J Med,* 1986, *80*(3):429-434.
7. Berg, R.L., & Cassells, J.S. (Eds.). *The second fifty years: Promoting health and preventing disability.* Washington, DC: National Academy Press, 1990.
8. Hindmarsh, J.J., & Estes, E.H. Falls in older persons: Causes and interventions. *Arch Intern Med, 1989,* 149(10):2217-2222.
9. Nickens, H. Intrinsic factors in falling among the elderly. *Arch Intern Med,* 1985, *145*(6):1089.
10. Parsons, M.T., & Levy, J. Nursing process in injury prevention. *J Gerontol Nurs,* 1987, *13*(7):36-40.
11. Isaacs, B. Are falls a manifestation of brain failure? *Age Ageing,* 1978, *7*(Supplement):97-111.
12. Wild, D., Nayak, U.S.L., & Isaacs, B. Description,

classification and prevention of falls in old people at home. *Rheum Rehab*, 1981, *20*(3):153.

13. Morse, J.M. *Preventing patient falls*. Thousand Oaks, CA: Sage, 1997.

14. Lach, H.W., Reed, A.T., Arfken, C.L., et al. Falls in the elderly: Reliability of a classification system. *J Am Geriatr Soc*, 1991, *39*(2):197-205.

15. Nevitt, M.C. Ascertainment and description of falls among older persons by self-report. In R. Weindruch, E.C. Hadley, & M.G. Ory (Ed.), *Reducing frailty and falls in older persons*. Springfield, IL: Charles C. Thomas, 1991, p. 476.

16. Cumming, R.G., Kelsey, J.L., & Nevitt, M.C. Methodologic issues in the study of frequent and recurrent health problems: Falls in the elderly. *Ann Epidemiol*,1990, *1*(1):49-56.

17. Cummings, S.R., Nevitt, M.C., & Kidd, S. Forgetting falls: The limited accuracy of recall of falls in the elderly. *J Am Geriatr Soc*, 1988, *36*(7):613.

18. Perell, K.L., Nelson, A., Goldman, R.L., et al. Fall risk assessment measures: An analytic review. *J Gerontol*, 2001, *56*(12):M761-M766.

19. Beers, M., Avorn, J., Soumerai, S.B., et al. Psychoactive medication use in intermediate-care facility residents. *JAMA*, 1988, *260*:3016-3020.

20. Campbell, A., Borrie, M.J., & Spears, G.F. Risk factors for falls in a community-based prospective study of people 70 years and older. *J Gerontol*, 1989, *44*(4):112.

21. Nevitt, M.C., Cummings, S.R., Kidd, S., & Black, D. Risk factors for recurrent nonsyncopal falls: A prospective study. *JAMA*, 1989, *261*(18):2663.

22. Tinetti, M.E., Speechley, M., & Ginter, S.F. Risk factors for falls among elderly persons living in the community. *New Engl J Med*, 1988, *319*(26):1701.

23. Blake, A.J., Morgan, K., Bendall, M.J., et al. Falls by elderly people at home: Prevalence and associated factors. *Age Ageing*, 1988, *17*:365.

24. Campbell, A., Reinken, J., Allan, B., et al. Falls in old age: A study of frequency and related clinical factors. *Age Ageing*, 1981, *10*:264-70.

25. Gabell, A., Simons, M.A., & Nayak, U.S.L. Falls in the healthy elderly: Predisposing causes. *Ergonomics*, 1985, *28*(7):965.

26. Mayo, N.E., Korner-Bitensky, N., Becker, R., & Georges, P. Predicting falls among patients in a rehabilitation hospital. *Arch Phys Med Rehab*, 1989, *68*(3):139.

27. Robbins, A.S., Rubenstein, L.Z., Josephson, K.R., et al. Predictors of falls among elderly people: Results of two population-based studies. *Arch Intern Med*, 1989, *194*:1628.

28. Wickham, C., Cooper, C., Margetts, B.M., & Barker, D.J.P. Muscle strength, activity housing and the risk of falls in elderly people. *Age Ageing*, 1989, *18*:47-51.

29. Janken, J.K., Reynolds, B.A., & Swiech, K. Patient falls in the acute care setting: Identifying risk factors. *Nurs Res*, 1986, *35*(4):215.

30. Wild, D., Nayak, U., & Isaacs, B. How dangerous are falls in old people at home? *Br Med J*, 1981, *282*:266-268.

31. Buchner, D.M., & Larson, E.B. Falls and fractures in patients with Alzheimer's type dementia. *JAMA*, 1987, *257*(11):1492.

32. Granek, E., Baker, S.P., Abbey, H., et al. Medications and diagnoses in relation to falls in a long-term care facility. *J Am Geriatr Soc*, 1987, *35*:503.

33. Prudham, D., & Evans, J. Factors associated with falls in the elderly: A community study. *Age Ageing*, 1981, *10*:141.

34. Buchner, D.M., & Larson, E.B. Transfer bias and the association of cognitive impairment with falls. *J Gen Intern Med*, 1988, *3*:254.

35. Morris, J. C., Rubin, E.H., Morris, E.J., & Mandel, S.A. Senile dementia of the Alzheimer's type: An important risk factor for serious falls. *J Gerontol*, 1987, *42*:412.

36. Tinetti, M.E. Performance-oriented assessment of mobility problems in the elderly. *J Am Geriatr Soc*, 1986, *34*(2):119.

37. Whipple, R.H., Wolfson, L.I., & Amerman, P.M. The relationship of knee and ankle weakness to falls in nursing home residents: An isokinetic study. *J Am Geriatr Soc*, 1987, *35*:13-20.

38. Perry, B. Falls among the elderly living in high-rise apartments. *J Fam Pract*, 1982, *14*(6):1069.

39. Adelsberg, S., Pitman, M., & Alexander, H. Lower extremity fractures: Relationship to reaction time and coordination time. *Arch Phys Med Rehab*, 1970, *70*:737.

40. Brocklehurst, J., Robertson, D., & Groom, J. Clinical correlates of sway in old age. *Age Ageing*, 1982, *11*:1-10.

41. Ring, C., Nayak, U.S.L., & Isaacs, B. Balance function in elderly people who have and who have not fallen. *Arch Phys Med Rehab*, 1988, *69*:261-264.

42. Tobis, J.S, & Reinsch, S. Postural instability in the elderly: Contributing factors and suggestions for rehabilitation. *Crit Rev Phys Rehab Med*, 1989, *1*(2):59-65.

43. Sorock, G.S., & Shimkin, E.E. Benzodiazepine sedatives and the risk of falling in a community-dwelling elderly cohort. *Arch Intern Med*, 1988, *148*:2441.

44. Guimaraes, R.M., & Isaacs, B. Characteristics of the gait in old people who fall. *Int Rehab Med*, 1980, *2*:177.

45. Imms, F., & Edholm, O. Studies of gait and mobility in the elderly. *Age Ageing*, 1981, *10*:147-56.

46. Wolfson, L.I., Whipple, R., & Amerman, P. Stressing the postural response: A quantitative method for resting balance. *J Am Geriatr Soc*, 1986, *335*:845.

47. Morse, J.M., Tylko, S.J., & Dixon H.A. Characteristics of the fall-prone patient. *Gerontologist*, 1987, *27*(4):516.

48. Ray, W.A., Griffin, M.R., Schaffner, W., et al. Psychotropic drug use and the risk of hip fracture. *New Engl J Med*, 1987, *316*(7):363.

49. Hendrich, A., Nyhuis, A., Kippenbrock, T., & Soja, M.E. Hospital falls: Development of a predictive model for clinical practice. *Appl Nurs Res*, 1995, *8*(3):129-139.

50. Corrigan, B., Allen, K., Moore, J., et al. Preventing falls in acute care. In Abraham, I., Bottrell, M.M., Fulmer, T., & Mezey, M.D., (Eds.), *Geriatric nursing protocols for best practice*. New York: Springer, 1999, p. 77-99.

51. Schmid, N.A. Reducing patient falls: A research-based comprehensive fall prevention program. *Military Med*, 1990, *155*(5):202.

52. Spellbring, A.M. Assessing elderly patients at high risk for falls: A reliability study. *J Nurs Care Qual*, 1992, *6*(3):30.

53. Oliver, D., Britton, M., Seed, P., et al. Development and evaluation of evidence based risk assessment

tool (STRATIFY) to predict which elderly inpatients will fall: Case-control and cohort studies. *BMJ*, 1997, *315*:1049.

54. Morse, J.M., Morse, R.M., & Tylko, S. Development of a scale to identify the fall-prone patient. *Can J Aging*, 1989, *8*(4):366.

55. Sheldon, J.H. On the natural history of fall in old age. *Br Med J*, 1960, *2*(2):1685.

56. Lucht, U. Prospective study of accidental falls and resulting injuries in the homes of elderly people. *Acta SocioÁmedica Scandinavica*, 1971, *2*(1):105.

57. Waller, J.A. Falls among the elderly: Human and environmental factors. *Accid Anal Prev*, 1978, *10*:21.

58. Morfitt, J.M. Falls in old people at home: Intrinsic versus environmental factors in causation. *Pub Health J London*, 1983, *97*(2):115.

59. Rubenstein, L.Z., Robbins, A.S., Schulman, B.L., et al. Falls and instability in the elderly. *J Am Geriatr Soc*, 1988, *36*(3):266.

60. Czaja, S., Hammond, K., & Drury, C. Accidents and aging: A final report. Washington, DC: Administration on Aging, 1982.

61. Morse, J.M. The patient who falls and falls again. *J Gerontol Nurs*, 1985, *11*(11):15-18.

62. Innes, E.M., & Turman, W.G. Evaluation of patient falls. *Qual Rev Bull*, 1983, *9*(2):30.

63. Berry, G., Fisher, R.H., & Lang, S. Detrimental accidents, including falls, in an elderly institutional population. *J Am Geriatr Soc*, 1981, *29*(7):322.

64. Lund, C., & Sheafor, M.L. Is your patient about to fall? *J Gerontol Nurs*, 1985, *11*(4):37-41.

65. Tinetti, M.E., & Speechley, M. Prevention of falls among the elderly. *New Engl J Med*, 1989, *320*(16): 1055.

66. Tideiksaar, R. *Falling in old age: Prevention and management.* New York: Springer, 1997.

67. Rodriguez, J.G., Sattin, R.W., Devito, C.A., et al. Developing an environmental hazards assessment instrument for falls among the elderly. In R. Weindruch, E.C. Hadley, & M.G. Ory (Ed.), *Reducing frailty and falls in older persons.* Springfield, IL: Charles C Thomas, 1991, p. 263.

68. Ryan, J.W., Dinkel, J.A., & Petrucci, K. Near falls incidence: A study of older adults in the community. *J Gerontol Nurs*, 1993, *19*(12):23.

69. Teno, J., Kiel, D.P., & Mor, V. Multiple stumbles: A risk factor for falls in community-dwelling elderly. *J Am Geriatr Soc*, 1990, *38*(12):1321.

70. Creason, N.S. Mobility: Current bases for practice. In S.G. Funk, E.M. Tournquist, M.T. Champagne, et al. (Eds.), *Key aspects of recovery: Improving nutrition, rest and mobility.* New York: Springer, 1990, p. 55.

71. Guralnik, J.M., Branch, L.G., Cummings, S.R., & Curb, J.D. Physical performance measures in aging research. *J Gerontol: Med Sci*, 1989, *44*(5):M141.

72. Tinetti, M.E., & Ginter, S.F. Identifying mobility dysfunction in the elderly. *JAMA*, 1988, *259*(8):1190.

73. Berg, K., Wood-Dauphinee, S., Williams, J.I., & Gayton, D. Measuring balance in the elderly: Preliminary development of an instrument. *Physiother Can*, 1989, *41*:304.

74. Hogue, C.C., Studenski, S., & Duncan, P. Assessing mobility: The first step in preventing falls. In S.G. Funk, E.M. Tournquist, M.T. Champagne, et al. (Eds.), *Key aspects of recovery: Improving nutrition, rest and mobility.* New York: Springer, 1990, p. 275.

75. Resnick, B., Corcoran, M, & Spellbring, A.M. Gait and balance disorders. In A. Adelman & M.P. Daly (Eds.), *Twenty common problems in geriatrics.* New York: McGraw Hill, 2001, 277-307.

76. Dayhoff, N.E. The postural control scale. In S.G. Funk, E.M. Tournquist, M.T. Champagne, et al. (Eds.), *Key aspects of elder care: Managing falls, incontinence, and cognitive impairment.* New York: Springer, 1992, p. 57.

77. VanSwearingen, J.M., Paschal, K.A., Bonino, P., & Yang, J.F. The modified gait abnormality rating scale for recognizing the risk of recurrent falls in community-dwelling elderly adults. *Phys Ther*, 1996, *76*(9):944-1002.

78. Shumway-Cook, A., Brauer, S., & Woollacott, M. Predicting the probability for falls in community-dwelling older adults using the timed up & go test. *Phys Ther*, 2000, *80*(9):896-903.

79. Podsiadlo, D., & Richardson, S. The timed "Up & Go": A test of basic functional mobility for frail elderly persons. *J Am Geriatr Soc*, 1991, *39*(2):142.

80. Roberts, B.L. Effects of walking on balance among elders. *Nurs Res*, 1989, *38*(3):180.

81. Roberts, B.L., & Mueller, M.G. The balance scale: Factor analysis and reliability. *Percept Motor Skills*, 1987, *65*(2):367.

82. Roberts, B.L., & Fitzpatrick, J.J. Improving balance: Therapy of movement. *J Gerontol Nurs*, 1983, *9*(3):151.

83. Rubenstein, L.Z., Robbins, A.S., & Josephson, K.R. Falls in the nursing home setting: Causes and preventive approaches. In P.R. Katz, R.L. Kane, & M.D. Mezey (Ed.), *Advances in long-term care.* New York: Springer, 1991, p. 28.

Appendix 35.1 Falls Classification Systems

Author/Theory	Characteristics
Isaacs:[11] The categorization of falls is based on the activity in which person is engaged at the time of the fall	Imposed (contact with a major external hazard) Judgmental error (occurring during hurried activity) Perceptual error (contact with an object that could have been avoided) Posture change (moving from lying, sitting, or standing with no external hazard) Walking (occurring during normal, unhurried walking with no external hazard) Standing (occurring while standing quietly)
Wild, Nayak, & Isaacs:[12] Falls are the result of uncorrected displacement of the body from its support base	Displacements either initiated (created by the subject himself) or imposed (unexpected events) Displacements have two magnitudes, either ordinary or extraordinary
Morse:[13] Identified three types of falls based on study of 200 hospitalized patients	Physiologic, anticipated: most prevalent (78%), involving patients who were disoriented, had a previous fall, had poor balance, impaired gait, or used walking aids Physiologic, unanticipated: least prevalent (8%) occurring in oriented patients who experienced drop attacks, seizures, dizziness, or fainting Accidental: (14%) occurring in oriented patients who tripped, slipped, or rolled out of bed
Lach et al.:[14] St. Louis Oasis Study Fall Classification system (based on 3-year, prospective study of 1358 community elders)	Extrinsic falls: includes falls due to slips, trips, and externally induced displacements, such as collision Intrinsic falls: due to impaired balance or mobility, sensory, or cognitive impairment or impaired consciousness Nonbipedal falls: person not standing on two feet, may have fallen out of bed or chair, or had failure of assistive device Unclassifiable falls: person unclear about what happened, no data

Appendix 35.2 Selected Intrinsic Risk Factors for Falls

Type of Risk Factor	Measure (Studies)	Strength of Evidence*
Demographic	Age > 80 Men (19–22)	Strong
	Female (22,23,28)	Inconsistent
General health & functioning	ADL, IADL, mobility impairment (6,21,22,24–28)	Strong
	Reduced physical activity/exercise (20–22)	Weak
	Past history of falls (6,20–22,29,30)	Strong
Medical conditions	Arthritis (6,21–23,27,31,32)	Moderate
	Stroke (20,21,26,33)	Moderate
	Parkinson's disease (20,21,32)	Strong
	Dementia (31,32,34,35)	Strong
	Incontinence (6,21,22,26,27,29)	Strong
	Postural hypotension (6,20–22,24,27)	Inconsistent
Musculoskeletal and neuromuscular	Reduced knee, hip, or ankle strength (6,20,21,27,30,31,36,37)	Strong
	Reduced grip strength (20,21,23,37)	Strong
	Foot problems (21–23,25,38)	Inconsistent
	Impaired knee/plantar reflexes (21,25,27)	Weak
	Slowed reaction time (21,25,39)	Weak
Sensory	Impaired visual acuity (6,20–22,24,27,38,40)	Strong
	Reduced depth perception (21)	Weak
	Visual perceptual error (20,41,42)	Weak
	Impaired lower-extremity sensory function (6,21,22,27,31,40,43)	Inconsistent
Other neurologic signs	Frontal cortex/release (6,27)	Weak
	Cerebellar, pyramidal, extrapyramidal (21,27)	Weak
Gait, balance, physical performance	Gait "abnormalities" (6,21,22,27,30,44)	Strong
	Reduced walking speed (20,21,44,45)	Strong
	Postural sway (20,21,40,41)	Moderate
	Impaired dynamic balance (6,21,22,27,30,41,46)	Strong
	Impaired tandem gait, one leg (21,22,31)	Moderate
	Difficulty rising from chair (20–22,36)	Strong
Cognitive, psychologic	Reduced mental status test score (21,22,24,27,29,31,33,34,47)	Strong
	Depression (6,21,22,24,32,47)	Strong
Medication use	Sedatives, hypnotics, anxiolytics (20,21,23,24,26,27,29,32,33,48)	Strong
	Antidepressants (21,23,24,26,48)	Moderate
	Cardiovascular (20,21,23,24,32,33)	Inconsistent
	National Health Interview Survey Supplement on Aging, 1984 (20,32)	Weak
	Number of medications (6,20,23,27,31,32)	Strong

ADL = activities of daily living; IADL = instrumental activities of daily living.

Numbers in parentheses correspond to studies cited in the References.

*Strong: association in multiple studies, at least two of which are prospective. Moderate: association in multiple studies, only one of which is prospective (some studies are negative). Weak: association in only a few studies, none of which are prospective (some studies are Negative). Inconsistent: generally conflicting and inconsistent findings in multiple studies.

Reprinted with permission from Berg, R.L., & Cassells, J.S. (Eds.), *The second fifty years: Promoting health and preventing disability*. Washington, DC: National Academy Press, 1990, pp. 270–271, 284–290. Courtesy of National Academy Press.

36

Measuring Nausea, Vomiting, and Retching

Roxanne W. McDaniel and Verna A. Rhodes

Although recent advances in pharmacology have improved the ability to prevent or control the symptoms of nausea, vomiting, and retching, they remain a problem for a variety of patients. Severe distress from these symptoms may decrease patients' quality of life and functional health status and may lead them to discontinue potentially life-saving treatment.[1-3] To use the findings of the increasing number of studies attempting to minimize these symptoms, it is important that the individual symptoms be accurately and appropriately measured.

Postoperative nausea and vomiting continue to occur in 20% to 70% of patients.[4,5] More than 70% of pregnant women may experience such symptoms,[6] which significantly influence their quality of life.[7] Nausea and vomiting continue to be some of the most disturbing side effects of cancer chemotherapy.[8] Up to 60% of patients report postchemotherapy nausea, and up to 50% report vomiting.[9-13] Anticipatory nausea and vomiting are problems for approximately 30% of the patients, but the figure has been reported to be as high as 57% among women receiving chemotherapy for breast cancer.[14,15] Radiation therapy patients also may experience the symptoms.[16]

Nausea, vomiting, and retching are separate concepts.[17] However, the interchangeable use of terms to describe them is confusing and diminishes the scientific knowledge base for practice, education, and research. *Nausea* is a subjective and unobservable phenomenon of an unpleasant sensation in the epigastrium and in the back of the throat that may or may not culminate in vomiting; it also is described as feeling "sick at the stomach." Nausea is an autonomic response that may have some objective elements, such as pallor, sweating, and feeling cold, and is usually known through self-report because of its intensity.[18-21] *Vomiting* is the forceful expulsion of the contents of the stomach, duodenum, and jejunum through the oral cavity as a result of changes in intrathoracic positive pressure. The vomiting center at the base of the medulla includes the chemoreceptor trigger zone (CTZ) that receives input from multiple peripheral and central afferent sources.[22] *Retching* is the attempt to vomit without expelling any material; it is also called *dry heaves*. The act of retching is regulated by the respiratory center in the brain stem.[23]

The increased attention to nausea and vomiting is demonstrated by the growing number of studies including these symptoms as outcome measures. A review by Penta et al.[24] showed more published research on nausea and vomiting and on the efficacy of antiemetics during 1980–1981 (31 studies) than in the preceding 20 years (26 studies from 1960 to 1979). An even more dramatic increase has taken place in the 1990s. A Medline search from 1997 to 2002 identified 4163 articles, including studies related to anesthesia, postoperative status, pregnancy, psychiatry, chemotherapy, radiation therapy, nausea, vomiting, and emesis. As in the early 1980s, most of this work was done by health professionals associated with oncology. There is little doubt that this increased interest results from the high prevalence and severity of the side effects associated with cancer chemotherapy and other cancer treatments. Although oncology health professionals have led this work, researchers in other health care areas also are examining the impact of nausea and vomiting on their patients.

Chemotherapy produces a variety of direct toxic effects on the body, and nausea and vomiting are among the most troublesome, challenging, and frequent. These problems often occur in anticipation of treatment through conditioned responses. The advent of more aggressive, multidrug, and higher-dose chemotherapy continues to make both direct (postchemotherapy) and anticipatory nausea and vomiting a significant problem. In addition to the psychologic stress caused by chemotherapy-induced nausea and vomiting, patients also may experience nutritional deficits, dehydration, electrolyte imbalance, weakness, and disruption in lifestyle.

Patients who often view the treatment and resulting discomfort as being worse than the disease may be reluctant to continue with repeated courses of treatment.[1-3] Because some patients stop or delay potentially curative treatment, nausea and vomiting could be considered a potentially fatal side effect if the disease is responsive to chemotherapy.[25]

Considering this negative impact, it is appropriate that considerable effort be used to develop and assess better pharmacologic and nonpharmacologic methods for controlling chemotherapy-related nausea and vomiting. Unfortunately, improvements in the assessment of nausea and vomiting have not kept pace with new interventions to alleviate the symptoms. Only very recently have investigators begun developing assessment and measurement methods that accurately reflect the range of important considerations for patients and providers.

Selecting an Instrument

Investigators should carefully select an instrument to measure nausea, vomiting, and retching and consider several dilemmas that exist in such measurement. Some of the major issues are:

- The use of observational assessment versus self-report
- Identification of specific symptoms and the components to be measured
- Reliability and validity
- Clarity, precision, and understandability of wording
- Format (appearance and readability)
- The timeframe for symptom recall
- Purpose for which instrument is intended (obstetrics, postoperative, postchemotherapy, or anticipatory symptoms)
- Ease of scoring

Global assessments of nausea, vomiting, and retching may have hindered the development of a scientific database. To obtain an accurate database, it is essential to have information about the individual symptoms. Interventions, both pharmacologic and non-pharmacologic, do not have uniform effects on these individual symptoms. Careful consideration of the issues listed is essential to measure accurately the individual phenomena, to determine symptom patterns, and to make comparisons.

Methods Available

The assessment of nausea and vomiting continues to evolve as an area of clinical research. Researchers and evaluators differentiate the separate symptoms rather than take a global or synonymous approach. As information increases in this area, new issues arise. Researchers must maintain a balance of obtaining accurate data about the specific symptom without putting an undue burden on the patient or clinical environment. Researchers also must take care not to direct suggestive attention to the symptom. Caution is required to avoid focusing on the incidence of the symptom because of the possibility of associative learning or conditioned responses that can occur in patients experiencing nausea and vomiting related to pregnancy, motion sickness, medications, or other psychologic or physical causes.

Many comprehensive instruments may include one or more of the components of nausea, vomiting, and retching. Some, such as the Adapted Symptom Distress Scale, measure multiple components.[26] Others measure either a single component, such as the Symptom Distress Scale,[27] or are global measures of the concepts. In this chapter only the instruments that specifically assess these symptoms are addressed. Appendix 36A provides a summary comparison of these instruments.

Counting Episodes of Nausea and Vomiting

The measurement of vomiting has been done simply by counting the number of emetic episodes and expressing them as an absolute number or by obtaining an average mean score per time unit (e.g., x/hour) for a defined observation period.[28,29] This approach accurately reflects vomiting and retching but is unable to reflect nausea accurately. Patients also must be able to provide accurate self-reports or must be continuously observed when this method is used.

Nausea and vomiting have been assessed by grouping the number of emetic and nausea episodes according to predefined criteria and then labeling the degree of severity of the side effect.[30] However, it is important to separate measures of nausea and vomiting because they are distinct symptoms. Nausea is a subjective experience that no objective method can measure. As it is not an observable phenomenon, nausea measurement must rely on patient self-report.

Duke Descriptive Scale (DDS)

The DDS grades nausea and vomiting from I to IV as follows, taking into account intensity, severity, and impairment in patient activity for a 24-hour period:[31,32]

    A. Nausea grades I to IV
       I: None
       II: Mild, activity not interfered with
       III: Moderate, activity interfered with
       IV: Severe, bedridden with nausea for more than 2 hours
    B. Vomiting grades I to IV
       I: No vomiting 24 hours after chemotherapy
       II: Mild, vomiting less than five times in the 24 hours after chemotherapy
       III: Moderate, 5 to 10 times in the 24 hours after chemotherapy
       IV: Severe, more than 10 times in 24 hours, patient bedridden, possible dehydration

C. Response will be graded as follows
   CR (complete response): Grade I, no nausea or vomiting
   PR (partial response): Grade II–III, nausea and vomiting
   NR (no response): Grade IV, nausea and vomiting
D. Source of response data
   PI: Patient interview
   NO: Nurse observation
   HCT: Other health care team

This easily administered scale lacks reported reliability and validity. In the highest grade (grade IV) it also has a low ceiling of 10 emetic episodes for a 24-hour period. Thus, patients who increase from 10 to 15 emetic episodes are evaluated as unchanged.[33]

Visual Analog Scales (VAS)

The VAS is a line, usually 100 mm in length (occasionally 150 or 160 mm long), with anchors at each end to indicate the extremes of the sensation under study (Figure 36.1). Traditionally, the VAS has been a horizontally oriented scale without indicators. However, more recently, it has been used as a vertical scale with or without markings.[34] The low endpoint is to the left in a horizontally oriented scale and at the base of a vertically oriented scale. Subjects indicate the point on the scale corresponding to the degree of sensation they are experiencing. Investigators score the intensity of the discomfort by measuring the millimeters from the low end of the scale to the mark.

Although the VAS avoids language descriptors to signify gradations of a subjective phenomenon, the anchor extremes require meaningful descriptors with tested reliability. For example, a vomiting VAS anchored at "none" on the low end of the continuum and at "constant retching" at the opposite end can link two different concepts. Administering analogue scales generally requires additional explanation.

When used properly, the VAS is a reliable, valid, and sensitive self-report tool for studying subjective symptoms. A study with 849 patients receiving chemotherapy found that analogue scales did not appear to offer a specific advantage of sensitivity over a simple discrete scale, regardless of the dimension of nausea considered.[35] In fact, these investigators found no advantage in using an analogue scale over a discrete scale. For subjective parameters such as nausea or toxicities of the antiemetics (e.g., sedation), VAS tools do not necessarily increase the quantitative accuracy of the assessment because respondents may be able to discriminate only between broad grades of a subjective sensation—none, mild, moderate, or severe.[36] Reliability and validity are strengthened when stable phenomena are being evaluated and measuring a single concept.[37] Caution must be taken when administering a VAS because it was designed for use with a seated subject marking the scale. Variations can affect the results, such as subjects responding from a supine position; when another individual marks the scale for the subject; when the subject marked a maximum rating, but later perceives the sensation to be greater; and accuracy of scoring must be ensured.

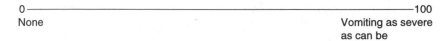

0 ——100
None   Vomiting as severe
                                              as can be

On this line mark how much vomiting you have had in the past 4 hours. At the left is zero, none. At the right is 100, vomiting as severe as can be.

Figure 36.1   Visual analogue scale for measuring vomiting severity.

Daily Diary

Daily diaries have been used in a variety of studies to record the incidence of nausea, vomiting, and retching. The diaries have been used for periods ranging from 24 hours to 15 days.[38-40] This method requires patient self-report and has been correlated to other measures, such as observation and the Functional Living Index.[41,42] Although reliability and validity are not reported, the diary card has the advantage of ease of administration and can be used in any setting. Comparison of findings among studies must be done with caution as there is no standardization of questions on the diary cards.

Morrow Assessment of Nausea and Emesis (MANE)

The MANE[25] and the Morrow Assessment of Nausea and Emesis Follow-Up (MANE-FU)[43-45] are self-report, Likert scales that measure post-treatment and anticipatory aspects of nausea and vomiting separately. These instruments provide data on onset, intensity, severity, and duration of nausea and vomiting. The frequency of anticipatory nausea and anticipatory vomiting are rated on a 5-point scale from "during and after every treatment" to "never after a treatment." Post-treatment nausea and post-treatment vomiting are rated on a 5-point scale ranging from "before every treatment" to "never before a treatment." The severity rating of nausea and vomiting is rated on a 6-point, equal-interval scale ranging from "very mild" to "intolerable." The time during which nausea and vomiting are worst is measured by a 6-point scale ranging from "during treatment" to "24 or more hours after treatment." An example of an item is: "The nausea is usually the worst" with response options ranging from 1 "during treatment" to 7 "no time is any more severe than any other time." Options 2 to 6 identify time periods from 2 "0–4 hours after treatment" to 6 "24 or more hours after treatment." The MANE-FU provides information about the effectiveness of medication for controlling nausea and/or vomiting.

Test–retest reliability for the MANE was determined with 20 randomly selected cancer patients who completed the instrument after each of four consecutive chemotherapy treatments. Correlations ranged from 0.72 (post-treatment nausea severity) to 0.96 (anticipatory nausea duration and post-treatment vomiting duration). Test–retest reliability also was determined with 18 patients who completed the MANE prior to the fourth treatment and approximately 7 months later. Correlations for this group ranged from 0.61 to 0.78. Content validity of the MANE was supported by the nonsignificant relationship between patient-reported anticipatory side effects and post-treatment side effects. Convergent validity was supported by the higher correlations of independent measures of nausea and vomiting than with other measures of chemotherapy side effects.[25]

Index of Nausea, Vomiting, and Retching (INVR)

The INVR measures the individual components of nausea, vomiting, retching, and associated distress. This 8-item, 5-point Likert pencil-and-paper tool measures patients' perceived (1) duration of nausea, (2) frequency of nausea, (3) distress from nausea, (4) frequency of vomiting, (5) amount of vomiting; (6) distress from vomiting, and (7) frequency of retching.[18,46,47] The original tool, INV-1, was developed and used by Rhodes et al. for a study to determine the reliability and validity of a self-report measure of nausea and vomiting.[18]

The INV-1 was compared to an adapted version of McCorkle and Young Symptom Distress Scale (ASDS).[18] Reliability of the INV-1 was determined employing a split-half procedure and Cronbach's alpha. Using the split-half procedure, reliability estimates of 0.83 to 0.99 were obtained.[18,48] Construct and concurrent validity were assessed by comparing family members' ratings to chemotherapy patients' ratings, yielding a correlation of $r = 0.87$. Psychometric properties of the original INV have been described in detail elsewhere. The investigators reported that both the INV-1 and ASDS were reliable and valid measures of post-treatment nausea and vomiting.[18,48]

The INV-1 was refined to include the occurrence and distress of dry heaves or retching and the distress from vomiting. This revised instrument, the INV-2, includes subscales for nausea, vomiting, and retching as well as for occurrence (intensity, duration, frequency and/or amount of distress). A numeric value is assigned to each response. These range from 0, the least amount of distress, to 4, the most distress. A total experience score from nausea, vomiting, and retching is calculated by summing responses to each of the eight items on the INV-2. The score range is from 0 to 32. The potential subscale scores are: nausea 0–12, vomiting 0–12, and retching 0–8. In a study of oncology patients, Cronbach's alpha for the INV-2 was 0.98.[20] The validity of the INV-2 was supported by a confirmatory factor analysis with a three-factor structure measuring nausea, vomiting, and retching.[49]

The INV-2 was originally developed for adult oncologic populations. However, it is appropriate for use with other populations because of its conceptual development. It has been used with oncologic, obstetric, cardiovascular, and postanesthesia patients.[50–52] A pediatric form has been pilot-tested with children ages 6 to 15 years. Correlations of 1.00 have been reported between the instrument and the observed and measured episodes of vomiting (M. Kachoyeamos, personal communication). An example of an item is: "During the last 12 hours, I have not felt any distress from nausea/sickness at my stomach"; "During the last 12 hours I have felt mild distress from nausea or sickness at my stomach"; "During the last 12 hours I have felt moderate distress from nausea or sickness at my stomach"; "During the last 12 hours I have felt great distress from nausea or sickness at my stomach"; "During the last 12 hours I have felt as severe distress from nausea or sickness at my stomach as can be." INVR was revised to improve readability by using introductory statements followed by five possible responses, presented in the same order as the complete sentences of the INV-2. The INVR has been used with different populations and has been translated into Chinese and Korean.[53,54]

Functional Living Index-Emesis (FLIE)

The 18-item FLIE, developed by Lindley et al., was designed for easy, repeated patient self-administration.[55] Although modeled after the Functional Living Index-Cancer, FLIE items deal specifically with the effects of nausea and vomiting on physical activities, social and emotional function, and the ability to enjoy food. Each FLIE item is answered in a Likert format ranging from 1 to 7, with 9 items for nausea, and 9 items for vomiting. A total score is created by adding the responses to the 18 questions. The range of total scores possible is between 18 (all 1 responses on the scale) and 126 (all 7 responses on the scale). Lower scores indicate a more negative impact of nausea and vomiting. An example of an item is: "How much nausea have you had in the past 3 days?"

The validity of the FLIE is supported by the difference in mean scores of subjects experiencing vomiting and those who were not experiencing vomiting. Content- and criterion-related validity were supported in the study by Lindley et al. Cronbach's alpha correlations support the reliability of the FLIE.

Summary

Although chemotherapy-related nausea, vomiting, and retching continue to be the most frequently investigated, researchers in other clinical areas are giving increased attention to these symptoms. The earliest techniques used to measure these symptoms have been simple and direct—usually counting episodes. Self-report tools used global terms that considered these symptoms as one, rather than as individual, symptoms. Norris's[17] work in the development of these individual concepts has helped to differentiate between objective and subjective experiences with varied conditions. This information was beneficial in the development of self-report measures of nausea, vomiting, and retching.

Instruments to measure nausea, vomiting, and retching have shown increased refinement and have demonstrated reliability and validity in various trials. Although progress has been made in the measurement of these symptoms, many studies continue simply to count the number of emetic episodes, ignoring the importance of the subjective experience of nausea. Measuring the human response to the occurrence of the symptom is critical to developing appropriate interventions.

Exemplar Studies

Zarate, E., Mingus, M., White, P.F., et al. The use of transcutaneous acupoint electrical stimulation for preventing nausea and vomiting after laparoscopic surgery. *Anesth Analges,* 2001, *92*(3):629-635.

The Functional Living Index-Emesis was used to measure the antiemetic efficacy of transcutaneous acupoint electrical stimulation (TAES) in a double-blind study of 221 outpatients undergoing laparoscopic cholecystectomy. An active ReliefBand device was placed at the P6 acupoint on experimental subjects and remained in place for 9 hours postoperatively. Comparison subjects had an inactive device applied at the P6 acupoint or the dorsal aspect of the wrist. The experimental group had significantly less nausea, but the incidence of vomiting was not significantly different. TAES was effective in reducing only postoperative nausea in this sample.

Dodd, M.J., Onishi, K., Dibble, S.L., & Larson, P.J. Differences in nausea, vomiting, and retching between younger and older outpatients receiving cancer chemotherapy. *Cancer Nurs,* 1996, *19*(3):155–161.

The Index of Nausea, Vomiting, and Retching was used in a longitudinal study conducted to determine if there were differences in chemotherapy-related nausea, vomiting, and retching (NVR) between individuals younger than 65 years and those 65 and older. Older individuals experienced less NVR 24 hours after chemotherapy than did the younger patients in later chemotherapy cycles. The higher incidence of NVR in younger individuals may be related to higher trait anxiety and greater expectations of being sick.

Monti, S., & Pokorny, M.E. Preop fluid bolus reduces risk of post op nausea and vomiting. A pilot study. *Internet J Adv Nurs Pract,* 2000, 4(2):1523-6064.

A pilot study compared the incidence of nausea and vomiting (NV) in women undergoing laproscopic gynecologic surgery. Forty-five women received a 1-liter fluid bolus preoperatively, and 45 women received standard fluids. All episodes of NV were recorded on a data flow sheet. Thirty percent of the control group had nausea and 5% experienced vomiting. There was a significant difference between groups for combined NV ($p = 0.001$), with 51% of the control group and 17% of the experienced group experiencing NV. The findings indicate that administering a liter of saline bolus decreases nausea and vomiting in this population.

Hickok, J.T., Roscoe, J.A., & Morrow, G.R. The role of patients' expectations in the development of anticipatory nausea related to chemotherapy for cancer. *J Pain Symptom Manage,* 2001, 22(4):843–850.

The relationship between expectation of nausea and the development of anticipatory nausea (AN) was examined in 63 women receiving their first course of chemotherapy. The

Morrow Assessment of Nausea and Emesis was used to measure nausea. Twenty women expected to experience nausea. The expectation of nausea predicted AN at cycle three (Spearman's $r = 0.41$, $p = 0.001$). Forty percent of patients who expected nausea and 13% of those who were uncertain if they would experience nausea had AN. Patients who did not expect nausea did not have AN. Expectation of nausea was the strongest predictor of AN ($X^2 = 13.15$; $p < 0.001$).

Carlsson, C.P.O., Axemo, P., Bodin, A., et al. Manual acupuncture reduces hyperemesis gravidarum: A placebo-controlled, randomized, single-blind, crossover study. *J Pain Symptom Manage*, 2000, 20(4):273–279.

The addition of acupuncture to standard treatment in improving hyperemesis gravidarum was examined with 33 women in a randomized, single-blind, crossover comparison study. Two methods of acupuncture, active (deep) PC6 acupuncture or placebo (superficial) acupuncture were used. The women estimated their degree of nausea on a visual analogue scale. Results indicated that there was a significantly faster reduction of nausea and vomiting after active acupuncture than after placebo acupuncture. The findings suggest that active PC6 acupuncture, in combination with standard treatment, could make women with hyperemesis gravidarum better faster than placebo acupuncture.

References

1. Bilgrami S., & Fallon, B.G. Chemotherapy-induced nausea and vomiting. Easing patients' fear and discomfort with effective antiemetic regimens. *Postgrad Med*, 1993, 94(5):55-58, 62-64.

2. Detmar, S.B., Muller, M.J., Schronagel, J.H., et al. Role of health-related quality of life in palliative chemotherapy treatment decisions. *J Clin Oncol*, 2002, 20(4):1056-1062.

3. Wampler, G., Schulz, J., Essig, L., et al. Virginia Oncology groups surgical adjuvant treatment Breast Carcinoma: A preliminary report. *Proc Am Assoc Cancer Res*, 1980, 21:412.

4. Gunta, K., Lewis, C., & Nuccio, S. Prevention and management of postoperative nausea and vomiting. *Orthop Nurs*, 2000, 19(2):39-48.

5. Cohen, M., Duncan, P., DeBoer, D., & Tweed, W. The postoperative interview: Assessing risk factors for nausea and vomiting. *Anesthes Analges*, 1994, 78(1):7-16.

6. Lacroix, R., Eason, E., & Melzack, R. Nausea and vomiting during pregnancy: A prospective study of its frequency, intensity, and patterns of change. *Am J Obstet Gynecol*, 2000, 82(4):931.

7. Gower, N.H., Rudd, R.M., Ruiz de Elvira, M.C., et al. Assessment of "quality of life" using a daily diary card in a randomized trial of chemotherapy in small-cell lung cancer. *Ann Oncol*, 1995, 6:575-580.

8. Morrow, G., Asbury, R., Hammon, S., et al. Comparing the effectiveness of behavioral treatment for chemotherapy-induced nausea and vomiting when administered by oncologists, oncology nurses, and clinical psychologists. *Health Psychol*, 1992, 11:250-256.

9. Chiara, S., Conte, P., Franzone, P., et al. High-risk early-stage ovarian cancer. Randomized clinical trial comparing cisplatin plus cyclophosphamide versus whole abdominal radiotherapy. *Am J Clin Oncol*, 1994, 17(1):72-76.

10. Du Bois, A., Meerpohl, H., Madjar, H., et al. Phase II study of pirarubicin combined with cisplatin in recurrent ovarian cancer. *J Cancer Res Clin Oncol*, 1994, 120(3):173-178.

11. Grunberg, S., & Hesketh, P. Control of chemotherapy-induced emesis. *N Engl J Med*, 1993, 329(24):1790-1796.

12. Thompson, H.J. The management of post-operative nausea and vomiting. *J Adv Nurs*, 1999, 29(5):1130.

13. King, C.R. Nonpharmacologic management of chemotherapy-induced nausea and vomiting. *Oncol Nurs Forum*, 1997, 24(7 Suppl):41.

14. Tyc, V.L., Mulhern, R.K., Barclay, D.R., et al. Variables associated with anticipatory nausea and vomiting in pediatric cancer patients receiving ondansetron antiemetic therapy. *J Ped Psychol*, 1997, 22(1):45-58.

15. Laszlo, J., & Cotanch, P. Managing chemotherapy-induced nausea and vomiting. *Cancer*, 1992, 70(4):1007-1011.

16. Grigsby, P., Vest, M., & Perez, C. Recurrent carcinoma of the cervix exclusively in the paraaortic nodes following radiation therapy. *Int J Radiation Oncol Biol Phys*, 1994, 28(2):451-455.

17. Norris, C.M. Nausea and vomiting. In C.M. Norris (Ed.), *Concept clarification in nursing*. Rockville, MD: Aspen, 1982, pp. 81-110.

18. Rhodes, V., Watson, P., & Johnson, M. Development of reliable and valid measures of nausea and vomiting. *Cancer Nurs*, 1984, 7(1):33-41.

19. Rhodes, V.A., & McDaniel, R.W. The Index of Nausea, Vomiting, and Retching (INVR): A new format of the Index of Nausea and Vomiting (INV). *Oncol Nurs Forum*, 1999, 26:889-894.

20. Rhodes, V., Watson, P., Johnson, M., et al. Patterns of nausea, vomiting, and distress in patients receiving antineoplastic drug protocols. *Oncol Nurs Forum*, 1987, 14(4):35-44.

21. Rhodes, V.A., McDaniel, R.W., Hanson, B., et al. Sensory perceptions of patients on selected antineoplastic protocols. *Cancer Nurs*, 1994, 17:45-51.

22. Veyrat-Follet, C., Farinotti, R., & Palmer, J.L. Physiology of chemotherapy-induced emesis and antiemetic

therapy: Predictive models for evaluation of new compounds. *Drugs*, 1997, *53*:206-234.

23. Guyton, A., & Hall, J. *Textbook of medical physiology* (9th ed.). Philadelphia: Saunders, 1996.

24. Penta, J., Poster, D., & Bruno, S. The pharmacologic treatment of nausea and vomiting caused by cancer chemotherapy: A review. In J. Laszlo (Ed.), *Antiemetics cancer chemotherapy*. Baltimore: Williams & Wilkins, 1983, p. 53.

25. Morrow, G. Assessment of nausea and vomiting: Past problems, current issues and suggestions for future research. *Cancer*, 1984, *53*(10):2267.

26. Simms, S.G., Rhodes, V.A., & Madsen, R.W. Comparison of prochlorperazine and lorazepam antiemetic regimens in the control of postchemotherapy symptoms. *Nurs Res*, 1993, *42*(4):235-239.

27. McCorkle, R. Non-obtrusive measures in clinical nursing research. In R. Tiffany (Ed.), *Cancer nursing update. Proceedings of the second international cancer nursing conference*. London: Balliere Tindall, 1981.

28. Fox, S., Einhorn, L., Cox, E., et al. Ondansetron versus ondansetron, dexamethasone, and chlorpromazine in the prevention of nausea and vomiting associated with multiple-day cisplatin chemotherapy. *J Clin Oncol*, 1993, *11*(12):2391-2395.

29. Bruera, E., Macmillan, K., Kuehn, N., et al. A controlled trial of megestrol acetate on appetite, caloric intake, nutritional status, and other symptoms in patients with advanced cancer. *Cancer*, 1990, *66*(6):1279-1282.

30. Bovbjerg, D., Redd, W., Jacobsen, P., et al. An experimental analysis of classically conditioned nausea during cancer chemotherapy. *Psychosom Med*, 1992, *54*:623-637.

31. Laszlo, J., Lucas, V., Hanson, D., et al. Levonantradol for chemotherapy-induced emesis: Phase I-II oral administration. *J Clin Pharmacol*, 1981, *21*(8, 9):515.

32. Cotanch, P. Relaxation training for control of nausea and vomiting in patients receiving chemotherapy. *Cancer Nurs*, 1983, *6*(4):277-283.

33. Cotanch, P. Measuring nausea and vomiting. In M. Frank-Stromberg (Ed.), *Instruments for clinical nursing research*. East Norwalk, CT: Appleton & Lange, 1988, pp. 313-321.

34. Bennett, B.B., & Hockenberry, M.J. An antiemetic study comparing halcion to ativan in children receiving cancer chemotherapy. *Oncol Nurs Forum*, 1989, *16*(2 Suppl):175.

35. Del Favero, A., Tonato, M., & Roila, F. Issues in the measurement of nausea. *Br J Cancer*, 1992, *66*(Suppl XIX):S69-S71.

36. Olver, I., Simon, R., & Aisner, J. Antiemetic studies: A methodological discussion. *Cancer Treat Rep*, 1986, *70*(5):555-563.

37. Grealish, L., Lomasney, A., & Whiteman, B. Foot massage. A nursing intervention to modify the distressing symptoms of pain and nausea in patients hospitalized with cancer. *Cancer Nurs*, 2000, *23*(3):237.

38. Baltzer, L., Kris, M., Tyson, L., et al. The addition of ondanstetron to the combination of metoclopramide, dexamethasone, and lorazepam did not improve vomiting prevention in patients receiving high-dose cisplatin. *Cancer*, 1994, *73*(3):720-723.

39. Buser, K., Joss, R., Piquet, D., et al. Oral ondansetron in the prophylaxis of nausea and vomiting induced by cyclophosphamide, methotrexate and 5-fluorouracil (CMF) in women with breast cancer. Results of a prospective, randomized, double-blind, placebo-controlled study. *Ann Oncol*, 1993, *4*(6):475-479.

40. Sung, Y.F., Wetchler, B.V., Duncalf, D., & Joslyn, A.F. A double-blind, placebo-controlled pilot study examining the effectiveness of intravenous ondansetron in the prevention of postoperative nausea and emesis. *J Clin Anesthes*, 1993, *5*(1):22-29.

41. Bleehen, N., Girling, D.J., Machin, D., & Stephens, R.J. A randomized trial of three or six courses of etoposide cyclophosphamide methotrexate and vincristine or six courses of etoposide and ifosfamide in small cell lung cancer (SCLC). II: Quality of life. Medical Research Council Lung Cancer Working Party. *Br J Cancer*, 1993, *68*(6):1157-1166.

42. Clavel, M., Soukop, M., & Greenstreet, Y. Improved control of emesis and quality of life with ondansetron in breast cancer. *Oncology*, 1993, *50*:180-185.

43. Anastasio, G., Robinson, M., Little, J., et al. A comparison of the gastrointestinal side effects of two forms of erythromycin. *J Fam Pract*, 1992, *35*(5):517-523.

44. Razavi, D., Delvaux, N., Farvacques, C., et al. Prevention of adjustment disorders and anticipatory nausea secondary to adjuvant chemotherapy: A double blind placebo-controlled study assessing the usefulness of alprazolam. *J Clin Oncol*, 1993, *11*(7):1384-1390.

45. Chin, S., Kucuk, O., Peterson, R., & Ezdinli, E. Variables contributing to anticipatory nausea and vomiting in cancer chemotherapy. *Am J Clin Oncol*, 1992, *15*(3):262-267.

46. Rhodes, V.A., Watson, P.M., & Johnson, M.H. Association of chemotherapy related nausea and vomiting with pretreatment and posttreatment anxiety. *Oncol Nurs Forum*, 1986, *13*(1):41-47.

47. Rhodes, V.A., Watson, P.M., & Johnson, M.H. Patterns of nausea and vomiting in antineoplastic postchemotherapy. *Appl Nurs Res*, 1988, *1*(3):143-144.

48. Rhodes, V.A., Watson, P.M., & Johnson, M.H. A self-report tool for assessing nausea and vomiting in chemotherapy. *Oncol Nurs Forum*, 1983, *10*(1):11.

49. Zhou, Q., O'Brien, B., & Soeken, K. Rhodes Index of Nausea and Vomiting—Form 2 in pregnant women: A confirmatory factor analysis. *Nurs Res*, 2001, *50*:251-257.

50. Belluomoni, J., Litt, R.C., Lee, K.A., & Katz, M. Acupressure for nausea and vomiting of pregnancy: A randomized blinded study. *Obstet Gynecol*, 1994, *84*(2):159-160.

51. Troesch, L., Rodehaver, C., Delaney, E., & Yanes, B. The influence of guided imagery on chemotherapy-related nausea and vomiting. *Oncol Nurs Forum*, 1993, *20*(8):1179-1185.

52. Stainton, M., & Mesf, E. The efficacy of seabands for the control of nausea and vomiting in pregnancy. *Health Care Women Int*, 1994, *15*(6):563-575.

53. Fu, M.R., Rhodes, B., & Xu, B. The Chinese translations of the Index of Nausea, Vomiting, and Retching. *Cancer Nurs*, 2002, *25*:134-140.

54. Kim, Y.J., Kim, J.Y., Choi, I.R., et al. The Index of Nausea, Vomiting, and Retching (Korean translation). *J Korean Acad Adult Nurs*, 2000, *12*(2):278-285.

55. Lindley, C., Hirsch, J., O'Neill, C., et al. Quality of life consequences of chemotherapy-induced emesis. *Qual Life Res*, 1992, *1*:331-340.

Websites

www.wlm.nih.gov/medlineplus/nauseaandvomiting.html. This website provides links to and information from many organizations, including the National Institutes of Health, Mayo Foundation, American Academy of Family Physicians, American College of Obstetricians and Gynecologists, and the National Cancer Institute. There is a general overview of nausea and vomiting, information about symptoms, nutrition, managing symptoms of nausea and vomiting, and clinical trial information.

Appendix 36A. Summary Comparison of Measures of Nausea, Vomiting, and Retching

Tool	Dimensions	Type	How Administered	Reliability/ Validity	Strengths/ Weaknesses
Duke Descriptive Scale (31–33)	Nausea and vomiting with frequency, severity, and activity combined	Check scale	Patient interview by nurse Observation Other health care worker	Unreported	Low ceiling may limit information
Visual Analog Scales (34–37)	May be devised for individual symptoms and their components: frequency, duration, severity, distress	A line usually 100-mm long with reliable anchor descriptors at extremes; self-report (mark when in sitting position)	Reliability is strength with stable phenomena	Unreported	Subjects' inability to discriminate between grades of sensation Requires more administrator time Inaccurate when marked by another or subject in supine position Unstated time frame
Morrow Assessment of Nausea and Emesis (25)	Post-treatment nausea and vomiting; onset, severity, intensity, duration	16-item, 5-point Likert scale (onset) 6-point Likert scale (severity-intensity)	Self-report	Test–retest reliability: 0.61–0.78 Validity: 0.72–0.96	Primarily used with antiemetic studies Long (> 24 hour) timeframe
Morrow Assessment of Nausea and Emesis Follow-up (43–45)	Anticipatory nausea and vomiting (frequency)	17-item, 5-point Likert scale (severity-intensity)	Self-report	Content and convergent validity supported	Assesses anticipatory nausea
Index of Nausea, Vomiting, and Retching (18,20,53,54)	Nausea, vomiting, retching, and the components of each symptom: frequency, amount, duration, severity, distress	8-item, 5-point Likert scale	Self-report	Split-half reliability: 0.83–0.99 Cronbach's alpha: 0.98 Validity: $r = 0.87$	12-hour timeframe Measure distress of symptom Totals symptom experience scale Subscales for triad and occurrence and distress Used with varied groups
Functional Living Index Emesis (55)	Effects of nausea and vomiting on physical activity, social and emotional functions, eating	18-item, 7-point Likert scale	Self-report	Content and criterion validity Internal consistency supported	Ease of use Provides information about the effect of nausea and vomiting on functional status

Numbers in parentheses correspond to studies cited in the References.

37

Assessing the Oral Cavity

Sharon Ann Hyland

Stomatitis, or oral mucositis, refers to the inflammatory reaction and sequelae that can occur in the mouth and oropharynx because of the effects of radiation therapy and certain chemotherapeutic agents.[1-4] Stomatitis can present as ulceration, oral pain, and/or infection. These symptoms can significantly alter the patient's performance status and compromise nutritional intake, airway status, and vocal ability and possibly lead to systemic infection. These symptoms may require therapy dose modification or delays in further chemotherapy and/or radiation treatment. Ultimately, stomatitis can increase the morbidity and mortality associated with cancer therapy.[5] The use of intensive chemotherapy during bone marrow transplant procedures and the resulting severe stomatitis that occurs increases the need to find successful mechanisms to allay this debilitating and potentially life-threatening side effect of treatment.

Clinicians have for some time recognized the need for accurate clinical assessment and effective interventions to identify and allay the symptoms associated with stomatitis. There is a need to have an adequate, consistent oral assessment guide to measure mucosal changes and oral complications associated with cancer therapy accurately and reliably. Standardized assessment is necessary to compare the effectiveness of various agents or clinical interventions used to treat mucositis.[6]

Risk Factors for Stomatitis

Stomatitis is one of the most common patient complaints during chemotherapy, with an incidence of 39%.[7] The likelihood of oral complications depends on the malignancy and its treatment. The incidence of stomatitis in patients with solid-tumor malignancies is about 12%; it is 33% in lymphomas and 50% among leukemia patients.[8]

The appearance of stomatitis is the result of complex interactions with a number of factors. Patient-specific factors include type of cancer (hematologic or solid tumor); nutritional state; condition of the oral cavity, teeth, and gums before cancer therapy; age (younger individuals having more risk); and underlying medical conditions. Predisposing factors include pretreatment oral health, dental caries, and periodontal disease. Oral irritants include ill-fitting prostheses, exposure to irritating chemicals (tobacco, alcohol), physical exposures (coarse foods), and thermal exposures (food temperature).[9]

The most important causative factor in stomatitis is the direct effect of the therapy. Certain types of chemotherapy are known to cause stomatitis, including antimetabolites (methotrexate, 5-FU), alkylating agents and natural products (daunorubicin, doxorubicin).[10–12] Head and neck radiation therapy causes some degree of mucositis. The combination of chemotherapy with head and neck radiation poses an increased risk for stomatitis.

A second treatment-related risk factor is dose of therapy. High doses are known to increase the risk and severity of stomatitis. About 75% of patients undergoing bone marrow transplant will experience significant stomatitis caused by the pretransplant chemotherapy dose.[10]

A third risk factor is prior therapy. Past and present drug therapy, including antibiotics and steroids, can affect the mucosa of the oral cavity, as can prior surgical intervention. "Recall" oral reactions from prior chemotherapy or radiation are common.

Immunocompetence significantly influences the potential for and duration of stomatitis. High-dose chemotherapy or dose intensification usually shortens the time interval before onset of stomatitis and increases the potential for infection. The degree and duration of neutropenia directly influences the probability and degree of oral complications.[13]

The drug dose, scheduling, and method of administration also may increase the frequency of occurrence of stomatitis. For example, giving a drug as a 24-hour infusion may result in stomatitis that is not experienced when the drug is given as an intravenous push. Patients with prior evidence of stomatitis are likely to experience recurrence if the same drug and dosage are administered without additional intervention. Methotrexate, even at standard dosing, can cause stomatitis. Subsequent courses at the same dose without citrovorum factor antidote or alteration in dose can result in severe stomatitis. Renal dysfunction may increase the risk of stomatitis, because drug clearance times are prolonged.

Physiologic Effects of Therapy

The oral cavity is a vulnerable environment for side effects from cancer therapy because it is an area of rapid cellular activity. There is a high rate of cell proliferation and turnover in the oral epithelium. It is one of the body's first lines of defense. Drugs act directly by interfering with the replication of epithelial cells, causing changes in the submucosal tissue. The most vulnerable areas to mucositis include the nonkeratinized mucosal surfaces (soft palate, cheeks, lips, ventral surface of the tongue, floor of the mouth). The gingiva, dorsal surface of the tongue, and hard palate are rarely affected (slower rate of turnover). The mucositis sites usually appear in the same locations. The most common histologic changes are epithelial hyperplasia and collagen degeneration. These changes can lead to spontaneous or traumatic ulceration. Any mucosal break can become secondarily infected. The immunocompromised patient carries the inherent risk of altered response to the large amount of microbial flora, both normal and opportunistic pathogens present in the oral cavity, which can cause severe primary or secondary infections.[14–18]

Symptoms can range from a dry, painful mouth, the result of a thinning of the epithelium, to life-threatening sepsis directly caused by oral microorganisms. Stomatitis can alter the individual's ability to ingest food and fluids, ranging from avoidance of irritating foods or fluids to a total inability to swallow. Oral ulcerations in the neutropenic patient can provide a source of bacterial and fungal flora that can invade the body. Mucositis can result in local bleeding. Severe ulceration and associated edema can affect the airway and make it almost impossible to eat.

Stomatitis generally follows a predictable pattern over four phases: (1) inflammatory/vascular, (2) epithelial, (3) ulcerative/bacteriologic, and (4) healing. The phases are interdependent and are related to multiple factors, including the direct effect of the chemotherapy agent on the epithelium, the oral bacterial flora, and the patient's bone marrow status. A series of actions are mediated by cytokines. The inflammatory phase occurs when cytokines are released from the epithelial tissue. These cytokines cause local tissue damage as the initiating event to mucositis. The epithelial phase occurs when the drug affects dividing cells of the oral basal epithelium, resulting in reduced epithelial renewal, atrophy, and ulceration. This is exacerbated by functional trauma and amplified by more cytokines. The ulcerative phase is mostly symptomatic. Erosions occur, which are covered by a fibrous pseudomembrane. Secondary bacterial colonization at the site occurs with mixed flora, which further stimulates cytokine release. This phase occurs at the time of the patient's maximum neutropenia. The healing phase is a renewal of epithelial proliferation and differentiation, normalizing of the white cell count, and reestablishment of the local microbial flora. When resulting from standard-dose chemotherapy, initial oral changes occur 7 to 10 days after drug administration. Stomatitis usually corresponds to a decrease in the granulocyte count. Healing occurs by the second to third week. The severity is usually mild to moderate without associated infection. Treatment involves the use of topical combination therapy with the primary use of analgesia for symptomatic relief. The goal of therapy is to maintain nutrition and hydration.[19]

The effects of radiation therapy depend on a number of factors and are primarily local. The radiosensitivity of the epithelial tissue varies throughout the oral cavity. The type of radiation fraction/dose, time between fractions, overall treatment time, cumulative dose, type of tissue irradiated, and field size affect the probability of stomatitis. The direct effect of radiation therapy results in a change in the epithelial characteristics, as the atrophic mucosa thins and an inflammatory reaction begins within the first week of treatment. The patient complains of a burning sensation, and there is decreased salivation in 7 to 10 days. The mucosa usually reddens and sometimes is white. The tongue may swell and develop a protective white coating, and there may be isolated ulcerations. Pseudomembranes may develop within 3 to 4 weeks of therapy, along with ulcerations and diminished taste sensation. Accelerated radiotherapy shortens the time to onset of mucositis by about 3 weeks. Because mucositis is more severe, treatment may need to be delayed. Healing occurs over weeks after therapy cessation.[17]

Severe stomatitis occurs commonly after bone marrow transplant conditioning regimens or extensive head and neck irradiation. Changes in the mucosal color (either red or white) occur from day 2 to 14. Mucosal atrophy is most marked between day 7 and 21. Painful, confluent ulceration results if neutropenia persists or when the adaptive resources of the patient are exhausted. With the recovery of the white blood cell count, stomatitis is self-limiting and resolves or reverses within 2 to 3 weeks. Dysphagia may be severe enough to result in an inability to swallow food and/or liquids. If there is a break in the mucosa and the blood counts are low, there is high risk for developing systemic infection. Stomatitis usually occurs near the nadir of the leukocyte count, and recovery from stomatitis precedes bone marrow recovery.[14]

Because neutropenic patients are at high risk of developing oral infections, such as candida or herpes simplex, it is important to differentiate whether the stomatitis is an oral infection or direct result of chemotherapy.[16] This requires direct visualization of the oral cavity on a regular basis. The patient's symptom report is not sufficient to determine accurately the cause of stomatitis. The sites of oral infections usually are the marginal, papillary, and attached gingiva. Secondary infection occurs when the leukocyte count is less than 1000. Infection can further result in opportunistic infections: bacterial, viral, and/or fungal. The classic signs of inflammation may be absent when the patient is severely neutropenic. It is important to perform oral cultures or other diagnostic techniques regularly.

The health professional cannot assume that all oral effects are the result of chemotherapy or radiation. The clinician must include all the following in an assessment: the overall systemic status of the patient, laboratory results, vital signs, presence of graft-versus-host disease, other medications, and associated local factors.

Additional sequelae of stomatitis include local bleeding, oral pain, and changes in the volume and consistency of the saliva. The pain can be severe enough to limit oral intake or even temporarily eliminate the ability to eat. Patients in this state require intravenous narcotics. Bleeding tends to be infrequent as long as the platelet count is adequate. Clinically, the saliva becomes more viscous.

All patients receiving chemotherapy should have an initial oral assessment, and the state of the oral cavity and teeth should be documented. The initial oral assessment includes a visual inspection with sufficient lighting to establish baseline data such as the state of the gums, the status of the teeth, and the use of any dental prostheses. Before bone marrow transplant, patients should have a dental consultation. All patients receiving chemotherapy and head and neck radiation should have a baseline oral examination even if the treatment they receive does not cause stomatitis.

Development of Oral Assessment Guides

Historically, there have been several approaches to the assessment and evaluation of oral complications of cancer therapy. The most common guidelines grade the clinical appearance of the oral cavity with or without the addition of functional input from the patient. The oral cavity is categorized into specific areas that are scored according to the severity of stomatitis. Another approach is to stage the stomatitis holistically. Each stage includes both the functional and objective aspects of stomatitis. Both of these approaches rely on direct visualization of the stomatitis. At present, such tools are hindered by the lack of observer standardization. Complications of stomatitis (edema, infection) can further confound the observer's findings. Soliciting the patient's assessment of symptom severity also can bring quite variable results. Therefore, the three goals of any instrument to assess mucositis should include clarity of wording and format, reliability, and ease/efficiency of use.

Early oral assessment tools lacked reliability and validity data[6,8,18] and they did not specifically assess the oral effects of cancer chemotherapy. Accurate descriptions of the mouth following chemotherapy treatment were lacking, as was a systemic pattern of assessment. Important categories to assess are voice, swallowing, lips, tongue, saliva, mucous membranes, gingiva, and teeth/dentures. Although early tools were tested with noncancer patients,[20] subsequent tools were developed providing detailed descriptors of potential oral signs and symptoms appropriate for patients receiving chemotherapy. However, severity was not adequately assessed. Manifestations of stomatitis complicated mucositis assessment and influenced the reliability of comparison assessment guides. For example, the amount and degree of edema may be more important than the size and number of the oral ulcerations. Presently, most oral assessment instruments include both subjective and objective information. Instruments that include only patient-reported functional status, such as voice changes and difficulty swallowing, are an inaccurate measurement of mucositis. Patient rating of severity will be variable regardless of observed oral changes. Other factors, such as infection, also may be influencing these symptoms.

Instruments and Guides for Assessing Stomatitis

Oral Mucositis Index (OMI)

The purpose of the OMI was to assess the types, patterns, and timing of oral mucosal changes after bone marrow transplantation. It is useful in a research setting to assess the effects of oral care protocols. Specific definitions of the appearance of stomatitis are listed here:[20]

Erythema. Increased redness of oral mucosa

Atrophy. Clinical impression of oral mucosa appearing atrophic and thin and/or exhibiting loss of keratinization

Vascularity. Clinically visible changes in apparent mucosal vascularity caused by an increase in the number of vascular elements detected and/or an increase in size of vascular elements that were seen

Ulceration. Frank ulcerations and/or surface erosions; severity of ulceration is rated according to number, depth, and surface area of lesions (e.g., the greater the number of lesions, the deeper the lesion, and/or the larger the surface area involved by the lesion, the higher the ulceration score)

Angular stomatitis. Inflammation and mucosal breakdown at the commissures of lips

Bleeding/crusted. Hemorrhage of oral cavity rated as active (bleeding) at time of examination or inactive (crusted) because of the presence of blood clots or dried blood

Saliva viscosity. Clinical impression of increased viscosity or thickness of saliva

Saliva xerostomia. Observer's impression of lack of saliva intraorally at time of evaluation

The OMI consists of 30 items. The oral cavity was divided into distinct anatomic regions: (1) lips, (2) labial mucosa, (3) buccal mucosa, (4) hard palate, (5) soft palate, (6) dorsal tongue, (7) ventral tongue, and (8) gingiva. Sites were assessed for changes from normal on a 0 to 3 rating scale (0, normal or no change; 1, mild change; 2, moderate change; 3, severe change). The items assess atrophy, erythema, edema, and pseudomembrane ulceration. Tissue changes rated included mucosa, color (increased whiteness or erythema), atrophy, vascularity, and ulceration. Other parameters assessed included the presence of angular stomatitis, oral bleeding, and salivary changes. Assessment of oral pain and dryness was rated on a visual analogue scale. The OMI was calculated by determining median scores of parameters that changed from baseline on specific examination days. The overall OMI score included the total of the oral mucosal changes for each anatomic region, plus the median salivary viscosity and xerostomia scores. The scores were plotted on a graph to portray oral changes over time. One examiner collected the data. Caution was advised in interpreting the data because multiple comparison tests were used. The OMI is internally consistent (Cronbach's alpha = 0.90–0.94; demonstrated test–retest reliability ($r = 0.31$–0.73, $p < 0.0001$).[21]

Oral Mucosa Rating Scale (OMRS)

The OMRS[20] provides comprehensive measurement of a broad range of oral tissue changes that occur with cancer therapy. The goal of the tool was to quantify the type and severity of clinically evident oral mucosal changes with a scale ranging from 0 to 3 (normal to severe).

The oral cavity was divided into seven distinct anatomic regions: (1) lips, (2) labial mucosa, (3) buccal mucosa, (4) tongue, (5) floor of the mouth, (6) palate, and (7) attached gingiva. Further subdivisions were made for upper and lower (lips and labial mucosa); right and left (buccal mucosa); dorsal, ventral, and lateral (tongue); or hard and soft (palate). Descriptive categories (erythema, atrophy, hyperkeratosis, lichenoid, ulceration, and edema) included common changes in the oral cavity after bone marrow transplant. The categories were rated on a 0 to 3 scale. Erythema, atrophy, hyperkeratosis, lichenoid, and edema are rated as 0 (normal/no change), 1 (mild), 2 (moderate), and 3 (severe). Ulceration and pseudomembrane scores were rated by estimating the involved surface area. The patient also rated mouth dryness and pain on a 1 to 10 visual analogue scale (1, no dryness/pain; 10, worst possible dryness/pain).

The OMRS was then tested with bone marrow transplant patients with the objective to develop an overall OMI relevant for patient care and research. The final OMI score included 34 items. Construction of the OMI was done on the basis of variance, low loading, and retention of items based on principal component analysis. Reliability was evaluated by internal consistency (Cronbach's alpha and Guttman split-half coefficient) and stability (test–retest). Validity data applied to this tool are supportive.[21] The tool is complex because of the total items assessed. It requires some training and additional time from a consistent observer, which limits its application in an ambulatory setting. The OMI uses only a partial subset of the accumulated data from the OMRS.

Mucositis with Radiation Therapy

Spijkervet and colleagues scored mucositis during radiation therapy of the head and neck by using both qualitative and quantitative parameters.[17] Table 37.1 lists these parameters. Local signs of mucositis were distinguished into five categories: (0) no mucositis, (1) whitish appearance of the oral mucosa, (2) erythema more pronounced than the red color of nonirradiated normal mucosa, (3) white or yellow plaques difficult to detach, and (4) complete loss of the mucosal layer. Mucositis was assessed at the following areas of the mouth: buccal mucosa (left and right), soft and hard palate, dorsum and border of the tongue (left and right), and mouth floor. The borders often overlapped. The degree of mucositis for each subarea was scored on an ordinal scale. The length of each subarea was measured by a modified pocket gauge and summed. The mucositis score of an area was defined as the sum of these products.

Table 37.1 Indices for Local Mucositis Symptoms and Indices for Length of Score Sum

Local Sign	k^*	Length (cm)	E
No mucositis	0		
White discoloration	1	< 1	1
Erythema	2	1–2	2
Pseudomembranes	3	2–4	3
Ulceration	4	> 4	4

*1,White appearance of oral mucosa; 2, redness more pronounced than the red color of nonirradiated normal mucosa; 3, white or yellow mucous plaques that are difficult to detach; 4, local complete loss of the mucosal layer.

Source: Spijkervet, F.K., VanSaene, H.F., Vermey, A., & Mehta, D.M. Scoring irradiation mucositis in head and neck cancer patients. *J Oral Pathol Med*, 1989, 18:167.

Although this assessment guide describes the local signs of mucositis, the scoring is of questionable clinical significance. There is no association with oral nutritional intake or associated oral pain. Measuring the size of oral ulceration is cumbersome and of limited clinical relevance.

WHO Index

The WHO Index is a simple, overall rating of mucositis. It often has been used as a general comparison index to other assessment scales.[22]

Grade 0. No change
Grade 1. Soreness, erythema
Grade 2. Erythema, ulcers, can eat solids
Grade 3. Ulcers, requires liquid diet only
Grade 4. Alimentation not possible

There are no reliability or validity data on the use of this guide. The grading does not capture the variety of oral changes that occur with cancer therapy. The descriptors of the grade are too ambiguous for consistent assessment. This tool focuses only on the status of the oral cavity, and the functional status of the patient is not well addressed.

Western Consortium for Cancer Nursing Research Staging System for Stomatitis

A panel of experts from nursing, dentistry, and medicine were solicited to develop criteria to evaluate the progressive severity of chemotherapy-induced stomatitis. The Western Consortium for Cancer Staging instrument was devised to measure the observable and functional dimensions of stomatitis.[23] The tool was compared with the Oral Assessment Guide (OAG) and WHO instruments. The WHO Index was found to be ambiguous when assessing oral fluid and food intake, as lack of oral intake often could be related to nausea rather than mucositis. The OAG descriptive ratings 2 and 3 were not always mutually exclusive when used to assess the mucous membrane.

This assessment guide provides a general description of the commonly associated characteristics of stomatitis, as well as its effects on the patient's nutritional intake and pain status. It provides an accurate, general assessment and aims to improve observer consistency. The stages in this guide provide a complete description of the progressive severity in chemotherapy-induced stomatitis. The functional dimensions include ability to eat, drink, and talk, which are influenced by the patient's pain perception. The observable dimensions are erythema, edema, presence of lesions, bleeding, and infection. There is less emphasis on specific anatomic sites and more emphasis on overall oral status and deviations from normal. The guide requires assessment by a clinician rather than relying on patient report only. The tool is brief and easy to use. The ratings are simple to record, and the descriptors are consistent with the clinical situation. The holistic approach may be preferable to measuring stomatitis and its specific dimensions through combining scores by simple summation.

Oral Assessment Guide (OAG)

The OAG was devised to meet the need for readily identifiable categories and easy descriptive ratings of the oral cavity in the clinical setting.[24] The instrument assesses functional impairment cause by mucositis. The OAG includes a chart with photographs showing deviations from normal. The categories were consensually validated by nursing staff and through review of the literature and include voice, talking, ability to swallow, lips, tongue, saliva, mucous membrane, gingiva, teeth, or dentures. Three levels of descriptors were identified for each of the eight categories. The descriptors were given a rating of 1, 2, or 3 (1, normal; 2, mild alteration without severe compromise of either epithelial integrity or systemic functioning; 3, definite compromise of either mucosal integrity or system function). The eight subscale scores are summed to obtain overall assessment score (possible range is 8 to 24, or they can be used alone as subscales). The tools for assessment and methods of measurement are identified and are shown in Table 37.2. The numeric ratings have brief descriptors listed with the corresponding category to provide consistency.

This assessment tool is clearly worded, but the potential for consistent results among different raters is high. The OAG is useful to obtain, record, and communicate oral cavity status and to determine changes secondary to chemotherapy and/or radiation as it includes voice and talking. Content validity was supported by an expert panel. However, the OAG does not include functional parameters in much detail. Interrater reliability is good (0.912). The percentage of agreement ranges from 70% to 100% across all eight subscales. Another criticism of the tool is that it assesses pain inadequately. The most pertinent clinical application for the OAG is in patients receiving high-dose radiation therapy and/or chemotherapy. The OAG would be useful when trying to identify oral care protocols or individuals at risk. Equal weight is given to the eight categories, which may not be consistent with the primary concerns of the patient. The tool combines functional performance with an objective examiner-rated evaluation.

The tool is readily available from the authors. Use in the outpatient setting requires modification because it relies on nursing observation and not necessarily on patient-reported symptoms. The exquisite detail makes it cumbersome to institute on a daily basis except in a research situation.

Summary

Stomatitis is an important and common side effect of chemotherapy and radiation therapy that warrants the identification of improved health care interventions. Developing appropriate and reliable oral assessment instruments is relevant to the evaluation of these interventions. The present tools have been used primarily in the bone marrow transplant setting because of the high incidence and severity of stomatitis. The health care researcher now has several tools that have been tested and compared. One needs first to determine the tool most appropriate to the setting. A quick, easy grading system that provides a summary of both functional and objective data is necessary for patients in ambulatory care and can be followed up by telephone interview. Tools that describe multiple categories of location and effect of stomatitis are applicable when the patient is receiving intensive, inpatient care.

Table 37.2 Oral Assessment Guide Example

Category	Tools for Assessment	Methods of Measurement	Numeric and Descriptive Rating		
			1	2	3
Voice	Auditory	Converse with	Normal	Deeper or raspy	Difficulty talking or painful

Eilers, J., Berger, A.M., & Peterson, M.C. Development, testing and application of the oral assessment guide. *Oncol Nurs Forum*, 1988, 15:327.

An initial visual assessment is key to determining whether the stomatitis is related to treatment or an infection so that proper treatment can be instituted as soon as possible. The instrument should include easily recognizable descriptions of the grading or staging of stomatitis. The grading should correlate with the known pattern of stomatitis progression. The difference between grades or categories should reflect this pattern and clearly correlate with distinct differences.

Finally, the grading system should include the functional status of the patient (ability to eat, drink, talk, or swallow, as well as a measure of the degree of pain). The goal of any oral assessment guide is to assist in the development of comprehensive oral care protocols to improve the patient's functional status, allay pain, and promote the patient's tolerance of chemotherapy or radiation. A team approach to care, in which the nurse, dentist, physician, pharmacist, and nutritionist participate, is best to accomplish this goal.

References

1. Carl, W. Oral complications in cancer patients. *Am Fam Physician*, 1983, 27(2):161-170.
2. NIH. Oral complications of cancer therapy: Prevention and treatment. *NIH Consens Develop Conf Statement*, April 1989, 7(7):17-19.
3. Bruya, N., & Madiera, N. Stomatitis after chemotherapy. *Am J Nurs*, 1975, 75(8):1349-1352.
4. Chabner, B. The clinical pharmacology of antineoplastic agents. *N Engl J Med*, 1975, 292:1107-1112.
5. Wujcik, D. Current research in side effects of high dose chemotherapy. *Semin Oncol Nurs*, 1992, 8(2):102-112.
6. Beck, S. Impact of a systemic oral protocol on stomatitis after chemotherapy. *Cancer Nurs*, 1979, 2(2):185-199.
7. Sonis, S.T., Sonis, A.L., & Lieberman, A. Oral complications in patients receiving treatment for malignancies other than of the head and neck. *J Am Dent*, 1978, 20:468-472.
8. Nieweg, R. The validity and reliability of an oral assessment instrument. *Oncol Nurs Forum*, 1993, 20(2):349.
9. Sonis, S.T., & Clark, J. Prevention and management of oral mucositis induced by antineoplastic therapy. *Oncology*, 1991, 5(12):11-22.
10. Peterson, D.E. Oral toxicity of chemotherapeutic agents. *Semin Oncol*, 1992, 19(5):478-491.
11. Dreizen, T. Stomatotoxic manifestations of cancer chemotherapy. *J Prosthet Dent*, 1978, 40:650-655.
12. Kostler, W.J., Hejna, M., Wenzel, C., & Zielinski, C.C. Oral mucositis complicating chemotherapy and or radiotherapy: Options for prevention and treatment. *CA Cancer J Clin*, 2001, 51:290-315.
13. Dodd, M., Miaskowski, C., Dibble, S., et al. Factors influencing oral mucositis in patients receiving chemotherapy. *Cancer Pract*, 2000, 8(6):291-297.
14. Zerbe, N.B., Parkerson, S.G., Ortlieb, M.L., & Spitzer, T. Relationships between oral mucositis and treatment variables in bone marrow transplant patients. *Cancer Nurs*, 1992, 15(3):196-205.
15. Poland, J. Prevention and treatment of oral complications in the cancer patient. *Oncology*, 1991, 5(7):45-62.
16. Kolbinson, D.A., Schubert, M.M., Flourney, N., & Truelove, E.L. Early oral changes following bone marrow transplantation. *Oral Surg*, 1988, 66(1):130-138.
17. Spijkervet, F.K., VanSaene, H.F., Vermey, A., & Mehta, D.M. Scoring irradiation mucositis in head and neck cancer patients. *J Oral Pathol Med*, 1989, 18:167-171.
18. McQuire, D., Yeager, K., Peterson, D., et al. Acute oral pain and mucositis in bone marrow transplant and leukemia patients: Data from a pilot study. *Cancer Nurs*, 1998, 21(6):385-393.
19. Sonis, ST. Mucositis is a biological process: A new hypothesis for the development of chemotherapy-induced stomatotoxicity. *Oral Oncol*, 1998, 34:39-43.
20. Schubert, M.N., Williams, B.E., Lloid, M.E., et al. Clinical assessment scale for the rating of oral mucosal changes associated with bone marrow transplant. Development of an oral mucositis index. *Cancer*, 1992, 69(10):2469-2477.
21. McQuire, D., Peterson, D., Muller, S., et al. The 20-item Oral Mucositis Index: Reliability and validity in bone marrow and stem cell transplant patients. *Cancer Invest*, 2002, 20(7&8):893-903.
22. WHO. *WHO Handbook for reporting results of cancer treatment* (Offset Publication No. 48). Geneva: World Health Organization, 1979, pp. 15-22.
23. Western Consortium for Cancer Nursing Research. Development of a staging system for chemotherapy-induced stomatitis. *Cancer Nurs*, 1991, 14(1):6-12.
24. Eilers, J., Berger, A.M., & Peterson, M.C. Development, testing and application of the oral assessment guide. *Oncol Nurs Forum*, 1988, 15:325-330.

38

Measuring Pain

Deborah B. McGuire, Hee-Ju Kim, and Xiaotao Lang

Pain is such an individual subjective experience that its measurement has long been a research challenge. Even a satisfactory definition of pain has remained elusive. Sternbach called pain "(1) a personal, private sensation of hurt; (2) a harmful stimulus which signals current or impending tissue damage; (3) a pattern of responses which operate to protect the organism from harm."[1] Melzack and Casey emphasized that pain is a sensory experience with motivational and affective properties.[2] Merskey and Spear described pain as an unpleasant experience primarily associated with actual tissue damage, described in such terms, or both.[3] Because of these many definitions of pain and the complexity of pain as a phenomenon, the International Association for the Study of Pain (IASP) developed a list of pain terms and definitions.[4] Pain was defined as "an unpleasant sensory and emotional experience associated with actual or potential tissue damage or described in terms of such damage."[4] This definition encompasses pain of pathophysiologic and psychologic origin and also accounts for the sensory, affective, and motivational aspects of the experience. In this same document,[4] the IASP published a list of additional pain terms, including definitions, descriptions of chronic pain syndromes, and a classification and coding schema for the syndromes. Studies of this coding schema demonstrate reasonable reliability for body location and etiology of pain[5] and evidence of clinical utility in deriving, coding, storing, and retrieving information on characteristics of pain.[6] In the years since the IASP formulated its definitions of pain and pain-related terms, it is relatively safe to conclude that these have been accepted by most clinicians and researchers in the field of pain.

Perception and Experience of Pain

The crucial point to remember when measuring pain is its highly subjective and unique nature. The IASP and others recognize the importance of viewing pain from the vantage point of those experiencing it.[3,4] A commonly used example of this precept is McCaffery's statement: "Pain is whatever the experiencing person says it is, existing whenever he [sic] says it does."[7]

Clinicians and researchers in the twentieth century developed a new concept of pain in which the perception of pain was determined by factors such as personality, previous experience, and culture.[8,9] In 1965, Melzack and Wall proposed the now-classic *gate control theory*.[10] This theory postulated that pain phenomena were determined by the interactions among three spinal cord systems. First, peripheral stimulation sent nerve impulses to the substantia gelatinosa in the dorsal horn of the spinal cord, where these cells modulated the afferent impulses (the gate control mechanism). Second, the afferent patterns in the fibers of the dorsal column acted as a central control trigger that activated selective brain processes, which in turn influenced the modulating gate control properties of the substantia gelatinosa. Third, central transmission cells in the dorsal horn activated neural mechanisms believed to be responsible for the perception of and response to pain. The gate control theory helped to explain many puzzling aspects of the phenomenon of pain and placed emphasis on the sensory and emotional components of pain perception. Although some of the proposed components of the theory have not been documented experimentally, there appears to be universal acknowledgment of the importance and value of the gate control theory in guiding pain research and clinical pain management.[11]

Following introduction of the gate control theory, a new conceptual model of pain, comprised of three dimensions, was developed by Melzack and Casey.[2] According to these authors, selection and modulation of incoming pain sensations in the neospinothalamic projection system provide the basis for the sensory/discriminative component of pain. The brain reticular formation and limbic systems drive the aversive and affective reaction to pain, forming the motivational/affective component of pain. Finally, higher central nervous system or central control activities become involved in the pain experience and response. This notion gradually evolved into a multidimensional concept of pain.

In the early 1980s, Ahles et al. described pain as a multidimensional experience consisting of physiologic, sensory, affective, cognitive, and behavioral aspects.[12] Although their conceptualization focused on cancer-related pain, it is generalizable to other types of pain for both research and clinical activities. McGuire[13] added a sociocultural dimension to this conceptualization and described specific, measurable components for each of the six dimensions.[14] Table 38.1 briefly describes each dimension and relevant components. A considerable body of research literature supports the existence of this multidimensional conceptualization in cancer pain as well as in other types of acute and chronic pain.[15] Researchers wishing to measure the experience of pain from this comprehensive, multidimensional standpoint should select instruments that tap dimensions relevant to their work.

Types of Pain

Pain can be arbitrarily categorized, but two commonly used methods are duration and cause. A primary distinction must be drawn between pain caused by experimental procedures in the laboratory and pain due to various organic processes (usually termed *clinical pain*). Researchers in the field of pain have long disagreed about whether both types of pain are directly comparable.[16] Experimental and clinical pain are generally not considered synonymous. The former is transient and manageable, whereas the latter may be persistent and uncontrollable.

This chapter focuses on the measurement of clinical pain for research purposes. A distinction based on duration can be made. Acute pain is associated with tissue damage. It decreases with healing and is generally of short duration, that is, days to weeks. Bonica defined acute pain as "a complex constellation of unpleasant sensory, perceptual, and

Table 38.1 Dimensions of Pain and Their Components

1. Physiologic
   a. Etiology/organic origin of pain
   b. Type of pain (duration)
   c. Endogenous opioids and neurotransmitters
   d. Psychophysiologic factors
   e. Location
2. Sensory
   a. Temporal pattern
   b. Intensity (severity)
   c. Quality
3. Affective
   a. Emotional responses (depression, mood, anxiety, worry, helplessness, fear)
   b. Suffering
   c. Psychiatric disorders
4. Cognitive
   a. Thought processes/views of self
   b. Meaning of pain
   c. Coping strategies
   d. Attitudes, beliefs, knowledge
   e. Influencing factors
   f. Level of cognition
   g. Pain relief
5. Behavioral
   a. Indicators of pain
   b. Pain control behaviors
   c. Communication of pain
   d. Associated symptoms (fatigue, sleep)
6. Sociocultural
   a. Demographic variables
   b. Cultural background
   c. Personal, family, and work roles
   d. Family factors
   e. Caregiver perspectives

emotional experiences and certain associated autonomic, psychologic, emotional, and behavioral responses."[17] He emphasized that noxious stimulation from injury to or disease involving cutaneous and deep tissues and abnormal function of visceral or musculoskeletal tissues were the two major causes of acute pain. Examples of acute pain are incisional discomfort following a surgical procedure, cholecystitis, and the unpleasant sensations that follow hitting one's thumb with a hammer.

Alternatively, chronic pain generally persists for 6 months or more. Real or impending tissue damage may or may not be a factor. Examples include inflammatory joint or degenerative disk disease, postherpetic neuralgia, and persistent cancer pain.

Some authors have developed subcategories of acute and chronic pain.[18,19] For example, acute pain may become subacute (or limited) in cases of prolonged healing, such as a crushing musculoskeletal injury. Acute pain also may be recurrent (or intermittent), such as migraine headaches or sickle cell crisis. Chronic pain can be subdivided as well. Chronic pain caused by cancer is sometimes called *intractable pain*. Another variant of chronic pain is persistent or chronic benign pain, such as low back pain or neuralgias. Finally, a classification schema for cancer pain that includes both acute and chronic pain caused by cancer, its treatment, or other causes has been developed by Foley.[20]

Measuring Pain

When considering the instruments available for measuring pain, the researcher must be deliberate in selection. The overall objective is to achieve useful and reliable data in the most expedient and sound manner possible. Several factors are important in the selection process:[14]

Research question or goal. Instrument must mesh with the researcher's measurement goals, e.g., a survey of prevalence of pain in a specific sample of patients requires a different tool than evaluation of a therapeutic intervention for pain.

Dimension(s) of pain being measured. Once the dimension(s) of the pain experience is determined, and perhaps the component of interest within the dimension, instrument selection is narrowed considerably.

Type of pain being measured. Tools used to measure acute pain may not be appropriate for measurement of chronic pain, and vice versa. Assess research that reports previous use of the instrument of interest. Some tools may be appropriate for acute and chronic pain in their original form or with minor modification. If modifications are made, psychometric reevaluation must occur.

Nature of patient population. Many characteristics can influence an individual's ability to complete the instrument. Consider education or literacy level, visual and hearing ability, motor coordination, cultural background and native language, diagnosis, type of pain, clinical environment, and acuity of illness. For example, use of a long and complex instrument is inappropriate in a sample of hearing-impaired people with acute pain; a short, simple pain intensity scale might be a better choice,.

Ease of administration and scoring. Respondent burden is a primary concern, particularly when the person is in pain. Minimize response time and effort. Burden on the researcher should also be considered, as should data entry and analysis capability.

Available data on reliability and validity of tools being considered. Data should be carefully evaluated as to benefits and limitations of using the instrument with a given sample. For many tools described in this chapter, authors are accessible and happy to provide more current information.

Regardless of the type of clinical pain to be measured, various problems will be encountered. Viewing the experience of pain from the subjective stance of the sufferer is the first major problem. Pain measurement may be influenced by individualized perceptions of and responses to pain. Thus, patients experiencing pain are not easily comparable, even when their pain has the same etiology. Verbal reports of pain may not be readily verifiable, and particular measures of pain may mean different things to different people. Finally, health professionals may differ in their responses to persons with pain, occasionally underestimating or overestimating its severity.[21-23] Despite these subjective problems, pain remains a uniquely individual experience that is private, depends on many factors, and varies between people but is consistent in each individual. When measuring clinical pain, these perspectives must be acknowledged and incorporated into any measurement strategy.

A variety of clinical and personal issues influence the measurement of pain as well. The type of pain, its etiology, and its duration are as important as the therapy employed. Patient characteristics, such as educational level, nature and acuity of physical illness, presence of affective disorders,[24] age,[13,25–27] motor coordination, visual ability, sociocultural background,[13] level of comfort of pain, hearing ability, and cognitive impairment from a variety of causes including opioid analgesics,[28] will influence not only the measurement of pain in particular populations but also the instruments selected. Situational factors also can create problems, such as the physical environment, the health care provider, or the presence or absence of family or friends.

Because pain is multidimensional, researchers must be clear which dimension of pain and which components are to be measured. They must examine the validity and reliability of appropriate tools before selecting instruments. Because much psychometric support for existing tools has been selectively gathered from specific groups, settings, and time periods, the expansion of these tools to other groups must be done cautiously and with appropriate modification and further psychometric evaluation.

The discussion of tools for measuring pain is limited to those that have been developed or used to measure clinical pain in adults. The multidimensional conceptualization of pain serves as this chapter's organizing framework. A number of instruments measure only one dimension of pain, others measure two dimensions, still others, more than two dimensions. Instruments are presented in two sections: unidimensional and multidimensional. Within these dichotomies, instruments are categorized by the dimension(s) they measure. Only tools that measure clinical pain from the perspective of the individual or family experience are discussed.

Several new developments and trends in pain measurement are incorporated into this edition. First, the rapid development of computer technology and biomedical informatics has stimulated researchers to develop computerized versions of older instruments (e.g., McGill Pain Questionnaire) or interactive computer animation programs to measure pain. Second, because there are many more psychometrically sound pain measurement instruments available today, researchers tend to focus more on their application to diverse patient samples rather than psychometric data analysis. For instance, researchers have compared pain instruments in specific groups (e.g., cancer patients, elderly) in order to determine the least burdensome yet most salient instrument(s) for measuring pain. Finally, not all general pain measurement instruments are appropriate for all possible patient populations. Thus, in another recent trend, pain researchers have focused on developing new instruments to meet the needs of people with specific types of pain (e.g., burns, cardiac, arthritis). Inclusion of these new developments and trends necessitated deletion of selected material from the previous edition that was deemed less useful today and/or for which there was little or no new research. Readers interested in this material should consult the previous edition of this text. Although the authors focus on measurement of pain for research purposes, it should be noted that many of the instruments are appropriate for clinical assessment in selected patient populations.

The instruments chosen are, for the most part, well established, have been used for research purposes, are particularly applicable or appropriate for clinical research, have been developed or revised fairly recently (with a few exceptions), and have evidence of reliability and validity. The chapter presents instruments that measure both acute and chronic pain, including types of pain that are very challenging to measure, such as pain in the critically ill, verbally or cognitively impaired, or terminally ill individuals. For each tool, the discussion includes the dimension(s) measured, a brief description of the tool, available psychometric data, examples of situations in which it has been used, recommendations for appropriate use in a research context, and advantages and disadvantages. Comparisons of scales and additional measures are presented in Appendices 38A to 38D.

Unidimensional Measurement Approaches

Physiologic Dimension

Very few clinical pain measurement instruments specifically address the physiologic dimension. It is difficult in the context of clinical settings to directly measure the etiology or organic origin of pain, levels of endogenous opioids and neurotransmitters, or other selected psychophysiologic factors. However, the more clinically salient components of this dimension of pain (location, duration, and type of pain) can be measured by selected items on standard pain instruments[29] or by more specific instruments that have been developed in recent years.

Weiner and colleagues[30] adapted a pain map (from the earlier work of Margolis and colleagues, reviewed in the previous edition) for use as a pain assessment tool in frail elders living in nursing homes. They defined the term *pain extensity* as the number of bodily areas noted on a pain map as painful, and explored test–retest reliability; convergent validity compared with pain intensity on a pain thermometer and on an 11-point graphic rating scale (GRS); and predictive validity with depression, functional impairment, and self-reported health. In phase one of their study, Weiner et al. studied 89 nursing home residents and 33 nurses, learning that there was very poor agreement between the two groups in sites of pain, except for lower-extremity phantom limb pain. In their second phase, they studied 115 nursing home residents. All were able to report locations of pain on the maps despite Mini Mental State Exam scores ranging from 6 to 30 (median 21). Fifty of the 115 had at least one painful area, and the mean number was 4.4. Test–retest reliability one hour apart on several different days was good to excellent (kappas ranged from 0.60 to 0.90). Convergent validity was only partially supported, with no association between pain maps and the GRS, but a significant association ($r = 0.37$, $p = 0.01$) between pain maps and the pain thermometer. There was no association between pain extensity and depression or physical disability, but there was a significant association between pain extensity and self-reported health, in that those with more extensive pain reported poorer health. The investigators concluded that the pain maps were simple to use, reliable, and valid and could serve as a useful clinical measure of pain. Future work should document the usefulness of this approach in the research arena, particularly for testing interventions.

Neuropathic pain, a specific type of pain associated with a variety of clinical conditions, can be measured specifically by the Neuropathic Pain Scale (NPS), developed by Galer and Jensen.[31] The NPS consists of two items assessing pain intensity and pain unpleasantness, eight items assessing specific qualities of neuropathic pain (sharp, hot, dull, cold, sensitive, itchy, deep, and surface pain), and an eleventh item assessing the temporal aspect of pain (intermittent increases, intermittent, or constant with fluctuation). Each of the eight quality items included a scale of 0 (no pain of this quality) to 10 (worst pain imaginable), as well as analogous words (e.g., hot = burning or on fire). Psychometric testing in two studies of 288 patients newly diagnosed with neuropathic pain and 78 patients receiving treatment for neuropathic pain revealed that the NPS had discriminant and predictive validity and was sensitive to treatments known to improve neuropathic pain. The authors noted that the NPS had potential and required further testing; it would be important to explore reliability since they did not address it.

Bennett[32] built on this work in his Leeds Assessment of Neuropathic Symptoms and Signs (LANSS) Pain Scale. The intent of this instrument is to estimate the probability that neuropathic mechanisms contribute to a patient's chronic pain experience. The instrument focuses on pain over the last week and asks patients whether any of five items match their pain (each is scored as no or yes). The items include what pain feels like, whether it makes the skin near the painful area look different, whether it makes it sensitive to touch, if the pain appears suddenly and for no apparent reason when still, and if the skin temperature in the painful area has changed abnormally. The LANSS Pain Scale also includes two items for sensory testing to determine allodynia and altered pinprick threshold, both answered in a no/yes format. Bennett described the derivation of a complex scoring system attached to the no/yes format for the seven items that results in a score range of 0 to 24. For a score of less than 12, the pain is unlikely to be due to neuropathic mechanisms, whereas for scores equal to or greater than 12, neuropathic mechanisms are likely to be contributing to the pain. He presented data suggesting that the LANSS Pain Scale had discriminant validity, internal consistency reliability, and interrater reliability. Interested readers should consult the original paper for more specific details.[32] This instrument offers an intriguing way to assess the physiologic dimension of neuropathic pain and may have potential for research use.

For measuring other components of the physiologic dimension, there are sophisticated cerebral measures of brain activity when pain is present. Although investigators have made some inroads on measuring pain with some of these procedures, it must be noted that most appear to focus on experimental pain. Pain intensity and pain threshold, for example, have been evaluated by measuring the nociceptive leg flexion reflex with an electrical stimulator and electromyelogram (EMG).[33] Another technique for measuring pain threshold is by requesting a yes/no response to electrical impulses administered in this research.[34] Positron emission tomography (PET) has been used to measure pain-evoked cerebral activity and the role of specific cortical areas related to multiple dimensions of pain perception, including the sensory and affective dimensions of pain and pain processing.[35]

Sensory Dimension

Scales are commonly used to measure this dimension, and the variable generally measured is pain intensity. Although quality and pattern of pain also are part of this dimension of pain, they usually are measured in the context of multidimensional instruments. Two major categories of scales are used to measure pain intensity: verbal descriptor scales and visual analogue scales. Additionally, other approaches to measuring pain intensity build on these more traditional methods or are alternate methods developed for specific pain problems or populations. These approaches include computerized pain instruments, facial pain scales, and thermometer pain scales.

Verbal Descriptor Scales (VDS)

VDS measure pain intensity, a major component of the sensory dimension of pain. They usually consist of three to five numerically ranked descriptors: (1) none, (2) mild, (3) moderate, (4) severe, and (5) unbearable. The number corresponding to the word chosen can be used to analyze the data on an ordinal level. The forerunner of VDS appears to have been Keele's Pain Chart, originally devised to assess responses to analgesics over a 24-hour time period[36] with descriptors ranging from agony to severe to moderate to slight to nil. Melzack's Present Pain Intensity Scale (PPI) on the McGill Pain Questionnaire (see later) is an additional type of VDS commonly found in the literature:[37]

_____ 0 No pain
_____ 1 Mild
_____ 2 Discomforting
_____ 3 Distressing
_____ 4 Horrible
_____ 5 Excruciating

Few authors using VDS have discussed reliability and validity, but most agree that an individual's subjective rating of the intensity of pain using word descriptors probably is a valid measurement. VDS are brief, easy to administer and complete, easy to score, and applicable to many types of patients and to acute or chronic pain. The data produced are probably reliable and valid. On the other hand, the word descriptors on a VDS may artificially categorize the intensity of pain and may not accurately reflect an individual's real sensory experience. Alternatively, researchers have indicated that the category words on a VDS do not divide the perceptual continuum of pain into equal segments, may lack sufficient sensitivity to measure pain intensity,[38] and require patients to "abstract an 'average' pain intensity for the requested duration."[39] This latter issue can be problematic when the researcher wishes to measure pain exactly at a specific point.

Visual Analog Scales (VAS)

VAS were first developed approximately 60 years ago to measure various subjective phenomena,[40] but the reference cited by most researchers using VAS is that of Clarke and Spear.[41] Gift[42] and Cline et al.[43] discussed a number of issues associated with using VAS to measure subjective phenomena (e.g., pain, depression, dyspnea) in research situations, including psychometric properties, advantages and disadvantages, and technical preparation and scoring. The patient is asked to place a mark through the line at the point that best describes how much pain is experienced at a particular moment. The VAS is called a Graphic Rating Scale (GRS) is descriptive words are placed along the line.[44]

No pain	Mild	Moderate	Severe	Pain as bad as it could possibly be

In pain research, VAS are generally used to measure the intensity of pain. The VAS usually consists of a 10-cm line with verbal anchors at either end:

No pain	Pain as bad as it could possibly be

Some researchers have focused on alternative formats for the VAS. One type is a mechanical format, generally described as a slide-rule type of plastic device showing a 10-cm horizontal VAS on the front with a movable tab that provides immediate feedback of numeric measures on its reverse side.[45,46] Another format is described as a "nonvisual" analogue scale[47] or a pain intensity number scale[48] that requests patients to score their pain on a scale from 0 (no pain) to 10 (the worst pain imaginable). The number selected by the patient, even if a fraction, is considered the pain intensity "score." Interval-level data are obtained on visual or graphic scales by measuring from the left end of the scale to the mark made by the patient. Price et al.[49] have validated the use of VAS as ratio-scale measures in chronic and experimental pain. VAS are considered more sensitive measures of pain intensity than VDS because they have a straight-line continuum rather than categorical responses. Many researchers using VAS have discussed reliability/validity issues in their published reports. Although these reliability data are somewhat varied, validity of the VAS seems to have been assumed, as with the VDS. Investigators testing mechanical and nonvisual formats of the VAS[45,46] examined concurrent validity of their new tools by comparing them to standard VAS and VDS, finding significant correlations that substantiated the validity of their newly formatted VAS. Grossman et al.[45] also examined test–retest reliability, demonstrating a high correlation ($r = 0.97, p < 0.001$) of repeated measures 5 minutes apart for a mechanical VAS. In general, subjective ratings of pain intensity may be considered reasonably valid regardless of the scale used.

Recent methodologic work has explored various aspects of administering, scoring, and interpreting VAS. In some patients a single measurement time point of "recalled average" pain intensity appears to be as reliable as multiple time points.[50] Distinct points on the VAS have now been linked to mild, moderate, and severe pain, which is important not only in understanding the link between verbal descriptors of intensity and VAS numeric values, but also in measuring pain intensity as an outcome in analgesic trials, so that comparability across studies is possible should investigators wish to perform meta-analyses.[51]

VAS have been used to measure pain intensity in a variety of patients, including people with cancer, patients with acute postoperative pain, patients with burn pain, people with arthritis, and others. Appropriate use of the VAS would encompass any group of patients with acute or chronic pain, provided such use was restricted to the measurement of pain intensity. The evaluation of treatment outcomes, particularly pharmacologic interventions, is a popular application of VAS in clinical research.

VAS are easy to administer and score. In addition, because VAS are considered to produce interval-level data, parametric statistics may be used in analysis. VAS have several disadvantages. Although it is unclear whether people prefer horizontal or vertical VAS format,[52] some people have difficulty conceptualizing a sensory phenomenon, such as pain intensity, in a straight-line continuum. They may place their marks near the anchor words, yielding data of questionable reliability and validity. Scott and Huskisson[53] believe that patient access to previous scores is important in obtaining accurate subsequent measures when administering the VAS repeatedly because previous ratings can be used for comparison. Careful instructions to research subjects regarding how to rate pain intensity on a VAS are imperative to proper understanding and use.

Computerized Pain Instruments

There are two approaches to computerized pain instruments. First, researchers have developed computerized versions of standard instruments, including the Seattle Angina Questionnaire and McGill Pain Questionnaire, among others. Feasibility and psychometric properties support these versions, as they are not significantly different from the originals, other than having subjects use the computer to rate their pain.[54,55]

The second approach consists of interactive computer animation, which more fully utilizes the capacity of computers to measure pain.[56] This technique uses computer-generated animations of symbolic visual representations of various aspects of the pain experience and is an alternative to fine verbal distinctions. It is composed of colored interactive animated (IA) images of four different categories of pain (pressure, burning, throbbing, and piercing) and an interactive version of a VAS (IVAS). The images were derived from a prior study on adult spontaneous pain drawings and were designed to express the lived pain experience of intensity and pattern of pain.

Swanston et al.[56] tested the utility of this system in 54 patients seen in a pain clinic by correlating the Short Form—McGill Pain Questionnaire (SF-MPQ), a paper-based VAS, and the Present Pain Index from the MPQ with IA and IVAS. All correlations for the overall patient group were significant ($0.297 < r < 0.877, p < 0.05$). However, when the researchers divided respondents into two groups (one category versus multiple categories of pain), they found that patients who chose more than one pain animation (e.g., burning and piercing) had no significant correlation between IA and the affective dimension of the SF-MPQ, whereas those who chose only one pain animation had no significant correlations between IA and the sensory dimension of the SF-MPQ nor between IVAS and the sensory and affective dimensions of the SF-MPQ. A majority (32 of 50) study participants also reported a preference for IA and IVAS. This instrument should be tested in various disease groups to establish its feasibility, and certainly, further psychometric evaluation is needed. Because of its high costs, formulation of recommendations for when and where it is most appropriately used will be important as well.

Facial Pain Scales

Facial scales, in which a spectrum of facial expressions is arranged in hierarchic order and assigned numbers to represent rank order from least to worst pain, were originally developed for measuring pain intensity or pain affect among children. Researchers have suggested that they can be used in adults, especially the elderly, who have difficulty using tools designed for adults, such as the VAS and numeric scales. Two widely used facial pain scales are discussed briefly.

Faces Pain Scale (FPS). The FPS was developed by Bieri and colleagues[57] to measure pain intensity in children and was based on faces drawn by children (grade 1, n = 195, mean age 6.7 years; grade 3, n = 358, mean age 8.7 years). There are seven faces with different facial expressions, including a neutral face for "no pain," a severely contorted face without tears for "worst pain," and five other facial expressions in between. On this scale, the oval faces are more adult in appearance, which may make the scale more acceptable to mature adults. None of the faces had tears in order to prevent bias introduced by personal beliefs related to pain expression.[58] Content validity was evaluated by having subjects rank-order the faces by severity when presented with all seven faces (grade 1 = 62%, grade 3 = 75%). Test–retest reliability data from a 2-week interval was r = 0.79, and the interrater correlation was 0.82 (n = 35). Herr and colleagues[58] tested the FPS with 168 adults 65 years of age or older. Construct validity was evaluated by examining whether the pictures represented some level of pain. Using a Likert-type scale (1 = strongly agree to 5 = strongly disagree), the authors asked the subjects (n = 33) to rate whether the faces represented pain, sourness, sadness, anger, boredom, and sleepiness. Mean ratings for these constructs were pain (2.09), sleeping (2.21), sadness (2.21), sourness (2.33), boredom (2.33), and anger (2.94), indicating that subjects felt the FPS represented pain more strongly than it did the other constructs. To further evaluate construct validity, 30 subjects were asked to place the seven faces (presented in random order) in order from most to least painful expression. Both initial and two-week-later tests were analyzed, revealing that Kendall's W (coefficient of concordance) and its significance test (equivalent to Friedman's two-way ANOVA for ranks) were 0.97 (p = 0.000) for the initial testing (indicating near-perfect agreement) and 0.96 (p = 0.000) for two weeks. There also was a trend toward decreased agreement as subjects became older, although all age groups demonstrated very high agreement coefficients (65–74 years, W = 0.99; 75–84 years, W = 0.97; ≥ 85 years, W = 0.94). Test–retest reliability was examined by rating a vividly remembered painful experience using the FPS in a 2-week interval, yielding a Spearman rank correlation coefficient of 0.94 (n = 41, p = 0.01). The mean pain score reported on initial testing was 4.78 (SD = 1.48) and 4.51 (SD = 1.64) on the repeat testing.

In additional work, Stuppy[59] examined concurrent validity with 60 hospitalized adults 55 years of age or older, looking at relationships between the FPS and the Pain Intensity Number Scale, VAS, and VDS. The FPS was strongly positively correlated with each of these when rating current level of pain (r = 0.81 to 0.95; p < 0.001), especially the number scale.

Wong-Baker Faces Scale (FACES)

The FACES scale was developed by Wong and Baker[60] to measure pain intensity or "amount of hurt" among children. It was drawn by children in pain as a way to convey their suffering as quickly and meaningfully as possible and without the requirements of literacy or conceptual ability.[61] The scale consists of six faces and is treated as a Likert scale ranging from 0 (happy face, no pain) to 5 (tearful face, worst pain). Wong and Baker[60] tested it with 150 hospitalized children aged 3 to 18, finding a concurrent validity of 0.60 and a test–retest reliability of 0.74. The scale has also been evaluated in adults. The concurrent validity was examined by Wong (cited in ref. 59) in 107 community volunteers receiving intradermal injections (21 to 67 years, mean = 38.2), using the FACES and a 0–5 number scale. The correlation of the scores of the two scales was 0.877 ($p < 0.05$). Cason and Grissom[62] examined correlations among FACES, VAS, and the Present Pain Intensity Scale (PPI) of the McGill Pain Questionnaire in the study of the effects of a sensory-based distraction intervention (kaleidoscope) on adults' perception of pain associated with phlebotomy. The correlations were 0.67 for FACES and VAS, and 0.79 for FACES and PPI ($n = 100$, 21–65 years old).

Although both of these facial pain scales were initially designed for children, they have shown sufficient validity and reliability in adults, except for lack of reliability data for the FACES scale. A meta-analysis indicated that the Wong-Baker FACES scale was the preferred scale among adults, children, parents, and nurses, compared with other well-established scales, such as numeric, verbal descriptor, visual analogue, color, photographic (the Oucher), and poker chip scales, possibly because of its clarity of meaning.[61] Thus, it clearly has potential for use in adults, but further research should address its reliability. Research is also needed to clarify whether the facial expressions (tears, smiles) and shape influence how adults rate their pain, particularly in studies comparing the scales within and across groups.

Thermometer Pain Scales

Visual Analog Thermometer (VAT). The VAT scale was developed by Choiniere and Amsel[63] to measure pain intensity. It was also intended as a way to overcome the limitations and disadvantages of the VAS, which can be difficult for people with perceptual/motor problems to complete, can be difficult for some people to understand conceptually, and requires additional time and effort to measure subjects' responses. The VAT is a device like a thermometer except that instead of measuring body temperature in degrees, it measures pain intensity. It consists of a white rigid plastic-encased cardboard strip with a horizontal black opening 10 cm long by 2 cm wide. The left and right extremes of this opening are identified by the expressions "no pain" and "unbearable pain." The opening is covered with a red opaque band that slides from left to right by means of a strip located on the back of the thermometer. On the back is a 10-cm ruler graduated to the nearest millimeter, with the extremities corresponding to the exact demarcation limits. As the strip is moved across the opening, the increasing intensity of pain is shown by the red band. The more intense the pain, the more the red band lengthens toward the limit of "unbearable." Although first used in burn patients, it has applicability for measuring pain intensity in other populations. Choiniere and Amsel[63] tested it in one group of 65 patients with chronic pain (median duration 27 months, range 6–390 months) such as back pain (66%), neuralgia (11%), reflex sympathetic dystrophy (8%), and other (15%). Concurrent validity was examined using scores from the VAT, standard VAS, and MPQ. Spearman correlation coefficients between the MPQ and VAT were positive and significant on all subscales, except sensory (sensory: $r = 0.17$, $p > 0.05$; affective: $r = 0.39$, $p < 0.01$;

evaluative: $r = 0.48$, $p < 0.01$; miscellaneous: $r = 0.56$, $p < 0.001$; total: $r = 0.37$, $p < 0.01$; present pain intensity: $r = 0.71$, $p < 0.001$). Correlations between VAT and VAS were 0.93, $p < 0.001$ for present pain; 0.78, $p < 0.001$ for pain at its worst in the last 7 day; 0.91, $p < 0.001$ for pain at its least; and 0.85, $p < 0.001$ overall. Construct validity was examined by assessing sensitivity for detecting changes in pain levels compared with the VAS; results demonstrated that significant differences existed among mean scores of patients' ratings for worst, least, and overall pain in the last 7 days. When patients were questioned about their scale preferences, 37% preferred the VAT, 26% preferred the VAS, and 37% had no preference. Comparison of mean ranks assigned to each scale revealed no significant difference between the VAT ($\bar{x} = 1.3 \pm 0.4$) and VAS ($\bar{x} = 1.4 \pm 0.5$).

It appears that the VAT is a simple and easy-to-use instrument for patients who have difficulties using other pain measurement instruments. Its design makes it suitable and valid for clinical use and research. Since test–retest reliability was not measured in this initial work, further research should address this area. In addition, research is needed to examine the validity and the reliability of the VAT across different age, cultural, and lingual groups. Finally, comparisons of the VAT and other similar instruments will be helpful in establishing criteria for selecting instruments for research or clinical use.

Comparisons of Scales

Because both VDS and VAS measure pain intensity, many researchers have compared the two in terms of sensitivity, reliability, validity, ease of administration and patient use, and patient preference. Studies of different forms of the VDS and VAS have been performed as well. These are described in Appendix 38A.[64–70] The results of these comparative studies indicate that the scales discussed are useful for measuring perceived pain intensity and, in general, correlate reasonably well. Their reliability is relatively well established, but any researcher using such scales must consider the individual characteristics of both patients and settings before choosing specific scales. For example, the VAS may be too abstract for patients with severe acute pain, lower educational levels, or impaired motor coordination. In such instances, a VDS may be easier to use and may produce more reliable data.

More recent work comparing scales has focused on clinical feasibility issues, application in specific populations, and identification of the best scales for determining outcomes in intervention research. Paice and Cohen[71] found that a verbally administered numeric pain intensity rating scale was a reliable and valid alternative to the VAS in cancer patients, particularly those whose pain ratings were obtained by phone. De Wit and colleagues[72] explored the use of a pain diary in cancer patients with chronic pain, assessing how well patients were able to record pain intensity over time using this approach. Results suggested that the pain diary was useful in capturing the day-to-day and within-day variability in pain and had a patient compliance rate of approximately 86%, even in those who were seriously ill. Vickers[73] compared a 100-mm VAS to a 7-point Likert scale in runners with muscle soreness, seeking to determine the relationship. He found that they were approximately linear, but that VAS responses for a zero-pain Likert score varied enormously. Thus, he suggested that researchers should not assume the lowest score meant zero pain.

Studies of scales in specific populations range across a number of groups. Gordon et al.[74] found that burn patients preferred faces and color scales to measure pain intensity, but recommended that further research address the potential impact of these preferences on pain interventions. Ramer et al.[75] addressed pain assessment in Hispanic, African American, and Anglo cancer patients, finding that the VAS, Memorial Pain Scale, and

Faces Scale were acceptable and performed well. In a study of patients with fibromyalgia, Bigatti and Cronan[76] tested several different scales, finding that the VAS was the most useful measure of pain. Pain assessment in cognitively impaired and unimpaired older adults is an important concern, and the focus of recent research. Krulewich et al.[77] found that the 6-item Pain Intensity Scale (using a response scale of 1 = not at all to 5 = extremely) performed best, particularly when used by both patient and caregiver. Interestingly, as patients' dementia progressed, this instrument was still used effectively by almost all caregivers. Chibnall and Tait[78] compared a 5-point verbal rating scale, a 7-point faces pain scale, a horizontal 21-point (0–100) box scale, and two vertical 21-point (0–20) box scales (measuring pain intensity and pain unpleasantness) in hospitalized older adults (mean age of 76 years). They examined accuracy, reliability, construct validity, postdictive validity, and bias susceptibility. Their findings supported the use of the 21-point box scale for pain assessment, including those who had mild to moderate cognitive impairment.

Finally, recent work examining the most appropriate pain instruments for evaluating outcomes of intervention research suggests that the answer is still unclear. In cancer patients receiving pain interventions, responses varied widely (16–91%) depending on which pain instruments were used to measure outcomes.[79] More work is clearly needed to establish optimal approaches for specific patient populations. In contrast, Lines et al.[80] found that in patients with migraine headache, a standard categorical four-grade scale (0 = no headache to 3 = severe pain) correlated highly with a VAS, but was easier to use and preferred by patients. In summary, these recent comparative studies have advanced our knowledge of how pain instruments perform in various populations and highlighted the need to consider clinical, demographic, and other factors when selecting an instrument for research.

Affective Dimension

The affective dimension involves how pain makes individuals feel and includes such variables as distress, anxiety, depression, and mood. Numerous instruments exist to measure these constructs, but few investigators have developed tools specifically to measure this dimension of pain, usually with VAS or VDS. Ahles et al.[81] used a 10-cm VAS to measure depression and anxiety in patients with cancer pain. The left anchor was "I am not depressed (anxious)" and the right anchor was "I am as depressed (anxious) as I can possibly imagine myself being." They found support for the validity of the VAS-depression through significant ($p = 0.05$) correlations with the Beck Depression Inventory ($r = 0.51$) and depression subscale of the Symptom Checklist-90 (SCL-90) ($r = 0.41$). The VAS-anxiety, however, was not significantly correlated with the anxiety subscale of the SCL-90 or the State Anxiety Inventory. The VAS for depression may provide a simple, valid, and clinically practical method for measuring this component of the affective dimension.

Price et al.[82] took a different approach to this dimension, measuring the "degree of unpleasantness" associated with pain intensity using a 15-cm VAS with word anchors "not bad at all" and "the most unpleasant feeling possible for me" at either end. Patients with different types of pain (experimental, low back pain, upper back pain, myofascial pain, causalgia, cancer pain, and labor pain) were studied. Their results demonstrated that, although many patients reported a wide range of sensory and affective ratings, in general VAS affective ratings were significantly higher than VAS sensory ratings ($p < 0.01$) in cancer patients. The overall findings clearly indicate the importance of distinguishing between sensory and affective dimensions of pain, particularly in certain types of pain.

Recent work has focused on the affective dimension of pain from the perspective of distress, or how bothersome, unpleasant, or upsetting the sensory dimension of pain is to those experiencing it, as well as on stress symptomatology associated with pain. Building on a substantial body of prior work by Johnson and colleagues, Good et al.[83] reported on the reliability, validity, and sensitivity of a VAS measuring pain sensation and a VAS measuring pain distress when compared to dual numeric rating scales (NRS) in a postoperative patient population. They found that test–retest reliability coefficients for their VAS on postoperative days 1 and 2, 15 minutes apart, were 0.73 to 0.82. Convergent validity was $r = 0.90$–0.92; construct validity of sensation and distress ranged from 0.72–0.85; and discriminant validity was 0.65–0.78. Both the sensation and distress VAS were significantly associated with reduction of pain after treatment ($p < 0.05$–0.01), which further supported construct validity. Good et al. recommended that these VAS be used in research studies since they produced continuous data that were amenable to parametric statistical analysis. In another study, Taal and Faber[84] reported on the relationship between perception of pain and post-traumatic stress in 43 burn patients. They assessed pain using Choiniere and colleagues' VAT and levels of stress symptomatology using the Impact-of-Event Scale. They found that high levels of post-traumatic stress were associated with higher pain scores during therapeutic procedures and when at rest. Although this study was primarily exploratory in nature, it provided strong evidence for the affective dimension of pain in burn patients and demonstrated that this dimension can be assessed by what might be considered nontraditional means (i.e., not a standard pain instrument).

Taal and Faber[85] also developed the Burn Specific Pain Anxiety Scale (BSPAS), a measure of anticipated or actual anxiety associated with burn pain. The original BSPAS consisted of nine items describing feelings of worry about wound healing, tension, and fear of losing control during dressing changes, anxious anticipation of pain during or after medical procedures, and generalized feelings of being "on edge" or "keyed up" because of continuing pain. In an initial study of 35 patients, the internal reliability coefficient was 0.94, and there was evidence of validity through statistically significant correlations with the State Trait Anxiety Scale-State and nurses' VAS scores of observed tension, and a high correlation between the BSPAS and procedural pain. In follow-up work with an abbreviated five-item BSPAS in a sample of 173 burn patients admitted to several burn centers, Taal et al.[86] found that the correlation between the original and abbreviated versions was high (0.96), and the coefficient alpha of the abbreviated BSPAS was 0.90; additionally, item-total correlations ranged from 0.67 to 0.81. Further validity testing revealed two highly correlated factors—anxiety during procedures and anticipatory anxiety—that had internal consistency coefficients of 0.89 and 0.79, respectively. An ANOVA across three groups of patients who had different extent and severity of burns showed a significant linear increase in average BSPAS subscale scores as burns became more extensive. Subsequent work by other researchers[87] revealed that the BSPAS was an accurate predictor of procedural pain levels, physical function, and medication use. Clearly, the BSPAS is a useful clinical and research instrument for those focusing on burn pain.

Cognitive Dimension

As shown in Table 38.1, the cognitive dimension includes numerous components. Some of these components, such as pain relief, are included in the selected multidimensional pain measurement instruments discussed later in this chapter. For example, the Brief Pain Inventory includes a pain relief item that asks respondents to report the extent (in percent) to which their pain is relieved by the pain interventions they are using. Other components of this dimension, such as factors that exacerbate or relieve pain, may not appear on formal pain measurement instruments but are easily assessed by interview. Still other components of this dimension, such as coping strategies, are measured with highly specific instruments. One relatively recent example is the Chronic Pain Coping Inventory (CPCI), which was developed to measure coping strategies that are a focus in pain treatment programs.[88] The authors reported initial evidence of reliability and validity and suggested that future research should confirm the CPCI's factor structure and explore both its predictive value for adjustment and ability to change in response to pain treatments. Another very important component of the cognitive dimension is attitudes, beliefs, and knowledge that influence an individual's response to pain and pain interventions (Table 38.1). Research over the past decade has resulted in an instrument to measure this component of the cognitive dimension, captured as a construct called *barriers*.

Barriers Questionnaire (BQ)

The BQ was developed by Ward and colleagues[89] to measure the extent to which individuals with cancer reported barriers to pain management. The authors defined *barriers* as erroneous beliefs or misconceptions about pain and pain medication. A comprehensive review of the cancer pain literature yielded eight important concerns: (1) fear of addiction, (2) concerns about tolerance, (3) concerns about side effects, (4) fatalism about experiencing uncontrolled cancer pain, (5) desire to be a "good" patient, (6) fear of distracting one's physician from treating the disease, (7) concern that pain meant disease progression, and (8) fear of injections. Two cancer pain management experts developed questions to measure these eight concerns, and then three additional pain experts and four researchers reviewed the items for clarity and categorized them into eight subscales. Each subscale had three items, except for the side effects subscale, which had six, for a total of 27 items. Subjects rated the extent to which they agreed with each of the items on a scale of 0, do not agree at all, to 5, agree very much. Mean scores for each subscale and the total mean score for the entire instrument were used in analyses, with higher scores reflecting more perceived barriers. Ward and colleagues'[89] initial psychometric evaluation in 270 persons with cancer yielded an internal consistency reliability coefficient of 0.89 for the total scale and the following coefficients for the subscales: addiction, 0.79; tolerance, 0.68; side effects, 0.72; fatalism, 0.54; being a good patient, 0.67; distracting the physician, 0.73; disease progression, 0.91; and fear of injection, 0.80. A panel of experts judged the BQ as having content validity, and there was a suggestion of construct validity through evidence that patients with higher BQ scores (i.e., more barriers) had less adequate pain management than those with lower scores. A follow-up study[90] demonstrated in 56 subjects that test–retest reliability over a one-week period was 0.90 for the total scale and ranged from 0.68 to 0.81 for the subscales, except for the fatalism subscale ($r = 0.60$). The data raise concern about the reliability of this particular subscale, given that it also had a lower internal consistency coefficient, but clearly the other subscales exhibited acceptable to excellent reliability, although the p values for the correlation coefficients were not provided.

More recently, Gunnarsdottir and colleagues[91] revised the BQ to reflect changes in pain management practices and because of input from patients in studies using the BQ. In their revision, the 27-item Barriers Questionnaire-II (BQ-II), they dropped two subscales: (1) concern that pain meant disease progression, and (2) fear of injections. They added two new subscales: (1) fear that analgesics impair the immune system, and (2) concern that analgesics may block ability to monitor illness symptoms. A group of six experienced oncology nurses generated items to address these barriers, and construct validity was then evaluated in two ways. First, based on the theoretical supposition that trained nurses would have lower barrier scores than would cancer patients, scores of these two groups were compared, and as predicted, the difference was statistically significant ($t = -2.16$, $p < 0.05$) in favor of the nurses. Second, a factor analysis revealed four factors: (1) physiologic effects (belief that side effects of analgesics were inevitable and unmanageable, concerns about tolerance, and concerns about not being able to monitor changes in one's body when taking strong pain medications); (2) fatalism (fatalistic beliefs about cancer pain and its management); (3) communication (concern that reports of pain distracted the physician from treating the underlying disease, and belief that "good" patients do not complain of pain); and (4) harmful effect (fear of becoming addicted to pain medication and belief that pain medications harm the immune system). The BQ-II total had an internal consistency reliability coefficient alpha of 0.89 ($n = 134$), and a range of 0.75–0.85 for the subscales. The mean score for the total scale was 1.53 (SD = 0.73). BQ-II scores were related to measures of pain intensity and duration, mood, and QOL, and patients who used adequate analgesics for their levels of pain had lower scores on the BQ-II than patients who used inadequate analgesics. These results support the validity and reliability (with the exception of test–retest reliability) of the BQ-II.

The BQ has been widely used. It is useful for measuring effectiveness of educational interventions in cancer patients and the population at large. It has also been used to measure barriers to cancer pain management in family caregivers in a hospice setting[92] and has been formatted into a computerized pain measurement software.[55] There is a Puerto Rican (Spanish-language) version (BQ-PR)[93] and a Taiwanese (Chinese-language) version (BQ-T),[94] both of which have good validity and reliability. Further research might focus on examining test–rest reliability of the BQ-II and also on relationships between the BQ-PR, BQ-T, and BQ-II, because it seems that they have not been compared yet to the revised BQ. In any case, these instruments offer a good method for assessing the attitudes, beliefs, and knowledge component of the cognitive dimension of pain.

Behavioral Dimension

The behavioral dimension has two major components: behaviors that are observable indicators of the presence and/or severity of pain (e.g., grimacing, nonverbal vocalizations, communication with others, guarding and splinting, fatigue), and behaviors that individuals engage in to decrease or control their pain (e.g., use of medications, positioning, sleep/rest/activity patterns). Many components of this dimension are measured within the context of multidimensional instruments such as diaries. A number of instruments, however, have been developed specifically to measure this dimension of pain in patients with acute pain who cannot complete self-report tools (such as those recovering from anesthesia) or in patients with chronic pain that affects numerous activities of daily living. Some instruments are reviewed in detail, and others are presented in Appendix 38B.[95–100]

Acute Pain

PACU Behavioral Scale. Mateo and Krenzischek[101] adapted the Chambers and Price Pain Rating Scale (Appendix 38B) to measure the behavioral manifestations of pain in patients recovering from general anesthesia with an instrument called the Post Anesthesia Care Unit (PACU) Pain Rating Scale. They retained the behaviors of restlessness, tense muscles, frowning or grimacing, and patient sounds. Each of these four pain behavior categories was measured with a scale having a zero base and clearly defined progression through ratings of 1, 2, and 3. Patient sounds were measured in this way:

0 = talking in normal tone or no sound
1 = sighs, groans, moans softly
2 = groans, moans loudly
3 = cries out or sobs

They ensured content validity through an expert panel: two clinical nurse researchers (one with expertise in pain assessment), a clinical nurse specialist in pain management, and several expert PACU nurses. The internal consistency of the PACU Behavioral Pain Rating Scale (BPRS) was assessed with coefficient alpha, which was 0.92. The investigators' interrater reliability across patients was measured with Pearson's correlation coefficient and ranged from 0.71 to 1.0. At the first timepoint (immediately after admission to the PACU), frowning or grimacing was significantly correlated with self-reports of pain intensity ($r = 0.69$, $p < 0.05$), but at the second timepoint (within an hour of admission), muscle tension and patient sounds ($r = 0.64$ and 0.63, respectively, $p < 0.05$) were significantly correlated with pain intensity.

In a subsequent study of 50 PACU patients who had undergone gastrointestinal surgery, the instrument was used to assess pain at two timepoints.[102] At time 1, frowning/grimacing, muscle tension, and sounds were correlated with self-reports of pain intensity ($r = 0.45$–0.63; $p \leq 0.01$), and at time 2, frowning/grimacing, muscle tension, and restlessness were correlated with self-reports of pain intensity ($r = 0.42$–0.52, $p \leq 0.01$).

Webb and Kennedy[103] substantiated the reliability and validity of the PACU BPRS in a sample of 36 postoperative gynecologic surgery patients who were all receiving patient-controlled analgesia. These investigators used the BPRS in an unaltered format but changed the pain intensity scale to 0 to 10 (to allow for more variance in pain scores), administering both scales five times to each patient within 6 hours of surgery. Their Cronbach's alphas ranged from 0.73 to 0.90. Correlations between patients' PACU BPRS and pain intensity scale scores ranged from $r = 0.56$ to 0.80 ($p < 0.05$), decreasing over time, with the highest scores within 2 hours of surgery. The PACU BPRS requires further evaluation for its psychometric properties, for its ability to measure changes resulting from pain interventions, and for its applicability to other cognitively impaired patients.

Checklist of Nonverbal Pain Indicators (CNPI). Another instrument designed to measure the behavioral dimension of acute pain is the CNPI, specifically intended for cognitively impaired elders because of the lack of reliable and valid instruments for measuring pain in this population.[104,105] Feldt modified the University of Alabama-Birmingham Pain Behavior Scale by eliminating selected items related to ambulation, posture, time in bed, and medications; by redefining restlessness to accommodate nonambulatory elders; and by adding an item on vocal complaints. The result was a six-item instrument that included vocalizations, grimaces, bracing, rubbing, restlessness, and verbal complaint, each of which was rated as present or absent. Feldt established face validity based on published pain behaviors of demented elders. She reported an interrater reliability of 93% agreement by two gerontologic nurse practitioners, who observed and rated pain behaviors in 12 of 88 patients participating in the study both while they were in bed and moving from bed to a chair (defined as pain during movement). The kappa statistic was 0.625–0.819 ($p = 0.019$–0.0057) for the observed behaviors. Feldt noted that some behaviors were not present at rest (bracing) or were present both at rest and with movement (restlessness and rubbing). The study included 88 elders admitted to three different hospitals with hip fractures. Patients were interviewed on the third postoperative day after surgical repair of their hip fracture using the Ferrell Pain Experience Interview, a VDS for pain severity, and the Mini-Mental State Examination (MMSE). At the end of the interview they were observed for nonverbal signs of pain behavior using the CNPI while in bed and while being transferred from bed to a chair by nursing staff. Over half the sample did not show any nonverbal signs of pain while at rest, but 62% showed nonverbal signs during movement. Fifty-three of the 88 patients were cognitively impaired ($\leq$ 23 points on the MMSE) and 35 were cognitively intact. The cognitively impaired group showed significantly more nonverbal indicators of pain ($p = 0.04$), although mean number of behaviors was low for both groups. Feldt[104] reported an alpha coefficient for the CNPI of 0.54 at rest and 0.64 during movement. She indicated that these low values might have resulted from the small number of items on the CNPI. The Spearman correlation coefficient between the CNPI scores and VDS scores for the 64 patients who had both was 0.372 at rest ($p = 0.001$) and 0.428 with movement ($p = 0.0001$). These data suggest evidence of validity, although Feldt did not specifically address validity in her report. In the conclusion, she indicated that "The CNPI proved to be an initially reliable and simple tool to measure pain behaviors in postoperative elders."[104,p19] Her recommendations for future research focused on the need for additional reliability testing, a larger and more diverse (acute and chronic pain) population, addition of items that would improve the internal consistency reliability, and comparison with other pain measures, which would allow examination of validity. Other investigators have used the CNPI to explore its feasibility in the inpatient and nursing home settings. Feldt reported (personal communication, March 3, 2003) that in one study, the CNPI was rated as easiest to use by inpatient nursing staff, and in another, it was feasible for use in cognitively impaired nursing home elders.[106] This instrument clearly shows potential for research use in cognitively impaired elders, but obviously, psychometric evaluation remains ongoing.

Chronic Pain

Selected instruments to measure the behavioral dimension of chronic pain are shown in Appendix 38C.[107-114] One new behavioral measure is described here.

Koho and colleagues[115] described an approach for assessing behavior related to chronic low back pain that relied on a functional video-based assessment system. Their goal was to develop a reliable assessment of pain behaviors during functional assessment by physical therapists. They videotaped patients as they sat; took a 5-minute walk; laid prone on the floor, rolled over 360 degrees, and stood up; bent and reached; filled, lifted, and carried a box of weights; and climbed stairs. Other measures included self-reports of pain (VAS) and disability, the Zung depression scale, modified somatic perception questionnaire, and fear of (re)injury (Tampa scale for kinesiophobia). Two observers rated the videotapes for eight specific pain behaviors on two occasions separated by four weeks. Intra- and interrater reliability achieved a high percentage of agreement, with the exception of facial expression and verbal report of pain. Deletion of facial expression improved the internal consistency coefficient to 0.73, so it was deleted, but deletion of verbal report did not, so it was retained. Scores on the eight pain behaviors were summed for a total pain behavior score. Correlations between this score and other variables revealed significant relationships with subjective pain report and disability ($p < 0.01$). Pain and pain behavior explained 48% of the variance in disability. The researchers concluded that their video-based assessment system was a reliable measure of pain behavior in patients with chronic back pain, but they cautioned that their sample was small and additional work was needed.

Sociocultural Dimension

This dimension has a number of components (see Table 38.1), most notably the ethnocultural and familial-social aspects of the pain experience. Additional components included in this dimension are the beliefs, attitudes, and values about pain held by lay and professional individuals. Discussion of tools that measure these concepts is beyond the scope of this chapter, as many of them take the form of survey questionnaires, lack rigorous psychometric evaluation, and are clinically oriented. Few instruments have been developed specifically to measure this dimension of pain, although numerous tools are available that measure related concepts, such as social support.

Family Pain Questionnaire

Ferrell and colleagues developed the Family Pain Questionnaire (FPQ) in tandem with a Patient Pain Questionnaire (see later) to measure knowledge and experiences of family members caring for patients with pain.[116-118] The FPQ was originally described as a 21-item linear analogue tool with knowledge items and experience items.[116] These two areas are encompassed within the cognitive and sensory dimensions of pain, but because they are asked of family caregivers, the tool is placed in the sociocultural dimension. Examples of knowledge and experience items, respectively, are:

Patients are often given too much pain medicine.

Agree _____ Disagree

How much pain is your family member having now?

No pain _____ A great deal

The published articles provide scant information on the psychometric development and evaluation of the tool, but another publication[119] provides some detail. The tool has an overall reliability of $r = 0.92$ ($p = 0.01$), evidence of content validity by expert review, and now has 13 items (9 knowledge, 4 experience). The authors will provide on request a copy of the FPQ and its scoring criteria. Readers who desire more specific information on the psychometric testing of the FPQ are advised to contact the primary author. This tool is helpful in ascertaining knowledge and experiences of family caregivers and could provide useful baseline information prior to initiating family-oriented intervention studies. Examples of further psychometric development are scant at present.

Multidimensional Approaches

The instruments reviewed thus far measure only one dimension of pain experience and are limited in their ability to provide a comprehensive picture of pain. For a number of research projects, however, unidimensional measurement of the pain experience may be quite appropriate and even desirable. The instruments now described were devised to measure more than one dimension of pain simultaneously. Appendix 38D briefly describes additional tools.[120-152]

The first five instruments were thoroughly described in the previous edition, thus the text below provides only a brief description and any relevant updates. Four instruments— Short-Form MPQ, Brief Pain Inventory, Pain-O-Meter, and Biobehavioral Pain Profile— are considered general multidimensional pain measures, whereas the Chronic Pain Experience Instrument was originally designed to measure arthritis pain but later expanded to include back pain and headache.

As noted in the introduction to this chapter, trends in pain measurement have included development of instruments to measure specific types of pain and to measure groups of symptoms simultaneously. Thus, the remaining instruments discussed in this section include one general measure (Glasgow Pain Questionnaire), one for rheumatoid arthritis pain (Rheumatoid Arthritis Pain Scale), and two for the pain of angina (Chest

Discomfort Diary and Seattle Angina Questionnaire). Because these instruments are newer, details of their development and evaluation are provided.

Short-Form McGill Pain Questionnaire (SF-MPQ)

In 1987 Melzack[153] introduced a short form of the MPQ, developed to provide a shorter and quicker multidimensional measure of pain in clinical settings than the original MPQ. This tool consisted of two sections. In the first one, 11 sensory words (throbbing, shooting, stabbing, sharp, cramping, gnawing, hot-burning, aching, heavy, tender, splitting) and 4 affective words (tiring-exhausting, sickening, fearful, punishing-cruel) were listed. These descriptor words were selected because they had been chosen by 33% or more of patients with labor, menstrual, headache, phantom limb, postherpetic, dental, cancer, arthritis, and low back pain in previous studies. Each word was accompanied by 0 to 3 severity ratings (0 none, 1 mild, 2 moderate, 3 severe). Three scores were derived by summing the intensity rank values of all selected words: a sensory score, an affective score, and a total score. In the second section, two measures of pain intensity were included: the Present Pain Intensity Index (PPI) from the original MPQ, and a 10-cm VAS with anchors of "no pain" and "worst possible pain." Melzack conducted two validation studies[153] of an English version of the tool as well as a Quebec French version. Dudgeon and colleagues[154] studied the tool in 24 patients with metastatic disease and chronic pain related to their cancer. Swanston et al.[56] described a method for assessing pain using interactive computer animation and validated it by comparing it to the SM-MPQ. McGuire and colleagues[155] used the SF-MPQ to assess acute oral pain in 48 patients receiving high-dose chemotherapy and bone marrow transplantation for their malignancies. Based on these studies and more, the SF-MPQ is clearly a reliable and valid, clinically feasible method for measuring the sensory and affective dimensions of pain. It is formatted in both paper-and-pencil and computerized versions. It is available in Dutch, French, German, Hebrew, Spanish, and Swedish versions, which have all been shown to be psychometrically sound.[156–160] It is also important to note that although the original Long-Form MPQ is rarely used anymore, it remains a very useful multidimensional instrument in some situations and now exists in reliable and valid Danish, Greek, and Norwegian versions.[161–163]

Brief Pain Inventory

Another multidimensional instrument for measuring pain, also modeled after the MPQ, is the Wisconsin Brief Pain Questionnaire,[164] now known as the Brief Pain Inventory (BPI).[165] It is a survey instrument originally constructed to measure pain caused by cancer and other diseases, such as rheumatoid arthritis and chronic orthopedic problems. Items on the BPI address pain history, etiology, intensity, location, quality, and interference with activities. With these items, the tool addresses the sensory, affective, cognitive, behavioral, and sociocultural dimensions of pain. An example of an intensity item (sensory dimension) is:

> Please rate your pain by circling the one number that tells how much pain you have right now:
>
> 0   1   2   3   4   5   6   7   8   9   10
> No Pain   Pain as bad as
>   you can imagine

A basic stem item is used to address the interference of pain with components of the affective, cognitive, behavioral, and sociocultural dimensions. For example: the individual is asked to "Circle the one number that describes how, during the past 24 hours, pain has interfered with your general activity: 0 (does not interfere) to 10 (completely interferes)." Additional items using this stem include mood, walking ability, normal work (inside and outside the home), relations with other people, sleep, and enjoyment of life.

The BPI can be used to measure pain in cancer and other conditions, although it is seen most frequently in studies of patients with cancer-related pain. The instrument is short, easily understood, designed for self-administration, and easy to score. Its readability level and comprehensive nature make it particularly suited for clinical research. It has clinical utility as well because it was recommended as a comprehensive assessment tool in the Clinical Practice Guidelines for Management of Cancer Pain.[29] The version in the guidelines is called the Brief Pain Inventory (Short Form) and consists of 9 items total (1 pain prevalence, 1 pain location, 4 pain intensity, 2 pain treatment, and 1 pain interference [with 7 subcomponents to tap multiple dimensions]). There are substantial reliability and validity data for both the original and shorter forms of the BPI that do not need to be reviewed here. Most researchers tend to use the pain severity subscale (pain now and at its worst, least, and average in the past 24 hours) and the pain interference subscale (activity, enjoyment of life, mood, relationships with others, sleep, walking, and work). The BPI has been used in descriptive studies of pain occurrence and as an outcome measure in interventions studies. In addition, Cleeland and colleagues[166] used it to explore how the cultural and linguistic backgrounds of cancer patients in four countries (China, France, Philippines, and the United States) affected relationships among their ratings of pain interference. The BPI is also available in Chinese, Hindi, Japanese, and Norwegian.[167–170]

Pain-O-Meter

The Pain-O-Meter (POM) was designed as a multidimensional measure of clinical pain, beginning with the exploration of verbal descriptors of painlike experiences (e.g., pain, ache, hurt) done in the mid-1980s.[171,172] The instrument is based on the gate control theory of pain and uses verbal descriptors from the McGill Pain Questionnaire. It is patented (U.S. patent #5,018,526) and is made of hard white plastic, 8 inches long, 2 inches wide, and 1 inch thick. It can be easily be held in one's hand. On one side of the current version of the POM[173] there are two lists of words—15 sensory words (e.g., cramping, splitting, shooting, crushing, stabbing, sharp) and 11 affective words (e.g., nagging, annoying, tiring, sickening, torturing)—as well as a vertical 10-cm VAS consisting of a marker that the patient can push between two anchors (no pain and worst possible pain) to indicate pain intensity. The other side of the POM includes an item for temporal pattern of pain (continuous or comes and goes), body diagrams (front and back) divided into grids so that patients can record location of their pain, and a 10-cm ruler for measuring the VAS rating. Thus, the POM measures physiologic, sensory, and affective dimensions of pain. Gaston-Johansson described the extensive reliability and validity work done on this instrument in 279 patients with pain, indicating that it had test–retest reliability and construct and concurrent validity. The patients had various types of pain and were recruited from a number of health care settings, thus increasing the generalizability of the findings. Gaston-Johansson proposed that the POM could be a useful assessment tool in clinical practice, but she did not address the utility of the POM for research purposes. This is an area that needs further research. Finally, since the POM is a patented device, its availability is unclear.

Chronic Pain Experience Instrument

The Chronic Pain Experience Instrument (CPEI) was developed to assess and measure accurately persistent, nonmalignant, chronic pain.[174] Davis[174] related that this instrument extended other tools for chronic pain by measuring personal responses to living with pain (e.g., frustration with ability to carry out activities) and provided a shorter, more feasible instrument than extensive multidimensional measures, such as the full-length, original MPQ with its clinical assessment questions.[175,176] This initial work on the assessment of chronic pain contributed to the content development of the CPEI. The instrument originally consisted of 33 items in a VAS format that were pilot-tested. Following the pilot test, a 24-item CPEI was constructed, consisting of 12 items from the original instrument, and 12 new or revised items.[174] Content validity was examined by two experts (patients with rheumatic disease), resulting in a content validity index of 1.0. The 24-item version was then tested in 160 individuals with rheumatic disease. Davis[174] reported an alpha coefficient of 0.85 overall, but only 9 items actually met her desired criterion of 0.50 to 0.70. Additional testing reduced the instrument to 16 items. The theta coefficient was 0.88. Stability was $r = 0.77$. Construct validity was assessed through factor analysis and predictive modeling. Results indicated that significant empirical relationships were in the direction predicted, thus supporting the CPEI's external construct validity. Davis[174] concluded that the CPEI demonstrated "high internal consistency, adequate stability, and moderate construct validity" in patients with rheumatic disease. She noted that additional psychometric work was needed, particularly in other groups of patients with chronic pain.

In subsequent work, Davis extended the psychometric evaluation of the CPEI and created two forms of the instrument, one for measuring arthritis and back pain (CPEI) and one for measuring headache (CPEI-H). Both have substantial reliability and validity. Because musculoskeletal conditions and headache are associated with very different pain experiences, Davis (personal communication, March 21, 2003) developed a new headache version (CPEI-HA) specifically to measure recurrent headache pain. Testing in 135 community-dwelling adults yielded a 16-item instrument with a Cronbach's alpha of 0.92 and three underlying dimensions (interference with core activities, helplessness, and stress, all ≥ 0.81). Correlations between the CPEI-HA and selected subscales of the SF-36 were moderate and in the predicted direction. Additional recent work by Davis (personal communication, October 28, 2002) addressed replicability of the arthritis/back pain CPEI in three arthritis groups (osteo, rheumatoid, and self-reported). Results supported internal consistency reliability, stability, and construct validity. Davis concluded that the CPEI was a promising clinical and research tool in arthritis populations, but she advocated additional psychometric work in various populations. Its use as an outcome measure in intervention studies also needs exploration.

Biobehavioral Pain Profile

The Biobehavioral Pain Profile (BPP) was developed to measure selected cognitive, behavioral, and physiologic reactions often associated with pain.[177] Using a stress-adaptation model, Dalton and colleagues noted that their methodologic study was aimed at developing and testing a pain measurement instrument that incorporated physiologic, personal, and environmental factors not addressed by other existing multidimensional pain measurement instruments. These factors were assumed to modulate nociception, coping, and pain-related behaviors, and thus to be important in guiding clinical treatment decisions.

The BPP was a 57-item questionnaire, with each item measured on a 0-to-7 Likert scale in which higher numbers represented more frequent or stronger influence of the item. Dalton et al.[177] studied three groups of patients representing different types of chronic pain: 274 persons with recurrent pain related to physical activities, such as dancing or physical education; 241 persons with chronic nonmalignant pain; and 102 persons with chronic cancer-related pain (n = 617). The analyses were quite extensive, covering construct and concurrent validity, internal consistency, and test–retest reliability. Dalton[178] concluded that the BPP's six subscales represented the multidimensionality of the pain experience and were able to provide information about psychologic and environmental factors related to pain. Such information could be useful in providing patient education and clinical care.

Glasgow Pain Questionnaire (GPQ)

Thomas and colleagues[179] developed the GPQ as a new generic measure of pain. They were specifically interested in subjective perceptions of the influence of pain on QOL and the burden that pain imposed. Based on the assumptions that existing pain measurement instruments did not adequately include QOL and that existing QOL instruments did not adequately include pain, they proposed an instrument that dealt with both constructs. Their objective was to develop a self-report instrument that could be useful in evaluating clinical care and in conducting community-based studies. Three criteria guided their work: (1) the instrument must be short and simple; (2) it must be multidimensional; and (3) it had to be relevant to people with different types and intensities of pain.

First, they conducted interviews with 230 lay people in ten locations (e.g., hospital inpatient unit, outpatient clinic, general practices, police offices, mother and baby groups) to obtain descriptions of pain, which they taped and transcribed. They then selected 59 statements based on more than 5000 descriptions of pain that they categorized into five areas: (1) types and causes of pain (e.g., location, illness, accidents, old age); (2) descriptions of pain (evaluative expressions and sensory feelings); (3) time (frequency, fluctuation); (4) emotion/coping/thoughts (ability to cope, emotions, theorizing about pain); and (5) mobility and restrictions of activity (activities, getting about, body movement). Sixty volunteers completed this initial instrument, scoring severity of pain in each pain description from 0 to 10, and answering yes or no to having had pain in the past month like the pain described in each item. Thomas et al.[179] weighted items based on pain severity ratings, asked 115 people to provide additional severity ratings on a 0–10 scale, and then calculated the median value of ratings for each item in order to derive its weight. They transformed the weights so that the sum total of weights in each of the five categories was 10. From the initial 59 items, they ended up with 24 items, each scored as yes or no. It is not clear how this reduction of items occurred. The items were divided into five categories: (1) pain frequency, (2) pain intensity, (3) emotional reactions, (4) ability to cope, and (5) restrictions of daily living. They did not provide a figure showing the final instrument nor did they provide complete examples of specific items. Scores were calculated by adding the weighted values for each item, with no category exceeding a sum of 10. They indicated that the total score was obtained by summing the category totals, thus presumably the maximum score could be 50.

The next step of their work focused on an evaluation of reliability, validity, and practical use. Three groups of subjects participated: (1) 100 patients with rheumatic disease, (2) 37 people attending an occupational health clinic, and (3) 294 chronic pain clinic patients. This last group also completed a VAS for pain intensity, and 80 patients who were randomly selected also completed the task of rating perceived severity as described above. Validity was tested in two ways. First, pain scores from the three groups were compared using the extreme groups method, with predictions that rheumatoid and pain clinic patients would have higher scores. Second, convergent validity was examined by comparing scores to pain measured by a VAS. Test–retest reliability was assessed in a sample of pain clinic patients who completed the GPQ twice, one month apart. Results indicated that pain scores were indeed significantly different among groups as hypothesized ($p < 0.001$, Kruskal-Wallace H statistic). Correlations between pain category scores and the VAS ranged from 0.26 to 0.61, and all were statistically significant ($p < 0.001$, Spearman's rank correlation). The authors justified the somewhat low correlations by noting that if they had been too high, the new measure would be redundant with existing measures. Finally, test–retest Spearman's rank correlations were all positive and statistically significant ($p < 0.001$). The authors concluded that their new instrument appeared to have good evidence of reliability and validity but required further psychometric evaluation. It appears to be a potentially useful instrument for clinical research; however, it would be important to explore whether additional psychometric data were available before proceeding.

Rheumatoid Arthritis Pain Scale (RAPS)

The RAPS was developed as a measure of pain in adults with rheumatoid arthritis for the primary purpose of using it in the clinical practice setting.[180] The underlying justification was that rheumatoid arthritis pain is "unique and different" (p. 317) from other types of chronic pain, and that an adequate instrument was not available. The author did not appear to be aware of the work of Davis, described above. The RAPS was based on the gate control theory of pain, which recognizes that pain is a multidimensional experience with sensory, motivational, affective, and cognitive elements. The instrument thus was composed of theoretical subscales that represented these elements from the unique perspective of the rheumatoid arthritis sufferer.

Anderson[180] began by interviewing patients to identify their experiences and extract commonalities. She then formulated subscales and defined them based on the gate control theory and the affective motivational model. The result was four subscales, purporting to measure major aspects of arthritis pain: (1) physiologic (morning stiffness, pain on motion, tenderness in joints, swelling in joints, level of fatigue and malaise); (2) affective (unpleasantness, distress, annoyance); (3) sensory-discriminative (intensity, duration, location, and quality of pain sensations); and (4) cognitive (longer-term aspects of having pain, such as depression, freedom, influence of pain on daily activity, self-esteem, memory, past experience). Items were scored using a seven-point Likert scale ranging from never to always.

Psychometric evaluation began with a pilot study in which the content validity of the initial 36-item instrument was assessed by six rheumatology experts; it was also completed by 59 patients with rheumatoid arthritis and pain of at least three months' duration. The content validity index, which measures how many items are judged relevant or very relevant, was 0.69. The coefficient alpha was 0.9239. Eleven items were deleted because experts did not judge them relevant enough; another item was deleted because patients found the wording to be confusing; and three items were reworded. One item endorsed by experts had an item-total correlation of only 0.3789 (less than the desired range of 0.4–0.7), but it was retained because of its high relevance ("I have swelling of at least one joint"). The revised RAPS consisted of 24 items.

Anderson[180] conducted full-scale psychometric testing in 120 rheumatoid arthritis patients seen in a large private practice in the southeastern United States. She tested ten hypotheses, all related to specific psychometric properties of the RAPS (e.g., all item-to-total correlations are between 0.4 and 0.7). Similar to the pilot study, each patient had had pain of at least three months' duration, items were scored using a seven-point Likert scale (never to always), and a higher score meant more severe pain. A rheumatologist performed a "joint count" (p. 319) using a modified VAS for pain. Data analysis focused on traditional psychometric tests. Cronbach's alpha coefficient for internal consistency reliability was 0.918 for the entire scale, and all items save two had item-total correlations between 0.4 and 0.7. Of the two, one (swelling in joints) was lower, at 0.299, and one (pain is severe) was higher, at 0.739. Internal consistency for each of the four subscales ranged from 0.64 to 0.86. The affective scale had the lowest alpha, probably because one item (pain described as annoying) was 0.295. Pearson correlations performed on the RAPS score, total joint count (TJC), and modified VAS were positively and significantly correlated ($p = 0.0001$). Furthermore, the shared variance among these measures ranged from 25% to 45.6%, thereby providing additional evidence of what the author called "concurrent criterion validity" (p. 320). To examine construct validity, Anderson conducted exploratory factor analyses using both the oblique method promax, which assumes factors are correlated, and the orthogonal method varimax, which assumes factors are uncorrelated. Three of the four originally proposed factors or subscales (Cognitive, Physiologic, Sensory) emerged and together explained 84% of the variance. None of the items on the Affective subscale loaded at the required value of 0.4 or higher, except pain described as annoying, and most of the items loaded on the sensory factor. Although Anderson did not confirm all ten hypotheses, the overall data do support the reliability and validity of the RAPS. She recommended that additional psychometric evaluation be undertaken to examine and refine specific items, explore convergent validity, and compile a normative profile for the RAPS. She concluded that in its present form, the instrument might be useful for clinicians who wanted to examine the effects of various treatments on pain. Researchers might use the RAPS in descriptive studies that examine occurrence and characteristics of rheumatoid arthritis pain, and could also explore it as an outcome measure in intervention studies, although this might be premature given Anderson's recommendations for refinement.

Chest Discomfort Diary (CDD)

The CDD is an instrument originally designed to assess pain in patients with coronary artery disease[181] with a predominant focus on the sensory dimension. Kimble and colleagues[182] attempted to use the CDD within the context of a study examining gender patterns of chronic angina. They discovered that the CDD was restricted in its ability to measure multiple dimensions of pain and was written at a ninth-grade level, which was deemed unacceptable for the many low-literacy-level subjects in their research. With the authors' permission, Kimble et al. embarked on a revision and psychometric evaluation of the instrument, which they termed the Chest Discomfort Diary-Revised (CDD-R).

The original CDD was a nine-item instrument designed for self-administration when anginal chest pain occurred. The items measured activity and mood before chest pain, pain location and intensity, pain descriptors, frequency and duration of pain, and pain relief measures. Kimble et al. revised the CDD extensively to include physiologic, affective, sensory, cognitive, and behavioral dimensions of pain. A panel of cardiac, pain, and medicine specialists endorsed the content validity of the CDD-R. In consultation with literacy experts, the instrument was written more simply and the reading level lowered to fourth grade. A pilot study of 20 subjects was then conducted to examine face validity. Because they expressed difficulty understanding some items, the instrument was revised again by placing similar items closer together and providing better instructions. This version of the CDD-R had 36 items that covered the dimensions noted above. Three subscales—other cardiac symptoms, emotional precipitants of angina, and extent of angina pain relief—accounted for 23 of the 36 items. Samples of single items include the following: Chest pain severity was measured with a Likert scale that had anchors of "no pain" and "as painful as it could be." Upset because of chest pain or discomfort was measured with a Likert scale that had anchors of "not at all upsetting" to "as upsetting as it could be." Scoring of the CDD-R is somewhat complex in that the three subscale scores are obtained by summing the Likert items; single items are analyzed individually; and ten items regarding physical activities that are negatively influenced by angina are summed. The 36 item CDD-R was then tested in 27 patients with a history of coronary artery disease (CAD), an episode of chest pain in the previous month, chest pain characteristic of angina, and a documented literacy level of fourth grade or higher. Each patient only completed the instrument once, usually without help from research assistants.

Data analyses addressed missing data and internal consistency reliability. The emotional precipitants subscale had 33–49% missing data, thought to be the result of poor directions and formatting. Internal consistency reliability coefficients for the cardiac symptoms subscale and emotional precipitants subscale were 0.88 and 0.86, respectively, and a coefficient could not be calculated for the third subscale. The CDD-R was useful in describing the characteristics and related factors of anginal pain. Greater emotional upset due to angina was associated with high chest pain severity ($r = 0.45$, $p = 0.02$) and worry about health ($r = 0.49$, $p = 0.01$). Kimble and associates concluded that the CDD-R performed well for a new instrument and appeared to have adequate initial psychometric properties. They recommended further testing with a larger sample and in fact went on to conduct another psychometric study in 130 patients with documented CAD (Kimble, personal communication, March 27, 2003). Patients completed the CDD-R as well as a battery of other generic and angina-specific pain instruments. The results demonstrated adequate internal consistency reliability (0.70) for the CDD-R subscales, and significant correlations between CDD-R and pain measurements of similar constructs. The authors concluded that the revised CDD-R was indeed reliable and valid. They further reduced the instrument to 16 items, but details were not provided about why or how. This instrument measures angina frequency, duration, severity, perceived seriousness of angina as a health problem, and emotional distress about having it. This instrument appears to have promise as a good multidimensional measure of anginal pain.

Seattle Angina Questionnaire (SAQ)

This instrument was developed by Spertus and colleagues[183] to measure functional status in CAD, but since it also measures frequency of chest pain and its impact on daily life, it can be considered a pain instrument. The SAQ contains five dimensions of coronary artery disease: (1) physical limitation (e.g., dressing); (2) anginal stability; (3) anginal frequency; (4) treatment satisfaction (e.g., how bothersome it is to take pills); and (5) disease perception (e.g., how much chest pain has interfered with enjoyment of life). The SAQ is 19-item self-administered questionnaire with five or six scales. The instructions for scoring indicate that each response is assigned an ordinal value, the scores within each of the subscales are summed and transformed into a 0–100 scale by subtracting the lowest possible score on the scale, dividing by the range of the scale, and multiplying by 100. Each subscale ranges from 0 to 100.

Spertus et al.[183] demonstrated the instrument's validity and reliability for patients with stable and unstable coronary artery disease. Validation of the physical limitation subscale was tested through correlation with duration of treadmill test performance. In an age-adjusted correlational analysis, the SAQ, Duke Activity Status Index, and Specific Activity Scale were associated with total exercise duration ($r = 0.36–0.42$, $p < 0.05$) and with each other ($r = 0.43–0.84$, $p < 0.001$). The SAQ showed the strongest correlation with treadmill performance ($r = 0.42$, $p < 0.001$). Validity of the anginal stability subscale was first tested by comparing anginal stability scores between groups of patients with and without unstable angina because the authors hypothesized that unstable angina patients would have lower stability than stable angina patients. The second validity test correlated anginal stability scores of stable angina patients and their global assessment of change after three months. Stable angina patients had higher stability scores than unstable angina patients. Significant correlation between the anginal stability scale and patients' perception of global change after three months was reported ($r = 0.70, p < 0.0001$). Anginal frequency scale was validated by correlating angina frequency scale with the number of nitroglycerin prescription refills for the previous year ($r = 0.31, p < 0.0006$). The treatment satisfaction scale was validated through correlation with scores for the American Board of Internal Medicine's Patient Satisfaction Questionnaire ($r = 0.67, p < 0.0001$). Finally, the disease perception scale was validated by correlation with the general health perceptions scale of the Short Form-36 ($r = 0.60, p < 0.0001$). Except for the angina stability scale ($r = 0.24$), correlation coefficients in a three-month-interval test–retest reliability were very high ($r = 0.76–0.83$).

One limitation of this initial work was the fact that the majority of the sample was elderly men. Dougherty and colleagues[184] extended the psychometric work, but again focused primarily on elderly men. Cronbach's alpha coefficients for subscales ranged from 0.66 to 0.89, except the angina stability subscale, which was excluded from analysis because it was composed of only one item. In a two-week interval for test–retest reliability, correlation coefficients were quite high (0.58–0.80), except for angina stability (0.33). Furthermore, the correlation coefficients for all subscales were statistically significant ($p < 0.001$). The researchers noted that the SAQ was a responsive instrument to anginal status and to clinical change in a trial of an antianginal drug. Subsequent work on the value of the SAQ as a prognostic indicator suggested that the SAQ was independently associated with one-year mortality and hospitalization for acute coronary syndrome.[185]

This instrument is concise and easily administered, but it also allows researchers to assess diverse effects of disease on patients and their activity limitations specific to coronary artery disease.[183] Validity and reliability in other diverse populations remains unclear. There is also a computer-assisted SAQ version. Bliven and colleagues[54] demonstrated high validity (correlation coefficient 0.84 to 0.90, $p < 0.001$); high correlation with a paper-based questionnaire (for all five dimensions $r = 0.84–0.93$); no practical time difference for completion between computer-assisted and paper-based; and an 82% patient preference rate for the computer-assisted SAQ. Garratt, Huchinson, and Russell[186] introduced a United Kingdom version of the SAQ (SAQ-UK) after changing some words and decreasing the instrument to 14 items that measured three dimensions: physical limitations, anginal frequency, and perception and treatment satisfaction. The investigators demonstrated reliability, validity, and responsiveness in 959 U.K. patients with stable angina, reporting internal reliability of 0.83–0.92, and test–retest reliability ($r = 0.63–0.81$). Validity was verified by significant correlations of the SAQ-UK with SF-12, the EuroQOL, and a health transition tool. Clearly, the SAQ has undergone extensive testing in a variety of populations, has good evidence of reliability and validity, and exists in multiple formats. It should be a useful tool in both descriptive and intervention research.

Summary

Although compromises must inevitably be made, a careful and deliberative selection process will help to ensure that the researcher selects appropriate instruments. The result should be reliable and valid data that assist in answering the research question(s). Given the long and painstaking process of instrument development, it may be more expedient for the researcher to use a tool that has been developed and assessed psychometrically or to revise such tools as needed. The repeated use of such instruments, with careful attention to psychometric issues, will help to refine and improve existing tools, resulting in better measures of clinical pain.

Websites

painsourcebook.ca
prc.coh.org
www.StopPain.org
www.iasp-pain.org
www.painbooks.org

References

1. Sternbach, R.A. *Pain—A psychophysiological analysis.* New York: Academic, 1960, p. 12.
2. Melzack, R., & Casey, K.L. Sensory, motivational and central control determinants of pain: A new conceptual model. In D. Kenshalo (Ed.), *The skin senses.* Springfield, IL: Chas. C. Thomas, 1968, pp. 423-439.
3. Merskey, H., & Spear, F.G. *Pain: Psychological and psychiatric aspects.* London: Balliere, Tindall, and Cassell, 1967.
4. International Association for the Study of Pain. Pain terms: A current list with definitions and notes on usage. *Pain,* 1986, *3*(Suppl):S216-S221.
5. Turk, D.C., & Rudy, R.E. IASP taxonomy of chronic pain syndromes: Preliminary assessment of reliability. *Pain,* 1987, *30*:177-189.
6. Brose, W.G., Cherry, D.A., Plummer, J., et al. IASP taxonomy: Questions and controversies. In M.R. Bond, J.E. Charlton, & C.J. Woolf (Eds.), *Proceedings of the VIth World Congress on Pain.* Amsterdam: Elsevier, 1991, pp. 503-507.
7. McCaffery, M. *Nursing management of the patient with pain.* Philadelphia: Lippincott, 1972, p. 8.
8. Beecher, H.K. Pain in men wounded in battle. *Ann Surg,* 1946, *123*:96-105.
9. Hardy, J.D., Wolff, H.G., & Goodell, H. *Pain sensations and reactions.* Baltimore: William & Wilkins, 1952.
10. Melzack, R., & Wall, P.D. Pain mechanisms: A new theory. *Science,* 1965, *150*(3699):971-978.
11. Weisenberg, M. Pain and pain control. *Psychol Bull,* 1977, *84*(5):1008-1044.
12. Ahles, T.A., Blanchard, E.B., & Ruckdeschel, J.C. The multidimensional nature of cancer-related pain. *Pain,* 1983, *17*(3):277-288.
13. McGuire, D.B. The multidimensional nature of cancer pain. In D.B. McGuire & C.H. Yarbro (Eds.), *Cancer pain management.* Philadelphia: Saunders, 1987, pp. 1-20.
14. McGuire, D.B. Comprehensive and multidimensional assessment and measurement of pain. *J Pain Symptom Manage,* 1992, *7*:312-319.
15. National Institute of Nursing Research. *6. Symptom Management: Acute Pain: A Report of the National Institute of Nursing Research Priority Expert Panel on Symptom Management: Acute Pain.* NIH Publication No. 94-2421. Bethesda, MD: U.S. Public Health Service, National Institute of Health, U.S. Department of Health and Human Services, 1994.
16. Wolff, B.B. Laboratory methods of pain measurement. In R. Melzack (Ed.), *Pain measurement and assessment.* New York: Raven, 1983, pp. 7-13.
17. Bonica, J.J. Definitions and taxonomy of pain. In J.J. Bonica (Ed.), *The management of pain* (ed. 2, vol. 1). Philadelphia: Lea & Febiger, 1990, p. 19.
18. Agnew, D.C., Crue, B.L., & Pinsky, J.J. A taxonomy for diagnosis and information storage for patients with chronic pain. *Bull LA Neurol Soc,* 1979, *44*:84-86.
19. Meinhart, N.T., & NcCaffery, M. *Pain: A nursing approach to assessment and analysis.* Norwalk, CT: Appleton-Century-Crofts, 1983.
20. Foley, K.M. The treatment of cancer pain. *N Engl J Med,* 1985, *313*:84-95.
21. Davitz, J.R., & Davitz, L.L. *Inferences of patients' pain and psychological distress: Studies of nursing behaviors.* New York: Springer, 1981.
22. Rankin, M.A., & Snider, B. Nurses' perceptions of cancer patients' pain. *Cancer Nurs,* 1984, *7*(2):149-155.
23. Grossman, S.A., Sheidler, V.R., Swedeen, K., et al. Correlation of patient and caregiver ratings of cancer pain. *J Pain Symptom Manage,* 1991, *6*:53-57.
24. Kremer, E.F., & Atkinson, J.H. Pain language as a measure of affect in chronic pain patients. In R. Melzack (Ed.), *Pain measurement and assessment.* New York: Raven, 1983, pp. 119-127.
25. Jeans, N.E. The measurement of pain in children. In R. Melzack (Ed.), *Pain measurement and assessment.* New York: Raven, 1983, pp. 183-189.
26. Ferrell, B.A., & Ferrell, B.R. Assessment of chronic pain in the elderly. *Geriatr Med Today,* 1989, *8*:123-134.
27. Harkins, S.W., Kwentus, J., & Price, D.D. Pain in the elderly. In C. Bendetti, C.C. Chapman, & G. Morrica (Eds.), *Advances in pain research and therapy* (vol. 7). New York: Raven, 1984, pp. 103-121.
28. Bruera, E., Macmillan, K., Hanson, J., et al. The cognitive effects of the administration of narcotic analgesics in patients with cancer pain. *Pain,* 1989, *39*:13-16.
29. Jacox, A., Carr, D.B., Payne, R., et al. *Management of cancer pain. Clinical practice guideline No. 9.* AHCPR Publication No. 94-0592. Rockville, MD: Agency for Health Care Policy and Research, U.S. Department of Health and Human Services, Public Health Service, 1994.
30. Weiner, D., Peterson, B., & Keefe, F. Evaluating persistent pain in long term care residents: What role for pain maps? *Pain,* 1998, *76*:249-257.

31. Galer, B.S., & Jensen, M.P. Development and preliminary validation of a pain measure specific to neuropathic pain: The Neuropathic Pain Scale. *Neurology*, 1997, *48*:332-338.

32. Bennett, M. The LANSS Pain Scale: The Leeds assessment of neuropathic symptoms and signs. *Pain*, 2001, *92*:147-157.

33. Guieu, R., Blin, O., Pouget J., & Serratrice, G. Nociceptive threshold and physical activity. *Can J Neurol Sci*, 1992, *19*:69-71.

34. Kurita, A., Takase, B., Uehata, A, et al. Differences in plasma β-endorphin and bradykinin levels between patients with painless or with painful myocardial ischemia. *Am Heart J*, 1992, *123*:304-309.

35. Hofbauer, R.K., Rainville, P., Duncan, G.H., & Bushnell, C. Cortical representation of the sensory dimension of pain. *J Neurophysiol*, 2001, *86*:402-411.

36. Keele, K.D. The pain chart. *Lancet*, 1948, *2*:6-8.

37. Melzack, R. The McGill Pain Questionnaire: Major properties and scoring methods. *Pain*, 1975, *1*(3):277-299.

38. Heft, M.W., & Parker, S.R. An experimental basis for revising the graphic rating scale for pain. *Pain*, 1984, *19*(2):153-161.

39. De Conno, F., Caraceni, A., Gamba, A., et al. Pain measurement in cancer patients: A comparison of six methods. *Pain*, 1994, *57*:161-166.

40. Maxwell, C. Sensitivity and accuracy of the visual analogue scale: A psycho-physical classroom experiment. *Br J Clin Pharmacol*, 1978, *6*(1):15-24.

41. Clarke, P.R.F., & Spear, F.G. Reliability and sensitivity in the self-assessment of well-being. *Bull Br Psychol Soc*, 1964, *17*(55):18A.

42. Gift, A.G. Visual analogues scales: Measurement of subjective phenomena. *Nurs Res*, 1989, *38*:286-288.

43. Cline, N.E., Herman, J., Shaw, E.R., et al. Standardization of the Visual Analogue Scale. *Nurs Res*, 1992, *41*:378-390.

44. Huskisson, E.C. Measurement of pain. *Lancet*, 1974, *2*(7889):1127-1131.

45. Grossman, S.A., Shielder, V.R., McGuire, D.B., et al. A comparison of the Hopkins Pain Rating Instrument with standard visual analogue and verbal descriptor scales in patients with cancer pain. *J Pain Sympt Manage*, 1992, *7*:196-203.

46. Price, D.D., Bush, F.M., Long, S., et al. A comparison of pain measurement characteristics of mechanical visual analogue and simple numerical rating scales. *Pain*, 1994, *56*:217-226.

47. Murphy, D.F., McDonald, A., Power, C., et al. Measurement of pain: A comparison of the visual analogue scale with a nonvisual analogue scale. *Clin J Pain*, 1988, *3*:197-199.

48. Wilkie, D., Lovejoy, N., Dodd, N., et al. Cancer pain intensity measurement: Concurrent validity of three tools—Finger dynamometer, pain intensity number scale, visual analogue scale. *Hospice J*, 1990, *6*(1):1-13.

49. Price, D.D., McGrath, D.A. Rafii, A., et al. The validation of visual analogue scales as ratio scale measures for chronic and experimental pain. *Pain*, 1983, *17*(1):45-56.

50. Forouzanfar, T., Kemler, M., Kessels, A.G.H., et al. Comparison of multiple against single pain intensity measurements in complex regional pain syndrome Type I: Analysis of 54 patients. *Clin J Pain*, 2002, *18*:234-237.

51. Collins, S.L., Moore, R.A., & McQuay, H.J. The visual analogue pain intensity scale: What is moderate pain in millimeters? *Pain*, 1997, *72*:95-97.

52. Scott, J., & Huskisson, E.C. Vertical or horizontal visual analogue scales. *Ann Rheumat Dis*, 1979, *38*:560.

53. Scott, J., & Huskisson, E.C. Accuracy of subjective measurements made with or without previous scores: An important source of error in serial measurement of subjective states. *Ann Rheumat Dis*, 1979, *38*:558-559.

54. Bliven, B.D., Kaufman, S.E., & Spertus, J.A. Electronic collection of health-related quality of life data: Validity, time benefits and patient preference. *Qual Life Res*, 2001, *10*:15-22.

55. Wilkie, D.J, Huang, H., Berry, D.L., et al. Cancer symptom control: Feasibility of a tailed, interactive computerized program for patients. *Fam Comm Health*, 2001, *24*(3):48-62.

56. Swanston, M., Abraham, C., Macrae, W.A., et al. Pain assessment with interactive computer animation. *Pain*, 1993, *53*:347-351.

57. Bieri, D., Reeve, R.A., Champion, G.D., et al. The Faces Pain Scale for the self-assessment of the severity of pain experienced by children: Development, initial validation, and preliminary investigation for ratio scale properties. *Pain*, 1990, *41*:139-150.

58. Herr, K.A., Mobily, P.R., Kohout, F.J., et al. Evaluation of the Faces Pain Scale for use with the elderly. *Clin J Pain*, 1998, *14*:29-38.

59. Stuppy, D.J. The Faces Pain Scale: Reliability and validity with mature adults. *Appl Nurs Res*, 1998, *11*(2):84-89.

60. Wong, D.L., & Baker, C.M. Pain in children: Comparison of assessment scales. *Pediatr Nurs*, 1988, *14*(1):9-17.

61. Wong, D.L., & Baker, C.M. Smiling face as anchor for pain intensity scales. *Pain*, 2001, *89*:295-300.

62. Cason, C.L., & Grissom, N.L. Ameliorating adults' acute pain during phlebotomy with a distraction intervention. *Appl Nurs Res*, 1997, *10*(4):168-73.

63. Choiniere, M., & Amsel, R. A visual analogue thermometer for measuring pain intensity. *J Pain Symptom Manage*, 1996, *11*:299-311.

64. Reading, A.E. A comparison of pain rating scales. *J Psychosom Res*, 1980, *24*:119-124.

65. Downie, W.W., Leatham, P.A., Rhind, V.M., et al. Studies with pain rating scales. *Ann Rheum Dis*, 1978, *37*(4):378-381.

66. Kremer, E., Atkinson, J.H., & Ignelzi, R.J. Measurement of pain: Patient preference does not confound pain measurement. *Pain*, 1981, *10*:241-248.

67. Jensen, M.P., Karoly, P., & Braver, T. The measurement of clinical pain intensity: A comparison of six methods. *Pain*, 1986, *27*:117-126.

68. Jensen, M.P., Karoly, P., O'Riordan, E.F., et al. The subjective experience of acute pain: An assessment of the utility of 10 indices. *Clin J Pain*, 1989, *5*:153-159.

69. Machin, D., Lewith, G.T., & Wylson, S. Pain measurement in randomized clinical trials. *Clin J Pain*, 1994, *4*:161-168.

70. Banos, J.E., Bosch, F., Canellas, M., et al. Acceptability of visual analogue scales in the clinical setting: A comparison with verbal rating scales in postoperative

pain. *Methods Find Exp Clin Pharmacol*, 1989, *11*(2):123-127.

71. Paice, J.A., & Cohen, F.L. Validity of a verbally administered numeric rating scale to measure cancer pain intensity. *Cancer Nurs*, 1997, *20*:88-93.

72. DeWit, R., van Dam, F., Hanneman, M., et al. Evaluation of the use of a pain diary in chronic cancer pain patients at home. *Pain*, 1999, *79*:89-99.

73. Vickers, A.J. Comparison of an ordinal and a continuous outcome measure of muscle soreness. *Int J Technol Transfer*, 1999, *15*:709-716.

74. Gordon, M., Greenfield, E., Marvin, J., et al. Use of pain assessment tools: Is there a preference? *J Burn Care Rehab*, 1998, *19*:451-454.

75. Ramer, L., Richardson, J.L., Cohen, M.Z., et al. Multimeasure pain assessment in an ethnically diverse group of patients with cancer. *J Transcult Nurs*, 1999, *10*:94-101.

76. Bigatti, S.M., & Cronin, T.A. A comparison of pain measures used with patients with fibromyalgia. *J Nurs Meas*, 2002, *10*:5-14.

77. Krulewich, J., London, M.R., Skakel, V.J., et al. Assessment of pain in cognitively impaired older adults: A comparison of pain assessment tools and their use by nonprofessional caregivers. *J Am Geriatr Soc*, 2000, *48*:1607-1611.

78. Chibnall, J.T., & Tait, R.C. Pain assessment in cognitively impaired and unimpaired older adults: A comparison of four scales. *Pain*, 2000, *92*:173-186.

79. DeWit, R., van Dam, F., Abu-Saad, H.H., et al. Empirical comparison of commonly used measures to evaluate pain treatment in cancer patients with chronic pain. *J Clin Oncol*, 1999, *17*:1280-1287.

80. Lines, C.R., Vandormael, K., & Malbecq, W. A comparison of visual analog scale and categorical ratings of headache pain in a randomized controlled clinical trial with migraine patients. *Pain*, 2001, *93*:185-190.

81. Ahles, T.A., Ruckdeschel, J.C., & Blanchard, E.B. Cancer related pain. II. Assessment with Visual Analogue Scales. *J Psychosom Res*, 1984, *28*(2):121-124.

82. Price, D.D., Harkins, S.W., & Baker, C. Sensory-affective relationships among different types of clinical and experimental pain. *Pain*, 1987, *28*:297-307.

83. Good, M., Stiller, C., Zauszniewski, J.A., et al. Sensation and distress of pain scales: Reliability, validity, and sensitivity. *J Nurs Meas*, 2001, *9*:219-238.

84. Taal, L.A., & Faber A.W. Burn injuries, pain and distress: Exploring the role of stress symptomatology. *Burns*, 1997, *23*:288-290.

85. Taal, L.A., & Faber A.W. The burn specific pain anxiety scale: Introduction of a reliable and valid measure. *Burns*, 1997, *2*:147-150.

86. Taal, L.A., Faber, A.W., van Loey, N.E.E., et al. The abbreviated burn specific pain anxiety scale: A multicenter study. *Burns*, 1999, *25*:493-497.

87. Aaron, L.A., Patterson, D.R., Finch, C.P., et al. The utility of a burn specific measure of pain anxiety to prospectively predict pain and function: A comparative analysis. *Burns*, 2001, *27*:329-334.

88. Hadjistavropoulos, H.D., MacLeod, F.K., & Asmundson, G.J.G. Validation of the Chronic Pain Coping Inventory. *Pain*, 1999, *80*:471-481.

89. Ward, S.E., Goldberg, N., Miller-McCauley, V., et al. Patient-related barriers to management of cancer pain. *Pain*, 1993, *52*:319-324.

90. Ward, S.E., & Gatwood, J. Concerns about reporting pain and using analgesics: A comparison of persons with and without cancer. *Cancer Nurs*, 1994, *17*:200-206.

91. Gunnarsdottir, S., Donovan, H.S., Serlin, R.C., et al. Patient-related barriers to pain management: The barriers questionnaire II (BQ-II). *Pain*, 2002, *99*:385-396.

92. Ward, S.E., & Berry, P.E. Barriers to pain management in hospice: A study of family caregivers. *Hospice J*, 1995, *10*(4):19-33.

93. Ward, S.E., & Hernandez, L. Patient-related barriers to management of cancer pain in Puerto Rico. *Pain*, 1994, *58*:233-238.

94. Lin, C., & Ward, S.E. Patient-related barriers to cancer pain management in Taiwan. *Cancer Nurs*, 1995, *18*:16-22.

95. Hanken, A. The measurement of pain. In M. Newton, W. Hunt, W. McDowell, & A. Hanken (Eds.), *A study of nurse action in relief of pain*. Columbus, OH: The Ohio State University School of Nursing, 1964.

96. Hanken, A., & McDowell, W. Development of a rating scale to measure pain. In M. Newton, W. Hunt, W. McDowell, & A. Hanken (Eds.), *A study of nurse action in relief of pain*. Columbus, OH: The Ohio State University School of Nursing, 1964.

97. Chambers, W.G., & Price, G.G. Influence of nurse upon effects of analgesics administered. *Nurs Res*, 1967, *16*(3):228-233.

98. Bruegel, M.A. Relationship of preoperative anxiety to perception of postoperative pain. *Nurs Res*, 1971, *20*(1):26-31.

99. Hagle, M.E. Diurnal variation in pain intensity of cancer patients. Unpublished master's thesis. University of Illinois at the Medical Center, Chicago, IL, 1980.

100. Bonnel, A.M., & Boureau, F. Labor pain assessment: Validity of a behavioral index. *Pain*, 1985, *22*(1):81-90.

101. Mateo, O.M., & Krenzischek, D.A. A pilot study to assess the relationship between behavioral manifestations and self-report of pain in postanesthesia care unit patients. *J Post Anesth Nurs*, 1992, *7*(1):15-21.

102. Mateo, O. Personal communication, July 1994.

103. Webb, M.R., & Kennedy, M.G. Behavioral responses and self-reported pain in postoperative patients. *J Post Anesth Nurs*, 1994, *9*(2):91-95.

104. Feldt, K.S. The checklist of nonverbal pain indicators (CNPI). *Pain Manage Nurs*, 2000, *1*:13-21.

105. Feldt, K.S. Improving assessment and treatment of pain in cognitively impaired nursing home residents. *Ann Long Term Care*, 2000, *8*(9):36-42.

106. Scherder, E., et al. Repeated pain assessment. *Alz Dis Dement Geriatr Cognitive Disord*, 2001, *12*:400-407.

107. Fordyce, W.E., Lansky, T., Calsyn, D.A., et al. Pain measurement and pain behavior. *Pain*, 1984, *18*(1):53-69.

108. Follick, M.J., Ahern, D.K., & Laser-Wolston, W. Evaluation of a daily activity diary for chronic pain patients. *Pain*, 1984, *19*:373-382.

109. Kremer, E.F., Block, A., & Gaylor, N.S. Behavioral approaches to treatment of chronic pain. The inaccuracy of patient self-report measures. *Arch Phys Med Rehab*, 1981, *62*(4):188-191.

110. Keefe, F.J., Wilkins, R.H., & Cook, W.A. Direct observation of pain behavior in low back pain patients during physical examination. *Pain*, 1984, *20*:59-68.

111. Richards, J., Nepomuceno, C., Riles, M., et al. As-

sessing pain behavior: The UAB pain behavior scale. *Pain*, 1982, *14*(4):393-398.

112. Keefe, F.J., Brantley, A., Manual, G., et al. Behavioral assessment of head and neck cancer pain. *Pain*, 1985, *23*(4): 327-336.

113. McDaniel, L.K., Anderson, K.O., Bradley, L.A., et al. Development of an observation method for assessing pain behavior in rheumatoid arthritis patients. *Pain*, 1986, *24*:165-194.

114. Keefe, F.J., & Block, A.R. Development of an observation method for assessing pain behavior in chronic low back pain patients. *Behav Ther*, 1982, *13*:363-375.

115. Koho, P., Aho, S., Watson, P., et al. Assessment of chronic pain behaviour: Reliability of the method and its relationship with perceived disability, physical impairment and function. *J Rehab Med*, 2001, *33*:128-132.

116. Ferrell, B.A., Rhiner, M., et al. Family factors influencing cancer pain. *Postgrad Med J*, 1991, *67*(Suppl):64-69.

117. Ferrell, B.R., Rhiner, N., Cohen, M.Z., et al. Pain as a metaphor for illness. Part I: Impact of cancer pain on family caregivers. *Oncol Nurs Forum*, 1991, *18*:1303-1309.

118. Ferrell, B.R., Cohen, M.Z., Rhiner, M., et al. Pain as a metaphor for illness. Part II: Family caregivers' management of pain. *Oncol Nurs Forum*, 1991, *18*:1315-1321.

119. Ferrell, B., Rhiner, M., & Rivera, L. Development and evaluation of the Family Pain Questionnaire. *J Psychosoc Oncol*, 1993, *10*(4):21-35.

120. Johnson, J.E. Effects of structuring patients' expectations on their reactions to threatening events. *Nurs Res*, 1972, *21*(6):499-504.

121. Johnson, E.E. Effects of accurate expectations about sensations on the sensory and distress components of pain. *J Pers Soc Psychol*, 1973, *27*(2):261-275.

122. Wells, N. The effect of relaxation on postoperative muscle tension and pain. *Nurs Res*, 1982, *31*:236-238.

123. Tursky, B. The development of a pain perception profile: A psychophysical approach. In M. Weisenberg & B. Tursky (Eds.), *Pain: New perspectives in therapy and research*. New York: Plenum, 1976, pp. 171-194.

124. Andrasik, F., Blanchard, E.B., Ahles, T., et al. Assessing the reactive as well as the sensory component of headache pain. *Headache*, 1981, *21*:218-221.

125. Urban, B.J., Keefe, F.J., & France, R.D. A study of psychophysical scaling in chronic pain patients. *Pain*, 1984, *20*:157-168.

126. Melzack, R., & Torgerson, W. On the language of pain. *Anesthesiology*, 1971, *34*(1):50-59.

127. Melzack, R., Katz, J., & Jeans, M.E. The role of compensation in chronic pain. Analysis using a new method of scoring the McGill Pain Questionnaire. *Pain*, 1985, *23*(2):101-112.

128. Graham, C., Bond, T.T., Gerkovich, M.M., et al. Use of the McGill Pain Questionnaire in the assessment of cancer pain: Replicability and consistency. *Pain*, 1980, *8*(3):377-387.

129. McGuire, D.B. Assessment of pain in cancer inpatients using the McGill Pain Questionnaire. *Oncol Nurs Forum*, 1984, *11*(6):32-37.

130. Klepac, R.K., Dowling, J., Rokke, P., et al. Interview vs. paper and pencil administration of the McGill Pain Questionnaire. *Pain*, 1981, *11*:241-246.

131. Byrne, M., Troy, A., Bradley, L.A., et al. Crossvalidation of the factor structure of the McGill pain questionnaire. *Pain*, 1982, *13*:193-201.

132. Reading, A.E. The internal structure of the McGill pain questionnaire in dysmenorrhoea patients. *Pain*, 1979, *7*(3):353-358.

133. Kremer, E., & Atkinson, J.H. Pain measurement: Construct validity of the affective dimension of the McGill Pain Questionnaire with chronic benign pain patients. *Pain*, 1981, *11*(1):93-100.

134. Burckhardt, C.S. The use of the McGill Pain Questionnaire in assessing arthritis pain. *Pain*, 1984, *19*(3):305-314.

135. Prieto, E.J., & Geisinger, K.F. Factor-analysis studies of the McGill Pain Questionnaire. In R. Melzack (Ed.), *Pain measurement and assessment*. New York: Raven, 1983.

136. Buren, J.V., & Kleinknecht, R.A. An evaluation of the McGill Pain Questionnaire for use in dental pain assessment. *Pain*, 1979, *6*:23-33.

137. Klepac, R.K., Dowling, J., Hauge, G., et al. Sensitivity of the McGill Pain Questionnaire to intensity and quality of laboratory pain. *Pain*, 1981, *10*:199-207.

138. Hunter, M., & Philips, C. The experience of headache—An assessment of the qualities of tension headache pain. *Pain*, 1981, *10*:209-219.

139. Reading, E.A. The McGill Pain Questionnaire: An appraisal. In R. Melzack (Ed.), *Pain measurement and assessment*. New York: Raven, 1983, pp. 55-61.

140. Reading, A.E. A comparison of the McGill Pain Questionnaire in chronic and acute pain. *Pain*, 1982, *13*:185-192.

141. Grushka, M., & Sessle, B.J. Applicability of the McGill Pain Questionnaire to the differentiation of "toothache" pain. *Pain*, 1984, *19*(1):49-57.

142. Dubuisson, D., & Melzack, R. Classification pain descriptions by multiple group discriminant analysis. *Exp Neurol*, 1976, *51*(2):480-487.

143. Reading, A.E., Everitt, B., & Sledmere, C.M. The McGill Pain Questionnaire: A replication of its construction. *Br J Clin Psychol*, 1982, *21*:339-349.

144. Turk, D.C., Rudy, T.E., & Salovey, P. The McGill Pain Questionnaire reconsidered: Confirming the factor structure and examining appropriate uses. *Pain*, 1985, *21*(4):385-397.

145. Wilkie, D.J., Savedra, M.C., Holzemer, W.L., et al. Use of the McGill Pain Questionnaire to measure pain: A metaanalysis. *Nurs Res*,1990, *39*:36-41.

146. Vanderiet, K., Adriaensen, H., Carton, H., et al. The McGill Pain Questionnaire constructed for the Dutch language (MPQ-DV). Preliminary data concerning reliability and validity. *Pain*, 1987, *30*:395-408.

147. Kiss, I., Muller, H., & Abel, M. The McGill Pain Questionnaire—German version. A study on cancer pain. *Pain*, 1987, *29*:195-207.

148. Maiani, G., & Sanavio, E. Semantics of pain in Italy: The Italian Version of the McGill Pain Questionnaire. *Pain*, 1985, *4*(3):377-387.

149. De Benedittis, G., Nassei, R., Nobili, R., et al. The Italian pain questionnaire. *Pain*, 1985, *33*:53-62.

150. Fishman, B., Pasternak, T., Wallenstein, S.L., et al. The Memorial Pain Assessment Card: A valid instrument for the evaluation of cancer pain. *Cancer*, 1987, *60*:1151-1158.

151. Kerns, R.D., Turk, D.C., & Rudy, T.E. The West Haven Yale Multidimensional Pain Inventory (WHYMPI). *Pain*, 1985, 23(4):345-356.

152. Turk, D. Personal communication, January 1994.

153. Melzack, R. The short-form McGill Pain Questionnaire. *Pain*, 1987, 30:191-197.

154. Dudgeon, D., Raubertas, R.F., & Rosenthal, S.N. The Short-Form McGill Pain Questionnaire in chronic cancer pain. *J Pain Symptom Manag*, 1993, 8:191-195.

155. McGuire, D.B., Altomonte, V., Peterson, D.E., et al. Patterns of mucositis and pain in patients receiving preparative chemotherapy and bone marrow transplantation. *Oncol Nurs Forum*, 1993, 20:1493-1502.

156. Waltz, M., Kriegel, W., & van't Pad Bosch, P. Social environment and health in rheumatoid arthritis: Marital quality predicts individual variability in pain severity. *Arthr Care Res*, 1998, 11:356-374.

157. Fleet, R.P., Dupuis, G., Marchand, A., et al. Panic disorder in emergency department chest pain patients: Prevalence, comorbidity, suicidal ideation, and physician recognition. *Am J Med*, 1996, 101:371-380.

158. David, Y.B., & Musgrave, C.F. Pain assessment: A pilot study in an Israeli bone marrow transplant unit. *Cancer Nurs*, 1996, 19:93-97.

159. McDonald, D.D., McNulty, J., Erickson, K., et al. Communicating pain and pain management needs after surgery. *Appl Nurs Res*, 2000, 13:70-75.

160. Lomi, C., Burckhardt, C., Norodholm, L., et al. Evaluation of a Swedish version of the Arthritis Self-Efficacy Scale in people with fibromyalgia. *Scand J Rheumatol*, 1995, 24:282-287.

161. Bajaj, P., Bajaj, P., Madsen, H., et al. A comparison of modality-specific somatosensory changes during menstruation in dysmenorrheic and nondysmenorrheic women. *Clin J Pain*, 2002, 18:180-190.

162. Mystakidou, A., Parpa, E., Tsilika, E., et al. Greek McGill Pain Questionnaire: Validation and utility in cancer patients. *J Pain Symptom Manage*, 2002, 24:379-387.

163. Kim, H.S., Schwartz-Barcott, D., Holter, I.M., et al. Developing a translation of the McGill Pain Questionnaire for cross-cultural comparison: An example from Norway. *J Adv Nurs*, 1995, 21:421-426.

164. Daut, R.L., Cleeland, C., & Flanery, R.C. Development of the Wisconsin Brief Pain Questionnaire to assess pain in cancer and other diseases. *Pain*, 1983, 17:197-210.

165. Cleeland, C.S. Measurement and prevalence of pain in cancer. *Semin Oncol Nurs*, 1985, 1(2):87-92.

166. Cleeland, C.S., Nakamura, Y., Mendoza, T.R., et al. Dimensions of the impact of cancer pain in a four country sample: New information from multidimensional scaling. *Pain*, 1996, 67:267-273.

167. Wang, X.S., Mendoza, T.R., Gao, S.Z., et al. The Chinese version of the Brief Pain Inventory (BPI-C): Its development and use in a study of cancer pain. *Pain*, 1996, 67:407-416.

168. Saxena, A., Mendoza, T., & Cleeland, C.S. The assessment of cancer pain in north India: The validation of the Hindi Brief Pain Inventory—BPI-H. *J Pain Symptom Manage*, 1999, 17:27-41.

169. Uki, J., Mendoza, T., Cleeland, C.S., et al. A brief cancer pain assessment tool in Japanese: The utility of the Japanese Brief Pain Inventory—BPI-J. *J Pain Symptom Manage*, 1998, 16:364-373.

170. Klepstad, P., Loge, J.H., Borchgrevink, P.C., et al. The Norwegian Brief Pain Inventory Questionnaire: Translation and validation in cancer patients. *J Pain Sympt Manage*, 2002, 24:517-525.

171. Gaston-Johansson, F. Pain assessment: Differences in quality and intensity of the words pain, ache, and hurt. *Pain*, 1984, 20:69-76.

172. Gaston-Johansson, F., & Allwood, J. Pain assessment: Model construction and analysis of words used to describe pain-like experiences. *Semiotica*, 1988, 71(1/2):73-92.

173. Gaston-Johansson, F. Measurement of pain: The psychometric properties of the Pain-O-Meter, a simple, inexpensive pain assessment tool that could change health care practices. *J Pain Symptom Manag*, 1996, 12:172-181.

174. Davis, G.C. Measurement of the chronic pain experience: Development of an instrument. *Res Nurs Health*, 1989, 12:221-227.

175. Davis, G.C. Measuring the clinical outcomes of the patient with chronic pain. In C.F. Waltz & O.L. Strickland (Eds.), *The measurement of nursing outcomes: Measuring client outcomes* (vol. 1). New York: Springer, 1988, pp. 160-184.

176. Davis, G.C. The clinical assessment of chronic pain in rheumatic disease: Evaluating the use of two instruments. *J Adv Nurs*, 1989, 14:397-402.

177. Dalton, J.A., Feuerstein, M., Carlson, J. et al. Biobehavioral Pain profile: Development and psychometric properties. *Pain*, 1994, 57:95-107.

178. Dalton, J.A. Personal communication, March 1994.

179. Thomas, R.J., McEwen, J., & Asbury, A.J. The Glasgow Pain Questionnaire: A new generic measure of pain; development and testing. *Int J Epidemiol*, 1996, 25:1060-1067.

180. Anderson, D.L. Development of an instrument to measure pain in rheumatoid arthritis: Rheumatoid Arthritis Pain Scale (RAPS). *Arthr Care Res*, 2001, 45:317-323.

181. Basilicato, S., Groves, M., Nisbet, L., et al. Effect of concurrent chest pain assessment on retrospective reports by cardiac patients. *J Cardiovasc Nurs*, 1992, 7(1):56-67.

182. Kimble, L.P., Dunbar, S.B., McGuire, D.B., et al. Cardiac instrument development in a low-literacy population: The revised Chest Discomfort Diary. *Heart Lung*, 2001, 30:312-320.

183. Spertus, J.A., Winder, J.A., Dewhurst, T.A., et al. Development and evaluation of the Seattle Angina Questionnaire: A new functional status measure for coronary artery disease. *J Am Coll Cardiol*, 1995, 25:333-341.

184. Dougherty, C.M., Dewhurst, T., Nichol, P., et al. Comparison of three quality of life instruments in stable angina pectoris: Seattle Angina Questionnaire, Short Form Health Survey (SF-36), and Quality of Life Index—Cardiac Version III. *J Clin Epidemiol*, 1998, 51:569-575

185. Spertus, J.A., Jones, P., McDonell, M., et al. Health status predicts long-term outcome in outpatients with coronary disease. *Circulation*, 2002, 106:43-49.

186. Garratt, A.M., Huchinson, A., & Russell, I. The UK version of the Seattle Angina Questionnaire (SAQ-UK): Reliability , validity and responsiveness. *J Clin Epidemiol*, 2001, 54:907-915.

Appendices 38A. Comparison of Scales

Researchers	Scales Compared	Findings
Scott and Huskisson (52)	6 different VAS and GRS to a simple VDS	Horizontal VAS and a horizontal GRS with descriptor words placed along the length of the line produced more uniform distributions, were more sensitive to perceived pain intensity, and were easier for patients to use
Reading (64)	3 scales: PPI scale (MPQ) (37), 10-cm VAS, and a 10-point horizontal numeric scale with anchor words (none, mild, moderately distressing, very distressing, unbearable)	Patient population studies: patients with episiotomy pain Wide variability in the distribution of ratings as well as in agreement between scale differences over time and subjective comparisons Correlations between VAS and VDS were significant ($r = 0.57$–0.71) Conclusion: insufficient psychometric analyses of scales had been performed; efficacy or usefulness of these scales may vary according to patient characteristics and setting
Downie et al. (65)	VAS, VDS compared to one another as well as to a 0–100 NRS	All scales correlated well and had similar loadings on factor analysis Conclusion: scales probably measured the same variable (i.e., pain intensity) 0–100 NRS preferred because it offered more choices than the VDS and was less confusing than the VAS
Kremer et al. (66)	Patient preference for VAS, NRS, or 5-adjective adaptation of PPI (37)	Most patients preferred the 5-adjective scale, and all were able to complete it VAS had an 11% failure rate NRS had a 2% failure rate Conclusion: VDS, such as Melzack's PPI, may be more reliable in certain circumstances
Jensen et al. (67)	6 scales: VAS, 100-point NRS, 11-point box rating scale (BS-11), 6-point BRS, and 4- and 5-point VRS	Patient sample: chronic pain Scales evaluated on (1) ease of administration and scoring; (2) rates of correct responding; (3) relative sensitivity as defined by number of response categories; (4) relative sensitivity as defined by ability to detect treatment effects; and (5) magnitude of relationship between each scale and a "best possible" combined measure of subjective pain intensity All scales similar in (2) correct responses, except for VAS (rate of incorrect responses increased with age) and in predictive validity (5), magnitude of relationship NRS surpassed all others on remaining criteria For current pain, correlation coefficients among the scales ranged from 0.65 to 0.88, ($p < 0.001$, two-tailed tests) Factor analysis: single factor for pain intensity with each scale correlating with the factor at 0.64 or above BRS correlated least, and the BS-11 and NRS the most Conclusion: scales were more similar than different, and were useful measures of pain intensity. NRS had practical advantages (ease of administration, scoring, high rate of correct response)

Appendices 38A. Comparison of Scales (*cont.*)

Researchers	Scales Compared	Findings
Jensen et al. (68)	10 scales and a linear combination of pain measures	Evaluated on (1) magnitude of relationship between them and a linear combination of pain measures and (2) rates of incorrect response in a sample of patients with acute pain 8 scales measured pain intensity (6 from previous study, a VRS-15, and a VRS-11 for pain intensity) 2 scales measured pain affect (again on a 15- and 11-point adjectival scale) Most subjects responded correctly to all scales (VAS 7.2%, NRS 5.8% were problematic) All scales were significantly correlated ($p < 0.001$, two-tailed tests); factor analysis revealed 1 factor, with all scales loading at 0.65 or higher BRS was least related to the construct of pain intensity (patients asked to rate pain in terms of effects rather than subjective intensity) Conclusion: 11-point box rating scale was most useful clinical measure; also noted need to explore pain affect scales further as only 1 factor was extracted rather than the anticipated 2 (intensity and affect)
Machin et al. (69)	VAS and FDS as measure of treatment effects	Focused on statistical methodology used for repeated measures of these scales in a clinical trial VAS and VDS may be measuring slightly different aspects of pain Conclusion: consider using both scales in clinical trials
Banos et al. (70)	VAS and VDS	Small, Spanish study of postoperative general, gynecologic, and orthopedic patients Scores highly correlated ($p < 0.001$) and not influenced by gender, age, surgical procedure, or hospital Patient ratings compared to physician ratings: at lower levels, correlations high; as pain scores increased (pain worsened) physicians rated the pain lower VAS offered a better measure of pain intensity than the VDS because of its sensitivity and lack of verbal descriptors, which might carry different meanings for different individuals
Grossman et al. (45)	Mechanical VAS to standard VAS and VDS	High correlations between Hopkins Pain Rating Instrument and the VAS and VDS in cancer patients with pain ($r = 0.99$ and 0.85, respectively; $p < 0.0001$) M-VAS offered reliable, valid, clinically useful measures of pain intensity; also, portable, easy to score, and free of potential bias from verbal descriptors

| Price et al. (46) | VDS and mechanical VAS (M-VAS) in terms of capacity to produce ratio-level measures of experimental pain | M-VAS provided consistent measures of both experimental and clinical pain intensity, was easy to administer and score
M-VAS offered reliable, valid, clinically useful measures of pain intensity; also portable and free of potential bias from verbal descriptors |
| De Conno et al. (39) | Compared 5 scales before and after pain treatment: VAS, 0–10 NRS, VRS, Italian Pain Questionnaire (PRI/Italian version of the MPQ), and the Integrated Pain Score (IPS) | Unidimensional measures (VAS, NRS, VRS) were more strongly associated with relief of pain than the multidimensional measures, but all were clinically interpretable
Patients' evaluation of pain relief was a more global concept, loosely related to measures of pain intensity
Conclusion: researchers must consider using pain relief scales as well as pain intensity scales when evaluating outcomes of pain treatments |

Abbreviations: VAS, Visual Analogue Scale; M-VAS, Mechanical Visual Analogue Scale; VDS, Verbal Descriptor Scale; NRS, Numerical Rating Scale; VRS, Verbal Rating Scale; BRS, Behavioral Rating Scale; PPI, Present Pain Intensity (from MPQ); MPQ, McGill Pain Questionnaire.

Numbers in parentheses correspond to studies cited in the References.

Appendix 38B. Additional Unidimensional Instruments to Measure the Behavioral Dimension of Acute Pain

Instrument/Study	Important Points	Psychometric Indices
Pain Rating Scale Developed by Hanken et al. (95,96) Modified by Chambers and Price (97)	Developed to measure postoperative pain 6 observable behaviors and physiologic parameters measured: attention to pain, anxiety, verbal statement of degree of pain, skeletal muscle response, characteristics of respiration, amount of perspiration Revised version (97): respiration deleted; added scales for sounds made by patient, nausea, muscle tension, and facial expression Advantages: focuses on anxiety, attention to pain, physiologic parameters; easy to administer and score Disadvantages (99): questionable construct validity; applicable to acute pain only; administration time 5–15 minutes	Construct validity: analyzed 289 nurse observations of 70 patients; correlation matrix of 6 parameters: positive relationships ($r = 0.44$–0.71) between attention, anxiety, stated degree of pain, skeletal muscle response Factor analysis (rotation): first factor was attention directed toward pain and stated degree of pain; both had highest factor loadings (96) Revised instrument (98): reported correlations between total scores and scores for verbal report of degree of pain ($r = 0.66$–0.87); validity reported: pain scores positively correlated with amount of analgesia ($r = 0.38$)
Behavioral Index for the Assessment of Labor Pain Developed by Bonnel and Boureau (100)	Study sample: 100 primiparous women Respiratory modifications, motor responses, and agitation measured Cumulative 5-point scale used (higher numbers indicated more behavioral manifestations of pain)	Validity: ratings made by obstetrician or midwife compared to patient's self-ratings to present pain intensity; global scores (entire labor period) significantly correlated ($r = 0.88$, $p < 0.001$) as were scores from different phases of labor (cervical dilations 3–10 cm, $r = 0.30$–0.50, $p < 0.01$–0.001) Further research warranted (physical parameters of labor progression and use of behavioral ratings as a potential index of self-control behaviors during labor)

Numbers in parentheses correspond to studies cited in the References.

Appendix 38C. Additional Unidimensional Instruments to Measure the Behavioral Dimension of Chronic Pain

Instrument/Study	Important Points	Psychometric Indices
Pain Diaries Fordyce et al. (107) Follick et al. (108)	Initially developed as a diary form for home recording of chronic pain: measures physical act, medications, pain intensity Hourly recording over 24 hours: whether individual is sitting, standing, walking, or reclining; kind and amount of medications used; pain rating (0, no pain, to 10, intolerable) Assesses functional impairment by timed activities, especially relation to consumption of pain, medications, and pain intensity Useful for home recording	Reliability studied chronic pain patients (108) Reliability coefficients for categories of daily-living were positive ($r = 0.44$–0.89) and significant ($p = 0.05$–0.01) Correlations between patient and spouse ratings (standing, walking, lying down, pain intensity, pill counts); also high and significant correlation between patient reports of lying down and electromechanical monitor measurements ($r = 0.94$, $p < 0.01$) Concerns: reliability, recall bias
University of Alabama-Birmingham (UAB) Pain Behavior Scale (109–111)	Objective assessment of 10 pain-related behaviors: verbal vocal complaints; time spent lying down; facial grimaces; standing posture; mobility; body language; use of visible, supportive equipment; stationary movement; medicine Simple, easy-to-use for health personnel or patient	Good interrater reliability ($r = 0.95$, $p < 0.01$) Good test-retest reliability ($r = 0.89$, $p < 0.01$) Validity not adequately tested
Behavioral Dysfunction Index (BDI) Developed by Keefe et al. (112)	Behavioral measure of chronic pain related to head and neck cancer (clinical assessment tool) Evaluates 6 quantitative areas: (1) motor pain behaviors, (2) specific painful activities, (3) general activity level, (4) pain-relieving methods, (5) pain medication intake, (6) weight loss Measures: motor pain behaviors: observers recorded; occurrence/nonoccurrence of 4 specific behaviors (guarded movement, grimacing, rubbing, sighing) while patients sat, stood, walked, reclined, rotated their heads, swallowed, coughed Remaining 5 areas: data collected by structured interview Behavioral Dysfunction Index (BDI) developed as composite measure for each patient (from observations, interview) Scoring: 0 no dysfunction, 1–3 mild to moderate dysfunction, 4–6 extreme dysfunction	BDI scores positively and significantly ($p < 0.05$) related to pain ratings on a 0–10 numeric scale (0, no pain; 10, pain as bad as it can be) Warrants further psychometric evaluation Limitation: time and skill required to administer the questions

Appendix 38C. Additional Unidimensional Instruments to Measure the Behavioral Dimension of Chronic Pain (*cont.*)

Instrument/Study	Important Points	Psychometric Indices
Observational Method for Rheumatoid Arthritis (RA) Pain McDaniel et al., Keefe & Block (113,114)	Method modified from earlier work by Keefe and Block in patients with chronic low back pain (114); 4 studies conducted to determine reliability and validity of behavioral observation method Study 1: assessed interobserver reliability of method and characteristics of patients' pain behaviors $n = 20$ adult patients with rheumatoid arthritis (RA) Patients identified painful joint or body area, and were observed and videotaped for 10 minutes while sitting, walking, standing, and reclining Videotapes scored by 2 trained research assistants (13 separate behaviors with operational definitions) 3 categories of behaviors recorded: (1) position: standing, sitting, reclining; (2) movement: pacing, shifting; (3) pain behavior: guarding, bracing, grimacing, sighing, rigidity, passive rubbing, active rubbing, self-stimulation Study 2: concurrent validity and objectivity of observation method examined $n = 53$ RA patients were observed and videotaped for 10 minutes during same activities as in Study 1; also completed Long form MPQ (LF-MPQ, [37]) 2- to 10-cm VAS (one, immediate pain level; one, unpleasantness of immediate pain level; anchors: "none/not at all <=> unbearable/extremely") Modified Health Assessment Questionnaire (HAQ) Depression Adjective Checklist (DAC) Trained observers viewed videotapes, recorded position, movement, pain behaviors	Observers' percentage agreements for all behaviors (96–100%) Reliability: kappa coefficients on each behavior (0.80–1.0) Guarding and rigidity were significantly associated with patients' reports on affected body sites ($r = 0.55$ and 0.73, respectively; $p < 0.01$) Study 1: guarding and rigidity significantly correlated with one another ($r = 0.55$, $p < 0.01$); patients had similar mean numbers of pain behaviors while moving or stationary Study 2: moderate and significant correlations observed between patients' pain behavior scores and the 2 VASs ($r = 0.26$, pain severity; $r = 0.32$ pain unpleasantness, both $p < 0.01$) Guarding only behavior related to VAS scores Total pain behavior scores significantly related ($r = 0.41$–0.45, $p < 0.001$) to patients' scores on certain MPQ indices: Number of words chosen (NWC), Sensory pain rating index (PRI), Affective PRI, and Total PRI Guarding most consistently related to total pain behavior scores significantly correlated with the HAQ daily function scores ($r = 0.49$, $p < 0.001$) and with DAC depression score ($r = 03.1$, $p < 0.05$) Patients' self-reports of depression correlated with the NWC and Affective and Total PRI scores (LF-MPQ)

Study 3: examined construct validity of behavioral observation method

11 psychology students reviewed 25 videotapes of RA patients engaged in described activities and made global estimates of severity or unpleasantness of patients' pain on 5 measures in counterbalanced order: 11-point categorical scale (0 no pain at all, 10 extreme pain)
10-cm VAS with anchors (no pain at all, unbearable pain)
11-point categorical scale (0 not at all unpleasant, 10 extremely unpleasant)
10-cm VAS with anchors (no unpleasantness at all, extreme unpleasantness)
Verbal descriptor scale: 15 sensory intensity (SI) items, 1 descriptor of no pain
Trained observer scored the 25 videotapes (as in study 1), blinded to students' ratings

Study 4: tested utility of the behavioral observation method as an indicator of treatment outcome

$n = 11$ patients with RA; observed for 10 minutes before, and after a cognitive–behavioral treatment program
Completed the MPQ-LF and 2 10-cm VASs (pain severity and unpleasantness) prior to and after the intervention
Conclusion: this behavioral observation method yielded useful, objective data about RA pain
Limitation: unknown effects of the presence of observers and videotaping on patients (patients reactivity)
Further research needed, particularly in other populations of patients with pain

Study 3: student ratings positively and significantly correlated ($r = 0.54$–0.57, $p < 0.01$) with patients' total behavior scores
Guarding and rigidity most highly associated

Study 4: significant decreases in total pain behavior scores and the specific behavior of passive rubbing found pre- and post-treatment ($t = 2.31$, 2.23, respectively, $p < 0.05$)
Significant decreases found in overall number of behaviors across different times of assessment; patients' self-reports of pain also decreased
Conclusion: Study 1: reliability supported; Study 2: concurrent validity supported, functional disability scores on HAQ related to total pain behavior scores; Study 3: construct validity supported; Study 4: further evidence of construct validity through responses pre- and postintervention

Numbers in parentheses correspond to studies cited in the References.

641

Appendix 38D. Additional Multidimensional Instruments to Measure Pain

Instrument/Study	Important Points	Psychometric Indices
Two-component scale Developed by Johnson (120,121) Used by Wells (122)	Separate scales for measurement of sensory and reactive (affective) components Subjects experiencing experimentally induced pain rated physical sensation on a 0–100 scale in terms of distress (slightly to moderately, very to just bearable): high pain intensity not always accompanied by high distress simple to use	Psychometric properties not described Requires further testing
Tursky's Pain Perception Profile (PPP) Developed by Tursky (123) Used by Andrasik et al. (124) and Urban et al. (125)	Goals to enable patients to scale pain by magnitude estimation (in equal-interval stimuli as compared to a standard pain statement) 3 sets of adjectives to measure intensity, sensory, and reactive (affective) components: (1) intensity list = 15 words (e.g., excruciating); (2) sensory list = 13 words (e.g., piercing); (3) reactive list = 11 words (e.g., agonizing) Subjects select 1 word from each list Advantages over VAS: fewer constraints on responses, enables investigator to test validity of responses with known reliable relationships	Tested with 56 college undergrads without clinical pain Intensity scale appears reliable (125)
Long Form McGill Pain Questionnaire (LF-MPQ) Developed by Melzack and Torgerson (37,126) in 1975 Analysis using new scoring method (conversion of rank values to weighted-rank values) (127)	Dimensions measured by scaled portion of LF-MPQ: sensory (location, pattern, intensity); affective; cognitive (evaluative); miscellaneous Other dimensions addressed in other items: behavioral; sociocultural; diagnosis; drug intake; pain and medical history; personal history; factors increasing or decreasing pain; effects on sleep, sexual activity, and work; least and worst pain Abbreviated version: (1) 4 parts: drawing of human body on which location(s) of pain documented; (2) 20 words or descriptors (2–6 words each) to measure sensory, affective, cognitive, and miscellaneous; (3) pattern of pain (brief, transient, intermittent, continuous); (4) present pain intensity (PPI) on scale from 0 (no pain) to 5 (excruciating pain) Scoring provides 3 pain indices: (1) Total Pain Rating Index (PRI-T): sum of rank value of words chosen from list: first word of list implies least pain (= 1); 20 lists are subdivided into 4 groups, each yielding subindex of pain (lists 1–10 PRI-sensory, 11–15 PRI-affective, 16 PRI-	Repeated reliability and consistency demonstrated across many subject groups, including cancer patients (128,129), experimentally induced pain (130), other medical, surgical diagnoses (37) Construct validity demonstrated for 3 major dimensions (sensory, affective, evaluative) in factor analytic studies of patients with low back pain (131,132), dysmenorrhea (132), chronic benign pain (133), and arthritis (134,135) Concurrent and predictive validity established in patients with dental pain (136), experimental pain (137), dysmenorrhea, headache (138), others (137,139) MPQ discriminates among groups of patients (acute and chronic pain [140]; different types of toothache pain [141], pain syndromes [142]) Reading et al. (143) attempted to replicate construction of MPQ word lists using multidimensional scaling and cluster analysis and provided evidence for reducing number of lists to 16 Turk et al. (144) confirmed 3 dimensions, but found them highly intercorrelated and without discriminant validity Metaanalysis performed (145)

642

	evaluative, 17–20 PRI-miscellaneous); technique available (145) to convert weighted-rank values to avoid loss of information about relative sensitivity of words chosen (2) Number of words chosen (NWC) from the 20 lists (not commonly analyzed) (3) Present Pain Intensity (PPI) or number + word combination selected from the 0 to 5 scale PRI and PPI data can be statistically analyzed Melzack considered MPQ a "rough instrument" Translated into Dutch (146), German (147), Italian (148) Italian investigators (149) developed culturally sensitive MPQ using same factor structure (3): 42 pain descriptors; 16 subclasses; quantitative data Caution in interpreting studies using MPQ (145) 5 versions, some researchers don't indicate which version used Derivation and examination of estimated normative mean scores of MPQ indices in 3624 subjects: scores no more than 50% of maximum possible score (? skewness to left); only 19 of 78 word descriptors selected by > 20% of all subjects Higher affective scores appeared related to chronic painful conditions (e.g., cancer, low back pain) Disadvantages: long and complex; can require intense concentration; takes up to 30 minutes to complete; some word descriptors may be hard to understand; scoring takes several minutes	Reliable, valid tool that can be used in a large variety of patient groups with different pain Useful in descriptive studies, evaluation of intervention outcomes, clarification of differences and similarities among pain types Wilkie (145) recommends to researchers using MPQ: (1) interpret their data in light of estimated normative scores (approach population mean); (2) report a common set of descriptive data (age, gender, ethnicity); (3) indicate version of MPQ used; (4) report percentage of sample using specific words and look at trends by painful condition
Memorial Pain Assessment Card (MPAC) Developed by Fishman et al. (150)	Measure of cancer pain and pain relief 8.5- × 11-inch card containing a VAS measuring pain relief, pain intensity, mood, and an adaptation of Tursky's pain adjective rating scale: example, Mood Scale (worst to best mood) Card folded in middle so that 4 sides can be presented separately and quickly to patients VAS Mood Scale is a compound measure of general psychologic distress MPAC is short, simple, easy to administer and score and may be used for a variety of clinical research purposes	In a study of 50 hospitalized cancer patients strong correlation found between the VAS pain and adjective rating scales and the MPQ ($r = 0.36$–0.45, $p = 0.005$–0.001) VAS pain relief scale appeared related to VAS mood scale ($r = 0.57$, $p < 0.001$) VAS mood scale correlated at varying degrees of significance with several subscales and total score from Profile of Mood States ($r = 0.31$–0.47, $p = 0.02$–0.001) as well as with the Hamilton Depression Scale ($r = -0.41$, $p = 0.005$) and Zung Depression Scale ($r = 0.44$, $p = 0.001$) Further studies of MPAC reliability and validity needed to substantiate use in cancer and other types of pain

Appendix 38D. Additional Multidimensional Instruments to Measure Pain (*cont.*)

Instrument/Study	Important Points	Psychometric Indices
West Haven-Yale Multidimensional Pain Inventory (WHYMPI) (151)	Based on cognitive/behavioral theory and developed specifically for patients with chronic pain (151) 52-item inventory divided into 3 parts: (1) perceived pain intensity and impact on various aspects of life; (2) perceptions of others' responses to pain and suffering; (3) involvement in common daily activities Patients record responses on 6-point and 7-point scales in each part (e.g., Part II: frequency with which others respond to patient's display of pain and suffering with a particular behavior [0 never to 6 very frequently]) Administration time is 15–30 minutes	Reliability and stability: coefficient alphas (internal consistency): 0.70–0.90 Pearson's product–moment correlations for test–retest reliability 0.62–0.92 Factor analysis: confirmed utility of scales within each part of the WHYMPI Factor analysis: documented construct validity Appears that WHYMPI is a reliable and valid tool for assessment of pain-related problems in a chronic pain population Cross-validation needed in other patient populations (initial sample, male veterans of U.S. Armed Services) Additional psychometric and utility data available (152)

Numbers in parentheses correspond to studies cited in the References.

39

Measuring Skin Integrity

Barbara J. Braden and Rita A. Frantz

The term *skin integrity* refers to the wholeness or intactness of the skin. For the clinical researcher, measurement issues related to skin integrity primarily revolve around etiologic factors in pressure sore development and healing of chronic and acute wounds.

Many instruments are available to the clinical researcher concerning skin integrity. Selecting one or more instruments will depend on the purpose of the inquiry. The common purposes of inquiry in this area are to identify patients at risk for skin breakdown and to determine the effectiveness of clinical modalities for preventing pressure sores and the effectiveness of treatment modalities to heal pressure sores and other wounds. Instruments available for these purposes can be divided into four categories: (1) measures of pressure and clinical determinants of pressure; (2) measures of clinical determinants of tissue tolerance for pressure; (3) measures of risk for developing pressure sores; and (4) measures of stage, size, and status of pressure sores, chronic wounds, or surgical wounds. Many instruments are discussed comprehensively, and additional measures of these categories are presented in Appendices 39A and 39B.

It is important to note that many factors contribute to the development and healing of pressure sores, and some probably remain to be discovered or adequately delineated. Certainly, many of these factors interact in ways that are not fully understood. Although it is expedient and wise to use the instruments currently available, the clinical researcher should be alert to other potentially relevant data. Furthermore, anecdotal data on a per-case basis may be enlightening. Clinicians providing direct care are important sources of this type of information, and their intuitive judgments about why pressure sores develop or heal in one patient and not in others should be solicited and evaluated.

Measurement Tools

Intensity and Duration of Pressure

Instruments measuring the intensity and duration of pressure usually measure pressure at the interface between a support surface (mattress, wheelchair pad) and a body surface. Such instruments may be used in various areas of inquiry, such as investigations into the effect of positioning on specific bony prominences, the effectiveness of therapeutic mattresses or wheelchair pads in reducing interface pressure, or comparison of the effects of differing or identical interface pressures on varying patient populations.

Continuous Pressure Monitor

Some studies have used relatively simple devices to measure pressure. The simplest of these, a Continuous Pressure Monitor, was used to study skin pressure measurements in cancer patients on various mattress surfaces.[1] This device has three components: (1) a pressure-sensing inflatable bladder with a 2-square-inch surface area, (2) a pump that inflates the bladder in response to internal pressures, and (3) a mercury manometer to measure the bladder pressure. The bladder is placed between the patient and the mattress at a bony prominence. The internal walls of the inflatable bladder have electrically conductive strips that are connected to the pump. When the bladder is flat, the conductive strips make contact and activate the pump. The pump inflates the bladder until the conductive strips separate. The separation occurs at a pressure that is equal to or slightly greater than the surface pressure between the patient and the mattress; this pressure is reflected on the mercury manometer. When the conductive strips separate, the pump is switched off and the bladder deflates until contact is reestablished. One group of researchers report the accuracy of this device to be ± 2 mm Hg at a pressure of 50 mm Hg mercury and below and ± 4 mm Hg from 50 to 80 mm Hg.[1] Instrument reliability is a problem, however, given that the bladder measures pressure over a very small area and the point of maximal pressure is not easily established. Positioning of the bladder and positioning of the patient (or subject) must be precisely the same if one is to obtain reliable comparisons. It is very difficult to achieve the degree of precision required to obtain reliable results with this instrument.

Purdue Pad

The Purdue Pad is the largest and most complex of the interface pressure instruments.[2] It is a full-body pressure mat that can sense pressure and subsequent changes in pressure every 5 seconds. The pressure mat is composed of two orthogonal arrays of silver-coated ribbonlike conductors, separated by open-cell natural latex foam for insulation. The points at which the horizontal and vertical conductors cross form 1536 pressure-sensitive nodes, each representing an area of 4 cm^2, arranged in a grid of 24 by 64. The system includes the electronically fitted pressure mat, a computer to process data, and a color video that displays the results as a false color map. This allows the researcher to view all areas of interface simultaneously and over time. The color map image can be frozen and copied to disk for further analysis. Repeated measurements may be obtained with a precision of 2 to 3 mm Hg. Calibration procedures can be accomplished in 30 minutes and will last for several days or until the ambient relative humidity changes. Because capacitance increases approximately 4% for every 1% change in relative humidity, the investigators are considering adding a moisture barrier, but they currently recommend use in a humidity-controlled environment. The Purdue Pad was developed under a contract from Hill-Rom Company, Batesville, IN, where it has been used to measure the effectiveness of support surfaces in reducing interface pressure and the variability that occurs in patients who differ by age, height, weight, and physical condition. It is not currently available for general use, but investigators whose research goals are congruent with those of Hill-Rom may be allowed to use this instrument under certain circumstances.

Computerized Insole Sensor System

An insole was developed by Randolph et al[3] that has an embedded computerized sensor system to measure pressure applied to the foot during walking. The insole consists of pressure-sensitive, resistive, and conductive silver-based cells that are embedded in a Mylar protective coating. These cells can be electronically scanned every 50–100 milliseconds to detect changes in pressure applied to the sole of the foot during the process of walking. Investigators used 10 healthy subjects to test mean peak pressures for each pair of four insoles. Intrasubject mean differences at the hindfoot, midfoot, and forefoot were calculated and tested. No statistical differences were found, suggesting that the insole sensor system has adequate reliability to compare data between and among subjects. This insole is manufactured by Tekscan, Inc., 307 West First Street, Boston, MA 02127.

Activity and Mobility

Measurement of activity and/or mobility commonly is associated with functional assessment or risk assessment tools. These tools, covered elsewhere in this book, are valuable in a number of different situations. It is important to remember, however, that the level of measurement provided by these tools is ordinal. The following instruments provide continuous data on activity/mobility and, as such, are more appropriate in certain research situations.[4]

Wheelchair Activity/Mobility

The Time-Logger Communicator (TLC) was developed by Merbitz et al.[5] to measure the number of times a patient lifts his or her body from a seated position for a period of time sufficient to relieve pressure. To prevent pressure sores, spinal cord-injured patients are taught to perform this maneuver every 15 to 20 minutes. This is referred to as *lift-off* behavior, and the TLC is a pocket-sized, battery-operated computer that is capable of continuously recording this behavior for up to 36 hours. The computer is equipped with a sensor apparatus that consists of a large, airtight vinyl bladder connected by tubing to a smaller vinyl bag. The smaller bag is inside an $8 \times 13 \times 26$-mm box that is mounted on the frame of the wheelchair alongside the computer and a lever. The larger air-filled bladder is placed between the seat cushion and the wheelchair's sling seat, and the system is designed so that a weight greater than 20 kg over the seat cushion forces air into the smaller bladder. This in turn moves the lever, which depresses a key that enters the event and the time of occurrence into the computer. When the weight over the seat cushion is reduced to 14 kg, a spring returns the lever, and this event as well as the time and duration of the occurrence are entered into the computer. Reliability and validity data are not reported for the TLC, but further information is available from the investigator.

Bed Mobility

Schnelle et al.[6] developed an instrument for monitoring gross body movement of bedridden patients that consists of strips of Kynar brand piezoelectric plastic film. These strips are the thickness and width of electrician's tape and are placed under the bed sheets across the full width of the bed. The strips are positioned at the level of the subject's hips and shoulders and attached to two channels connected to a bedside monitor. Movement creates electrical signals transmitted to the bedside monitor and digitized from each channel more than 100 times per second. The monitor then subtracts the lowest reading from the highest reading every 2 minutes, recording the peak activity for that 2-minute period. Large body moves are considered to have taken place when large moves of the hip and the shoulder are recorded in the same 2-minute interval.

Because the instrument is sufficiently sensitive to record movement from respirations and movement from extremities, investigators tested it against direct observation, using two observers. The interrater reliability (percent agreement) between these two observers for identifying large body movements (at least 45 degrees movement of body off the bed surface) was 92%. Behavioral observations (large movement, yes/no) were compared with the 424 instrument readings (large movement, other movement), and sensitivity and specificity were calculated to establish the validity (decisional accuracy) of the readings. The sensitivity for hip and shoulder movements was 83% and 84%, respectively, and the specificity was 93% and 92%. For both the hip and the shoulder, the total percent correctly classified was 92%. These investigators also used technology to detect light and sound in conjunction with body movement data, so that caregiver-initiated body turns could be distinguished from patient-initiated turns.

Sensory Perception

The intensity and duration of pressure that patients tolerate is related to their ability to perceive pain and other noxious stimuli and to respond to remove the noxious stimulus. Instruments in this section help both the clinician and the researcher develop semiobjective data related to sensory perception as it relates to the cutaneous sensation. Such instruments have been used in studies of peripheral neuropathies and might be helpful in studies of the interaction between peripheral neuropathies and other factors implicated in the etiology of chronic wounds.

Three-Point Esthesiometer

The three-point esthesiometer is a millimeter ruler with a slide placed on it. The zero end of the ruler has two spikes, one of which is placed at the end of the ruler in an axial direction that is used to apply a one-point stimulus. The second spike is placed perpendicular to the ruler below the zero line and, in conjunction with a third spike attached to a movable slide, is used to apply a two-point stimulus. Measurement of two-point discrimination is determined by applying the spikes in two trials to either one or two stimulus points and asking the subject whether two stimulus points were applied in the first or second trial. If the subject answers correctly, the distance between the two points is diminished by 1 mm and reapplied in successive trials until the subject cannot discriminate. The threshold is the smallest measurement distance between the two spikes at which the person can discriminate.

Researchers should keep in mind that inter- and intrainvestigator differences in pressure applied can influence the reliability and validity of the findings. One group of investigators found a high degree of consistency in the evaluation of five serial tests over 22 sites but did not specify whether these measures were obtained by one person or different people.[7] They also found that the threshold for two-point discrimination increased with age but did not differ between men and women. Reviewing the paper by Werner and Omer[8] will help potential investigators to standardize procedures and temper interpretations. See Appendix 39A for additional instruments.[7,9]

Clinical Determinants of Tissue Tolerance

Tissue tolerance refers to the ability of the skin and supporting structures to withstand the effects of pressure without adverse sequelae. The amount and duration of pressure required to damage the skin can be mediated by intrinsic and extrinsic factors that alter the ability of the tissues to tolerate pressure. The instruments covered in this section measure either the effects of varying tissue tolerance or the mediating intrinsic or extrinsic factors. See Appendix 39A for additional instruments.[10–14]

Hard Instrumented Seat to Measure Shear and Pulsatile Blood Flow

The Hard Instrumented Seat measures shear and pulsatile blood flow as well as pressure. This device consists of a hard, clear plastic seat containing flush-mounted sensors capable of monitoring all three variables. The pressure and shear sensors consist of a combination of cantilever beams and strain gauges. These sensors straddle the blood flow device at a known lateral separation that allows both average pressure and the pressure gradient over the blood flow device to be determined. The blood flow device is a photoplethysmograph, which has the disadvantage of lacking an absolute calibration procedure and limits usage to intercomparison data. It has been used to determine differences in pressure, shear, and pulsatile blood flow among paraplegic, geriatric, and normal subjects in a sitting position.[15] This device has limited applications in clinical research because it cannot be used inside soft, pressure-relief mattresses or cushions and is prone to certain types of quantification errors. Nevertheless, it has several unique qualities for researchers with special interest in this area.

Compound Sensor for Biomechanical Analyses of Buttock Soft Tissue in Vivo

A compound sensor was developed for use in an enhanced Computer Automated Seating System (CASS) to enable researchers to measure pressure, force, tissue layer thickness, and orientation of the CASS sensor head.[16] The sensor is on a swiveling head with a pressure transducer in the center, surrounded by four ultrasonic transducers. This instrumentation can be used to examine differences in intrinsic soft tissue mechanical characteristics (tissue tolerance) under conditions of pressure and to determine which responses to pressure are most predictive of pressure ulcer development.

Magnetic Resonance Imaging and Computed Tomography Scanning

Research on the effects of external forces on soft tissue have previously been limited because of an inability to adequately visualize the deformation of these internal structures. The emergence of magnetic resonance imaging (MRI) and computer-augmented x-rays has expanded the potential to analyze the anatomic changes caused by external forces imposed on bony prominences. Although the equipment needed for these measurements is expensive and often not easily accessible for clinical research, efforts to incorporate these methods in such studies could produce profound insights regarding the dynamics of pressure-induced soft-tissue injury. MRI provides a noninvasive method of measuring tissue shapes in vivo. The technique employs magnetic energy sources to create cross-sectional images of the human anatomy without using radiation. Atomic nuclei, contained in a magnetic field created by the magnetic resonance machine and stimulated by specific radio frequencies, emit measurable radio signals that are influenced by the type and condition of tissue composed of these nuclei. The radio signals are captured and converted to a visual display on a computer monitor. By monitoring the response of atomic nuclei in magnetic fields, longitudinal and transverse views of internal tissue structures from the skin surface to underlying bony prominences can be reconstructed.[17] Reger, McGovern, and Chung[18] describe the results of using MRI to measure soft-tissue deformation in five subjects (2 normal, 3 paraplegic) seated on various support surfaces. They found distinct anatomic differences in soft tissues underlying bony prominences between the paraplegic subjects and controls. This preliminary work suggests that the measurement capability of MRI in assessing soft-tissue deformations makes it an instrument well suited to evaluating the effects of pressure on soft tissue.

Computed tomography (CT) scanning has recently been applied to in vivo study of the effects of shearing forces on soft tissue underlying bony prominences. CT scanning uses x-rays augmented with a scanning system and computer to measure the attenuation of tissue. Conner and Clack[19] employed CT scanning to evaluate the soft tissue–skeletal relationship at the ischial tuberosity in three healthy subjects lying on various support surfaces. Using measurements derived from the pelvic CT scans, the investigators were able to calculate shear stress and shear strain. This study provides a model for future efforts to quantify the effects of external forces on the anatomic configuration of human tissue.

Skin Hydration

Recent advances in technology have enhanced the precision with which skin hydration can be measured noninvasively. Among the devices most applicable to clinical nursing research are the hydrometer (Skicon-100™), the electrical capacitance monitor (Corneometer CM 420), and the evaporimeter (Servo Med EPI™). The hydrometer measures the hydration of the stratum corneum via electrical conductance.[20] It consists of a main recorder and a probe with two concentrically arranged brass electrodes. The probe is applied to the skin, allowing high-frequency current to flow between the two electrodes. The conductance is registered and displayed digitally, expressed as reciprocal impedance in measures of 1 micro ohm. The electrical capacitance monitor is equipped with a probe containing a circular brass grid covered with plastic foil (Schwarzhaupt GmbH, Cologne, West Germany). The skin surface below this electrode acts as the other electrode. The probe is applied to the skin, and the capacitance is expressed digitally in arbitrary units. The evaporimeter measures water evaporation for the skin surface.[21] The probe consists of a cylindrical chamber mounted with sensors for measurement of relative humidity and temperature. The transepidermal water loss (TEWL) is calculated automatically and digitally displayed in terms of $g/m^2/hour$. Blichmann and Serup[21] compared the three methods of measuring skin hydration on 10 healthy subjects using test sites on the forearm and palm of the hand. They found that the hydrometer was more sensitive in measuring increased hydration but the electrical capacitance monitor was more highly sensitized to decreased hydration. There were no significant inter- and intraindividual variations. Reproducibility testing revealed that the electrical capacitance monitor was more accurate than the hydrometer. The investigators concluded that both the hydrometer and the electrical capacitance monitor provided valid assessments of skin hydration.

Risk for Skin Breakdown

Several instruments designed to predict the risk of skin breakdown have been reported.[22,23] These instruments use summative rating scales based on observations of factors contributing to skin breakdown and specify critical scores for identifying patients at risk. Because the panel of experts convened by the Agency for Healthcare Research and Quality[24] found that only the Norton Scale and the Braden Scale had sufficient evidence of reliability and validity to warrant clinical use, discussion is limited to these instruments.

Researchers or clinicians considering the use of these instruments should be reminded that they are designed to measure risk for skin breakdown rather than to predict with absolute accuracy the occurrence of skin breakdown. It also is important to note that these instruments were tested using almost exclusively hospitalized and institutionalized elderly subjects. It would, therefore, be unwise to expect predictive values to be similar to those previously reported when these instruments are used to study younger populations.

Norton Scale

The Norton Scale has been studied extensively. This tool consists of five parameters: physical condition, mental state, activity, mobility, and incontinence, each of which is rated from 1 to 4, with one- or two-word descriptors for each rating. The sum of the ratings for all five parameters yields a score that can range from 5 to 20, with lower scores indicating increased risk. From data collected among elderly patients, Norton et al. concluded that a score of 14 indicated the "onset of risk" and a score of 12 or below indicated high risk for pressure sore formation.[22]

The Norton Scale was used by Roberts and Goldstone[25] in a study of 59 pressure sore–free patients over age 60 admitted to an orthopedic ward. Thirty-two patients received scores below 14, and 12 of these at-risk patients developed pressure sores deeper than stage I. Using 14 as a cutoff score, the following values can be calculated from these data: sensitivity of 92%, specificity of 57%, a predictive value of a positive test of 37.5%, and a predictive value of a negative test of 96%. These investigators trained a team of nurses to rate the patients, but they do not report data regarding interrater reliability.

In a later study Goldstone and Goldstone[26] used only one rater in an apparent attempt to control the reliability of the scores. Among patients over age 60 admitted to an orthopedic ward, 30 of 40 were judged to be at risk, and 16 of these at-risk patients developed pressure lesions. This resulted in a sensitivity of 89%, a specificity of 36%, a predictive value of a positive test of 53%, and a predictive value of a negative test of 80%. Goldstone and Goldstone do not define pressure lesions, but they likely classified skin erythema as a pressure lesion, which may account for the improvement in the predictive values.

Lincoln and her associates[27] also conducted an evaluation of the Norton Scale and reported very poor (0%) sensitivity and predictive value of a positive test. The sample size was so small, however, that these results should be considered with caution. Lincoln also tested for interrater reliability, using data from 73 patients who were rated on four separate occasions by two registered nurse investigators. They reported a low percent agreement among RN raters (39.7%). There also was disagreement among experts concerning face validity. The exact nature of these concerns was not reported, but another panel of experts convened by the Agency for Health Care Policy and Research found this scale to have enough validity and reliability to recommend it for clinical use.[24]

Braden Scale

The Braden Scale was developed in 1983 to predict the risk for pressure sore development.[23] The Braden Scale is composed of six subscales that conceptually reflect degrees of sensory perception, skin moisture, physical activity, nutritional intake, friction and shear, and ability to change and control body position. All subscales are rated from 1 to 4, with the exception of the friction and shear subscale, which is rated from 1 to 3. Each rating is accompanied by a brief description of criteria for assigning the rating to facilitate consistency in rating. Potential scores range from 4 to 23, and lower scores indicate higher risk.

This instrument has undergone extensive testing. Content validity has been established by expert opinion. Two studies of reliability have been carried out in two extended care facilities.[23] The purpose of the first study was to estimate interrater reliability between a graduate student research assistant and registered nurses trained in the use of the tool. The Pearson's product–moment correlation among 84 pairs of observation scores was $r = 0.99$ ($p < 0.001$) and the percent agreement was 88%. In no case did the total score assigned by the two raters differ by more than 1 point. The purpose of the second study was to determine the reliability of the scale when used by licensed practical nurses and nurse aides who were not trained in the use of the tool. Pearson's product–moment correlations among 53 pairs of scores ranged from $r = 0.83$ to 0.87 ($p < 0.001$), but percent agreement ranged from 11% for those on the day shift to 19% for those on the evening shift.

Studies of predictive validity have been conducted using patient populations admitted to a general nursing unit, a critical care stepdown unit, and an adult intensive care unit, all in tertiary care settings. In the two studies conducted outside the intensive care unit ($n = 99, n = 100$)[23], the tool demonstrated 100% sensitivity and predictive value of a negative test in both groups and 90% and 64% specificity, respectively, at a cutoff score of 16. However, the predictive value of a positive test diminished to 50% and 19%, respectively, in these two studies.

In the study of predictive validity among 60 subjects admitted to an adult intensive care unit,[28] a critical cutoff score of 16 or below demonstrated a sensitivity of 83%, a specificity of 64%, a predictive value of positive a test of 61%, and a predictive value of a negative test of 85%. Preliminary results of a related study of subjects admitted to a skilled nursing facility indicate that a score of 18 produced a sensitivity of 79%, a specificity of 74%, a 54% predictive value of a positive test, 90% predictive value of a negative test, and 75% correct classification rate.[29]

The differences in predictive validity when using the tool in different settings probably occur as a result of variances in age and severity of illness among subjects, as well as variance in caregiver-to-patient ratios in all three settings. For example, in areas that have low caregiver-to-patient ratios, patients who are identified as at risk may receive more attention to preventive strategies and thus some pressure sores may be prevented, which could result in lower levels of specificity. This may have been occurring in the step-down and intensive care units as the primary nurses participated in rating the patients.

Other investigators have tested the Braden Scale with various degrees of rigor and differing results. Salvadalena, Snyder, and Brogdon[30] reported significantly lower indices of predictive validity, but the method for identifying stage I ulcers may have led to the discrepancy with previous results.[31] Hergenroeder, Mosher, and Sevo[32] found that nurses' judgment was as reliable in predicting pressure sore risk (yes/no answer) as the Braden Scale. The wide difference in mean Braden Scale score between patients at risk (14.45) and patients not at risk (20.24) leaves open the question of whether nurses would be able to discriminate among patients who were more homogeneous in relation to risk or differed less in degree of risk. Xakellis et al.[33] found that the nurses base their judgment of risk on patients' diminished mobility and increased exposure to friction and shear. Although diminished mobility and increased friction and shear may identify those most obviously at risk, other factors measured in both the Norton Scale and the Braden Scale have been found to improve prediction.[34,34]

Xakellis et al.[33] also compared the Norton Scale and the Braden Scale to determine whether these tools would predict the same patients to be at risk. The Cohen's kappa for agreement between the two tools was 73. The Norton Scale identified 38% of the patients as being at risk, and the Braden Scale predicted 27% of the patients to be at risk. Because this study was cross-sectional rather than prospective, one cannot draw conclusions about which tool was more accurate. It could be said, however, that the Braden Scale was more conservative than the Norton in identifying patients at risk.

Pressure Sore Status
Staging

Many staging systems have been proposed, but one four-stage classification has achieved the highest degree of consensus among professionals:

Stage I. Nonblanchable erythema of intact skin, that heralds lesion of skin ulceration.

Stage II. Partial thickness skin loss involving epidermis and/or dermis. The ulcer is superficial and presents clinically as an abrasion, blister, or shallow crater.

Stage III. Full-thickness skin loss involving damage or necrosis of subcutaneous tissue that may extend down to, but not through, underlying fascia. The ulcer presents clinically as a deep crater with or without undermining of adjacent tissue.

Stage IV. Full-thickness skin loss with extensive destruction, tissue necrosis, or damage to muscle, bone or supporting structures (for example, tendon or joint capsule).

The clinical researcher should know that wound staging cannot be confirmed when the wound is covered with eschar or full of necrotic tissue. This staging system provides only a gross assessment of the severity of a pressure sore. It is sufficient for studies of the epidemiology of pressure sores, but it is too global to be of use for wound healing studies. Tools that are somewhat more helpful in describing the severity of pressure sores are presented in Appendix 39B.[36,37,38,39]

Tissue Reflective Spectroscopy (TRS)

TRS is a noninvasive instrument to quantify skin color and may also be used to detect erythema in darkly pigmented skin.[40] The instrument works by beaming a white light at the skin and measuring the light returned. The light passes through the epidermis and is reflected back by collagen in the lower dermis. The output is affected by hemoglobin, oxyhemoglobin, and melanin, and accurate results depend on the means used to correct the signal for melanin and a sensitive erythema-detection algorithm. The investigators describe and test six methods for making these adjustments and compare sensitivity and specificity from tests on 20 subjects.

Pressure Sore Surface Area

Meticulous and accurate measurement of pressure sore surface area is probably most important in studies related to the effectiveness of therapeutic modalities in enhancing healing. Several methods are reported in the literature, some requiring more sophisticated equipment than others.

Acetate Tracings

Three common methods of using acetate tracings to determine pressure sore surface area have been described by Bohannon and Pfaller.[41] The materials for tracing are sterilized transparency film and a fine-tip transparency marker. To obtain the tracing, the investigator places the sterilized transparency film over the sore and traces the perimeter with the transparency marker. The tracing then is cut from the transparency film and quantified by one of three methods. The first method used by Bohannon and Pfaller involved placing the tracing over metric graph paper and counting the square millimeters within the perimeter; the second method consisted of weighing the tracing on a gram balance scale; and the third method required the edges of the tracing to be retraced with an electronic planimeter.

To determine the accuracy of each method in their study, Bohannon and Pfaller used multiple tracings of the same sore obtained by two different clinicians, resulting in 10 pairs of tracings. Mean differences in the area mass identified by each of the three methods were then calculated in the 10 pairs. The mean difference with the weighing technique was 4.4%, 3.9% with the counting technique, and 3.6% with the planimetry. According to these investigators, the greatest percentage differences were found in the tracings of small wounds, but the differences were of no greater magnitude than the difference between larger tracings. They reported that the greatest difference found in the calculated areas of tracings of the same wound by two different clinicians was 8.8%, or 0.81 cm^2.

Thomas and Wysocki[42] compared acetate tracing to methods involving photography and the Kundin Wound Gauge, a measurement device involving length and width rulers placed at right angles to each other with a recommended formula for calculating surface area.[43] Both the photographs and the acetate tracings were digitally analyzed by an image analysis system (Zeiss Interactive Digital Analysis System). These investigators found that the results of all three methods were strongly correlated, but the acetate tracing reportedly resulted in the most accurate measure of surface area. No information was given on the image analysis system regarding standard error for readings.

Photography

Photography has been used for clinical documentation of wounds and wound progress, but quantification problems can occur that may be unacceptable in measurement of certain outcomes. Many variables must be optimized and held constant, including distance from the wound, lighting for the photograph, the type of lens, the f-stop of the lens aperture, and the type of film.

Thomas and Wysocki[42] used a 35-mm camera (Nikon, FE2) equipped with a 120-mm medical lens (Nikkor) with built-in ring flash and reproduction ratio imprinting feature. They used color slide film (EKtachrome, ASA 100) and calculated wound area from the slide film image by placing the image on a digitizing table and using a stylus to trace the wound margins. They found a strong correlation ($r = 0.99$, $p = < 0.0001$) between measurements obtained by the photography and acetate tracings. A significant difference between surface areas obtained by these methods was found using a repeated-measures analysis of variance, however, and these investigators concluded that acetate tracings were more accurate.

Pressure Sore Volume

Measures of surface area of pressure sores have become more sophisticated but, as two-dimensional measures, they are not sensitive to progression or regression of deeper wounds. Three-dimensional measures are necessary to accurately estimate greater wound volume and changes in deeper wounds. These measures are useful in testing the effectiveness of various treatments (e.g., topical applications, pressure-reducing or pressure-relieving surfaces) in promoting wound healing (Appendix 39B).[43-47]

Status of Surgical Wounds

Measuring wound status in closed surgical wounds requires tools that are different from those used to describe pressure sores or other open, chronic wounds. Siddall[48] outlines nine criteria for external assessment of the surgical wound as follows: (1) apposition, (2) capillary fill, (3) temperature, (4) healing ridge, (5) scab, (6) drainage, (7) discoloration, (8) swelling, and (9) pain. These characteristics seem to describe the most relevant attributes of a surgical wound, but no tool could be found that offered a realistic or replicable method for quantifying these characteristics. Some tools measured only a few of these characteristics, and others were designed to measure internal markers of healing. Instruments used to measure surgical wounds are shown in Appendix 39B.[49-54]

Exemplar Studies

Bergstrom, N., & Braden, B. A prospective study of pressure sore risk among institutionalized elderly. *J Am Geriatr Soc*, 1992, 40(12):747–752.

This study exemplifies measurement of many of the variables related to the etiology of one disturbance in skin integrity, pressure sores. The design is prospective, and most of the variables associated with the development of pressure sores are measured with particular attention to nutritional variables. The methods are rigorous and explained in detail.

The instruments used had been previously tested for reliability and validity, and procedures were used to ensure continued reliability and validity throughout the 3 years of the study. One of these instruments, the Braden Scale, is described in this chapter, and the computer program, Nutritionist III, is described in the chapter on nutritional measures. Because the etiology of pressure sores is multivariate, appropriate multivariate analyses were used to determine the relative contribution of multiple factors in predicting pressure sore development.

Allman, R., Walker, J., Hart, M., et al. Air-fluidized beds or conventional therapy for pressure sores. *Ann Intern Med*, 1987, *107*(5):641–649.

This study exemplifies measurement of treatment outcomes for one disturbance in skin integrity, pressure sores. This is a randomized clinical trial comparing healing rates of persons nursed on two different support surfaces. The methods are rigorous and described in excellent detail. The Norton Scale was used to recognize the fact that the same factors that contribute to etiology of pressure sores can contribute to maintenance and degeneration of that wound. Other factors related to pressure sore etiology, regeneration, or degeneration also were measured. The measures used to determine healing rate were acetate tracings and serial color photographs. The investigators used rigorous methods to ensure the reliability of this outcome measure. Usual care was controlled, observed, and described.

References

1. Berjian, D., Douglass, H., Holyoke, E., et al. Skin pressure measurements on various mattress surfaces in cancer patient. *Am J Phys Med*, 1983, *62*(5):217-226.
2. Babbs, C., Bourland, J., Graber, G., et al. A pressure-sensitive mat for measuring contact pressure distributions of patients lying on hospital beds. *Biomed Instrum Technol*, 1990, *24*(6):363-369.
3. Randolph, A.L., Nelson, M., Akkapeddi, S., et al. Reliability of measurements of pressures applied on the foot during walking by a computerized insole sensor system. *Arch Phys Med Rehab*, 2000, *81*(5):573-8.
4. Merbitz, C., Morris, J., & Grip, J. Ordinal scales and foundations of misinference. *Arch Phys Med Rehab*, 1989, *70*(4):308-312.
5. Merbitz, C.T., King, R.B., Bleiberg, J., & Grip, J.C. Wheelchair push-ups: Measuring pressure relief frequency. *Arch Phys Med Rehab*, 1985, *66*(7):433-438.
6. Schnelle, J., Ouslander, J., Simmons, S., et al. Nighttime sleep and bed mobility among incontinent nursing home residents. *J Am Geriatr Soc*, 1993, *41*(9):910-914.
7. Halar, E., Hammond, M., LaCava, E., et al. Sensory perception threshold measurement: An evaluation of semiobjective testing devices. *Arch Phys Med Rehab*, 1987, *68*(8):499-507.
8. Werner, J., & Omer, G. Evaluating cutaneous pressure sensation of the hand. *Am J Occup Ther*, 1970, *24*(5):347-356.
9. Arezzo, J., Schaumburg, H., & Laudadio, C. Thermal Sensitivity Tester: Device for quantitative assessment of thermal sense in diabetic neuropathy. *Diabetes*, 1986, *35*(5):590-592.
10. Shepherd, A., Riedel, G., Kiel, J., et al. Evaluation of an infrared laser-Doppler blood flowmeter. *Am J Physiol Gastrointest Liver Physiol*, 1987, *252*(6):G832.
11. Holloway, G., & Watkins, D. Laser Doppler measurement of cutaneous blood flow. *J Invest Dermatol*, 1977, *69*(3):306-312.
12. Huch, R., Lubbers, D., & Huch, A. Quantitative continuous measurement of partial oxygen pressure on the skin of adults and newborn babies. *Pflugers Arch*, 1972, *337*:185-192.
13. Bader, D., & Grant, C. Changes in transcutaneous oxygen tension as a result of prolonged pressures at the sacrum. *Clin Phys Physiol Meas*, 1988, *9*(1):33-37.
14. Coleman, L., Dowd, G., & Bentley, G. Reproducibility of tcO^2 measurements in normal volunteers. *Clin Phys Physiol Meas*, 1986, *7*(3):259-263.
15. Bennett, L., Kavner, D., Lee, B., et al. Skin stress and blood flow in sitting paraplegic patients. *Arch Phys Med Rehab*, 1984, *65*(4):186-190.
16. Wang, J., Brienza, D.M., Yuan, Y., et al. A compound sensor for biomechanical analyses of buttock soft tissue in vivo. *J Rehab Res Dev*, 2000, *37*(4):433.
17. Crooks, L.E. An introduction to magnetic resonance imaging. *IEEE Engineer Med Biol*, 1985, *4*(3):8-12.
18. Reger, S., McGovern, T., & Chung, K. Biomechanics of tissue distortion and stiffness by magnetic resonance imaging. In D.L. Bader (Ed.), *Pressure sores: Clinical practice and scientific approach*. London: Macmillan, 1990.
19. Conner, L., & Clack, J. In vivo CT scan comparison of vertical shear in human tissue caused by various support surfaces. *Decubitus*, 1993, *6*(2):20-26.
20. Tagami, H., Ohi, M., Iwatsuki, K., et al. Evaluation of the skin surface hydration in vivo by electrical measurement. *J Invest Dermatol*, 1980, *75*(6):500-507.
21. Blichmann, C., & Serup, J. Reproducibility and variability of transepidermal water loss measurement: Studies on the Servo Med evaporimeter. *Acta Dermatol Venereol (Stockh)*, 1987, *67*(3):206-210.

22. Norton, D., McLaren, F., & Exton-Smith, A. *An investigation of geriatric nursing problems in hospital.* Edinburgh: Churchill Livingston, 1975.

23. Bergstrom, N., Braden, B., Laguzza, A., & Holman, V. The Braden Scale for predicting pressure sore risk. *Nurs Res*, 1987, *36*(4):205-209.

24. Panel for the Prediction and Prevention of Pressure Ulcers in Adults. *Pressure ulcers in adults: Prediction and prevention. Clinical practice guideline, No. 3.* AHCPR Publication No. 92-0047. Rockville, MD: Agency for Health Care Policy and Research, Public Health Service, U.S. Department of Health and Human Services, 1992.

25. Roberts, B.V., & Goldstone, L.A. A survey of pressure sores in the over sixties on two orthopaedic wards. *Int J Nurs Stud*, 1979, *16*(5):355-359.

26. Goldstone, L.A., & Goldstone, J. The Norton score: An early warning of pressure sores? *J Adv Nurs*, 1982, *1*(5):419-425.

27. Lincoln, R., Roberts, R., Maddox, A., et al. Use of the Norton pressure sore risk assessment scoring system with elderly patients in acute care. *J Enterostomal Ther*, 1986, *13*(4):17-23.

28. Bergstrom, N., Demuth, P.J., & Braden, B. A clinical trial of the Braden Scale for predicting pressure sore risk. *Nurs Clin North Am*, 1987, *22*(2):417-421.

29. Braden, B., & Bergstrom, N. Predictive validity of the Braden Scale for Pressure Sore Risk in a nursing home population. *Res Nurs Health*, 1994, *17*(6):459-470.

30. Salvadalena, G., Snyder, M., & Brogdon, K. Clinical trial of the Braden Scale on an acute care medical unit. *J Enterostomal Ther Nurs*, 1993, *19*(5):160-165.

31. Bergstrom, N. Braden Scale and clinical judgement. *J Enterostomal Ther Nurs*, 1993, *20*(3):133-136.

32. Hergenroeder, P., Mosher, C., & Sevo, D. Pressure ulcer risk assessment—simple or complex. *Decubitus*, 1992, *5*(7):47-49.

33. Xakellis, G., Franz, R., Arteaga, M., et al. A comparison of patient risk for pressure ulcer development with nursing use of preventive interventions. *J Am Geriatr Soc*, 1992, *40*(12):1250-1253.

34. Bergstrom, N., & Braden, B. A prospective study of pressure sore risk among institutionalized elderly. *J Am Geriatr Soc*, 1992, *40*(8):747-758.

35. Goldstone, L.A., & Roberts, B.V. A preliminary discriminant function analysis of elderly orthopaedic patients who will or will not contract a pressure sore. *Int J Nurs Stud*, 1980, *17*(1):17-23.

36. Bates-Jensen, B. New Pressure Ulcer Status Tool. *Decubitus*, 1990, *3*(3):14-17.

37. Bates-Jensen, B., Vredevoe, D., & Brecht, M. Validity and reliability of the Pressure Sore Status Tool. *Decubitus*, 1992, *5*(6):20-25.

38. Ferrels, B., Artinian, B.M., & Sessing, D. The Sessing Scale for assessment of pressure ulcer healing. *J Am Geriatr Soc*, 1995, *43*(1):37-40.

39. Knighton, D., Fiefel, V., Austin, L., et al. Classification and treatment of chronic nonhealing wounds. *Ann Surg*, 1986, *204*(3):323-325.

40. Riordan, B., Sprigle, S., & Linden, M. Testing the validity of erythema detection algorithms. *J Rehab Res Dev*, 2001, *38*(1)13-22.

41. Bohannon, R.W., & Pfaller, B.A. Documentation of wound surface area from tracings of wound perimeters. *Phys Ther*, 1983, *63*(10):1622-1624.

42. Thomas, A., & Wysocki, A. The healing wound: A comparison of three clinically useful methods of measurement. *Decubitus*, 1990, *3*(1):18-23.

43. Kundin, J. A new way to size up a wound. *Am J Nurs*, 1989, *89*(2):206-208.

44. Eriksson, G., Eklund, A.E., Torlegard, K., & Dauphin, E. Evaluation of leg ulcer treatment with stereophotogrammetry. *Br J Dermatol*, 1979, *101*(2):123-125.

45. Bulstrode, C.J.K., Goode, A.W., & Scott, P.J. A prospective controlled trial of topical irrigation in the treatment of delayed cutaneous healing in human leg ulcers. *Clin Sci*, 1988, *75*(6):637-640.

46. Franz, R., & Johnson, D. Stereophotography and computerized image analysis: A three-dimensional method of measuring wound healing. *Wounds*, 1992, *4*(2):58.

47. Resch, C., Kerner, E., Robson, M., et al. Pressure sore volume measurement: A technique to document and record wound healing. *J Am Geriatr Soc*, 1988, *36*(5):444-449.

48. Siddall, S. Wound healing: An assessment tool. *Home Healthcare Nurse*, 1983, *5*:35-37.

49. Holden-Lund, C. Effects of relaxation with guided imagery on surgical stress and wound healing. *Res Nurs Health*, 1988, *11*(4):235-241.

50. Wilson, A., Treasure, T., Sturridge, M., & Gruenenberg, R. A scoring method (ASEPSIS) for postoperative wound infections for use in clinical trials of antibiotic prophylaxis. *Lancet*, 1986, *1*(8476):311-313.

51. Viljanto, J. Assessment of wound healing speed in man. In A. Barbul (Ed.), *Clinical and experimental approaches to dermal and epidermal repair.* New York: Wiley-Liss, 1991, p. 279.

52. Raekallio, J., & Viljanto, J. Regeneration of subcutaneous connective tissue in children. A histological study with application of the Cellstic device. *J Cutan Pathol*, 1975, *2*:191-197.

53. Viljanto, J. Cellstic: A device for wound healing studies in man. Description of the method. *J Surg Res*, 1976, *20*(2):115-119.

54. Goodson, W., & Hunt, K. Development of a new miniature method for the study of wound healing in human subjects. *J Surg Res*, 1982, *33*(5):39-43.

Appendix 39A. Additional Instruments to Measure Skin Integrity

Instrument	Description	Psychometric Indices
Measures of Intensity and Duration of Pressure		
Semmes-Weinstein Pressure Aesthesiometer Measures sensory perception	Used to establish the threshold of light touch to deep pressure Investigator uses a series of 20 calibrated nylon monofilaments that exert pressure ranging from 1.65 to 6.65 mg of pressure Pressure exerted is a function of the length and diameter of each monofilament Calibration of the monofilaments provides quantification of cutaneous sensibility	Reliability established by 5 serial measurements made over 22 sites without significant differences in sensory perception thresholds (7) Instrument relatively impervious to error when used to obtain quantifiable results; requires skilled investigator in eliciting and interpreting patient responses in qualitative determinations
Thermal Sensitivity Tester Measures sensory perception	Measure of skin temperature and thermal perception thresholds at the distal portion of upper and lower limbs providing quantifiable measurement of small-fiber nerve function Portable device consisting of two 25-cm^2 nickel-coated copper plates, each connected to separate power units and perfused with water in series Temperature of each plate can be changed at a rate >1°C/sec over a 50.0°C range (accurate to within 0.1°C) Thresholds determined by a series of trials where subject contacts each plate for 2 seconds and indicates which plate is colder Temperature of finger or toe should be maintained between 28°C and 34°C Plate contact should blanch the nail	Thermal threshold means (n = 100, normal subjects) (9): index finger: 0.67 C (SD, 0.31°C); great toe: 1.01°C (SD, 0.61°C); both threshold and variance increase with age Repeatability tested with varied results (7,9)
Optacon Tactile Tester Measures sensory perception	Portable device used to determine vibration thresholds as an index of large-fiber nerve function Stimulator pad consists of 144 miniature rods organized into a 24 × 6 matrix Subjects positioned so rods come into contact with ventral surface of index finger pad Rods have a 2-mm horizontal and 1-mm vertical interrod spacing and protrude through a contoured plastic plate Rods vibrate continuously at 230 Hz; amplitude varies as a function of voltage During testing, vibration is manipulated and interspersed with sham stimuli	100 normal subjects studied: mean vibratory threshold: 4.54 V (SD, 1.09 V); thresholds and variance increased with age Test–retest reliability (1-week interval, 5 subjects tested for 3 trials): no significant difference in threshold (7)

Appendix 39A. Additional Instruments to Measure Skin Integrity (*cont*)

Instrument	Description	Psychometric Indices
	Subjects wear earphones (continuous white noise) and eye shielding to mask changes in voltage (accompanied by noise and movement in the area of intensity knob/voltimeter) Testing period is < 5 minutes	
Measurements of clinical determinants of tissue tolerance		
Laser Doppler velocitometry	Measure of physiologic consequences of compressive pressure on tissue Consists of central unit containing a laser diode light source, photodetector, electronic signal filter board, microprocessor, continuous LED digital display, probe connected to central unit by optical fiber (Vasamedics Inc, St. Paul, MN) Laser light emitted from the probe penetrates the skin to a 1-mm depth Light is scattered by soft-tissue components Scatter produced by flowing red blood cells is Doppler shifted relative to that produced by stationary soft tissue Frequencies of returned light collected by probe sensor are analyzed and expressed in mL/min/100 g of tissue	Reliability established in animal studies (linear relationship between total flow and laser Doppler blood flow on liver surface ($r = 0.98$) and gastric mucosa ($r = 0.98$) (10) Comparative measurements of cutaneous blood flow obtained by (133) Xenon clearance technique and laser Doppler; Y on X linear regression coefficient of 0.89 ($p < 0.001$, $n = 16$) (11) Artifact eliminated by preventing movement and stimulation
Skin oxygen sensor	Transcutaneous oximetry measures partial pressure of oxygen at skin surface, providing indirect indication of tissue tolerance Uses Clark polarographic electrode with oxygen-permeable membrane containing a heating element and thermistor Electrode attached to skin by adhesive ring and gel Electrode heated to present temperature (43–45°C) Stimulates maximal vasodilation, increased skin pore opening, and release of oxygen from hemoglobin molecule, producing oxygen tensions at skin surface Approximates arterial oxygen tension (12) Novametrix Medical Systems Inc, Wallingford, CT Used in studies (13)	Reliability is a function of accurate system calibration and application of the electrode; requires frequent recalibration All bubbles must be removed when applying electrode to skin 15-minute calibration is needed after electrode application to ensure maximal vasodilation Inaccurate measure of tissue oxygen values, especially in poor perfusion states Variations of 10% from the mean in average daily measurement can be avoided by consistent placement of electrode in same anatomic location (14)

Numbers in parentheses correspond to studies cited in the References.

Appendix 39B. Measurement of Pressure Sore Status

Instrument	Description	Psychometric Indices
Measures of pressure sore status		
Pressure Sore Status Tool	Measure of the status of pressure sores (35) that is composed of 13 subscales, each rated from 1 to 5 Subscale represents a physical attribute of pressure sore (e.g., size, depth, color) Scores range from 13 to 65; lower scores associated with lesser severity and improved healing; higher scores associated with greater severity and problems with healing	Delphi process involving expert clinicians used in tool development and refinement Content validity established: index 0.91 Interrater reliability (20 pairs of observations made by 2 enterostomal therapists at 2 separate observations): $r = 0.91$ and 0.92 ($p < 0.001$), respectively; rater 1: $r = 0.99$; rater 2: $r = 0.96$ ($p < 0.001$) (36)
Sessing Scale	Measure of pressure sore status Ratings range from 0 (normal skin) to 6 (severe, heavily infected) Ratings accompanied by description of wound characteristics After initial rating, wound progress described with gain scores Charts progress of wound healing in testing of pressure sore treatments (37)	Content validity index: 100% (38) Test–retest validity: 0.90 (weighted kappa) (38) Interrater reliability: 0.8. (weighted kappa) (38) Additional validity tests conducted (38)
Wound Severity Score	Quantifiable measure of severity of chronic nonhealing cutaneous wounds (39) Measures 3 groups of variables (1) Clinical: rated none (0), mild (2), or marked (4); edema, wound purulence, wound fibrin, limb pitting edema, limb brawny edema, wound granulation Wound purulence and limb brawny edema more heavily weighted (mild = 3, marked = 6) Wound granulation is reversed scored (none = 4, marked = 0) (2) Anatomic Exposed to bone (yes = 10, no = 0) Exposed tendon (yes = 7, no = 0) Dorsalis pedis and post tibial pulses (0–1+ = 5; 2+ = 2; 3–4+ = 0)	Correlation between initial wound severity score and time to 80% healing ($r = 0.29$, $p = 0.03$); time to 100% healing ($r = 44$, $p = 0.002$) No tests of interrater reliability performed includes observations of periwound erythema, periwound

Appendix 39B. Measurement of Pressure Sore Status (*cont.*)

Instrument	Description	Psychometric Indices
	(3) Measured wound, patient variables Size (cm^2), scored 1–10 for sizes ranging to > 30 cm^2 Depth (mm), scored 1–10 for depths ranging to > 20 mm Undermining: scored 3–8 for depth ranges to > 5 mm Duration, scored 1–10 for duration up to > 10 years Wound severity score: total range 0–97; found to decline over time in relation to wound healing, declining sharply as healing approaches 100%	
Measures of pressure sore volume		
Kundin Wound Gauge	Measures wound on either 2 (length, width) or 3 (length, width, depth) dimensions (42) Ruler used to measure depth and is placed in center (flat wound) or deepest part of crater Length and width rulers slide down until edges of wound reached; distances recorded Must use same positions for all measurements Formulae used to determine surface area or wound volume Single-use item (sterile), costing approximately $2.00	Validity of wound surface area obtained using gauge compared to acetate tracings and photography (41) Highly correlated when wounds small, circular or elliptically shaped Kundin consistently underestimated surface area of large or irregularly shaped wounds No validation testing of wound volume or interrater reliability Difficulties in exact placement of gauge make repeated measurements subject to error

Stereophotography	Designed to overcome distortion in measurement of 3-dimensional multiplanar surfaces
	Method of applying optical triangulation to produce 3-dimensional photographs
	Noninvasive method to document topical surface and internal configuration of ulcer
	3 systems
	  (1) 2 cameras on a supporting bar (43)
	    Light beam projected along optical axis of each camera, and beam intersection establishes camera positioning in in relation to ulcer surface (slightly < 2 meters)
	    Measurements made of surface area, perimeter, volume, maximum depth
	    Utility limited by distance between cameras and ulcer, so inadequate for full-thickness ulcers, and wound edge determination subject to error
		Initial testing of remote stereophotogrammetry system as in (3), using sample of 144 pairs of pressure ulcers
		Technical error of measurements range: +1.00 mm (depth) and +5.6 mm^2 (surface area)
		Interrater reliability: 0.99 (circumference); 0.96 (depth)

(2) Stereophogrammetric camera apparatus linked to computer (44)

Focus and field of view remain constant

More accurate than direct tracing or simple photography

Useful only for ulcers on flat surfaces that can be positioned under camera frame, and smaller surfaced area ulcers so as to require no magnification adjustment

(3) Remote 3-dimensional measurement by 2 simultaneously taken photographic slides (45)

Lighting system projects grid on ulcer surface that accommodates to the contours of the wound surface, establishing points of reference for computer

Slides scanned and converted to PICT image and analyzed by image analysis software

Generates circumference, surface area, volume, maximum depth

Able to monitor full-thickness wound repair

Wounds Volume Molds	Dental mold substance specifically formulated for moist tissues used as a rapid, safe, and simple measurement Alginate compound mixed with water to form liquid plaster (Jeltrate Alginate Impression, L.D. Caulk Co, Div of Dentply Internat'l, Milford, Delaware) Wound quickly filled using syringe for craters, spatula for flat surfaces Molds removed, rinsed, placed in airtight container Mold weighed, volume estimated by dividing weight by density (1.13 g/cc) (46)	Potential sources of error: excessive dessication of the mold prior to weighing; variations in leveling procedure (error in shallow wounds); may disrupt healing process (injure fragile epithelial cells in wound base)

Measure of the status of surgical wounds

Wound Assessment Inventory	Developed for use in a study of effects of relaxation on postoperative wound healing (48) Summated rating scale: 3 subscales: edema, erythema, exudate, each rated 0 (absent) to 3 (marked) Primarily a measure of local tissue inflammation in early surgical wounds	Content validity established Interrater reliability 0.70 (2 graduate nurses in 12 pairs of ratings)
ASEPSIS	Measure of wound healing developed for use in clinical trial comparing efficacy of antibiotics (49)	Scoring: > 40 agree with findings of other investigators when severe infection present; intermediate scores: provides information other tests do not

661

39B. Measurement of Pressure Sore Status (*cont.*)

Instrument	Description	Psychometric Indices
ASEPSIS (*cont.*)	Points alloted for: A: Additional treatment (antibiotics, 10 points) S: Serous discharge (drainage of pus, 5 points) E: Erythema (rated 1–5 depending on size, amount) P: Purulent exudate (same as E) S: Separation of deep tissues (same as E) I: Isolation of bacteria (10 pts) S: duration of inpatient Stay (> 14 days, 5 points)	Interrater reliability not tested
Cellstic	Measure of healing rate Small, silastic catheter with internal jaws holds viscose cellulose sponge to collect wound cells Catheter placed in one end of surgical incision and later removed to monitor events in healing cascade Harvested wound cells analyzed histologically, biochemically, or cytologically	Developed through years of animal and human studies Demonstrates differences in healing rates with aging and shift in collagen types with wound maturation (50) Testing has involved 1,766 subjects to determine ideal procedures and materials (51,52)
PTFE tubing	Developed to evaluate healing potential of preoperative patients (53) Insertion of small tube of expanded polytetrafluoroethylene (PTFE) in lower lateral portion of upper arm; tube interstices become filled with connective tissue; tube removed after 7 days, and amounts of hydroxyproline/cm of tubing analyzed	Animal studies conducted to determine complication rates, optimal tube, and pore size Appears to be a safe, minimally invasive method for measuring healing potential; has high patient acceptability

Numbers in parentheses correspond to studies cited in the References.

40

Assessing Vaginitis

Sue B. Davidson and Marcia M. Grant

Vaginitis is a common and distressing health problem experienced by women. Three separate but overlapping perspectives on this problem are held by (1) the staff, office, or clinic nurse; (2) the advanced practice nurse, whether a clinical nurse specialist, nurse midwife, or nurse practitioner; and (3) the nurse researcher. The staff, office, or clinic nurse is focused on the best way of preparing the patient for vaginal examination, providing self-care instruction, and coaching patients about achievement of adherence with the medication regimen. The advanced practice nurses in primary care are concerned about diagnostic accuracy, helping patients manage the distressing symptoms of vaginitis (such as pruritis or discharge), and prescribing and evaluating treatment effectiveness. The clinical nurse specialist focuses on reducing symptom distress in patients and on improving the outcomes of care through integration of evidence-based standards of care with nurses and in the system. The nurse researcher selects specific and reliable methods and measurement approaches to explore causal relationships, test alternative or innovative interventions, and identify meaningful outcomes or experiences pertinent to the study of vaginitis. The authors' perspective is primarily that of researchers of a problem that is embedded in the clinical nursing care of women with diabetes mellitus. We became interested in vaginitis as a recurrent and distressing clinical problem for women with diabetes and were interested in testing the effectiveness of a noninvasive and nonpharmacologic approach to symptom management.[1]

Because of our combined clinical and research perspectives, our approach blends practice with research, and it should have meaning for staff, advanced practice, and research nurses. In this chapter, the following definitions of selected terms related to vaginitis assessment are important:

Sensitivity: The probability that test results will be reactive if the specimen is truly positive.

Specificity: The probability that test results will be nonreactive if the specimen is truly negative.

Precision or accuracy: The degree of accuracy of a microscope.

Incidence: The number of new cases that develop in a given population during a defined period.

Prevalence or point prevalence: The number of cases present in the population at risk at a specific time.

Scope of the Problem

Vaginitis is one of the 25 most common reasons for which women seek health care in the United States.[2] Since 1992, vaginitis has accounted for over 10 million office visits per year to health care professionals in primary care.[3] Three common vaginal infections have been identified: bacterial vaginosis (BV), vulvovaginal candidiasis (VVC), and trichomoniasis. In family, private practice, and student health clinic settings, BV is the most common form (40% to 50%); VVC (20% to 25%) and trichomoniasis (15% to 20%) are less common forms.[2,4]

Vaginitis is costly, but the explanation of its cost is complicated. For example, reimbursement by Blue Cross Blue Shield for one year for vaginitis visits to physicians in North Carolina totaled $300 million.[5] Drugs used to treat fungal vaginal infection became available over the counter (OTC) in 1990 and by 1995, $369 million in sales of these products had been reached.[6] Women who believed they had fungal vaginitis bought OTC antifungal vaginitis medications, but this cost may have been offset because less time was lost from work and cost savings were achieved within the health system from fewer visits and tests. It is estimated the savings are about $45 million per year.[7] However, there is emerging evidence that women who use OTC medications for vaginitis may never have seen a health care professional for an initial diagnosis of the causative organism, do not read drug insert instructions, and may be not diagnosing themselves accurately (e.g., treating symptoms when there is no actual infection, treating vaginitis caused by bacteria or protozoa with an inappropriate agent).[8] For these and other reasons, one group estimates that, despite OTC availability of antifungal vaginal medications, the cost of vaginitis from other causes rose to an estimated $1.8 million in 1995.[7]

Appreciation of the serious problems that can result from insufficient treatment or nontreatment is emerging. For example, women with BV also tend to have pelvic inflammatory disease. If women are untreated for BV before abdominal and gynecologic surgeries, cuff infections and other postoperative infections may occur. Pregnant women with BV are associated with preterm rupture of membranes and preterm birth, and about one third may have postpartum endometritis.[9,10] An association between BV and HIV has been identified. Similar relationships (preterm birth, premature rupture of membranes) have been found in pregnant women with trichomoniasis. Clearly, these particular vaginal infections are a significant source of morbidity unless treated.[2]

Vaginitis can be difficult to diagnose and treat. As many as 50% of women will experience symptoms of vaginal infection without corresponding objective evidence. Some women have no subjective symptoms but do have objective evidence of vaginitis. Diagnostic methods to analyze vaginal secretions vary in sensitivity and specificity. Treatment difficulties may result from the presence of an infection caused by several different organisms, the presence of resistant strains, or local topical reaction to the treatment. Providers should, but often do not, use a systematic or thorough process for evaluating subjective symptoms and objective data for the causative organism.[11,12] Alternative interventions, sometimes less costly than traditional therapy, have been explored to treat vaginitis, but their efficacy is unknown. For example, ingestion of exogenous lactobacillus or vaginal instillation of yogurt have been cited as a way of improving lactobacilli levels in the vagina.[13–15] Others have found that biotherapeutics have no effect.[16–21] Few research studies have been published to support or refute these options.[20]

The recurrence of vaginitis is common. Many factors can influence adherence and treatment outcomes. These include a woman's knowledge of her anatomy and the treatment, the timing and frequency of drug administration, the length of the course of treatment, dosage form, and ease or difficulty of the regimen in relation to daily routines.[21] If these are not part of the decision making and planning of therapy for women with vaginitis, the infection may recur. In two of the major vaginal infections, BV and trichomoniasis, recurrence is a significant problem. For example, within 3 months of treatment, infection recurs in 30% of women experiencing BV, whereas less than 5% of women with candida have recurrence.[10,22] Numerous theories exist about the mechanisms of the differing subjective and objective phenomena in vaginitis.

In a few instances, nurses have published research dealing with some aspects of vaginitis. For example, Deitch and Smith[23] evaluated 30 women with chronic vaginitis to see whether the use of colposcopy would clarify why the infection was not responding. Although there are conceptual, sampling, and methodologic issues of concern in this study, it is important to note that these nurse practitioners were using research processes to answer a very difficult clinical problem. Others have tested novel approaches to the diagnosis of vaginitis and cystitis in military women in the field.[24] Other nurses in advanced practice have published protocols for the management of vaginitis,[25,26] and another explored the decision making of women with vaginal symptoms.[27] The nurse practitioner, clinical nurse specialist, and nurse researcher will find multiple opportunities for research in this area.

Definition and Theoretical Description

Vaginitis is an inflammation of the vulvar and vaginal tissues. It is usually associated with changes in the vaginal environment (pH) and in the usual distribution of microbes and/or the presence of abnormal pathogenic organisms. Vaginosis describes vaginal changes that are not accompanied by inflammation of vaginal tissues or leukocytosis. This term is applied most frequently to bacterial vaginosis. The definition and theoretical description of vaginitis can be better understood within the framework of the physiology of the vaginal environment.

Vaginal Environment

A great variety of microorganisms coexist in the vagina. Particular groups of organisms are found in different areas (e.g., vaginal flora differ from cervical flora). In addition, the relationship among these organisms (the vaginal ecosystem) is complex. This ecosystem is sensitive and responsive to changes in a woman's physiologic status. When physiologic status changes, the numbers and types of organisms change, which change the vaginal environment. For a number of years, researchers have reported efforts to describe the vaginal flora and the relationships between microorganisms. Some of that research is flawed because researchers did not recognize differences between the various sites in the vagina, subjects were not homogeneous, specimen collection techniques were imperfect, and specimen transport and culture techniques varied widely.[14] Armed with this knowledge and more sophisticated identification techniques, Brown, Sautter, and Pickrum (as cited in Redondo-Lopez et al.)[18] sampled a cohort of healthy women nine times over three menstrual cycles. They found that there were four major groups of vaginal organisms. The first and most common group were gram-positive rods, of which the *Lactobacillus* species were most frequent, followed by *Corynebacterium* (in 37% of healthy women), and finally the *Propionibacterium*, *Bifidobacterium*, and *Eubacterium* species. The second most frequently observed microorganisms are gram-positive cocci such as

Staphylococcus epidermidis, which was isolated in 62% of the healthy women. Anaerobic forms of gram-positive cocci also are found in 20% to 80% of healthy women. Gram-negative rods (*Gardnerella vaginalis*, the *Mobiluncus* species, and the *Bacterioides* species) also may be cultured from vaginas of health women (rates of 14% to 40%). The last group—yeasts such as *Candida albicans* and *Torulopsis glabrata*, are detected vaginally in 15% to 20% of healthy women.[28] The purpose of the bacteria is to keep vaginal pH between 3.8 and 4.2 through metabolism of glycogen, which yields lactic acid and hydrogen peroxide, thus fostering the growth of acid-tolerant vaginal microorganisms and suppressing growth of anaerobes. Although evidence is mixed as to whether flora of the vagina vary significantly during the menstrual cycle, other factors such as stress, number of sexual partners, and feminine hygiene practices (e.g., douching) have been shown to affect it.[29]

The vaginal epithelium is renewed from the basal toward the luminal layer. The outermost cells are sloughed along with the microorganisms that are attached to them. The vaginal epithelium is nourished by nutrients derived from the circulation to this area of the body and intercellular channels in the vaginal epithelium. Some intracellular nutrients of vaginal epithelium become available for microorganism growth by the enzymatic degradation of sloughed cells and menstrual blood and from secretions of glands in the vagina. The thickness of the vaginal epithelium is regulated by levels of estrogen. When estrogen levels are increased, glycogen deposition in the vaginal epithelium is promoted.[30]

The vagina also produces a fluid in the amount of 1 to 4 ml/day. This secretion contains vaginal epithelial cells, mucus, and discharge from the Skene's and Bartholin glands. The volume and consistency of this fluid varies with the phase of the menstrual cycle and is directly related to circulating estrogen levels. Vaginal fluid, collected from tampons worn four different days during a typical menstrual cycle, has been studied. The fluid is permissive to some strains of *Lactobacillus* (*L. crispatus, L. vaginalis*) but killed *L. Jensenii*, a different strain of lactobacillus, as well as *E. coli* and group B streptococci. Antimicrobial proteins such as calprotectin, lysozyme, and histone were found, as were two defensins, HNP1–3 and HBD-2. It is hypothesized that these molecules have an antimicrobial function when lactate levels are low and the pH of the vagina is high.[31,32]

Interactions occur among the normal flora inhabiting the vaginal environment. A complementary interaction occurs when the product of metabolism of one organism is used by another for growth; an antagonistic interaction occurs when the products of metabolism of one species retard the growth of another. For example, prevalence studies of microorganisms have shown that in pregnancy, conditions that favor the presence of lactobacillus in the vagina also favor the presence of vaginal candida colonization.[17] This could be the result of a synergistic interaction. This information makes it difficult to interpret studies that focus on single microorganisms that may cause symptoms of vaginitis. Future research needs to consider synergistic interactions between flora.

Basal and laminal layers of the vaginal epithelium and the cervix contain cells that provide immune functions. Macrophages, lymphocytes, mast cells, Langerhans cells, and eosinophils can be found in the laminal layer. The levels of these appear to be stable through phases of the menstrual cycle.[30] The presence of these lymphocytes and of immunoglobulin (Ig)G- and IgA-producing cells located in the vaginal epithelium strongly suggests that the vagina is able to produce antibodies.[31] The vagina can absorb substances, including drugs and other protein-like materials, such as sperm, potentially producing overt or subacute inflammatory responses. As Witkin suggests, it seems very likely that vaginal T cells present antigens that are formed in response to inflammation caused by vaginal Langerhans cell activity. If vaginal T cells are activated chronically, this process could be an underlying mechanism of increased risk for developing vaginal infections.[31]

Vaginal flora may be altered. When this occurs, it can change the way the vaginal flora express virulence. A cascade of events is hypothesized, although the sequence of these events is not yet clear. It is assumed that one of the first events is a change in vaginal pH. Subsequently, microorganism adherence is increased, possibly because of an increase in the numbers of receptors on vaginal epithelial cells or through changes in cell surface charge that create a gradient between the host and the bacterial cell surface.[18] As more microorganisms adhere, colonization is likely to occur. It does not always follow that colonization leads to symptoms.

Three common factors can alter vaginal flora, although the research base for these factors is still emerging: (1) damage to mucosal barriers resulting from self-care practices such as douching or individual sexual practices such as receptive oral sex or a greater number of sexual partners; (2) presence of foreign bodies such as a diaphragm, intrauterine device (IUD), certain tampons, and use of spermicides, especially those containing nonoxynol-9;[33] and (3) alterations in immune status caused by steroid use or diabetes, among other things. These changes may exist alone or, more frequently, in combination. When these alterations occur, specific varieties or combinations of vaginitis may result.

Vaginitis

The three most common are BV, VVC, and trichomoniasis. A description of each of these vaginal infections provides the basis for considering how vaginitis is assessed.

Bacterial Vaginosis

Bacterial vaginosis is characterized by an overgrowth of several species of facultative anaerobic bacteria. A unique characteristic of BV is that it represents a disturbance of the vaginal microbial flora rather than being a tissue-based infection. In the past, it has been known variously as nonspecific vaginitis, *Gardnerella* vaginitis, anaerobic vaginitis, or anaerobic vaginosis. The incidence (new cases that appear in a specific period of time) of BV varies in different populations. For example, Sobel et al.[10] indicates that in sexually transmitted disease (STD) clinics, the incidence of BV is between 33% and 64%, a figure that is higher than previous reports; in family planning and obstetrics clinics, the incidence is around 23% to 29%. The incidence of BV is lowest in asymptomatic college student populations.

The following sequence explains how BV occurs.[10] Vaginal pH increases because of a reduction of hydrogen peroxide–producing species of lactobacilli, replacing them with species such as *G. vaginalis*; *Mycoplasma hominis*; anaerobic gram-negative rods; *Prevotella*, *Porphyromona*, and *Bacterioides*; and anaerobic *Peptostreptococcus* species. Organisms that are usually repressed begin to flourish and produce *aminopeptidases*, or enzymes that break down peptides into various amino acids. Part of this chain reaction involves the formation of amines such as trimethylamine, which in the presence of an alkaline pH produces strong odors. Amines are associated with vaginal transudation and vaginal epithelial cell sloughing, which creates clue cells.

The most typical subjective symptoms that women with BV report is a mild vulvar itch, possibly some burning, and a fishy vaginal odor (Table 40.1). This odor may be more noticeable right after intercourse because the alkaline semen reacts with the vaginal secretion to produce amines. Approximately 50% of women with BV are asymptomatic.

Since the mid-1980s, a system for increased accuracy of diagnosis of BV was proposed and tested and is now accepted as a standard for diagnosis of BV. The Amsel system focuses on four objective signs of BV: thin vaginal secretions, vaginal pH above 4.5, presence of clue cells when vaginal secretion is examined under a microscope, and positive findings of strong odor when secretions are combined with potassium hydroxide. Three of the four signs must be present for the diagnosis of BV to be confirmed.[34] In addition, one of two approaches are used to evaluate and rate gram stain findings: the Hay/Ison or the Nugent approach.[35] The Hay/Ison system proposed three grades (normal, intermediate, and bacterial vaginosis) based on the numbers and types of cells found on microscopic examination of the slide. The Nugent system estimates the proportions of morphotypes such as lactobacilli, *G. vaginalis*, and/or *Mobiluncus* species to give a score between 0 and 10. A score of < 4 is normal, 4–6 is intermediate, and > 6 signifies the diagnosis of BV.[36]

The pH of vaginal secretions in women with BV is nearly always greater than 4.5 or 5.0. Thus, a vaginal pH exceeding 5.0 is a very specific indicator of BV, but it has weak sensitivity because vaginal pH can also be altered by the presence of blood, semen, and alkaline douches or creams. The vaginal discharge of a woman with BV is usually present at the introitus, is malodorous, and looks gray; it has a thin, homogeneous consistency. It adheres to, but can be easily wiped from, the vaginal wall. Samples of secretions should be taken from the mucosa along the vaginal walls and vault. The whiff test can be done on vaginal secretion that pools in the speculum or is put on a glass slide. Several drops of 10% potassium hydroxide (KOH) solution are added to the secretion and the sample is smelled for the development of a fishy odor. Vaginal secretion, mixed with normal saline, is then examined under microscopy (10X and 40X objectives and subdued light). Clue cells and epithelial cells that have been sloughed with fuzzy or ill-defined borders may be seen. The indistinct borders of these cells are caused by the collection of bacteria clinging to the cell borders. Another form that may be seen are curved rods with corkscrew motility; these signify the presence of *Mobiluncus*, another causative organism of BV. Gram stain can provide more definitive identification and reveals many small coccobacilli sticking to the clue cell's surface. Unlike other vaginal infections, culture of vaginal secretion is not recommended, because it will add little additional information.[10,37–39]

The main risk factors for BV are use of intrauterine devices, douching, nonwhite ethnicity, and prior pregnancy.[10,40–42]

Vulvovaginal Candidiasis

Vulvovaginal candidiasis (VVC) is a vaginal infection caused mostly by *Candida albicans*. Other organisms, such as *Candida glabrata* or *Candida tropicalis*, have also been implicated in this vaginal infection. Most (80–85%) of VVC is caused, however, by *C. albicans*. This form of vaginitis has two other characteristics. The first is that the diagnosis of VVC cannot be made on the basis of symptoms alone. For example, sometimes women with vaginitis have symptoms but no corresponding positive findings on microscopic examination or by culture; conversely, the woman can have positive findings and not be symptomatic. The second characteristic is that there is a small (< 5%) but important group of women who have repeated episodes of VVC, defined as having four or more symptomatic episodes of VVC per year. Whether this is caused by recurrence or relapse of VVC has been difficult to determine. Clinicians who identify women in this group struggle to find effective treatment for them.[14,37]

Incidence and prevalence of VVC are not reportable in the United States; thus, accurate estimates are not available. Consequently, the overall incidence (point prevalence) of VVC is estimated at 25%. It is estimated that 75% of all women will have at least one

Table 40.1 Symptom Patterns in Three Vaginal Infections

Symptoms and Signs	Bacterial Vaginosis	Vulvovaginal Candidiasis	Trichomoniasis
Subjective			
Itch	Mild	Intense, especially at night	Mild
Discharge	Mild to moderate	Scant to moderate	Mild
Odor	Fishy; stronger after intercourse	Minimal	Present
Vulvar excoriation	Absent	Present, can be severe	Absent
Dysuria	Mild	Present	Present
Dyspareunia	Not usual	Present	Present
Objective/vaginal inspection			
pH of secretions	> 4.5	4.0–4.5	> 4.5; usually 5–6
Discharge	Thin, homogenous, gray	Varies, thin to curdlike	Yellow-green; gray
Odor	Fishy	Not usually present	Very mild
Vulva and labia	No inflammation	Edema and redness	Cervical erythema
Vaginal vault	No inflammation	May see white plaques	Cervical erythema
Objective/laboratory			
Whiff test	Positive	Negative	Negative
Gram stain	Positive	Negative	Negative
Cells that will be seen on saline or KOH microscopy	Clue cells or motile curved rods	Budding hyphae; WBCs; no protozoa, and no clue cells	Pear-shaped cells flagellae; PMNs and no clue cells
Culture	Not recommended	Recommended	Recommended
Papanicolaou test	Not recommended	Not recommended	Recommended

Key: KOH = potassium hydroxide; WBC = white blood cell; PMN = polymorphonuclear leukocytes

episode of VVC and one half will have more than one episode. Five percent will experience relapse and recurrence over a period of many years. The incidence of self-reported VVC is greater in African American women than in Caucasians, suggesting that there are differences among ethnic groups.[6]

The physiologic mechanisms whereby VVC occurs are not fully defined. The contemporary view is that *C. albicans* is a commensal (normal resident) *and* a pathogen; *Candida* can and does exist in low levels among the vaginal flora of many women. What appears to tip the balance in the direction of VVC is a change in the host or in the host environment. When the balance is changed, the yeast is able to adhere to vaginal tissue and germination of the yeast and development of hyphae will occur, leading to colonization. *Candida* is then able to engage in the process of switching, whereby cell strains that are less pathogenic are switched into more pathogenic strains through replication and division; in short, the virulence of the yeast is enhanced.[43] The final result of switching is that a cell strain is produced that penetrates tissue, probably via proteases or other enzymes. Once this occurs, even blastophores, the early nonbudding form of *Candida*, can penetrate tissue. This phase signals a loss of local defenses in the vaginal tissue.

Generally, the most common symptom of VVC is perianal and vulvar itching (pruritis), usually more intense at night (Table 40.1). In addition, women with VVC may have dysuria, or postvoiding dysuria from urine spreading on the surface of the perianal skin where scratching and excoriation has occurred. There may be vaginal discharge, although this is not a usual symptom, or it may be very minimal. There is minimal odor and it is not offensive. There may dyspareunia (pain upon vaginal penetration during sexual intercourse). Unfortunately for the clinician and the researcher, the typical subjective symptoms that women with VVC present are highly variable.

The mechanisms of these symptoms includes a yeast overgrowth with an inflammatory response in the walls of the vagina. At the same time, yeast interacts with glucose that may be present in several forms: in the form of glycogen in vaginal tissue that is converted to glucose or in the form of glucose in urine and vaginal secretion if the woman has diabetes. Either way, the yeast combines with glucose to produce an alcohol, which, when it spreads over the skin, is irritating and initiates the redness and inflammation commonly seen.

On examination for objective signs of VVC, the clinician or researcher will find vulvar and labial edema and redness; these signs may extend to the groin and thighs (Table 40.1). When examining the vaginal introitus, canal, and vault, vaginal plaques may be seen. The vaginal discharge varies; it may be thin, clear, and watery or thick, white, and curdlike 20–25% of the time. The curds, if seen, may be white or yellow and are usually adherent. These curds consist of clumps of sloughed vaginal epithelium and parts of the hyphae of the yeast. Red satellite lesions may be seen on the thighs; sometimes, these red lesions have a scalloped outer edge. The vaginal pH is usually lower than 5.0 (e.g., 4.0–4.5).

Other objective signs may be seen during the wet-mount slide examination by using 10% KOH and normal saline (Table 40.1). After the vaginal pH is checked, KOH is added to the vaginal smear or secretion. In VVC, when the slide or secretion is smelled, there should be no fishy odor, meaning that the woman does not have BV. The addition of KOH to the slide serves to alter the shape of the yeast cells, making their borders more visible. What should be seen, if the woman has VVC, is budding hyphae of the yeast cells; few, if any, leukocytes; and no trichomonads or clue cells. Because noncandidal varieties of yeasts can also cause vaginitis, the presence of a large number of spores with no hyphae should raise the index of suspicion that vaginitis was caused by *Torulopsis glabrata*. Another slide made from a mixture of vaginal secretion and normal saline should then be viewed. According to two nurse practitioners, the viewing of both slides can produce a 70–89% sensitivity in detecting vaginitis caused by candida.[14] Because as many as 50% of women with yeast infections may have negative microscopy, cultures are recommended as the last step in diagnosing VVC (Table 40.2).

A variety of predisposing host factors have been identified for VVC. A recent course of antibiotic therapy with agents such as tetracycline, ampicillin, or oral cephalosporins can predispose to VVC by eliminating the protecting anaerobic and aerobic lactobacilli. The use of high-estrogen birth control pills or corticosteroids can also predispose to VVC. Uncontrolled diabetes is a risk factor, although the mechanism has not been clearly described. Another predisposing factor is pregnancy, especially in the third trimester; frequency of sexual intercourse or anal/oral/genital sexual intercourse is linked with predisposition to VVC. Finally, women who have had a transplant and take immunosuppressive drugs, have HIV, or are stressed for other reasons may be predisposed to VVC because of a reduction of T lymphocytes and increased levels of T-cell suppressors. Anecdotally, some clinicians believe that tight, restrictive clothing; nylon underwear; the use of commercial douches, perfumed toilet paper, and feminine hygiene sprays; and swimming in chlorinated pools are predisposing factors for VVC. Recurrent VVC is linked to reservoirs such as the gut and/or sexual partners who carry yeasts. Few research studies to confirm these factors have been reported.

Table 40.2 Comparison of Sensitivity and Specificity of Diagnostic Methods for Vaginitis

Method	Sensitivity (%)	Specificity (%)
Bacterial vaginosis		
pH	84–97	92
Microscopic	93	70
Vulvovaginitis		
Microscopic (KOH)	61	77
Culture (Nickersons)		
24 hours	31	99
48 hours	72	97
Culture with Microstick-CA		
24 hours	51	97
48 hours	83	96
Trichomoniasis		
Microscopic	99.8	100
Culture	90–98.5	95
Papanicolaou test	57	97
Monoclonal antibodies	86	99

Trichomoniasis

Trichomoniasis, an STD, is a vaginal infection caused by anaerobic protozoa. It is considered the most prevalent cause of STD in the United States, with 8 million new cases every year.[4] The prevalence varies with the setting in which it is diagnosed and the frequency of sexual activity. For example, the prevalence of trichomoniasis is estimated to be 5% in family planning clinics, 39–40% in STD clinics, and between 50% and 75% among prostitutes. In the United States, the highest trichomoniasis frequency is found in the South, the lowest in the Western regions. The National Disease and Therapeutic Index survey found that African American women were treated for trichomoniasis about four times more frequently than white women, even though about 60% of physician visits for this infection occurred in white females. These facts illustrate the complex patterns of women seeking help for vaginitis and some of the health policy issues involved in targeted treatment groups of women at high risk for vaginitis. Both of these issues may be of interest to nurse researchers and nurse epidemiologists.

The prevalence of trichomoniasis is declining in countries such as Denmark and Sweden; this trend appears to be related to a 20-year policy of treating without diagnosis partners of women infected with trichomoniasis.[44] In addition, reduced sexual activity resulting from fear of contracting AIDS and increased condom use may have contributed to this reduced prevalence. Although prevalence of trichomoniasis is declining in family planning and student health clinics in the US, it is rising in STD clinics where women with HIV have a reinfection rate of up to 36%.[45]

A picture of the pathogenesis of trichomoniasis is emerging. At first contact, these protozoa swim over the cell, layering, clumping, and then adhering by means of microfilaments to its surface. As the filaments adhere, the cells retract and lyse, possibly because of the production of free lactic or acetic acid by the protozoa themselves. The trichomonad requires multiple nutrients, such as carbohydrates, amino acids, and fatty acids. These macronutrients may be supplied by macromolecules such as plasminogen or fibrinogen, and other molecules such as ferritin, albumin and transferrin, which bind to the parasite's surface. Other in vivo mechanisms that enable the trichomonad to live include interaction with growth-stimulating factors in the tissue of the host. This mechanism may account for the vaginal epithelial hyperplasia seen in trichomoniasis.[46,47]

In symptomatic women, the most typical symptoms of trichomoniasis are vulvovaginal irritation and pruritus (~50%) and pain on intercourse (~50%) (Table 40.1). Symptoms may occur during or right after menstruation. The reason for this may be that the trichomonad flourishes in an iron-rich milieu, such as occurs during a menstrual period. In men, there may be urethral discharge or urethral inflammation. On examination, vaginal discharge may be yellow/green[4,39] or gray.[2] The vaginal pH is generally above 4.5 and is usually between 5.0 and 6.0. Under colposcopy, a procedure that enables the magnification of tissues being examined, as much as 45–50% of women with trichomoniasis will demonstrate a reddened and inflamed strawberry cervix.[2]

Other objective signs may be seen during wet-mount examination of vaginal discharge (Table 40.1). Once a sample has been obtained from the posterior vaginal fornix, the sample should be mixed with normal saline or acridine orange (KOH kills the protozoa). Identification of the organism may be assisted by keeping the sample warm (having the patient hold the specimen tube in her hand) and by reducing sources of lighting that affect the field of view. What is seen are pear-shaped cells with flagellae; some of the cells may be moving, or the cells may be stationary, but the flagellae are moving. A concentration of 10^4 or 10^5 of the organism is needed in the vaginal discharge; if this is not found, visualization may be compromised. Other methods of increasing visualization of the trichomonad are to view at least 10 microscopic fields or to focus on clumps of white blood cells where the protozoa tend to cluster.[48,49] Gram staining is not used in diagnosing trichomoniasis. As with the diagnosis of other vaginitis by microscope, time, skill, and well-maintained equipment increase diagnostic accuracy. Culture is the most sensitive commercially available method of diagnosis.[48,49]

In summary, in symptomatic women, microscopic methods have a sensitivity of around 60–70% in diagnosing women with trichomoniasis; cultures (read at 46–98 hours) have a sensitivity of 90–95%.[2] As with other vaginitis, there are multiple considerations in choosing a diagnostic method for trichomoniasis that affect both the advanced practice nurse and the researcher. Sensitivity and specificity, cost, skill at microscopy, and time influence decision making. Lossick[50] discusses the various trade-offs to be considered by advanced practice nurses and nurse researchers when diagnosing trichomoniasis. Although cultures for trichomoniasis are not a perfect gold standard, they have an estimated sensitivity of between 86% and 97%. Newer methods of transport and culture (the plastic envelope, InPouch) for trichimoniasis also hold promise of improving identification of this organism.[51,52] The Papanicolaou smear has been used to diagnose trichomoniasis, but because of a nearly 50% error rate (false positives and false negatives), this approach has less appeal for diagnostic work with this type of vaginitis.

Several situations emerge as risk factors for trichomoniasis.[46,48] As with VVC, high level of sexual activity and multiple sex partners increase the likelihood of developing trichomoniasis. Age (older) and gender (women) are factors in the development of trichomoniasis, although there is rising incidence of trichomoniasis in men.[45] Other less clear risk factors for trichomoniasis include race (African Americans are more likely to develop it), previous history of STD, and coexistent gonorrhea or HIV.[45,46]

Other Vaginal Infections

Women may contract other serious vaginal infections, such as chlamydia, gonorrhea, and herpes.[53,54] The causative pathogens and locus of infection may differ from the vaginal infections already described. However, issues related to measurement and diagnosis for nurses in advanced practice and nursing research are much the same for nearly all kinds of vaginitis.

Other Techniques to Diagnose Vaginitis

A variety of approaches have been developed that augment wet-mount, gram-stain, and culture techniques to identify the causative organisms of vaginitis. The following new techniques are emerging in the assessment of vaginitis:

1. Immunologic function-based tests
   a. Enzyme-linked immunosorbent assay (ELISA), including monoclonal antibodies[55]
   b. Proline aminopeptidase assay
   c. Latex agglutination[2]
2. DNA probe-based tests
   a. Nucleic acid hybridization[58,59]
   b. Polymerase chain reaction[60]

These methods, their uses, sensitivity and specificity, and applications are reviewed in Appendix 40A.

These new methodologies for diagnosing vaginitis offer greater specificity in populations of women with higher rates of a particular type of vaginitis. They offer potential to the nurse researcher because of their high sensitivity and specificity. Drawbacks are cost and the need for special equipment and, potentially, trained personnel.

Issues Related to Assessment Approach and Instrument Selection

In most studies of vaginitis, the purpose is to examine the incidence of the problem in a population in general or to test specific approaches to prevention and/or treatment. The development of an instrument to measure vaginitis has been the focus of a few publications. Most studies have compared incidence rates using different methods for identification of organisms and different sets of signs and symptoms; in these studies, the assessment approach has been related to the known characteristics of specific organisms that cause vaginitis. This has had implications for the building of an evidence base for knowledge about vaginitis, although evidence bases exist for treatment guidelines of vaginitis caused by various organisms.

Three types of information are used to assess vaginitis: (1) pathogenic organisms, (2) subjective symptoms, and (3) observations of objective signs. For each type of information, advanced practice nurses and researchers may select different methods and different parameters, depending on sensitivity and reliability as well as cost and availability.

An expanded group of assessment parameters is emerging from recent studies.[33,41] Culhane et al.[41] looked at the relationship between the context of the study participant and the incidence of BV. Context included adequacy of housing, interpersonal conflict, material hardship, neighborhood danger, perceived stress, use of a shelter, and incidence of assault. The rationale for linking incidence of BV with these expanded variables is that if context is viewed by the woman as stressful and if the community in which she lives is stressful, this activates the stress response, which leads to alterations in the neuroendocrine system and further alterations in the immune responses. In the Culhane study, African American women rated all the contextual variables as more stressful compared to the other subjects (Hispanics, white women), and she postulates that this may explain why the rates of BV are four times greater in African American women than other ethnic groups. Another study[33] shifted assessment data collection to subjects who were asked to maintain a daily written diary and collect a daily vaginal swab for the study period of 6 weeks. Here, the data collection burden for accuracy and completeness relied heavily on the subject. This may explain why the findings from this study confirmed some but not all the extant knowledge about variations in vaginal flora, thus suggesting that these approaches may be more susceptible to missing data or collection errors, while reflecting actual vaginal flora that lead to vaginitis over the course of time. These two studies illustrate some of the considerations that must be taken into account in the conduct of research on vaginal infections.

Identification of Pathogenic Organisms

Performing the vaginal examination to obtain a specimen and conducting the wet-mount examination of vaginal fluids are assessments that are done by nursing, medical, and other health care personnel. Such assessments are consistent with the knowledge and competencies of staff nurses in a women's health specialty area and of nurses in advanced practice.

The wet-mount or immediate microscopic examination is done right after the collection of vaginal secretions and the vaginal examination. A slide is prepared and examined under the microscope for characteristics of suspected pathogens. In the second method, secretions obtained during the vaginal examination are transferred onto various culture media. They are incubated for at least 48 hours, after which the pathogenic organisms are identified.

A variety of culture media are used for transport and inoculation of the specimen on media, depending on the organism identified. Here is a list of suggested culture media used to identify vaginal pathogens:[61-63]

Media for organisms causing BV
    Transport: Amies Transport Medium, Stuart Transport Medium
    Culture: Columbia Blood Agar, G. Vaginilis Specific, Human Blood Tween™ Bilayer Medium (HBT)
Media for organisms causing VVC
    Transport: Bismuth Sulfite Glucose Glycerin Yeast Extract Agar (BIGGY; also known as Nickersons Medium), Stuart Transport Medium
    Culture: Corn Meal Agar, Mycosel Agar, Sabourand Dextrose Agar, Sabourand Difco Mycotic Media
Media for organisms causing trichomoniasis
    Transport: Diamonds Modified Medium, Stuart Transport Medium
    Culture: Diamonds Cysteine Trypticase™ Agar, Modified Columbia Agar Broth

Two variations in collection procedures for vaginal specimens are being reported.[24,33,62] The first variation is that subjects are collecting the vaginal specimens. In two studies, the reason was that women were living in isolated areas or in military environments where there were logistical constraints on travel. In Lowe and Ryan-Wenger's study,[24] the subjects received a kit that included a diagnostic algorithm for candidiasis, BV, and cystitis. The kit also included a sterile swab, pH paper, a tube of KOH solution, and a pencil. After using the algorithm to confirm subjective symptoms, the subject was guided through steps for obtaining a vaginal specimen, testing with pH paper, and putting the swab into the tube of KOH to complete the sniff test associated with trichomoniasis. The clinical decision of the subject was compared to that of the advanced practice nurse. The second study evaluated urine, swab, and tampon vaginal specimens and endocervical vaginal specimens for three common vaginal infections. The self-collected vaginal swab and tampon had 100% positive predictive value. It should be noted that this study did not confirm the diagnosis of vaginitis using wet mount or cultures, but instead conducted DNA-probe testing for *Trichomonas vaginalis*.

The second variation in collection procedures is that new products are emerging that contain both the transport and culture medium for an organism in one pouch (Affirm VP III, MicroProbe Corporation, Bothell, WA; Affirm VP III Ambient Temperature Transport System (ATTS), Becton Dickenson & Company, Sparks, MD). The pouch has a collection swab, transport tube, and dropper containing preservative so that the specimen is stable up to 48 hours. These products are used to diagnosis trichomoniasis, organisms found in BV, and VVC.

Validity and reliability of the various methods of identifying the microbes involves comparing results across the various methods and various preparations and comparing results obtained among various investigators. When comparing immediate wet-mount and microscopic examination to culture and subsequent examination, results show that greater numbers of organisms occur when culture results are added to data obtained from immediate microscopic examination. In practical terms, treating patients without culture confirmation of pathogenic organisms usually is based on expediency; that is, the patient has acute symptoms that are typical and treatment is not held up for 3 days to await culture results. In addition, the cost of cultures using various media and requiring laboratory identification procedures can be prohibitive.[42]

Subjective Symptoms

The second type of assessment used to assess vaginitis involves the subjective symptoms obtained during patient interview. The most frequently reported symptoms include pruritis, discharge, odor, dyspareunia, dysuria, vaginal pressure, soreness, and burning.[2,4,10] However, use of symptoms alone or combined with historic data is of limited value in the accurate diagnosis of vaginal infections.[63] Approximately half the women presenting with vaginal symptoms generally are given a specific microbiologic diagnosis of their vaginitis when subjective symptoms are combined with objective signs and examination for specific organisms.

Observation of Objective Symptoms

The third type of assessment of vaginitis includes the objective signs obtained during patient examination. The external genitalia may be examined for erythema, lesions, and secretions. Secretions can be tested for pH and glucose. Typical signs for each type of vaginitis are described in Table 40.1. The standard procedure for clinical diagnosis is to accept three typical signs (e.g., pH, discharge characteristics, and odor) as acceptable evidence of vaginitis. This method, however, still results in a sensitivity of only 60–72%.[63] Combining culture with objective and subjective information to assess vaginitis clearly is the best current way to obtain the most accurate diagnosis.

Behaviors and Environment

As demonstrated by others,[33,41] the use of vaginal self-care diaries, self-collected vaginal swabs, estimates of perceived stress, and estimations of the individual's home and community may be included in the assessment. These variables may explain vaginal infection rates that are unexpectedly high, resistant to therapy, or recurrent.

Assessment Tools and Treatment Protocols

Assessment tools and treatment protocols have been developed to assist advanced practice nurses in the diagnosis and differentiation of the different kinds of vaginitis. Several of these are highlighted in Appendix 40B.[26,53,54,64]

Summary

Assessment of vaginitis may involve four kinds of information: identification of pathogenic organisms, subjective symptoms, objective signs, and a review of the environment and self-care behaviors. Different combinations of information are useful depending on whether the staff nurse, nurse practitioner, clinical nurse specialist, or nurse researcher is involved in the assessment. Most studies dealing with the validity and reliability of the variables have focused on methods of organism identification. Continuing issues in assessment of vaginitis include testing predisposing factors, the problem of mixed infections, recurrence of the infection, successful management of symptoms, and the need for increased specificity and sensitivity of organism identification methods. These issues illustrate the need for a more thorough assessment of the patient rather than attenuated clinical assessment approaches that are being reported in the cost-driven health care environment.

For nurse researchers, the variables used in assessment often are most valuable when they are standardized and understood. For the nurse working with patients clinically, management of symptoms is an important focus. One way to enrich this clinical practice area would be to supplement the tools already developed for assessing vaginitis with some qualitative information; for example, examining what relationships occur between vaginitis and sexual function, personal hygiene, and types of clothing. In this way, tools developed via a qualitative methodology could be used to assess, measure, and diagnose the responses of women with vaginitis and help to identify additional variables to be explored in other research projects.

Website

www.guideline.gov

References

1. Grant, M., & Davidson, S. *Effects of perineal care on diabetic vulvovaginitis: Final report of project.* Washington, DC: Division of Nursing, Bureau of Health Manpower, Health Resources Administration, Department of Health and Human Resources, 1984.

2. Haefner, H. Current evaluation and management of vulvovaginitis. *Clin Obstet Gynecol*, 1999, 42(2):184-195.

3. American College of Obstetricians and Gynecologists. Vaginitis. *ACOG Techn Bull*, 1996, 226(7):886-893.

4. Sobel, J.D. Current concepts: Vaginitis. *New Engl J Med*, 1977, 337(26):1896-1903.

5. Gwyther, R.E., Addison, C.A., Spottswood, S., et al. An innovative method for specimen autocollection in the diagnosis of vaginitis. *J Fam Pract*, 1986, 23:487-488.

6. Foxman, B., Barlow, R., D'Arcy, H., et al. Candida vaginitis: Self reported incidence and associated costs. *Sex Trans Dis*, 2000, 27(4):230-235.

7. Lipsky, M.S., Waters, T., & Sharp, L.K. Impact of vaginal antifungal products on utilization of health care services: Evidence from physician visits. *J Am Bd Fam Prac*, 2000, 13(3):178-182.

8. Ferris, D.G., Nyirjesy, P., Sobel, J.D., et al. Over-the-counter antifungal drug misuse associated with patient-diagnosed vulvovaginal candidiasis. *Obstet Gynecol*, 2002, 99(3):419-425.

9. Koumans, E.H., & Kendrick, J.S. Preventing adverse sequelae of bacterial vaginosis: A public health program and research agenda. *Sex Transm Dis*, 2001, 28:292-297.

10. Sobel, J.D. Bacterial vaginosis. *Ann Rev Med*, 2000, 51:349-356.

11. Wisenfeld, H.C., & Macio, I. The infrequent use of office-based diagnostic tests for vaginitis. *Am J Obst Gynecol*, 1999, 181(1):39-41.

12. Allen-Davis, J.T., Beck, A., Parker, R., et al. Assessment of vulvar vaginal complaints: Accuracy of telephone triage and in-office diagnosis. *Obstet Gynecol*, 2002, 99(1):18-22.

13. Fredericcson, B., Englund, K., Weintraub, L., et al. Ecological treatment of bacterial vaginosis. *Lancet*, 1987, 1:276.

14. Carcio, H.A., & Secor, R.M.C. Vulvovaginal candidiasis: A current update. *Nurse Pract Forum*, 1992, 3(3):135-144.

15. Hilton, E., Isenberg, H.D., Alperstein, P., et al. Inges-

tion of yogurt containing *Lactobacillus acidophilus* as prophylaxis for candidal vaginitis. *Ann Intern Med*, 1992, *116*:353-357.

16. Kaufman, R.H., & Hammill, H.A. Vaginitis. *Primary Care*, 1990, *17*:115-125.

17. Larsen, B. Vaginal flora in health and disease. *Clin Obstet Gynecol*, 1993, *36*(1):110-121.

18. Redondo-Lopez, V., Cook, R.L., & Sobel, J.D. Emerging role of lactobacillus in the control and maintenance of the vaginal bacterial microflora. *Rev Infect Dis*, 1990, *12*(5):856-872.

19. Summers, P.R., & Sharp, H.T. The management of obscure or difficult cases of vulvovaginitis. *Clin Obstet Gynecol*, 1993, *36*(1): 206-214.

20. Hilton, E., Isenberg, H.D., Alperstein, P., et al. Ingestion of yogurt containing *Lactobacillus acidophilus* as prophylaxis for candidal vaginitis. *Ann Intern Med*, 1992, *116*:353.

21. Nixon, S.A. Vulvovaginitis: The role of patient compliance in treatment success. *Am J Obstet Gynecol*, 1991, *165*:1207-1209.

22. Odds, F.C. Candidosis of the genitalia. In F.C. Odds (Ed.), *Candida and candidosis* (2nd ed.). London: Balliere Tindal, 1988, p. 124.

23. Deitch, K.V., & Smith, J.E. Symptoms of chronic vaginal infection and microscopic condyloma in women. *J Obstet Gynecol Neonatal Nurs*, 1990, *19*(2):133-138.

24. Lowe, N.K.U., & Ryan-Wenger, N.A. A clinical test of women's self-diagnosis of genitourinary infections. *Clin Nurs Res*, 2000, *9*(2):144-160.

25. Gietl, K.A. Role of the nurse practitioner in the management of vaginitis. *Am J Obstet Gynecol*, 1988, *158*:1009-1111.

26. Schodde, G. A vaginitis protocol that helps teach. *Nurs Pract*, 1985, *1*(2):64-68.

27. Theroux, R. Bypassing the middleman: A grounded theory of women's self-care for vaginal symptoms. *Health Care Women Int*, 2002, *23*(5):417-431.

28. Levison, M.E., Corman, L.C., Carrington, G.R., et al. Quantitative microflora of the vagina. *Am J Obstet Gynecol*, 1977, *127*:80-85.

29. Eschenbach, D.A., Thwin, S.S., Patton, D.L., et al. Influence of the normal menstrual cycle on vaginal tissue, discharge, and microflora. *Clin Infect Dis*, 2000, *30*:901-907.

30. Patton, D.L., Thwin, S.S., Meier A., et al. Epithelial layer thickness and immune cell populations in the normal human vagina at different stages of the menstrual cycle. *Am J Obstet Gynecol*, 2000, *183*(4):967-973.

31. Witkin, S.S. Immunology of the vagina. *Clin Obstet Gynecol*, 1993, *36*(1):122-128.

32. Valore, E.V., Park, C.H., Igreti, S.L., et al. Antimicrobial components of vaginal fluid. *Obstet Gynecol*, 2002, *187*(3):561-568.

33. Schwebke, J.R., Richey, C.M., & Weiss, H.L. Correlation of behaviors with microbiological changes in vaginal flora. *J Infect Dis*, 1999, *189*:1632-1637.

34. Amsel, R., Totten, P.A., Spiegel, C.A., et al. Nonspecific vaginitis. *Am J Med*, 1983, *74*:14-22.

35. Nugent, R.P., Krohn, M.A., & Hillier, S.L. Reliability of diagnosing bacterial vaginosis is improved by a standardized method of gram stain interpretation. *J Clin Microb*, 1991, *28*(2):297-301.

36. Association for Genitourinary Medicine; Medical Society for the Study of Venereal Diseases. 2002 national guidelines for the management of bacterial vaginosis. Released August 1999; updated 2002. Access date March 3, 2003. www.guideline.gov/.

37. Workowski, K.A., & Levine, W.C. Sexually transmitted diseases treatment guidelines, 2002. *MMWR Morb Mortal Wkly Rep*, 2002, *51*(RR-6):1-78.

38. Andrist, L.C. Vaginal health and infections. *J Obstet Gynecol Neonatal Nurs*, 2000, *30*(3):306-315.

39. Cullins, V.E., Dominguez, L., Guberski, T., et al. Treating vaginitis. *Nurs Pract*, 1999, *24*(10):46-63.

40. Ness, R.B., Hillier, S.L., Richter, H.E., et al. Douching in relation to bacterial vaginosis, lactobacilli, and facultative bacteria in the vagina. *Obstet Gynecol*, 2002, *100*(4):765-772.

41. Culhane, J.F., Rauh, V., Farley, K., et al. Exposure to chronic stress and ethnic differences in rates of bacterial vaginosis among pregnant women. *Am J Obstet Gynecol*, 2002, *187*(5):1272-1276.

42. Holzman, C., Levethan, J.M., Qiu, H., et al. Factors linked to bacterial vaginosis in nonpregnant women. *Am J Pub Health*, 2001, *91*(10):1664-1670.

43. Sobel, J.D., Faro, S. Force, R., et al. Vulvovaginal candidiasis: Epidemiologic, diagnostic and therapeutic considerations. *Am J Obstet Gynecol*, 1998, *178*(2):203-211.

44. Dragsted, D.M., Farholt, S., & Lind, I. Occurrence of trichomoniasis in women in Denmark. *Sex Transm Dis*, 2001, *28*(6):326-329.

45. Niccolai, L.M., Kopicko, J.J., Kassie, A., et al. Incidence and predictors of reinfection with *Trichomonas vaginalis* in HIV-infected women. *Sex Transm Dis*, 2000, *27*(5):284-288.

46. Petrin, D., Delgaty, K., Bhatt, R., et al. Clinical and microbiological aspects of *Trichomonas vaginalis*. *Clin Microb Rev*, 1998, *11*(2):300-317.

47. Graves, A., & Gardner, W.A. Pathogenicity of *Trichomonas vaginalis*. *Clin Obstet Gynecol*, 1993, *36*(1):145-152.

48. Association for Genitourinary Medicine, Medical Society for the Study of Venereal Disease. 2002 national guidelines on the management of *Trichomonas vaginalis*. Released 1993, revised May 10, 2002. Access date: March 8, 2003. www.guideline.gov/.

49. Centers for Disease Control and Prevention. Diseases characterized by vaginal discharge. Sexually transmitted diseases treatment guidelines 2002. Released 1993, revised May 10, 2002. Access date: March 8, 2003. www.guideline.gov/.

50. Lossick, J.G. The diagnosis of vaginal trichomoniasis. *JAMA*, 1988, *259*(8):1230.

51. Briselden, A.M., & Hillier, S.L. Evaluation of Affirm VP microbial identification test for *Gardnerella vaginalis* and *Trichomonas vaginalis*. *J Clin Microb*, *32*(1):148-152.

52. Brown, H.L., Fuller, D.D., Davis, T.E., et al. Evaluation of the Affirm Ambient Temperature Transport system for detection and identification of *Trichomonas vaginalis*, *Gardnerella vaginalis*, and *Candida* species from vaginal fluid specimens. *J Clin Microb*, 2001, *39*(9):3197-3199.

53. Summers, P.R., & Sharp, H.T. The management of obscure or difficult cases of vulvovaginitis. *Clin Obstet Gynecol*, 1993, *36*(1), 206-214.

54. Eschenbach, D.A., & Mead, P.B. Managing problem vaginitis. *Patient Care*, 1992, *26*(14):137-140,145, 149-152.

55. Krieger, J.N., Tam, M.R., Stevens, C.E., et al. Diagnosis of trichomoniasis: Comparison of conventional wet-mount examination with cytologic studies, cultures, and monoclonal antibody staining of direct specimens. *JAMA*, 1988, *259*(8):1223-1227.

56. Schoonmaker, J.N., Lunt, B.D., Lawellin, D.W., et al. A new proline aminopeptidase assay for diagnosis of bacterial vaginosis. *Am J Obstet Gynecol*, 1991, *165*:737-742.

57. Eschenbach, D.A., & Hillier, S.L. Advances in diagnostic testing for vaginitis and cervicitis. *J Repro Med*, 1989, *34*(suppl 8):555-565.

58. Obata-Yasuoka, M., Ba-Thein, W., Hamada, H., et al. A multiplex polymerase chain reaction-based diagnostic method for bacterial vaginosis. *Obstet Gynec*, 2002, *100*:759-764.

59. Wendel, K.A., Erbelding, E.J., Gaydos, C.A., et al. *Trichomonas vaginalis* polymerase chain reaction compared with standard diagnostic and therapeutic protocols for detection and treatment of vaginal trichomonas. *Clin Infect Dis*, 2002, *35*(1):576.

60. Ferris, D.G., Hendrich, J., Payne, P.M., et al. Clinician-performed tests compared with a rapid nucleic acid hybridization test. *J Fam Pract*, 1995, *41*(6):575-581.

61. Atlas, R.M., & Parks, L.C. *Handbook of microbiological media* (2nd ed.). Boca Raton, FL: CRC Press, 1997.

62. Knox, J., Tabrizi, S., Miller, P., et al. Evaluation of self-collected samples in contrast to practitioner-collected samples for detection of *Chlamydia trachomatis*, *Neisseria gonorrhoeae*, and *Trichomonas vaginalis* by polymerase chain reaction among women living in remote areas. *Sex Transm Dis*, *29*(11):747-754.

63. Schaaf, V.M., Perez-Stable, E.J., & Borchardt, K. The limited value of symptoms and signs in the diagnosis of vaginal infections. *Arch Intern Med*, 1990, *150*:1929-1933.

64. Greenfield, S., Friedland, G., Scifers, S., et al. Protocol management of dysuria, urinary frequency, and vaginal discharge. *Ann Intern Med*, 1974, *81*(4):452-457.

Appendices 40A. Assessment Tools and Treatment Protocols for Vaginitis

Instruments	Description	Psychometric Indices
Assessment Tools		
Grant and Davidson Vaginitis Assessment Form (1)	Designed for use with diabetic patients Tests effectiveness of a perineal care technique to prevent and manage vaginitis Subjects followed for one month Form includes: subjective symptoms, objective signs, laboratory findings	Content validity established by a panel of nurse practitioner experts familiar with assessing vaginitis Sensitivity and reliability by random, weekly exam assessment of 143 subjects Cronbach's alpha: history: 0.78; external exam: 0.97; internal vaginal exam: 0.82; total of all variables: 0.92 Some consistency within subscale and total scale Relationship between occurrence of vulvovaginal symptoms and positive cultures Comparison of 90 subjects having positive vulvovaginal symptoms at beginning of study (64%) vs 90 subjects with positive cultures for *Candida, Trichomonas,* and/or *Gardnerella* (13%) High incidence of patients with positive symptoms and negative cultures leads to need for assessment tool that includes signs, symptoms, and culture data
Summers and Sharp Vaginitis History Form (53)	Targets information needed for obscure or difficult cases Data elicited: occurrence of symptoms; medications; other symptoms (e.g., rashes, dry skin, painful joints); sexual history General guidelines described, including situations to refer to a dermatologist	Reliability and validity reports not included
Lowe and Ryan-Wenger Vaginitis and Cystitis Decision Making Guide (24)	Designed for use by women in isolated areas (due to job, recreation, missionaries, military) Guides women in self-diagnosis of VVC, BV, and UTI Includes diagnostic algorithm and testing procedure Data elicited for three types of vaginitis: itch, pH, whiff, odor, consistency of vaginal fluid, color Data elicited for cystitis: burning, frequency, urgency, continued urge Temp-a-Dot, sterile swab, pH paper, small tube of KOH, pencil provided in kit	Content validity procedures for both vaginitis and cystitis guide used; reliability report not included Positive predictive values of each sign/symptom calculated Sensitivity of Vaginitis and Cystitis Decision Making Guide reported for VVC, BV, and cystitis Error rates between self-diagnosis of subjects and APN diagnosis calculated with result that some subjects would have treated when they should not have

Appendices 40A. Assessment Tools and Treatment Protocols for Vaginitis (*cont.*)

Instruments	Description	Psychometric Indices
Treatment Protocols Schodde Protocol (26)	Includes: subjective symptoms (e.g., odor, burning after urination); objective physical exam (e.g., vulvar inflammation, vaginal discharge); laboratory tests; area for interpreting the assessment data and planning the follow-up treatment	None reported
Greenfield et al. Protocol (64)	Used in management of dysuria, urinary frequency, and vaginal discharge · Uses branching logic format, including history, physical exam, and laboratory criteria	Logic format validated by medical consultants. Effectiveness tested on 146 patients: group 1 (patient seen by nurse using the protocol form, then by MD with usual medical approach); group 2 (patient seen by physician using usual medical approach) Agreement: Medical history: 136/146 (6/7 discrepancies = physician error); physical exam: 136/146; lab data: similar Criteria validated by demonstrating that patients received protocol-directed treatment obtained same high degree of symptom relief as those treated by physician Reliability of nurse identification of *Candida* in 9/39 positive cases Summary: tool criteria has initial reliability and validity and includes parameters relative to dysuria, frequent urination, and vaginitis
Eschenbach and Mead Protocol (64)	Branching patient flowchart leading practitioner through steps needed: begins with patient's report signs/symptoms, pH of vaginal secretions, and gram staining Treatment based on findings; includes first-line therapy as well as recommendations for persistent infections or recurrences	No reliability or validity reported
Summers and Sharp Protocol (53)	Organized approach to treatment of obscure or difficult cases, history form, physical exam approaches, subjective symptoms, objective signs, and therapeutic options	No reliability or validity reported

Numbers in parentheses correspond to studies cited in References.

Appendix 40B. New and Emerging Objective Techniques to Diagnose Vaginitis

Diagnostic Test/ Microorganism	Description	Psychometric Indices/ Advantages/Disadvantages
Immunoassays Enzyme-Linked Immunosorbent Assay (ELISA) (55)	Basis for a number of tests measuring the response of vaginal fluid to test antigen or antibody systems Vaginal fluid is mixed with a specific antibody and antigens are formed; another substances is added (e.g., antigen-enzyme sensitive to antibody/antigen reaction); the substance interacts with original antibody-antigen complex; dyes attached to the enzyme develop color indicating a positive response ELISA may be used with monoclonal antibodies, direct or indirect immunofluorescence, or fluorescein-tagged monoclonal antibodies Organisms: *Trichomonas vaginalis*	Sensitivity: 91–96% (59) Sample of 60 patients with incidence of trichomoniasis of 13%: sensitivity 86%; specificity 99%; positive predictive value: 96% Advantages: requires little time to perform; standard preparation for cytologic evaluation Disadvantages: requires special reagents, high-quality microscopes, and trained personnel; predictive value drops when used on low-risk populations
Proline Aminopeptidase (56)	Detects enzyme proline aminopeptidase that is produced in vitro by wide variety of bacteria (e.g., lactobacillus, *Mobiluncus*, and *Candida* Vaginal samples are washed and combined with L-proline β naphthylamide or L-proline ρ nitroanilide, which acts as a color developer Enzyme reaction measured by color intensity either visually or by spectrophotometer Organism: *Lactobacillus, Candida,* organisms found in BV	Compared to other methods (e.g., culture, gram stain): sensitivity: 54.3%; specificity: 93.6% Advantages: has highest specificity of any diagnostic test for BV Disadvantages: time-consuming, expensive
Latex Agglutination Test (2,57)	Polystyrene latex particles, coated with purified immunoglobulins, are exposed to purified derivatives of the cell wall of *C. albicans* (serotypes A, B) and *Torulopsis glabrata* Vaginal swab added to the sensitive latex on black cardboard slide and mixed Swab washing added to latex cardboard that does not contain immunoglobulins, serving as control Positive reaction is a coarse clumping within the prescribed time (antigen/ antibody reaction to the organism) Organisms: *C. albicans, T. glabrata*	Sensitivity of 72.7% in study with 137 symptomatic and asymptomatic women with *C. albicans* (lower than sensitivity of KOH method, 90%) (2,59)
DNA Probe Testing Polymerase Chain Reaction (PCR) (58,59)	DNA sequences of a known infectious agent are cloned, synthesized, and used as a probe; probes hybridize with DNA and RNA targets in a clinical specimen Probes can be labeled with enzyme, luminescent tags, or radioisotopes so they can be detected Specificity depends on the size and composition of the probe and original specimen	

Appendix 40B. New and Emerging Objective Techniques to Diagnose Vaginitis (*cont.*)

Diagnostic Test/ Microorganism	Description	Psychometric Indices/ Advantages/Disadvantages
Nucleic acid hybridization (60)	DNA polymerase elongates the 3′ end of a primer, which joins with a long sequence of DNA in the target (specimen). When two primers bind to a target DNA, the sequence between the two primer sites is amplified. A number of amplifications are completed until there are detectable amounts of the target sequence. Various methods and modifications of PCR: reverse transcription, nested, and multiplex PCR Detection of the organism's DNA done through agarose gel electrophoresis with a staining, radio-labeled or fluorescein labeled Gel exposed to x-ray film where the hybridization products are identified by dark bands FDA required to approve PCR products Organisms: *Trichomonas vaginalis, C. albicans*, organisms found in BV	Sample of 501 symptomatic patients comparing traditional methods (saline/KOH wet mount, whiff test, pH) with nucleic acid hybridization. Sensitivity and specificity for BV and trichomoniasis > 95% with PCR compared to 75–80% with traditional methods. Advantages: Shorter time between collection and specific diagnosis of vaginitis; procedure adaptable to other organisms; laboratories have access to a library of organisms, DNA from genome project Disadvantages: Some organisms have a high amount of phenotypic variations; contamination of specimens leading to false-positives/negatives; cannot be used if causative organism not known; concerns that presence of an identified sequence may not be related to actual disease; requires careful specimen handling

Index

A

Ability tests
  item difficulty or preference indexes of, 78
  for projective testing in children, 46
ABS (Affects Balance Scale), 369
Acculturation, 59–60
  readings on, 62
Accuracy, physiologic measurement and, 67
Acetate tracings, of pressure sore surface area, 653–654
Actigraphic Scoring Analysis, for sleep studies, 301
Actigraphy, 301, 309
Actillume, for sleep studies, 301
Action, definition of, 431, 439
Active coping, 200
Activities of Daily Living—Household Activities Scale (ADL-HAA), 89
Activities of Daily Living—Multiple Sclerosis (ADL-MS), 89
Activity Index, 89
Activity measurement, for sleep studies, 300–301
Acute pain, 604–605. *See also* Pain
  tools for measuring, 618–620
Adjustment disorders with depressed features, 377, 380
ADL Scale, 90
Adolescent-Family Inventory of Life Events and Changes (A-FILE), 205–206, 214
Adolescents. *See also* Children and adolescents
  hope perceptions in, 218
  measurement strategies for, 40
Advanced activities of daily living (AADL), measurement of, 84
Affective disorders, permissive amine hypothesis of, 378
Affective evaluations of life quality, 154
Affects Balance Scale (ABS), 369
A-FILE (Adolescent-Family Inventory of Life Events and Changes), 205–206, 214

Age. *See also* Children and adolescents; Elderly
  fall risk and, 582
  fatigue and, 545
  sleep stages and, 293, 294
Age of understanding, informed consent and, 34–35
Agency for Healthcare Research and Quality, 430, 650
Ageusia, 474
AIDS. *See also* HIV
  exemplar study on hope and spiritual well-being with, 240–241
  QOL measures in, 153
AIDS Discussion Strategy Scale, 271
AIDS Empathy Scale, 271
AIDS Psychosocial Scale, 268
AIMS (Arthritis Impact Measurement Scales), 90, 319–320
Alabama-Birmingham Pain Behavior Scale, 619, 639
Alameda County Study of Health and Ways of Living, 404
Albumin test, 287
Alcoholism
  changes in taste or smell from, 476
  sleep disorders and, 295
Allebeck et al. Apparatus for Measuring Disturbances in Size and Shape, 255
Allergic rhinitis, changes in taste or smell from, 476
Alpha, 8
Alternate forms reliability, 7
Althof et al. Semistructured interview, 277
Alzheimer's disease, naming ability and, 103
Ambulatory polysomnography, 299–300
American Cancer Society, 340, 429–430
American College of Gastroenterology, 430
American Geriatrics Society, 571
American Heart Association, on Korotkoff sounds, 501
American Journal of Health Promotion, 402